Paul and Juhl's

ESSENTIALS OF
Radiologic Imaging

Edited by

John H. Juhl, M.D.

Professor Emeritus
Department of Radiology
University of Wisconsin Medical School
Madison, Wisconsin;
Professor Emeritus
Department of Radiology
University of New Mexico School of Medicine
Albuquerque, New Mexico

Andrew B. Crummy, M.D.

Chief of Angio-Interventional Radiology
Professor of Radiology
University of Wisconsin Medical School
Madison, Wisconsin

With 13 Contributors

Paul and Juhl's

ESSENTIALS OF
Radiologic Imaging

Sixth Edition

J. B. LIPPINCOTT COMPANY
Philadelphia

Acquisitions Editor: Charles McCormick, Jr.
Sponsoring Editor: Kimberley Cox
Project Editor: Bridget Hannon Thatch
Indexer: Alexandra Nickerson
Art Director: Susan Hermansen
Cover Designer: Tom Jackson
Production Manager: Caren Erlichman
Production Coordinator: David Murphy
Compositor: Circle Graphics
Printer/Binder: Arcata Graphics/Kingsport

6th Edition

6   5   4   3   2   1

Library of Congress Cataloging-in-Publication Data

Paul and Juhl's essentials of radiologic imaging / edited by John H.
  Juhl, Andrew B. Crummy ; with 13 contributors.—6th ed.
      p.   cm.
  Includes bibliographical references and index.
  ISBN 0-397-51099-3
  1. Diagnostic imaging.   I. Juhl, John H.   II. Crummy, Andrew B.
III. Title: Essentials of radiologic imaging.
  [DNLM: 1. Radiography.   WN 200 P3232]
RC78.7.D53P38   1993
616.07′57—dc20
DNLM/DLC
for Library of Congress   92-49091
                                                              CIP

The authors and publisher have exerted every effort to
ensure that drug selection and dosage set forth in this
text are in accord with current recommendations and
practice at the time of publication. However, in view of
ongoing research, changes in government regulations, and
the constant flow of information relating to drug therapy
and drug reactions, the reader is urged to check the
package insert for each drug for any change in indications
and dosage and for added warnings and precautions. This
is particularly important when the recommended agent is
a new or infrequently employed drug.

Contributors

Murray G. Baron, M.D.
Professor of Radiology
Emory University School of Medicine
Associate Chairman
Department of Radiology
Emory University Hospital
Atlanta, Georgia

Andrew B. Crummy, M.D.
Professor of Radiology
University of Wisconsin School of Medicine
Director of Angiography and Interventional
Radiology
University of Wisconsin Hospitals and Clinics
Williams S. Middleton Veteran's Administration
Hospital
Madison, Wisconsin

Michael Davis, M.D.
Professor of Radiology
University of New Mexico Medical Center
Chief, Gastrointestinal Radiology
University of New Mexico Hospital
Albuquerque, New Mexico

John H. Juhl, M.D.
Professor Emeritus
Department of Radiology
University of Wisconsin Medical School
Madison, Wisconsin
Professor Emeritus
Department of Radiology
University of New Mexico School of Medicine
Albuquerque, New Mexico

Charles A. Kelsey, Ph.D.
Professor of Radiology
Division of Biomedical Physics
University of New Mexico School of Medicine
Albuquerque, New Mexico

Fred T. Lee, Jr., M.D.
Assistant Professor of Radiology
University of Wisconsin Medical School
University of Wisconsin Clinical Science Center
Madison, Wisconsin

Mary Ellen Peters, M.D.
Professor of Radiology
University of Wisconsin Medical School
Madison, Wisconsin

Lee F. Rogers, M.D.
Doctors Frederick J. Bradd and William Kennedy
Professor
Northwestern University Medical School
Chairman
Department of Radiology
Northwestern Memorial Hospital
Chicago, Illinois

Joseph F. Sackett, M.D.
Professor
University of Wisconsin Medical School
Professor and Chairman
University of Wisconsin Hospital and Clinics
Madison, Wisconsin

Charles M. Strother, M.D.
Professor of Radiology, Neurology and Neurosurgery
University of Wisconsin Medical School
Madison, Wisconsin

John R. Thornbury, M.D.
Professor of Radiology
University of Wisconsin Medical School
Chief, Section of Body Imaging
University of Wisconsin Hospital
Madison, Wisconsin

June M. Unger, M.D.
Professor of Radiology
University of Wisconsin Medical School
Diagnostic Radiology
University of Wisconsin Hospital and Clinics
Madison, Wisconsin

Jeffrey D. Wicks, M.D.
Clinical Professor of Radiology
University of Colorado Health Sciences Center
School of Medicine
Staff Radiologist
St. Anthony Hospital
Denver, Colorado

Preface

The goal of the 6th edition continues to be a single volume presentation of the basics of Radiology for residents, medical students and interested physicians from the other specialties.

The continued rapid advance in the new methods of diagnostic imaging has prompted us to revise the text to include them. Magnetic Reasonance Imaging is now being expanded to evaluate bone and joint lesions as well as the mediastinum, the pelvis and the cardiovascular system. It is now a standard modality in CNS diagnostic studies. Its ultimate place in a number of areas awaits further research and experience.

There has been extensive revision of the chapters on the central nervous system. The same is true in the musculoskeletal system and heart, where MRI is now included. The chapters on the gastrointestinal tract have been expanded, using many more illustrations to demonstrate the use of CT. In the urinary and genital tracts, ultrasound in the examination of prostate and testis has been added, in addition to MRI of the pelvis. The coverage of ultrasound in obstetrics has also been extended. More emphasis has been placed on the use of MRI and CT in the study of trauma and of neoplastic-diseases of the sinuses, facial structures and upper airway. Some examples of the use of high resolution thin-section CT in interstitial and other pulmonary conditions have been included.

As in the past, we have updated the references by adding material from recent literature and must again acknowledge our debt to the authors of books and articles cited or quoted in the text.

We wish to thank all of the contributors in this sixth edition of Essentials of Diagnostic Imaging who have worked diligently and submitted their sections in timely fashion. I (JHJ) wish to thank in particular Dr. Fred Mettler, who supported my efforts in many ways, and also Dr. June Unger and Dr. Julie Mitby for providing new illustrations in the Chest section. We also appreciate the efforts of the many secretaries and typists who aided the contributors and editors in preparing the manuscripts. Without their help, we would still be on first base with little hope of getting home.

We also thank the publisher's staff who have been tolerant, helpful and patient.

John H. Juhl, MD
Andrew B. Crummy, MD

From Preface to First Edition

In preparing this volume, it has been our aim to organize and to set down as concisely as possible what we consider to be the basic facts of roentgen interpretation. Designed to bridge the gap between the elementary text and the multiple-volume reference work, it will, we believe, serve equally well as a review source for the practicing physician and surgeon, for those taking postgraduate training in one of the specialties, and as a textbook for the undergraduate medical student.

We have discussed briefly the roentgen anatomy of the various divisions of the body. The descriptions of disease processes are concise, with discussions of clinical and pathologic features limited to the information necessary to clarify the roentgen observations. The emphasis necessarily is restricted to roentgen diagnosis. All the common and most of the unusual conditions and diseases with positive roentgen findings are included. Roentgen differential diagnosis has been emphasized in the more common diseases. Methods of roentgen examination are described, particularly those dealing with the more complicated diagnostic procedures such as bronchography and myelography. The care of the patient before and after such investigations is important, and the referring physician should have some idea of what the examination entails and the way in which it is conducted. Technical methods are likely to vary somewhat from one institution to another; those described here are used by us at University Hospitals and give a general concept of the procedures and what they entail. We have avoided discussions of controversial matters, indicating only either the existence of controversy or the present lack of knowledge about some subjects.

Because of the variable patterns and the changing character of disease processes, often from day to day, it is possible only to illustrate the signs most frequently encountered. The illustrations have been chosen to present as many facets as possible, but the reader should be aware that only infrequently can a single roentgenogram portray all of the possible variants.

References have been selected carefully to direct the reader to a wide range of literature; books and articles have been chosen that contain more extensive bibliographies than it would be advisable to include in a book of relatively restricted size as this.

We have been fortunate in having a group of associates who have been willing to give freely of their time to aid us in many ways. Dr. Edgar S. Gordon has reviewed two chapters (on the osseous system and the abdomen and gastrointestinal tract) and offered valuable criticism. Dr. D. Murray Angevine has done the same in the chapter dealing with diseases of the joints. Dr. Theodore C. Erickson kindly read two chapters covering diseases of the brain and spinal cord; Dr. Helen Dickie reviewed the chapters dealing with diseases of the lungs, and Dr. Richard H. Wasserburger, the cardiovascular system. To these and many others who gave us advice and encouragement go our most heartfelt thanks.

Dr. Margaret Winston prepared several drawings. Dr. Arthur Chandler, Jr. prepared those for the chapters dealing with diseases of the cardiovascular system and the lungs. Other members of our staff who aided us in many ways during the preparation of the manuscript and the selection of illustrative material include Drs. Charles Benkendorf, Robert F. Douglas, Joyce Kline, Lee A. Krystosek, M. Pinson Neal, Jr., and John F. Siegrist. The photographic work has been under the supervision of Mr. Homer Montague, who has personally prepared most of the illustrations. To him goes the credit for the faithful reproduction of the roentgenograms. The typing has been done by Miss Lorena Carmichael with assistance from Mrs. Charlotte Helgeson. Their careful workmanship has made our tasks easier.

Finally, we wish to thank the publisher, Mr. Paul B. Hoeber, for his many courtesies and the excellent cooperation we have received at all times. In particular, Mrs. Eunice Stevens of the publisher's staff deserves our gratitude. Her enthusiasm and her skillful guidance have been invaluable aids.

Lester W. Paul, M.D.
John H. Juhl, M.D.

ix

Contents

Paul and Juhl's

ESSENTIALS OF
Radiologic Imaging

Paul and Juhl's Essentials of Radiologic Imaging,
Sixth Edition, edited by John H. Juhl and
Andrew B. Crummy. J.B. Lippincott Company,
Philadelphia, © 1993.

Introduction

Charles A. Kelsey

X-RAY PROPERTIES

X-rays, which are a form of electromagnetic radiation, travel with the speed of light: 3×10^8 meters per second (6.7×10^8 miles per hour). Figure I-1 illustrates the location of x-rays in the electromagnetic spectrum. Only x-rays and gamma rays have enough energy to produce an ion pair by separating an orbital electron from its parent atom. The amount of radiation present is measured by detecting such ionization. Exposure is measured either in units of coulombs per kilogram (C/kg) or in roentgens (1 R = 258 μC/kg). Although the roentgen is no longer an official scientific unit, it is still widely used in radiology.

RADIATION UNITS

When a patient undergoes a diagnostic x-ray, most of the radiation passes through the patient's body and strikes the film. The roentgen (or C/kg) measures how many x-rays were present. From the patient's point of view, the more interesting quantity is the number of x-rays that stop in the body and how much energy is deposited by those x-rays. The radiation dose is a measure of the energy deposited. One gray (Gy) is the new Système International d'Unites (SI) unit of dose and is defined as 1 joule per kilogram (J/kg). The former unit of dose is the rad. One rad represents a deposition of 100 ergs per gram. One gray equals 100 rad.

Some other types of radiation found near nuclear power reactors or in physics laboratories produce different amounts of biologic effect. Differences in biologic effectiveness are included in the dose equivalent units: the sievert (Sv), which is the SI unit of dose equivalent, and the rem. Table I-1 illustrates the relation between units of exposure, dose, and dose equivalent.

THE X-RAY GENERATOR

Figure I-2 presents a schematic view of an x-ray generator circuit. The circuit consists of a high-voltage transformer, rectifiers to change the AC current to DC, and a filament supply to control the temperature of the filament, which produces the current in the x-ray tube. The efficiency of x-ray production and the penetration of the x-rays strongly depend on the voltage waveform used to produce the x-rays.

Figure I-3A illustrates a single-phase waveform with voltage plotted as a function of time. When a rectifier circuit is added, a full-wave rectified single-phase (two-pulse) waveform, shown on the bottom of Figure I-3B, is obtained. The average value of the applied voltage is 71% of the peak voltage.

When two more waveforms are added, each 180° out of phase, a three-phase (six-pulse) waveform is ob-

High-energy	Gamma rays
	X-rays
	Ultraviolet
	VISIBLE LIGHT
	Infrared
	Microwaves
	Radar
Low-energy	Radio

Figure I–1. The electromagnetic spectrum.

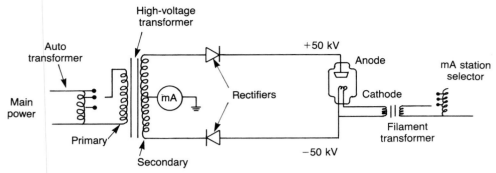

Figure I–2. Schematic diagram of x-ray generator with 100 kV applied across the x-ray tube.

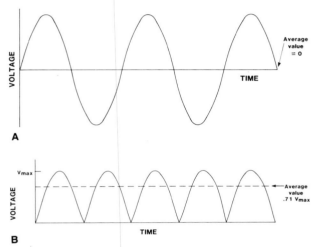

Figure I–3. **(A)** Single-phase voltage waveform, unrectified. **(B)** Full-wave rectified voltage waveform.

tained. Figure I-4 illustrates a three-phase waveform. The average value of the voltage is 95% of the maximum voltage in a three-phase, six-pulse circuit.

Three-phase circuits (six-pulse) have higher voltage and higher average current values than single-phase (two-pulse) circuits. X-ray production is more efficient at higher voltages. The higher average voltage of the three-phase circuit produces more x-rays per milli-ampere than can be obtained with a single-phase circuit with the same average current. Three-phase circuits are more complex, more expensive to purchase, and more difficult to repair than single-phase circuits.

THE HIGH-VOLTAGE TRANSFORMER

The high-voltage transformer consists of primary and secondary wire coils wrapped around an iron core. The secondary winding has many more turns than the primary winding. The difference in windings produces a higher secondary voltage but a lower secondary current. Modern high-voltage transformers are sealed in an oil tank to provide additional insulation and cooling. The kilovolt peak (kVp) measures the voltage across the x-ray tube. Increasing the kVp increases the x-ray output (number of x-rays) and the maximum energy, as well as the average energy, and therefore increases penetration of the x-ray beam. The milliamperes (mA) measures the tube current, and the time in seconds (s) measures the duration of the current. Different values of mA and time (s) that have the same product (the same milliampere seconds [mAs]) produce the same number of x-rays (same exposure).

X-ray generators are connected with a center tap ground so that the high-voltage cables to the anode and cathode are required to withstand only half of the total voltage across the x-ray tube. For example, a center tap

Table I–1. Radiation Units

QUANTITY	UNIT		CONVERSION FACTOR
	CONVENTIONAL	SI	
Amount or exposure	Roentgen (R)	Coulomb per kilogram (C/kg)	1 R = 2.6 × 10^{-4} C/kg
Dose	Rad	Gray (Gy)	1 Gy = 100 rad
Dose equivalent	Rem	Sievert (Sv)	1 Sv = 100 rem
Activity	Curie (Ci)	Becquerel (Bq)	1 Ci = 3.7 × 10^{10} Bq

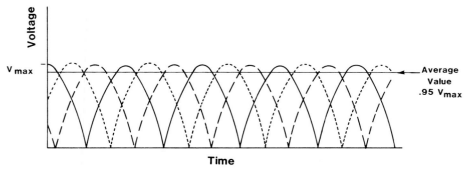

Figure I–4. Three-phase voltage waveform.

generator can apply 100 kVp across an x-ray tube by putting $+50$ kV on the anode and -50 kV on the cathode.

By convention, the power rating of a generator is the product of the kVp and maximum mA allowed at 0.1 s at 100 kV. For example, a generator capable of delivering 500 mA at 0.1 s and 100 kVp would be rated as a 50-kilowatt (kW) generator.

$$500 \text{ mA} \times 100 \text{ kVp} = 50,000 \text{ watts, or } 50 \text{ kW}$$

FILAMENT TRANSFORMER

The filament transformer provides insulation for the large negative voltage applied to the cathode and also controls the current through the filament. The filament temperature and electron current are controlled by the filament current.

AUTOMATIC EXPOSURE TERMINATION

An automatic exposure termination circuit is designed to halt the x-ray production when the proper number of x-rays has passed through the patient and reached the x-ray film cassette. A radiation detector is located between the patient and the x-ray film cassette and is connected to a generator on-off circuit. The proper exposure for the film-screen combination in use is always achieved. If a heavier patient is being examined, the x-ray beam remains on for a longer time.

X-RAY TUBES

Figure I-5 illustrates schematically the operation of a modern x-ray tube. Electrons boiled off the heated filament are accelerated to the anode, and a small percentage of the electron energy is converted into x-ray energy.

The recessed cathode shown in Figure I-6 shapes the electric field to focus the electron beam on the anode focal spot. Some tubes have the cathode cup insulated from the rest of the tube. Applying a negative voltage to the insulated focusing cup prevents electrons from traveling from the cathode to the anode. Such a grid control x-ray tube is used in angiography and in other applications when a very short exposure time is required or it is necessary to synchronize the x-ray pulses with a cine camera.

The anode is tilted about 15° in the direction of the x-ray beam, as shown in Figure I-7. The heat produced by the electron beam stopping in the anode is spread over a larger area than is projected on the patient. The effective or apparent focal spot size is always smaller than the actual focal spot size.

Modern x-ray tubes have rotating anodes to spread the heat over the circumference of the anode. The heat capacity of the tube puts a limit on the peak tube

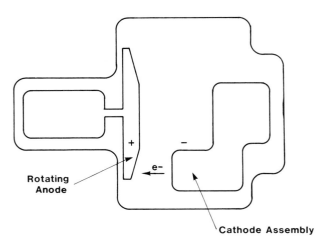

Figure I–5. Schematic view of x-ray tube with a rotating anode and a cathode assembly containing the filaments and focusing cap.

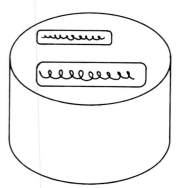

Figure I–6. Cathode assembly with filaments recessed into focusing surfaces.

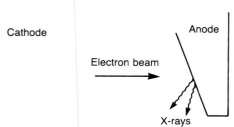

Figure I–7. Tilted anode surface spreads the heat over a larger area.

current as well as time and number of x-ray exposures. Too high a tube current (mA) or too short a time can damage the focal spot. Too many exposures in too short a time can damage the anode or the entire x-ray tube. The heat capacity of a tube is measured in heat units (HU). For a single-phase generator, one heat unit equals kV × mA × s. Because of the difference in waveforms, three-phase generators deposit 1.35 times as many heat units as do single-phase units with the same kVp and mAs. The heat units from a three-phase unit are given by the following equation:

$$HU \ (3\phi) = 1.35 \times kVp \times mAs$$

X-RAY PRODUCTION

When the high-energy electron beam strikes the rotating anode, x-rays are produced by both bremsstrahlung and characteristic x-ray production. About 95% of the electron energy is deposited as heat in the anode, and only about 5% is expended in the production of x-rays. Figure I-8 illustrates a typical x-ray spectrum plotted as intensity of x-ray photons having energy (E) as a function of energy (E) for a tube that has a tungsten target and an applied voltage of 110 kVp.

Many low-energy x-rays produced in the x-ray tube cannot penetrate the x-ray tube housing and so have no clinical importance. The peaks in x-ray production are due to characteristic x-ray production.

VARIATION OF X-RAY OUTPUT

Changes in the mA (tube current) produce changes only in the number of x-rays but not in the shape of the energy spectrum. That is, neither the energy distribution, the maximum energy, nor the penetration of the x-rays changes. Figure I-9 illustrates x-ray spectrum changes resulting from changes in mA. Increasing the mA only increases the number of x-rays.

CHANGES IN X-RAY SPECTRA WITH CHANGES IN FILTRATION

Adding filtration to the x-ray beam eliminates more of the low-energy than the high-energy x-rays from the beam. This tends to increase the average energy, and thus the penetration of the x-ray beam. Figure I-10 illustrates the effect of adding filtration to the x-ray beam. The average energy of the x-ray beam increases because low-energy photons are selectively removed. The maximum x-ray energy does not change with changes in filtration. At least 2.5 mm of aluminum filtration is required for x-ray beams whose energy is higher than 90 kVp.

INTENSITY VARIATION WITH CHANGES IN kVp

Changing the kVp changes the intensity of the x-ray beam, and both the average energy and the maximum energy of the x-ray beam are altered. Figure I-11 illustrates the effect of changing kVp on the x-ray spectrum. The "average" energy of the x-ray beam is about one third the applied voltage. The variation of intensity with kVp depends on filtration, and kVp produces the same effect as a factor of 2 change in mAs.

HALF-VALUE LAYER

The half-value layer (HVL) is the thickness of material that will reduce an x-ray beam to half of its original intensity. Figure I-12 shows the results of an experiment in which layers of attenuator material are added to the x-ray beam. The resulting curve is not a straight

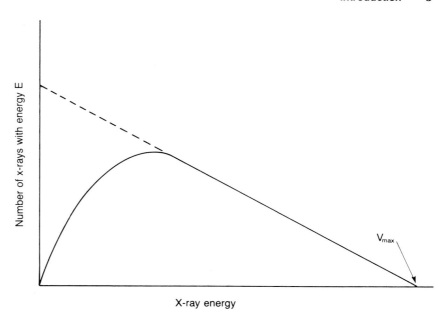

Figure I–8. X-ray production for an applied voltage V_{max}. The dotted line represents x-rays produced inside the x-ray tube but filtered out of the beam by the x-ray tube walls.

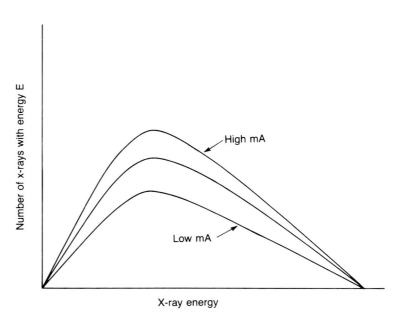

Figure I–9. Variation of x-ray spectra with changes in mA.

line, because the heterogeneous x-ray beam contains many energies. The addition of the attenuator material selectively removes the less penetrating, lower-energy x-rays. The resulting beam is made up of more penetrating, higher-energy x-rays. For this reason, the second HVL is always greater than the first HVL. Typical diagnostic x-ray beams have an HVL in tissue of about 5 cm. Only about 1% of the incident x-rays emerge from a patient who is 30 cm thick.

X-RAY INTERACTIONS

X-rays that pass through a patient are attenuated by absorption and scattering, as shown in Figure I-13. The intensity (I) after passing a distance (d) through a material is given by

$$I = I_o exp - (\mu d)$$

where I_o is the original intensity and μ is the linear

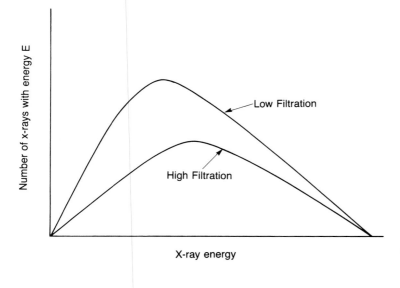

Figure I–10. Variation of x-ray spectra with changes in filtration.

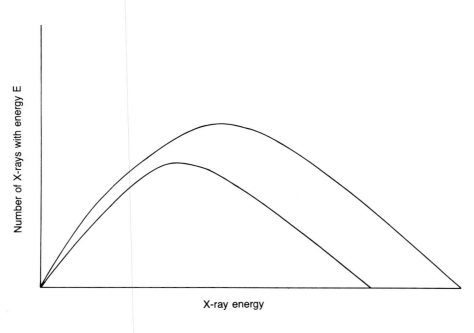

Figure I–11. Variation of x-ray spectra with changes in kVp.

attenuation coefficient. The linear attenuation coefficient is related to the mass absorption coefficient by

$$\mu_m = \mu/\rho$$

where ρ is the mass density of the material in g/cm^3. Mass attenuation coefficients are useful because the effect of density has been removed. As an example, the mass attenuation coefficient of water has a single value for a specific energy, but the linear attenuation coefficients, μ, are different for steam, ice, and water.

X-RAY INTERACTIONS INSIDE THE BODY

Inside a patient's body, diagnostic x-rays can interact through either photoelectric absorption or Compton scattering. Photoelectric absorption, shown schematically in Figure I-14, involves the complete interaction and absorption of the incident x-ray photon by the atom. The incoming photon energy is given to one of the orbital electrons, which is ejected as a photo-

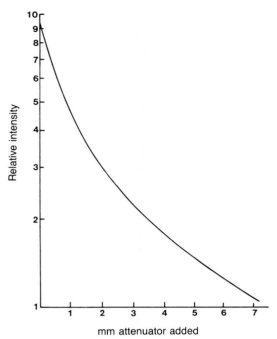

Figure I–12. Transmitted intensity as a function of added absorption material.

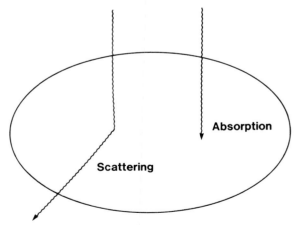

Figure I–13. Scattering and absorption interactions within a patient.

electron. The ejected electron leaves a vacancy in one of the orbital electrons, which is ejected as a photoelectron. The ejected electron leaves a vacancy in one of the inner orbits, and this vacancy is immediately filled by and outer-orbit electron. The difference in binding energies between the outer and inner orbits is released as a characteristic x-ray. The energy ($h\nu$) of the

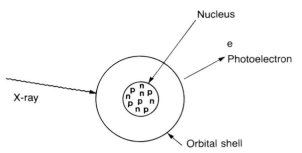

Figure I–14. Photoelectric scattering.

incident photon is shared between the characteristic x-ray energy ($E_{x\text{-ray}}$) and the energy of the photoelectron ($E_{electron}$), as shown in the following equation:

$$h\nu = E_{x\text{-ray}} + E_{electron}$$

The mass attenuation coefficient of the photoelectric effect has a dependence on atomic number and energy given by

$$(\mu/\rho)_{PE} = Z^3/E^3$$

The photoelectric interaction decreases rapidly with increasing energy and increases rapidly with increasing atomic number. This is why lead is such an effective shield in protective aprons and why bone has more absorption than soft tissue.

COMPTON SCATTERING

In Compton scattering, the incident x-ray knocks an electron from an outer orbit, producing a scattered x-ray and a scattered electron. The incident photon gives some of its energy to the scattered electron, which has a range of less than 1 mm in tissue.

At low photon energies (less than about 60 kVp), photoelectric interactions predominate; at about 140 kV, the photoelectric and Compton interactions transfer equal energy to tissue, and above about 200 kVp, most of the energy transfer to tissue is through the Compton interaction.

IMAGE FORMATION STATISTICS

The detection of x-ray photons in a digital imaging system, in a computed tomographic (CT) scanner, or in an image-intensifier tube is a random process. The number of photons collected in a particular 1-mm-square area of an image intensifier is not the same from second to second. Figure I-15 shows the random distribution of photons collected in one second. Note that most of the time, the number of photons collected in

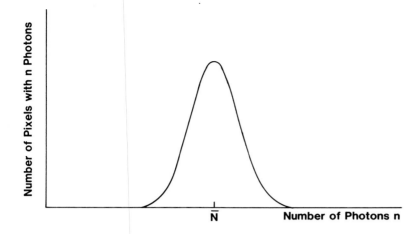

Figure I–15. Random distribution of x-rays.

one second is very close to the average number of photons, $\overline{N}$. The standard deviation, σ, is a measure of the difference between the average value $\overline{N}$ and the measured values. The standard deviation can be calculated by

$$\sigma = \sqrt{\overline{N}}$$

The shape of the distribution curve is described by σ. The percentage of standard deviation is given by

$$\% \ \sigma = \frac{\sigma}{\overline{N}} \times 100$$

$$\% \ \sigma = \sqrt{\overline{N}}/\overline{N} \times 100$$

The percentage of standard deviation is a measure of the statistical noise or quantum noise of an imaging system. As an example, an imaging system that collects an average number of 2000 counts per pixel per exposure has a statistical noise level of

$$\sigma = \sqrt{2000}$$

$$\sigma = 44.7$$

$$\% \ \sigma = \frac{44.7}{2000} \times 100$$

$$\% \ \sigma = 2.2\%$$

As more counts per pixel are collected, the percentage of standard deviation and the statistical noise decrease and the fluctuations on the image decrease. This is true for all digital imaging systems, including CT and magnetic resonance (MR) scanning.

IMAGE QUALITY

An x-ray image is formed through differences in x-ray transmissions through various parts of the body. Differences in patient thickness or density give rise to differences in x-ray transmission called subject contrast.

Subject contrast is defined as

$$C = \frac{N_o - N_s}{N_s}$$

where N_o is the number of photons transmitted through the object and N_s is the number of photons transmitted through the surrounding tissue. Subject contrast depends on thickness, density, material composition, and kVp and beam filtration.

Portions of the body with greater thickness or density have greater contrast than thinner areas or areas with lesser density. Material with high atomic numbers (Z) have higher contrast because of the photoelectric effect. The difference in transmission depends on the filtration and kVp of the x-ray beam. Contrast materials use their high Z components to improve x-ray absorption and improve contrast.

Higher kVp values result in lower subject contrast because there is less difference between areas of similar density. Low kVp examinations are inherently examinations of higher contrast than are studies of higher kVp.

SPATIAL RESOLUTION

Spatial resolution measures the minimum separation between two objects when they can just be distinguished as two separate objects rather than as a single object. Spatial resolution is measured in line pairs per millimeter (lp/mm) and is related to pixel size in digital, CT, and MR imaging. One line pair consists of one dark and one light line. Two objects separated by a distance equal to half the reciprocal of the resolution in lp/mm can be resolved as two objects. In all radiographic imaging systems, unsharpness or blur will cause a point to be imaged as a spot. There are four major sources of unsharpness in radiography: focal spot penumbra, absorption blur, motion blur, and detector blur.

Focal spot penumbra is caused by the finite size of the focal spot. Smaller focal spots produce smaller penumbras and can be used to image smaller objects. Absorption blurring results because most in vivo objects have curved rather than straight edges. The differences in absorption near the edge cause a gradual blurring of the edge rather than a sharp edge. Motion blurring occurs when the object is moving during the x-ray exposure.

Motion blurring can be reduced by decreasing the exposure time. As exposure time is reduced, the load on the anode focal spot increases, so there is a limit to the amount of exposure time reduction permitted in real clinical systems. Detector blur is produced either by a spreading of light in the film screen cassette or by the finite size of the radiation detectors in digital imaging systems.

MEASURES OF IMAGE QUALITY

The modulation transfer function (MTF) measures how faithfully the input signal is reproduced at the output display. MTF is measured in terms of spatial frequency. One hundred percent MTF means that the display signal faithfully reproduces the input signal. The MTF of a complex imaging system is made up of the product of MTFs of the individual systems. Thus, the MTF of an entire image-intensifier system can be calculated from the MTF of the input phosphor, the focusing electrodes, the output phosphor, the focusing lenses, and the TV system. Each of these can be measured individually and combined to produce an overall MTF of the system. Figure I-16 illustrates the individual MTF values of the components of an imaging system.

RECEIVER OPERATING CHARACTERISTIC TESTS

Receiver operating characteristic (ROC) tests evaluate observer performance and hence evaluate the effectiveness of different imaging systems. ROC tests mea-

Table I–2. Possible Responses

| | PATIENT CONDITION | |
OBSERVER RESPONSE	DISEASE PRESENT	DISEASE ABSENT
Yes—disease present	True-positive TP	False-positive FP
No—disease absent	False-negative FN	True-negative TN

sure the characteristic curve of each observer for a given imaging system. Table I-2 presents all possible observer responses depending on whether a disease is present or absent. The sensitivity or true-positive fraction (TPF) is given by

$$\text{Sensitivity} = \frac{TP}{TP + FN}$$

where TP is the number of true-positive responses and FN is the number of false-negative responses.

The TPF is the number of true-positive responses divided by the total number of positive cases. The specificity, or true-negative fraction (TNF), is given by

$$TNF = \frac{TN}{FP + TN}$$

TNF is the number of true-negative responses divided by the number of normal or negative cases. The accuracy is the fraction of correct responses given by

$$\text{Accuracy} = \frac{TP + TN}{TP + FP + TN + FN}$$

The ROC curve plots true-positive responses as a function of false-positive responses.

Figure I-17 gives an ROC curve for a typical observer. Image perception theories predict that each observer has an individual characteristic curve that

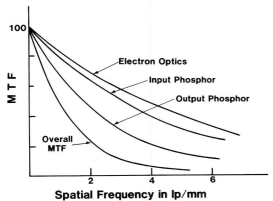

Figure I–16. MTF of image-intensifier system.

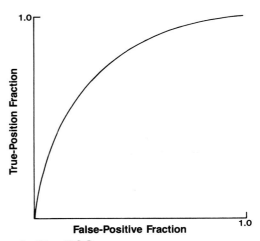

Figure I–17. ROC curve.

does not change without additional training and experience. The observer can change the shape of the curve. For example, an observer might decide to reduce the number of false-positive responses but can do this only while simultaneously reducing the number of true-positive responses. Similarly, any increase in the number of true-positive responses results in a corresponding increase in the number of false-positive responses.

X-RAY FILM

X-ray film is the most common detector and display medium used in radiology today. In film radiography, the detector and the display medium are identical. To change the display characteristics, a different type of film must be used. X-ray film consists of a film emulsion containing silver halide crystals coated on a blue-tinted plastic base. After development, the areas that have been exposed to x-rays appear darker than those that were not exposed to x-rays. The darkness of the x-ray film is measured in units of optical density (OD), where OD is defined as the logarithm of the ratio of incident to transmitted visible light intensities as given by

$$OD = \log (I_o/I)$$

Clinical radiographs usually have ODs ranging from 0.3 to 2.5 OD. The response of film to different levels of x-ray film is measured in units of OD, where OD is defined as the logarithm of the ratio of incident to transmitted visible light intensities as given by

$$T = \frac{D_2 - D_1}{\log E_2 - \log E_1}$$

which is the slope of the characteristic curve. A typical characteristic curve is shown in Figure I-18 which plots the film optical density against the logarithm of the relative exposure. Film speed is defined as a reciprocal of the exposure in roentgens required to produce an OD of 1.0 above base fog. Film latitude describes the range of exposure over which an acceptable radiograph can be obtained. Films with low contrast and low gamma have wide latitude.

INTENSIFYING SCREENS

In modern film-screen systems, about 98% of the film OD results from visible light produced in intensifying screens located on both sides of the film. The other 2% is by direct exposure of the film by x-rays. In an intensifying screen, fluorescent crystals are uniformly mixed in a transparent plastic binder coated on top of a reflective layer. The amount of light intensification is de-

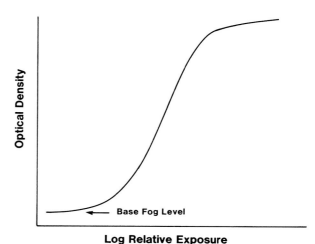

Figure I–18. Characteristic curve of film-screen combination.

scribed by the screen speed. Thicker screens have higher speed, but because the screen light can diffuse laterally, they have poorer resolution. Intensifying screens are constructed either of calcium tungstate ($CaWO_4$) or of rare earth materials. Rare earth materials have higher absorption efficiency or higher conversion efficiency. Compounds with higher absorption efficiencies are more efficient in absorbing x-rays. Compounds with a higher conversion efficiency are more efficient at converting x-rays to light energy. Rare earth screens can be constructed to be two to ten times faster than the conventional $CaWO_4$ screens. This results in lower tube loading and shorter exposures so that patient motion blurring is reduced. Many rare earth screens give off a lower-energy green light and therefore require a film with different sensitivity.

SCATTER

Photons undergoing Compton scattering change direction but lose only a small fraction of their energy. Thus, many Compton-scattered photons reach the detector system after having suffered only a change in direction. These scattered photons carry no diagnostic information and only reduce the contrast. Figure I-19 illustrates the effect of scatter on contrast. The amount of scatter is directly proportional to field size. Important reductions in scatter can be obtained by reducing the field size. Grids are also used to reduce scatter. Grids are thin sheets constructed of thin strips of lead and plastic. The alternate lead and plastic strips permit the unscattered radiation to pass through but attenuate the scattered radiation. Figure I-20 illustrates the use of a grid to reduce scatter. The ratio of the height to the separation between the lead strips is defined as the grid ratio given by

$$GR = h/D$$

where h is the height of the grid and D is the distance between the lead strips.

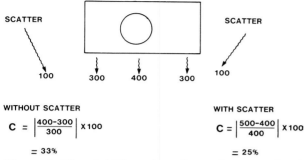

WITHOUT SCATTER

$$C = \left|\frac{400\text{-}300}{300}\right| \times 100$$

$$= 33\%$$

WITH SCATTER

$$C = \left|\frac{500\text{-}400}{400}\right| \times 100$$

$$= 25\%$$

Figure I–19. Addition of scatter reduces contrast.

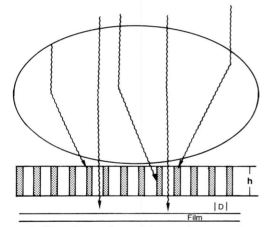

Figure I–20. Use of a grid to reduce scatter.

Bucky grids move the grid to blur out the grid lines. With 100 lines per inch or greater, the grid lines are so fine that they are hardly noticeable and moving of grids is not as necessary.

FLUOROSCOPIC IMAGING

Figure I-21 shows schematically the operation of an image-intensified fluoroscopy unit. After passing through the patient, x-rays interact with the input phosphor of the image intensifier tube. The input phosphor converts the incident x-rays into visible light, which causes the photocathode to emit electrons. These electrons are accelerated and focused by electrodes within the image intensifier onto the output phosphor to produce visible output light. The output light can be viewed directly through an optical system or by a TV system. The output image is considerably brighter than the input because the high-voltage acceleration of the electrons and minification of the output image produce a net gain in brightness.

DUAL-MODE IMAGE INTENSIFIERS

Dual-mode image intensifiers can switch the focal properties of the intensifier tube so that only the central portion of the input face is imaged on the output. This produces a magnified image of a smaller field of view but requires a higher patient dose.

FLUOROSCOPIC IMAGE RECORDING

Fluoroscopic images can be recorded either on film or on videotape. Cineradiographs recorded on film provide better spatial resolution but must be processed

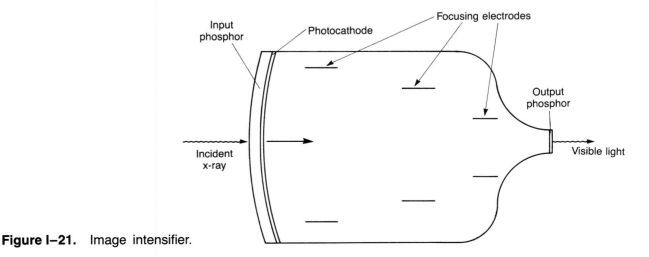

Figure I–21. Image intensifier.

before viewing and result in a higher patient dose than videotape recording.

TV RECORDING

TV images are obtained by coupling the image-intensifier output to a TV system using either a vidicon or a plumbicon TV tube. Plumbicon systems are more desirable than vidicon tubes because when the light levels change rapidly they have less image lag.

DIGITAL IMAGING

Analog-to-digital converters (ADC) produce digital signals by sampling the time-varying analog voltage at regular times called sampling intervals. Higher sampling frequencies (shorter sampling intervals) are required to digitize higher-frequency signals. Figure I-22 illustrates an analog signal and the resulting digital signal from the output of the ADC.

RESOLUTION IN DIGITAL IMAGING

Two types of resolution are important in digital imaging, spatial and contrast, or gray scale, resolution.

SPATIAL RESOLUTION

Spatial resolution describes the separation at which two objects merge into a signal image. Spatial resolu-

tion depends on the picture element (pixel) size. The pixel size is measured in millimeters. Spatial resolution is expressed in line pairs per millimeter (1p/mm). One line pair consists of one bright and one dark line. At least two pixels are required to display one line pair. Pixel size is calculated by dividing the length of an image side measured in millimeters by the number of pixels along that side.

CONTRAST RESOLUTION

Contrast resolution measures how great a contrast difference must exist between two areas to be reliably perceived as distinctly different areas. The number of gray levels and the overall system noise determine the contrast resolution.

JUST NOTICEABLE DIFFERENCE IN CONTRAST

In a noiseless system, the minimum detectable contrast, or just noticeable difference (JND), is one gray scale level. The amount of contrast represented by one gray level depends on the number of gray levels. The number of gray levels depends on the number of bits used to represent contrast in the computer. A bit can be considered an on-off switch or a single power of two. Eight bits are combined to form a byte. A word in a computer represents the maximum number of bits that is used at one time. Eight-, 16-, and 32-bit words are common. Table I-3 presents the number of bits, the number of gray levels, and the minimum detectable contrast step for each choice of bits. Notice that for high-contrast resolution, at least 6 and preferably 8 bits must be devoted to signal contrast. Medical experience indicates that more than 16 shades of gray are rarely required.

SIGNAL/NOISE

The total noise of a digital imaging system consists of quantization noise from the ADC, electronic noise in the TV electronic chain, and quantum noise due to x-ray input fluctuations. Electronic noise is expressed

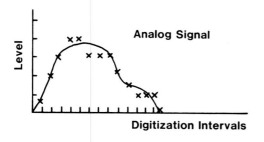

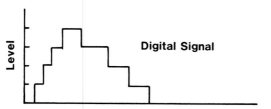

Figure I–22.   Analog signal, digitization levels, and resulting digital signal.

Table I–3. Bits, Gray Levels, and Minimum Detectable Contrast Levels

BITS	GRAY LEVELS	MINIMUM DETECTABLE CONTRAST
4	16	6.25%
5	32	3.1%
6	64	1.6%
7	128	0.8%
8	256	0.4%

in terms of the signal-to-noise ratio, which is the ratio of the object contrast to the background noise. Signal-to-noise ratios of 500 to 1 or 1000 to 1 are typical. This means that the noise is 0.002 or 0.001 times the full-scale input signal.

Digitization errors arise because an ADC assigns a signal value to one of two adjacent gray levels. The ADC does not round off the analog value. The quantum noise depends on the number of photons per pixel at the entrance to the image intensifier and is directly related to patient dose. A well-designed imaging system always has the image noise dominated by quantum noise. This ensures the most efficient use of radiation, because if some other part of the imaging system were the major contributor to image noise, it would mean that we could reduce the patient dose without changing the final image noise.

NOISE, PATIENT DOSE, AND NUMBER OF GRAY LEVELS

If the number of photons per pixel does not change (i.e., constant patient dose), an increase in the number of gray levels results in a decrease in the signal-to-noise ratio because the same number of photons is spread over a larger number of gray levels. To maintain the same signal-to-noise ratio, the patient dose must be increased when the number of gray levels is increased.

TEMPORAL AVERAGING

Temporal averaging reduces the noise and improves the signal-to-noise ratio by combining the signals from several TV frames using signal averaging. The noise decreases by the square root of the number of frames averaged. Although temporal averaging reduces quantum noise, it introduces uncertainties because of patient motion. Temporal averaging over several frames produces improved contrast resolution because of the decreased noise but suffers from a loss of spatial resolution if the patient moves during the averaging time.

COMPUTED TOMOGRAPHY

CT scanning obtains cross-sectional images of a patient rather than the conventional shadow images of conventional radiography. Figure I-23 schematically illustrates CT scanner operation. Confusing and distracting overlying structures are eliminated. In x-ray CT scanning, a fan x-ray beam from a source rotating about the patient passes through the patient, and the exit transmission intensity is monitored by a series of detectors. The x-ray beam "cuts a slice" about 10 mm thick through the patient. The transmission at any angle can

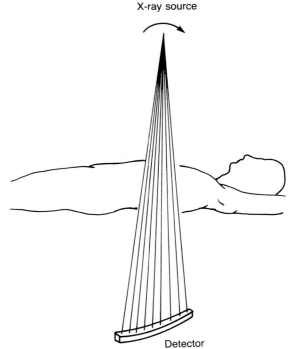

Figure I–23. Schematic view of CT scanning geometry.

be used to calculate the average attenuation coefficient along the length of the x-ray beam. By measurement of the transmission at many angles around the patient, a complex group of mathematical equations can be solved to calculate and determine the mass attenuation coefficient of small (about 1 mm × 1 mm × 10 mm) volume elements (voxels). The final cross-sectional image is then made up of a display of the gray scale value of every voxel. For historical reasons and convenience, the attenuation coefficients are reported in terms of Hounsfield units. In Hounsfield units, bone and other dense materials are +1000, water is equal to 0, and air is equal to −1000. CT scanning, like digital radiography, can separate spatial and contrast resolution.

The matrix or memory size measures how large the computer memory is and how many pixels can be stored in the memory. For a given picture size, memory and pixel size are inversely related. To store an image of a given diameter, a larger matrix will be able to store more pixels and each individual pixel will represent a smaller area of the object. Similarly, a scanfield of smaller diameter will result in the same number of pixels imaging a smaller field. Each pixel then images a smaller area with correspondingly better resolution. The contrast or density resolution depends directly on the number of counts recorded per pixel.

The difference in counts per pixel between two areas must be larger than the statistical fluctuations (quantum noise) for the two areas to be recognized as distinct. The signal is usually about five times larger than the background or surrounding noise in order for a human observer to reliably recognize the difference as real.

Density or contrast resolution depends on radiation dose and scan time. As the radiation dose or the scan time increases, the number of photons collected in each pixel increases and the statistical noise decreases. This results in an increased signal-to-noise ratio or a decrease in the signal required to achieve the just visible signal-to-noise ratio. Increasing either the pixel size or the voxel size (larger slice thickness) results in more counts per pixel collected and a corresponding decrease in the statistical noise. This results in the improved signal-to-noise ratio and an improved contrast resolution.

MAMMOGRAPHY

Mammography must image fibrous, glandular connective tissues of low subject contrast as well as microcalcifications as small as 0.1 mm in diameter. Excellent spatial and contrast resolution is required. Mammography uses applied voltages in the range of 25 to 40 kVp, where most of the interactions are photoelectric, resulting in a very high contrast imaging technique. A molybdenum (Mo) anode x-ray tube with a 0.03-mm Mo filter operated at about 30 kVp produces an x-ray beam whose energy is slightly less than 20 kilo electron volts (keV).

Modern mammographic systems use a vacuum cassette to hold the x-ray intensifying screen against the single emulsion x-ray film. Breast compression should always be used during mammography because it reduces the thickness of the breast near the chest wall and reduces the overall thickness of the breast as well. The reduced thickness results in less scatter and improved contrast. Special low-ratio grids have been used with high-speed film-screen combinations to produce an image with reduced scatter, improved contrast, and an acceptable patient dose of radiation. Typical radiation doses for modern mammographic film-screen systems are approximately 500 mrem per film.

CONVENTIONAL TOMOGRAPHY

Body section or conventional tomography uses motion blurring to eliminate unwanted images. Both the x-ray tube and the film cassette are moved during the exposure. Objects above or below the plane of focus or focal

plane appear to be blurred out and disappear. Objects lying within the plane of focus appear to be unaffected by the motion. Figure I-24 illustrates how objects above and below the plane of the cut are blurred out by being spread over the entire film-screen cassette. The tomographic cut thickness can be changed by altering the amount or range of motion. Tomographic motions that have been used in medicine are linear, circular, elliptical, and hypocycloidal.

DIAGNOSTIC ULTRASONOGRAPHIC IMAGING

Ultrasonography is made up of increases and decreases in pressure with frequency above 20,000 hertz (cycles per second). A transducer converts electric energy into ultrasonic energy. Figure I-25 shows a plot of pressure as a function of distance in front of the transducer. The wavelength is the distance between two corresponding maxima or minima in the ultrasound wave. The

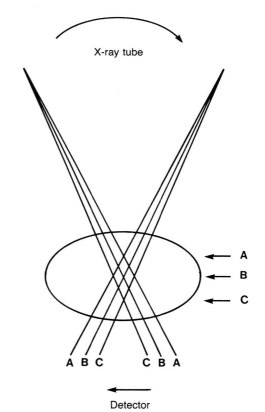

Figure I–24. Conventional tomography blurs objects in levels **A** and **C** while objects in the plane of focus (**B**) remain unblurred.

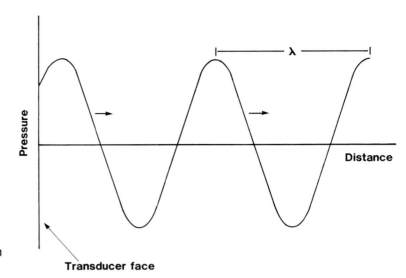

Figure I–25. Pressure distribution in front of ultrasonographic transducer.

frequency of an ultrasound wave is the number of cycles that pass a point each second. The period of a wave is the time of one cycle. The velocity of an ultrasound wave is related to its frequency, f, and wavelength, λ, by

$$v = f\lambda$$

Pulsed ultrasonographic imaging sends an ultrasonic pulse into the body and measures the time of echo return. The distance to the reflecting surface is related to the time of echo return. Ultrasonic reflections are produced whenever there is a change in acoustic impedance, Z, which is defined as

$$Z = \rho V$$

where ρ the physical density in grams per cubic centimeter and V is the velocity of sound in centimeters per second. The acoustic impedance, Z, is measured in rayls.

The reflected intensity, I_r, is related to the incident intensity, I_o, by

$$I_r = RI_o$$

where the reflection coefficient is given by:

$$R = \left| \frac{Z_1 - Z_2}{Z_1 + Z_2} \right|^2$$

Note that tissues with large differences in acoustic impedance (i.e., physical density or velocity) produce reflections of almost 100%. Tissue–air and muscle–bone interfaces always give large reflections. A coupling fluid must be used between the ultrasonic trans-

ducer and the patient's skin to avoid 100% reflection from the transducer–air interfaces.

DOPPLER ULTRASONOGRAPHY

Doppler ultrasonography uses the frequency shift in the reflected ultrasonic beam to detect and monitor moving surfaces and fluids in the body.

MAGNETIC RESONANCE IMAGING

Figure I-26 presents the essential components of an MR imaging system. A large cylindrical magnet with an internal diameter large enough to accept the human body provides an external magnetic field along the body axis. Gradient coils add a smaller identification field. The external magnetic field, together with the gradient field, provides a net external magnetic field, B_o. The radio frequency (RF) coil provides a force to rotate the spins away from the direction of the external magnetic field. As the nuclear spins precess back toward the direction of the external magnetic field, they emit RF signals. These RF signals can be combined to form an image. Depending on the pulse sequences, the image can form maps of the proton density or can be used to form information regarding the local magnetic fields of the nuclear spins. By varying the RF pulse sequence, the image can be made up of predominantly T1 information or predominately T2 information. T1 is known as the spin lattice relaxation time. Images formed using T1 information are most heavily weighted

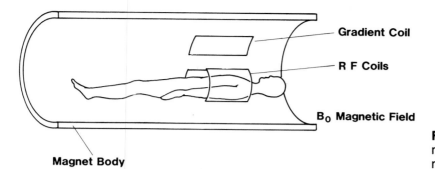

Figure I–26. MR imaging: schematic view of a patient inside magnetic field coils.

toward proton density. T2, called the spin-spin interaction, forms images that provide information on tissue differences.

RADIATION PROTECTION

The three ways to reduce radiation exposure are to

1. Reduce the time of exposure
2. Increase the distance from the radiation source
3. Provide radiation shielding between the individual and the radiation source.

The maximum permissible dose for radiation workers is given in Table I-4 in both SI units (millisieverts [mSv]) and in traditional units (rem). All medical institutions are required to subscribe to ALARA (as low as reasonably achievable) principles. The entries in Table I-4 are to be considered maximum values, and radiation exposure should be reduced to ALARA. The values in Table I-4 are for exposures other than natural background and medical exposures. Medical exposures and natural background are not included in the values in Table I-4. Radiation levels to nonradiation workers are limited to exposure values of less than 500 mrem/year (5 mSv/year). The recommendation for pregnant women is to limit the fetal dose during pregnancy to no more than 500 mrem (5 mSv).

RADIATION DETECTORS

Gas-filled detectors apply a voltage across a gas-filled space and collect all the ions formed by the radiation in the region. At applied voltages of a few hundred volts, all the ions can be collected in an ionization chamber. In a Geiger-Müller counter, which uses a higher voltage of approximately 1500 volts, the ionized electrons gain enough energy to produce secondary ionizations and a larger output signal. Such a Geiger-Müller counter has very high sensitivity and can be used to survey regions for lost or spilled radioactive material.

THERMOLUMINESCENT DOSIMETERS

Thermoluminescent dosimeters undergo changes in their crystal structure when irradiated. Electrons formed by the ionizing radiation are captured in traps within the crystal and are held until the crystal is heated to greater than 200°C. The heating of the crystal releases the trapped energy, which appears as visible light. The amount of light released is a measure of the radiation dose.

SCINTILLATION DETECTORS

Scintillation detectors give off light immediately when hit by x-ray photons. They do not need to be heated. Sodium iodide (NaI), cesium iodide (CsI), and bismuth germinate (BGO) are commonly used scintillation crystals. The scintillation crystal is connected to a photomultiplier tube, which converts the light from the crystal into an electric signal. Scintillation crystals are used in CT scanners.

RISK FACTORS IN DIAGNOSTIC RADIOLOGY

Radiation produces either somatic or genetic effects. Long-term somatic effects are cancer and leukemia induction and cataract production. Data on low-dose

Table I–4. Maximum Permissible Doses for Radiation Workers

	ANNUAL LIMIT
Whole body	5 rem
	50 mSv
Hands or feet	75 rem
	750 mSv

Table I–5. Estimates of Cancer Induction and Mortality (due to a dose of 1 rad [0.01 Gy] to a population of one million persons)

	CANCERS INDUCED	CANCER DEATHS
Unirradiated population	330,000	164,000
Linear response	340	170
Linear-quadratic response	160	80

radiation effects have been obtained by extrapolation from high-dose data estimates. There is some controversy about what is the best way to extrapolate from the high-dose data to the low-dose region of interest in diagnostic radiology. The linear quadratic seems to fit the animal data best, but the linear hypothesis is more conservative and has been used to set limits and make estimates of radiation effects. It is the more conservative because the linear extrapolation probably overestimates the number of cancers and leukemias induced per rad. Table I-5 presents the best estimate of cancer and leukemia induction. The numbers in Table I-5 can be interpreted to mean that if one million individuals received a whole-body radiation dose of 1 rad over the lifetime of the individuals, 300 cancers would be induced as a result of the radiation dose and about 150 people would die from these induced cancers. By comparison, there will be 165,000 cancer deaths in the lifetime of one million individuals who did not receive any radiation dose. Table I-6 presents typical radiation doses from selected radiologic examinations.

IN UTERO EXPOSURE AND THE 10-DAY RULE

Irradiation effects during the first 2 weeks of pregnancy are believed to be an all-or-nothing phenomenon. Any radiation damage to the embryo during this interval will produce a spontaneous abortion. If there is no damage, the fetus develops normally. No radiation effects to the fetus have been observed at radiation doses less than 10 rad. At one time, there was an effort to restrict abdominal examination of potentially pregnant women to the 10-day interval following the onset of menses. Current expert opinion is opposed to postponing any examination of a potentially pregnant female. A female either is or is not pregnant when she appears for an examination. If she is not pregnant, there is no sense in postponing the examination. If she is pregnant, then the examination should either be postponed until the end of pregnancy or performed as soon as possible. If the examination can be postponed

Table I–6. Estimated Whole-Body Radiation Doses from Common Diagnostic Procedures

PROCEDURE	ESTIMATED WHOLE-BODY DOSE (MREM)
Dental	2
Chest	10
Skull	40
C spine	50
Cholecystogram	70
IVP	120
Lumbar spine	130
CT head	200
T spine	240
KUB	450
Mammogram	450
Upper GI*	750
Barium enema*	1100

* Includes fluoroscopy.

until the end of pregnancy, it probably should not be ordered at all.

The American College of Radiology has stated that interruption of pregnancy is never justified because of the radiation risk to the fetus from a diagnostic x-ray examination.

RELATIVE RISKS FROM RADIATION AND OTHER COMMON HAZARDS

An easily understood way to assess risk is to relate the hazards from x-ray examinations to other common hazards faced every day.

A chest radiograph, for example, increases the patient's chance of dying from a radiation-induced cancer

Table I–7. How to Increase Your Chances of Death by One in a Million

ACTIVITY	CAUSE
1 chest x-ray	Radiation
2 months in Denver	Radiation
2 months in stone building	Radiation
150 miles travel by car	Accident
1000 miles by jet airplane	Accident
Smoking 1.5 cigarettes	Cancer/cardiovascular disease
Living 2 months with a cigarette smoker	Cancer/cardiovascular disease
Eating 100 charcoal-broiled steaks	Cancer
Drinking 30 cans of diet soda	Cancer
Drinking 500 ml of wine	Cirrhosis

by about one in a million. Table I-7 presents other common hazards that present a one-in-a-million chance of death. By referring to Tables I-6 and I-7, a physician can relate any radiographic study to hazards that the patient can easily understand. For example, a barium enema gives a whole-body radiation dose of 1100 mrem. This is 110 times as much as a chest examination, and so the chances for a cancer-induced death due to the barium enema would be 110 per million. This is, then, equivalent to living for 18 years in Denver or driving 17,000 miles in a car.

SELECTED READINGS

CURRY TS, DOWDY JE, MURRY RC: Christensen's Introduction to the Physics of Diagnostic Radiology. Philadelphia, Lea & Febiger, 1984

HENDY WR: Medical Radiation Physics. Chicago, Year Book Medical Publishers, 1979

JOHNS HE, CUNNINGHAM JR: The Physics of Radiology. Springfield, IL, Charles C Thomas, 1978

METTLER FA, MOSELEY RD: Medical Effects of Ionizing Radiation. New York, Grune & Stratton, 1985

The Osseous System

Paul and Juhl's Essentials of Radiologic Imaging, Sixth Edition, edited by John H. Juhl and Andrew B. Crummy. J.B. Lippincott Company, Philadelphia, © 1993.

CHAPTER *1*

Introduction to Skeletal Radiology and Bone Growth

Lee F. Rogers

Radiographic examination is the key to the diagnosis of many skeletal abnormalities. It is essential that each bone be examined in its entirety, including the cortex, medullary canal (cancellous bone or spongiosa), and articular ends. The position and alignment of joints are determined. In children, the epiphysis and epiphyseal line or physis must be observed. The adjacent soft tissues are examined. Obliteration of normal soft-tissue lines and the presence of a joint effusion are of particular importance. When disease is present, it is important to determine whether the process is limited to a single bone or joint or whether multiple bones or joints are involved. The distribution of disease is also a consideration. The presence and type of bone destruction and bone production, the appearance of the edges or borders of the lesion, and the presence or absence of cortical expansion and periosteal reaction are also noted. The radiographic findings are then correlated with the clinical history and the age and sex of the patient to arrive at a logical diagnosis. The diagnosis may be firm in some instances; in other cases, a differential diagnosis is offered since the exact diagnosis cannot be determined.

SKELETAL SCINTIGRAPHY

Skeletal scintigraphy or bone scanning is a valuable adjunct to standard film radiography (Fig. 1-1).[10] Bone-seeking radionuclides are taken up in areas of increased bone turnover. This occurs normally at the growth plate in children and at abnormal sites in tumors, infections, and fractures; in sites of reactive bone for-

mation in arthritis; and in periostitis regardless of the etiology. Technetium-99m-labeled polyphosphates are the most common radiopharmaceuticals used, particularly technetium-99m methyldiphosphonate (^{99m}Tc-MDP). Fifteen to 20 millicuries (mCi) is injected intravenously, and a scan is obtained two hours later. The radiation-absorbed dose is very low, since the total body dose is 0.009 rad/mCi. The agent is excreted in the kidneys and collects in the bladder. The target organ—that is, the organ receiving the highest dose—is the wall of the bladder, exposed to approximately 0.275 rad/mCi. Bone scanning is more sensitive to areas of bone turnover and destruction than plain film radiography or tomography. The bone scan may be positive in the presence of a normal radiograph, well before the radiograph becomes abnormal. However, the bone scan is less specific than the radiograph. Areas of increased activity are detected, but the cause of the increase often cannot be stated with certainty, and correlation with plain film radiographs or computed tomography and magnetic resonance imaging is necessary to establish a correct diagnosis.

COMPUTED TOMOGRAPHY

Computed tomography (CT) is advantageous in the evaluation of the skeletal system. It allows visualization of adjacent soft-tissue structures and also the marrow in the medullary cavity. The position of surrounding vascular structures can be determined by the use of contrast media. CT has the added advantage of being more sensitive to the detection of bone destruction than

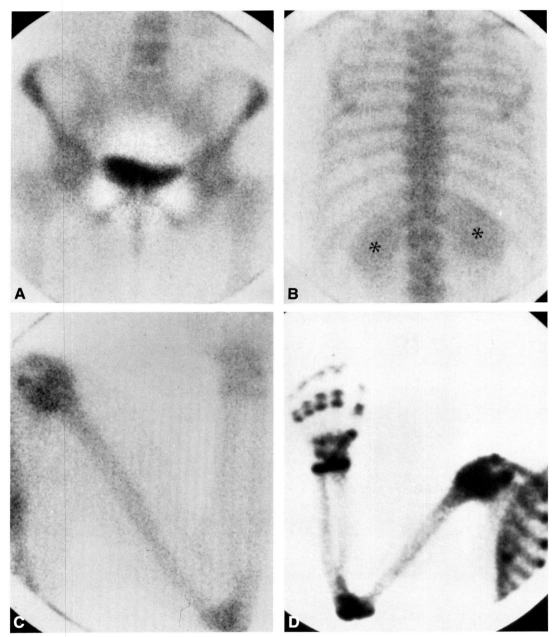

Figure 1–1.   Normal bone scan. (**A**) Normal bone scan of 23-year-old woman. Anterior view of the pelvis. The bones of the pelvis, lower lumbar spine, and proximal femurs are visualized but are poorly defined. The greatest concentration of radioactivity is within the bladder. (**B**) Posterior view of the thoracolumbar spine. The scapulae, vertebrae, and ribs are demonstrated. Radioactivity is identified within the kidneys (*asterisk*). (**C**) Anterior view of the left upper extremity. The humerus, ulna, radius, and bones of the hand are seen. Diffuse activity is present in the carpus, but the individual carpal bones are not discernible. (**D**) Normal bone scan of the right upper extremity of a 10-year-old girl. Note the band of increased radioactivity in the region of the growth plates, seen particularly well at the distal radius and ulna, metacarpals, and proximal phalanges.

plain film radiography or standard tomography. CT images are displayed in the axial or horizontal plane, and even sagittal and coronal planes, with image reconstruction. Unfortunately, image reconstruction degrades the image. Images are displayed with both bone and soft-tissue windows. The soft-tissue window setting allows visualization of surrounding soft tissue but is suboptimal for the bony skeleton (Fig. 1-2A). The bone window setting maximizes the visualization of cortical and medullary bone (Fig. 1-2B).

MAGNETIC RESONANCE IMAGING

Magnetic resonance (MR) imaging is of great value in the evaluation of the skeletal system, particularly in the detection and evaluation of tumors, infection, bone infarction, and ischemic necrosis.[3, 17] Because the image is dependent on the presence of hydrogen, which is abundant in marrow fat, MR imaging visualizes the bone marrow exquisitely. However, the hydrogen content of cortical bone is very low, and MR imaging

therefore is not as sensitive as CT for the evaluation of cortical bone. MR imaging has the added advantage of displaying the anatomy in any plane, including the coronal and sagittal planes, which are distinctly advantageous in the demonstration or visualization of abnormalities within bone and their relationship to surrounding soft tissue (Fig. 1-3). Discrimination between and differentiation of various soft tissues and pathologic processes may be enhanced by varying the technical parameters used for the examination. Furthermore, vascular structures are demonstrated and are clearly visualized without the necessity of contrast media injection.

SKELETAL GROWTH AND MATURATION

OSSIFICATION OF THE SKELETON

The process of bone formation in cartilage is known as *endochondral ossification*, which causes bones to grow in length. Some bones are formed in membrane, known as *membranous bone formation*. The bones of

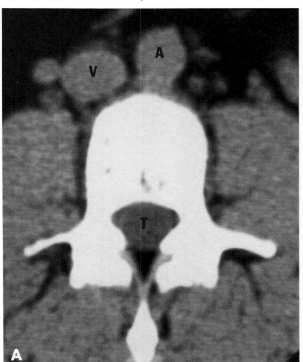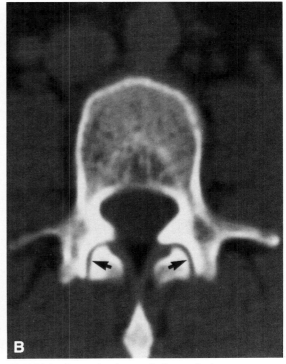

Figure 1–2. CT of the third lumbar vertebra. **(A)** Within the spinal canal, the soft-tissue window setting demonstrates the paraspinous muscles, the aorta (*A*), the vena cava (*V*), and the thecal sac (*T*) and its contents. **(B)** Bone window setting. This is the same slice shown in Figure 1-2A, but the window setting is set to accentuate bone. The cortex and intramedullary portion of the vertebral body are readily identified. Note the cortex of the pedicles and transverse processes. At this setting, the facet joints (*arrows*) are visualized but are not identifiable on the soft-tissue setting of Figure 1-2A.

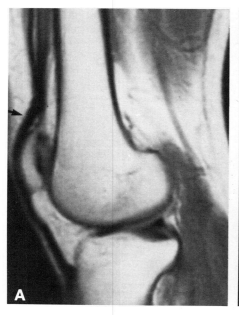
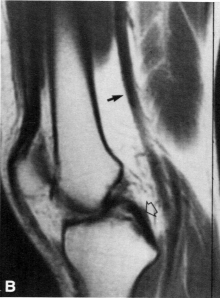

Figure 1–3. MRI of the knee in the sagittal plane. (**A**) Note the black lines of the cortex and the white signal of the intramedullary bone and marrow. Muscle is seen as a streaky gray density. The subcutaneous fat and infrapatellar fat pad emit a strong signal because of the high content of hydrogen in fat. The quadriceps tendon is readily identified (*arrow*). (**B**) Sagittal section obtained more medially demonstrates the popliteal artery (*arrow*) and the posterior cruciate ligament (*open arrow*).

the cranial vault are the principal example. Ossification occurs in both cartilage and membrane in the mandible and clavicle. The tubular bones grow in their transverse diameters by bone formation within the osteogenic cells of the inner layer of the periosteum. This could be considered a form of membranous bone formation.

At birth, the shafts of the long tubular bones are ossified, but both ends (epiphyses), with a few exceptions, consist of masses of cartilage. Cartilage is relatively radiolucent as compared with bone, having the same density as soft tissue on a conventional radiograph. Thus, at birth the ends of the bones are separated by radiolucent spaces representing the cartilaginous epiphyses. At variable times after birth, one or more ossification centers appear in the epiphyses (the epiphyseal ossification centers). Exceptions occur at the distal femur and proximal tibia epiphyses, where ossification centers appear during the last 1 or 2 months of intrauterine life. The short tubular bones are similar to the long bones except that they have an epiphysis at only one end. The carpal bones are cartilaginous at birth. In the tarsus, ossification centers are present at birth in the calcaneus, cuboid, and talus. The remaining tarsal bones are cartilaginous. Three ossification centers are present in each vertebra, one in the body and two in the arch. Shortly after birth, the two halves of the laminae fuse. Union of the arches to the bodies begins at age 3 and is completed at about age 7. The cranial bones are ossified at birth but remain separated by fibrous tissue sutures. The individual pelvic bones

are present but are separated by cartilaginous plates, the Y-shaped triradiate cartilage of the acetabulum.

The distal femur and proximal tibia epiphyseal ossification centers can be used as indicators of fetal maturity. Formerly, radiographs of the mother's abdomen were obtained to visualize these centers as evidence of fetal maturity during the last month of gestation prior to induced labor or cesarean section. Fetal maturity is now determined by ultrasonographic examination, which is highly advantageous.[11, 13] Because it does not use ionizing radiation, it can be employed throughout pregnancy and is safe, accurate, and free of side effects.

After an epiphyseal ossification center appears at or near the center of the epiphysis, it gradually enlarges and takes on a shape distinctive for that particular bone (Fig. 1-4). In some areas, there is more than one ossification center—for example, in the distal humerus. They appear at different times and eventually fuse. The ossified epiphysis remains separated from the shaft by a cartilaginous disc or plate known as the epiphyseal plate, growth plate, or physis. The epiphyseal plate gradually becomes thinner as growth proceeds until it finally ossifies, the epiphysis fuses to the shaft, and growth in length is complete.

The times of appearance of the various epiphyseal ossification centers are good indicators of skeletal age during infancy and early childhood.[8, 9, 12, 15, 16] Similarly, the times of fusion of the epiphyses can be used as indicators of skeletal age during late adolescence.

The flared end of bone is known as the metaphysis, and the tubular midportion of the shaft the diaphysis.

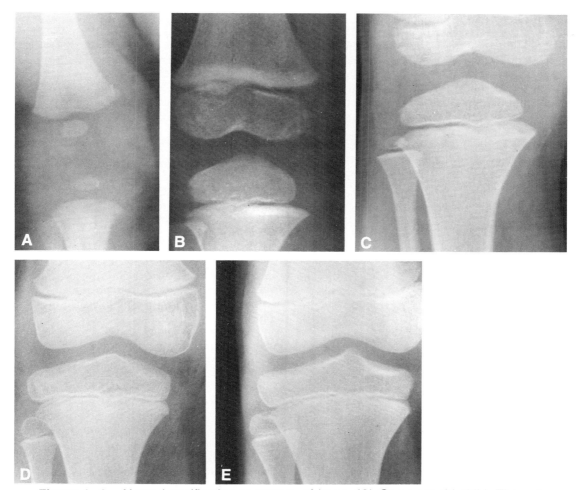

Figure 1–4. Normal ossification sequence of knee. (**A**) One-year-old child. The epiphyses are largely cartilaginous, but there are small ossification centers for the femur and tibia. (**B**) Child 2 years of age. The ossification centers have grown considerably. The zone of provisional calcification produces the wide transverse lines at the metaphyses. Note the normal irregularity of the medial margin of the distal femoral epiphysis. (**C**) Child 5 years of age. The epiphyses have developed to a point where the ends of the bones resemble those of an adult. A cartilaginous plate (termed the *physis, epiphyseal line,* or *growth plate*) remains between the epiphysis and metaphysis. (**D**) In this 8-year-old child, the epiphyseal line remains distinct and the femoral condyles approach the adult configuration. (**E**) In this 10-year-old child, there has been further ossification in the physis (epiphyseal line). Longitudinal growth continues until the epiphysis fuses to the metaphysis and the physis disappears.

Between the metaphysis and epiphysis lies the physis or cartilaginous growth plate consisting of four distinct zones—the resting zone, the proliferating zone, the hypertrophic zone, and the zone of provisional calcification. In the zone of provisional calcification, mineral salts are temporarily deposited around the degenerating cartilage cells. Blood vessels subsequently grow into the lacunae left by the degenerated cartilage cells, bringing with them osteoblasts, specialized connective tissue cells whose main function is the production of osteoid. Osteoid is the organic matrix in which mineral salts are deposited to make bone. Osteoid is relatively radiolucent and, when present in large amounts, will cause bone to appear more radiolucent than normal. As osteoid is formed, the zone of provisional calcification is replaced by trabecular bone.

It is rather common to see one or more thin opaque lines crossing the shaft near its ends. These are commonly known as "growth lines" and, while there may be other causes for them, it is probable that in most cases they indicate a temporary cessation of orderly ossification brought about by one or more episodes of systemic illness.

The following are definitions of some terms used in describing the bones during infancy and childhood (Fig. 1-5):

Epiphysis: The cartilaginous end of a bone.

Physis: The cartilaginous zone between the epiphysis and the calcified cartilage, also known as the growth plate or the epiphyseal plate. When it becomes thin, in late adolescence, it is sometimes called the epiphyseal line.

Metaphysis: The flared end of the shaft of a tubular bone.

Diaphysis: The tubular shaft of a long bone.

Epiphyseal ossification center: The ossified portion of an epiphysis.

Zone of provisional calcification: The zone of deposition of mineral salts at the end of the shaft that serves as a framework for the deposition of osteoid. It is seen in roentgenograms as a thin white line or narrow zone.

Osteoid: The organic matrix that is formed by the osteoblasts and that, when mineralized, becomes bone.

Endochondral ossification: The process by which bone is formed from cartilage.

Intramembranous ossification: The process by which bone is formed from membrane without a cartilaginous stage; periosteal and endosteal growth are included.

Apophysis: An accessory ossification center that forms a protrusion from the end or near the end of the shaft of a long bone. Apophyses function as growth centers at nonarticular margins of bone, i.e., the greater trochanter of the femur or ischial tuberosity of the pelvis. They serve as attachments for muscles or ligaments and do not contribute to the length of a long bone.

SKELETAL MATURATION

The radiographic determination of bone age is useful in the determination of physiologic age, growth potential, and prediction of adult stature.[4, 14] Variations between physiologic age as identified by the maturity of the skeleton and chronologic age are clinically important. Childhood diseases and disorders causing growth abnormalities show differences between the bone age and chronologic age.[7] Deficiencies of thyroid and growth hormones cause the most severe degree of bone age retardation. Conditions such as thyrotoxicosis, sexual precocity, and even simple exogenous obesity advance bone age.

The most well-known and widely accepted method of determining skeletal bone age or skeletal maturation is that of Greulich and Pyle, described in their book *Radiographic Atlas of Skeletal Development of the Hand and Wrist.*[8] This method is particularly helpful after the age of 2 years. The accuracy of this method for the American population is such that its use as the sole method of assessment is sufficient in most instances. The determination of skeletal age is based on the comparison of a radiograph obtained on the case in question and the standard radiographs for age and sex in the text. The age is based on the presence or absence of ossification centers and their configuration (Figs. 1-6 and 1-7). Its accuracy can be enhanced by attention to detail. As a rule, the metacarpal and phalangeal centers correlate with the chronologic age more accurately than the carpal centers. The appearance of carpal centers is more variable than that of the metacarpals and phalanges, and carpal centers are more commonly affected by congenital disorders.[14]

The appearance and fusion time of various centers in the hand, wrist, and other bones are listed in Tables 1-1 and 1-2.

Skeletal maturation is determined in part by the chronologic age and sex of the individual. Girls tend to mature faster than boys, and therefore it is mandatory to use the standards that are appropriate for the sex. Furthermore, there are distinct racial and ethnic differences in skeletal maturation. Standards developed in American children may not be applicable to English and European children. Skeletal maturation of black American children generally exceeds that of white American children by approximately 0.5 stan-

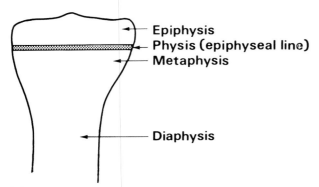

Figure 1–5. Normal anatomic divisions of the end of a typical growing bone.

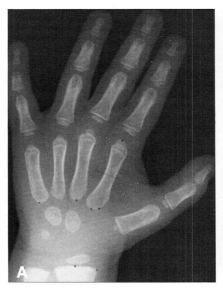

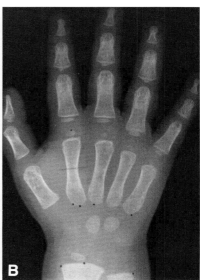

Figure 1–6. (**A**) Hand of a normal 2-year-old girl. (**B**) Hand of a normal 2-year-old boy. The differences in the appearance of the bones are quite subtle at this age. Note that the epiphyseal ossification centers of the proximal phalanges and distal radius of the girl in Figure 1-6*A* are larger than those of the corresponding epiphysis of the boy in Figure 1-6*B*. Epiphyseal ossification centers are present in the distal phalanx of the third and fourth fingers of the girl in Figure 1-6*A* but are not present in the boy.

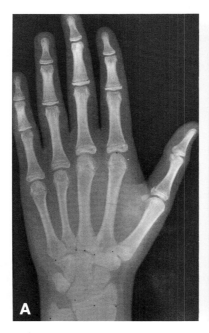

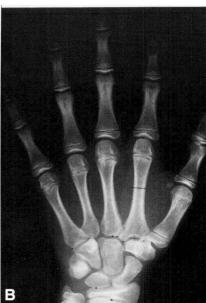

Figure 1–7. (**A**) Hand of a normal 13¹/₂-year-old girl. (**B**) Hand of a normal 13¹/₂-year-old boy. The principal differences are in the width of the epiphyseal plates, the relative size of the carpal ossification centers, and the configuration of the epiphyses. Note in Figure 1-7*A* that there is almost complete fusion of the proximal epiphysis of the first metacarpal and the distal epiphysis of the second and third metacarpals. Compare with the corresponding epiphysis of the male in Figure 1-7*B*.

dard deviations in each site under consideration.[6] This racial difference is seen in both boys and girls.

Prior to age 9, the changes in the appearance of the ossification centers of the hand are minimal and it is difficult to determine the skeletal age with sufficient accuracy by the Greulich and Pyle method. Standards described by Garn and colleagues are useful in infants and young children.[5] These are based on the appear-

ance time of various ossification centers. Figure 1-8 shows the centers of maximum predictive value and ranks them in order of the greatest correlation value for both boys and girls.

Standard radiographic atlases have been compiled by Pyle and Hoerr[15] for the knee and by Hoerr and colleagues[9] for the foot and ankle, which are of value in the assessment of the skeletal age in younger children.

Table 1–1. Ossification Time Table (Females)

CENTERS PRESENT	HAND AND WRIST	FUSION (IN YEARS)	OTHER BONES	FUSION (IN YEARS)
At birth	Capitate (birth to 3 mo) Hamate (birth to 3 mo)		Distal femur Proximal tibia Proximal humerus (occasionally) Calcaneus Talus Cuboid	17 16 to 17 17½ to 20
End of 1 yr	Prox. phalanges II, III, IV Metacarpal II, III Distal radius (9 to 12 mo)	15 15 17	Coracoid, scapula Capitellum Proximal femur (1 to 6 mo) Distal tibia (1 to 7 mo) Distal fibula (1 to 7 mo) Cuneiform III (3 mo)	14 to 16 14 to 15 16 to 17 16 to 17 15½ to 17
End of 2 yr	Triquetrum (18 to 24 mo)* Prox. phalanges I, V Mid. phalanges II, III, IV Dist. phalanges I, III, IV, V Metacarpals I, IV, V	 15 14½ 13½ 15	Metatarsals Prox. phalanges, toes (1 to 2½ yr) Mid. phalanges, toes (½ to 2½ yr)	17 to 20 18 18
End of 3 yr	Dist. phalanx II Mid. phalanx V Lunate (30 to 36 mo)	13½ 15	Proximal fibula (2 to 4 yr) Cuneiform I, II (½ to 2½ yr) Tarsal navicular (1 to 3 yr) Dist. phalanges, toes (1½ to 4 yr) Greater trochanter (1½ to 3 yr)	17½ to 20 18 16
End of 4 yr	Trapezium (36 to 42 mo)* Trapezoid (42 to 50 mo)* Scaphoid (42 to 50 mo)*		Med. epicondyle humerus (2 to 5 yr) Patella (2 to 3½ yr)	 20
End of 6 yr	Distal ulna	16½	Proximal radius (3 to 5½ yr)	14 to 15
End of 8 yr	Pisiform (variable and unreliable)		Trochlea humerus (7 to 9 yr) Calcaneal apophysis (5 to 12 yr)	14 12 to 22
End of 10 yr			Less. trochanter (9 to 14 yr) Tibial tuberosity (10 to 13 yr) Olecranon (8 to 11 yr)	16 19 14 to 15
End of 13 yr			Lat. epicondyle, humerus (11 to 14 yr)	 20
End of 15 yr			Inner border scapula Secondary centers pelvis	20 21+
End of 17 yr			Medial end clavicle	25

NOTE: Figures in parentheses indicate range of normal variation in time of appearance.
* Usual range but highly variable.

Kuhns and Finnstrom's method will be found to be useful in premature infants and newborns.[12]

PREDICTION OF ADULT HEIGHT

In general, the most important factor in the determination of the ultimate adult height of an individual is parental height, the height of the individual's parents. The maturity of an individual should not be confused with the size or height of an individual. The relative degree of depression or acceleration of skeletal maturation is compared with present height to determine the ultimate height of an individual. If the skeletal maturation is more advanced and the present height is normal, the individual will ultimately be small. If maturation is retarded and the present height is normal, the individual will ultimately be taller than normal.

Many methods have been developed for the prediction of adult height.[8, 18, 19] The standards have largely been based on the growth of normal children whose heights fall within a relatively restrictive range on either side of normal or mean stature. In clinical practice, it is the very tall or short children for whom a prediction is most often needed. In these cases, the standards are found to have limited reliability. The older the chronologic age, the more accurate the prediction. Therefore, in some situations it is not possible to predict the ultimate adult height of young children with the desired accuracy.

Greulich and Pyle have reproduced the Bayley and

Table 1–2. Ossification Time Table (Males)

CENTERS PRESENT	HAND AND WRIST	FUSION (IN YEARS)	OTHER BONES	FUSION (IN YEARS)
At birth	Capitate (birth to 3 mo) Hamate (birth to 3 mo)		Distal femur Proximal tibia Proximal humerus (occasionally) Calcaneus Talus Cuboid	18 to 19 18 to 19 21
End of 1 yr	Distal radius (12 to 15 mo)	18	Coracoid, scapula Capitellum, humerus Proximal femur (2 to 8 mo) Distal tibia (1 to 7 mo) Distal fibula (1 to 7 mo) Cuneiform III (6 mo)	14 to 16 14 to 15 18 17½ to 19 17½ to 19
End of 2 yr	Prox. phalanges II, III, IV, V Mid. phalanges III, IV Dist. phalanx I Dist. phalanges III, IV Metacarpals II, III, IV	17 16 to 17 15 15½ 17	Prox. phalanges, toes (1 to 2½ yr)	17 to 18
End of 3 yr	Triquetrum (24 to 32 mo)* Mid. phalanx II Prox. phalanx I Metacarpal I Metacarpal V Lunate (24 to 36 mo)	 16 17 15½ 17	Metatarsals Mid. phalanges, toes (1 to 4 yr) Cuneiform I, II (1 to 3½ yr)	18 to 20 18
End of 4 yr	Mid. phalanx V Dist. phalanges II, V Trapezium (40 to 48 mo)*	16 15¼	Great. trochanter (2½ to 4 yr) Prox. fibula (2½ to 5 yr) Tarsal navicular (1½ to 5½ yr)	16 19
End of 6 yr	Trapezoid (60 to 66 mo)* Scaphoid (60 to 66 mo)* Distal ulna (60 to 66 mo)	 17½	Medial epicondyle (5 to 7 yr) Patella (2½ to 6 yr) Dist. phalanges, toes (3½ to 6½ yr) Prox. radius (3 to 5½ yr)	20 18 15
End of 8 yr	Pisiform (variable and unreliable)		Trochlea, humerus (7 to 9 yr)	14
End of 10 yr			Less. trochanter (9 to 13 yr) Olecranon (8 to 11 yr) Calcaneal apophysis (5 to 12 yr)	16 14 to 15 12 to 22
End of 13 yr			Tibial tuberosity (10 to 13 yr) Lat. epicondyle, humerus (11 to 14 yr)	19 20
End of 15 yr			Secondary centers, pelvis Inner border scapula	21+ 18 to 20
End of 17 yr			Medial end clavicle	25

NOTE: Figures in parentheses indicate range of normal variation in time of appearance.
* Usual range but highly variable.

Pinneau Tables for predicting adult height using the skeletal age as determined by the Greulich and Pyle Hand Standards and the height and chronologic age of the individual.[8] This is reasonably accurate as an American standard.

Tanner and associates also have devised a method for use in English and European populations for assessing skeletal maturity along with predicting adult height.[19] The method is very complex and too time-consuming for regular clinical use, but it may be employed as an alternative in difficult situations, particularly for pre-dicting height. Their new system (TM Mark 2) is based on the samples that include very tall and very short children and may prove useful in these situations.

DISTURBANCE IN SKELETAL GROWTH AND MATURATION

The relationship of the endocrine glands to skeletal growth and maturation is very important. Roentgen examination of the growing skeleton may give valuable information concerning thyroid, pituitary, and gonadal

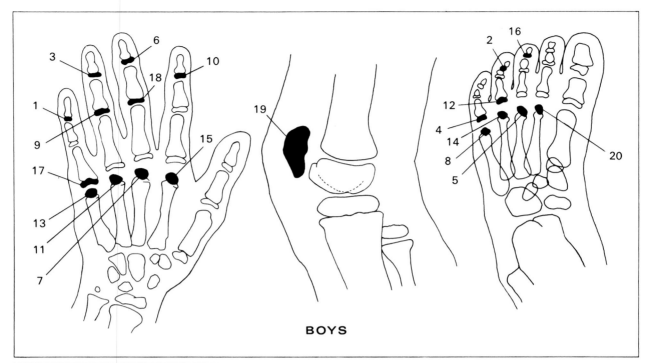

BOYS

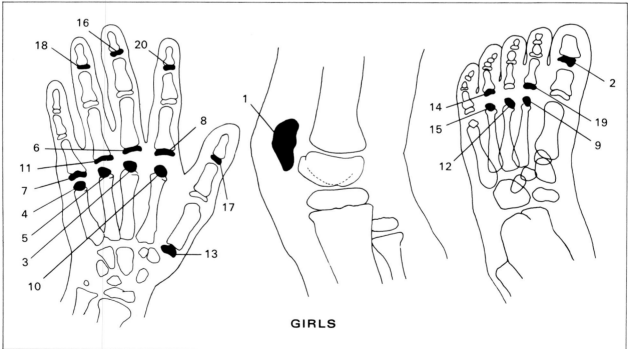

GIRLS

Figure 1–8.   Predictive values of various ossification centers. The centers marked in black have the highest predictive value. The numbers represent the order of predictive value of these centers. (Garn SM: Medical Radiography and Photography. Radiography Markets. Rochester, New York, Eastman Kodak Company, 1967. With permission of Stanley M. Garn, Ph.D.)

disturbances. Delay in appearance or fusion or retardation of epiphyseal centers may result from deficient secretion by one or more of these glands. Hypersecretion may accelerate these processes. Table 1-3, prepared by Graham, indicates a number of glandular

disturbances and their effect on skeletal maturation.[7] Chapter 6 describes radiographic findings other than changes in skeletal maturity in each of these conditions.

Acceleration or deceleration of growth may be gen-

Table 1–3. Abnormalities of Skeletal Maturation*

CONDITION	BONE AGE	STATURE	COMMENTS
CENTRAL AND GENERAL			
Hyperpituitarism (giantism)	N or (↓), may fuse late	↑ ↑	Eosinophilic adenoma, acromegalic if late
Hypopituitarism (pan-, pituitary dwarfism)	↓ ↓ may never fuse	↓ ↓	? "Normal" early
Primordial dwarfism (genetic, constitutional)	N or (↓)	↓	
CNS disorders			(2° to neoplasm or other disease)
Pinealoma	↑	↑, adult ?N	Especially males
Fibrous dysplasia	↑	↑, adult ?N	Especially females
Craniopharyngioma	↓	↓	
Hypothalamic dysfunction	↑ or ↓	↑ or ↓	Many associations, e.g., obesity
Exogenous obesity	N or (↑)	N or (↑), adult N	
Malnutrition and/or chronic disease	(↓)	(↓), adult may be N	
Chondro-osseous dysplasias and syndromes	↓ occasionally	↓ ↓ occasionally	Rarely advanced, many die early
GONADS			
Hypergonadism (hyperplasia, neoplasm)	↑ ↑, fuse early	↑ ↑, adult ↓	
Hypogonadism			
Eunuchoidism	N or (↓), fuse late	↑, long extremities	Intrinsic, castration, 2° to disease
Pituitary	N	↓	Not panhypopituitarism
Gonadal "dysplasia"			
Turner's syndrome	N or (↓), fuse late	↓	XO types, hypomineralization
Kleinfelter's syndrome	N or (↓), fuse late	↑, long extremities	XXY types
Abnormal sexual differentiation	(N)	(N)	Pseudohermaphrodite types
Sexual developmental variations			
Delayed adolescence	(↓), then N	↓, adult N	
Premature pubarche	(↑), then N	↑, adult N	
Premature thelarche	N or ? (↑)	N	
Constitutional precocity	(↑), then N	↑, adult N	
ADRENALS			(May be 2° to ACTH ↑ ↓)
Cortical insufficiency (Addison's disease)	(↓)	(↓)	Like a chronic disease
Cortical hyperactivity (Cushing's disease)	↓ occasionally	↓	Cortisol ↑, hypomineralization
Adrenogenital syndrome (hyperplasia, neoplasm)	↑ ↑ ↑, fuse early	↑ ↑, adult ↓	Usually masculinizing, rarely feminizing
THYROID			
Hypothyroidism	↓ ↓ ↓ ↓	↓ ↓ ↓, infantile	Epiphyseal dysgenesis
Congenital (cretinism)			Hypermineralization
Acquired	↓	↓	
Hyperthyroidism	(↑)	(↑), adult N	? Hypomineralization
PARATHYROIDS			
Hyperparathyroidism (1° or 2°)	(N)	(N)	Hypomineralization
Hypoparathyroidism	(N)	(N)	Hypermineralization
Pseudohypoparathyroidism	(N)	↓	Associated with XO types

* Modified from Graham CB: Assessment of bone maturation methods and pitfalls. Radiol Clin North Am 10:198, 1972
Legend: N = normal   ↑ = advanced   ↓ = retarded
             (N) = probably normal   (↑) = possibly advanced   (↓) = possibly retarded

eralized and may involve all ossification centers, or it may be focal and limited to one ossification center.

Generalized acceleration of skeletal maturation is usually associated with precocious development and early puberty. Among the conditions in which this is found are the following:

Albright's Syndrome. Albright's syndrome consists of widespread osseous lesions of fibrous dysplasia and pigmented areas (café-au-lait spots) in the skin. In females, there may be precocious sexual development, rapid skeletal growth, and early fusion of the epiphyses. As a result, the patients usually show some degree of dwarfism. These latter changes do not usually occur in males.

Granulosa Cell Tumor of the Ovary. Granulosa cell tumor of the ovary causes precocious puberty, and the skeletal system responds by early closure of the epiphyses.

Hyperfunction of the Adrenal Cortex in Childhood. Hyperfunction of the adrenal cortex may affect both sexes. In females, it causes virilism; in males, sex characteristics are intensified and puberty develops early. The epiphyses fuse prematurely and the patients tend to be dwarfed.

Several rare syndromes have also been recorded in which there is accelerated skeletal maturation. Most affected persons have multiple defects such as facial abnormalities, motor inadequacy, and mental deficiency.

Generalized delayed maturation of the skeleton can occur as a result of hypofunction of the gonads, pituitary, and thyroid glands. Delay in maturation also occurs in association with severe cyanotic heart diseases, dietary deficiencies, and a number of chronic illnesses, including renal disease and celiac disease.

Focal increases in maturation are usually due to an increased blood supply or local hyperemia, associated with rheumatoid arthritis, tuberculous arthritis, hemophilia, or healing fractures adjacent to the joint. Focal decreases in maturation may occur following infection, burns, frostbite, radiation therapy, or trauma, particularly epiphyseal separations. These all impair the growth potential of the physis either by destroying the resting cells or by disrupting the blood supply, and growth may cease. Premature closure of the epiphysis may also occur as the result of bone infarcts, particularly in sickle cell disease.

REFERENCES AND SELECTED READINGS

1. BUCKLER JHM: How to make the most of bone ages. Arch Dis Child 58:761, 1983
2. EDMUND CS: Development of the musculoskeletal system. Clinical symposia. Ciba Found Symp 33:2, 1981
3. EHMAN RL, BERQUIST TH, McLEOD RA: MR imaging of the musculoskeletal system: A 5-year appraisal. Radiology 166:313, 1988
4. GARN SM: Neuhauser lecture. Contributions of the radiographic image to our knowledge of human growth. AJR Am J Roentgenol 137:321, 1981
5. GARN SM, ROHMANN CC, SILVERMAN FN: Radiographic standards for postnatal ossification and tooth calcification. Med Radiogr Photogr 43:45, 1967
6. GARN SM, SANDUSKY ST, NAGY JM, ET AL: Advanced skeletal development in low-income Negro children. J Pediatr 80:965, 1972
7. GRAHAM CB: Assessment of bone maturation methods and pitfalls. Radiol Clin North Am 10:185, 1972
8. GREULICH WW, PYLE SI: Radiographic Atlas of Skeletal Development of the Hand and Wrist, 2nd ed. Stanford, CA, Stanford University Press, 1959
9. HOERR NL, PYLE SI, FRANCIS CC: Radiographic Atlas of Skeletal Development of the Foot and Ankle. Springfield, IL, Charles C Thomas, 1962
10. HOLDER LE: Radionuclide bone-imaging in the evaluation of bone pain: Current concepts review. J Bone Joint Surg [Am] 64:1391, 1982
11. JEANTY P, ROMERO R: Estimation of the Gestational Age. Semin Ultrasound CT MR 5:121, 1984
12. KUHNS LR, FINNSTROM O: New standards of ossification of the newborn. Radiology 119:655, 1976
13. LANGE IR, MANNING FA: Fetal biophysical assessment: An ultrasound approach. Semin Ultrasound CT MR 5:269, 1984
14. POZNANSKI AK: The Hand in Radiologic Diagnosis, 2nd ed. Philadelphia, WB Saunders, 1984
15. PYLE SI, HOERR NL: A Radiologic Standard of References for the Growing Knee. Springfield, IL, Charles C Thomas, 1969
16. ROCHE AF, FRENCH NY: Differences in skeletal maturity levels in the knee and hand. Am J Roentgenol 109:307, 1970
17. SARTORIS DJ, RESNICK D: MR imaging of the musculoskeletal system: Current and future status. Am J Roentgenol 149:457, 1987
18. TANNER JM, LANDT KW, CAMERON N, ET AL: Prediction of adult height from height and bone age in childhood. Arch Dis Child 58:767, 1983
19. TANNER JM, WHITEHOUSE RH, MARSHALL WA, ET AL: Assessment of Skeletal Maturity and Prediction of Adult Height (TW2 Method). London, Academic Press, 1975

*Paul and Juhl's Essentials of Radiologic Imaging,
Sixth Edition*, edited by John H. Juhl and
Andrew B. Crummy. J.B. Lippincott Company,
Philadelphia, © 1993.

CHAPTER *2*

Traumatic Lesions of Bones and Joints

Lee F. Rogers

Although a fracture may be obvious on clinical examination, roentgenograms are essential for precisely defining the nature and severity of the injury. In many instances, the clinical findings are questionable and a roentgen examination is necessary to determine whether or not a fracture is present. As a general rule, a roentgen examination should be performed if there is the slightest doubt concerning the possibility of a fracture or dislocation. Following reduction of a fracture, roentgenograms are required to evaluate the accuracy of reduction and subsequently to monitor the progress of healing. No set rules can be given for the frequency of follow-up examinations because the indications vary widely depending upon the type of fracture, the bone involved, the method of treatment employed, and the age of the patient. A fracture treated by skeletal traction may require daily examinations, whereas a satisfactorily reduced and casted fracture may only be examined immediately after the application of the cast and at intervals of several weeks thereafter until healing is complete.

METHODS OF EXAMINATION

ROENTGENOGRAMS

An accurate assessment requires at least two views made at right angles, usually an anteroposterior and a lateral projection. At times the fracture line may be visible in only one of several projections (Fig. 2-1). A fracture cannot be ruled out solely on the basis of a roentgenogram in a single projection. Two views are also necessary to obtain a true perspective of the spatial relationships of the fragments (Fig. 2-2). An additional oblique projection is usually required to accurately assess trauma in the region of a joint. Because of superimposition, it is not possible to obtain technically satisfactory direct lateral radiographs of either the hip or shoulder. Some form of oblique projection is mandatory. The radiographic examination of a long bone should always include the entire length of the bone, from the joint above to the joint below. Although this may not always be true of injuries involving the ends of the bone, it is certainly true for those involving the shaft or diaphysis. Fractures of the shaft may be associated with injuries of an adjacent joint, particularly the proximal joint, and if this joint is not included in the radiographic examination, such injuries may be overlooked.

FLUOROSCOPY

At one time, fluoroscopy was widely used to aid in the reduction of fractures because it enabled the orthopaedic surgeon to manipulate the fragments under direct fluoroscopic vision. The danger of radiation overexposure to the person performing the reduction is real. Many physicians in the past have developed severe reactions from repeated or prolonged exposure of the hands during the fluoroscopic manipulation of fractures. If fluoroscopy is used, certain precautions are

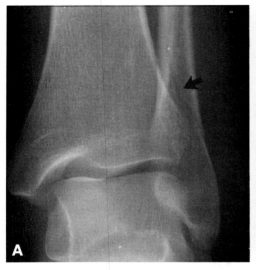
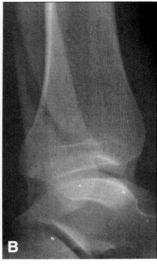

Figure 2–1. Fracture of lateral malleolus identified with certainty on only one of two views. (**A**) AP view of the ankle demonstrates soft-tissue swelling about the lateral malleolus and a faint fracture line (*arrow*). (**B**) Lateral view demonstrates obvious long oblique fracture of the lateral malleolus.

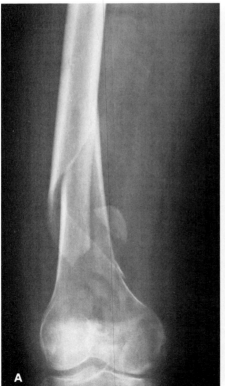
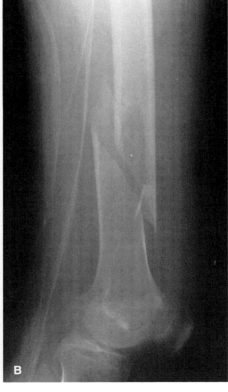

Figure 2–2. Spiral fracture of the femur. (**A**) AP view. (**B**) Lateral view. The distal fragment is angulated medially and offset posteriorly. There is minimal comminution of the fracture distally. The relationship between the fracture fragments is best appreciated by viewing the fracture in two planes, preferably at 90° to each other.

essential: (1) The person operating the fluoroscope must be fully aware of the amount of radiation being delivered and equally aware of methods of protection. (2) A timing device should be incorporated in the roentgen-ray circuit to shut off the current automatically after a predetermined amount of time has elapsed. (3) All manipulation should be done with the fluoroscope turned off, and it should be turned on for quick visual inspection only when the surgeon's hands have been removed from the field of exposure.

RADIOISOTOPE BONE SCANNING

Technetium-99m can be used in the assessment of skeletal trauma. The examination is obtained 2 hours following the intravenous injection of the isotope. The isotope is localized in areas of increased bone turnover, and thus is concentrated at the margins of a fracture. Radioisotope bone scanning is more sensitive, though less specific, than a roentgenographic examination of the skeletal system. Therefore, the isotope examination may disclose fractures that are not apparent on radiographic examination (Fig. 2-3). It is used under the following circumstances: (1) in stress fractures[31] in which the radioisotope scan may be positive as much as 6 weeks before the stress fracture is evident on radiographic examination; (2) in otherwise occult injuries following trauma, particularly in the assessment of scaphoid and other carpal injuries; (3) in establishing the diagnosis of a battered child; and (4) in the assessment of the full extent of injury in the patient with multiple injuries. The principal objective of the isotopic examination is to identify fractures not apparent on radiographic examination. If there is no evidence of increased radioactivity, then a fracture can be safely ruled out, except in elderly individuals who have a slow metabolic rate of bone turnover. In the elderly, a repeat scan may be required as late as 72 hours following the injection of the isotope to identify the fracture site. The isotopic bone scan is nonspecific; areas of increased activity are also caused by tumors, arthritis, and metabolic bone disease. These must be ruled out before the diagnosis of fracture is accepted.

COMPUTED TOMOGRAPHY

Computed tomography (CT) has distinct advantages in the assessment of skeletal trauma at certain sites. Because of the unique display of anatomy in the axial projection, these sites are usually difficult to evaluate by plain film radiography. CT is particularly useful in the evaluation of facial, spinal (see Fig. 2-31), pelvic, and acetabular[13] fractures because it displays various components in isolation, free of overlap by surrounding structures, i.e., bony margins of sinuses, spinal canal, sacroiliac joint, sacral ala, hip joint, and anterior and posterior rims of the acetabulum. It is also useful in the evaluation of the sternoclavicular joint and carpal and tarsal[10] bones (see Fig. 2-64). The greatest limitation is the difficulty in determining the relationship of one axial image to another in the sagittal or coronal planes. This problem may be overcome by image reconstruction in the appropriate plane. To do so requires both thin sections and the absence of patient movement between slices. The latter is often difficult in the acutely injured patient; they often cannot hold still.

MAGNETIC RESONANCE IMAGING

Magnetic resonance imaging (MRI)[7, 11, 17] provides direct visualization of soft-tissue structures, including ligaments, tendons, joint capsule, menisci, and joint cartilage (Fig. 2-4); structures which are impossible to see on plain film radiographs and often not clearly distinguishable by CT. It has the added advantage of displaying these structures in any longitudinal plane,

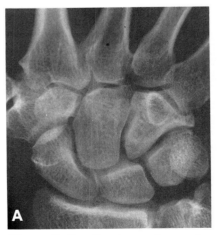
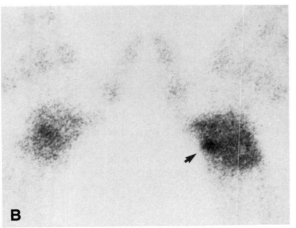

Figure 2–3. Fracture of carpal scaphoid. **(A)** There is no obvious fracture of the scaphoid. **(B)** Technetium bone scan demonstrates focus of increased radioactivity in the region of the scaphoid (*arrow*) and a general increase in the carpal joints due to traumatic synovitis. (Courtesy of Khalil Shirazi, M.D., Ann Arbor, Michigan)

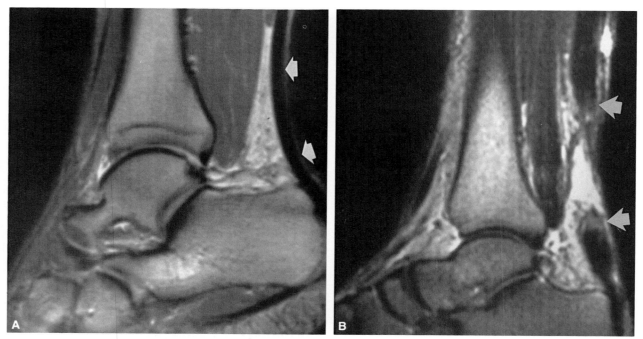

Figure 2–4. MRI of the Achilles tendon. (**A**) Normal T1-weighted image demonstrates the uniformly low signal Achilles tendon (*arrows*). This is sharply defined anteriorly by the pre-Achilles fat pad. (**B**) T2-weighted image of a patient with a torn Achilles tendon demonstrates an area of high signal interposed between the two ends of the torn tendon (*arrows*). The high signal is due to a hematoma. The margins of the tendon are widened and contain irregular signal consistent with hemorrhage.

i.e., sagittal, parasagittal, coronal, or oblique, in addition to the axial plane.

MRI has proved to be the method of choice in the assessment of internal injuries of the knee (see Figs. 2-56 through 2-58). With refinements in surface coils, MRI has also proved valuable in the assessment of the carpus. It is also used in the evaluation of the shoulder, spine, and various tendon injuries at other sites, particularly the Achilles tendon (Fig. 2-4).

MRI can detect intraosseous injuries that are not apparent on plain film radiography (see Fig. 2-6).[7, 11] These have been termed *bone bruises* and are discussed later in this chapter. MRI can also detect stress, insufficiency, and other obscure fractures, e.g., femoral neck, that are not apparent on plain films.

TYPES OF FRACTURES

There are several ways in which fractures can be classified. They are easily divided into two major groups, open and closed fractures. An open fracture, previously known as a compound fracture, denotes a frac-ture in which there is a perforation, laceration, or avulsion of the overlying skin and soft tissues. The importance of an open fracture lies in the possibility of infection because of contamination at the time of injury. This possibility must be taken into account when follow-up roentgenograms of an open fracture are being evaluated. A closed fracture, one in which the overlying skin and soft tissues are intact, may be converted into an open fracture by the need for open surgical reduction and internal fixation with metallic plates, bone grafts, or other fixation devices. Although infrequent with good surgical technique, infection is always possible subsequently.

DESCRIPTION OF FRACTURE—TERMINOLOGY

When describing displacement of fracture fragments, it is customary to refer to the displacement of the distal fragment in relation to the proximal, the latter being considered as the stationary part. Thus, one speaks of a posterior displacement of the distal fragment of the tibia in relation to the proximal fragment rather than an anterior displacement of the proximal in relation to the distal. The same method is used in describing dislocations, the distal portion of the extremity being considered to be the dislocated one. For example, all dislocations of the elbow joint are displacements of the bones of the forearm on the humerus. In describing angular deformity, the distal fragment should be considered as being angled in relation to the proximal fragment. Thus, a fracture of the distal tibia with lateral displacement of the foot would be described as lateral angulation of the distal fragment. As an alternative, the angulation may be defined at the fracture site. In the case given with lateral displacement of the foot, there would be medial angulation at the fracture site. The most common use is to describe the angulation of the distal fragment. Apposition, overlap or overriding, and number of fragments are other important observations.

The following groupings of fractures are useful for descriptive purposes, and the terms are those used in the roentgen and clinical evaluation. Some fractures will not fit into a specific group because they show mixed features. For example, a compression fracture may also show evidence of comminution; the line of demarcation between an impacted fracture and a compression fracture is not sharp; a Colles' fracture at the wrist is usually comminuted as well as impacted. These limitations must be kept in mind when one attempts to classify any specific fracture.

Complete and Incomplete Fractures

The term *complete* is used to designate a fracture that caused a complete discontinuity or disruption of bone with separation into two or more fragments. An *incom-*

plete fracture does not extend across the entire width of the bone.

Occult Fractures

Occult fracture describes a fracture strongly suspected by physical examination but not visualized roentgenographically on the initial evaluation. At times these fractures may be demonstrated on a subsequent radiographic examination because of the deossification that occurs along the edge of the fracture line (Fig. 2-5), making the fracture more readily visible on roentgenographic examination. Such fractures may be detected by bone scanning prior to their demonstration by radiographic examination (see Fig. 2-3).

Bone Bruise

MRI evaluation of suspected meniscal or ligamentous injuries of the knee has revealed incidental intraosseus abnormalities that have been termed occult, intraosseous fractures[11] but are popularly referred to as bone bruises. They appear as irregular areas of high signal intensity on T2-weighted images within the subchondral medullary space. T1-weighted and proton density images (Fig. 2-6) show ill-defined, speckled areas of low signal intensity in these same areas. Occasionally, a linear or branching band of signal void is identified within the same area. Radioisotopic bone scans may show increased activity. These abnormalities can be identified in both the medial and lateral femoral condyles and tibial plateaus.

Bone bruises are presumed to represent hemor-

Figure 2–5. Occult fracture of the lateral condyle of the humerus in a 4-year-old girl. (**A**) AP view demonstrates no definite fracture. (**B**) Repeat examination 8 days later demonstrates a linear, hairline fracture of the lateral condyle (*arrow*). This is classified as a Salter-Harris type IV epiphyseal injury.

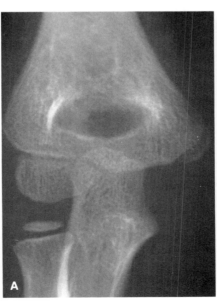
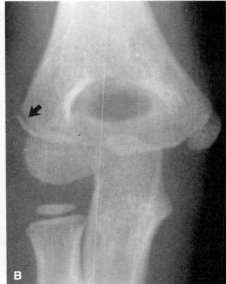

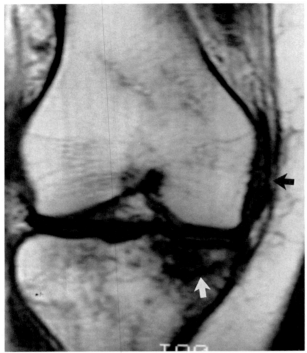

Figure 2–6. Bone bruise or occult intraosseous fracture. The irregular area of low signal in the medial tibial plateau on this T1-weighted image indicates the presence of an intraosseous hemorrhage or bone bruise. Compare this signal with that of the lateral plateau and femoral condyles. Note also the irregular linear density in the midst of the surrounding irregular densities (*white arrow*). This represents a crack or undisplaced fracture. This injury was associated with a complete tear of the anterior cruciate ligament and a partial tear of the medial collateral ligament (*black arrow*). Compare with Figure 2-58*B*.

rhage and edema associated with trabecular microfractures sustained as the result of compression or impaction forces applied to the joint surface. They are often associated with meniscal or ligamentous injuries but may occur as isolated findings. Similar lesions may occur in the joint margins of other bones.

Hairline Fractures

A hairline fracture is an undisplaced fracture with minimal separation of the fracture fragments. The fracture line is so fine that it is compared to the width of a single hair (see Fig. 2-36).

Comminuted Fractures

A comminuted fracture is composed of more than two fragments. Occasionally the bone may be extensively shattered, but more often comminution is less severe and the fracture has a fairly distinct pattern. For instance, a triangular-shaped fragment at one margin of a shaft fracture is referred to as a butterfly fragment (Fig. 2-7A). Fractures that are at the end of the bone and that extend intra-articularly commonly do so in a T-, V-, or Y-shaped pattern, and these letters are used to describe the nature of the comminution. For instance, a T-shaped fracture in the lower end of the femur consists of a transverse fracture extending across the width of the bone in the supracondylar area, with a vertical extension into the knee joint between the two condyles (Fig. 2-7B).

Avulsion and Chip Fractures

An avulsion fracture consists of a fragment of bone pulled away or avulsed from a tuberosity or bony process at the end of a bone at sites of ligament or tendon attachments (Fig. 2-8A). When the fragment is very small, it may be referred to as a chip or sprain fracture. These small cortical avulsions, also known as flake fractures, frequently occur in the ankle as a result of ankle sprains (Fig. 2-8B) and are also commonly encountered in the finger, where the fragments are often tiny (see Fig. 2-33).

Segmental Fractures

Two or more complete fractures may involve the shaft of a single bone. These differ somewhat from the more common form of comminuted fracture in that each is complete, leaving a segment of intact shaft between them. These are known as segmental fractures. In the common comminuted fracture, one or more small fragments have been separated along the line of a major fracture, but these pieces as a rule do not include the entire width of the bone.

Impacted Fractures

In an impacted fracture, the fragments are driven into one another, either along the entire line of fracture or only along one side. A radiolucent fracture line may not be seen, since impaction completely obscures it. Instead, the line of impaction is denser than normal because of the condensed bony trabeculae within it. In addition, an impacted fracture can be recognized by the disruption of normal bone trabeculae at the site of

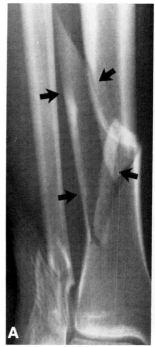
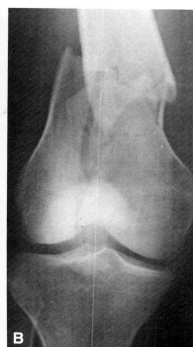

Figure 2–7. **(A)** Comminuted fracture of distal tibia with large butterfly fragment (*arrows*) and an associated fracture of the lateral malleolus. **(B)** Comminuted T-shaped fracture of the distal end of the femur. In addition to the irregular transverse fracture through the shaft, there is a vertical fracture extending to the articular surface within the intercondylar notch.

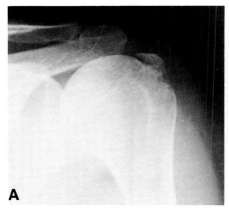
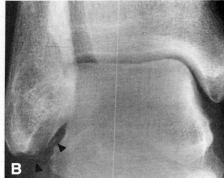

Figure 2–8. **(A)** Avulsion fracture of the greater tuberosity of the humerus. **(B)** Soft-tissue swelling over the lateral malleolus is associated with small avulsion fractures (*arrows*) from the tip of the lateral malleolus. This is known as a sprain fracture.

impaction and by the sharp angulation of the cortical margin at least on one side of the fracture. Two of the more frequent impacted fractures are the Colles' fracture of the distal radius (see Fig. 2-35) and the subcapital fracture of the neck of the femur (see Fig. 2-53A). Impacted fractures are also frequent in the vertebral bodies (see Fig. 2-25) and os calcis (see Fig. 2-63), where they are usually referred to as compression fractures.

Greenstick Fractures

Greenstick fractures occur almost exclusively during infancy and childhood. The appearance of such a fracture is similar to that obtained by trying to break a green twig. There are three basic forms of greenstick fractures.[23, 24] In the first, a transverse fracture occurs in the cortex, extends into the midportion of the bone, and then becomes oriented along the longitudinal axis

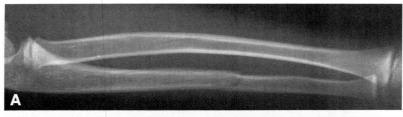

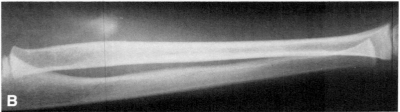

Figure 2–9. Bow and greenstick fractures of the distal radius and ulna. **(A)** Lateral view demonstrates anterior bowing of the radius without an obvious fracture line associated with a greenstick fracture of the midshaft of the ulna. **(B)** Lateral view of opposite normal side for comparison.

of the bone without disrupting the opposite cortex (Fig. 2-9). The second form is a torus or buckling fracture (Fig. 2-10). This is due to impaction. The cortex is buckled and overlapped, but there is no distinct disruption of the cortex. The third form is a bow fracture, in which the bone becomes curved along its longitudinal axis but without either a distinct buckle or break in the cortex (Fig. 2-9).[3] The bow fracture is most commonly encountered in the forearm, less commonly in the fibula, and rarely in the femur, clavicle, and humerus.

Epiphyseal Fractures

During childhood, a fracture may extend either in part or completely through the epiphyseal plate at the end of a long bone and may lead to displacement of the epiphysis on the shaft. This most commonly occurs at age 10 through 16 years and is most frequently encountered in the distal end of the radius, in the phalanges, and in the lower end of the tibia.[24–26] If the line of fracture is limited to the cartilage, it will not be directly visible and its detection rests upon the evidence of epiphyseal displacement or upon variation in width of the epiphyseal line. In the absence of displacement, detection of a pure epiphyseal plate fracture is difficult; comparison with the opposite extremity is helpful in doubtful cases. In most cases, the fracture does not remain confined to the cartilaginous plate but angles sharply into the bone so that a corner fragment of the metaphysis remains attached to and displaced with the epiphysis. If there is no displacement, the oblique fracture line in the metaphysis indicates the nature of the injury.

Since the epiphysis is responsible for bone growth, injuries involving the epiphyseal growth plate may result in an alteration in length of the involved bone. In children, dislocations and ligamentous tears are uncommon. Injuries that cause these conditions in adults produce epiphyseal separation in the younger age group. The extent of the injury is important in assessing the likelihood of growth alterations. Prognosis depends on the degree of vascular damage, with growth

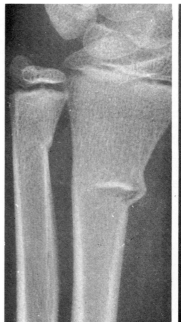
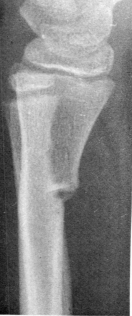

Figure 2–10. Torus fractures of the distal radius and ulna. There is anterolateral buckling of both the radius and ulna, but despite the slight angulation of the distal fragments, the fracture line does not extend across the width of the shaft.

disturbance paralleling the degree of arterial disruption. The Salter-Harris classification is commonly used in describing injuries of the epiphyseal plate (Fig. 2-11A).[25, 26] Radiographic findings are distinct for each type, and prognosis usually varies with each type. In general, injuries involving the lower extremity have a much more serious prognosis than those of the upper extremity, irrespective of the type. The classification is as follows:

Type I: Pure epiphyseal separation. The line of cleavage is confined to the zone of hypertrophic cells within the epiphyseal plate. Since the fracture line is in the cartilage, it is not visible radiographically; displacement of the epiphyseal ossification center is the only positive radiographic sign. The prognosis is generally favorable, with no alterations in growth in most instances.

Type II: A fragment from the metaphysis accompanies the displaced epiphysis, separating a segment of bone on the metaphyseal side (see Fig. 2-11). This is by far the most common injury, accounting for approximately 75% of cases. The most common site is the distal radius, which accounts for up to one-half of all epiphyseal injuries. The distal tibia, distal fibula, distal femur, and ulna are involved in decreasing order of frequency. The prognosis is generally favorable except at the ankle or knee.

Type III: The fracture runs vertically through the epiphysis and through the growth plate. A portion of the epiphysis is detached and displaced. Usually the displacement is minimal, without an associated fracture of the metaphysis. The most frequent site is the distal tibia. The prognosis is good if the fragment is replaced properly so that the joint surface does not become irregular.

Type IV: This is a vertically oriented fracture extending through the epiphysis and growth plate and into the metaphysis. The fracture fragment consists of a portion of metaphysis, growth plate, and epiphysis. The most common sites are the lateral condyle of the humerus in patients under age 10 years and the distal tibia in those over age 10. Growth arrest and joint deformities are the distinct hazard in this type of injury, although the incidence is reduced by proper reduction and surgical fixation.

Type V: This rare injury is a result of crushing-type force, usually directed to the distal femoral or proximal or distal tibial epiphyseal centers. These are more commonly associated with fractures of the shaft of the femur or tibia. There is no immediate visible radiographic alteration within the epiphyseal complex. Subsequently, some shortening or angulation occurs. Premature closure of an epiphyseal line and a slowing of the growth rate are the factors that result in deformity. Patients must be observed for a minimum of 2 years before the possibility of these complications can be ruled out.

Pathologic Fractures

A pathologic fracture is one occurring through diseased bone, characteristically resulting from a relatively trivial injury. Most are encountered in adults and are associated with foci of metastatic carcinoma (Fig.

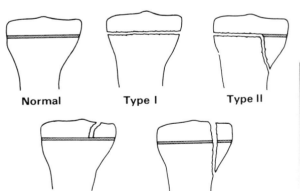
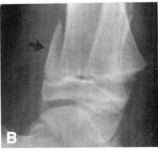
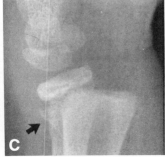

Figure 2–11. Fractures of the epiphysis. (**A**) Diagram of the Salter-Harris classification of epiphyseal fractures. Type V injury is not included, since there are no radiographic abnormalities at the time of the initial injury. (**B** and **C**) Salter-Harris type II fracture of the distal tibia and radius. Note the large, triangular, metaphyseal fragment, the "corner sign" (*arrow*). There is an associated fracture of the distal fibula (**B**). Dorsal displacement of the distal radial epiphysis accompanied by a small triangular fragment (*arrow*) from the dorsal surface of the metaphysis (**C**).

2-12*A*) or much less frequently with a benign cause such as Paget's disease or benign tumor, particularly an enchondroma of the phalanges (Fig. 2-12*B*). The lesions responsible for most pathologic fractures in children are benign. Simple bone cysts of the proximal humerus or other sites often present with a pathologic fracture. Osteogenesis imperfecta is subject to frequent fractures.

Pathologic fractures are often transversely oriented at right angles to the longitudinal axis of the long bone. The ends of the fragments are often smooth or slightly irregular. Comminution is infrequent. In the presence of such a fracture, the fragment should be observed carefully for evidence of bone destruction, endosteal erosion, or periosteal new-bone formation that gives evidence of a preexisting lesion.

Pseudofractures

Pseudofractures are transverse fissurelike defects that extend partly or completely through the bone. They are frequently seen in osteomalacia and are sometimes called *looser zones* or *umbauzonen*. They are infractions of bone in which osteoid is formed in the defect but with failure of calcium deposition. Healing is delayed, and the fissure persists as a roentgenographically visible defect. Multiple pseudofractures of this type were described by Milkman in 1930, and the condition sometimes is designated as Milkman's syndrome. Most investigators now believe that this represents osteomalacia in which the pseudofractures happen to be a particularly prominent part of the disease (see Osteomalacia in Chapter 6).

A similar type of transverse fracture is seen in Paget's disease, fibrous dysplasia, and osteogenesis imperfecta. Some authorities contend that these differ from the pseudofractures of osteomalacia in that they are true fractures that have healed by fibrous or cartilaginous union. Roentgenographically they are similar to the pseudofractures of osteomalacia, but the basic change of the underlying bone disease (e.g., Paget's disease) is different and should lead to the correct diagnosis. A pseudofracture may become complete following an injury and may lead to displacement of fragments and the clinical signs and symptoms of fracture.

Birth Fractures

Fractures of the fetal skeletal system occasionally occur during birth, particularly during difficult deliveries.[24] The most common site of fracture is the clavicle (Fig. 2-13). Occasionally the shaft of a long bone is fractured. Epiphyseal separations may also occur. These have been termed *pseudodislocations* because clinically they are mistaken for dislocations. The difficulty is

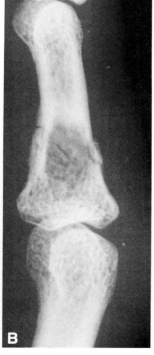

Figure 2–12. Pathologic fractures. **(A)** Carcinoma of the lung metastatic to the proximal radius. A transverse fracture has occurred through a lytic focus of metastatic disease. Note the endosteal erosion. **(B)** Pathologic fracture through a phalangeal enchondroma.

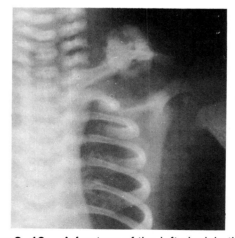

Figure 2–13. A fracture of the left clavicle that occurred during birth. Examination at 2 weeks of age demonstrates a large amount of callus at the fracture site.

compounded by the radiographic appearance. The fractures most commonly involve the proximal humerus, proximal femur, and distal humerus. Since none of the epiphyses are ossified at birth, the radiographic diagnosis may be difficult. True dislocations in newborns are unusual, however. Ultrasonography, MRI or arthrography may be necessary to establish the diagnosis with certainty. The injuries usually occur in high-weight babies who are born to diabetic mothers and who present in unusual positions such as breech presentation and who undergo a difficult delivery.

Apophyseal Injuries

Apophyses are the growth centers for bony projections and tuberosities and serve as attachments for muscles, tendons, and ligaments. They may be avulsed by the pull of the attached muscle or tendon. These most commonly occur about the pelvis, particularly the ischial tuberosity and the medial epicondyle of the elbow.

Stress Fractures

Stress or fatigue fractures occur in normal bone of healthy individuals in response to the stress of repeated activities. They were first described in military recruits with painful feet and thus were termed *march fractures*. The majority have been reported in military recruit populations,[9] but more recently it has been recognized that they occur in athletes or, at least, the athletically inclined.[29] The radiographic examination is within normal limits initially, and no evidence of fracture is usually identified until 10 to 20 days following the onset of symptoms. A fracture may be visualized as a thin line of transverse or oblique radiolucency, as fluffy or compact periosteal callus without an obvious underlying fracture (Fig. 2-14), or as a band of increased density indicating healing and possibly compression of medullary bone (Fig. 2-15). The most common sites of occurrence are at the distal shaft of the metatarsals (Figs. 2-14A and B), the tuberosity of the calcaneus (Fig. 2-15), the shafts of the tibia (Fig. 2-14C) and fibula, the neck of the femur, and the pubic rami.[9, 29]

Bone scanning is useful in the diagnosis of stress fractures (Fig. 2-15).[15, 31] The bone scan is often positive before the radiographic findings are apparent.

In cases with considerable periosteal callus formation, the lesion may be easily mistaken for a tumor—particularly an osteoid osteoma or even osteosarcoma—or for evidence of infection. When such a lesion is encountered, it is necessary to inquire about a history of athletic participation or unusual activity to avoid an error in diagnosis.

Insufficiency Fractures

Insufficiency fractures are the result of normal activity in weakened bone as opposed to fatigue or stress fractures, which are the result of unusual activity in normal bone.[5, 6, 27] The most distinctive variety occurs in the pelvis of elderly osteoporotic women.[5, 6] Similar fractures occur with rheumatoid arthritis, with renal osteodystrophy, with steroid use, and after pelvic irradiation. Patients present with a history of pain, and the plain film findings are often obscure. Occasionally, an ill-defined sclerosis can be seen in the sacral alae, or an obvious healing fracture of the pubic ramus may be evident (see Fig. 2-51A). The body of the pubis may show patchy areas of lucency and sclerosis and on occasion an obvious loss of bone volume. The diagnosis can be confirmed by CT, which demonstrates patchy sclerosis, often with fissurelike fractures and no associated soft-tissue mass (see Fig. 2-51C). The lack of a soft-tissue mass aids in distinguishing insufficiency fracture from metastatic disease, which is often a clinical consideration in these patients.[18]

Peculiar forms of fractures are identified in the lower extremity, and these result from no more than normal activity, particularly in rheumatoid arthritis, whether or not steroids are used. At times these fractures may follow resumption of ambulation after periods of prolonged bed rest. They often present as linear bandlike densities in the metaphysis paralleling the joint surface and are similar in appearance to stress fractures in the same location.

Similar fractures have also been described after joint replacement for osteoarthritis in osteoporotic individuals. Such fractures also occur in patients treated with fluorides for osteoporosis. Insufficiency fractures of the sternum occur in osteoporotic individuals with severe dorsal kyphosis.

HEALING OF FRACTURES

UNION OF FRACTURES

When a fracture occurs, the soft tissues are lacerated, the periosteum is torn, and vascular channels in the adjacent soft tissues are opened.[23, 24] A hematoma forms about the fracture site. Since the blood supply to the cells adjacent to the fracture is interrupted, these cells die. The edges of the fracture then consist of dead bone back as far as the junction of collateral vascular channels. A network of fibrin is precipitated in the clot, and collagenoblasts penetrate the hematoma from the adjacent mesenchymal tissues. A network of endothelial buds is formed, and the hematoma is organized into a mass of granulation tissue. Viable osteoblasts begin to produce osteoid, and new fibroblasts mature

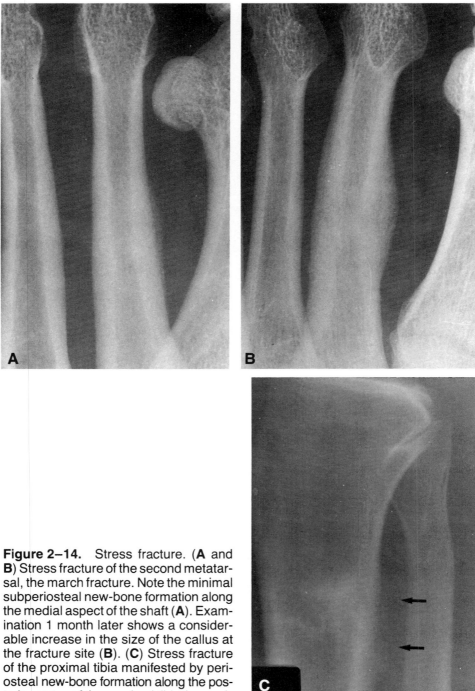

Figure 2–14. Stress fracture. (**A** and **B**) Stress fracture of the second metatarsal, the march fracture. Note the minimal subperiosteal new-bone formation along the medial aspect of the shaft (**A**). Examination 1 month later shows a considerable increase in the size of the callus at the fracture site (**B**). (**C**) Stress fracture of the proximal tibia manifested by periosteal new-bone formation along the posterior cortex of the proximal tibia (*arrows*).

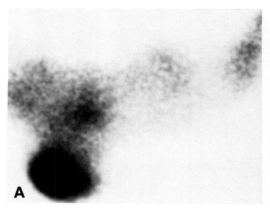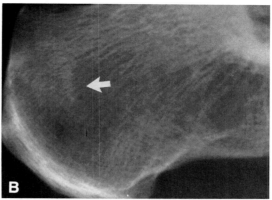

Figure 2–15. Stress fracture of the calcaneus. **(A)** Technetium bone scan reveals increased radioactivity in the posterior margin of the tuberosity of the calcaneus. **(B)** Lateral radiograph demonstrates area of increased density due to endosteal callus formation at the site of stress fracture (*arrow*). (Courtesy of Joseph Norfray, M.D., Springfield, Illinois)

into osteoblasts and chondroblasts. Osteoid is laid down. There is also production of new bone between the periosteum and the old cortex, and a solid mass of bone also replaces the marrow tissue. This new bone extends toward the fracture line and meets with the similar bone produced on the opposite side of the fracture. All of this new bone is termed *callus*.

At first the bone composing the callus is largely woven bone, which must be replaced with compact adult bone before it can withstand functional stresses. Lines of stress determine the reformation of bone so that angulations or malpositions may be corrected during the healing process. However, rotational deformity cannot be corrected. Subsequently, there is a decrease in the bulk of the callus as the stronger adult bone replaces the weaker woven bone. Healing is delayed when there is significant destruction of the periosteum. Movement of the fracture edges tends to delay the healing process. Motion of the fracture site also increases the size of the callus.

Roentgenographic Evidence of Bone Union

A fracture that may have been very difficult to visualize initially will usually become more obvious within a week or two because of resorption along the fracture edges (see Fig. 2-5).

Uncalcified osteoid is not visible roentgenographically. Failure to visualize calcified callus therefore does not necessarily indicate that the fragments are not held together. Eventually, the callus becomes more dense and compacted. Ultimately in normal healing the callus from the margins of the fracture joins and obliterates the fracture line. Clinical union often occurs before there is complete obliteration of the fracture line (Fig. 2-16). Clinical union is determined by the absence of tenderness and the ability to bear weight and use the extremity. Satisfactory progress of healing is shown by the changes described in the following paragraphs.

The amount of visible periosteal callus varies greatly in different fractures. It is more extensive when there is displacement of fragments than when there has been accurate replacement and a close apposition of fragments. It is more prominent beneath large muscle masses. In bones covered with little or no muscle, periosteal callus will be slight. This is noted in fractures of the phalanges, which often unite with little evidence of periosteal callus. It also is observed in fractures of the tibial shaft, where heavy calcified periosteal callus may form along the posterior and outer side of the fracture but with very little over the anterior surface. The intra-articular portion of bone is not covered by periosteum, and therefore, intra-articular fractures such as those of the femoral neck do not form periosteal callus. Fractures of the skull also do not form callus because the periosteum of the cranial bones does not have osteogenic properties.

The amount and character of periosteal callus are the principal indicators of when the part may be removed from traction or cast. The radiographic findings must be interpreted in light of the clinical findings. The absence of tenderness and the ability to use the part without pain are excellent indicators of satisfactory

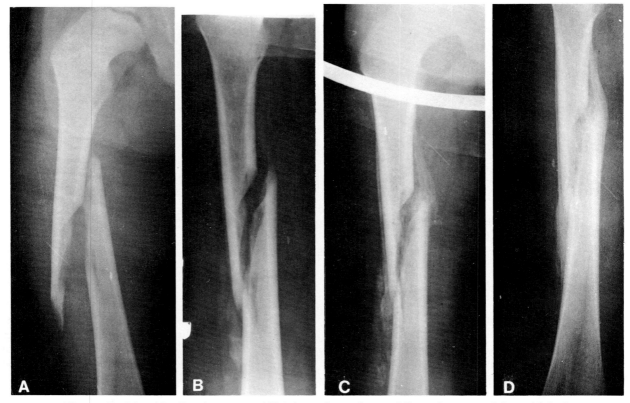

Figure 2–16.   Healing fractures. **(A)** Injury shows long, oblique fracture of the midshaft of the femur. **(B)** In 2 weeks, some hazy callus formation is identified at the margins of the fracture. **(C)** At 4 weeks, considerable callus is evident. **(D)** Three months after injury, there is a solid bridge of callus between fragments along the external surfaces. The fracture line is disappearing, indicating presence of endosteal callus. (Courtesy of Ralph C. Frank, M.D., Eau Claire, Wisconsin)

healing. There usually is clinical evidence of union before the healing process has completely obliterated radiographic evidence of the fracture line.

DELAYED UNION AND NONUNION FRACTURES

General Aspects

Fractures unite more slowly in the aged than in younger adults and always heal more slowly in adults than they do in infants and children. The rapidity of callus formation and bone union in fractures occurring during birth is striking. For example, a birth fracture of a clavicle may develop a fusiform area of dense periosteal callus that is easily visualized in roentgenograms within 5 to 7 days after the injury (see Fig. 2-13).

The term *nonunion* refers to a failure of bony union. When the rate of progress of healing of a fracture is slower than normal for the age of the patient and partic-

ular type of fracture under consideration, it is termed *slow* or *delayed union*. Some causes of nonunion may also be responsible for delay in union. The principal difference between the two is that in a delayed union, healing eventually takes place. Some fractures fail to undergo bony union but may unite with fibrous union, and in certain areas this may be sufficient for practical purposes. In weight-bearing bones, fibrous union is not adequate.

Fractures in certain areas are noted for the frequency with which delayed union or nonunion occurs. These include fractures of the junction of the middle and lower thirds of the tibia, the carpal navicular or scaphoid, the central third of the shaft of the humerus, and the lower third of the ulna.

The causes of delayed union and nonunion include the following: (1) infection, (2) distraction of fragments (Distraction refers to a separation or pulling apart of the fragments, leaving a gap between them. It is

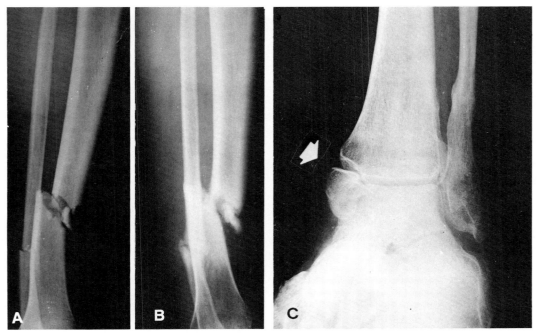

Figure 2–17. Fracture nonunion. **(A)** Comminuted tibial fracture and transverse fibular fracture 3 weeks after injury without callus formation. **(B)** Eight months later there is partial union of the fibula, but no definite callus bridges the tibial fracture. There is some eburnation of bone adjacent to the tibial fracture site. **(C)** Old ununited fracture of the medial malleolus (*arrow*).

usually caused by excessive traction.), (3) injury to the blood supply of one or both fragments, (4) improper fixation, and (5) interposition of soft tissues between the fragment ends. Other causes include local bone disease at the site of fracture and certain generalized conditions, such as osteomalacia, neuropathic bone, and joint disease.

Roentgenographic Observations

Roentgenographic findings suggesting nonunion include one or more of the following (Figs. 2-17 and 2-18):[23, 24]

Smoothness at Fracture Margins. At first the ends of fracture fragments are ragged and irregular. A fracture that is not going to unite often shows, as first evidence, the development of smoothness of the margins of the fracture.

Absence of Peripheral Callus. In most shaft fractures some periosteal callus becomes visible, and its presence is a good indicator that union is commencing. Failure to demonstrate peripheral callus formation in a

normal anticipated time for the site of fracture is an indication of delayed union. In atrophic nonunion, little or no peripheral callus may ever appear. More commonly, however, callus formation occurs along the peripheral margins of the fragments but never bridges across the line of fracture. An irregular translucent line

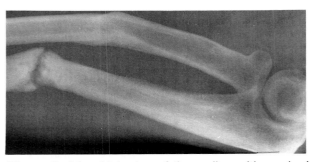

Figure 2–18. Malunion of the radius with marked volar angulation at the fracture site associated with pseudoarthrosis of a fracture of the midshaft of the ulna. Note the bony eburnation at the fracture site and the formation of a false joint.

remains between the callus and appears to be an extension of the fracture line.

Eburnation of Fragments. The fragment ends may undergo increasing sclerosis and eburnation when bony union fails to take place. The amount of eburnation varies from case to case, but the occurrence of sclerotic density in the fragment ends is often the first evidence that bony union will fail to occur. The longer the duration of nonunion, the more eburnated the fragments become.

Motion Between Fragments. In the absence of bony union, motion can be demonstrated when roentgenograms are obtained with and without the application of stress. This is an excellent way to demonstrate absence of union in patients in whom the clinical examination gives indefinite results. Care should be exercised when pressure is made in an attempt to elicit motion so that early callus not be disrupted or that the bone not be refractured.

Pseudarthrosis. With rounding and eburnation of the fragments and continued motion at the fracture site, a false joint may be formed in the fracture line. The ends of the fragments are plugged with cortical bone, and the fracture line is filled with fibrous tissue. With sufficient motion, a cleft may appear in the fibrous tissue, simulating a joint cavity (see Fig. 2-18).

OTHER COMPLICATIONS

Disuse Osteoporosis and Sudeck's Atrophy (Reflex Sympathetic Dystrophy)

Simple immobilization of bone will result in a loss of osseous tissue known as disuse osteoporosis. This process begins at and extends distal to the fracture. Occasionally, after a fracture and sometimes after relatively minor trauma without fracture, a more severe and painful form of osteoporosis known as Sudeck's atrophy (reflex sympathetic dystrophy) develops. These conditions also are discussed in Chapter 6 (see Fig. 6-12). The roentgenographic findings in the two conditions are quite similar, although the findings tend to be more severe in reflex sympathetic dystrophy. The distinction between the two conditions is made on the basis of clinical findings. In reflex sympathetic dystrophy, the patient experiences pain and demonstrates evidence of edema and atrophic changes in the skin, whereas none of these findings are present in simple uncomplicated disuse osteoporosis. Simple disuse osteoporosis causes a minimal to moderate degree of increased radiolucency of bone, often more pronounced in the regions of the metaphysis in children or at the site of the previous epiphyseal growth plate in adults. This is probably because of an increased vascularity in this region. The bone loss develops gradually and is usually noted after several weeks of immobilization. The loss in density is more commonly uniform, but it may assume a spotted or mottled appearance in the tarsal and carpal bones and at the ends of long bones.

Osteomyelitis

Osteomyelitis is a relatively common complication of open fractures and is seen in a small percentage of closed fractures following open reduction and internal fixation. Osteomyelitis is extremely rare in closed fractures that have been treated by closed means. The radiographic indications of osteomyelitis are periosteal new-bone formation, irregular destruction of bone, and eventually the formation of sequestra as described in Chapter 5, Infections and Inflammations of Bone. The clinical evidence of infection is often obvious, but it may take 10 days to 2 weeks for radiographic signs to develop. The roentgenograms serve to establish the extent of the involvement and the progress of the disease.

Traumatic Arthritis

When a fracture enters the articular surface, injury to the articular cartilage occurs and may be followed in time by the development of degenerative changes within the joint. This is particularly true in the weight-bearing joints, most frequently in the ankle and knee. This condition is sometimes referred to as traumatic arthritis, but it is pathologically quite similar to degenerative joint disease or osteoarthritis. See Chapter 3, Diseases of the Joints, for further consideration of this abnormality.

FRACTURES OF THE SKULL

Injuries of the intracranial contents—the brain, vascular system, and meninges—are much more important than any injury of the cranial bones. The demonstration of a skull fracture does not indicate the presence of an intracranial injury, nor does the absence of a skull fracture rule out the presence of an intracranial injury. The only plain film findings that indicate the possibility of an associated intracranial injury are a shift in the calcified pineal and a depressed skull fracture. If there is serious concern about the possibility of an intracranial injury based upon the clinical findings, a CT examination should be obtained. This is an extremely sensitive method of identifying intracranial hematomas, depressed skull fractures, and fractures involving the base of the skull. Only approximately 20% of linear fractures of the skull are demonstrated by CT, but in the absence of intracerebral injury these fractures are of little or no clinical significance; therefore, the inability of CT to demonstrate them is not a serious deficiency.

The percentage of skull examinations following trauma and revealing a fracture is, in large measure, dependent upon the clinical findings.[24] If there has been a loss of consciousness or other neurologic signs or symptoms, the percentage approaches 40% or more. When there are no neurologic signs and symptoms or positive physical findings and the examining physician is doubtful that a fracture exists, then a fracture will be identified in significantly less than 5% of patients.

TYPES OF FRACTURES

Linear Fractures

A linear fracture is visualized as a sharp, dark, translucent line, often irregular or jagged and occasionally of branching character (Fig. 2-19). Linear fractures often extend into the base of the skull, and their inferior terminations become invisible. A linear fracture must be distinguished from suture lines and vascular grooves. A vascular groove usually has a smooth, curving course and is not as sharp or distinct as a fracture line. An old fracture that occurred 6 months or more previously may closely resemble a vascular groove, and at times it is difficult or impossible to be certain about the nature of such a line. Suture lines generally have serrated edges. Occasionally, the sagittal suture will appear as a straight, dark line when viewed end-on in anteroposterior roentgenograms. The sutures between the temporal, parietal, and occipital bones may also resemble fracture lines. The bilateral and symmetrical nature of the lines and their positions should enable the examiner to recognize them.

A linear fracture will be more sharply defined when it is on the side that is closer to the film. For instance, a fracture involving the right parietal bone will be visualized as a sharp line on the right lateral view of the skull, but it is slightly wider and less well defined on the left lateral view of the skull.

Ordinarily, linear fractures without depression and without clinical signs of disturbed sensorium or neurologic findings are of little significance.

Depressed Fractures

After more severe trauma, particularly if the force has been localized to a small area of the skull, one or more fragments of bone may be separated and depressed into the cranial cavity. Such fractures are often stellate, with multiple fracture lines radiating outward from a central point and with one or more comminuted pieces present. When viewed *en face*, the line of fracture may appear more dense than normal bone because of overlap or tilting of fragments (Fig. 2-20). This effectively increases the thickness of bone and therefore increases its radiographic density. Tangential views are essential to determine the amount of depression. If the underlying dura is torn, surgery is indicated; the greater the depression, the more likely an associated dural tear. However, the exact amount of depression indicating the need for surgery is a subject of some dispute. Depressed fractures are easily and advantageously evaluated by CT (Fig. 2-20C).

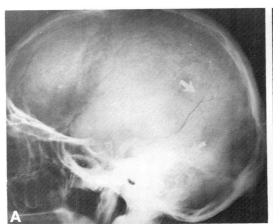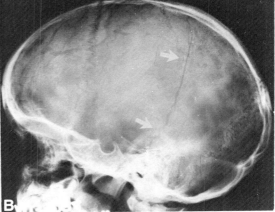

Figure 2–19. Linear fracture of the skull. (**A**) A linear fracture of the parietal bone extends posteriorly toward the occipital bone (*arrow*). (**B**) In this patient, a linear fracture line extends into the posterior temporal bone from the parietal area (*arrows*).

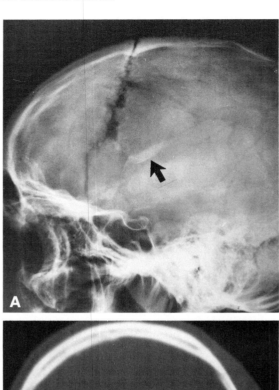

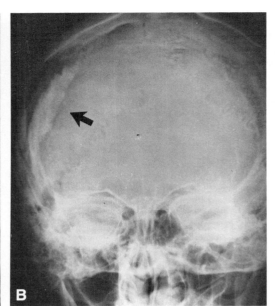

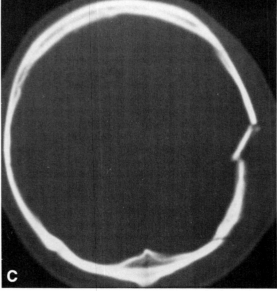

Figure 2–20. Depressed comminuted skull fracture. (**A**) Lateral view shows an irregular fracture line with overlapping causing increased density (*arrow*). (**B**) AP view demonstrates the extent of depression. Note the inward displacement of the large bone fragment (*arrow*). (**C**) CT of another case demonstrating typical findings of a depressed fracture.

Diastatic Fractures

A linear fracture may extend into a suture and separate it along at least a part of its course (Fig. 2-21). Less commonly there is a separation of the suture without an associated linear fracture. This type of fracture is seen most frequently during infancy and childhood and most commonly involves the lambdoid or sagittal suture. Separation of a suture causes widening so that the suture stands out more clearly than normal. Occasionally, a normal coronal or lambdoid suture will ap-pear slightly wider than its mate because of a slight tilting of the head from the true anteroposterior plane. Sutures that are separated by 1 to 2 mm and that are wider than their opposite mate indicate fracture.

Basal Skull Fractures

Fractures limited to the base of the skull are very difficult to visualize by roentgenographic examina-tions, including the basal view of the skull. Although the base of the skull can be shown in various radio-

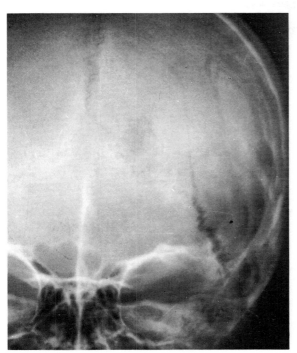

Figure 2–21. Diastatic fracture. A linear fracture of the parietal bone extends into the lambdoidal suture, with obvious widening of the suture line.

graphic projections, the detail is poor and the anatomic structures composing the base add to the difficulty in recognizing a fracture line. Many basal fractures will extend into the vault for at least a short distance, and part of the fracture may be visible. A basal skull fracture often involves the sphenoid sinus, and when lateral roentgenograms are obtained using a horizontal beam, an air–fluid level or complete opacification of the sinus may be demonstrated. Basal skull fractures are much more easily and satisfactorily demonstrated by CT; therefore, when there is a serious question of a basal skull fracture, a CT examination should be obtained (Fig. 2-22).

RADIOGRAPHIC INTERPRETATION OF SKULL ROENTGENOGRAMS FOR TRAUMA

The principal radiographic features to be determined when evaluating a traumatized skull are the presence or absence of fracture, the presence of a depressed fracture and the degree of depression (this may require a tangential view), the presence and the position of the pineal if calcified (when shifted this is strongly suggestive of an intracerebral hematoma), and the presence of pneumocephalus (the air is most commonly identified in the subarachnoid cisterns or about the sella turcica,

but it may be found over the convexity or within the ventricular system). The most significant findings are a depressed fracture, a shift of the pineal, and air within the cranial vault.

Pneumocephalus

If a fracture has extended through the frontal, ethmoid, or sphenoidal sinuses or the mastoids, air may enter the cranial cavity. If the dura and arachnoid have been torn, the air may find its way into the subarachnoid space and eventually reach the ventricles. This condition is known as *post-traumatic pneumocephalus* (see Fig. 2-22). It is an uncommon but serious complication and can be recognized easily on CT scans and roentgenograms because of the transparency of the air in contrast to the density of the surrounding brain tissue and cerebrospinal fluid.

Cephalohematoma

Cephalohematoma is found in newborn infants as a result of birth trauma, usually caused by the application of forceps. Injury to the external fibrous tissue covering the skull is followed by formation of a hematoma beneath it. This forms a localized mass that subsequently undergoes calcification. It is then visible in roentgenograms as an area of increased density. When viewed tangentially, the typical cephalhematoma is visualized as a homogeneous shadow of soft-tissue density showing a sharply demarcated convex outer border, which, in time, is marginated by a fine rim of calcification, the margins merging smoothly with normal bone (Fig. 2-23). The bone beneath the area of calcification usually is normal. With the passage of time, a cephalohematoma tends to undergo gradual decrease in size and disappears completely if small, or at the most it leaves only an area of slightly thickened bone.

COMPLICATIONS OF SKULL FRACTURE

Leptomeningeal Cyst

If the dura is torn beneath an area of fracture, it may become adherent to the bone along the margins of the fracture and allow the cerebral cortex to come into contact with the bone. An accumulation of cerebrospinal fluid may form in this space and develop into a leptomeningeal cyst. In other instances, both cerebral cortex and dura adhere to the bone. Either condition predisposes to a gradual erosion of the bone overlying the cyst or cicatrix, apparently caused by the pulsating pressure of the blood vessels along the surface of the cortex. This condition is seen most frequently in infants

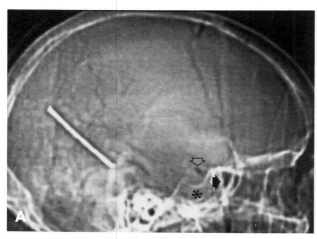

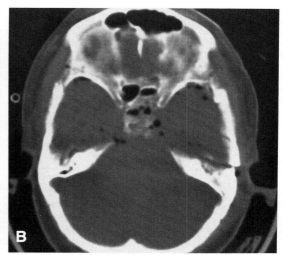

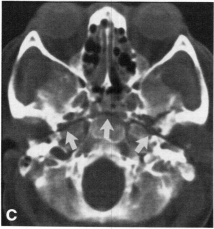

Figure 2–22. Basal skull fracture with pneumocephalus. (**A**) A digital radiograph of the skull demonstrates opacification of the sphenoid sinus (*asterisk*), air–fluid level in the posterior ethmoid sinuses (*closed arrow*), and pneumocephalus in the basal cisterns (*open arrow*). The linear metallic density is a hairpin that was left on the patient at the time of the examination. (**B**) CT demonstrates small bubbles of air within the subarachnoid space of the middle cranial fossa and opacification of the sphenoid and posterior ethmoid sinuses with air–fluid levels. (**C**) An arcuate, transverse fracture of the base of the skull is visualized (*arrows*).

and young children. It occurs most commonly in the parietal area following a diastatic type of fracture. The fracture may heal satisfactorily at first, but within a few months erosion of bone along the line of fracture becomes apparent (Fig. 2-24). The bone is often destroyed sufficiently for a soft-tissue mass to bulge through the defect and to be obvious on inspection and palpation.

HEALING OF SKULL FRACTURES

The time required for the disappearance of a skull fracture is extremely variable. A fracture in a young child usually heals promptly. The fracture line fades gradually and may disappear completely within several months. Fine hairline fractures heal more rapidly than those with a greater separation of surfaces. In older individuals, the fracture lines tend to remain visible for longer periods and in some cases never completely

disappear. It is therefore difficult to date or determine the age of skull fractures with certainty on the basis of radiographic examination. Usually after several months the sharp edge of bone along the fracture line becomes indistinct. Gradually some reossification occurs and portions of the fracture become obliterated. A residual defect may remain more or less permanently as a hazy, dark line that is easily mistaken for a vascular groove.

INJURIES OF THE SPINE

Fractures and dislocations of the spine are most common in the lower cervical region from C4 through C7, at the thoracolumbar junction between the tenth dorsal and the second lumbar vertebrae, and at the craniovertebral junction.[24] Fractures usually involve the vertebral body with or without associated fractures of the posterior elements of the affected vertebra. The impor-

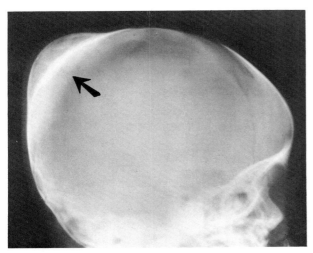

Figure 2–23. Calcified cephalohematoma (*arrow*) following birth trauma. The dense, calcified mass shown here gradually decreases in size and eventually disappears.

tant diagnostic observations in spinal trauma are to determine whether or not the height of the vertebral bodies is maintained; the alignment of the spine is normal; the distances between the vertebrae at the intervertebral disc space, facet joints, and spinous process remain normal; and the contiguous surfaces of the joints and vertebral end-plates remain parallel.[24] Fractures and dislocations are manifested by a loss of vertebral body height, disruption of the cortical margins of the posterior elements, malalignment of the spine, and a loss of the parallel apposing cortical surfaces of bone at the facet joints or intervertebral disc spaces. Fractures limited to the vertebral body or the posterior elements are considered stable. Those fractures that involve both the vertebral body and posterior elements are considered unstable. Paraspinous hematomas may point to an otherwise obscure fracture or dislocation in the cervical or thoracic spine. The hematomas present as retropharyngeal masses in the cervical spine and as paraspinous masses on the frontal projection in the dorsal spine.

RADIOGRAPHIC EXAMINATION OF SPINAL INJURY

Great care is needed in handling patients with suspected spinal injuries so as not to cause more extensive cord injury than may already be present. Therefore, it is wise to secure the lateral film for examination before additional views are obtained. Once it is determined that there is no subluxation or dislocation, anteroposterior and oblique views may be obtained. Often CT is necessary to verify fractures.[21] CT is particularly useful

Figure 2–24. A leptomeningeal cyst or growing fracture caused by meningeal adhesions to the inner margins of an old linear fracture. Swelling was noted over the region of previous fracture several months following injury. The elongated, slightly elliptical lucency with slightly sclerotic margins is characteristic of a leptomeningeal cyst.

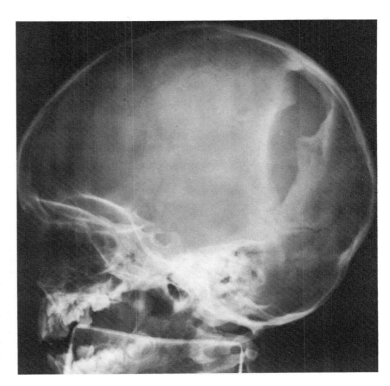

in the demonstration of bony fragments impinging on the spinal canal and, therefore, possibly on the spinal cord or nerve roots. It is also useful in the demonstration of fractures of the posterior elements. Horizontal fractures—fractures in the plane of tube movement—may not be disclosed by this method because of volume averaging. Reconstruction in either the sagittal or coronal plane is required.

FRACTURES

Compression Fractures

A compression fracture is manifested by an anterior wedge deformity of the vertebral body or a depression limited to the vertebral end-plate, usually the superior end-plate. The fracture is caused by a flexion of the spine. The degree of deformity is dependent upon the severity of the forces involved. A minor degree of depression may be difficult to recognize, since it consists of only a slight depression of the superior end-plate of the vertebra coupled with a bulging irregularity of the anterosuperior margin of the vertebra as seen on the lateral projection. A faint band of sclerosis is identified just beneath the deformed end-plate, indicating a zone of bony impaction. With a more severe degree of injury, there is a very definite narrowing of the anterior height of the vertebra (Fig. 2-25). Rarely the injury is limited to the inferior end-plate of the vertebral body. With severe compression injuries, a portion of the vertebral body may be displaced into the spinal canal, compromising the spinal cord or nerve roots. This is most commonly encountered in the form of a teardrop fracture in the cervical spine and in burst fractures at the thoracolumbar junction.[1, 24] Whenever a severe compression fracture is encountered, retropulsion of a fragment of the vertebral body must be considered.

Fracture-Dislocations

Fracture-dislocations occur most commonly in the lower cervical spine and at the thoracolumbar junction. Usually the upper vertebral body is displaced anteriorly, relative to the lower vertebral body. There is often an anterior wedge compression fracture of the lower vertebral body and fractures involving the laminae, facets, or spinous processes. Alternatively, there may be disruption of the joint capsule of the facet joints and interspinous ligament without associated fractures. At times, there may be no significant fracture associated with a dislocation, since the injury is limited to the intervertebral disc, facet joint capsules, and intervening ligaments. This commonly occurs in the cervical spine. The degree of dislocation is variable. If minimal, it is often referred to as a subluxation, whereas dislocation is used to indicate a more extensive or complete displacement of one vertebra relative to the other. Complete displacement—that is, a total dislocation of one segment of the spine relative to the other—is quite uncommon.

Fractures of the Posterior Elements

Fractures of the posterior elements do not commonly occur without accompanying fractures of the vertebral bodies, except for fractures of the transverse processes of the lumbar spine, the neural arches of the first and

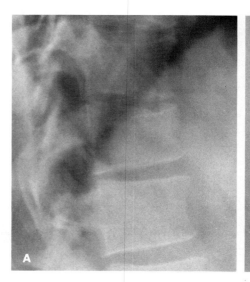
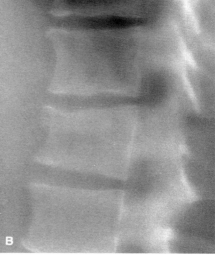

Figure 2–25. Compression fracture of the 12th thoracic vertebra. (**A**) Lateral view demonstrates anterior wedged compression of the 12th vertebral body. The anterosuperior margin of this vertebra is irregular. The posterior wall of the vertebra remains intact. (**B**) Tomogram demonstrates the findings with clarity. Note the zone of increased radiodensity in the upper portion of the vertebral body representing impaction of bone.

second cervical vertebrae, and the spinous processes at the cervicothoracic junction. Isolated fractures of the vertebra at other locations are often difficult to diagnose and require tomography or CT to establish with certainty.

CERVICAL SPINE INJURIES

In patients with potential injuries of the cervical spine, it is important to be certain that all seven cervical vertebrae are included on the film (Fig. 2-26).[24] Failure to visualize the seventh cervical vertebra is the most common error made in the radiographic assessment of cervical spine injury. Retropharyngeal hematomas point to underlying fractures or dislocations of the cervical spine. In adults, the soft tissues anterior to the arch of C1 measure approximately 10 mm; anterior to C4, 4 to 7 mm; and anterior to C6, 16 to 20 mm. Measurements of soft tissue in excess of these amounts should alert one to the possibility of underlying fracture or dislocation. Measurements anterior to the mid-cervical spine on films obtained in the emergency room are quite variable, and in fact, measurements up to 7 mm are quite common. If the measurement is much greater than 7 mm, a fracture is likely and the neck should be immobilized until a fracture is identified or the situation is clarified. Under those circumstances, the injury is often ultimately found at

either extreme—the craniovertebral or cervico-thoracic junction.

Fractures of the first cervical vertebra or atlas are relatively uncommon. The most common is a fracture involving the posterior neural arch because of hyperextension of the head upon the neck. These fractures are commonly undisplaced and bilateral. Care must be taken to differentiate these fractures from gaps in the neural arch that occur as normal variations. Direct forces in the axial direction may split the vertebra both anteriorly and posteriorly, with resultant lateral displacement of the two fragments. This is termed a *bursting* or *Jefferson fracture* (Fig. 2-27). Characteristically it is identified by a bilateral offset of the lateral masses of C1 relative to C2 on the frontal projection. Tilting or rotation of the head may cause a unilateral offset, but this should be associated with a corresponding inset of the lateral masses on the contralateral side. Whenever there is a bilateral offset, a Jefferson fracture is suggested. Often the fractures of the anteroposterior arch cannot be identified on the plain radiographs. CT is the best means of visualizing the fracture sites.

Fractures of the axis, C2, are produced by a hyperextension force such as that commonly experienced when the head or face hits the windshield or steering wheel in a motor vehicle accident. This may result in bilateral fractures of the neural arch anterior to the inferior facets. This is the same fracture caused by judicial

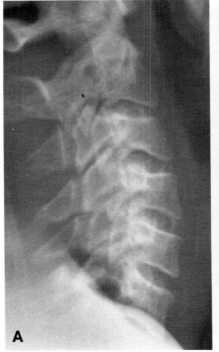 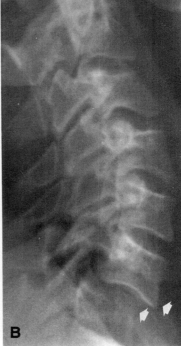

Figure 2–26. All seven cervical vertebrae must be seen on the film. (**A**) Initial cross-table lateral view demonstrates only six cervical vertebrae without apparent injury. (**B**) Repeat lateral view while pulling down on the arms demonstrates a fracture-dislocation of C6–C7 (*arrows*).

hanging, and it is therefore often referred to as a *hangman's fracture* (Fig. 2-28A).[24] The fracture lines are usually oblique and tend to be relatively symmetrical and often associated with dislocation of C2 on C3. There may be an avulsion fracture of the anteroinferior margin of C2. Fractures of the odontoid are also quite common. These commonly are transversely oriented and situated at the base of the odontoid (Fig. 2-28B). There may be anterior or posterior displacement, depending upon the nature of the injuring force.[24]

In the remainder of the cervical spine, flexion injuries commonly produce anterior compression fractures that are usually readily visualized on the lateral roentgenograms. Severe compression fractures with posterior displacement of the upper spine and a characteristic triangular or quadrilateral fragment arising from the anteroinferior surface of the vertebral body are often termed *teardrop fractures* (Fig. 2-29B). These are usually associated with spinal cord injury and are often the result of diving into shallow water.

Flexion injuries may disrupt the intervertebral disc, facet joints, and interspinous ligaments with little or no fracture of the vertebral bodies. These are the result of hyperflexion without axial compression and are often

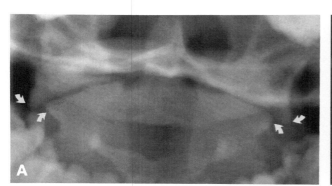
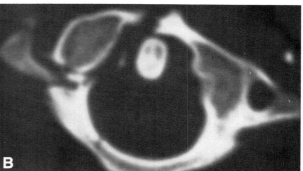

Figure 2–27. Jefferson fracture of C1. (**A**) Open-mouth view demonstrates lateral displacement of the lateral masses of C1 in relation to C2 (*arrows*). No fracture is evident, however. Normally, the lateral masses of C1 should align with the lateral masses of C2. (**B**) CT reveals a fracture of the anterior arch of C1 and of the junction of the posterior arch with the lateral mass and an incomplete fracture of the posterior arch.

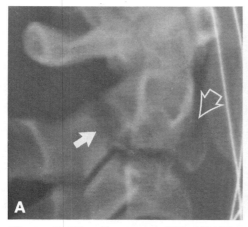
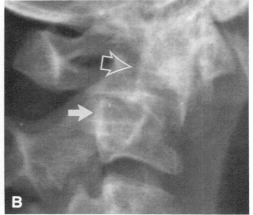

Figure 2–28. Fractures of C2. (**A**) Hangman's fracture of C2. Note the fractures of the neural arch (*arrow*) associated with fracture of the inferior margin of the vertebral body (*open arrow*) and overlying soft-tissue swelling. (**B**) Fracture of the dens with anterior displacement. Note the relationship of the posterior cortical margin of the dens (*open arrow*) with the posterior cortical margin of the vertebral body (*arrow*).

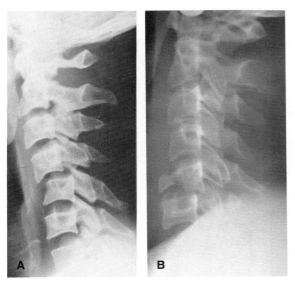

Figure 2–29. Fractures of the lower cervical spine. **(A)** Hyperflexion strain of the fourth on the fifth cervical vertebra. The fourth cervical vertebra is displaced anteriorly upon the fifth, and the facet joints are disrupted. **(B)** Teardrop fracture of C5. Note the characteristic triangular anterior fragment and the posterior displacement of C5 relative to C6.

referred to as *hyperflexion strains* (Fig. 2-29A). Characteristically the interspinous distance is increased, the facet joints are disrupted, and the intervertebral disc is narrowed anteriorly at the involved level with an angulation of the spine at the same level. At times there may be subluxation or even complete dislocation (see Fig. 2-26). If the superior facets come to rest anterior to the inferior facets, this is referred to as a *bilateral locking of the facets* (Fig. 2-30A). *Unilateral locking* of the facets may occur because of a rotation and flexion injury (Fig. 2-30B). This may be a diagnostic problem. Characteristically, one vertebra is displaced 25% of its width upon the inferior vertebra. The vertebral bodies below this level are seen in lateral profile, whereas those above are in oblique profile. The distance between the posterior cortex of the lateral mass and the spinolaminar junction above the dislocation is decreased or there is an overlap of these structures. Close examination will demonstrate that one of the facets above is anterior to the facet below, whereas the opposite facet remains in normal alignment.

Fractures are at times limited to the posterior elements. A fracture of the spinous process of C7 or T1 may occur because of rotational injury. This is known as a *clay shoveler's fracture*. Fractures of the lateral mass may occur. These commonly reorient the facet such that the joint surface of the facet is evident on the anteroposterior projection.

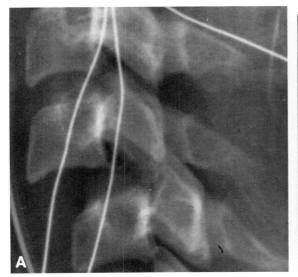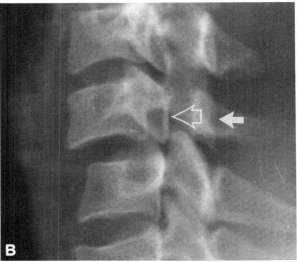

Figure 2–30. Facet locking of the cervical spine. **(A)** Bilateral facet locks. Anterior displacement of C4 on C5 exceeds 50% of the width of the vertebral body. The facets of C4 have come to rest in front of the facets of C5. **(B)** Unilateral facet lock. There is anterior displacement of C5 on C6 approximating 25% of the width of the vertebral body. The vertebral bodies below the dislocation are in lateral profile, whereas those above are in oblique profile. The *closed arrow* points to the undisplaced facet and the *open arrow* to the rotated and locked facet.

Older patients with spondylosis of the cervical spine may sustain a spinal cord injury as a result of a simple fall.[24] Hyperextension of the head upon the neck causes the cord to be pinched between posterior vertebral osteophytes and the hypertrophied ligamentum flavum, resulting in a spinal cord injury. This is often associated with a retropharyngeal hematoma secondary to a disruption of the anterior longitudinal ligament. On occasion you may notice a small fracture of the anteroinferior surface of the vertebra as a result of an avulsion fracture at the site of the tear in the anterior longitudinal ligament.

Whiplash Injury

The so-called whiplash injury of the cervical spine is of considerable importance because of its legal implications. The injury is caused by a sudden deceleration of the body, as when an automobile is stopped suddenly by collision or when a stationary automobile is struck from behind by a moving vehicle. The head is thus snapped back and forth—whiplashed. There is considerable difference of opinion about the importance of the whiplash injury as a cause of clinical complaints and disability. With a definite compression fracture or subluxation, the evidence of injury is obvious. When no fracture exists but the supporting ligaments have been injured, the diagnosis becomes more difficult and it may be impossible to state from roentgenographic evidence alone whether or not an injury exists. The cervical spine may be straightened or the curve of the spine reversed because of cervical muscle spasm. Minor degrees of reversal of the cervical lordotic curve can be seen in normal individuals. A careful evaluation of the roentgenographic appearances with a consideration of the age of the patient, the duration of the injury, and the character of the clinical findings and complaints is necessary in cases of this nature. In our experience, minor degrees of reversal of the cervical curve as well as minimal offset of one cervical vertebra on another may be produced by voluntary muscle contraction and therefore presumably can be produced by muscle spasm secondary to pain without any actual ligamentous injury of the cervical spine. This adds to the difficulty in assessing the significance of minor variations in the cervical spine. Care should be taken not to overemphasize these variations.

THORACOLUMBAR SPINE FRACTURES

Most fractures of the thoracic and lumbar vertebrae tend to be anterior compressions, which are usually readily observed in the lateral projections (see Fig. 2-25) and may be evident on the frontal projection because of loss of height or obliteration of the superior end-plate of the involved vertebra. Fractures of the upper thoracic spine are usually associated with violent muscular action such as in convulsion or high-impact motor vehicle accidents. In the absence of such injury, compression of one of the upper four thoracic vertebrae should raise the possibility of an underlying pathologic condition such as a tumor or metabolic disease. On the other hand, fractures of the lower thoracic and upper lumbar spine are caused by flexion injuries.

Burst fractures are common at the thoracolumbar junction.[1] In this injury, a fragment from the superoposterior margin of the vertebral body is displaced into the spinal canal (Fig. 2-31) and may cause a neurologic injury of the spinal cord, conus medullaris, or nerve roots. Every compression fracture should be closely examined for evidence of a retropulsed fragment. CT is an excellent means of visualizing such fragments.

Horizontal fractures may occur with little or no compression of the vertebral body. These are known as *Chance fractures* or *seat belt fractures*, since they are commonly associated with the wearing of seat belts. At times, a horizontal fracture of the posterior elements may be associated with a horizontal fracture through the vertebral body, or alternatively there may be a disruption of the ligaments and intervertebral discs without fracture (Fig. 2-32A). The cause of these injuries is a flexion of the trunk over an object that serves as a fulcrum, such as a seat belt. The fulcrum of the flexion forces is displaced forward to the object over which the body is flexed, and therefore, the compression forces are removed from the vertebral body and no significant compression fracture results from such injuries.

Fracture-dislocations are commonly encountered at the thoracolumbar junction with compression fractures of the involved lumbar vertebral body and associated fractures of the posterior elements, including the superior facet, laminae, and disruptions of the apophyseal joints (Fig. 2-32B). The full evaluation of such injuries requires tomography or CT.

Fractures of transverse processes may occur in association with severe injury anywhere in the spine, but in the lumbar area there may be an isolated injury due to local trauma, the result of either muscle pull or direct local injury. Radiolucent lines simulating fracture of transverse processes may be produced by the psoas shadow, intra-abdominal gas, or ununited ossification centers.

FRACTURES AND DISLOCATIONS IN SPECIAL AREAS

Most fractures and dislocations are easily recognized on roentgenograms and cause little difficulty in diagnosis. For a detailed analysis of the various types of fractures and dislocations, the mechanical principles involved,

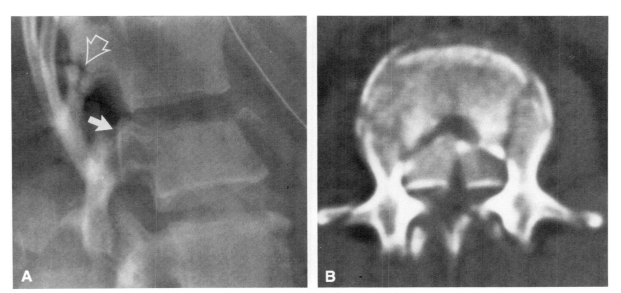

Figure 2–31. Burst fracture of the second lumbar vertebra. **(A)** Lateral view demonstrates the anterior wedged compresson of the second lumbar vertebral body. Note the retropulsion of the posterosuperior margin of the vertebral body (*arrow*), which compromises the spinal canal. There is also a horizontal fracture through the lamina of L1 (*open arrow*). **(B)** Retropulsion of a split fragment, with marked compromise of the spinal canal. There is also a fracture of the left lamina. The superior surface of the vertebral body is comminuted. Fractures of the transverse processes are also present.

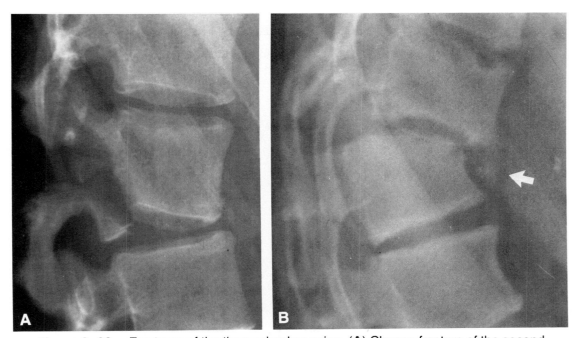

Figure 2–32. Fractures of the thoracolumbar spine. **(A)** Chance fracture of the second lumbar vertebra. Note the absence of compression of the vertebral body. A horizontal fracture has extended through the lamina, the base of the pedicles, and the inferior, posterior margin of the vertebral body. The L2–L3 disc is disrupted. **(B)** Fracture-dislocation of T11–T12. Anterior displacement of T12 and a characteristic small triangular fragment displaced from the anterosuperior margin of T12 (*arrow*).

complications, methods of treatment, and the processes of repair, the reader should consult one of the texts dealing specifically with these problems.[23, 24] Only those features of importance from the standpoint of roentgen examination and diagnosis will be considered in this section.

THE HAND

The Phalanges

Crushing injuries to the tips of the fingers may result in compression fractures of the ungual tuft. Dislocations of the interphalangeal and metacarpophalangeal joints are common. They are the result of hyperextension and are often associated with small avulsion fractures from the volar surface of the joint margin of the displaced phalanx. Hyperextension injury of an interphalangeal joint, more commonly the proximal than the distal, may also cause such an avulsion without an associated dislocation (Fig. 2-33*A*). The fracture fragment is often quite small, even minute. Avulsion fractures occur on the dorsal surface of the base of the distal phalanx with or without flexion deformities of the distal interphalangeal joint (Fig. 2-33*B*). These are known as *baseball* or *mallet fingers*.

Fractures of the Metacarpals

Fractures of the neck of the fourth and fifth metacarpal are referred to as *boxer's fractures*. Characteristically there is volar angulation of the distal fragment (Fig. 2-33*C*). Fractures are also common at the base of the first metacarpal, where they may traverse across the width of the shaft or extend into the joint with an associated dislocation of the metacarpal. The latter are known as *Bennett's fractures* (Fig. 2-34).

THE WRIST

Most injuries of the distal forearm and carpus are due to a fall on the outstretched hand. The age of the patient is an excellent indicator of the site of resultant injury. Before the age of 10 years, transverse or greenstick fractures of the distal radius and ulna are common; between the ages of 11 and 16, separations of the distal radial epiphysis occur; between the ages of 14 and 40, fractures of the scaphoid; and after the age of 40, Colles' fractures of the distal radius are most common. Fractures of the carpal bones are very uncommon before the age of 12 years and after the age of 45. In general, fractures of the forearm bones are ten times more common than those of the carpal bones.

The pronator quadratus fascial plane, seen on the lateral radiograph anterior to the distal shafts, is a sensitive indicator of underlying fracture of the distal forearm. The fascial plane may bulge outward or may be partially or completely obliterated by hemorrhage as a result of the underlying fracture.

Colles' Fracture

Colles' fracture involves the distal 2 or 3 cm of the radius, with dorsal angulation of the distal fragment (Fig. 2-35). The deformity is usually obvious on clinical

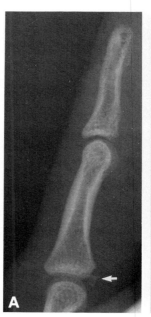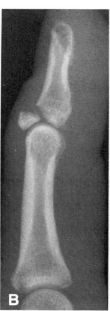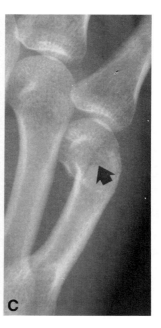

Figure 2–33. Fractures of the phalanges. (**A**) Volar plate avulsion from the base of the middle phalanx (*arrow*). The fragment is characteristically quite small. (**B**) Baseball finger, with characteristic fracture of the dorsal surface at the base of the distal phalanx. (**C**) Boxer's fracture of the neck of the fifth metacarpal (*arrow*), with characteristic volar displacement of the distal fragment.

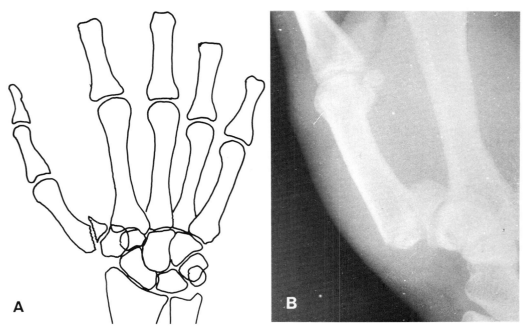

Figure 2–34. Bennett's fracture of the first metacarpal. (**A**) Diagram illustrating the characteristic deformity. (**B**) Radiograph showing lateral displacement of the shaft and characteristic oblique fracture of the base of the metacarpal.

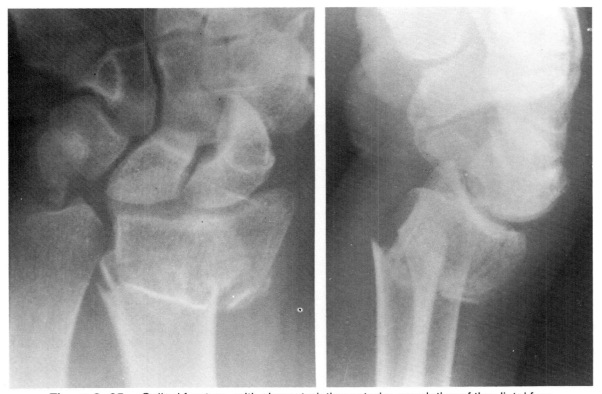

Figure 2–35. Colles' fracture, with characteristic posterior angulation of the distal fragment. Note the comminution and posterior lateral impaction. The ulnar styloid has been avulsed and is faintly seen lateral to its normal position.

examination and has been described as a *silver fork deformity*. The fracture is usually impacted, with comminution along its dorsal aspect. Frequently there is an associated avulsion fracture of the styloid process of the ulna.

Occasionally a fracture is encountered with anterior displacement of the distal fragment. This is a reverse Colles' or Smith fracture. Rarely a fracture is limited to either the anterior or posterior rim of the distal radius. Undisplaced transverse fractures occur, and they may be difficult to identify. Changes in the pronator quadratus fascial plane are helpful clues to these injuries.

Injuries of the Carpus

Three-fourths of all fractures of the carpus involve the scaphoid, and 15% involve the triquetrum. The majority of the remainder involve either the trapezium or hamate. Fractures of the remaining carpal bones are rare.

Fractures of the Scaphoid. This is the most common fracture of the carpal bones. The majority are transversely oriented and occur in the central part or waist of the scaphoid. Displacement is minimal, and therefore the visualization of the fracture line may be difficult (Fig. 2-36, and see Fig. 2-3). The best view to demonstrate the fracture is a posteroanterior projection with the hand in as much ulnar deviation as possible. The scaphoid is then seen in profile. The other fractures of the scaphoid occur in either the distal or proximal pole. After fracture of the scaphoid, the proximal fragment may become avascular because the principal blood supply enters through the dorsal surface of the distal fragment. Ischemic necrosis of the proximal fragment becomes apparent as disuse osteoporosis develops in the bones around it. The proximal fragment, having no blood supply, remains of normal density and is therefore more dense than that of the surrounding viable bone.

Triquetral Fracture. The common triquetral fracture is a small avulsion from its dorsal surface visualized on the lateral radiograph of the wrist (Fig. 2-37). It is usually not evident on the posteroanterior projection.

Other Carpal Fractures. Isolated fractures of the trapezium commonly occur because of abduction of the thumb. This results in a vertical fracture through the lateral margin of the trapezium. Fractures of the dorsal surface of the hamate occur commonly and are seen in the lateral view of the wrist. These are often associated with a dislocation of the metacarpohamate joint. Post-traumatic aseptic necrosis of the lunate, lunatomalacia, or Keinböck's disease, is occasionally encountered. The lunate is small, and fractures of the bone are commonly identified when a tomographic examination is performed.

Combinations of carpal fractures may occur as a result of severe injuries. The most common is the associa-

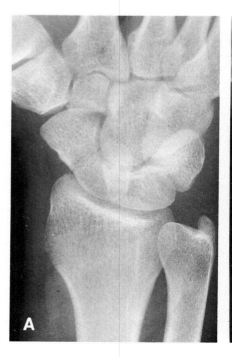 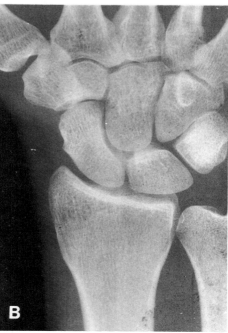

Figure 2–36. Fracture of the carpal scaphoid. Note that the fracture line is observed on the oblique projection (**A**) but not on the posteroanterior view (**B**).

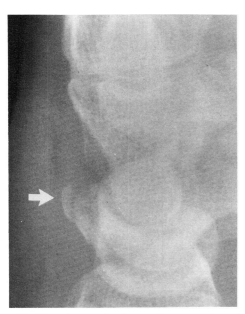

Figure 2–37. Lateral view of the wrist demonstrates characteristic small avulsion of the dorsal surface of the triquetrum (*arrow*) and overlying soft-tissue swelling.

tion of fractures of the scaphoid and those of the capitate, the so-called naviculocapitate (scaphocapitate) syndrome. Multiple fractures or fracture-dislocations are often heralded by displaced or angulated fractures of the scaphoid (see Fig. 2-39).

Dislocations

Dislocations at the wrist usually involve the lunate.[8, 23, 24] The lunate may be dislocated anteriorly from the radius and surrounding carpal bones. This is referred to as an *anterior lunate dislocation*, and it is most obvious on the lateral radiograph (Fig. 2-38). More commonly there is a posterior displacement of the distal carpus relative to the lunate. This is termed a *perilunate dislocation*. Usually the displacement is dorsal, the capitate being displaced posterior to the lunate, which remains in normal position, and thus it is more accurately called a *posterior perilunate dislocation* (Fig. 2-39). These dislocations are usually associated with transverse fractures of the waist of the scaphoid and are also best recognized on the lateral radiograph of the wrist.

Rotatory subluxation of the scaphoid is quite rare.[8] On the anteroposterior radiograph, the scaphoid appears foreshortened and a gap is present between the scaphoid and the lunate, commonly measuring more than 4 mm. The scaphoid is foreshortened because it is tilted on its longitudinal axis. When the scaphoid is tilted in this fashion, the cortical margins of the distal pole often have the appearance of a ring. On the lateral view, the long axis of the scaphoid will be seen in a more horizontal orientation.

Dislocations of the metacarpal joints most commonly involve the fourth and fifth metacarpals. The displacement may be either dorsal or volar. The distal radioulnar joint may also dislocate. This more commonly

Figure 2–38. Anterior dislocation of the lunate. In the posteroanterior view (**A**), disruption of the normal joint space between the proximal and distal rows of the carpus is noted. On the lateral view (**B**), the lunate is displaced anteriorly (*arrow*) and has the profile of a quarter moon.

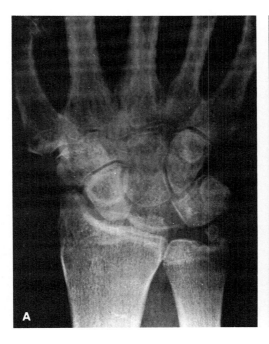

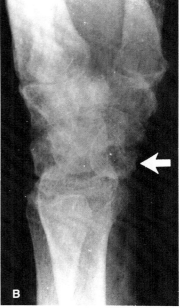

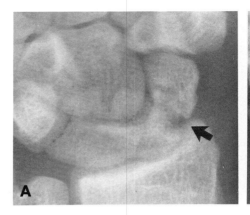
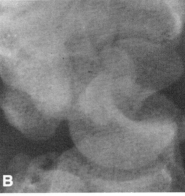

Figure 2–39. Transscaphoid, posterior perilunate dislocation. (**A**) Posteroanterior view of the wrist demonstrates a widely displaced fracture of the scaphoid (*arrow*) and an apparent overlap of the distal and proximal rows of the carpal bones. (**B**) Lateral view demonstrates posterior displacement of the distal carpal row relative to the proximal carpal row, with slight tilting of the lunate.

occurs with an angulated or overriding fracture of the distal radius.

THE FOREARM AND ELBOW

Midshaft Fractures

When a fracture or dislocation involves one of paired bones, there is usually a fracture or dislocation of the other, most commonly fractures of the shafts of both bones. Less often there is a fracture of one bone associated with dislocation of the other. A common example of this principle is Monteggia's fracture. A Monteggia's fracture is a fracture of the proximal ulna, associated with a dislocation of the proximal radius at the elbow joint. The ulnar fracture is either angulated or overriding and is immediately obvious, but if the examiner is unaware of this possibility, the associated dislocation of the radial head can easily be overlooked (Fig. 2-40). Angulated fractures of the distal radioulnar shaft are associated with dislocations of the distal radioulnar joint. This is known as the Galeazzi's fracture.

Isolated fractures of one of paired bones may occur as a result of direct blows. The most common form is the nightstick fracture of the distal third of the ulna, resulting from a direct blow to the forearm. These fractures are typically transverse and undisplaced without angulation of the fracture fragment. A similar fracture may occur from a direct blow to the radius.

Elbow Fat Pads

Injuries to the ends of the bones forming the elbow joint are accompanied by joint effusions. Normally there is a small accumulation of fat adjacent to the anterior surface of the lower end of the humerus. If the joint capsule is distended by fluid, this fat pad will be displaced forward and upward.[2, 19] There is a similar fat pad along the posterior surface of the humerus, but in the normal individual it lies largely within the olecra-

non fossa and is not visible on lateral views of the elbow. If the joint capsule is distended by fluid, the pad is elevated and displaced posteriorly and can then be visualized (Fig. 2-41, and see Fig. 2-43*B*). Recognition of the abnormal position of the fat pad should cause the observer to search carefully for bone injury if it is not

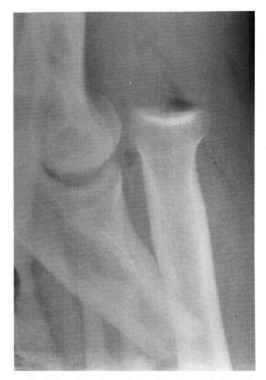

Figure 2–40. Monteggia's fracture-dislocation of the elbow. There is an angulated fracture of the proximal third of the ulna, with overriding of the fracture fragments associated with anterior dislocation of the radius. This is an open injury evidenced by air within the joint and soft tissues.

Figure 2–41. Impacted fracture of the radial head with hemarthrosis. **(A)** The fat pads are identified as lucencies anterior and posterior to the lower humeral shaft. In the absence of a joint effusion, the posterior fat pad should not be seen. Visualization of the posterior fat pad is referred to as a "positive fat pad sign." **(B)** An impacted fracture of the neck of the radius is identified as a linear band of density at the junction of the radial head and neck.

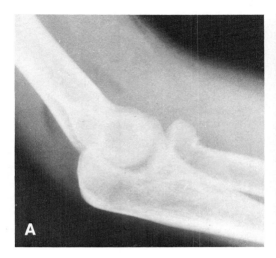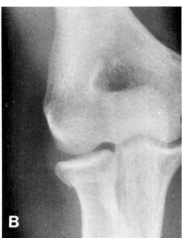

readily apparent.[2, 19] Displaced fat pads are a sign of joint distention and thus, in addition to trauma, could occur in any disease or condition in which there is synovitis (e.g., rheumatoid arthritis).

In the absence of joint disease, no abnormal fat pads are ordinarily seen. Therefore, a positive fat pad sign almost always indicates trauma, and in our experience, fracture of the radial head or proximal ulna is present in the vast majority of these patients. We obtain oblique views when no fracture is visible on anteroposterior and lateral projections in patients with a positive fat pad sign, and we suggest a 2- to 3-week follow-up film when no fracture is evident.

Fractures of the Elbow—Adults

The most common fracture of the elbow in adults involves either the head or neck of the radius. The fracture is often a simple vertical fracture extending through the outer margin of the articular surface, and it is usually best visualized on the anteroposterior or oblique projection (Fig. 2-42). Fractures involving the neck are of the impaction type, manifested by a slight buckling or angulation at the cortical junction of the head and neck (see Fig. 2-41). This may be visualized on either the anteroposterior or the lateral projection. Oblique views of the elbow are often required to visualize subtle fractures of the radial head and neck.

Olecranon fractures extend from the joint to the adjacent posterior cortex of the ulna, with variable degrees of separation of the fracture fragments. Less common fractures are avulsions of the coronoid or olecranon processes of the ulna. Severe forces may result in fractures of the distal humeral shaft and condyles, which often extend to the joint surface.

Fractures of the Elbow—Children

A knowledge of the sequence of appearance of the various ossification centers is essential to avoid diagnostic errors. If you are unfamiliar with the developmental process, you should consult standard charts.[24] In doubtful cases, it may be necessary to obtain a radiograph of the opposite normal elbow joint for comparison.

The most common fracture of childhood is a supracondylar fracture of the humerus. This is usually the result of a fall on the outstretched hand with the elbow partially flexed. Typically there is a backward displacement or angulation of the condylar fragment in relationship to the humeral shaft (Fig. 2-43). Displaced fractures are easily diagnosed but are potentially a therapeutic problem. Care must be taken to avoid

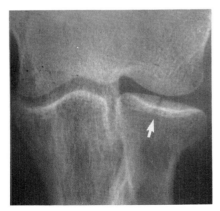

Figure 2–42. A characteristic linear fracture of the radial head (*arrow*).

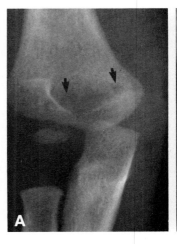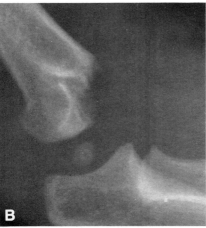

Figure 2–43. Supracondylar or transcondylar fracture of the humerus in a child 19 months old. (**A**) AP view demonstrates transverse fracture line (*arrows*). (**B**) Lateral view reveals incomplete greenstick fracture, with posterior displacement of the articular margin.

compression of the brachial artery against the proximal fragment, compromising the arterial circulation to the forearm and leading to the feared complication of Volkmann's contracture. At times the fractures are incomplete. Normally the distal humeral surface is angulated approximately 140° with the shaft of the ulna. A line drawn down the anterior humeral surface, (the anterior humeral line), should pass through the middle third of the capitellum.[24] In the presence of a subtle incomplete supracondylar fracture, this line will pass through the anterior third or even anterior to the capitellar center.

Fractures frequently involve the lateral condyle (see Fig. 2-5). These are Salter-Harris type IV injuries, the fracture line running through the lateral margin of the metaphysis and extending into the trochlear groove. Since the extensor muscles of the forearm are attached to the lateral condyle containing the capitellum, this fragment is frequently displaced laterally and posteriorly. Open reduction and pin fixation are usually required to avoid elbow instability or deformity.

The medial epicondyle is often avulsed by a pull of the flexor pronator tendon. When there is wide displacement, open reduction and pin fixation are required. Less commonly, as a result of a valgus injury of the elbow, the medial epicondylar ossification center may become entrapped in the medial joint space. In every child's elbow the presence and location of the medial epicondylar ossification center should be noted. The center usually appears around age 5 and is always present by age 7. Entrapment of the center may also occur following the reduction of elbow dislocations in children.

Dislocations of the Elbow Joint

Complete dislocation of the elbow joint almost invariably consists of a posterior or posterolateral dislocation of the radius and ulna on the humerus. These disloca-

tions may be associated with small avulsion fractures, particularly of the coronoid process, in adults. Complete dislocations of the joint are also common in children and are often associated with an avulsion of the medial epicondylar ossification center. As the joint is reduced, the epicondylar ossification center may become entrapped within the joint. It is therefore important to localize the medial epicondylar ossification center on both the pre- and postreduction radiographs of elbow dislocations in children.

Elbow joint dislocations may be complicated by the subsequent occurrence of calcification in and around the elbow joint—a post-traumatic myositis ossificans or periarticular ossification—which may lead to considerable impairment of function, even though the anatomic relationships of the bones have been restored.

Isolated dislocations of the head of the radius are reported in infants and children. Care must be taken to rule out a Monteggia's fracture-dislocation before accepting this diagnosis. At times the associated fracture of the ulna is a simple bow fracture without a disruption in the cortex. Isolated dislocations of the head of the radius are extremely rare in adults. Most are congenital dislocations. When a dislocation of the radial head is encountered, the entire ulnar shaft should be examined to rule out the presence of a fracture.

THE SHOULDER

Dislocations

Dislocations of the shoulder are of two principal types: anterior and posterior. The anterior is by far the most common, accounting for 90% of all shoulder dislocations. The posterior dislocation is much less frequent, accounting for only 2% to 4%, but it is of importance because the diagnosis is difficult and these dislocations are overlooked in as many as 50% to 60% of cases.[4]

In an anterior dislocation, the humeral head is displaced forward anterior to the glenoid and comes to rest beneath the coracoid process of the scapula (Fig. 2-44). This is also known as a *subcoracoid dislocation*. The radiographic diagnosis is not difficult because of the characteristic location of the humeral head. It is the most frequent dislocation of any joint in the body. Recurrent anterior dislocations are quite common, particularly in younger individuals, and may be associated with the Hill-Sachs defect, an impaction fracture having the appearance of an indentation or groove on the posterolateral aspect of the humeral head (Fig. 2-44*B*).[24] Less commonly there is a fracture of the anterior rim of the glenoid.

About one-half of posterior dislocations are the result of epileptic convulsive seizures, and the remainder are produced by direct blows to the anterior aspect of the shoulder. Whenever a posterior dislocation is encountered, the possibility of epilepsy must be considered. With a posterior dislocation, the head of the humerus is locked in internal rotation with the articular surface facing posteriorly. Since the findings are quite subtle, the major problem lies in recognizing the possibility of a posterior dislocation on the anteroposterior radiographs (Fig. 2-45).[24] Normally two views of the shoulder are obtained, one in internal and one in external rotation. Whenever a shoulder is fixed in internal rotation, the possibility of a posterior dislocation must be considered. The second most common sign of posterior dislocation is an impaction fracture of the medial joint surface manifested by a vertical line of cortical bone paralleling the medial cortex of the humerus. This has been called the *trough line*.[4] The third sign is widening of the joint, termed a *positive rim sign*. Normally the space between the anterior glenoid rim and the medial aspect of the humeral head measures 6 mm or less. In posterior dislocations, this is often widened. Once a posterior dislocation is suspected, axillary (Fig. 2-45*B*) and anterior oblique radiographs of the shoulder should be obtained to confirm this diagnosis. The 60° anterior oblique view of the shoulder is easily obtained and quite helpful. This is sometimes known as the Y view because the scapula appears as a Y in this projection. The acromion process is the posterior limb, the coracoid process is the anterior limb, and the body of the scapula is the vertical limb of the Y. The glenoid is represented as a circular density at the junction of the limbs overlaid by the humeral head. In a posterior dislocation, the head faces posteriorly and lies below the acromion; in an anterior dislocation, it is in a subcoracoid position. Posterior dislocations are nicely dis-

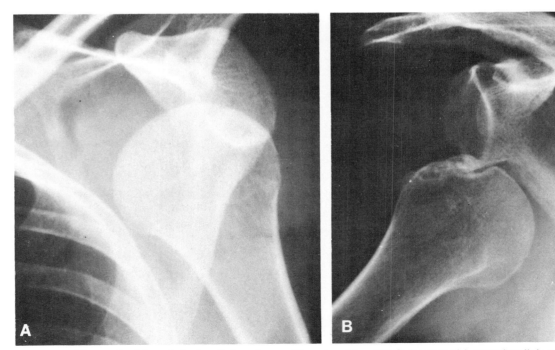

Figure 2–44.   Anterior dislocations of the shoulder. (**A**) Subcoracoid, anterior dislocation with characteristic displacement of the humeral head. The head lies anterior to the glenoid and beneath the coracoid process of the scapula. (**B**) A chronic anterior dislocation of the shoulder. Note the indentation of the humeral head (Hill-Sachs) caused by impaction against the rim of the glenoid.

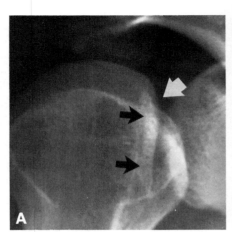 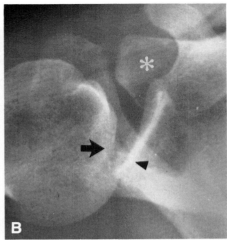

Figure 2–45.   Posterior dislocation of the shoulder. **(A)** AP view demonstrates that the humeral head is held in internal rotation, characteristic of a posterior dislocation. Note the impaction fracture manifested by a notch on the medial margin of the humeral head (*white arrow*) and the "trough line" (*black arrow*). **(B)** Axillary view demonstrates the impaction fracture of the humeral head (*arrow*) and posterior displacement of the humeral head in relation to the posterior rim of the glenoid (*arrowhead*). An *asterisk* marks the lateral margin of the clavicle.

played by CT. The real problem, however, is to consider the diagnosis in the first place.

Approximately 20% of shoulder dislocations have an associated fracture. An avulsion of the greater tuberosity or injury of the anterior lip of the glenoid commonly accompanies an anterior dislocation, whereas an avulsion of the lesser tuberosity is common in posterior dislocations.

Comminuted fractures of the humeral head and neck result in large hemarthroses. With a large joint effusion, the head is frequently displaced inferiorly and laterally, widening the joint space with an obvious incongruity of the joint surfaces. The joint appears to be dislocated, but this is not in fact a true dislocation (Fig. 2-46A). It has been termed a *pseudodislocation*. When the joint is evacuated, the normal relationships are restored. Pseudodislocation of the shoulder may also occur in hemophilia and acute suppurative arthritis.

Arthrography of the shoulder is used to demonstrate tears in the rotator cuff (see Fig. 3-60), the contrast extending superiorly and laterally from the joint capsule into the subacromial bursa and surrounding tissues. Arthrography is also used to evaluate the glenoid labrum and cartilaginous surface of the joint. With the use of CT and axilliary projections, tears in the cartilaginous labrum and associated fractures of the glenoid rim can be demonstrated.

Fractures of the Humerus

Fractures of the proximal end of the humerus are frequent in the elderly. They involve the anatomic neck, surgical neck, greater tuberosity, and lesser tuberosity, either alone or in varying combinations. The most common is a fracture of the surgical neck, often accompanied by an avulsion of the greater tuberosity (Fig. 2-46). All types of fractures occur in the shaft of the humerus. A pathologic fracture is a common presentation of a unicameral bone cyst in the proximal humeral metaphysis in children.

Fractures of the Clavicle

Fractures of the middle third of the clavicle are most common and may be of a greenstick variety in children. Fractures in the outer end are less common but may be associated with disruption of the coracoclavicular ligaments or may extend into the acromioclavicular joint.

Fractures of the Scapula

Isolated fractures of the scapula are uncommon, but they are usually not difficult to recognize in radiographs of the shoulder. They are frequently associated with crushing injuries of the chest and may be overlooked on the initial examination. Fractures usually

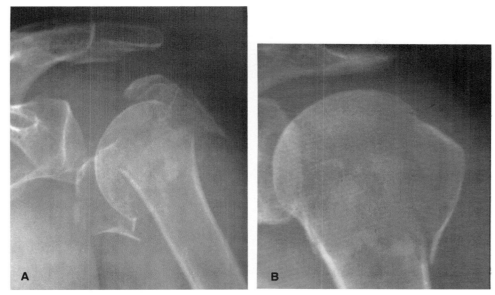

Figure 2–46. Fractures of the proximal humerus. (**A**) Comminuted fracture with pseudodislocation. Note that there are fractures of the surgical neck and avulsions of both the greater and lesser tuberosities. The humeral head is laterally and inferiorly displaced because of a large hemarthrosis. This gives the false appearance of a dislocation and thus is designated a pseudodislocation. (**B**) Impacted fracture of the surgical neck of the humerus, with avulsion of the greater tuberosity.

occur in the neck or body of the scapula and less commonly involve the inferior angle, acromion, or glenoid. Fractures at the base of the coracoid process are difficult to detect. These may be associated with acromioclavicular injuries, particularly in adolescents. An anteroposterior view with a steep cephalic angulation of the x-ray beam of 40° or more is required to demonstrate these fractures. Stress fractures at the base of the coracoid have been described in trapshooters.

Acromioclavicular Joint Injuries

Subluxations or complete dislocations of the acromioclavicular joint are frequent injuries, particularly in athletes, and are caused by a fall on the shoulder. These injuries are sometimes called acromioclavicular separations. The dislocation may be incomplete, in which case the lesion is termed a *subluxation.*

There are two principal considerations in the evaluation of acromioclavicular injuries (Fig. 2-47): first, the status of the acromioclavicular joint, and second, the status of the coracoclavicular ligaments that extend between the inferior, outer margin of the clavicle and the coracoid process of the scapula. Normally the distance between these two structures measures less than 1.2 cm with intact ligaments. When this distance is

increased, the coracoclavicular ligaments are disrupted. The status of these ligaments should be determined in every case of potential injury of the acromioclavicular joint. Acromioclavicular separations may not be evident on routine films and often require comparison with upright anteroposterior views obtained with 15- to 20-pound weights in each of the patient's hands. Stress films are required in every suspected case of acromioclavicular joint injury, unless a complete disruption of the acromioclavicular joint and of the coracoclavicular ligaments is demonstrated on the initial radiograph. Incomplete injuries widen the joint, but there is little or no upward displacement of the clavicle on the acromion process. The normal joint measures 3 to 5 mm in width. When dislocation is complete, the clavicle is displaced upward on the acromion and the ligaments attaching the clavicle to the coracoid process are ruptured. In evaluating the presence or absence of subluxation, the relationship of the undersurface of the clavicle to that of the acromion is important. The relative thickness of the acromion and clavicle varies in different individuals, and the superior borders of these bones cannot be relied upon to indicate normal or abnormal relationships. The inferior surfaces, however, usually lie in the same plane. As with many other injuries, comparison with the opposite shoulder may

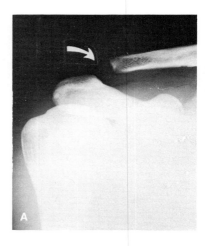
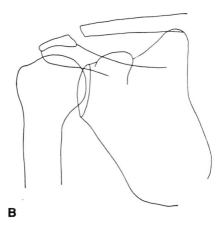

Figure 2–47. Third-degree acromioclavicular separation. (**A**) The joint is widened (*arrow*) and the clavicle displaced superiorly. There is also an abnormal separation between the clavicle and the coracoid, indicating a disruption of the coracoclavicular ligaments. (**B**) A line drawing of this injury.

be very helpful in determining whether or not minor deformity exists.

Dislocations of the Sternoclavicular Joints

Dislocation of the sternoclavicular joint is uncommon and may be difficult to diagnose on plain radiographs. Retrosternal dislocation of the clavicle is less common, but prompt diagnosis is important because the posteriorly displaced clavicle may compress the trachea and vascular structures, producing a considerable amount of morbidity, including cough, dyspnea and dysphagia, voice change, and vascular compromise. On the other hand, anterior dislocation does not compromise the mediastinal structures and is usually readily diagnosed clinically by the presence of a palpable mass surrounding the anteriorly displaced clavicle. The diagnosis is difficult on plain film radiography. Displacement can be identified with 35° to 40° cephalic angulation in the anteroposterior projection. With an anterior dislocation the clavicle will appear above, and with posterior dislocation it will appear below the level of the normal clavicle. CT precisely defines the anatomy and will disclose abnormalities with certainty. Since CT is the best means of evaluating the sternoclavicular joint, it should be used whenever there is a clinical question of injury or other abnormality of the sternoclavicular joint.

STERNUM AND RIBS

Fractures of the Sternum

Fractures of the sternum are usually transverse, are often relatively undisplaced, and are best demonstrated in the lateral projection. A surrounding hematoma may lead to the recognition of an otherwise obscure fracture. Many of these injuries result from automobile accidents, in which the driver is thrown against the steering wheel column, and they are often associated with myocardial contusions.

Fractures of the Ribs

Displaced, complete fractures of the ribs usually can be identified without difficulty on roentgenograms obtained to show rib detail. Incomplete or undisplaced fractures are more difficult to recognize. The surrounding hematoma, an extrapleural sign, will often point to an underlying fracture. Hairline fractures are very difficult to visualize and, in some cases, may not be evident for several days after the injury, becoming evident as the fracture line is resorbed and the fragments are displaced by the muscular action of breathing. Others may not be evident until a delayed reexamination demonstrates the presence of callus formation. The visualization of undisplaced fractures is facilitated when the exact site of the suspected injury is known and oriented tangentially at the margin of the radiographs so as to reveal the surrounding hematoma and thus disclose the underlying fracture.

One or more fatigue fractures may occur in the lower ribs as a result of repeated and severe coughing spells. These usually develop in the axillary arcs of the seventh, eighth, or ninth ribs and may or may not be a cause of pain. They have been discovered in roentgenograms of the chest in patients who have had no complaints referable to the fracture. As with fatigue fractures elsewhere, the line of fracture may be very indistinct at first and may only become obvious after several weeks, when periosteal callus begins to form. These are termed *cough fractures.*

Stress fractures occur in the lateral margin of the first rib. These have been found in military recruits after long marches while carrying heavy packs and in hikers and baseball pitchers. The stress of repeated throwing or carrying of a heavy pack leads to a fatigue or stress fracture in the midportion of the bone. Radiographically, they are evidenced by periosteal callus formation and a lucent fracture line.

FRACTURES OF THE PELVIS

Fractures of the pelvis may be conveniently divided into stable and unstable injuries.[23, 24] The stable injuries generally result from moderate trauma such as those that occur in a fall or athletic injury, whereas unstable injuries are the result of more severe forces such as those that occur in motor vehicle accidents. Since the pelvis is essentially a ring of bone, fracture in one area should alert the observer to the possibility of an associated second fracture or, alternatively, a subluxation of the pubic symphysis or sacroiliac joints. The ring of the pelvis is conveniently divided into an anterior arch extending across the pubic bones from one acetabulum to another and a posterior arch, extending from one acetabulum to the other through the sacroiliac joints and sacrum. Stable fractures involve one portion of the ring or the margins of the bony pelvis. Unstable fractures generally involve both the anterior and posterior ring, usually a fracture through the pubic rami, and a fracture of the sacrum or dislocation of the sacroiliac joint on the same side of the pelvis.[20] Occasionally, injuries involving both rings are on opposite sides of the pelvis.

The most common stable fracture of the pelvis involves the pubic ring. It may involve one or both rami or the body of the pubis (Fig. 2-48). Transverse fractures of the sacrum and coccyx and fractures of the iliac wing or apophyseal avulsions are uncommon.

Unstable fractures consist of fractures involving both the anterior and posterior arches of the pelvis. These may be due to anterior or lateral compression or vertical shearing.[20] The classic pelvic fracture as described by Malgaigne consists of a fracture of both pubic rami and an oblique fracture of the sacrum on the same side with vertical displacement of the hemipelvis (Fig. 2-49). Anterior compression causes an opening of the pubic symphysis and of the sacroiliac joints. This has been termed an *open-book injury*. Lateral compression injuries do not cause significant displacements. They may cause bilateral fractures of the pubic bones, and the sacral component of the injury is often obscure. The deformity of the sacral fracture often is manifested by an irregularity of one or more of the sacral neural foramina.[12, 24]

Pelvic fractures often involve the acetabulum, with or without an associated dislocation of the hip. The important considerations are the position of fracture fragments, the location of the femoral head, and the possibility of entrapment of bony or cartilaginous fragments within the hip joint. The entrapped fragment is often difficult to see on the plain roentgenogram but is readily identified by CT, which is also of value in defining injuries around the sacroiliac joint (Fig.

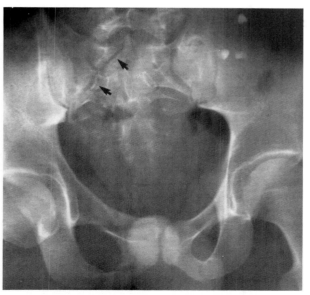

Figure 2–49. Malgaigne's fracture of the pelvis. Fractures of the pubis and an oblique fracture extending through the right sacral ala (*arrows*) disrupt the sacral foraminal lines. Note the intact foraminal lines in the left sacral ala.

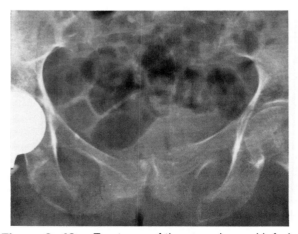

Figure 2–48. Fractures of the superior and inferior pubic rami. The inferior pubic ramus fracture is impacted.

2-50).[13, 18] If there is any question of injury on the basis of the plain films, a CT examination should be obtained.[24] This very clearly demonstrates disruptions of the sacroiliac joint and fractures of the adjacent margins of the sacrum or iliac bone.

A number of avulsion injuries in the region of the pelvis and hips usually occur as a result of muscle traction, particularly in young track athletes (e.g., sprinters, hurdlers, and even cheerleaders). Anterosuperior iliac spine avulsions result from the pull of the sartorius muscle, anteroinferior iliac spine avulsions are due to the rectus femoris, and the abdominal muscles may avulse fragments of the iliac crest. The hamstrings cause ischial tuberosity avulsion, whereas pull of the adductor muscles may produce injury in the region of the symphysis pubis and along the medial aspect of the inferior ischial ramus. Lesser trochanteric avulsions result from iliopsoas muscle traction.

Stress fractures occur in the medial aspect of the inferior pubic ramus and are manifested by a transverse band of sclerosis.

Transverse fractures of the sacrum and coccyx are the result of falls on the buttocks and can usually be identified without much difficulty in the lateral roentgenogram. In some individuals, the coccyx points directly forward to form a right angle or occasionally even an acute angle with the sacrum. This is a normal developmental variant, and it should not be confused with traumatic displacement.

Insufficiency fractures of the pelvis occur in elderly individuals, particularly postmenopausal women.[5, 6, 27] Patients characteristically present with pain of one to several months duration, localized to the sacrum, to the low back, or within the groin. A history of trauma is denied or minimal. Most fractures are associated with osteoporosis, but a few have been related to hyperparathyroidism, radiation osteitis, or osteoporosis complicated by the administration of steroids.[147, 164] Osteoporosis complicated by steroid use is more likely the case in men or in those with rheumatoid arthritis. The fractures are more commonly located within the pubis or sacrum but have also been reported just above the acetabulum and within the iliac bone. Multiple sites of involvement are generally present.

The radiographic findings are often subtle and easily overlooked but seen in retrospect after the lesions are identified by bone scanning. They are manifest by poorly defined patchy sclerosis in the affected site (Fig. 2-51A).

Fractures may occur in either the body of the pubis at the symphysis or the pubic rami.[6] They are more common in the body and often bilateral. Radiographically, they are evidenced by irregular lysis and patchy sclerosis (Fig. 2-51A). There is usually a distinct loss of bone volume as seen by comparing one side with the other or with previous films should both sides be affected. The pubis may be affected alone.

Insufficiency fractures may be identified on radionuclide bone scans before they are evident on radiographs.[5, 6, 27] Multiple foci of increased activity are the

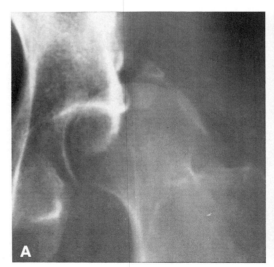
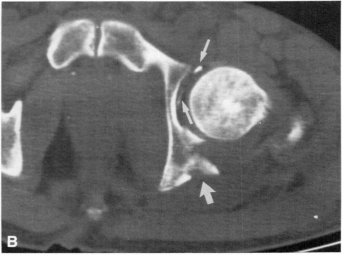

Figure 2–50. Posterior dislocation of the hip. **(A)** AP view demonstrates characteristic posterosuperior displacement of the femoral head, with numerous surrounding fragments from the posterior wall of the acetabulum. **(B)** CT obtained after reduction of the fracture demonstrates fractures of the posterior rim of the acetabulum (*large arrow*) and small fragments entrapped within the joint (*small arrows*).

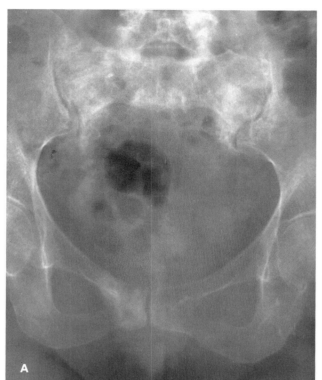

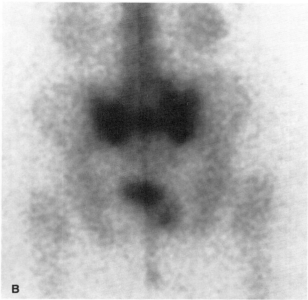

Figure 2–51. Insufficiency fractures of the pelvis. (**A** and **B**) Case 1: An 82-year-old osteoporotic woman with low back pain. AP film (**A**) demonstrates mottled sclerosis of the sacrum and body of the right pubic bone. Bone scan (**B**) demonstrates typical "H-type" pattern in the sacrum and increased radioactivity in the right pubis beneath the bladder. (**C**) Case 2: CT scan of insufficiency fracture of the sacrum in a 71-year-old osteoporotic woman. A linear, lucent fissure is in the right sacral ala (*arrow*) surrounded by sclerosis. Note the absence of a soft-tissue mass. There is also a small insufficiency fracture in the anterior portion of the left sacral ala.

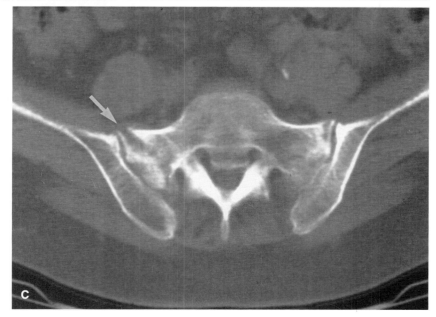

rule and tend to suggest metastatic disease to the unwary. However, the location and appearance are sufficiently distinctive to allow a correct diagnosis by the informed. In the sacrum, the classic pattern is a broad band of increased radioactivity in both sacral alae, connected by a linear transverse band across the body of the sacrum (Fig. 2-51B). This has been termed the H-type, butterfly pattern, or the Honda sign, the latter because it resembles the logo for Honda cars. On occasion, there is only a single or double vertical band without the transverse component. In the pubis there is increased activity over the body, either unilaterally or bilaterally, that is easily obscured by activity in the bladder.

The fractures may be confirmed by CT (Fig. 2-51C). This is particularly useful when there is a previous history of malignancy and the diagnosis of metastatic disease is a consideration. An insufficiency fracture is confirmed by identifying sclerosis in the appropriate location and visualizing fractures when present. The characteristic distribution, absence of a soft-tissue mass, and cortical disruption, other than the fracture and loss of bone volume sometimes identified with healing, distinguish insufficiency fractures from metastatic deposits.

DISLOCATIONS OF THE HIP

Dislocations of the hip may occur either posteriorly or anteriorly. The posterior dislocations are more common and are frequently associated with fractures of the posterior rim of the acetabulum (see Fig. 2-50). One or more fragments may become entrapped in the hip joint. Widening of the joint space or incongruity of the hip joint surfaces should suggest the possibility of an entrapped fragment and warrants a CT examination.[13] The femoral head is displaced superiorly in a posterior dislocation and inferiorly into the obturator foramen in an anterior dislocation. The displacement of an anterior dislocation is usually obvious, but on occasion the displacement in a posterior dislocation may underlie the acetabulum and may be manifested only by a slight incongruity of the joint surfaces. CT is warranted following reduction of every hip dislocation to disclose or rule out entrapped fracture fragments and to identify any associated fracture of the femoral head.

FRACTURES OF THE PROXIMAL FEMUR

Fractures of the proximal femur are quite common in the elderly but are unusual prior to age 50. The strength of bone is considerably weakened by osteoporosis, and most fractures result from simple falls. When femoral fractures occur in younger individuals, they are the result of severe forces sustained in motor vehicle accidents or falls from great heights. The various types of fractures affecting the proximal femur are shown in Figure 2-52. Subcapital and intertrochanteric fractures are the most frequent. The subcapital fracture may be either impacted or displaced (Fig. 2-53). When displaced, the leg is held in external rotation. Intertrochanteric fractures are often comminuted, with fractures involving either the lesser or greater trochanters or both (Fig. 2-54). Mid- and basicervical fractures are rare. Subtrochanteric fractures are frequently pathologic, through a focus of metastatic disease or in association with Paget's disease.

The radiographic diagnosis of most fractures is made

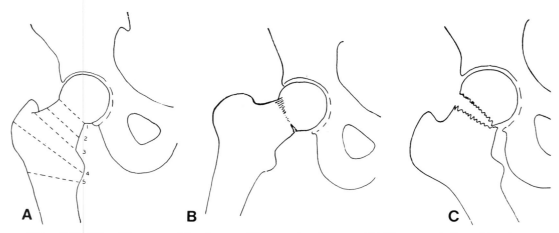

Figure 2–52.   Diagram of fractures of the proximal femur. **(A)** The usual sites of fracture: 1, subcapital; 2, transcervical; 3, basicervical; 4, intertrochanteric; and 5, subtrochanteric. **(B)** Displaced subcapital fracture. **(C)** Nonimpacted subcapital fracture.

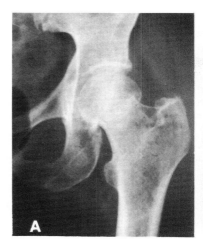
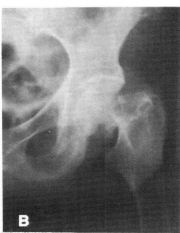

Figure 2–53. Two fractures of the femoral neck. **(A)** Impacted subcapital fracture. Note the characteristic distortion of the superolateral margin of the junction of the head and neck, with a vague zone of increased density due to impaction along the course of the subcapital fracture. **(B)** Nonimpacted subcapital fracture. The shaft is drawn proximally and is externally rotated. The margins of the fracture are not in apposition.

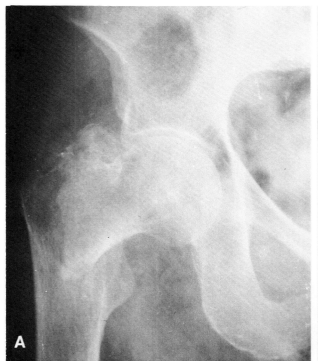
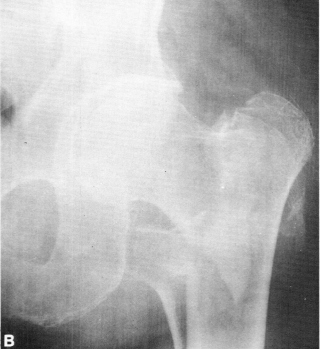

Figure 2–54. Two intertrochanteric fractures. **(A)**There is a comminution of the greater trochanter. **(B)** This fracture involves the lesser trochanter and is highly unstable.

without difficulty except for the impacted subcapital fracture (see Fig. 2-49A). In such a fracture, a distinct fracture line is not present and diagnosis depends upon recognizing a line of sclerosis along the zone of impaction and a valgus deformity of the head in relation to the neck. Stress fractures involving the femoral neck usu-

ally present as a band of sclerosis traversing the medial aspect of the base of the femoral neck.

The principal blood supply of the femoral head enters at the lateral margin of the junction of the head and neck. Displaced subcapital fractures disrupt the blood supply, and nonunion is an inevitable consequence.

Impacted fractures, on the other hand, usually leave the blood supply intact. Impacted fractures are therefore treated by the placement of multiple pins, whereas displaced fractures are treated by prosthetic replacement of the femoral head. Intertrochanteric fractures leave the blood supply intact but must be stabilized by internal fixation to mobilize the patient. A nail fixed to a plate placed along the lateral margin of the femoral shaft is commonly used.

Fractures of the hip in the elderly are frequently associated with simultaneous fractures of the distal forearm and proximal humerus. Whenever a fracture is identified in one of these sites, the other sites should be closely examined for evidence of injury.

FRACTURES OF THE FEMORAL SHAFT

All forms of fractures occur throughout the entire length of the femoral shaft (see Figs. 2-2 and 2-16). They are often the result of severe trauma and frequently occur in young individuals. Subtrochanteric fractures should suggest the possibility of metastatic disease, and the fracture site should be examined closely.

The principal diagnostic difficulty with the fractures of the femoral shaft is their frequent association with injuries around the hip, such as simultaneous fractures of the femoral neck or posterior fracture-dislocations of the hip. Similarly there is a frequent association with fractures of the patella and ligamentous injuries around the knee and fractures of the proximal tibia. To avoid diagnostic oversights, it is essential that the entire length of the femur, including the hip and knee, be included on the initial radiographic examination.

FRACTURES AND DISLOCATIONS OF THE KNEE

Fractures involving the distal femoral metaphysis are termed *supracondylar fractures*, and they should be closely examined for vertical components extending into the knee joint (see Fig. 2-7B). These usually lie between the condyles. Similarly, fractures involving the proximal tibia should be evaluated for vertical or oblique intra-articular extensions involving the tibial plateau.

The knee joint may be dislocated anteriorly or posteriorly. Fractures of the distal femur and proximal tibia and dislocations of the joint are frequently associated with injuries and occlusions of the popliteal artery. Angiography may be required.

Lipohemarthrosis

Most fractures and dislocations are readily identified on the standard anteroposterior, lateral, and oblique radiographs of the knee. Lipohemarthrosis serves as a clue to otherwise obscure fractures involving the articular surfaces.[24] Intra-articular fractures allow fat from the marrow to extrude into the joint space. When the joint is aspirated, the fat in the aspirate will float on the blood. Radiographically this can be identified by using a horizontal beam while obtaining a lateral radiograph of the knee. The fat–fluid level is identified in the suprapatella bursa (Fig. 2-55). The radiolucent fat floats on the blood in the joint and is observed as a relative lucency. Lipohemarthrosis may also be identified in other joints in the presence of an intraarticular fracture, particularly the shoulder and elbow, but it is most commonly identified in the knee. When a fat–fluid level is identified, it usually indicates that there is a fracture extending into the joint. It is possible that on occasion a fat–fluid level could be found in association with a severe injury of the soft tissues without fracture.

Magnetic Resonance Imaging of the Knee

MRI affords excellent visualization of the menisci, cruciate and collateral ligaments, and cartilaginous joint surface.[17] On T1-weighted images the meniscus is of low signal and homogeneously black (Fig. 2-56). Subcutaneous fat and bone marrow are depicted as relatively high intensity structures. The articular cartilage is significantly higher in intensity than the adjacent meniscus or cortical bone.

The menisci are slightly elongated triangles in profile and uniformly black or of low signal intensity (Fig. 2-56A). With aging, a variable degree of signal often

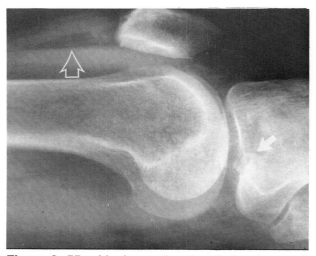

Figure 2–55. Lipohemarthrosis of the knee. A cross-table lateral view with a horizontal beam demonstrates a fat–fluid level in the suprapatellar bursa (*open arrow*) due to a fracture of the lateral tibial plateau (*arrow*).

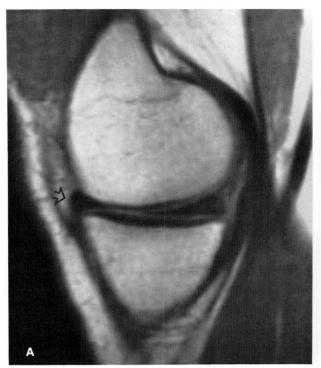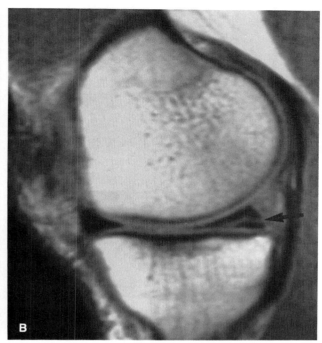

Figure 2–56. MRI of the medial meniscus. **(A)** Normal medial meniscus. Note the typical triangular shape of the anterior (*arrow*) and posterior horns of the medial meniscus. There is a very low signal within the medial meniscus that does not extend to the joint surface. This is a normal finding. Note the medium signal of the joint cartilage and the high signal of the intermedullary bone. **(B)** Torn posterior horn of the medial meniscus. Linear, low signal extends through the substance of the meniscus to the joint surface (*arrow*). The inferior portion of the meniscus is not easily seen by arthroscopy, and this tear could be easily overlooked.

appears within the meniscus. Only those signals extending to and through the surface of the menisci represent tears (Fig. 2-56*B*), (i.e., an intrameniscal signal that unequivocally extends to the articular surface of the meniscus.) Changes in the profile or shape of the menisci are also important. Truncation and irregular elongation in shape are suspect.

The anterior cruciate ligament (ACL) and posterior cruciate ligament (PCL) are distinctive not only in their location and course, but also in the difference in their normal signal. The ACL is best seen in the sagittal plane with 10° to 20° of external rotation of the knee. Without such rotation the entire length of the ligament will not be captured on one image. The normal ACL is depicted as a low signal band, commonly as two or three separate fiber bundles, extending from the anterior tibial plateau to the medial surface of the lateral femoral condyle (Fig. 2-57*A*). The ACL is the most frequently torn knee ligament. In those who sustain sufficient injury to result in a hemarthrosis, 70% will have had a tear of the ACL. In an acute tear as depicted

on MRI, either the ACL is obviously disrupted or its anterior margin is wavy or concave and not straight as when intact (Fig. 2-57*B*).

The PCL is usually readily identified by MRI (Fig. 2-58*A*) as a solid black band of low signal intensity that extends in a smooth, convex arc from the posterior surface of the medial femoral condyle to the posterior, intercondylar surface of the tibia. Tears usually appear as foci of increased signal intensity often accompanied by widening of the ligament. Complete tears, manifested by separations of the margins of the ligament, are less common.

The collateral ligaments are visualized as thin, linear, dark bands of low signal intensity on both T1- and T2-weighted images (Fig. 2-58*B*). The medial collateral ligament (MCL) consists of a superficial and deep portion. Complete tears are depicted by discontinuity and serpiginous irregularity. This appearance is accompanied by surrounding hemorrhage and edema of intermediate signal on T1, which increases in signal on T2. Associated bone bruise of the lateral femoral con-

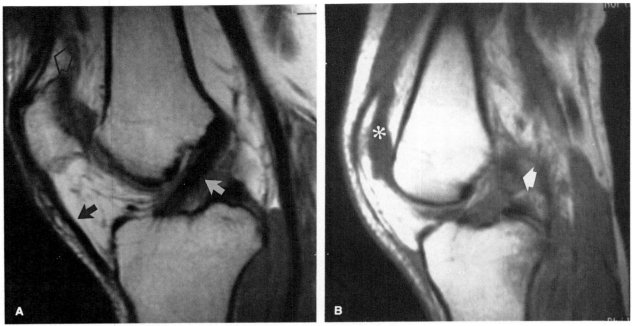

Figure 2–57. MRI of the anterior cruciate ligament. **(A)** T1-weighted image demonstrating normal ligament (*white arrow*). Note also the infrapatellar ligament (*black arrow*) and the quadriceps tendon (*open arrow*). **(B)** Torn anterior cruciate ligament. There is no clear demonstration of the substance of the tendon. The normal signal of the tendon is replaced by an ill-defined mass of intermediate signal (*arrow*). Note also the presence of a joint effusion in the suprapatellar bursa (*asterisk*).

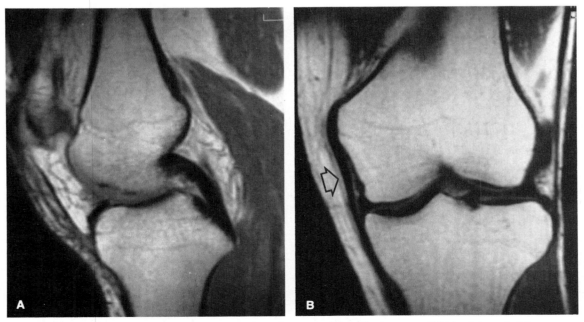

Figure 2–58. Normal posterior cruciate ligament identified as a solid black band of low intensity that extends in a smooth convex arc from the posterior surface of the medial femoral condyle to the posterior intercondylar surface of the tibia. **(B)** Normal medial collateral ligament (*arrow*) visualized as a thin, linear, dark band of low signal extending from the medial femoral condyle to the medial surface of the tibial plateau.

dyle and tears of the ACL and menisci are frequent. Sprain of the ligament without tears leaves the ligament intact, but its margins are blurred by surrounding edema and hemorrhage.

The lateral collateral ligament (LCL) is less commonly injured. It is a thin, linear dark band similar in low signal intensity to that of the ACL. The LCL extends from the lateral surface of the femoral condyle to insert on the head of the fibula. The course is oblique from anterosuperior to posteroinferior, and therefore, the entire ligament is usually not seen on a single image as is the MCL. The appearance of sprains and tears is similar to that of the MCL.

The quadriceps and infrapatellar tendons (see Fig. 2-57A) are similar in intensity to the PCL, MCL, and LCL. Complete tears are manifest by retraction and wavy contours of the separated margins, a mass of intermediate signal on T1, and increased signal on T2-weighted images surrounding the site of the tear.

Fractures of the Tibial Plateau

A valgus injury of the knee may result in a fracture of the lateral tibial plateau. At times these fractures are difficult to identify and are obvious only on oblique radiographs. The fractures consist of either a vertical split through or a depression of a portion of the joint surface (Fig. 2-59). There may be an associated fracture of the neck of the fibula. When the fracture involves the lateral margin of the plateau or is associated with a

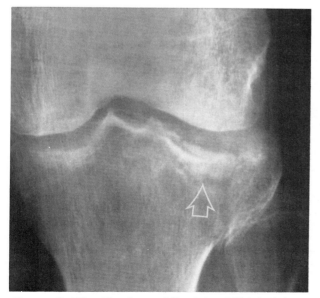

Figure 2–59. Fracture of the lateral tibial plateau. There is a vertical component laterally and a depression of the joint surface (*arrow*).

fracture of the neck of the fibula, an accompanying disruption of the medial collateral ligament is likely.

Fractures of the Tibial Eminence

The ACL is attached to the anterior tibial spine. On occasion, a fracture is identified through the base of the tibial spine. This may be incomplete and undisplaced or complete with elevation and on occasion even reversal of the avulsed fragment. When it is displaced or reversed, surgical reattachment is required.

Fractures of the Patella

Most fractures of the patella are transverse, and separations of fragments may be severe because of the pull of the quadriceps muscle on the upper fragment. Infrequently the line of fracture is vertical, and it may be visualized with difficulty unless oblique or tangential views are obtained. In dealing with injuries to the patella, care must be used not to confuse a bipartite or multipartite patella for a fracture (Fig. 2-60). This anomaly consists of one or several unfused ossification centers that remain along the upper outer quadrant of the bone. The rounded corners of an anomalous center and the generally smooth cortical borders are in contrast to the irregular edges of a fracture fragment. The condition is bilateral in about 80% of cases.

The patella may dislocate laterally. The dislocation may be transient or complete. In either event, the dislocation is usually reduced before a radiographic examination is obtained. The importance of this diagnosis is recognizing that the dislocation is often associated with an osteochondral fracture of the joint surface, as described subsequently.

Osteochondral Fractures

Injuries may be limited to the surface of the joint, resulting in fragments that contain cartilage or cartilage and a small portion of subchondral bone.[16] Pure cartilage fragments cannot be identified on a plain radiograph; however, those containing subchondral bone may be visualized. The bony fragment is often quite small.

Most osteochondral fractures are caused by a transient or complete dislocation of the patella. The medial facet of the patella impacts against the lateral condyle of the femur as the patella is dislocated. An osteochondral fracture may result from either of these two surfaces. An axial or sunrise projection of the patella is usually required to demonstrate the fracture. Although the fragment may be visualized, it is difficult, if not impossible, to identify its site of origin.

The joint cartilage can be identified and injuries visualized by MRI. Osteochondral injuries are best

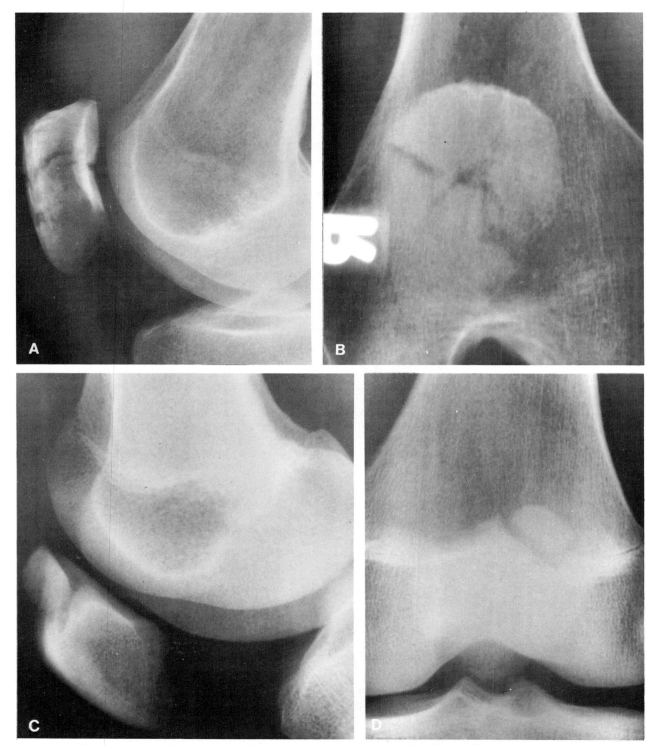

Figure 2–60.   (**A** and **B**) Undisplaced fracture of the patella. (**C** and **D**) Bipartite patella showing smooth cortical surfaces and characteristic location on the superolateral margin of the patella. The margins are not as sharply defined as in fracture.

demonstrated on gradient echo or T2-weighted images, which result in a high signal from joint fluid contrasting with the intermediate signal of cartilage, allowing visualization of defects in the joint surface. This may also disclose osteochondral fragments free within the accompanying joint effusion.

When an injury of the knee is suspected but not immediately evident on the radiograph, one should search closely for evidence of small bony fragments indicating an osteochondral fracture, look closely at the lateral tibial plateau for evidence of fracture, and look at the base of the tibial eminence for evidence of fracture. Of course, there is no plain film radiographic evidence of the common injuries of the menisci, and MCL.

In adolescents, all types of epiphyseal separations of ACL, the distal femur or proximal tibia may occur, although Salter-Harris type II is the most common.

THE ANKLE AND FOOT

Achilles Tendon Injuries

Injuries of the Achilles tendon may be suspected on plain film by widening of the tendon, obliteration of the pre-Achilles fat pad, and a rather abrupt change in the contour of the tendon. However, such injuries are exquisitely demonstrated and confirmed by MRI in the sagittal and axial planes. The tear in the low signal tendon is directly visualized and contrasted with the higher signal hematoma within and about the torn tendon (see Fig. 2-4).

Fractures and Dislocations of the Ankle

The ankle is a combination of bones and ligaments, and the injuries commonly involve both components. Fractures commonly involve the lateral malleolus of the distal fibula, the medial malleolus of the distal tibia, and the posterior malleolus of the distal tibia (Fig. 2-61).[23, 24] The most common fracture is a spiral or oblique fracture of the lateral malleolus (see Fig. 2-1). Most ankle injuries are thought to be due to external rotation of the foot, relative to the leg. In actual practice, the leg is likely rotated internally relative to the fixed foot as the injury occurs.

Ankle effusions, including hemarthroses, may be detected on lateral radiographs of the ankle by observing a teardrop-shaped density extending anteriorly from the ankle joint over the neck of the talus.[30] These may occur as the result of either bone or ligamentous injury.

Because there is no direct evidence of ligamentous injury, it must be inferred from the relative position of adjacent bony structures. The ankle mortise measures

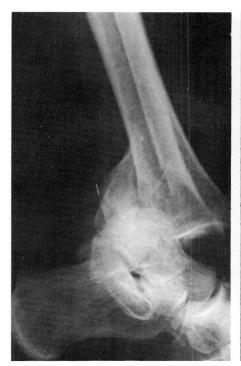
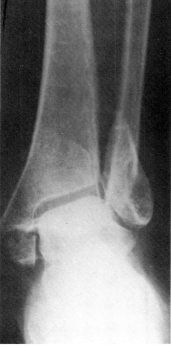

Figure 2–61. Fracture-dislocation of the ankle. There are fractures of the medial and lateral malleolus and the posterior malleolus (posterior tubercle) of the tibia. The malleolar fragments are characteristically displaced posteriorly with the foot.

3 to 4 mm over its entire surface. Separation of the medial margin of the talus from the lateral surface of the medial malleolus by more than 6 mm would indicate the presence of a deltoid ligament rupture. Normally the syndesmosis extending between the inferior tibia and fibula measures no more than 5½ mm. Measurements in excess of this would indicate a rupture of the syndesmosis. Generally, the syndesmosis is ruptured to the lowest point of the fibular fracture. Therefore, in those fractures that lie proximal to the joint margin there is some degree of rupture of the syndesmosis.

Flake Fractures

Ankle sprains are manifested radiographically by soft-tissue swelling. The ligament is usually ruptured in its midportion, and therefore there are no radiographic changes within the adjacent bone. On occasion, the ligament is ruptured at its origin or insertion and avulses off a small fragment of bone (see Fig. 2-8*B*). This avulsion fracture is sometimes known as a *sprain* or *flake fracture*. These fractures occur at the tips of the medial and lateral malleolus and the adjacent surfaces of the talus and calcaneus.

There are many accessory ossicles around the ankle and foot. These may easily be mistaken for fractures. An accessory ossicle usually has rounded margins, is bounded by cortex around its entire periphery, and is separated from the major part of the bone by a space of relatively uniform width. A fracture, on the other hand, will show irregularity of the margin without a distinct cortex. Accessory centers of ossification occur at very predictable sites, particularly at the tips of both malleoli, the lateral margin of the cuboid bone, the dorsal surface of the distal talus and navicular, and the proximal pole of the navicular among others (see Chapter 8, Normal Variants).

When there is a clinical suggestion of instability but no radiographic evidence of displacement, stress films are sometimes obtained to confirm the clinical diagnosis of a ligament injury. Stress films demonstrate excessive movement of the talus within the ankle mortise. Generally, stress films are obtained with both inversion and anterior traction of the foot.

Children and adolescents may sustain epiphyseal separations of either the distal tibial or distal fibular epiphysis.[14, 28] These separations are evidenced by widening of the growth plate or associated fractures of the margin of the metaphysis but may be difficult to recognize if there is little or no displacement. All types of epiphyseal separations occur at the distal tibia (see Fig. 2-11*B*), the most common of which are Salter-Harris II and Salter-Harris III. The latter may involve either the medial or lateral margin of the epiphysis. Salter-Harris IV injuries involve the medial malleolus. Injuries of the distal fibular epiphysis are the adolescent counterpart of the common ankle sprain. These are either Salter-Harris type I or II injuries.

Fractures of the Os Calcis

Compression fractures of the os calcis occur as a result of a fall from a height, with the patients landing on their feet. The more severe injuries are visualized without difficulties on the lateral radiograph, because of the extensive crushing and comminution. Lesser degrees of compression may be difficult to recognize unless one is completely familiar with the normal appearance. It may be necessary to compare the injured side with the opposite normal foot. Böhler's angle is of value in the determination of fractures of the os calcis (Figs. 2-62 and 2-63). This angle is formed by drawing two lines, one from the anterosuperior margin of the bone and the other from the posterosuperior margin, to the highest point of the articular surface. In a normal individual the complement of this angle is 20° to 40°. When there is impaction, this angle is reduced and may become zero or even reversed. In many fractures there is an injury to the subastragalar joint. The extension of the fracture into the posterior facet of this joint can be demonstrated on an axial view. CT in the coronal and longitudinal planes precisely defines the degree of comminution, the involvement of the joint surface, and the displacement of the fracture fragments (Fig. 2-64).[10] Various types of avulsion fractures occur at the margins of the os calcis without affecting Böhler's angle. These fractures may involve the tuberosity, the anterior process, or the lateral margin of the calcaneus. They are visualized in the lateral and axial views of the calcaneus and the anteroposterior and oblique views of the foot.

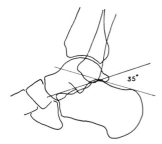

Figure 2–62. Böhler's angle, the tuber-joint angle of the calcaneus. Diagram illustrates the method for determining this angle, normally between 20° and 40°.

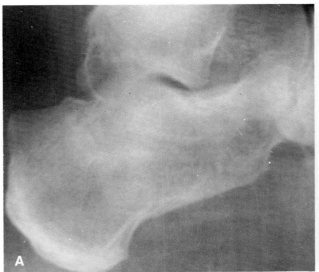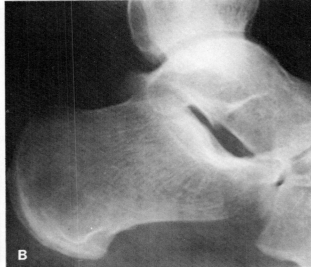

Figure 2–63. Compression fracture of the os calcis. **(A)** Note the characteristic loss of Böhler's angle and impaction of fracture fragments manifested by an increase in density without an obvious line of fracture. **(B)** Normal os calcis for comparison.

Fractures of the Talus

Simple avulsion fractures occur from the dorsal surface of the head to the neck of the talus and must be differentiated from accessory centers of ossification. Vertical fractures occur through the neck just distal to the tibial articular surface. These are often followed by ischemic necrosis of the articular fragments since the principal blood supply to the bone enters through the neck (see Fig. 7-23).

Fractures of the Navicular

Fractures of the navicular are relatively infrequent and usually are undisplaced. The fracture may be either vertical or horizontal through the body of the bone or may involve the proximal pole situated on the medial side of the foot. The latter must be differentiated from an accessory center of ossification, the os tibiale externum.

Isolated fractures of the cuneiform and cuboid are rare. The os peroneum lies on the lateral margin of the cuboid and should not be mistaken for a fracture.

Fractures of the Metatarsals and Phalanges

All types of fractures occur in the metatarsals and phalanges, with or without dislocation of adjacent joints. They are commonly the result of crushing injuries or stubbing of the toe.

Fractures involving the proximal tuberosity of the fifth metatarsal are frequent and usually follow an inversion injury of the foot (Fig. 2-65). These may masquerade clinically as injuries of the ankle. It is essential that the base of the fifth metatarsal be included on every lateral radiograph of the ankle to rule out this common injury. Characteristically the fracture line extends transversely across the proximal end of the bone, with separation of a triangular fragment. This fracture must not be confused with the normal apophysis that occurs on the outer edge of the tuberosity and is oriented with the long axis of the bone, as opposed to the transverse orientation of a fracture (see Chapter 8, Normal Variants).

Fatigue or stress fractures of the metatarsals involve the neck or shaft of the second, third, or fourth metatarsals. They are manifested by an undisplaced transverse line of fracture or fluffy periosteal callus formation (see Fig. 2-14). These are commonly seen in military recruits, runners, and less often following surgery to the foot.

Dislocations of the Foot

There are a number of foot dislocations; any joint may be involved, but some are more common than others. The radiographic diagnosis is usually not difficult. The dislocations are often associated with avulsions or other types of fractures of adjacent bone.

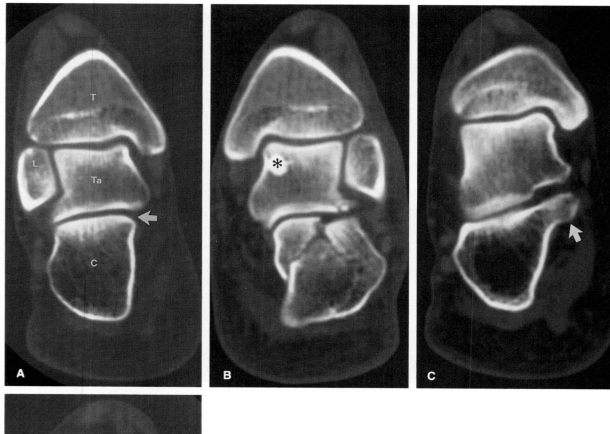

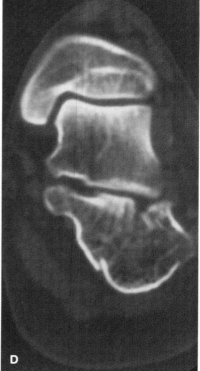

Figure 2–64.   Comminuted fracture of the left calcaneus examined by CT in the axial plane. (**A**) Normal right calcaneus at the level of the posterior facet of the subtalar joint (*arrow*). (**B**) Comminution of the left calcaneus that extends into the posterior facet. A small bone island is present within the talus (*asterisk*). (**C**) Scan through the normal right sustentaculum (*arrow*). (**D**) Corresponding image on the left demonstrates a fracture separating off the sustentaculum tali. There is also a comminuted fracture of the lateral wall of the calcaneus. *T*, tibia; *L*, lateral malleolus of fibula; *Ta*, talus; *C*, calcaneus.

In a subtalar dislocation the talus remains in place within the ankle mortise but the subtalar joint is disrupted and the bones of the foot are usually displaced medially. These are frequently accompanied by fractures of the neck of the talus or malleoli.

Dislocations of the tarsometatarsal joints are known as *Lisfranc's fracture-dislocations*. The dislocation usually involves two or more metatarsals. The most common is a lateral displacement of all five metatarsals or a lateral displacement of the second through fifth metatarsals and medial displacement of the first metatarsal. The deformity is best recognized on the anteroposterior and oblique views of the foot (Fig. 2-66). There is usually a fracture of the recessed base of the second metatarsal and other smaller fractures at the margins of the joint. Normally, the first metatarsal is aligned with the medial cuneiform and the second metatarsal with the middle cuneiform, the third with the lateral cuneiform, and the medial margin of the fourth metatarsal with the medial border of the cuboid. These relationships are best determined on the anteroposterior and oblique views of the foot.

Dislocations of metatarsophalangeal and interphalangeal joints are quite common and are often associated with fractures of the apposing joint surfaces.

Lisfranc's and other fracture-dislocations of the tarsus are a common manifestation of neurotrophic arthritis in diabetics (see Fig. 3-43). Unusual fractures or dislocations of the ankle or tarsus and those without a history of trauma should suggest this possibility.

THE BATTERED CHILD SYNDROME

The hallmark of this syndrome is clinical and radiographic evidence of repeated injury in children frequently under 2 and usually under 6 years of age.[22] The skeletal changes may be extensive and rather bizarre. These changes are often discovered while examining the infant for some totally unrelated condition, and a history of injury may be unobtainable from the parents. In some cases, this may be a deliberate misrepresentation; in others, the traumatic episode may not have been noticed by other members of the family. The possibility of deliberate mistreatment of the infant by a psychotic or an alcoholic parent must be borne in mind. The condition is known as the *battered child syndrome*.

The infant skeleton responds to trauma more easily and more rapidly than that of the older child or the adult. The lesions vary considerably in their roentgenographic appearance (Fig. 2-67).[22] There may be separation of one or more small fragments from the corner of a metaphysis. Characteristically the metaphyseal

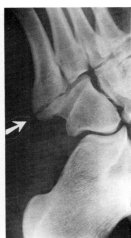
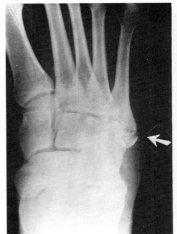

Figure 2–65. Fracture of the base of the fifth metatarsal. Arrows indicate a typical transverse fracture without significant displacement.

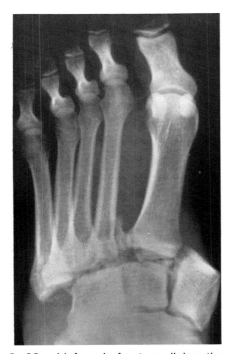

Figure 2–66. Lisfranc's fracture-dislocation of the tarsal–metatarsal joints, with lateral displacement of all metatarsals and numerous small fractures at the margins of the joint including the base of the second metatarsal.

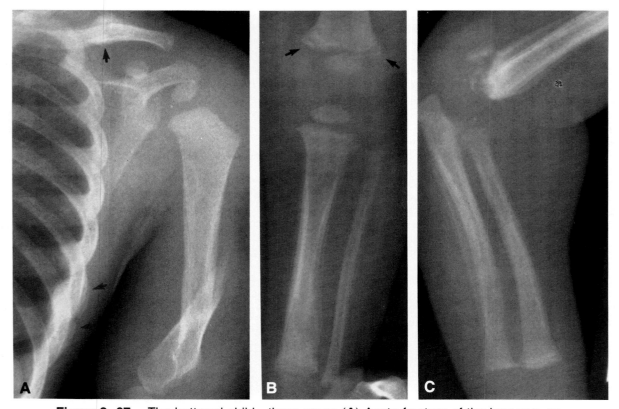

Figure 2–67. The battered child—three cases (**A**) Acute fracture of the humerus associated with healing fractures of the sixth and seventh ribs and clavicle (*arrows*) in a 19-month-old girl. (Courtesy of Mary Ann Radkowski, M.D., Chicago, Illinois) (**B**) Corner fractures of the distal femoral epiphysis (*arrows*), periosteal new-bone formation along the shafts of the tibia and fibula, and a bucket-handle fracture of the distal tibial metaphysis in an 8-month-old girl. (**C**) Metaphyseal, corner fracture of the distal humerus and periosteal new-bone formation along the shafts of the humerus, radius, and ulna in a 10-month-old boy.

margin of one or more bones may show an irregular or serrated appearance, probably representing the effects of previous metaphyseal infractions. Skull fractures may be found in some and are often complicated by subdural hematoma. Lung contusions and lacerations can be found in association with rib fractures. Subluxation of one or more of the epiphyses, extensive subperiosteal callus, and frank shaft fracture showing evidence of callus may all be present in the individual case. Although the metaphyseal fractures and epiphyseal separations are classic manifestations of the disease, in fact, shaft fractures and skull fractures are more common. Typically the lesions are likely to be found in multiple bones, although there is no particular symmetry to the distribution and they may vary in

severity from one area to the other. Characteristically there is evidence of trauma of varying duration—some recent, some old and well healed. The proper diagnosis in the absence of a history depends on the irregular distribution of the lesions in the skeleton, the otherwise normal density and texture of the bones involved, and the lack of clinical signs of infection or other serious disease. When the diagnosis of a battered child is considered on clinical grounds or suspected on the basis of radiographic evaluation, bone scanning may be helpful in disclosing other sites of more obscure skeletal injury. The life of the child may depend on establishing the diagnosis so that the child may be removed from the environment and protected from future harm.

CONGENITAL INDIFFERENCE TO PAIN

This is a rare disorder characterized by a congenital insensitivity to pain. The skeletal lesions are a reflection of this and consist of gross fractures or healing fractures, various forms of osteochondrosis or ischemic necrosis apparently due to repeated minor traumas, or osteomyelitis in its various phases. In some cases the roentgenographic evidence of trauma is similar to that noted in battered children, with metaphyseal infractions or "corner" fractures and periosteal callus formation. The inflammatory lesions are usually those of an infection of low virulence, with abscess formation. Necrosis of the distal phalanges has been reported, evidently the result of persistent cutaneous infections of the fingers. Other lesions that have been described include hydrarthrosis and subluxations.

REFERENCES AND SELECTED READINGS

1. ATLAS SW, REGENBOGEN V, ROGERS LF, KIM KS: The radiographic characterization of burst fractures of the spine. Am J Roentgenol 147:575, 1985
2. BOHRER SP: The fat-pad sign following elbow trauma. Its usefulness and reliability in suspecting "invisible" fractures. Clin Radiol 21:90, 1970
3. BORDEN SIV: Roentgen recognition of acute plastic bowing of the forearm in children. Am J Roentgenol 125:524, 1975
4. CISTERNINO SJ, ROGERS LF, STUFFLEBAM BC, ET AL: The trough line: A radiographic sign of posterior shoulder dislocation. Am J Roentgenol 130:951, 1978
5. COOPER KL, BEABOUT JW, SWEE RG: Insufficiency fractures of the sacrum. Radiology 156:15, 1985
6. DESMET AA, NEFF JR: Pubic and sacral insufficiency fractures: Clinical course and radiologic findings. Am J Roentgenol 145:601, 1985
7. DEUTSCH AL, MINK JH, WAXMAN AD: Occult fractures of the proximal femur: MR imaging. Radiology 170:113, 1989
8. GILULA LA, WEEKS PM: Post-traumatic ligamentous instabilities of the wrist. Radiology 129:641, 1978
9. GREANEY RB, GERBER FH, LAUGHLIN RL, ET AL: Distribution and natural history of stress fractures in U.S. Marine recruits. Radiology 146:339, 1983
10. GUYER BH, LEVINSOHN EM, FREDERICKSON BE, BAILEY GL, FORMIKELL M: Computed tomography of calcaneal fractures: Anatomy, pathology, dosimetry, and clinical relevance. Am J Roentgenol 145:911, 1985
11. LEE JK, YAO L: Occult intraosseous fracture: Magnetic resonance appearance versus age of injury. Am J Sports Med 17:620, 1989
12. JACKSON H, KAM J, HARRIS JH JR, et al: The sacral arcuate lines in upper sacral fractures. Radiology 145:35, 1982
13. MACK LA, HARLEY JD, WINQUIST RA: CT of acetabular fractures: Analysis of fracture patterns. Am J Roentgenol 138:407, 1982
14. MACNEALY GA, ROGERS LF, HERNANDEZ R, ET AL: Injuries of the distal tibial epiphysis: Systematic radiographic evaluation. Am J Roentgenol 138:683, 1982
15. MEURMAN KO, ELFVING S: Stress fracture in soldiers: A multifocal bone disorder. Radiology 134:483, 1980
16. MILGRAM JW, ROGERS LF, MILLER JW: Osteochondral fractures: mechanisms of injury and fate of fragments. Am J Roentgenol 130:651, 1978
17. MINK JH, DEUTSCH AL: MRI of the musculoskeletal system: A teaching file. New York, Raven Press, 1990
18. MONTANA MA, RICHARDSON ML, KILCOYNE RF, HARLEY JD, SHUMAN WP, MACK LA: CT of sacral injury. Radiology 161:499, 1986
19. MURPHY WA, SIEGEL MJ: Elbow fat pads with new signs and extended differential diagnosis. Radiology 124:659, 1977
20. PENNAL GF, TILE M, WADDELL JP, ET AL: Pelvis disruption: Assessment and classification. Clin Orthop 151:12, 1980
21. POST MJD, GREEN BA: The use of computed tomography in spinal trauma. Radiol Clin North Am 21:327, 1983
22. RADKOWSKI MA, MERTEN DF, LEONIDAS JC: The abused child: Criteria for the radiologic diagnosis. Radiographics 3:262, 1983
23. ROCKWOOD CA JR, GREEN DP: Fractures. 3rd ed, Vols 1, 2, 3. Philadelphia, JB Lippincott, 1991
24. ROGERS LF: Radiology of Skeletal Trauma. 2nd ed. New York, Churchill-Livingstone, 1992
25. ROGERS LF: The radiography of epiphyseal injuries. Radiology 96:289, 1970
26. SALTER RB, HARRIS WR: Injuries involving the epiphyseal plate. J Bone Joint Surg [Am] 45:587, 1963
27. SCHNEIDER R, YACOVONE J, GHELMAN B: Unsuspected sacral fractures: Detection by radionuclide bone scanning. Am J Roentgenol 144:337, 1985
28. SPIEGEL PG, MAST JW, COOPERMAN DR, ET AL: Triplane fractures of the distal tibial epiphysis. Clin Orthop 188:74, 1984
29. SULLIVAN D, WARREN RF, PAVLOV H, ET AL: Stress fractures in 51 runners. Clin Orthop 187:188, 1984
30. TOWBIN R, DUNBAR JS, TOWGIN J, ET AL: Teardrop sign: Plain film recognition of ankle effusion. Am J Roentgenol 134:985, 1980
31. WILCOX JR JR, MONIOT AL, GREEN JP: Bone scanning in the evaluation of exercise-related stress injuries. Radiology 123:699, 1977

Paul and Juhl's Essentials of Radiologic Imaging, Sixth Edition, edited by John H. Juhl and Andrew B. Crummy. J.B. Lippincott Company, Philadelphia, © 1993.

CHAPTER *3*

Diseases of the Joints

Lee F. Rogers

The ends of apposing bones, as portrayed on a roentgenogram, are separated by a space commonly referred to as the *joint space.* This space is occupied by articular cartilage and a small amount of synovial fluid, both of which have the same radiodensity and are therefore indistinguishable from each other. Loss of articular cartilage is manifested radiographically as a decrease in the width of the joint space. The joint capsule of the normal joint is of the same density as the surrounding soft tissue and is usually difficult to visualize. However, when the joint is distended by fluid, its outer limits may be seen if there is sufficient fat in the periarticular tissues to offer contrast (see Figs. 3-15, 3-16A, and 3-18). This is particularly true of the peripheral joints: the interphalangeal (IP) and metacarpophalangeal (MCP) joints of the hand, the ankle, the wrist, the elbow, and the suprapatellar bursa of the knee. However, it is difficult to identify distention of the major proximal joints—the shoulder, hip, and axial skeleton. Periarticular edema or hemorrhage tends to obliterate the fat and tissue planes. Close observation of periarticular soft tissues will often permit the detection of early signs of inflammatory disease in the joint or adjacent structures.

Radiographs are used in diseases of the joints to confirm the clinical diagnosis of joint disease, determine the type of joint disease, and evaluate the extent of clinically known disease.[20] The radiographic findings may be either consistent or inconsistent with the clinical diagnosis. If inconsistent, an alternative diagnosis should be made on the basis of the radiographic appearance of the disease process. On other occasions, joint disease is observed on a radiograph obtained for some other reason, such as for peripheral trauma; on a chest radiograph demonstrating changes in the spine or pectoral girdle; or on radiographs of the abdomen and pelvis revealing abnormalities of the spine, sacroiliac joints, or hips. In the latter situations, the joint disease should be categorized and included in the radiographic report.

There are four principal radiographic signs of joint abnormalities or joint disease. These are (1) abnormalities of the apposing margins of both bones at a joint, (2) change in the width of the joint space, usually narrowing, but occasionally widening because of an increase in synovial fluid, (3) malalignment of the joint (subluxation or dislocation with the joint margins no longer in apposition), and (4) periarticular swelling due to distention of the joint capsule. The most common findings are narrowing of the joint space and abnormalities of the apposing articular margins of bone.

Each joint disease has a more or less specific pattern of radiographic abnormalities. This pattern is based on the radiographic characteristics at each individual joint, the distribution of joint involvement, and the presence or absence of other ancillary radiographic findings.[11, 29] When the characteristic pattern is coupled with the clinical history, physical findings, and laboratory examinations, the correct diagnosis can be established with reasonable certainty.

The distribution of joint involvement is extremely important. To begin a diagnostic evaluation, it should be determined whether or not the process is limited to one joint (monoarticular) or involves multiple joints (polyarticular). Each joint disease has a characteristic distribution of joint involvement (Fig. 3-1) more likely to involve certain joints than others, and to involve those joints either symmetrically (simultaneous in-

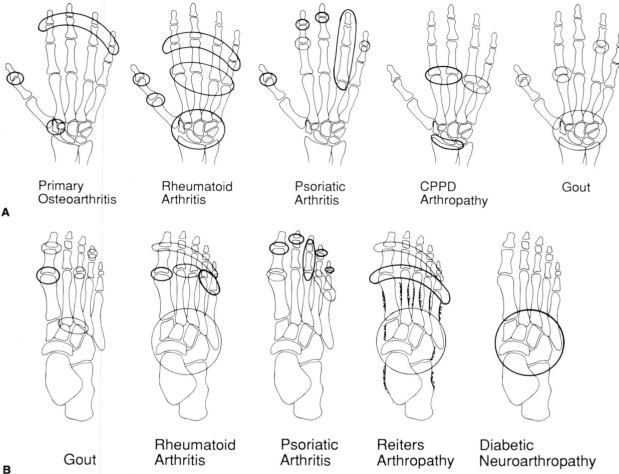

A

Primary Osteoarthritis   Rheumatoid Arthritis   Psoriatic Arthritis   CPPD Arthropathy   Gout

B

Gout   Rheumatoid Arthritis   Psoriatic Arthritis   Reiters Arthropathy   Diabetic Neuroarthropathy

Figure 3–1. Sites and distribution of common arthrides of the hand (**A**) and foot (**B**). The more common sites are encircled with heavy lines and the less common sites with lighter lines. Note the periosteal reaction or new-bone formation classically identified in Reiter's disease and psoriasis. Note also the potential for "sausage digit" distribution in psoriasis. When joints are encircled in isolation, the distribution is random and may be isolated to any joint.

volvement of similar joints of both extremities) or asymmetrically (involvement of a joint on one side without simultaneous involvement of the corresponding joint on the opposite side).

The specific radiographic characteristics of importance in establishing or confirming the diagnosis often are (1) whether or not the joint space narrowing is symmetrical or asymmetrical, (2) whether or not soft-tissue swelling is present and if it is symmetrical (indicating a joint effusion) or asymmetrical (indicating the presence of a periarticular mass), and the presence or absence of (3) periarticular osteoporosis, (4) periarticular erosions, and (5) spur formation.

Ancillary radiographic findings include the presence or absence of periosteal reaction of bones in the vicinity of the involved joint and the character of calcification or ossification of ligamentous attachments or tendinous attachments about the joint. Such calcifications and ossifications are referred to as *entheses*, and their diffuse presence in the skeletal system is known as an *enthesopathy*. Finally, the presence or absence of calcification within the joint cartilage (*chondrocalcinosis*) is to be noted. This finding is characteristic of certain joint disorders.

The clinical findings of importance are the age and sex of the patient, a history of previous trauma, the clinical appearance of the joint or joints involved, the presence or absence of associated diseases (particularly skin disease, uveitis, urethritis, and diarrhea), and identifiable tophaceous deposits. Laboratory values of importance are the erythrocyte sedimentation rate; the presence or absence of serum rheumatoid factor; the white blood cell count; and the serum calcium, phosphorus, alkaline phosphatase, and uric acid levels. The radiographic diagnosis is greatly aided by knowledge of the clinical and laboratory findings, and the opposite is equally true: the radiographic diagnosis of joint disease may be severely handicapped in the absence of knowledge of clinical and laboratory examinations.

Joint disease is classified in Table 3-1.

INFECTIOUS ARTHRITIS

ACUTE AND CHRONIC PYOGENIC ARTHRITIS OF THE PERIPHERAL JOINTS

The source of infection resulting in pyogenic arthritis may be hematogenous from other infections of the skin, respiratory tract, or urinary system; a direct extension from a focus of adjacent osteomyelitis; or a consequence of bacterial contamination resulting from surgical procedures or open injuries of the joint. The course of the disease may vary considerably. In some cases, it is relatively mild and subsides without residua. In others, a purulent infection ensues, causing pyarthrosis with rapid destruction of joint surfaces. In still others, it follows a comparatively indolent and chronic course from the outset.

In children, infection more commonly involves the major peripheral joints, and the source of infection is very likely to be an infection of the skin, upper respiratory tract, or lungs. In adults, the source is more likely to be trauma or surgery secondary to vascular disease, particularly in the feet of diabetic patients. Bacterial spondylitis is more common in adults than in children and is often associated with a urinary tract infection or follows catheterization or other manipulative procedures of the bladder and urethra.

Unusual sites of pyogenic infection occur in intravenous drug abusers. These include the sternoclavicular and sacroiliac joints, and infections are often due to gram-negative organisms. Septic arthritis may also complicate intra-articular injection of steroids.

ROENTGENOGRAPHIC OBSERVATIONS

The radiographic findings described subsequently occur in an untreated or inadequately treated infection of virulence.[11, 29] With present-day therapeutic measures, most cases of acute pyogenic joint infection can be brought under control before appreciable damage occurs within the joint.

Table 3–1. Classification of Joint Disease

I. Infectious arthritis
  A. Acute infectious arthritis (pyogenic or septic arthritis)
  B. Chronic infectious arthritis
    1. Pyogenic
    2. Tuberculous
    3. Other
II. Arthritis of collagen disease
  A. Rheumatoid arthritis
    1. Adult
    2. Juvenile type (Still's disease)
  B. Rheumatoid variants (seronegative spondylo-arthropathies)
    1. Ankylosing spondylitis
    2. Psoriatic arthritis
    3. Reiter's syndrome
    4. Colitic arthritis
  C. Connective tissue diseases
    1. Systemic lupus erythematosus (SLE)
    2. Dermatomyositis and polymyositis
    3. Scleroderma
    4. Mixed connective tissue disease
    5. Jaccoud's arthropathy (chronic postrheumatic fever arthritis)
III. Degenerative joint disease (osteoarthritis, osteoarthrosis)
  A. Primary osteoarthritis
  B. Secondary osteoarthritis
    1. Previous trauma
    2. Previous infection
    3. Preexisting arthritis
  C. Diffuse idiopathic skeletal hyperostosis (DISH, Forestier disease)
IV. Neuropathic joint disease (neuroarthropathy)
  A. Primary neurologic disease
  B. Diabetes
V. Metabolic disease
  A. Gout
  B. Pseudogout (calcium pyrophosphate deposition disease, CPPD)
  C. Hemochromatosis
  D. Hyperparathyroidism
  E. Ochronosis
  F. Wilson's disease
VI. Primary synovial disease
  A. Pigmented villonodular synovitis
  B. Synovial osteochondromatosis
  C. Idiopathic synovitis
VII. Miscellaneous
  A. Amyloidosis
  B. Hemophilia
  C. Lipoid dermatoarthritis (reticulohistiocytosis)
  D. Idiopathic chondrolysis
  E. Relapsing polychondritis
  F. Hypertrophic osteoarthropathy

Soft-Tissue Swelling

In the first few days of infection, the only roentgenographic changes are those of soft-tissue swelling and distention of the joint capsule by fluid (Fig. 3-2). This causes an increase in soft-tissue density about the joint (Fig. 3-3). Periarticular edema tends to obliterate the tissue planes around the joint and often extends into the subcutaneous fat. In the absence of trauma, such

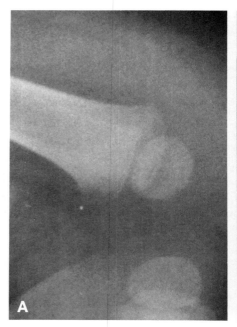 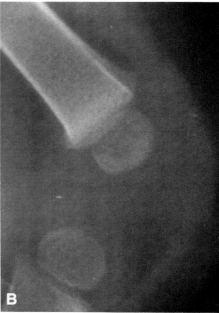

Figure 3–2. Acute pyogenic arthritis of the left knee in an 18-month-old boy. **(A)** Lateral radiograph of the left knee. Soft-tissue swelling, joint distention, and obliteration of fascial planes is evident. There are no bony abnormalities. Compare with normal right knee. **(B)** Lateral view of normal right knee.

findings, particularly in a febrile child with pain or tenderness in the area, strongly suggest the diagnosis of septic arthritis. Soft-tissue changes of this type are not specific of course, and at this stage of the disease needle aspiration should be promptly performed to establish the diagnosis or rule out the possibility of infectious arthritis. The diagnosis of infectious arthritis should not await the appearance of radiographic changes.

Joint-Space Narrowing

Purulent organisms excrete proteolytic enzymes that destroy articular cartilage (Fig. 3-4), resulting in a decrease in the width of the joint space. In a virulent infection, this may become evident in a week or 10 days following the onset of disease. If the infection is untreated or inadequately treated, the narrowing progresses rapidly and the joint space may disappear completely within several weeks. Early in the course of acute infection, the bones about the joint maintain normal density; however, if the infection becomes subacute or chronic, osteoporosis will become evident. Joint narrowing and destruction in the absence of osteoporosis are indicative of a highly virulent infection.

Bone Destruction

Bone destruction is manifested by irregularity of the subchondral bone at the apposing margins of the joint (Figs. 3-3 and 3-4B). The destruction may initially be focal, but it eventually extends across the entire joint surface. Since bone destruction does not occur for 8 to 10 days, this sign is of no value in the early diagnosis of joint infection.

Ankylosis

If the articular cartilages are completely destroyed, bony ankylosis usually follows. Eventually, bone trabeculae form across the ends of the bones, and in time all evidence of the joint may disappear.

When antibiotic treatment is ineffective or is discontinued too quickly, the acute infection may be transformed into a chronic indolent process with a slowly progressive course extending over months. In this case, there is gradual decrease in the joint space, the articular ends of the bone become roughened, and sequestra may form. As the infection subsides, the bones gradually regain density and bony ankylosis may occur. If the infection continues, fibrous or bony ankylosis may occur, so there may be little or no joint motion (Fig. 3-4C).

Neonatal Infections

Septic arthritis frequently occurs as a complication of neonatal osteomyelitis. Such infections occur in premature and term infants who have had catheterization of umbilical vessels. In the neonate, the blood supply of the epiphysis is contiguous with that of the metaphysis, and extension of an infectious process into the joint is

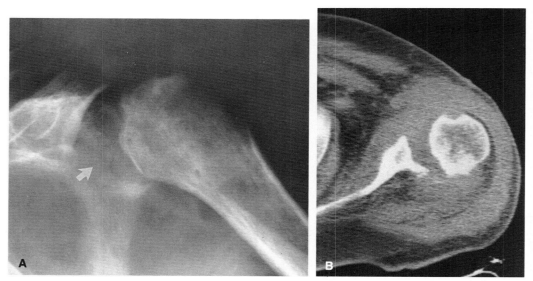

Figure 3–3. Subacute suppurative arthritis of the shoulder. (**A**) AP view demonstrates destruction of the opposing margins of the joint. Note the irregularity of the humeral head and the poor definition of the glenoid rim (*arrow*). The joint space appears widened. (**B**) CT scan confirms the widening of the joint space and irregularity and destruction of the opposing margins of the joint. Note the joint distention and surrounding soft-tissue swelling with obliteration of fascial planes and partial obliteration of the subcutaneous fat.

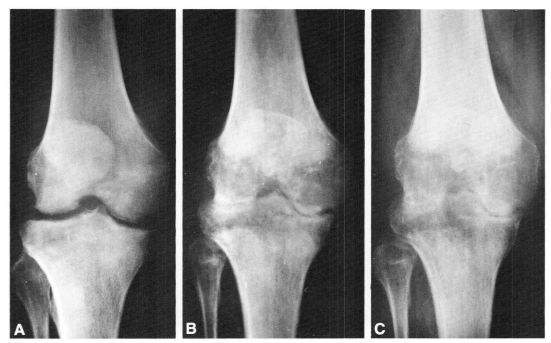

Figure 3–4. Chronic infectious arthritis of the knee. (**A**) On the initial examination, erosion of the bony articular surfaces is identified medially and is associated with narrowing of the joint space both medially and laterally. (**B**) In 4 months, further destruction of bone and the virtual absence of the joint space are evidenced, indicating destruction of the joint cartilage. (**C**) Nine months after the onset, the infection has subsided and there is early bony ankylosis. Note that periarticular osteoporosis has persisted.

therefore very likely (Fig. 3-5). Multiple sites of infection are the rule, and septic arthritis is quite common. The hip is involved in 45% of cases, the knee in 35%, and the remaining sites are the shoulder, elbow, and ankle. When the hip is involved, the joint distention may be sufficient to result in a dislocation accompanied by a large surrounding soft-tissue mass (Fig. 3-6).

Neonatal osteomyelitis may also occur in those who have not had umbilical catheterization. Under these circumstances, the signs are often vague and there is only a single focus of disease.

TUBERCULOSIS OF THE PERIPHERAL JOINTS

Tuberculosis of the joints is a chronic indolent infection having an insidious onset and a slowly progressive course. It usually affects a single joint (monoarticular). The joint disease may result from hematogenous dissemination to the synovial membrane or may be secondary to a tuberculous abscess in the neighboring

bone. The latter is common in childhood. Pathologically, tuberculosis usually begins as a synovitis. Proliferation of inflammatory granulation tissue, known as pannus, begins at the perichondrium and spreads over the joint surfaces. It interferes with nutrition of the cartilage, resulting in degeneration and destruction. In weight-bearing joints, and to a lesser degree in non-weight-bearing joints, there is a tendency for preservation of the joint cartilages at sites of maximum weight bearing or close apposition of cartilage. This is in contrast to pyogenic infections, in which the joint exudate contains proteolytic enzymes that rapidly destroy the entire cartilaginous joint surface.

ROENTGENOGRAPHIC OBSERVATIONS

Tuberculous Arthritis

The earliest evidence of tuberculous arthritis of a peripheral joint is a joint effusion. In time, often after several months, the bones adjacent to the joint become osteoporotic. The degree of osteoporosis is often severe

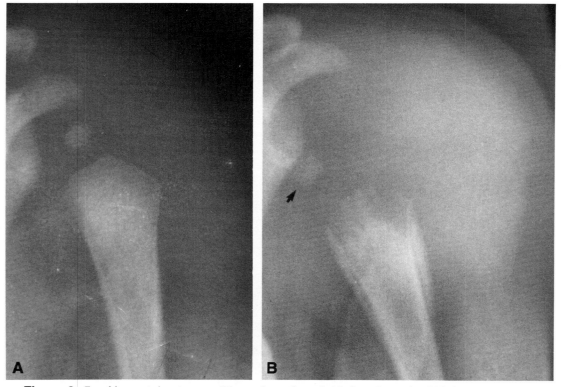

Figure 3–5.   Neonatal osteomyelitis and septic arthritis in a 2-week-old infant. **(A)** Initial examination demonstrates only soft-tissue swelling around the shoulder. **(B)** A repeat examination 13 days later demonstrates poorly defined destruction in the metaphysis, with surrounding periosteal reaction and marked distention of the shoulder joint with pseudodislocation. Note the inferior displacement of the epiphysis (*arrow*).

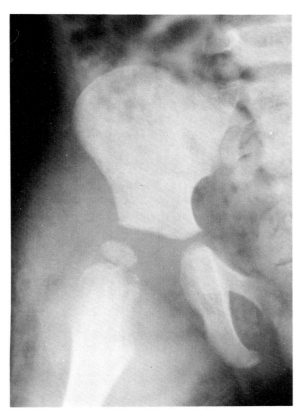

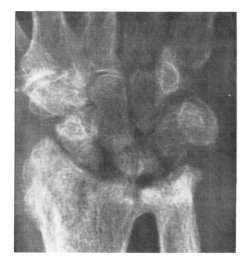

Figure 3–7. Tuberculous arthritis of the carpus in an 82-year-old woman. Diffuse osteoporosis is present, with narrowing of the radiocarpal and midcarpal joints and erosion and destruction of their opposing margins. The metacarpohamate joint is also involved. The distal margin of the ulna including the styloid is eroded.

Figure 3–6. Acute osteomyelitis of the proximal metaphysis of the femur, with secondary involvement of the hip joint. There is a small focus of bone destruction in the medial margin of the metaphysis. The femur is displaced laterally by the large joint effusion. Note the marked soft-tissue swelling in the upper thigh.

and probably is caused by a combination of hyperemia and disuse (Fig. 3-7). Eventually, destruction of articular cartilage is manifested by narrowing of the joint and erosion of bone. In the weight-bearing joints, there is a tendency for preservation of cartilage at the point of maximum weight-bearing (Fig. 3-8). The earliest evidence of bone destruction is the appearance of erosions at the margins of the joint. These marginal defects are sharply circumscribed and closely resemble erosions seen in rheumatoid arthritis. Marginal erosions gradually extend across the joint surface. With further progression, gross disorganization of the joint may occur. The articular cartilage disappears, ragged destruction of the articular ends of the bone occurs, and separation of dead fragments (sequestra) is noted (Fig. 3-8C). Very little reactive sclerosis is observed in untreated tuberculosis.

Caries sicca is a relatively uncommon form of tuberculosis that is characterized by a very chronic and indolent course, with an absence of joint effusion. Except for the lack of fluid and associated swelling of soft tissues, the roentgenographic findings in this type of disease differ little from those described in the foregoing. This type occurs most frequently in the shoulder.

Unilateral abnormalities of the sacroiliac joint should suggest the possibility of tuberculosis. Bacterial infections of this joint are also encountered in drug abusers. The radiographic findings are destruction of the joint margins, with some degree of reactive sclerosis.

In tuberculosis there is little tendency for spontaneous healing, and bony ankylosis seldom develops without surgical intervention.

The principal differential diagnosis of tuberculous arthritis includes acute and chronic pyogenic arthritis and rheumatoid arthritis. In acute pyogenic arthritis, there is early destruction of joint space and an absence of osteoporosis. In chronic pyogenic arthritis, the findings are very similar. Bony ankylosis is much more likely in a pyogenic infection than in tuberculosis. In a given joint, the differentiation between tuberculosis and rheumatoid arthritis may be difficult. However, the polyarticular nature and distribution of rheumatoid arthritis should distinguish it from tuberculosis, which is almost always monoarticular.

Fungal Infections

Joint involvement is rare in fungal infections. However, blastomycosis, histoplasmosis, actinomycosis, coccidioidomycosis, and cryptococcosis joint infections are occasionally observed. They are similar in appearance to tuberculosis. Diagnosis must be based on recovery of the causative organism.

INFECTIOUS SPONDYLITIS

Infections of the spine are initiated by hematogenous spread of organisms. These may be of arterial or paravertebral venous plexus origin. The latter is very likely the source of infections of the spine associated with infections of the urinary tract or following urinary tract manipulations. The bacteria lodge beneath the end-plate of a vertebra, usually anteriorly, and quickly extend into the adjacent intervertebral disc and then into the inferior end-plate of the adjacent vertebral body (Fig. 3-9).[29] From here, the infection may extend out of the vertebra, along the spine, beneath the paravertebral ligament, thus forming soft-tissue masses and abscesses.

The radiographic findings indicative of infectious spondylitis are (1) narrowing of the disc space, (2) erosion and destruction of adjacent vertebral end-plates, and (3) a paravertebral soft-tissue mass (Figs. 3-10 and

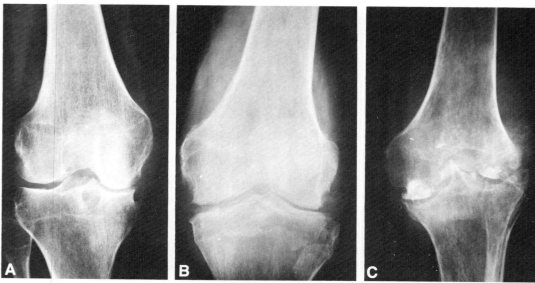

Figure 3–8.   Tuberculosis of the knee in three different patients. **(A)** The joint space is intact, but there are marginal erosions on the medial margin of the tibia and fibula, and a subchondral radiolucency is present in the tibia just beneath the tibial spine. **(B)** The disease is more extensive than in **A**, manifested by greater narrowing of the joint space and marginal erosions. **(C)** Advanced disease is manifested by multiple sequestra producing the dense white bony fragments and considerable destruction of bone, particularly in the lateral tibial plateau.

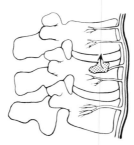
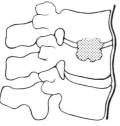
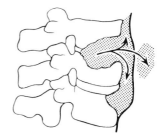

Bacterial
Embolization

Involves Disc
and Adjacent
Vertebra

Subligamentous
Extension

Figure 3–9.   Diagram of infectious spondylitis.

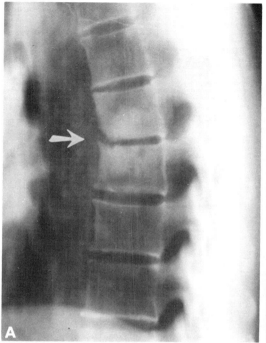

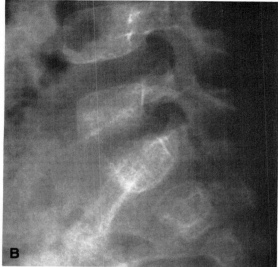

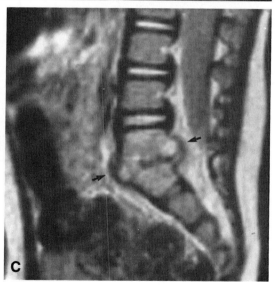

Figure 3–10. (**A**) Infectious spondylitis. Tomogram demonstrates erosion of the opposing margins of adjacent vertebral bodies anteriorly (*arrow*), with some underlying sclerosis of bone. Note the minimal disc space narrowing. (**B** and **C**) AP and lateral views of infectious spondylitis of L5–S1 in a 10-month-old girl, more advanced than **A**, as manifested by greater destruction of opposing margins of the vertebral bodies. The disc space is nearly obliterated. The intervertebral disc space (**B**) is narrowed with destruction of the opposing margins of the vertebrae. T2-weighted sagittal MRI (**C**) reveals destruction of the intervertebral disc and opposing margins of the vertebrae with surrounding soft-tissue mass of increased signal intensity (*arrows*). (Case courtesy of Andrew Poznanski, M.D., Chicago)

3-11). In the cervical spine, the soft-tissue mass is identified on the lateral radiograph as an enlargement of the retropharyngeal soft tissues and, in the thoracic spine, as a paravertebral soft-tissue mass that is best seen on the anteroposterior radiograph of the chest or thoracic spine (Fig. 3-11A). The soft-tissue mass associated with an infection of the lumbar vertebral bodies is usually difficult if not impossible to see on the anteroposterior radiographs of the lumbar spine. In all locations, both the paraspinous soft-tissue mass and the degree of vertebral body destruction are readily identified by computed tomography (CT) (Fig. 3-12). In questionable cases, polytomography is the best method of evaluation because it clearly demonstrates the end-plates of the adjacent vertebral bodies. Magnetic resonance imaging (MRI) demonstrates all of the findings quite satisfactorily, including any encroachment upon or compression of the spinal cord (see Figs. 3-10

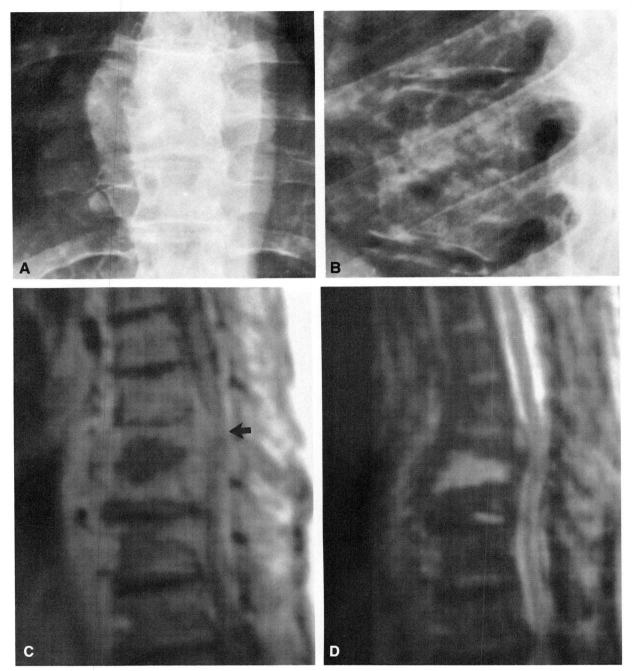

Figure 3–11. (**A** and **B**) Tuberculosis of the spine. Note that the paraspinal mass (**A**) is more localized on the right than on the left. There is a loss of disc space. Lateral projection (**B**). Obliteration of joint space and destruction of the adjacent vertebral end-plates are demonstrated. (**C** and **D**) Another case demonstrated by MRI. T1-weighted image (**C**) demonstrates soft destruction of opposing margins of two vertebrae with surrounding soft-tissue mass that bulges anteriorly and extends posteriorly to compress the spinal cord (*arrow*). There is an area of decreased signal in the region of the destroyed intervertebral disc between the two involved vertebrae. On the T2-weighted image (**D**) the area in the midst of the soft-tissue mass now emits a high signal. The spinal cord compression is clearly depicted.

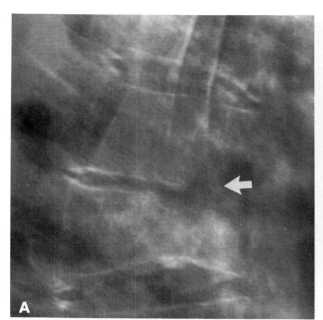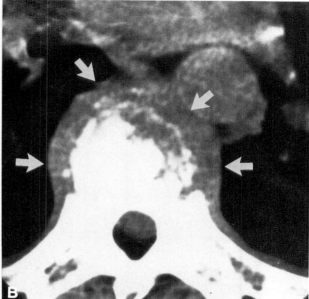

Figure 3–12. Infectious spondylitis of T6–T7. (**A**) Lateral view demonstrates obvious disc space narrowing and destruction of the adjacent margins of the vertebral bodies anteriorly (*arrow*). (**B**) CT demonstrates paraspinous mass (*arrows*) and destruction of the anterior margin of the vertebral body. Note that the process does not extend to the spinal canal.

and 3-11). Rarely, an infectious process is limited to the vertebral body or posterior bony elements and presents as a focus of destruction. In general, the posterior elements are not involved by the infectious process.

PYOGENIC SPONDYLITIS

Infectious spondylitis caused by pyogenic organisms has a tendency to be confined to one interspace, and the paraspinous soft-tissue masses are not as large as those seen with tuberculosis (see Figs. 3-11 and 3-12). The earliest roentgenographic sign is a decrease in the height of the disc space. CT or polytomography may be necessary to confirm destruction of the adjacent endplates. The infections tend to be subacute, and the destructive process often has a sclerotic margin.

JUVENILE SPONDYLOARTHRITIS

Calcification of one or more intervertebral discs in childhood is a rare disorder. Afflicted children are usually between 2 and 11 years old, with a predominance of boys. Patients usually complain of pain, with limitation of motion, muscle spasm, tenderness, and torticollis. Roentgenograms show calcification in one or more intervertebral discs, usually in the cervical area.

The disease tends to be self-limited, and the calcifications gradually disappear over a period of several months. It has been regarded as an infection by some observers. However, there is evidence to indicate that some cases are of traumatic origin. Calcification in the disc of adult patients is usually found in the thoracic spine. This is quite common and appears to be a degenerative change related to the aging process.

TUBERCULOUS SPONDYLITIS

Tuberculous spondylitis has a greater tendency than infectious spondylitis to spread along the spine (Figs. 3-11 and 3-13). The spread occurs beneath the paraspinous ligaments, both above and below the initial site of infection. This spread forms an elongated paravertebral soft-tissue mass. Radiographically, the soft-tissue mass may be accompanied by irregular erosions or smooth, saucerized defects or scalloping of the anterior borders of several adjacent vertebral bodies. On other occasions, there is minimal radiographic evidence of disc disease but extensive paravertebral soft-tissue masses are present, there is little or no vertebral collapse, and the intervertebral discs appear to be preserved. In long-standing cases, calcification may occur in the paravertebral abscesses. These calcified or

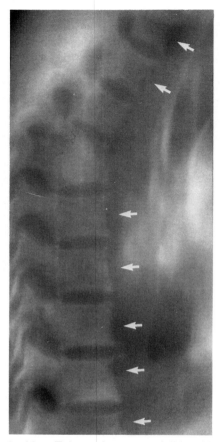

Figure 3–13. Tuberculous spondylitis with subligamentous extension. There is obliteration of the disc space and destruction of adjacent vertebral endplates in the middorsal spine. Note the superior and inferior subligamentous extension manifested by erosions of the anterior margin of the vertebral bodies (*arrows*).

partially calcified abscesses remain throughout life. With quiescence and healing of the disease, the bones regain a more normal density and bony ankylosis may occur across the involved disc. In very old cases of tuberculous spondylitis, several contiguous vertebrae may have been destroyed to such an extent that their individual outlines are no longer recognizable and all evidence of the intervening disc space may have disappeared. The resultant angled deformity of the spine is known as a *gibbus* (a Latin term meaning *hump*).

FUNGAL SPONDYLITIS

Involvement of the spine occasionally occurs in actinomycosis, blastomycosis, and coccidioidomycosis. Most lesions resemble those of tuberculosis. Coccidioi-

domycosis has a tendency to involve bony protuberances and may present as isolated destructive foci in the posterior elements.

RHEUMATOID ARTHRITIS

Rheumatoid arthritis affects adults between the ages of 20 and 60 years, with the highest incidence between the ages of 40 and 50 years. Females are affected much more frequently than males. The clinical course of the disease varies. Most cases begin insidiously and then either run a protracted and progressive course or undergo remissions of variable length. In most cases, the disease eventually leads to a variable degree of deformity of the affected joints. In the typical case, the disease begins in the peripheral joints, usually the proximal IP and MCP joints of the hand and the carpal joints of the wrist. There is a tendency for symmetrical involvement of the joints when comparing the right and left sides. This tendency is stronger in women than men. As the disease progresses, it affects more proximal joints, advancing toward the trunk in all extremities until finally almost every joint in the body is involved. The disease may become arrested at any stage.

Pathologically, rheumatoid arthritis begins as synovitis. In the early stages there is edema and inflammation of the synovium and the subsynovial tissues. Joint effusion accompanies the synovial changes. If the disease advances, the synovium becomes greatly thickened, with enlargement of the synovial villi. This is followed by proliferation of fibrovascular connective tissue known as pannus. Pannus is responsible for the characteristic marginal erosions that first occur in the so-called bare areas between the peripheral edge of the joint cartilage and the insertion of the joint capsule (Fig. 3-14). Ultimately, pannus grows over the surface of the articular cartilage, interfering with normal nutrition, which results in cartilage degeneration, and destroying foci of underlying articular bone. In advanced cases the joint becomes filled with pannus, articular cartilage disappears, and fibrous ankylosis results, frequently followed by bony ankylosis. As these changes are occurring in the joint, the adjacent bone undergoes osteoporosis and muscles atrophy from disuse.

ROENTGENOGRAPHIC OBSERVATIONS

Radiographic findings vary with each stage of the disease. The initial manifestations are soft-tissue swelling, symmetrical narrowing of the joints, periarticular osteoporosis, and marginal erosions (Fig. 3-15). Radiographic manifestations of the disease are present in 66% of patients 3 to 6 months after the onset of disease and in 85% of those affected for 1 year. The distribution of joint involvement is characteristic. The disease be-

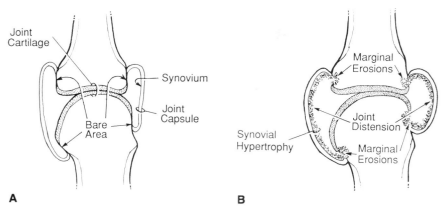

Figure 3–14. Marginal erosions in rheumatoid arthritis. (**A**) The normal metacarpophalangeal joint. Note the so-called bare area between the site of insertion of the joint capsule and the peripheral margin of the joint cartilage. (**B**) Synovial hypertrophy results in increased joint fluid, joint distention, and soft-tissue swelling and ultimately leads to marginal erosions beginning in the bare areas, the first site of bone destruction in rheumatoid arthritis.

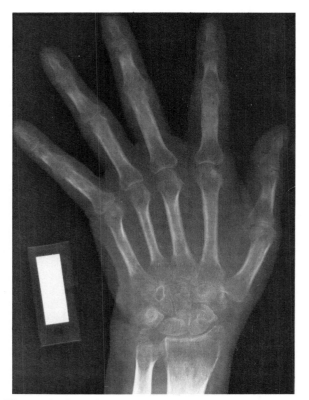

Figure 3–15. Early rheumatoid arthritis. Periarticular osteoporosis is identified. Soft-tissue swelling is present around the PIP and MCP joints. Small erosions are present at the radial side of the base of the proximal phalanx of the index finger.

gins in the proximal interphalangeal (PIP), MCP, and carpal joints (see Fig. 1A) with a more or less symmetrical distribution when comparing the right with the left extremity. In some cases the joints of the hand and wrist are equally affected, but in others the destructive process may be much more severe in the hand than in the carpus (Fig. 3-16). In still others, it may be more severe in the carpus than in the hand, even extensive in the carpus and yet minimal in the MCP and IP joints (Fig. 3-17). In the foot (see Fig. 1B), the metatarsophalangeal (MTP) joints, particularly the fourth and fifth, are often involved in the initial stage of the disease process. In fact, characteristic changes of erosion may be present in the heads of the fourth or fifth metatarsal when the radiographic changes of the hand are minimal or nondiagnostic (Fig. 3-18). Therefore, it is important to examine not only the hands but also the feet in the initial evaluation for rheumatoid arthritis.

Soft-Tissue Swelling

The earliest roentgenographic evidence of the disease is periarticular soft-tissue swelling, characteristically symmetrical and fusiform (see Fig. 3-15). This is easily identified in the PIP joints and to a lesser extent in the MCP and MTP joints. Joint distention can also be identified in the knee, ankle, and wrist. The joint effusion is caused by the synovitis.

Periarticular Osteoporosis

Local demineralization of bone occurs adjacent to the involved joint. In the metacarpals and phalanges, this

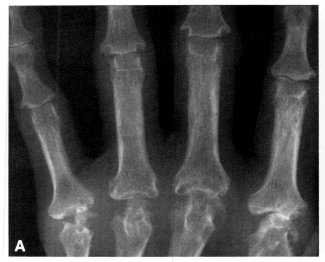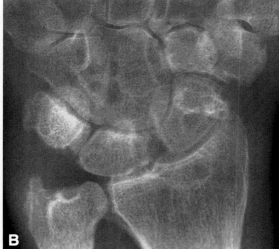

Figure 3–16. Advanced rheumatoid arthritis. **(A)** Joint distention is evidenced by capsular swelling at the MCP joints. There are extensive erosions of the heads of the metacarpals and small erosions of the base opposing margins of the proximal phalanges. The PIP joints are symmetrically narrowed, and distinct marginal erosions are seen. **(B)** Narrowing of the radiocarpal and midcarpal joints, with erosions of the opposing margins, particularly of the ulnar styloid with overlying soft-tissue swelling.

involves the base and heads of the bone but spares the diaphysis (see Fig. 3-15). In the wrist, all the carpal bones are involved, as are the distal margins of the radius and ulna and the bases of the metacarpals. The bones in the affected area are more radiolucent because of loss of bone mineral. In early cases, this finding is often rather striking because of the symmetry of the process.

In advanced disease, generalized osteoporosis develops, involving all portions of the skeleton. This is in part due to the disease process and in part due to disuse and may be compounded by the use of steroids.

Symmetrical Joint Space Narrowing

Narrowing of the joint space results from degeneration of the articular cartilages as pannus spreads across the joint surfaces (see Fig. 3-15). Typically this diminution in the joint is uniform, the joint space is symmetrically narrowed as opposed to the asymmetrical narrowing characteristic of osteoarthritis. The narrowing may progress gradually until the ends of the bones practically impinge on one another.

In the hip, thinning of the central aspect of the joint space causes displacement of the femoral head in an axial direction—that is, it moves upward and inward (Fig. 3-19). The joint space is characteristically symmetrically narrowed. The acetabulum may become

deepened, eventually leading to characteristic changes of protrusio acetabuli (Otto pelvis) (Fig. 3-19). Rheumatoid arthritis of the knee characteristically involves all compartments—medial, lateral, and patellofemoral. When the knee is involved, there is an even or symmetrical narrowing of the joint space in all compartments, particularly medial and lateral.

Joint-space narrowing also occurs in osteoarthritis, but it differs in some ways (see Figs. 3-34 through 3-36). In osteoarthritis the joint-space narrowing is characteristically asymmetrical. In the hip joint space, narrowing is more marked superiorly, and in the knee joint space, narrowing is commonly limited to the medial compartment. These and other findings such as the absence of osteoporosis and the presence of subchondral sclerosis of bone, subchondral cyst, and marginal spur formation should facilitate the distinction between rheumatoid arthritis and osteoarthritis.

Marginal Erosions

After a variable interval, bony erosions occur as a result of the development of granulation tissue (pannus) at the peripheral margin of the joint cartilage (see Figs. 3-15 through 3-18). These appear as small foci of destruction along the margins of the articular ends of the bones. They may be very minute but represent one of the most significant roentgenographic observations of

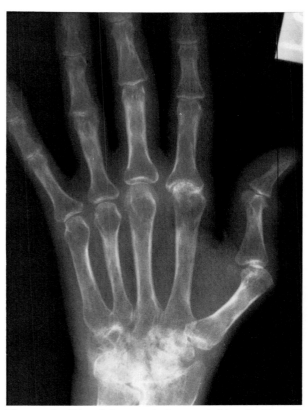

Figure 3–17. Advanced rheumatoid arthritis with carpal predominance. Note that the destructive process is much more marked in the carpal joints than in the peripheral joints of the hand. The hyperextension deformity of the interphalangeal joint of the thumb is typical of rheumatoid arthritis and is termed the hitchhiker's thumb.

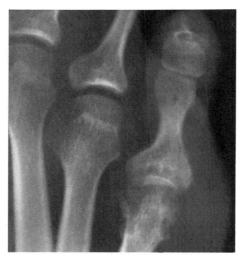

Figure 3–18. Rheumatoid arthritis of the fifth MTP joint. Note the erosive process involving the head of the fifth metatarsal and the opposing proximal phalanx. There is little or no identifiable destruction of the third and fourth MTP joints. On occasion, erosions are more obvious in the heads of the metatarsals than in the hand, as in this case.

early disease. The use of a magnifying lens is helpful when searching for the smallest erosion. The most common sites are the radial sides of the heads of the first, second, and third metacarpals; the heads of the fourth and fifth metatarsals; the margins of radiocarpal joint; the distal ends of the proximal third and fourth phalanges; and the ulnar styloid, as well as the adjacent margins of the distal radioulnar joint. The initial manifestation of the erosion may be simply a loss of the articular margin or an interruption of the articular margin. The smooth, continuous articular margin may be disrupted intermittently, causing a dot and dash pattern, or it may be completely resorbed, giving rise to a bare appearance of the underlying subarticular trabeculae. Characteristically, the distal IP joints are spared. Erosions occur at the sites of tendinous attachments, such as the Achilles tendon on the calcaneus and the plantar fascial attachment on the plantar surface of the os calcis.

Joint Malalignment

The degree of malalignment varies with the extent of the disease—the worse the disease, the greater the malalignment. Ulnar deviation of the phalanges with or without associated subluxation or dislocation is characteristic. The distal phalanx of the thumb is characteristically hyperextended, giving rise to the "hitchhiker thumb" deformity (see Fig. 3-17). The carpus is characteristically rotated ulnarward. Other carpal subluxations may occur, such as a scapholunate dislocation. With advanced disease, the carpus is markedly foreshortened by a combination of a rotational displacement and erosions of bone (see Fig. 3-17).

Joint Destruction

Marginal erosions and joint destruction are more common in the smaller peripheral than in the proximal major joints. In fact, marginal erosions may be difficult to identify in the hip and knee despite the severe joint involvement manifested by narrowing and marked osteoporosis. In smaller joints, deep excavations may occur. This is particularly common in the base of the proximal phalanx, often associated with destruction of

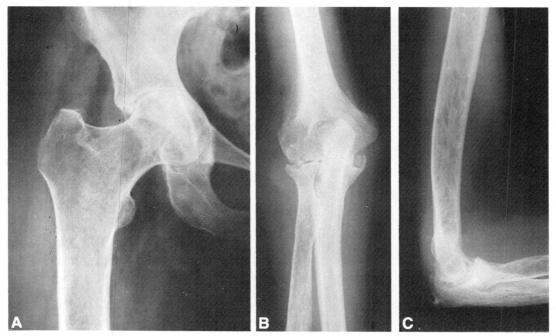

Figure 3–19. Rheumatoid arthritis. (**A**) There is uniform thinning of joint space and deepening of the acetabular cavity, causing a moderate degree of protrusio acetabuli. (**B** and **C**) Note the destructive lesions of the joint surfaces of the radius and ulna, the symmetrical narrowing of the joint space, and periarticular soft-tissue swelling. The bones are osteoporotic.

the head of the metacarpal, giving rise to the "pencil-in-cup" deformity. The ends of the metatarsals, metacarpals, and phalanges may be sharpened almost to a point, like a pencil. Extensive destruction of the articular ends of the bones in the hands, wrists, and feet is often referred to as *arthritis mutilans*.

Resorption of the distal end of the clavicle is common in severe to moderately severe rheumatoid arthritis. This can often be detected on the chest roentgenogram and may confirm or suggest the diagnosis. Other causes of absorption of the distal clavicles include hyperparathyroidism, scleroderma, gout, and post-traumatic osteolysis.

Bony Ankylosis

Destruction of articular cartilages may lead to the development of bony ankylosis. This is particularly frequent in the intercarpal and radiocarpal joints of the wrist. After all cartilage has been destroyed, bony trabeculae form across the previous joint space, and the end result is a complete obliteration of the joint and formation of a solid bony fusion.

Spinal Involvement

Spinal involvement in rheumatoid arthritis is usually limited to the cervical spine and more particularly to the craniovertebral junction. One of the characteristic changes is erosion of the odontoid process of the second cervical vertebra (Fig. 3-20). At times the dens is almost completely destroyed. Atlantoaxial subluxation may occur (Fig. 3-21) in rheumatoid arthritis.[35] Normally the distance between the posterior aspect of C1 and the dens is no more than 2.5 mm in adults, and it remains constant in flexion. The subluxation occurs because of a laxity of the transverse ligament, which holds the odontoid in position, and the presence of pannus about the dens. In these patients the distance is increased, but a lateral view in flexion may be required to demonstrate this abnormality. It may be reduced in extension. There may also be upward displacement of C2 or, more accurately, settling of the skull and C1 about C2. This is identified radiographically by an abnormally low position of the anterior arch of C1 in relation to the base of the vertebral body of C2. Either process may give rise to neurologic symptoms because of impingement on the upper cer-

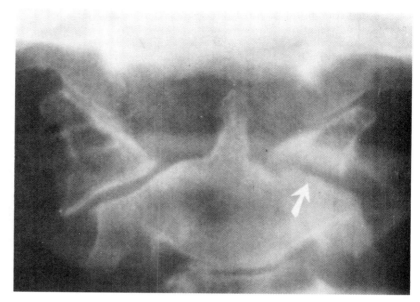

Figure 3–20. Rheumatoid arthritis of the upper cervical spine demonstrating erosion and thinning of the odontoid process and lateral subluxation of C1 on C2. There are marginal erosions of the facet joints of C1 on C2 on the left (*arrow*).

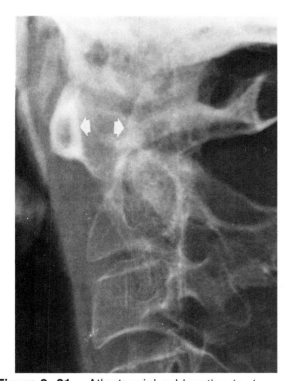

Figure 3–21. Atlantoaxial subluxation in rheumatoid arthritis. Note the increased distance between the posterior margin and the anterior arch of C1 and the anterior margin of the dens (*arrows*). The odontoid process is eroded.

vical cord or medulla. This is more likely when the subluxation measures 9 mm or more, or when the anterior arch of C1 appears to articulate with the lower half of the odontoid or the body of C2. The entire spectrum of abnormalities is nicely displayed by MRI.[28] The facet joints of the cervical spine may also be involved. This is most commonly evidenced by small erosions, but in some cases the involvement leads to ankylosis of the facet joints (see Fig. 3-24). This is much more frequent in the juvenile form of rheumatoid arthritis. In adults, disc-space narrowing may be identified with or without associated subluxation. The disc-space narrowing characteristically is not associated with subchondral sclerosis or spur formation, as seen in osteoarthritis or spondylosis.

Unusual Manifestations of Rheumatoid Arthritis

Giant Bone Cysts. Subarticular bone "cysts" or geodes are uncommon but not rare. They may become 8 to 10 cm or more in diameter, usually occur in a subarticular position, and may expand the cortex and lead to pathologic fracture. They may be caused by synovial fluid that is under pressure and that extends into the subarticular bone by way of a defect in the articular surface, particularly in the upper tibia. Some authors have reported that the geodes contain rheumatoid granulation tissue, which may be an extension of pannus through an articular surface defect, and in certain instances geodes may be caused by intramedullary rheumatoid nodules.

Rheumatoid Synovial Cysts. Increased intra-articular pressure may enlarge a joint capsule and produce cystlike extensions. Alteration in connective tissue of the capsule may also be a factor. This has been reported adjacent to a number of different joints in rheumatoid arthritis. Cysts about the knee are the most common. Popliteal cysts may dissect into the calf, where they may present clinical signs resembling those of deep vein thrombosis. Arthrography and ultrasonography are used to make the diagnosis. Such cysts may occur in a number of other diseases associated with joint effusion. They are rare in children with Still's disease.

"Robust" Rheumatoid Arthritis. Robust rheumatoid arthritis is a form of rheumatoid arthritis encountered in individuals who characteristically remain active despite the presence of severe arthritis. It is uncommon, occurs more frequently in men than women, and characteristically lacks osteoporosis. Marginal erosions are more likely to be asymmetrical and worse on the dominant side.

"Unilateral" Rheumatoid Arthritis. Central or peripheral neurologic deficits in patients with rheumatoid arthritis may lead to a sparing of the paralyzed side. The degree of protection tends to be directly proportional to the amount of paraplegia. The cause is not clear.

JUVENILE RHEUMATOID ARTHRITIS

The terminology for chronic arthritis in children is confusing. The term *Still's disease* is used by some to indicate all forms of rheumatoid arthritis in children, but others reserve the designation of Still's disease to that form that begins in infancy with systemic symptoms of fever and rash and findings of hepatosplenomegaly and lymphadenopathy, often with pericarditis, muscle wasting, and ultimate dwarfism. As a rule, systemic manifestations are more severe in the juvenile than in the adult form of rheumatoid arthritis. There is often a period of 2 years or more in which the systemic symptoms are present before the roentgenographic features of joint-space narrowing and marginal erosions are observed.

In general, the younger the patient, the more likely the disease is to be monoarticular, particularly involving a large joint such as the knee (Fig. 3-22), ankle, or wrist. The disease may be limited to a few major joints. If the disease begins in an older child, there is more likely to be symmetrical involvement of the smaller peripheral joints, as in an adult. The disease is most

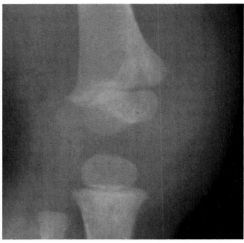

Figure 3–22. Juvenile rheumatoid arthritis. The lateral radiograph of the knee demonstrates soft-tissue swelling with joint effusion without evidence of bone destruction (compare with Fig. 3-2). At this stage, the correct diagnosis is dependent on joint aspiration.

often manifested by joint effusions, soft-tissue swelling, and periarticular osteoporosis.[11, 23, 29] Joint-space narrowing and erosion may not be visualized for many months. Periosteal reaction of the small bones of the hand is much more common than in the adult form of the disease. There is interference with skeletal maturation, usually manifested as acceleration of maturation, most likely secondary to hyperemia with premature fusion of ossification centers. The premature fusion leads to shortening of the bones involved (Fig. 3-23). This is clinically manifested as shortening of the digits. Extensive growth retardation may lead to short stature. Involvement of the spine is much more common in children than in adults. The involvement may be manifested by atlantoaxial subluxation and erosions and eventual bony ankylosis of the facet joints (Fig. 3-24).

RHEUMATOID VARIANTS (SERONEGATIVE SPONDYLOARTHROPATHIES)

The term *rheumatoid variants* refers to a group of inflammatory arthritides differing immunologically, clinically, and radiographically from rheumatoid arthritis. The diseases are ankylosing spondylitis, psoriatic arthritis, Reiter's disease, and colitic arthritis. Afflicted persons usually have a negative rheumatoid factor, but a significant percentage have the HLA-B27 antigen. The diseases are more common in males and usually cause symptoms in the axial skeleton. This in contrast to rheumatoid arthritis, which is more com-

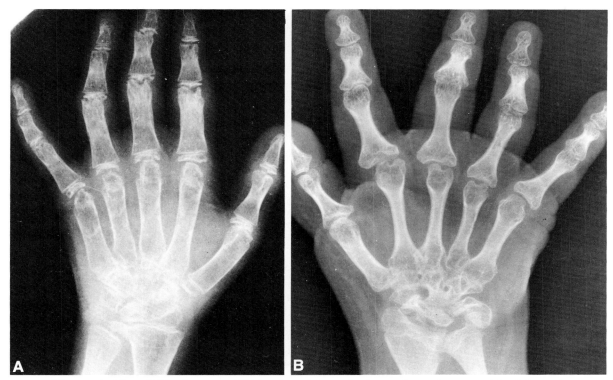

Figure 3–23. Still's disease. **(A)** Erosion of the articular surfaces in most of the joints of the hand and wrist, as well as severe osteoporosis, is demonstrated. **(B)** In this older patient, Still's disease has resulted in marked shortening of the digits, deformity of the carpal bones, and erosions of the head of the metacarpals.

mon in females and involves the distal appendicular skeleton. Radiographically, these diseases differ from rheumatoid arthritis in the absence or mild nature of periarticular osteoporosis or demineralization, the frequent occurrence of periostitis or periosteal new-bone formation, and the asymmetrical involvement of the peripheral skeleton.[26,29]

Ankylosing Spondylitis

Ankylosing spondylitis is typically a disease of young adult males, with a ratio of about 15 to 1 males to females. The onset of the disease in females is later in life. The earliest clinical manifestation is usually persistent low back pain of insidious onset. The disease initially involves the sacroiliac joints and then the spine, progressively from the lumbar to the cervical area. The disease may remain confined to the spine, but in 30% of patients, peripheral joint manifestation will occur, principally in the major proximal joints of the hips, shoulders, and knees.

Ankylosing spondylitis of juvenile onset differs somewhat from the usual form in the adult. Most of these patients present with complaints of pain in appendicular joints: hips, knees, or shoulders, with the more distal joints affected in decreasing frequency. Radiographically the peripheral joint changes predominate early in the disease. Eventually the typical axial manifestations of sacroiliitis and spondylitis occur.

Roentgenographic Observations. The initial manifestation is in the sacroiliac joints. All patients with this disease have sacroiliac involvement. The absence of sacroiliac disease rules out this diagnosis. The process is characteristically symmetrical and manifested by blurring and irregularity of the joint margins (Fig. 3-25). The process involves both the iliac and sacral side of the joint, although it may appear more severe on one side or the other. The joints may appear irregularly widened. Eventually there is sclerosis and complete obliteration of the joint. Ninety percent of patients will demonstrate changes in the sacroiliac joint at the time of initial presentation. Although this initially may be unilateral, the process characteristically is bilateral and

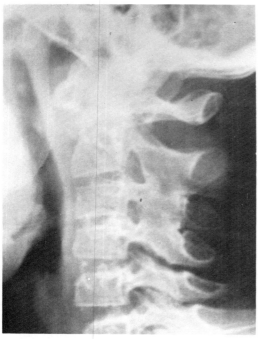

Figure 3–24. Still's disease of the cervical spine. Note the ankylosing of the apophyseal joints between C2, C3, and C4.

symmetrical. Every young male who presents with chronic low back pain should be closely examined for radiographic evidence of sacroiliac disease.

Bony irregularity of the margins of the pelvis are common. This "whiskering" is caused by inflammation and periostitis at the attachments of tendons. These occur in the ischial tuberosities, in the femoral trochanters, and on the iliac wings. Erosive changes may also occur at the symphysis pubis.

The initial radiographic manifestation of spinal involvement is squaring of the vertebral bodies, referring to the appearance of the vertebral body on the lateral view (Fig. 3-26). The superior and inferior corners of the vertebrae are almost square, without the normal concavity. This is caused by a subligamentous erosive process involving the anterosuperior and anteroinferior margins of the vertebral bodies. Later, syndesmophytes form from ossification in the outer layers of the annulus fibrosis of the intervertebral disc. These tend to be thin, vertically oriented, and symmetrical, arising from the peripheral margin of the vertebral body immediately adjacent to the end-plate (Fig. 3-27). When extensive, they are responsible for the typical "bamboo" spine appearance of this disease. The apophyseal joints become ankylosed, and the interspinous and paraspinous ligaments ossify. Atlantoaxial subluxation and erosions of the dens may also occur in ankylosing spondylitis.

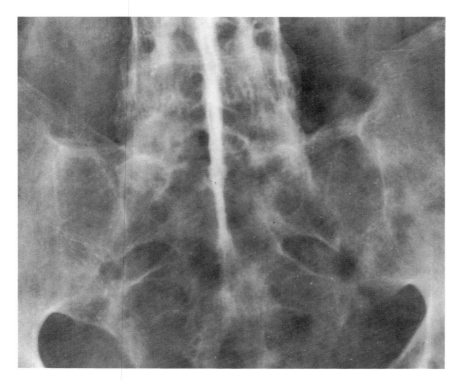

Figure 3–25. Ankylosing spondylitis. There is complete bony ankylosis of the sacroiliac joints and calcification and ossification of the interspinous ligaments in the lower lumbar spine.

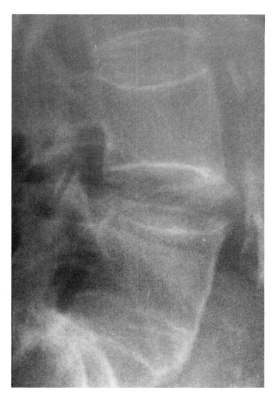

Figure 3–26. Ankylosing spondylitis. The lateral view of the lumbar spine demonstrates squaring of the vertebral bodies, characteristic of this disease. Note the loss of concavity of the anterior margin of the vertebrae. There is also a syndesmophyte at the L5–S1 disc space.

As the joints fuse, the spine and pelvis become osteoporotic. The spine then becomes susceptible to fractures that occur through the ankylosed intervertebral disc and posterior elements. Dislocations and spinal cord injuries are frequent.

Occasionally a destructive process is identified at a disc space and is manifested by narrowing of the disc space and erosion of the adjacent margins of the vertebrae, thus mimicking an infectious spondylitis. The erosive process may have a poorly defined sclerotic border. This may be focal, involving only the anterior central margin of the end-plate, or diffuse across the entire disc space. This process is most likely initiated by trauma, possibly the result of a stress fracture. Motion at the site then causes the formation of pseudoarthrosis. Despite its similarity in appearance to an infectious spondylitis, there is no evidence of bacterial growth on culture of the tissues.

Involvement of the extremities is uncommon, and when it occurs, it tends to be confined to the proximal major joints—hip, shoulder, and knee. The small peripheral joints are rarely involved; when they are involved, the process is isolated and transient, without destruction. The peripheral disease is rarely symmetrical and is not associated with osteoporosis but frequently shows evidence of erosion and periostitis. Erosions and periostitis on the plantar and posterior surface of the calcaneus are common in ankylosing spondylitis, just as in other rheumatoid variants.

Psoriatic Arthritis

Less than 10% of patients with psoriasis develop a peculiar form of arthritis, a smaller percentage develop classic rheumatoid arthritis, and an even smaller number develop some combination of the two. Psoriatic arthritis is a rheumatoid variant in which the serum is negative for rheumatoid factor. The extent of the arthritis does not correlate with the degree of skin disease. On occasion, the arthritis may even precede the skin manifestations by several years.

Psoriatic arthritis tends to involve the small joints of the hands and feet (Figs. 3-1, 3-28 and 3-29).[24] The process is characteristically asymmetrical and is not associated with periarticular osteoporosis. The most characteristic involvement is in the distal interphalangeal (DIP) joints of the hands and toes, usually in association with psoriatic changes of the nails. At times the asymmetrical involvement is confined to a single digit, sometimes referred to as a "sausage digit," with involvement of both IP joints and at times the MCP joint of one digit of one hand. Ankylosis of the IP joints is also common (see Figs. 3-28 and 3-29). This is rarely encountered in the other rheumatoid variants or rheumatoid arthritis. Also characteristic is a peculiar destruction of the IP joints that results in widening of the joint space, with sharply demarcated bony margins. This is not found in other forms of arthritis. Periostitis with periosteal reaction is frequent in the small bones of the hand and on the plantar surface of the calcaneus, as in other rheumatoid variants. Resorption of the tufts of the terminal phalanges may occur. In advanced cases, bone resorption and destruction result in arthritis mutilans.

Sacroiliitis is common and resembles that seen in ankylosing spondylitis except that it is often asymmetrical (see Fig. 3-30).[29] Spondylitic changes are less common. The syndesmophytes in psoriatic spondylitis are typically broad, coarse, and asymmetrical (see Fig. 3-30). Vertebral squaring and apophyseal joint ankyloses are also less common than in ankylosing spondylitis.

Reiter's Syndrome

Reiter's syndrome is characterized by urethritis, conjunctivitis, and mucocutaneous lesions in the oro-

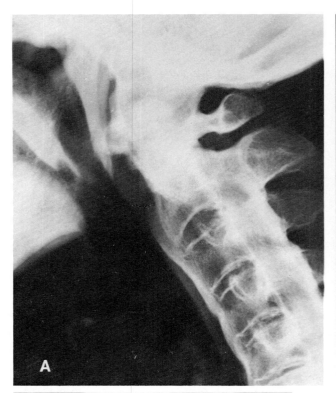

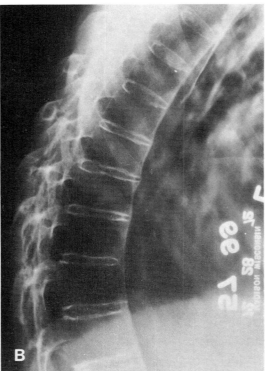

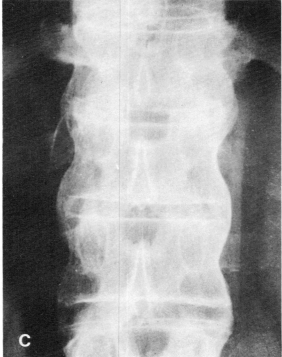

Figure 3–27. Ankylosing spondylitis. (**A**) Note the complete ankylosis of the apophyseal joints and dense ossification of the anterior spinal ligament. (**B**) Typical subligamentous ossification and syndesmophyte formation in the thoracic spine. (**C**) Similar changes, noted on this AP view of the lower thoracic and upper lumbar spine, are sometimes referred to as a "bamboo" spine.

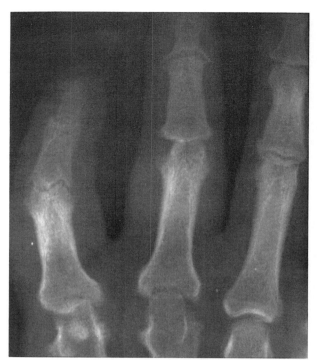

Figure 3–28. Psoriatic arthritis. There are erosions and fine periosteal new-bone formation at the margins of several joints. Note involvement of the distal IP joints of the index and middle fingers and bony ankylosis of the DIP joint of the index finger. The DIP joint of the middle finger appears somewhat widened.

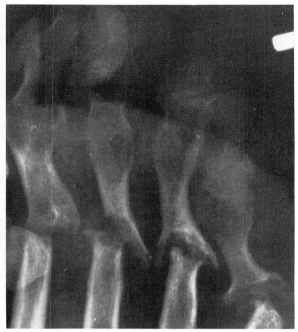

Figure 3–29. Psoriatic arthritis. There is a mutilating destruction of the MTP joints and ankylosis of the PIP joints.

pharynx, tongue, glans penis, and skin, as well as arthritis. This is probably a postinfectious syndrome following certain enteric or venereal infections. Arthritis occurs in 50% of sufferers. Joint involvement is frequently asymmetrical when comparing one side with the other. In general, the radiographic manifestations are similar to those of psoriatic arthritis, except that the axial skeleton is not as commonly involved and changes in the upper extremity are rare.[11, 22, 29] The major joint involvement is the lower extremities, particularly the feet (Figs. 3-1B and 3-31). The sacroiliac joint changes tend to be asymmetrical. Spinal involvement is much less common than in psoriatic arthritis. The most dramatic radiographic finding is usually periostitis, particularly the exuberant, fluffy, or whiskerlike periostitis at the site of tendon insertions, most frequently at the attachment of the plantar fascia, forming a poorly defined spur on the plantar surface of the calcaneus (see Fig. 3-31C). The destructive process may involve the IP, MTP, and tarsal joints. Involve-

ment of the ankle and knee is less common. Periosteal reaction is also found in metatarsal shafts (see Fig. 3-31B) and on the surfaces of the tarsal bones in the distal tibia and fibula. Periarticular osteoporosis is sometimes seen in contrast to other rheumatoid variants.

Colitic Arthritis

Arthritis occurs in approximately 10% of patients with chronic inflammatory bowel disease,[3] more commonly in ulcerative colitis than in Crohn's disease. The most common manifestation is sacroiliitis, similar to but not as extensive as ankylosing spondylitis and usually symmetrical.[29] Patients are rarely symptomatic, and the radiographic findings of sacroiliitis are often noted incidentally on abdominal radiographs obtained as part of a small bowel or colon examination (Fig. 3-32). Joint effusions and soft-tissue swelling are occasionally encountered in proximal major joints as a result of transient synovitis, but deforming arthritis is rare. The axial skeletal disease is not related to the activity of the underlying process. Peripheral arthritis, when present, tends to parallel the activity of the inflammatory bowel disease.

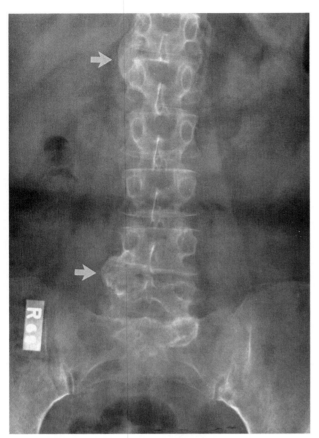

Figure 3–30. Psoriatic spondylitis and sacroiliac joint disease. Irregular destruction of both margins of the sacroiliac joints and slight widening of the joint space are evident. Note also the characteristic syndesmophytes (*arrows*), which are broad, coarse, and asymmetrical in this disease.

ARTHRITIS ASSOCIATED WITH CONNECTIVE TISSUE DISEASES

DERMATOMYOSITIS AND POLYMYOSITIS

The most characteristic radiographic finding in dermatomyositis and polymyositis is soft-tissue calcification in the subcutaneous tissues and fascial planes. Bone and joint changes are rare.[21] Severe flexion contractures occur in late stages of the disease, and osteoporosis secondary to disuse and steroid therapy is common.

SYSTEMIC LUPUS ERYTHEMATOSUS

Arthralgia is a very common complaint in systemic lupus erythematosus (SLE), but radiographic findings occur in only one-third of cases, usually nonspecific changes of soft-tissue atrophy and osteoporosis. The most characteristic radiologic finding is an abnormality of joint alignment without articular erosions.[6, 21] Involvement of the IP joints results in a "swan neck" deformity of the digit, consisting of extension of the PIP and flexion of the DIP joints. Involvement of the MCP joints and IP joint of the thumb leads to ulnar deviation of the digit. Many sufferers are able to correct their deformities voluntarily. Similar alignment abnormalities occur in patients with Jaccoud's arthritis. Avascular necrosis of bone is common but is more likely related to steroid treatment than to SLE itself.

SCLERODERMA

Scleroderma is commonly associated with characteristic roentgenographic changes in the hand. These include atrophy of soft tissue in the tips of the fingers giving them a tapered appearance, resorption of bone in the terminal tufts resulting in a pointed appearance of the phalanx (termed *acro-osteolysis*), and small punctate calcific deposits in the soft tissues, especially in the tips of the fingers (Fig. 3-33). These changes may be associated with a variable degree of osteoporosis. Joint-space narrowing occurs occasionally in the intercarpal and radiocarpal joints and, rarely, there is intra-articular calcification. A peculiar tendency to involve the first metacarpocarpal joint with extensive erosions and dislocation of the joint has been noted.[21, 29]

MIXED CONNECTIVE TISSUE DISEASE

Mixed connective tissue disease combines features of scleroderma, SLE, polymyositis, and rheumatoid arthritis. The radiographic findings are varied, consisting of diffuse and periarticular osteoporosis, soft-tissue swelling, erosive changes, narrow joint space, terminal tuft resorption, soft-tissue atrophy, and, occasionally, subluxations.[34] There is clinical variation ranging from no symptoms to features of scleroderma or rheumatoid arthritis.

JACCOUD'S ARTHROPATHY (CHRONIC POSTRHEUMATIC FEVER ARTHRITIS)

This is a migratory polyarthritis in which there is an insidious, painless onset of joint deformity after resolution of the active polyarthritis of acute rheumatic fever. Patients have rheumatic valvular heart disease. The joint deformities consist of ulnar deviation, flexion deformity, or subluxations of the MCP joints that are reducible early but later become fixed. The PIP joints are hyperextended. The toes may be involved with hallux valgus and subluxation of the great toe. Roent-

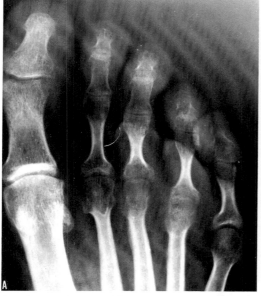

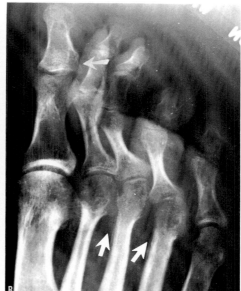

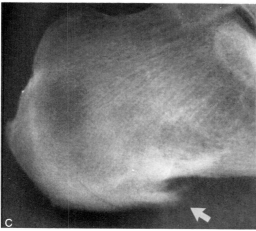

Figure 3–31. Reiter's syndrome. (**A** and **B**) Anterior and oblique views of the fore-foot. Note the periarticular osteoporosis and erosions of several of the MTP and IP joints. Fine periosteal new-bone formation is demonstrated on the distal margins of the third and fourth metatarsals (*arrows*). (**C**) A lateral view of the calcaneous demonstrates a typical fluffy, poorly defined, plantar spur (*arrow*), characteristic of this disorder.

genograms showing changes of severe deformity with minimal, if any, bone destruction should suggest the diagnosis in a patient with a history of rheumatic fever.

DEGENERATIVE JOINT DISEASE (OSTEOARTHRITIS)

Pathologically degenerative joint disease is characterized by degeneration and shredding of articular cartilage. It is not an inflammatory lesion, and therefore the term *arthritis* is a misnomer. Some authorities prefer the use of the term *osteoarthrosis*, which removes reference to inflammation.[2, 15] It is mainly a disease of older individuals, affecting IP joints of the fingers, particularly the DIP joints (see Fig. 3-1A) and the weight-bearing joints of the spine, hips, and knees. Degenerative joint disease occurs in two major forms, primary and secondary. The primary form may be a generalized disease affecting all of the aforementioned joints. The cause is unknown, but it appears to be the result of aging, the effects of wear and tear. The secondary form develops in joints disrupted by previous intra-articular trauma or other joint disease. It most commonly follows an intra-articular fracture or fracture-dislocation. In the hip, it may follow or complicate dysplasia of the acetabulum or Legg-Perthes disease or epiphysiolysis. The roentgen signs and pathologic changes are similar in the two forms. The primary form may be symmetrical, whereas the secondary form is

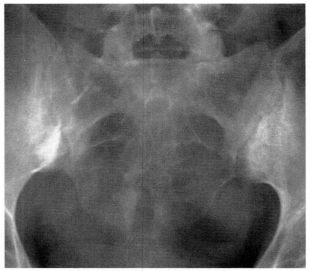

Figure 3–32. Colitic arthritis involving the sacro-iliac joints. The marginal erosions and sclerosis of the SI joints were an incidental finding on radiographs of the abdomen obtained for the evaluation of possible bowel obstruction in this patient with a long history of Crohn's disease.

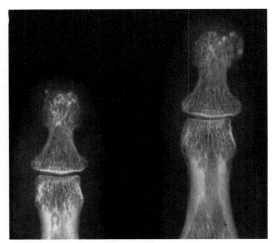

Figure 3–33. Scleroderma. There is minimal tapering of the distal soft tissues and punctate soft-tissue calcifications, changes characteristic of scleroderma.

limited to the joint or joints affected by either trauma or another primary disease process.

ROENTGENOGRAPHIC OBSERVATIONS

The principal radiographic features of osteoarthritis are asymmetrical joint-space narrowing, subchondral sclerosis of bone, marginal osteophytes, and subchondral cysts (Figs. 3-34 through 3-36).

Asymmetrical Joint-Space Narrowing

One of the principal characteristics of osteoarthritis is asymmetrical narrowing of the joint space. In contrast to that of rheumatoid arthritis, the narrowing of the joint space in osteoarthritis is almost invariably uneven and more pronounced in that portion of the joint where weight-bearing strains are greatest. In extreme cases, the cartilage may be completely destroyed and the articular ends of the bones then form the opposing surfaces of the joint. In general, the greater the degree of narrowing, the more severe the associated findings of subchondral sclerosis and spur formation.

Osteophyte Formation

One of the earliest changes is the development of small bony spurs or osteophytes on the apposing surfaces of bone at the peripheral margins of the joint. Osteo-

phytes in the spine may become particularly large (see Fig. 3-38).

Subchondral Sclerosis

Subchondral sclerosis or eburnation refers to the increase in density of the subchondral surface of bone. In weight-bearing bones, this is often extensive.

Subchondral Cysts

Subchondral cyst formation is much more pronounced in larger joints and is frequently more prominent on one side of the joint than on the other. The cysts extend to the articular surface and may communicate with the joint (see Fig. 3-34). In the superior margin of the acetabulum, they are commonly 1 cm or less in diameter but may reach a diameter of several centimeters in some cases. The cysts have a sclerotic border.

Loose Bodies

Calcified or ossified fragments of bone termed *loose bodies* may be identified within the joint but are particularly common in the knee. They represent calcified or ossified detached fragments of cartilage. In some instances, they may be formed by fragments of hypertrophied synovium.

OSTEOARTHRITIS OF SPECIFIC JOINTS
The Fingers

Primary osteoarthritis principally involves the DIP joints of the fingers and the first metacarpocarpal joint

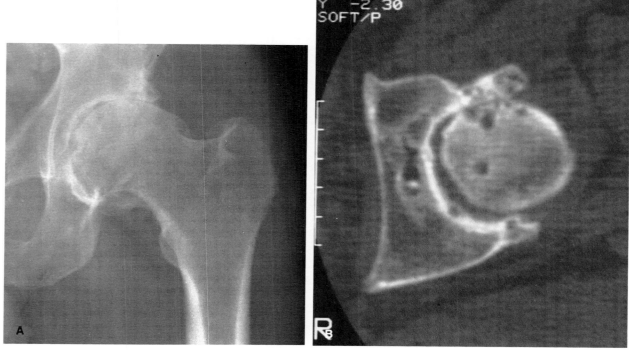

Figure 3–34. Osteoarthritis of the hip. (**A**) Characteristic joint changes consist of asymmetrical narrowing of the joint space, marginal spurs, subchondral sclerosis, and subchondral cyst formation. (**B**) CT scan more clearly identifies the subchondral cyst formation and the marginal spurs anterior and posterior rims of the acetabulum. Note also the subchondral sclerosis and asymmetrical joint space narrowing.

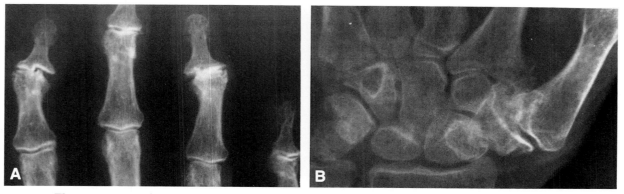

Figure 3–35. Osteoarthritis of the hands. (**A**) Characteristic changes of the DIP joints consisting of asymmetrical narrowing, subchondral sclerosis, and marginal spur formation, with minimal subluxation. Note the relative sparing of the PIP joint. (**B**) Osteoarthritis of the first metacarpocarpal joint. Notice the subluxation, subchondral sclerosis, and spur formation.

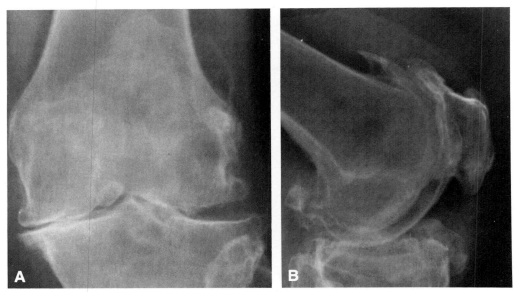

Figure 3–36. Osteoarthritis of the knee. **(A)** The medial compartment is narrowed, with marginal spur formation. A genu varum ("bowleg") deformity of the knee is present. **(B)** Lateral view demonstrates prominent spur formation of the patellofemoral joint and posteior margin of the femoral condyles. The joint space is narrowed, with subchondral sclerosis.

of the thumb (see Fig. 3-35). The PIP joints may also be involved, but never as severely as the DIP joints. The early findings consist of asymmetrical joint-space narrowing, with small, marginal osteophytes. These enlarge gradually to form well-defined, bony protuberances that cause an irregular, visible, and palpable knobby thickening known as Heberden's nodes, the most significant clinical diagnostic feature of the disease. The largest spurs form on the dorsal edges of the terminal phalanx and are best demonstrated on the lateral view. Eventually the joint surfaces become irregular and minimally malaligned, but the bony eburnation is never pronounced. The first metacarpocarpal joint at the base of the thumb is characteristically narrowed, with subchondral sclerosis and spur formation, with or without subluxation of the joint. In some cases, the changes are more severe here than in the DIP joints. The scaphotrapezoid joint is involved, in some cases, with or without involvement of the first metacarpocarpal joint.

Erosive Osteoarthritis. Erosive osteoarthritis is an inflammatory form of osteoarthritis occurring in postmenopausal women. It is usually limited to the IP joints of the hand. Clinically the joints are acutely inflamed, and marginal erosions are prominent and are superimposed on the standard radiographic features of

osteoarthritis. Erosions are often more pronounced at the PIP joints. The radiographic appearance may resemble rheumatoid arthritis at any given joint, but involvement of the DIP joints is very uncommon in rheumatoid arthritis and allows a distinction between the two processes.[24] The involved joints may eventually undergo bony ankylosis, which rarely occurs in the more common form of primary osteoarthritis. This must be distinguished from ankylosis occurring in the IP joints in psoriatic arthritis.

The Hip

The early and classic signs of osteoarthritis of the hip are superior joint-space narrowing, subchondral sclerosis of bone, and marginal spur formation (see Fig. 3-34). In contrast to rheumatoid arthritis, the decrease in the joint space in degenerative disease of the hip is characterized by its asymmetry, and because of weight-bearing it is confined to the superior portion of the joint in most cases. The joint space may eventually be completely obliterated. In far-advanced cases, the femoral head appears flattened and the hip is subluxated superiorly and laterally. As the femoral head migrates, the acetabulum is enlarged and bone is laid down around the medial and inferior margins of the femoral head. The medial cortex of the femoral neck is thickened.

The apposing joint surfaces become markedly eburnated. A prominent osteophyte forms on the superolateral margin of the acetabulum, and a smaller spur rims the entire femoral head but is best seen in profile on its medial and lateral margins. Subchondral cysts develop on both margins of the joint and may be quite large on the acetabular side of the joint. Less commonly, the hip migrates medially or in an axial direction and may form an acetabular protrusio in some cases.[29]

The Knee

Degenerative joint disease is the most common type of arthritis encountered in the knee. This may be secondary to previous trauma, particularly to some combination of the menisci and cruciate and collateral ligaments. The earliest sign is narrowing of the medial compartment of the joint (see Fig. 3-36). This is followed by subchondral sclerosis of the apposing margins of this compartment, the medial femoral condyle and medial tibial plateau. Marginal spur formation occurs on the medial margin of the joint. Spur formation may also occur on the tibial spine. Characteristically the lateral compartment composed of the lateral femoral condyle and lateral tibial plateau is not involved, and the lateral joint space remains normal. The patellofemoral surface of the joint is frequently involved to a variable degree. Changes in the patellofemoral compartment are visualized on the lateral radiograph and are manifested by narrowing of the joint space and marginal spur formation on the superior and inferior joint margins of the patella.

Eventually a varus or "bowleg" deformity develops. The medial compartment narrowing and the varus deformity may be better visualized on anteroposterior radiographs obtained with the patient standing or bearing weight.

Joint effusions are frequent. The fluid is demonstrated in the suprapatellar bursa, seen on the lateral radiograph anterior to the distal femoral shaft just proximal to the patella. Subchondral cysts are infrequent. Loose bodies are a common feature of the disease in this joint.

The Shoulder

Degenerative arthritis is a common occurrence in elderly patients, particularly in association with tears of the rotator cuff. Few patients seem to be overtly symptomatic since most cases are encountered as incidental findings on chest radiographs. The characteristic findings are superior displacement of the humeral head such that it articulates with the inferior surface of the acromion, subchondral sclerosis, glenohumeral joint-

space narrowing, and marginal spur formation on the humeral head (Fig. 3-37). When combined with periarticular calcification, the condition has been referred to as the *Milwaukee shoulder*.[25]

The Spine

An almost universal finding in patients beyond middle age is hypertrophic spur formation along the anterior and lateral margins of the vertebral bodies (Fig. 3-38). This is the most common manifestation of degenerative arthritis or osteoarthritis (osteoarthrosis) of the spine. These marginal osteophytes are particularly prone to develop in the lower cervical and lower lumbar spine. In addition to the spurs, small calcific or bony deposits may form in the spinal ligaments or in the anterior margin of the annulus fibrosis, with or without attachments to the adjacent vertebra. In all but the most mild forms of the disease, some degree of thinning of the

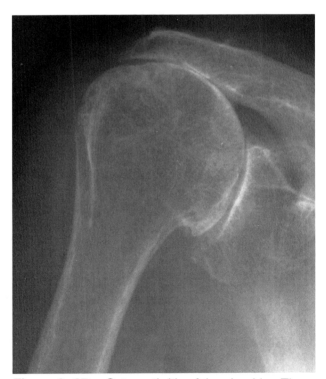

Figure 3–37. Osteoarthritis of the shoulder. There is superior migration of the humeral head that articulates with the undersurface of the acromion. The glenohumeral joint is asymmetrically narrowed. There is slight subchondral sclerosis and marginal spur formation in the inferior aspect of the humeral head. The superior migration of the humeral head implies a tear of the rotator cuff.

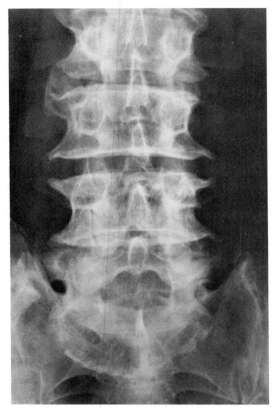

Figure 3–38. Degenerative joint disease of the spine manifested by marginal osteophytes of the vertebral bodies.

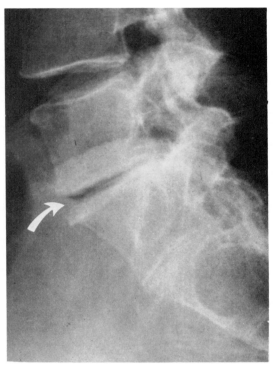

Figure 3–39. Degenerative disc disease of the lumbar spine. The L-5, S-1 interspace is markedly narrowed, with subchondral sclerosis of bone and marginal spur formation. Note the vacuum disc manifested by a thin, dark translucency within the disc space (*arrow*).

intervertebral disc space is present, particularly in the lower cervical and lower lumbar spine and commonly involving the lumbosacral joint. The narrowing of the disc space is usually uniform (Figs. 3-39 and 3-40). Occasionally a thin, waferlike translucent space is visualized within one or more discs severely involved by degenerative disease (Fig. 3-39). This is called the "phantom disc" or "vacuum phenomenon" (see later discussion). In scoliosis, osteophytic spurs and disc-space narrowing are more severe along the concave side of the curvature.

The apophyseal joints may or may not be involved in the process. When they are involved, the changes consist of thinning of the joint space, marginal spur formation, and bony hypertrophy. These changes are best identified on axial CT examinations. Subluxation of the vertebra may occur as a result of severe degenerative changes in facet joints. With facet joint disease, the uppermost vertebra slips forward on the vertebra below. This is referred to as a *spondylolisthesis*, and it is a common manifestation of degenerative disease in the

spine. Spondylolisthesis more commonly occurs in the lumbar spine but may occur on occasion in the cervical spine as well (see Fig. 3-40A). Retrolisthesis, posterior displacement of the vertebra above, relative to the vertebra below, may occur in association with severe disc narrowing. This is usually minimal, amounting to no more than 2 or 3 mm.

In the cervical spine, spurs on the posterior margin of the vertebra may be of sufficient size to compress the spinal cord or nerve roots and give rise to neurologic symptoms. Spur formation at the joint of Luschka or oncovertebral joint may give rise to nerve root symptoms (see Fig. 3-40B). This joint is located in the posterolateral margin of the intervertebral disc, and the spurs extend into the adjacent intervertebral foramen, impinging on the exiting nerve root. These changes are best visualized in oblique radiographs of the cervical spine.

Vacuum Phenomena. Under certain circumstances, a radiographic examination of a joint reveals a thin,

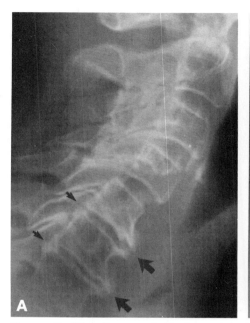 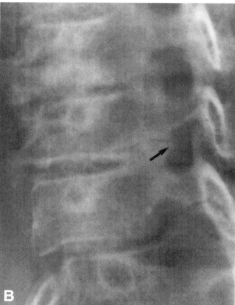

Figure 3–40. Osteoarthritis (spondylosis) of the cervical spine. **(A)** Degenerative arthritis of the cervical spine. The C5–C6 and C6–C7 interspaces are narrowed, with subchondral sclerosis of bone and marginal spur formation both anteriorly and posteriorly (*arrows*). There is also very minimal anterior subluxation or spondylolisthesis of C4 on C5 secondary to the degenerative disease within the facet joints. Note the narrowing and subchondral sclerosis of the upper cervical facet joints. **(B)** Oblique view of the cervical spine demonstrates osteophytic spur formation at the joint of Luschka or oncovertebral joints at C6–C7 (*arrow*), with encroachment on the adjacent intervertebral foramen.

translucent dark line or space between the articular cartilages (see Figs. 3-39 and 3-57). This most commonly occurs in the lumbar spine in association with severe degenerative disease of one or more intervertebral discs. This has been called a phantom or vacuum disc. A similar appearance has been noted in the symphysis pubis of women during pregnancy. On other occasions, the vacuum phenomenon is produced by traction of the joint. This is most frequently seen in the shoulder and is particularly common in chest radiographs of children. It is not entirely clear whether this space represents a vacuum or whether it is filled with the gas liberated from the blood and surrounding tissues. Most consider this to be nitrogen gas.

Traumatic Arthritis

The term *traumatic arthritis* should be reserved to designate that form of secondary degenerative joint disease initiated by trauma, either as a single episode or as the result of repeated injuries. Traumatic arthritis

may develop following a dislocation or fracture that extended into the joint, or it may follow a severe sprain or recurrent injuries to the supporting structures of the joint. In general, the roentgenographic findings are similar to degenerative joint disease or osteoarthritis, the difference being that the arthritic process is limited to a single joint previously affected by trauma. Because the diagnosis of traumatic arthritis may have medicolegal implications, it is not wise to use this term unless it can be established with reasonable certainty that the joint was normal prior to trauma.

DIFFUSE IDIOPATHIC SKELETAL HYPEROSTOSIS (DISH, FORESTIER DISEASE)

Diffuse idiopathic skeletal hyperostosis (DISH) is a disease of older individuals characterized by extensive hyperostosis or massive ossification of the paraspinal ligaments anteriorly and laterally, bridging the inter-

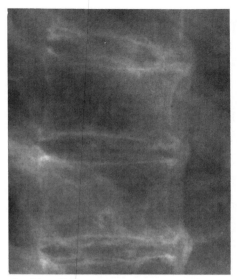

Figure 3–41. Diffuse idiopathic skeletal hyperostosis of the lower thoracic spine. Note the typical ossification of the anterior longitudinal ligament applied to the anterior surface of the vertebral bodies. The underlying anterior cortex of the vertebra can still be distinguished. Minimal spurs are present on the anterior margins of the vertebra, beneath the ligamentous ossification.

vening disc spaces (Fig. 3-41). It tends to be more pronounced in the lower cervical and thoracic spine than elsewhere. Minor expressions of this disorder are common, usually identified in the middorsal spine on lateral radiographs of the chest. Bony bridging may be continuous or discontinuous. The anterior cortex of the vertebral body can be visualized within the ossification. Skeletal hyperostosis is also characterized by the tendency to ossify the ligaments or tendon insertions, to form entheses elsewhere in the body.[30] They appear as a regular outgrowth or whiskering of the iliac crest; the ischial tuberosites; the greater trochanters; and the margins of the acetabulum, sacroiliac joint, and symphysis pubis.[29] They also may be seen about the patella and the posterior and plantar surface of the os calcis. Ossification may occur in the iliolumbar and sacrotuberous ligaments and, in fact, in any muscular ligamentous attachment to bone.

The radiographic appearance bears a superficial resemblance to ankylosing spondylitis. The appearance of the spinal ossification is very irregular and unlike that of the thin, vertical syndesmophytes seen in ankylosing spondylitis.[29] The relative absence of changes in the lumbosacral spine and the absence of changes in the sacroiliac joint should differentiate DISH from an-

kylosing spondylitis. DISH is seen in older individuals of both sexes, whereas ankylosing spondylitis is characteristically a disease of young males.

NEUROTROPHIC ARTHROPATHY

Tabes dorsalis, syringomyelia, diabetic neuropathy, leprosy, transsection of the spinal cord, and peripheral nerve injury impair the sensation of joints, rendering them susceptible to repeated trauma that may lead to severe disorganization of the joint. The resulting arthropathy is known as a Charcot's joint. The weight-bearing joints of the lower extremities are the most frequently affected in tabes dorsalis. Less commonly there is involvement of the lower lumbar spine. Neuropathic arthropathy in the upper extremities is much less common but when encountered is usually due to syringomyelia. The identification of characteristic changes of a neuropathic joint in an upper extremity should suggest this diagnosis (Fig. 3-42). Diabetic neuropathic joints occur in the feet and ankles.

Pathologically, the source of the arthropathy appears to be repeated infractions, often of a minor degree but eventually resulting in fragmentation of the articular cartilages and the apposing margin of bone. Hemorrhage occurs into the joint and surrounding soft tissues.

The principal radiographic features of neuropathic arthropathy are soft-tissue swelling, bone fragmentation, and sclerosis of bone at the margins of the joint (see Fig. 3-42).[7, 11] In the early stages, the roentgenographic findings are usually limited to soft-tissue swelling due to joint effusions. The apposing margins of bone may become eburnated and fragmented. These changes are followed by a general breakdown of the joint structures, eventually resulting in considerable disorganization (Figs. 3-42 and 3-43). The progress may be very rapid (see Fig. 3-42). Multiple ossific fragments are found in and about the joint and in some instances are very quickly reabsorbed. The fragments may be so small that they suggest soft-tissue calcification. The debris may break through and extend out of the joint capsule by dissecting along fascial planes. Subluxation is frequent and may occur early. The rapidity of development of these changes is variable, but in some cases relatively advanced disease may occur within 1 to 6 weeks after roentgenograms have demonstrated a normal joint. In the spine, the vertebral bodies develop a marked increase in density and tend to undergo some degree of compression and fragmentation as well as alterations in alignment. Thinning or disappearance of the intervertebral disc accompanies these changes.

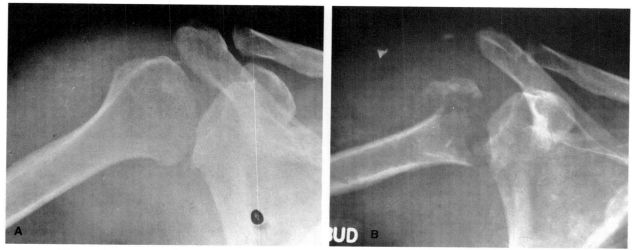

Figure 3–42. Neurotrophic arthropathy of the shoulder secondary to syringomyelia. **(A)** There is disintegration of the joint. Note the numerous small fragments of bone within both the joint and the soft tissues lateral to the humeral head. The humeral head is flattened and the joint is subluxated inferiorly. **(B)** Repeat examination 1 week later demonstrates complete disintegration of the humeral head with multiple fragments of bone in and about the shoulder joint. The bony fragments are more widely dispersed than on the previous examination. Rapid dissolution of the joint may occur in neuropathic arthropathies. (Case courtesy of Jerome Wiot, M.D., Cincinnati)

DIABETIC OSTEOARTHROPATHY

Diabetic osteoarthropathy differs somewhat from the other neurotrophic arthropathies. It is confined almost exclusively to the ankle and foot (see Fig. 3-43), rarely involving the hands, femur, and tibia. The principal radiographic features are fractures and dislocations, fragmentation, sclerosis, osteolysis, and periosteal reaction.[8] Calcification of the smaller arteries of the foot is a frequent and important clue to the presence of underlying diabetes but may not always be evident. At times, destructive changes are extensive, leading to absorption of the distal ends of the metatarsals with pencil-point narrowing and arthritis mutilans. The role of infection in the destructive process is not clear, but the two processes may coexist in some instances. This is discussed in Osteomyelites in the Diabetic Foot in Chapter 5, Infections and Inflammations of Bones.

Fractures or fracture-dislocations of the tarsals or metatarsals are particularly common manifestations of diabetic neuropathic joints (see Figs. 3-1*B* and 3-43*B*). Often such fractures or dislocations are incidental findings on radiographs obtained for the evaluation of infections of the foot or complaints of swelling without a history of trauma. Less commonly, the neuropathic process appears to be initiated by a traumatic event that

results in a fracture or dislocation. The subsequent radiographs may demonstrate the absence of normal healing, extensive fragmentation, sclerosis, and the other changes associated with neuropathic joint disease.

METABOLIC JOINT DISEASE

GOUT

Gout is a metabolic abnormality of unknown etiology, predominately affecting males. It is characterized by intermittent acute attacks of arthritis, an increase in the serum uric acid, and deposition of sodium urate in joints, bones, and periarticular tissues. Irregular, superficial, soft-tissue masses of varying size eventually appear. Known as tophi, they represent accumulations of monosodium urate monohydrate crystals. The tophaceous deposits occur in articular cartilages and tendinous and capsular insertions about the joint and in bones adjacent to the joint. As they enlarge, they create localized, punched-out defects at the margins of the joints and in the ends of the bone.

Classically, the first MTP joint is the joint most often affected (see Fig. 3-1*B*). The clinical expression of the disease in this location is known as *podagra*. Other

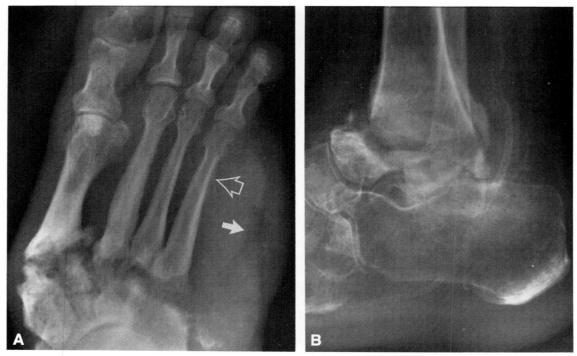

Figure 3–43. Diabetic neuroarthropathy. (**A**) Note the disorganized fragmentation and sclerosis about the metatarsotarsal joints. The fifth toe and metatarsal have been amputated. Soft-tissue swelling is present, with a radiolucency within it, indicating the presence of an ulcer in the soft tissues (*solid arrow*). Periosteal new-bone formation is also identified along the distal lateral margin of the fourth metatarsal (*open arrow*). (**B**) The ankle joint is practically completely destroyed. Note the marked and almost complete destruction of the talus, subchondral sclerosis of bone, fragmentation, and periosteal new-bone formation about the distal tibia. There is calcification of the posterior tibial artery, characteristic of diabetes.

joints of the feet are often affected. The hands (see Fig. 3-1A), wrists, elbows, ankles, knees, and even the spine may be involved. Involvement of the metatarsotarsal and metacarpocarpal joints is frequent. Joint involvement is characteristically asymmetrical, both within any given joint and when comparing joints on both sides of the body.

Radiographic findings of gout do not occur until the disease has been present for as much as 6 to 8 years. Thus, a negative roentgenogram does not rule out the possibility of gout. The principal radiographic features[5] of the disease are periarticular marginal erosions, asymmetrical periarticular soft-tissue masses with or without calcification, preservation of the joint space, and an absence of osteoporosis (Fig. 3-44).

The margins of the erosion are characteristically rather sharply defined, are of variable size, are asymmetrical, and are often defined by a sclerotic margin with an overhanging edge or hook of bone at their periphery. When the deposit is entirely within bone, it may have the appearance of a cyst. When the deposit is at the margin of the joint, there is a minimal periosteal reaction, which forms a characteristic hook or spurlike projection of cortical bone at the peripheral margin of the erosion.

The soft-tissue masses, or tophi, are characteristically asymmetrical and often contain flecks of calcification. These soft-tissue masses appear at the margins of the joints of the foot and hand and in bursae, particularly the olecranon bursa, where they may be associated with underlying erosion of the olecranon.

Characteristically, the bones maintain a normal density without evidence of osteoporosis. Disuse osteoporosis does not develop, because the joints are relatively free of symptoms between acute exacerbations.

The joint space is often well maintained despite the presence of sizable erosions. Because of the deposition of urate deposits within the articular cartilage, eventually there is some thinning or degeneration of the articular cartilage, resulting in narrowing of the joint

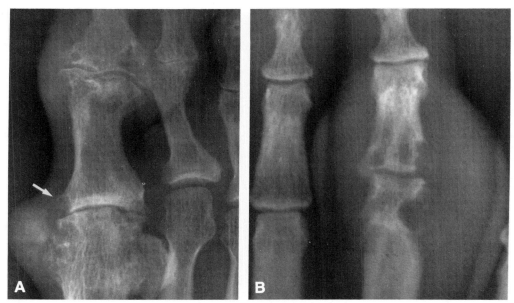

Figure 3–44. **(A)** Gout. Asymmetrical soft-tissue masses containing calcification are identified at the peripheral margins of both the MTP and IP joints of the great toe. These are typical of gout. Erosions are present at the margins of the involved joints. Note the typical overhanging edge at the base of the proximal phalanx (*arrow*). Associated degenerative arthritic changes are present in the MTP joint, but the IP joint space is preserved. Note also the absence of osteoporosis. **(B)** Gout of the PIP joint of the middle finger. There is a large, asymmetrical soft-tissue mass. Erosions are present at the margins of the joint, but the joint space is well preserved. The margins of the erosions are slightly sclerotic and have overhanging margins. This was a monoarticular process. The remaining joints in the hand are normal.

space. However, this does not occur early nor is it particularly severe.

The diagnosis of gouty arthritis is largely clinical in the early stages of the disease. When far advanced, it may be radiographically confused with rheumatoid arthritis because of marginal erosions and soft-tissue swelling. The difference in distribution of the marginal erosions and the appearance of the soft-tissue swelling is the key to the differential diagnosis. Characteristically, in rheumatoid arthritis there is periarticular osteoporosis and symmetrical involvement of the PIP, MCP, and radiocarpal joints, and the soft-tissue swelling about the joints is symmetrical. In contrast, gouty arthritis initially involves the feet, specifically the MTP or IP joints of the great toe, tophaceous deposits appear as asymmetrical soft-tissue masses, and there is no evidence of osteoporosis.

CHONDROCALCINOSIS

Chondrocalcinosis is a descriptive term designating the presence of intra-articular calcium-containing salts within hyaline and fibrocartilage. It is a generic term,

not a specific diagnosis. Calcium within the fibrocartilage is characteristically somewhat irregular, as seen in the menisci of the knee (Fig. 3-45) or the triangular fibrocartilage of the wrist (Fig. 3-46). The articular surface is composed of hyaline cartilage and, when calcified, appears as a fine, linear radiodensity closely paralleling the bony margins of the joint. Chondrocalcinosis is most commonly encountered in and characteristic of calcium pyrophosphate dihydrate deposition disease (CPPD), or pseudogout, but also occurs in hyperparathyroidism, hemochromatosis, ochronosis, Wilson's disease, and occasionally gout and degenerative arthritis.[29]

CALCIUM PYROPHOSPHATE DISEASE (CPPD, PSEUDOGOUT)

Deposition of calcium pyrophosphate dihydrate crystals in the joint cartilage and periarticular tissues occurs in elderly individuals, usually manifested in the sixth and seventh decades by the radiographic demonstration of chondrocalcinosis, calcifications in the fibrocartilage, and hyaline cartilage of the knees and wrists.

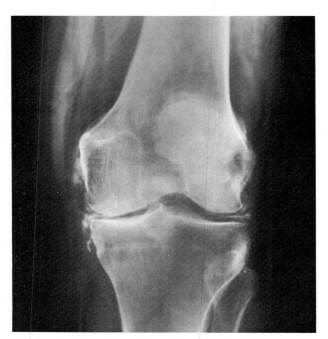

Figure 3–45. Chondrocalcinosis of the knee. Note the extensive calcification of the menisci.

Many afflicted persons are asymptomatic, but in others a spectrum of clinical presentations may be encountered.[29] These include (1) intermittent acute attacks of arthritic pain associated with a joint effusion resulting from an acute synovitis caused by the presence of crystals within the joints, (2) continuous acute attacks of arthritic pain, (3) progressive chronic arthritic pain with acute exacerbations, and (4) progressive chronic pain without acute episodes. The acute disease predominates in men and the chronic in women. Acute attacks and superimposed degenerative changes may occur without radiographically visible calcification in the joint cartilage. The correct diagnosis is established by the identification of typical calcium pyrophosphate crystals in the synovial fluid.

The most commonly involved joints are the knee, the radiocarpal joints of the wrist, the MCP joints of the hand, the shoulder, and the hip.

Chondrocalcinosis characteristically appears in the triangular ligament of the wrist (see Fig. 3-46A), the menisci of the knee, the symphysis pubis (see Fig. 3-46B), and the hyaline cartilage of the hip joint and shoulder.[16] Calcification may also appear in the periarticular tendons and bursa. Linear calcification may also occur in the capsules of the small joints of the hand.

Eventually, the changes of secondary osteoarthritis appear. These include narrowing of the joint, subchondral sclerosis of bones, subchondral cysts, and marginal spur formation. Involvement of the MCP joints, particularly the second and third MCP joints, is characteristic of this disorder (see Fig. 3-1A).[29] The radiographic findings include narrowing of the joint, subchondral sclerosis of bone, and peculiar broadbased osteophytes arising on the margins of the heads of the metacarpals. Hemochromatosis also affects these joints in a similar fashion. Primary osteoarthritis is uncommon in those joints frequently involved in CPPD. Therefore, the possibility of CPPD must be considered whenever the radiographic changes of de-

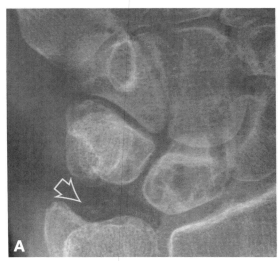

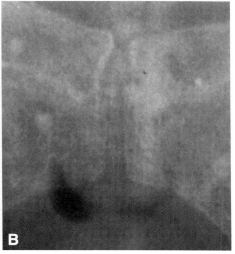

Figure 3–46. Calcium pyrophosphate disease (CPPD, pseudogout). **(A)** Typical calcification in the triangular cartilage (*arrow*). There is also a cyst within the lunate. **(B)** Chondrocalcinosis involves fibrocartilage of the symphysis pubis.

generative arthritis are encountered in unusual locations such as the radiocarpal (see Fig. 3-1A),[29] shoulder, elbow, or patellofemoral joint.

Subchondral cyst formation is occasionally so severe that it leads to bony collapse and fragmentation, with loose-body formation. These changes are more commonly seen in the hip and may be so severe as to resemble neuropathic arthropathy.[17]

HEMOCHROMATOSIS

Hemochromatosis is characterized by signs of cirrhosis, diabetes, and brown pigmentation of the skin. The disease is frequently associated with an arthropathy, which may antedate the other signs of disease. The joint involvement is very similar if not identical to that encountered in CPPD.[29, 33] Osteopenia is characteristic. Chondrocalcinosis is common, particularly in the knees and wrists, and is due to the deposition of calcium pyrophosphate.

HYPERPARATHYROIDISM

Primary and secondary hyperparathyroidism is sometimes accompanied by radiographic manifestations of arthritis in addition to the characteristic subperiosteal resorption of the radial aspect of the phalanges and erosive changes in the ungual tufts. These include chondrocalcinosis and capsular calcifications similar to those noted in CPPD, together with subchondral erosion of bone in the sacroiliac, sternoclavicular, and acromioclavicular joints; in the symphysis pubis and discovertebral junctions; and to a lesser extent in the MCP joints of the hand.[11, 29] Spontaneous ruptures or avulsions of tendons may occur, usually involving the quadriceps and infrapatellar tendons.

OCHRONOSIS

Ochronosis is a rare disorder of metabolism in which there is an abnormal accumulation of homogentisic acid in the blood and urine owing to a lack of homogentisic oxidase. It usually goes unrecognized until the fourth or fifth decade of life, when arthropathy appears. The urine is either very dark on voiding or becomes black after standing or after it is alkalized. The deposition of homogentisic acid results in degeneration of the articular cartilages. The most significant roentgenographic observation is the extensive calcification of the intervertebral discs, especially in the thoracolumbar region.[11, 29] Extensive calcification of multiple intervertebral discs should arouse the suspicion of ochronosis. In addition, the intervertebral disc degenerates and the disc space becomes quite thin, often accompanied by a vacuum phenomenon. Subchondral sclerosis occurs in the vertebral end-plates, but characteristically

spur formation is minimal despite the marked thinning of the disc. Calcifications, subchondral destruction, and fusion of the symphysis pubis may be seen. Destructive changes are also encountered in the knee, shoulders, and hips but are rare in the more peripheral joints. This destructive process may be quite rapid and characteristically occurs in the shoulders.

WILSON'S DISEASE (HEPATOLENTICULAR DEGENERATION)

Wilson's disease is an autosomal recessive disorder that is characterized by retention of excess amounts of copper. Osteoporosis or demineralization occurs in about 50% of sufferers. Bone and joint involvement is otherwise unusual. Joint manifestations include subarticular cysts and fragmentation of subchondral bones, chiefly in the hands, feet, wrists, and ankles.[11, 29] The fragments are small and resemble accessory ossifications. The cysts are small and occur mainly in the small joints of the hands, wrists, feet, and ankles. Other findings include osteochondritis dissecans, irregularity of the vertebral end-plates, squaring of the vertebral bodies, and vertebral body wedging. Periarticular calcification may occur at the insertion of tendons and ligaments. The earliest articular changes usually take place in the MCP joints, especially the second and third, manifested by joint-space narrowing, small subchondral cysts, and broad-based osteophyte formation—all findings quite similar to those seen in idiopathic chondrocalcinosis or CPPD. Cyst formation, erosions, and osteophytes may also occur in the carpal joint and less commonly elsewhere. A generalized osteopenia may be seen.

PRIMARY SYNOVIAL DISEASE

PIGMENTED VILLONODULAR SYNOVITIS

Pigmented villonodular synovitis is a disease of unknown etiology occurring in young adults and characterized by villous and nodular hyperplasia of the synovium either in joints or in tendon sheaths. It is monoarticular, involving the knee in 80% of cases. Other joints affected, in decreasing order of frequency, are the hip, ankle, small joints of the hands and feet, shoulder, and elbow.[9] The clinical complaint is pain. Joint aspirates are characteristically serosanguineous. Soft-tissue swelling is the most common radiographic finding, manifested in the knee by distention of the suprapatellar bursa. Osteoporosis is not a feature of this disease, and the joint space is maintained. Sharply marginated cortical and subchondral erosions occur in the majority of cases in joints with tight capsules such as the hip[12, 13, 29] (see Fig. 3-47A) but are relatively uncommon in the knee (less than 25%). CT may dem-

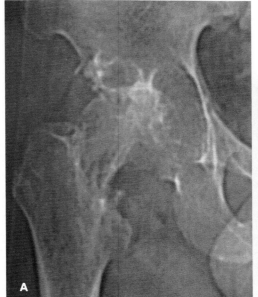

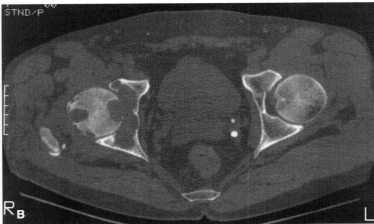

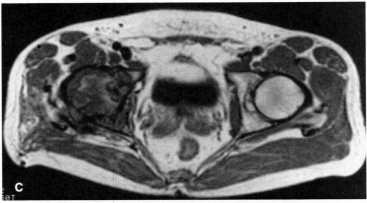

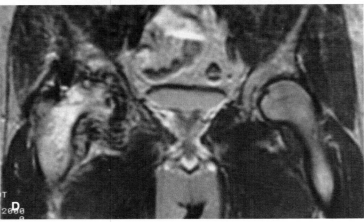

Figure 3–47. Pigmented villonodular synovitis (PVNS). (**A**) AP digital radiograph demonstrates marked erosions of both the acetabulum and femoral neck and head. Most erosions have a fine sclerotic rim. There is no evidence of osteoporosis. (**B**) CT scan confirms the presence of erosions with a fine sclerotic rim. The joint space apears normal. The joint itself is distended. (**C**) T1-weighted MRI demonstrates marginal sclerosis with variable areas of low signal filling and distending the joint space. (**D**) Coronal T2-weighted image demonstrates variable low signal of the masses filling the joint space. The findings of low signal on both T1 and T2 are due to hemosiderin deposition within the hypertrophied synovial villi and are characteristic of PVNS.

onstrate both erosions and nodular soft-tissue masses within the joint (Fig. 3-47*B*). MRI is an elegant means of establishing the diagnosis.[19] The synovial proliferations characteristically are of low to medium signal on both T1- and T2-weighted images (Fig. 3-47*C, D*) owing to the hemosiderin content. In contrast, other synovial diseases are of high signal on T2, with the single exception of synovial osteochondromatosis, which is also hypointense but easily distinguished in most cases by the characteristic calcification of loose bodies on plain films, a finding counter to the diagnosis of pigmented villonodular synovitis.

SYNOVIAL CHONDROMATOSIS (OSTEOCHONDROMATOSIS)

Synovial chondromatosis is a rare disorder of the joint, tendon sheath, or bursa and is characterized by proliferation of synovial villi and cartilage formed by chondrometaplasia of the subsynovial connective tissue.[13, 29] These masses may become detached and lie free within the joint, forming loose bodies. In larger joints they measure approximately 1 cm in diameter but are smaller in smaller joints. The disease is encountered most frequently in the knee and elbow and occasionally in the shoulder and small peripheral joints. Calcification or ossification of the masses is common,

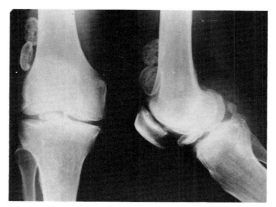

Figure 3–48. Osteochondromatosis of the knee. There are typical laminated, calcific densities within the suprapatellar bursa and both anteriorly and posteriorly within the joint space.

characteristically having a laminated appearance (Figs. 3-48 and 3-49). Usually there are multiple bodies, but at times only a few or less commonly one or two are present. Often there is an associated joint effusion, and degenerative arthritis may occur. The loose bodies may cause pressure erosions of the bone at the margins of

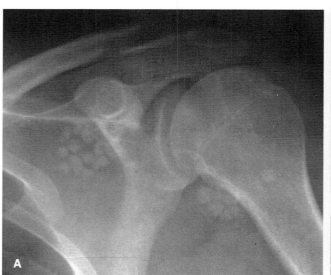
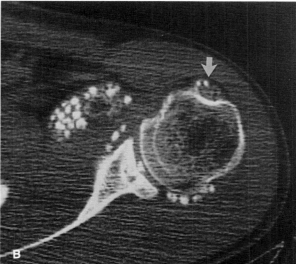

Figure 3–49. Synovial osteochondromatosis of the shoulder. (**A**) AP view of the shoulder demonstrates numerous irregular ossific radiodensities inferior to the coracoid process lying within the axillary pouch of the joint space. Other similar densities lie inferior to the medial aspect of the humeral head. (**B**) CT scan in a second case demonstrates irregular ossific radiodensities in and about the shoulder joint. Note also that a few densities lie within the tendon sheath of the long head of the biceps muscle (*arrow*). (Case courtesy of Col. David K. Shelton, M.C., Travis Air Force Base, California)

the joint.[27] In a third of cases, there is no calcification and the diagnosis may be established by arthrography or MRI, which demonstrates the hypertrophied villi as irregular masses within the joint.

LOOSE BODIES

Intra-articular loose bodies may arise from multiple causes. Among these are (1) synovial chondromatosis, as previously mentioned, (2) degenerative joint disease, (3) osteochondral fracture, an intra-articular fracture with separation of a fragment of cartilage with or without underlying bone, (4) fragmentation of the meniscal cartilage in the knee, and (5) osteochondritis dissecans. Injuries account for the majority of loose bodies and occur most frequently in the knee. If composed only of cartilage, the fragment cannot be visualized on a roentgenogram but may be seen on an arthrogram or by MRI. Cartilaginous bodies become radiopaque as they calcify and then are easily visualized. The appearance of a loose body on MRI is variable (see Figure 3-55A). If composed purely of cartilage, the loose body has the same signal intensity as joint fluid on T1-weighted images but is of lower signal than joint fluid on T2. If composed of cortical bone or calcified, it is of low signal on both T1 and T2, and if composed of intramedullary bone, it has a signal similar to that of fat, with a higher signal on T1 than T2. Most have mixed characteristics. Calcified loose bodies are formed in degenerative joint disease as a result of fragmentation of the articular cartilage. Joint bodies are also seen in neuropathic joints.

TRANSIENT SYNOVITIS OF THE HIP

Transient synovitis of the hip characteristically occurs in children under the age of 10. The principal clinical manifestations are pain and limping. The thigh is held in flexion. The disease is self-limited and leaves no sequelae. A joint effusion may be evident, manifested by widening of the joint space.[14] A secondary synovitis occurs in association with intra-articular osteoid osteomas. In this situation, the pain is long-standing, joint contractures may be present, and periarticular osteoporosis and joint effusion are common (see Osteoid Osteoma, Chapter 4).

SYNOVIOMA

Synovioma is an uncommon tumor most frequently arising in young adults, usually originating in the vicinity of a large joint in the periarticular soft tissue just beyond the confines of the joint capsule, most commonly around the knee and foot.[11, 36] In fact, it may be

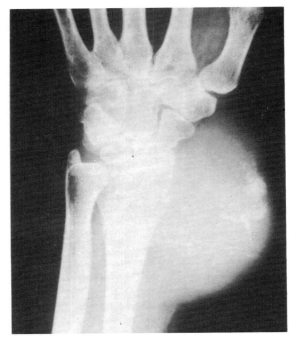

Figure 3–50.   Synovial sarcoma. The large soft-tissue mass adjacent to the distal radius contains irregular plaques of calcification. Note the absence of bone involvement.

found at some distance from the joint, and it is unusual for this tumor to arise within a joint. The degree of malignancy is variable. The lesion is visualized on a radiograph as a mass of soft-tissue density adjacent to a joint (Fig. 3-50). The outer margins of the mass are usually well demarcated from adjacent soft tissues. Hazy deposits or linear streaks of calcification are frequently seen within the tumor. Initially the underlying bone may be normal, but as the tumor increases in size the underlying bone may be eroded or actually invaded, with irregular destruction.

MISCELLANEOUS ARTHRITIDES

AMYLOIDOSIS

Amyloidosis is a rare disease characterized by the deposition of amyloid in various organs, including the bones and joints. The arthropathy of amyloidosis usually occurs in elderly individuals and most frequently involves the shoulders and hips and, less frequently, the wrists and elbows; it tends to be bilateral. Patients present with painful joints and a dramatic enlargement of the periarticular soft tissues. The swelling of the shoulders gives the appearance that the patient is wearing shoulder pads.[11, 14, 29] Bilateral carpal tunnel syndrome frequently accompanies wrist involvement. The radiographic appearance is characterized by juxta-articular osteoporosis, soft-tissue swelling, well-defined subchondral cysts (often large), and pressure erosions from synovial hypertrophy. Joint spaces are preserved until late in the disease. Pathologic fractures may occur through large subchondral cysts in the femoral neck.

LIPOID DERMATOARTHRITIS (MULTICENTRIC RETICULOHISTIOCYTOSIS)

Lipoid dermatoarthritis is a rare disorder affecting skin and synovium; it causes an erosive polyarthritis. Roentgen findings include the following: striking symmetry of clearly defined erosive changes, spreading from joint margins to the articular surfaces; IP joint predominance; early and severe atlantoaxial disease; minimal or no periosteal reaction; minimal osteoporosis; and soft-tissue nodules in skin, subcutaneous tissues, and tendon sheaths.[13, 29]

IDIOPATHIC CHONDROLYSIS OF THE HIP

Idiopathic chondrolysis of the hip is a rare condition occurring in adolescence; girls are more frequently affected than boys. The clinical course is variable. There is an insidious onset of hip pain, which in mild cases lasts for 6 to 12 months. The radiographic manifestations are periarticular osteoporosis and progressive narrowing of the hip joint space.[14, 29] Spontaneous recovery may occur in 6 to 12 months. In other cases, the disease progresses, with subchondral cysts, osteophyte formation, joint irregularity, and finally ankylosis.[4] The rheumatoid factor is negative, and the cause of the disease is unknown.

RELAPSING POLYCHONDRITIS

Relapsing polychondritis is an intense inflammatory and degenerative process that may result from altered immunity or hypersensitivity. Joints of the hands, wrists, and feet are involved by erosion of articular surfaces accompanied by soft-tissue swelling.[14, 29] Sacroiliac joints may also show erosive change resulting in irregularity of the joint space and partial obliteration of the space in some areas. Also, bony end-plates of vertebral bodies may show areas of erosion with sclerosis of adjacent bone. Cartilage dissolution in the ear, nose, trachea, and bronchi may also occur, leading to a saddle nose, respiratory disease, and death. Calcifications may appear in the ear cartilage.

HEMOPHILIAC ARTHROPATHY

Recurrent hemorrhage into the joints occurs in more than 50% of those afflicted with hemophilia. The knee, elbow, and ankle are more frequently affected, but any joint may be involved.[11, 13, 29] Joint involvement is usually asymmetrical. As a result of repeated hemorrhages and the irritating effect of blood, a synovitis develops, ultimately resulting in degeneration of the articular cartilage and erosion of the bony surfaces.[32]

The initial radiographic finding is a joint effusion. Eventually, after repeated hemorrhages, the soft tissues become thickened (Fig. 3-51). In chronic cases, the deposition of iron pigment in the tissues leads to a cloudy increase in density. Hemorrhage into the articular ends of the bones forms subchondral cysts. The joint margins are eroded and irregular (Fig. 3-52). In the knee, enlargement of the intercondylar notch of the femur is characteristic (Fig. 3-52): the joint disorder is nicely defined by MRI.[37] Synovial hypertrophy is displayed as areas of low to intermediate signal intensity on T1- and T2-weighted images with occasional foci of increased signal on T2.

Acceleration of epiphyseal growth from chronic irritation leads to an enlargement of the ends of bones. This is similar to that seen in other chronic inflammatory diseases with hyperemia, such as juvenile rheumatoid arthritis and tuberculosis. Occasionally a hemorrhage may occur within a bone some distance from a joint and may result in the formation of a cystlike radiolucent expansile cavity termed *pseudotumor of hemophilia* (Fig. 3-53). The ilium and calcaneus are frequently reported sites of this lesion.

STERNOCOSTOCLAVICULAR HYPEROSTOSIS

This disorder is characterized by hyperostosis and soft-tissue ossification between the clavicles and the adjacent anterior ribs and manubrium.[29, 31] The majority of cases are bilateral. Men are more commonly affected than women and are typically 30 to 50 years of age. They present with pain or swelling in the affected area. The condition may be associated with ankylosing spondylitis or DISH.

HYPERTROPHIC OSTEOARTHROPATHY

Periosteal reaction occasionally occurs on the long tubular bones in association with or as a result of diseases of the lungs or other conditions. The periosteal reaction may be a source of pain and arthralgia. This condition is known as hypertrophic osteoarthropathy. Osteoarthropathy most often occurs in association with intrathoracic neoplasms, especially bronchogenic carcinoma

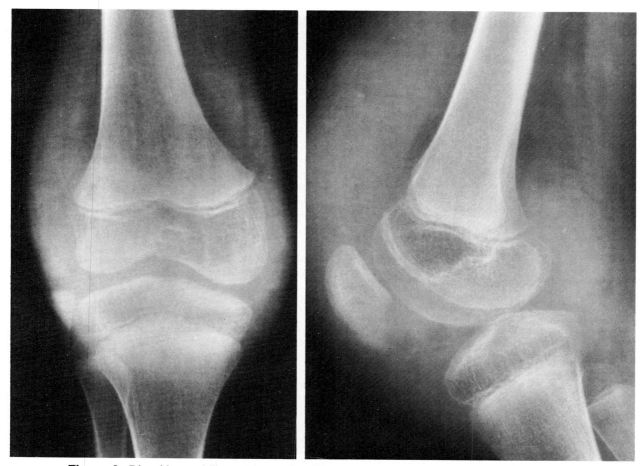

Figure 3–51. Hemophiliac arthropathy. This child had repeated episodes of hemarthrosis. Note the massive, dense joint effusion caused by accumulation of iron in the soft tissues, minimal loss of joint space, and a slight irregularity of the joint surface.

and mesotheliomas of the pleura. For this reason, the condition was known in the past as hypertrophic pulmonary osteoarthropathy. However, it is now recognized that this condition may also occur in association with gastrointestinal diseases, particularly ulcerative colitis and Crohn's disease.

Hypertrophic osteoarthropathy presents radiographically as a fine, linear periosteal reaction along the external surface of the long bones.[11, 29] Multiple bones are usually involved. The radius and ulna and the tibia and fibula are most frequently affected, and less commonly the metacarpals, metatarsals, and proximal and middle phalanges. As hypertrophic osteoarthropathy progresses, the periosteal reaction becomes thick and dense, and its outer surface develops a wavy outline (Fig. 3-54). The process often extends along the entire length of the diaphysis and metaphysis, but on other occasions shorter segments of the bone may be in-

volved. Characteristically, the intramedullary and cortical bone are otherwise normal. No other condition in adults is likely to cause periosteal reaction involving multiple long bones of both the upper and lower extremities with perfectly normal underlying cortical and medullary bone. The principal differential diagnosis in adults is periosteal reaction secondary to venous stasis. This, of course, is identified only in the lower extremity and is limited to the tibia and fibula. The wavy, compact nature of the periosteal reaction is very similar in appearance to that associated with hypertrophic osteoarthropathy, however. Radioisotopic bone scans, usually obtained to evaluate the possibility of metastatic disease in a patient with carcinoma of the lung, may demonstrate linear areas of increased activity paralleling the cortices of the affected bones, mirroring the radiographic findings of periosteal reaction.

Pachydermoperiostosis is a rare disease, a familial

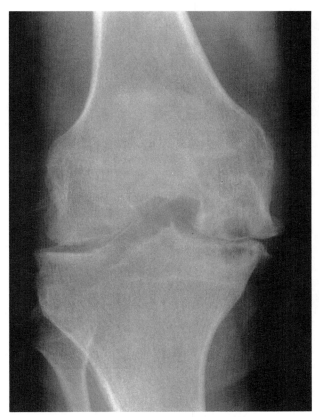

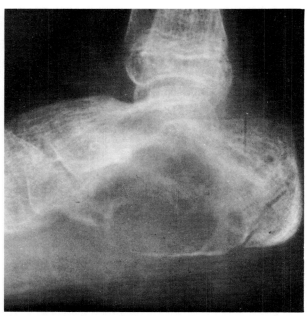

Figure 3–53. Hemophiliac pseudotumor. Note the large, expanding cystlike cavity in the os calcis.

Figure 3–52. Hemophiliac arthropathy in a 25-year-old man. The joint surfaces are irregular with marginal osteophyte formation and subchondral cysts, but there is no discrete subchondral sclerosis. Of importance is widening of the intercondylar notch of the distal femur, characteristic of hemophiliac arthropathy.

condition transmitted as an autosomal dominant trait with variable penetrance. It is essentially an idiopathic type of hypertrophic osteoarthropathy. In some patients, there is an associated thickening of the skin of the forehead and the face, with prominent creases and folds. This idiopathic form shows essentially the same radiographic features as described for hypertrophic osteoarthropathy; however, the bone scan is characteristically normal despite the presence of the periosteal reaction on the radiographic examination.

Clubbing of the digits is a related condition that is more common than hypertrophic osteoarthropathy. Clubbing consists of thickening of the soft tissues of the ends of the fingers. It usually follows chronic pulmonary disease, particularly suppurative lesions such as bronchiectasis and lung abscess or congenital cardiovascular diseases. Radiographs of the hands and feet

demonstrate soft-tissue enlargement, but the bones are entirely normal. On occasion, clubbing may coexist with hypertrophic osteoarthropathy.

MISCELLANEOUS CONDITIONS

POPLITEAL CYSTS

Popliteal cysts, or Baker's cysts, present clinically as a mass behind the knee (Fig. 3-55A). They are synovial cysts formed in association with any knee joint abnormality that results in distention of the joint, most commonly occurring in osteoarthritis and rheumatoid arthritis. A true popliteal cyst communicates with the joint and has a constant location arising between the tendons of the medial head of the gastronemius and semimembranous muscles (Fig. 3-55B). These cysts may contain loose bodies (Fig. 3-55A) or pannus. Popliteal cysts must be differentiated from aneurysms of the popliteal artery, a distinction easily accomplished by ultrasonography.

OSTEITIS CONDENSANS ILII

Osteitis condensans ilii is found almost exclusively in females during childbearing and almost always follows one or more pregnancies. It appears as a zone of dense sclerosis within the ilium along the iliac side of the

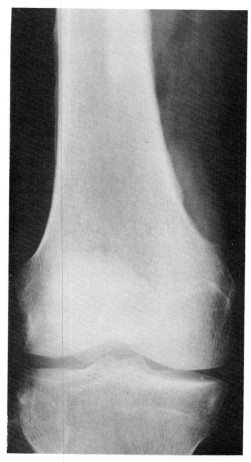

Figure 3–54.   Hypertrophic osteoarthropathy. Note the irregular, wavy periosteal new-bone formation of the distal femur.

Osteitis condensans ilii must be differentiated from a sacroiliitis associated with arthritis, particularly ankylosing spondylitis and the other spondyloarthropathies. Sacroiliitis affects the joint space and the articular surfaces of the apposing bones on both sides of the joints. Characteristically, the joint margins become blurred and eventually ankylose. Osteitis condensans ilii is confined to the ilium, and the sacroiliac joint remains normal.

A similar type of sclerotic reaction is observed in the pubic bones adjacent to the symphysis (Fig. 3-57). This too is seen almost exclusively in women who have borne children, and both pubic and iliac sclerosis may be seen in the same individual.

HALLUX VALGUS

Hallux valgus is a deformity of the great toe consisting of a lateral deviation of the phalanges and prominent soft-tissue thickening over the medial surface of the head of the first metatarsal, commonly referred to as a bunion (Fig. 3-58). It is often bilateral. The deformity usually develops after the age of 35 years. Osteoarthritic changes of the first MTP joint occur only after the deformity has been present for some time. There is often an associated widening of the forefoot, seen radiographically as an increase in the soft tissue between the heads of the metatarsals.

HALLUX RIGIDUS

Hallux rigidus is, as the name implies, a loss of flexibility of the great toe as a result of osteoarthritic or degenerative changes in the first MTP joint (Fig. 3-59). It is usually unilateral and is distinguished from hallux valgus by the lack of angular deformity (the alignment remaining normal) and the prominence of the osteoarthritic changes at the dorsal surface of the joint, asymmetrical joint-space narrowing, subchondral sclerosis, marginal spurs, and, at times, rather large subchondral cysts.

ARTHROGRAPHY

Arthrography is the radiographic examination of the internal structures of joints accomplished by injecting contrast medium into the joint and obtaining multiple radiographic views under fluoroscopic control. The radiographic examination must be performed promptly after the injection because the contrast material is rather rapidly absorbed. A water-soluble contrast medium and air are used as the contrast materials. Use of water-soluble contrast alone is referred to as single-contrast arthrography. Single-contrast examinations

sacroiliac joint. It is usually bilateral and symmetrical, although some variation in intensity may be observed between the two sides (Fig. 3-56). The joint space is not affected, and the sacrum is normal. The areas of sclerosis may be slight and may fade into the normal bone, or they may be several centimeters in width and sharply demarcated from adjacent normal bone. The cause of the condition is unknown, but it seems to be related to pregnancy and may represent the bony reaction to abnormal stresses occurring during pregnancy and delivery. It is discovered incidentally when a radiographic examination is performed to evaluate the abdominal or pelvic organs. The lesion probably disappears spontaneously in most cases, since sclerotic changes of this type are found very infrequently in older women.

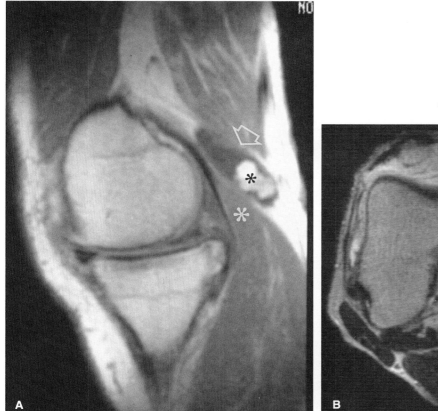
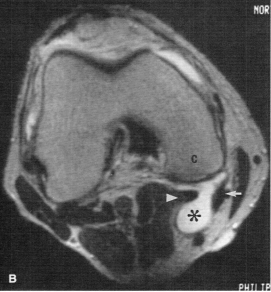

Figure 3–55. Two popliteal cysts. (**A**) T1-weighted sagittal image in a man with osteo-arthritis. Note the oviod area of low signal (*arrow*) overlying the medial head of the gastrocnemius muscle (*white asterisk*). The cyst contains loose bodies of higher signal marginated by a fine rim of low signal (*black asterisk*). Degenerative arthritis is present, manifested by narrowing of the articular cartilage and marginal spur formation, and there is a tear of the posterior horn of the medial meniscus. (**B**) Axial T2-weighted image in a separate case demonstrates a posterior protrusion of a popliteal cyst (*asterisk*) character-istically situated between the semimembranous tendon (*arrow*) and the medial head of the gastrocnemius (*arrowhead*). The Baker's cyst is contiguous with the joint space overlying the medial femoral condyle (**C**).

are used in the hip, wrist, ankle, and elbow. Double-contrast arthrography uses both water-soluble contrast material and air and is preferred by many authorities for the evaluation of the knee and shoulder. Arthrography of the knee has been essentially replaced by MRI.

Arthrography of the shoulder is commonly used to detect tears of the rotator cuff (Fig. 3-60) and disruptions of the biceps tendon and to verify reductions in the capacity of the joint. Arthrography of the hip is used to evaluate prostheses in adults and to verify the position of the femoral head in children. Arthrography

of the wrist is used to evaluate the integrity of the triangular ligament and the compartments of the carpus (Fig. 3-61).

RADIOGRAPHIC EVALUATION OF JOINT PROSTHESES

Radiography is essential in the evaluation of prosthetic devices. Joint prostheses are commonly used in the treatment of severe forms of arthritis of the hip and

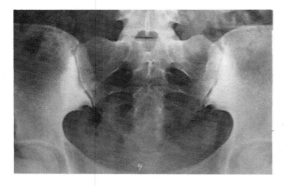

Figure 3–56.   Osteitis condensans ilii. Sclerosis is present on the iliac sides of the sacroiliac joint. The joint space and margins of the joint are normal. There is no sclerosis within the sacrum.

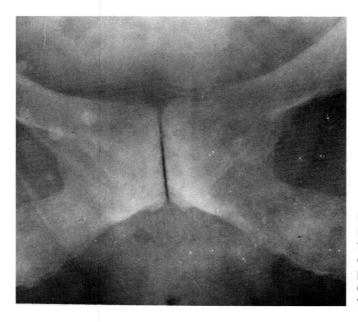

Figure 3–57.   Osteitis pubis. The symphysis is narrowed, with subchondral sclerosis of bone at the apposing margins and a thin radiolucency indicative of a vacuum phenomenon within the symphysis. Although not shown here, some cases demonstrate erosions of the apposing margins of the pubis.

knee and less commonly in the MCP and proximal IP joints and elsewhere. The prosthetic devices are made of some combination of a radiolucent high-density polyethylene and a nonferrous metal alloy.

The hip is the most common joint to be replaced by a prosthesis. The indications for replacement are severe degenerative arthritis, rheumatoid arthritis, avascular necrosis, and displaced fractures of the femoral neck. The complications of prosthetic replacement include fractures of the prosthetic device, the surrounding bone cement, or the surrounding femoral shaft; dislocations of the prosthetic joint; heterotopic ossification about the joint; and, most common of all, loosening and infection.

Loosening or infection is usually manifested clinically by the onset of pain. Radiographic evaluation consists of plain films, isotopic scanning, and arthrography. Unfortunately, the radiographic findings of loosening and infection are very similar and cannot be distinguished with certainty. On plain films, at the interface between the cement and bone there is normally a thin lucent line measuring no more than 1 mm. A line that is 2 mm or more wide is strongly suggestive of infection or loosening (Fig. 3-62A).[10] Periosteal newbone formation along the cortex is more indicative of infection; however, this is an infrequent finding.

Loosening and infection may be present in the absence of an increase in this radiolucency along the cement–bone interface. In these situations, isotopic bone scanning and arthrography may be required. Increased activity is normally observed on the isotope scan up to 6 to 8 months following surgical implanta-

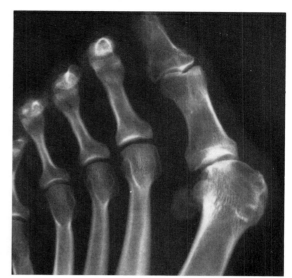

Figure 3–58. Hallux valgus. Note the typical valgus deformity of the first MCP joint. The proximal phalanx is subluxated laterally. There is minimal, if any, associated osteoarthritis. Separation of the heads of the first and second metatarsas is characteristic of this disorder.

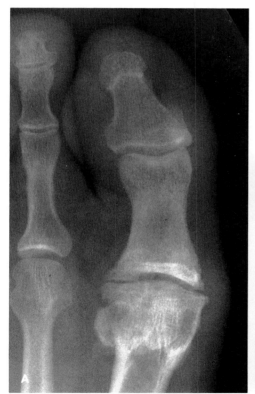

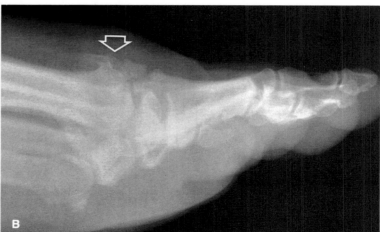

Figure 3–59. Hallux rigidus. (**A**) AP view of the great toe demonstrates marginal spur formation, subchondral sclerosis, and asymmetrical narrowing of the first MCP joint. There is no angular deformity of the joint. (**B**) Lateral view demonstrates characteristic large dorsal osteophytes at the margins of the joint (*arrow*). There has been a fracture at the base of the spur arising from the proximal phalanx.

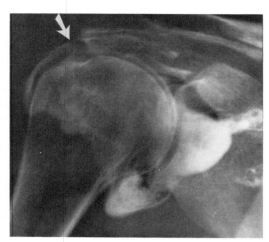

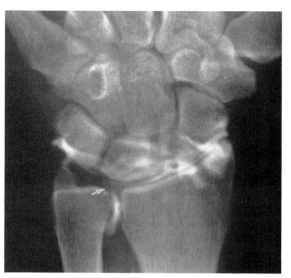

Figure 3–60.   Shoulder arthrogram. Note that the contrast material extends superiorly to rest just beneath the acromion (*arrow*), indicative of a tear in the rotator cuff.

Figure 3–61.   Wrist arthrogram. Contrast material injected into the radiocarpal joint extruded through a tear in the triangular fibrocartilage (*arrow*) into the distal radioulnar joint.

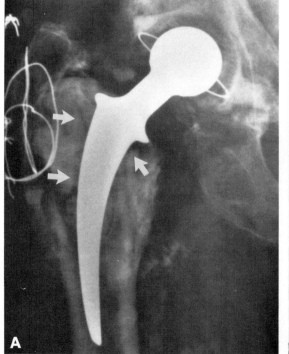

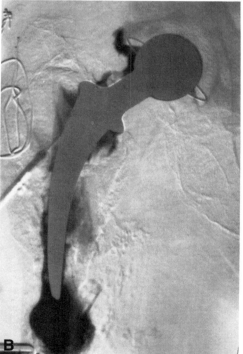

Figure 3–62.   The loosening of a hip prosthesis. (**A**) Note the wide radiolucency bordering the stem of the femoral component (*arrows*). The homogeneous radiodensity surrounding the metallic component is methyl methacrylate. Wire sutures are present in the greater trochanter. (**B**) A Subtraction film of a hip arthrogram demonstrates contrast material extruded from the joint space around the stem of the prosthesis, indicative of loosening.

tion. After this, the image should return to normal. Diffuse increased activity and focal increased activity adjacent to the tip of the femoral stem are the most common patterns associated with loosening. Gallium scanning may be of value in differentiating an infection from loosening.

The arthrogram of the prosthetic joint begins with an aspiration of the joint and culture of the fluid to diagnose or rule out infection.[10, 18] An arthrogram is then obtained. Normally the contrast material should be confined to the pseudocapsule of the joint. An abnormal hip arthrogram demonstrates a seepage of contrast material between the methacrylate and bone of either the acetabular or femoral components or between the metal and methacrylate of the femoral component (Fig. 3-62*B*). Abscess cavities or fistulous tracts may occur with infection and can be demonstrated by the arthrogram.

The evaluation of complications of prosthetic implants in other joints is similar to that in the hip. Loosening and infection are suggested by the presence of a radiolucent line at the margins of the prosthesis at either the cement–bone or implant–cement interfaces. Other plain film radiographic findings suggestive of loosening or infection are migration of the component or a change in the alignment of the component.

REFERENCES AND SELECTED READINGS

1. ADAMSON TC III, RESNIK SC, GUERRA J JR, ET AL: Hand and wrist arthropathies of hemochromatosis and calcium pyrophosphate deposition disease: Distinct radiographic features. Radiology 147:377, 1983

2. ALEXANDER CJ: Osteoarthritis: A review of old myths and current concepts. Skeletal Radiol 19:327, 1990

3. BJORKENGREN AG, RESNICK D, SARTORIS DJ: Enteropathic arthropathies. Radiol Clin North Am 25:189, 1987

4. BLECK EE: Idiopathic chondrolysis of the hip. J Bone Joint Surg [Am] 65:1266, 1983

5. BLOCK C, HERMANN G, YU TF: A radiologic reevaluation of gout: A study of 2,000 patients. Am J Roentgenol 134:781, 1980

6. BRAUNSTEIN EM, WEISSMAN BN, SOSMAN JL, ET AL: Radiologic findings in late onset systemic lupus erythematosus. Am J Roentgenol 140:587, 1983

7. BROWER AC, ALLMAN RM: The neuropathic joint: A neurovascular bone disorder. Radiol Clin North Am 19:571, 1981

8. CLOUSE ME, GRAMM HF, LEGG M, ET AL: Diabetic osteoarthropathy. Clinical and roentgenographic observations in 90 cases. Am J Roentgenol 121:22, 1974

9. DORWART RH, GENANT HK, JOHNSTON WH, ET AL: Pigmented villonodular synovitis of synovial joints: Clinical, pathologic, and radiologic features. Am J Roentgenol 143:877, 1984

10. DUSSAULT RG, GOLDMAN AB, GHELMAN B: Radiologic diagnosis of loosening and infection in hip prostheses. J Can Assoc Radiol 28:199, 1977

11. EDEIKEN J: Roentgen Diagnosis of Diseases of Bone, Vol 1, 3rd ed. Baltimore, Williams & Wilkins, 1981

12. FLANDRY F, MCCANN SB, HUGHSTON JC, KURTZ DM: Roentgenographic findings in pigmented villonodular synovitis of the knee. Clin Orthop 247:208, 1989

13. FORRESTER DM, BROWN JC: The Radiology of Joint Disease, Vol 2, 3rd ed. Philadelphia, WB Saunders, 1987

14. GOLDMAN AB: Some miscellaneous joint diseases. Semin Roentgenol 17:1, 60, 1982

15. HAMERMAN D: The biology of osteoarthritis. N Engl J Med 320:1322, 1989

16. HELMS CA, VOGLER JB, SIMMS DA, ET AL: CPPD crystal deposition disease or pseudogout. Radiographics 2:40, 1982

17. HELMS CA, CHAPMAN GS, WILD JH: Charcot-like joints in calcium pyrophosphate dihydrate deposition disease. Skeletal Radiol 7:55, 1981

18. HENDRIX RW, WIXSON RL, RANA NA, ET AL: Arthrography after total hip arthroplasty: A modified technique used in the diagnosis of pain. Radiology 148:647, 1983

19. JELINEK JS, KRANSDORF MJ, UTZ JA, ET AL: Imaging of pigmented villonodular synovitis with emphasis on MR imaging. Am J Roentgenol 152:337, 1989

20. KAYE JJ: Arthritis: Roles of radiography and other imaging techniques in evaluation. Radiology 177:601, 1990

21. LAWSON JP: The joint manifestations of connective tissue disease. Semin Roentgenol 17:1, 25, 1982

22. MARTEL W, BRAUNSTEIN EM, GOOD AE, ET AL: Radiologic features of Reiter disease. Radiology 132:1, 1979

23. MARTEL W, HOLT JF, CASSIDY JT: Roentgenologic manifestations of juvenile rheumatoid arthritis. Am J Roentgenol 88:400, 1962

24. MARTEL W, STUCK KH, DWORIN AM, ET AL: Erosive osteoarthritis and psoriatic arthritis: A radiologic comparison in the hand, wrist and foot. Am J Roentgenol 134:125, 1980

25. MCCARTHY DJ, HALVERSON PB, CARRERA GF, ET AL: "Milwaukee Shoulder"—association of microspheroids containing hydroxyapatite crystals, active collagenase, and neutral protease with rotator cuff defects. Arthritis Rheum 24:464, 1981

26. NANCE PE JR, KAYE JJ: The rheumatoid variants. Semin Roentgenol 17:1, 16, 1982

27. NORMAN A, STEINER GC: Bone erosion in synovial chondromatosis. Radiology 161:749, 1986

28. PETTERSSON H, LARSSON EM, HOLTAS S, ET AL: MR imaging of the cervical spine in rheumatoid arthritis. AJNR 9:573, 1988

29. RESNICK D, NIWAYAMA G: Diagnosis of Bone and Joint Disorders with Emphasis on Articular Abnormalities, 3rd ed. Philadelphia, WB Saunders, 1991

30. RESNICK D, NIWAYAMA G: Entheses and enthesopathy. Anatomical, pathological and radiological correlation. Radiology 146:1, 1983

31. SARTORIS DJ, SCHREIMAN JS, KERR R, ET AL: Sternocostoclavicular hyperostosis: A review and report of 11 cases. Radiology 158:125, 1986

32. STEIN H, DUTHIE RB: The pathogenesis of chronic haemophilic arthropathy. J Bone Joint Surg [Br] 63:601, 1981

33. TWERSKY J: Joint changes in idiopathic hemochromatosis. Am J Roentgenol 124:139, 1975

34. UDOFF EJ, GENANT HK, KOZIN F, ET AL: Mixed connective tissue disease: The spectrum of radiographic manifestations. Radiology 124:613, 1977

35. WEISSMAN BNW, ALIABADI P, WEINFELD MS, ET AL: Prognostic features of atlantoaxial subluxation in rheumatoid arthritis patients. Radiology 144:745, 1982

36. WRIGHT PH, SIM FH, SOULE EH, ET AL: Synovial sarcoma. J Bone Joint Surg [Am] 64:112, 1982

37. YULISH BS, LIEBERMAN JM, STRANDJORD SE, ET AL: Hemophilic arthropathy: Assessment with MR imaging. Radiology 164:759, 1987

Paul and Juhl's Essentials of Radiologic Imaging, Sixth Edition, edited by John H. Juhl and Andrew B. Crummy. J.B. Lippincott Company, Philadelphia, © 1993.

CHAPTER *4*

Bone Tumors and Related Conditions

Lee F. Rogers

Primary tumors of bone are relatively uncommon, whereas metastatic disease of bone is encountered daily. Because of the rarity of these tumors, physicians are often unfamiliar with them and feel uncertain about their diagnosis and treatment. The application of certain basic principles should allow a correct diagnosis or at least a reasonable differential diagnosis in most cases.

Bone tumors are not easily classified. The classifications in common use are related more to the microscopic characteristics of the tumor and its presumed tissue of origin than to the radiographic appearance of the lesion.[8, 11, 19] The initial pathologic diagnosis is usually based on a small portion of tissue that may well suggest the tissue of origin, but the radiographic manifestations of the process are often a better clue to the aggressiveness of the lesion. Therefore, the final diagnosis of most bone tumors should be based on a combination of both the microscopic and radiographic characteristics. The development of classifications is also hindered by the fact that benign lesions do not necessarily have malignant counterparts. Lesions are either benign and remain benign or are malignant from their inception. Very few primary bone lesions convert from a benign to a malignant character. The classification of tumors in Table 4-1 serves as a guide to the radiographic characteristics of lesions.

RADIOGRAPHIC ANALYSIS OF BONE TUMORS

The radiologist's role is to identify and characterize the lesion.[19] A few benign types of bone tumors are quite characteristic in appearance, and they require no treatment. Dr. Harold Jacobson[32] has characterized these as "leave me alone lesions," lesions so commonly encountered and characteristic in appearance that a diagnosis can be made with absolute assurance on the basis of radiographic characteristics alone. These lesions are osteoma, bone island, and nonossifying fibroma. In other cases, the radiographic manifestations are sufficiently characteristic to allow a diagnosis with a high degree of probability. In the remainder, it may be difficult to establish a tissue diagnosis with assurance. In these situations, one should attempt to determine whether the lesion is benign or malignant and to differentiate tumors from infectious, metabolic, or dysplastic processes.

The extent or limits of the lesion must be determined. In general, the diagnosis of the lesion is based on plain film radiography and is further defined by tomography. Computed tomography (CT) and magnetic resonance imaging (MRI) do not add to the tissue characterization of the lesion but are useful in evaluating the extent of the lesion by determining the pres-

Table 4–1. Classification of Primary Bone Tumors

I. Cartilaginous
  A. Benign
    1. Osteochondroma (exostosis)
    2. Chondroma (enchondroma)
    3. Parosteal (juxtacortical) chondroma
    4. Chondroblastoma
    5. Chondromyxoid fibroma
  B. Malignant
    1. Chondrosarcoma
      a. Primary
      b. Secondary
II. Osseous
  A. Benign
    1. Osteoma
    2. Bone island
    3. Osteoid osteoma
    4. Osteoblastoma (giant osteoid osteoma)
  B. Malignant
    1. Osteosarcoma
    2. Parosteal (juxtacortical) osteosarcoma
    3. Periosteal osteosarcoma
    4. Osteosarcomatosis
III. Fibrous (fibrogenic, histiocytic)
  A. Benign
    1. Nonossifying fibroma (fibrous cortical defect, xanthoma)
    2. Desmoplastic fibroma
    3. Ossifying fibroma
  B. Malignant
    1. Fibrosarcoma
    2. Malignant fibrous histiocytoma
IV. Cystic
  A. Benign
    1. Simple bone cyst (unicameral bone cyst)
    2. Giant cell tumor
    3. Aneurysmal bone cyst
      a. Isolated
      b. Associated with other tumors
    4. Intraosseous ganglion
    5. Synovial cyst
    6. Epidermoid cyst
    7. "Brown tumor" of hyperparathyroidism
  B. Malignant
    1. Giant cell tumor
V. Myelogenous (round cell)
  A. Malignant
    1. Myeloma
      a. Multiple myeloma
      b. Solitary myeloma
    2. Reticulum cell sarcoma (malignant lymphoma)
    3. Ewing's tumor
VI. Miscellaneous
  A. Benign
    1. Hemangioma
    2. Lipoma
    3. Synovioma
  B. Malignant
    1. Chordoma
    2. Adamantinoma
    3. Synovial sarcoma
    4. Hemangiosarcoma

ence or absence of soft-tissue extension outside of bone and intramedullary extension within bone.

The best site for biopsy should be determined on the basis of the radiographic characteristics. The most active or aggressive portion of the lesion can usually be identified, and tissue that best characterizes the lesion is likely to be found at this site.

As a broad generalization, a benign lesion is sharply defined, the overlying cortex is intact, and there is no associated soft-tissue mass. In contrast, a malignant lesion is poorly defined, the overlying cortex is disrupted, and there is an associated soft-tissue mass.

DIAGNOSTIC CRITERIA

The specific characteristics of value in the determination of a specific diagnosis are the age of the patient,[11] whether the lesion is single or multiple, the location of the lesion in relation to both the long axis and central axis of the bone, the bone in which the lesion is located, the character of the internal margins of the lesion,[24] the presence or absence of periosteal reaction and its character,[35] the presence or absence of tumor matrix calcification and its character,[39] and the presence or absence of a previous history of malignancy particularly in patients older than 40 years.

AGE

The age of the patient alone is an excellent indicator of the type of tumor encountered.[11] For instance, metastatic neuroblastoma is the most common malignant-appearing tumor before the age of 1 year, whereas between the ages of 1 and 20 Ewing's tumor is encountered in tubular bones. Between the ages of 10 and 30, osteosarcoma and Ewing's tumor are encountered in flat bones. After the age of 40, metastatic carcinoma, multiple myeloma, and chondrosarcoma are more likely.

LOCATION

Different types of tumors occur in relatively characteristic locations within the skeletal system (Fig. 4-1). Location in relation to the long axis of bone is of primary importance. Certain tumors arise in the metaphysis, others in the diaphysis or within the epiphysis. Location in relation to the central axis is likewise important. Some tumors arise centrally, in the central axis; some arise eccentrically, off the central axis; still others arise within the cortex or the surface of the cortex, referred to as parosteal. When lesions of long tubular bones that are characteristically eccentric in position occur in the smaller tubular bones, such as the fibula or metacar-

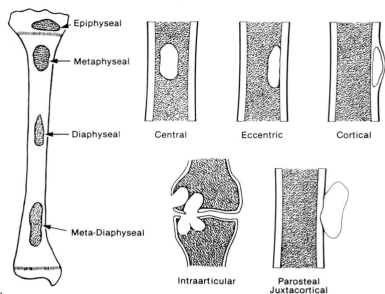

Figure 4–1. Location of tumors.

pals, they may easily involve the entire width of the shaft and lead to a ballooned expansion of the involved bone (see Fig. 4-16). This is particularly true of nonossifying fibromas, giant cell tumors, and aneurysmal bone cysts.

SPECIFIC BONE

To a lesser extent, the bone in which the tumor is located is also of importance. Some tumors are more likely to arise in a specific bone than others. For instance, the most common site of an osteoblastoma is the posterior elements of the vertebral body, whereas adamantinomas arise in the tibia.

INTERNAL MARGINS

The internal margin of a lesion relates to the radiographic appearance of the tumor–bone interface, the interface between the tumor and the bone from which it arises.[24] This is dependent on the nature of the disturbance of the endosteal surface of the cortex and the pattern of medullary destruction.

Medullary destruction may be geographic, confined to a relatively specific area that is more or less easily defined; moth-eaten, irregular patches of medullary destruction; or permeative, rather poorly defined areas of destruction (Fig. 4-2).

The margin of the lesion may be sharply defined by a thin or thick wall of sclerotic bone (Fig. 4-2). Some lesions, although sharply defined, have no reactive

bone formation about them and are said to be "punched out." Others are poorly marginated and less well defined, with the margin of the lesion more or less blending imperceptibly into the surrounding intramedullary bone.

Zone of transition refers to the border between the lesion and normal surrounding bone. Well-defined lesions are said to have a sharp zone of transition, and those that are poorly defined are said to have a broad zone of transition.

The aggressiveness of a bone lesion is manifested radiographically by the tumor–bone interface. Indolent or slow-growing tumors are marginated by sclerotic bone, whereas those with more rapid growth lack a sclerotic margin. Should growth be even more aggressive, the margin becomes progressively less well defined. A rapid growth rate may be encountered in benign as well as malignant lesions, and the opposite is also true—that is, some malignant lesions are slow growing and have sharply defined margins. Therefore, although the radiographic appearance of the tumor–bone interface indicates the aggressiveness and growth rate of a bone lesion, the interface does not in and of itself indicate benignancy or malignancy. Eosinophilic granuloma, aneurysmal bone cyst, most giant cell tumors, and chondromyxoid fibroma may have an aggressive radiographic appearance and yet be benign. Conversely, solitary myeloma, adamantinoma, and juxtacortical osteogenic sarcoma are slow growing and radiographically nonaggressive but in fact are malignant.

A lesion may affect the cortex in several ways (Fig. 4-3). It may expand the cortex outward, distorting the

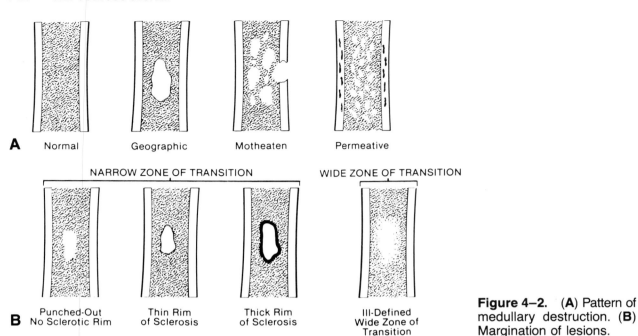

Figure 4–2. **(A)** Pattern of medullary destruction. **(B)** Margination of lesions.

normal outline of the bone with the cortex remaining intact. This type of lesion is said to be expansile or ballooned. It may erode and scallop the endosteal surface, referred to as endosteal scalloping. Some lesions have an invisible peripheral margin of cortical bone. In these, the peripheral margin is so fine that it cannot be identified on a plain film but may be visualized by tomography or CT. This is characteristic of aneurysmal bone cyst, chondromyxoid fibroma, and eosinophilic

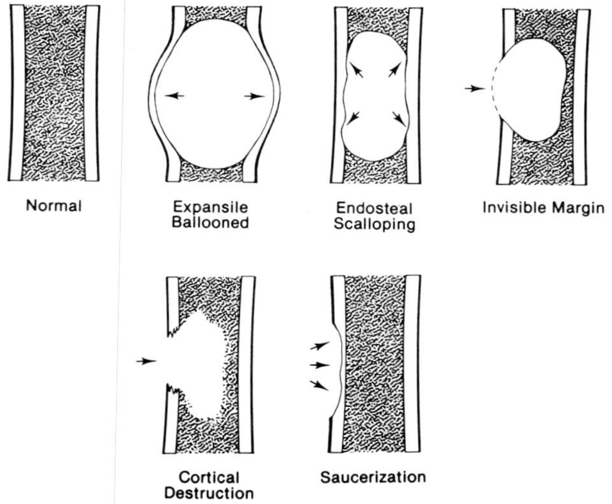

granuloma, particularly in a young child. Malignant tumors and infections lead to cortical destruction manifested by an irregular loss of cortical bone. Lesions arising in the periosteum or adjacent to the cortex cause a shallow erosion of the external surface of the cortex referred to as saucerization. However, saucerization may also occur in Ewing's tumor and periosteal osteosarcoma.

The lesion may also be further characterized by the presence or absence of septation (Fig. 4-4). Certain lesions either are or appear to be divided by thin walls or septa of cortical bone. A lesion without any evidence of internal septa is said to be nonseptated. This is characteristic of a unicameral bone cyst. Other lesions appear to contain multiple septa and are said to be multiseptated. In some, this is because true septa extend throughout the lesion; in others, the septation is actually due to an erosion or scalloping of the endosteal surface, with the ridges of bone between the scallops giving the false appearance of septa when viewed radiographically.

PERIOSTEAL NEW-BONE FORMATION

The presence and character of periosteal new-bone formation or periosteal reaction lend important clues to the nature of an underlying lesion (Fig. 4-5).[34]

A single layer of periosteal reaction (lamellar) is a faint radiodense line of 1 to 2 mm width paralleling the cortical surface. This is a hallmark of a benign process;

Figure 4–3.   Patterns of cortical disturbance.

it is usually seen in acute osteomyelitis and is rarely encountered in neoplasms.

Solid or wavy periosteal reaction is a solid reaction with an undulant outer margin. This is typical of long-standing peripheral vascular disease (varicosities) of the lower extremities and pulmonary osteoarthropathy.

Solid, compact, or thick periosteal reaction represents multiple successive layers of new bone applied to the cortex overlying a lesion. This may also be referred to as cortical thickening or hyperostosis. It is encountered in osteoid osteomas, chronic osteomyelitis, eosinophilic granulomas, and central chondrosarcomas of long bones.

A combination of lamellar and nodular periosteal reaction is typical of a benign process and is often associated with cortical bone abscess.

Layered or laminated periosteal reaction created by several parallel concentric layers or lamellae of periosteal new bone is often referred to as "onionskin" reaction. It implies a more aggressive process but is

encountered in both benign and malignant disease. It is most characteristic of Ewing's tumor (Ewing's sarcoma) but may be found in osteosarcoma, acute osteomyelitis, stress fractures, and eosinophilic granuloma in very young patients.

Uniform, fine, parallel linear shadows oriented perpendicular to the cortex form the "hair-on-end" pattern, characteristic of Ewing's tumor. A "sunburst" or divergent periosteal reaction is characteristic of osteosarcoma. The spicules of bone are more irregular and coarser than those encountered in the hair-on-end pattern. Periosteal reaction that is irregular and otherwise unclassifiable is typical of bone sarcoma and is often encountered in osteosarcoma.

Periosteal new-bone formation may be interrupted and may incompletely cover the surface of a lesion, as is often the case with osteosarcomas. A triangle consisting of several layers of periosteal reaction may form at the margin of the lesion. This is known as Codman's triangle. Codman's triangle was at one time thought to be pathognomonic of bone sarcomas but in fact is also

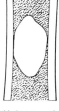 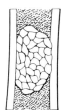 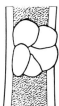 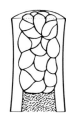 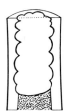

| Unicameral Nonseptated | Honeycomb Multiseptated | Soap Bubble | True Septation | Ridging |

Figure 4–4. Septation in bone lesions.

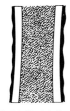 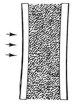 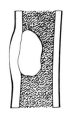 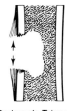 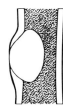

| Lamellar Solid, Thin, Fine | Solid, Undulating, Wavy | Solid, Thick | Codman's Triangles | Buttress |

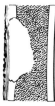 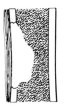 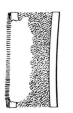 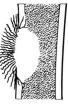 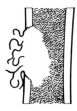

Figure 4–5. Periosteal new-bone formation.

| Onion-Skin Layered | Lamellar Nodular | Hair-on-end Spiculated | Sunburst Divergent | Irregular |

encountered in osteomyelitis. The triangle is composed entirely of periosteal reaction and is usually free of tumor; therefore, it should be avoided as a site for biopsy.

Periosteal new-bone formation associated with slow-growing lesions may result in a somewhat similar triangle of more compact and sometimes solid bone at the margin of the lesion. This is known as a buttress and is characteristic of benign lesions. Buttress formation is often associated with those lesions that have an invisible cortical margin, such as aneurysmal bone cyst, chondromyxoid fibroma (see Fig. 4-11), and eosinophilic granuloma in young patients.

TUMOR BONE FORMATION (MATRIX CALCIFICATION)

Calcification occurring within the matrix of a tumor, particularly osteoid and chondroid tumors, occurs in patterns that are characteristic[39] of the tissue of origin (Fig. 4-6).

Calcification of osteoid characteristically creates a cloudlike, amorphous, homogenous opacity (see Figs. 4-44 and 4-45). On the radiograph, it appears as if painted or "chalked in" in white.

Calcific densities characteristic of chondroid matrix in small tumors are stippled or punctate, whereas in larger tumors nodules, flocculent (popcornlike) rings, and arcs of calcific density are noted (see Figs. 4-7 through 4-9).

Reactive new bone forms in some tumors and at the margins of infections. The new bone forms on existing normal trabeculae at the border of chronic bone abscesses and in the presence of certain malignant cells, particularly metastatic malignancies of the breast and lung (see Figs. 4-33 and 4-34). The osteoblastic response in these tumors is not due to ossification of the tumor but to reactive new-bone formation surrounding the tumor. Reactive new bone is characteristically homogenous and amorphous.

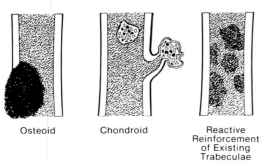

Osteoid   Chondroid   Reactive Reinforcement of Existing Trabeculae

Figure 4–6. Tumor bone formation, matrix calcification.

IMAGING TECHNIQUES IN BONE TUMORS

TOMOGRAPHY

Tomography is used to augment the plain film and provides useful information in selected cases. It more clearly delineates and defines the lesion than plain films and may be helpful in the demonstration of matrix calcification and cortical destruction.

COMPUTED TOMOGRAPHY

In most cases, CT adds little to the specific histologic diagnosis of a bone tumor beyond that of the plain radiograph, but it does give a better indication of the extent of the lesion both within the intramedullary canal and surrounding soft tissues and its relationship to adjacent vascular structures (see Fig. 4-43).[35] Both bone and soft-tissue windows demonstrate the extent of cortical destruction, but soft-tissue windows better demonstrate the extent of soft-tissue disease and involvement of the marrow. The normal marrow is of fat density and usually -20 to -40 Hounsfield units. When tumor involves the marrow, its density is increased to that of soft tissue, well into the positive range. Because CT is more sensitive than plain films, CT can delineate lesions indicated by a positive bone scan but inapparent on a radiograph (see Figs. 4-27 and 4-28). This is particularly helpful in the disclosure of metastatic lesions in the spine and pelvis and less commonly in the peripheral skeleton. CT can also identify fine bony margins of a lesion that are inapparent on plain films (see Fig. 4-20). CT displays calcified and bony matrix within lesions much better than MRI.

MAGNETIC RESONANCE IMAGING

MRI demonstrates the extent of soft-tissue and marrow involvement and also defines the relationship of the tumor to the surrounding vessels.[31, 35] The direct sagittal and coronal images of MRI permit a more accurate assessment of the relationship of the tumor to adjacent normal structures along the longitudinal axis of the bone, particularly the neurovascular structures, spinal cord, joints, and physis.

Most malignant bone tumors are inhomogeneous on both T1- and T2-weighted images. The degree of inhomogeneity varies with the type of tumor matrix and the extend of homorrhage and necrosis. T1-weighted images are best for determining the extent of marrow involvement (see Fig. 4-45B), and T2 images are more useful in evaluating cortical bone destruction and soft-tissue extension (see Fig. 4-45C). MRI is not as useful in the evaluation of cortical bone because of the absence of signal. Matrix and marginal calcification and

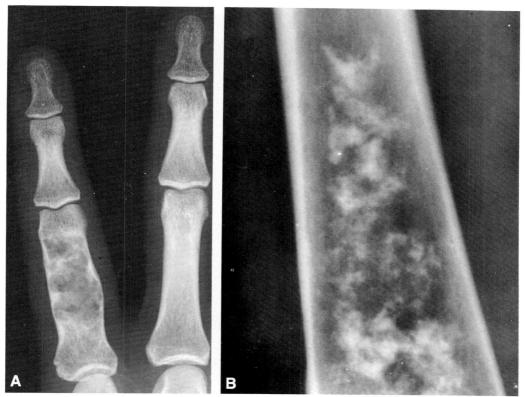

Figure 4–7. (**A**) Enchondroma of the proximal phalanx of the fifth digit. Note the small calcifications distally, typical of cartilaginous tumors. (**B**) Closeup view of the lower femur showing characteristic chondroid calcification within the medullary canal. Note the lack of boundary rim of sclerosis and the small, rounded areas of lucency representing islands of uncalcified cartilage. Note also the absence of endosteal erosion and cortical thickening (compare with Fig. 4-49, chondrosarcoma, and Fig. 7-24, bone infarction).

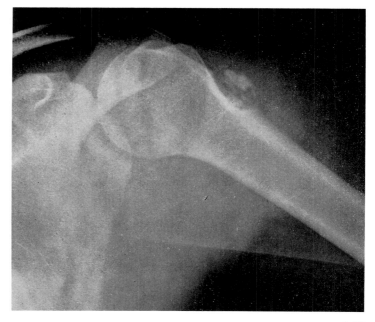

Figure 4–8. Parosteal chondroma. The base of the lesion is bounded by a zone of sclerosis. Note the buttress at the distal margin of the lesion, the scalloping of the cortex, and the chondroid calcification within the lesion.

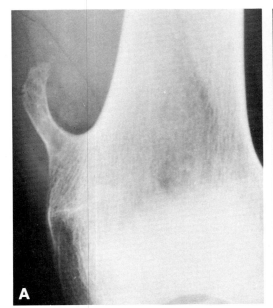
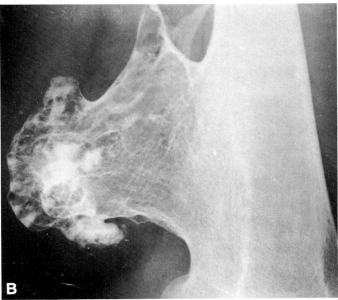
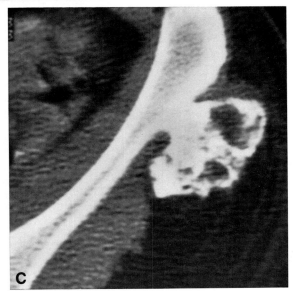

Figure 4–9. **(A)** Osteochondroma (exostosis) arising from the medial aspect of the distal femur. The pedicle is composed of cortical bone that merges with and is continuous with the normal femoral cortex. The medullary bone within the stalk of the lesion is likewise continuous with the medullary canal of the femur. **(B)** Broad-based osteochondroma arising from the posterior cortex of the lower femur. The periphery of the tumor is composed of a mixture of cartilage, calcified cartilage, and bone. Note the characteristic chondroid calcification in the distal portion of the lesion. **(C)** CT of osteochondroma arising from the iliac bone. The lesion is sharply defined without an overlying soft-tissue mass. The cortex of the lesion is contiguous with the cortex of the iliac bone (compare with Fig. 4-50).

subtle cortical changes may be more obvious on CT. The hydrogen content of cortical bone is very low and therefore gives no signal on MRI, whereas the fat in marrow contains a high hydrogen content and gives a pronounced signal on T1-weighted images. The replacement of marrow fat by tumor, infection, or hemorrhage reduces the strength of the signal. MRI affords superior soft-tissue contrast, allowing better delineation and differentiation of soft tissues than is possible by CT (see Fig. 4-45). For these reasons, MRI has largely replaced CT in the evaluation of bone and soft-tissue tumors.

ISOTOPE SCANNING

Bone scanning is performed with ^{99m}Tc-labeled phosphate compounds, most commonly technetium-99m methyldiphosphonate (^{99m}Tc-MDP). Fifteen to 20 millicuries (mCi) is administered intravenously, and 2 hours later a scan is obtained of the entire skeletal system. The radiopharmaceutical is taken up in all sites of active bone turnover irrespective of cause—tumor, infection, fracture, or metabolic. The increased radioactivity occurring at such sites is referred to as a positive bone scan. The bone scan is several times more sensitive than film radiography, and therefore activity may be demonstrated on bone scan in the face of normal x-ray findings (see Figs. 4-27 and 4-28). It is said that approximately 50% of trabecular bone must be removed from a given site before it is evident on a radiograph, whereas only 5% to 15% must be removed before it can be identified on a bone scan.

Increased radioactivity occurs at practically all sites of primary or metastatic bone tumors, with the exception of multiple myeloma. Bone scanning is unreliable in the evaluation of patients with multiple myeloma, since the avidity of the tumor for the radiopharmaceutical is unpredictable and often nonexistent. Negative bone scans may be obtained in as many as 40% of sites of multiple myeloma. Bone scans are particularly useful in the detection of skeletal metastatic disease from tumors arising out of the skeletal system, such as lung, breast, and prostatic cancers (see Fig. 4-33). Bone scanning is less useful in primary tumors but should be used in the evaluation of Ewing's tumors and osteosarcomas that are likely to metastasize to other bones. Bone-to-bone metastasis in other primary bone tumors is most unlikely.

ANGIOGRAPHY

Angiography is necessary in selected cases to determine the vascularity of the lesion and the position of adjacent vascular structures to aid the surgeon in the design of the surgical approach to a lesion. This can usually be accomplished by CT or MRI, however.

NEEDLE BIOPSY

Percutaneous needle biopsy is used to establish the diagnosis of metastatic disease or infection. Its use in the diagnosis of primary bone tumors remains controversial, and the success rate is somewhat less than that for metastatic tumors.

Bone tumors that are obviously benign and are characteristic in appearance often need not be evaluated by anything more than a plain radiograph. When surgery is contemplated, tomography or CT and MRI may be required to further evaluate the extent of the lesion.

In primary malignancies of bone, the extent of the lesion must be determined. Usually this requires a CT scan or MRI (see Fig. 4-46) and occasionally angiography. In primary bone tumors in which an amputation is contemplated, a CT examination of the chest should be obtained to rule out pulmonary metastasis. CT is much more sensitive to the presence of lung nodules than is the plain radiograph or standard tomography. An amputation is not performed in the presence of metastatic disease in the lung except under unusual circumstances.

BENIGN BONE TUMORS

BENIGN CARTILAGINOUS TUMORS

Enchondroma

An enchondroma is a benign cartilaginous tumor arising from cartilage cell rests within the medullary cavity. It is the most common tumor encountered in the bones of the hand, its usual location. Enchondroma also occurs in the ribs, pelvis, and occasionally the long bones.

Roentgenographic Features. An enchondroma is a central lesion originating within the medullary cavity, usually at or near the epiphysis. The mass is radiolucent and usually contains calcification characteristic of chondroid matrix (see Figs. 4-6 and 4-7). It is stippled or nodular in the small bones; in the flat bones and long tubular bones, it is nodular and flocculent, with rings and arcs of ossification.

In the small bones of the hand the tumor grows slowly, and as it enlarges, expands and thins the cortex (see Fig. 4-7A). The endosteal surface of the cortex is scalloped. The lesion is geographic, usually clearly defined, and marginated by a thin rim of sclerotic bone. Pathologic fractures may occur.

Enchondromas occurring in the long bones arise within and are generally limited to the medullary cavity and contain typical chondroid calcification (see Fig. 4-7B). Many are manifested only by chondroid calcification without an apparent surrounding lucency or sclerotic rim. These must be differentiated from bone infarcts. The principal distinction is the characteristic nature of the chondroid calcification. Calcification in bone infarct is plaquelike and occurs on the surface of the infarct (see Fig. 7-24A), whereas chondroid matrix calcification occurs within the central portion of the lesion.

When the tumor occurs in the hands or feet, it is rarely malignant; but in the flat bones such as the ribs and ilium and in the long bones of the extremities, malignancies are always a possibility. Changes indicating malignancy include a loss of marginal definition, cortical disruption, overlying periosteal reaction, and the growth of the previously identified enchondroma. Normally a patient experiences no pain from a benign enchondroma. When pain is present in the area, the possibility of malignancy must always be considered.

In the long bones, an enchondroma is usually confined to the medullary cavity without affecting the surrounding cortex. Therefore, the presence of endosteal scalloping or thickening of the overlying bone suggests the possibility of a malignancy.

Ollier's disease is a congenital osseous dysplasia characterized by the occurrence of multiple enchondromas at the ends of the long bones, very commonly in the hands, often in only one extremity or in the extremities on one side of the body. When this condition is associated with multiple cavernous hemangiomas, the rare combination is termed *Maffucci's syndrome* (see Chapter 9).

Parosteal Chondroma (Juxtacortical)

Parosteal chondroma develops in the periosteum or soft tissue immediately adjacent to the outer surface of the cortex. Ordinarily the lesion is relatively small. The most common site is the phalanges of the hand, but the lesion may occur at the ends of the long bones of the extremities and rarely in the carpal bones. It produces a small, saucerlike erosion of the underlying cortex, with a rather dense rim of reactive bone beneath the erosion (see Fig. 4-8). One or both of the margins may demonstrate a buttress of compact bone. The tumor does not invade the medullary cavity. Typical chondroid calcification may be found within the soft-tissue mass. The outer margin of the mass is not defined by a rim of bone. In some lesions, there may be no chondroid calcification, but the cortical defect is sufficiently typical to suggest the diagnosis.

Osteochondroma (Exostosis)

Osteochondroma is a benign tumor composed of cartilage, calcified cartilage, and bone in variable amounts. The term *exostosis* is synonymous with osteochondroma. The lesion most likely represents a local dysplasia of cartilage at the epiphyseal growth plate. It retains a cartilage cap that cannot be recognized radiographically except by the presence of chondroid calcification within it. These tumors begin during early childhood, grow slowly, and cease growth when the skeleton matures at puberty. They occur frequently in the distal ends of the long tubular bones, particularly the lower end of the femur and the upper and lower ends of the tibia, but they may occur in any part of the skeleton preformed in cartilage. When practically all the bones are involved, this condition is known as osteochondromatosis or hereditary multiple exostosis. It is discussed in Chapter 9.

Roentgenographic Features. The tumor arises from the cortex and grows outward, pointing away from the nearest joint. It is usually pedunculated and cauli-

flower shaped, the pedicle merging smoothly with the normal cortex of the bone (see Fig. 4-9). The cortical and cancellous bone of the stalk of the lesion is contiguous with that of the bone from which it arises. Occasionally the lesion is flat and broad but has the other features of an osteochondroma. The tip of the osseous stalk contains chondroid elements and, in the absence of chondroid calcification, may be invisible. When the lesion is mature, its peripheral margin is distinct and bounded by a thin rim of bone. As a rule, single lesions are asymptomatic unless the mass becomes large enough to interfere with function. Any osteochondroma is capable of becoming malignant, developing into a chondrosarcoma. When an osteochondroma begins to enlarge or becomes painful after a period of stationary size, malignant degeneration should be suspected. This has been reported to occur in approximately 5% of cases. Pain may also result from a fracture of the stalk of an osteochondroma or inflammation within a bursa over the surface of the lesion.

Chondroblastoma

Chondroblastoma is a rare, benign variety of cartilaginous tumor arising in the epiphysis.[8, 38] The growth plate may have closed by the time the tumor is first discovered. The tumor is usually encountered between the ages of 10 and 20, with occasional cases in the first, third, and fourth decades of life. The usual locations are in the epiphyses of the proximal humerus, distal femur, proximal tibia, and proximal femur, and a few have been reported in the tarsal bones, around the acetabulum, and elsewhere.

Roentgenographic Features. A chondroblastoma (Fig. 4-10) presents as a well-defined geographic area of bone destruction that may contain stippled or small nodules of chondroid calcification.[26] The lesion is characteristically located in the epiphysis, but as it enlarges it may extend into the metaphysis. The tumor often extends into the articular surface but rarely into the joint. The lesion is often small and located eccentrically, and it sometimes has a scalloped appearance. There may be slight expansion of the cortex, and periosteal reaction is sometimes encountered (Fig. 4-10B). The margin of the lesion is usually well defined by a thin rim of sclerosis, but the appearance is dependent upon the aggressiveness of the lesion. When indolent, the lesion has a sharply defined rim of sclerosis, and when aggressive, it may expand bone with less sharply defined margins and overlying periosteal reaction.

Chondromyxoid Fibroma

Chondromyxoid fibroma is a relatively rare, benign tumor of bone most frequently found in the metaphysis

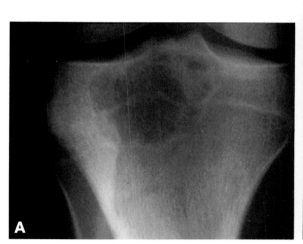
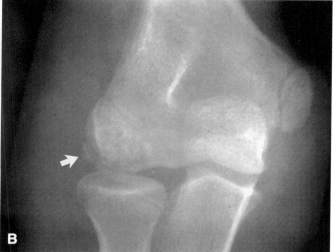

Figure 4–10. Two cases of chondroblastoma in 14-year-olds. **(A)** Sharply defined lobulated lesion located in the proximal tibia epiphysis. The lesion is bordered by a thin rim of sclerosis. **(B)** Slightly lobulated lesion with a sclerotic margin located eccentrically in the distal humeral epiphysis. It contains punctate chondroid calcification, and periosteal reaction (*arrow*) is noted at the lateral margin.

of long bones.[40] Patients usually present in the second and third decades of life but on occasion may be encountered under 10 or over 30 years of age. The proximal tibia is the most common site, followed by the distal femur and distal tibia, the tibia accounting for approximately one-third of all cases. Two-thirds occur in long tubular bones, but the tumor may also arise in the small bones of the hands and feet and the pelvis, with sporadic examples in the vertebrae, ribs, scapula, and skull.

Roentgenographic Features. The classic lesion arises eccentrically in the metaphysis as a sharply circumscribed zone of rarefaction that occasionally causes expansion of bone (Fig. 4-11). The lesion may abut the growth plate or be a variable distance from it. It is often elongated, with its long axis oriented with the long axis of the bone. Its margin is scalloped, and the sclerosis may vary somewhat in thickness in different areas of the lesion. In smaller bones, the lesion will be located more centrally and will expand the bone. In the long bone, the lesion usually causes a local thinning and expansion of the overlying cortex. In some patients, the outer cortex may be invisible and appear completely destroyed; however, a thin shell of overlying bone will be evident pathologically. A buttress of new bone may be found at the margin of the lesion. Although calcification may be evident microscopically, it is rarely visible on a radiograph.

BENIGN OSSEOUS TUMORS

Osteoma

Osteomas are small, flat, bony growths of cortical bone believed to be localized exaggerations of intramembranous ossification. They appear as small, dense, structureless masses of cortical bone that are usually found in the skull, most often in the frontal or ethmoid sinuses (Fig. 4-12), but occasionally on the surface of the outer table. Less frequently they arise from the inner table, but in this position they suggest the possibility of enostoses secondary to an underlying meningioma. The tumors show little tendency to enlarge and are rarely of clinical significance. Rarely an osteoma in the paranasal sinuses will enlarge sufficiently to cause bulging of the walls of the sinus or obstruct the orifice and lead to retention of secretions and sinusitis. Osteomas occasionally arise on the surface of long bones or ribs.

When multiple osteomas are encountered or a single osteoma is encountered in an unusual site, an examination of the colon is warranted because of the possibility of Gardner's syndrome. The syndrome consists of skin nodules, desmoid tumors, osteomas, and colonic polyps, the polyps having a high potential for malignant degeneration. The osseous lesions frequently precede the appearance of clinical and radiographic evidence of intestinal polyps.

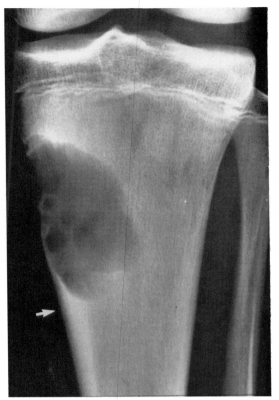

Figure 4–11.   Chondromyxoid fibroma in an 11-year-old boy. An eccentric, sharply defined lesion arising in the metaphysis of the proximal tibia is partially marginated by a thin rim of sclerosis. Note the buttress inferiorly (*arrow*). The medial margin of the cortex is completely destroyed, and the medial margin of the lesion is invisible. (Courtesy of Arthur Newburg, M.D., Boston)

Bone Islands

Bone islands, or enostoses, are asymptomatic, benign, radiodense nodules of compact cortical bone and have little clinical significance other than that they must be distinguished from other pathologic processes. They are probably not true neoplasms. They appear on a radiograph as ovoid, round, or oblong sclerotic areas of variable size but often less than 1.5 cm in diameter, with discrete margins (Fig. 4-13).[16] Thorny, radiating bony spicules extend from the periphery of the lesion, intermingling with the surrounding trabeculae. The lesions do not protrude from the cortical surface of the involved bone. They are most commonly found in the pelvis, proximal femur, and ribs, and occasionally the vertebral bodies.[35] When found in the long bones, they usually occur in the epiphysis. Most

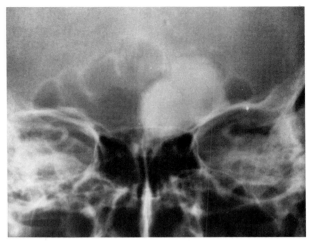

Figure 4–12.   Osteoma of the frontal sinus. A homogeneously dense, sharply marginated, slightly lobulated mass lies in the left frontal sinus. The location, density, and configuration are typical of an osteoma. This lesion is larger than average.

appear to be static; occasionally they may grow and sometimes recede and disappear. In most cases, the bone scan is normal—that is, without increased uptake in the region of the radiographic abnormality.[17] The principal diagnostic consideration is a sclerotic, metastatic focus. The typical radiographic appearance of a bone island, the lack of growth, and a normal bone scan are helpful in the differential diagnosis. Multiple small nodules of sclerotic bone are characteristic of osteopoikilosis, discussed in Chapter 9.

Osteoid Osteoma

Osteoid osteoma is a benign osteoid-forming lesion that in many ways resembles a low-grade chronic bone abscess. Most investigators now consider it to be a reactive process, possibly inflammatory in origin, but its pathogenesis is unknown. About 75% of cases occur between the ages of 11 and 26 years. It is more than twice as common in males. The tibia and femur are frequent sites of involvement, but the lesion may be found in any tubular bones, as well as in the pelvis and vertebrae.[32] The patient complains of pain, usually of mild and intermittent character, worse at night, and characteristically relieved by aspirin. In some patients, pain may be severe and virtually intractable.

The central nidus of tumor is 1.5 cm or less in diameter and made up of irregular masses of osteoid in a vascular fibrous matrix, which may calcify. The histologic appearance is very similar to that of a benign osteoblastoma (giant osteoid osteoma).[8] The distinction is made on the basis of the greatest diameter of the lesion; if less than 1.5 cm, the lesion is an osteoid osteoma; if greater, it is an osteoblastoma. Most osteoid osteomas arise in the cortex but occasionally occur in the periosteum or in the medullary cavity within or adjacent to a joint.[21]

Roentgenographic Features. The cortical osteoid osteoma is seen as a small lucent area surrounded by a dense, compact sclerosis (Fig. 4-14A). The lucency or cavity is often no more than a few millimeters in diameter and may be difficult if not impossible to identify on plain radiographs. Usually the sclerotic reaction is in-

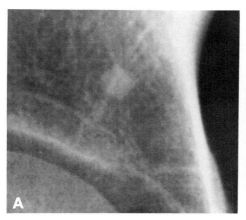

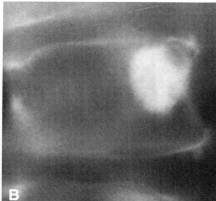

Figure 4–13. Bone island. **(A)** A typical small, dense nodule above the right acetabulum. **(B)** Tomogram demonstrating a radiodense nodule of cortical bone with a sharply defined though slightly irregular peripheral margin in the second lumbar vertebral body.

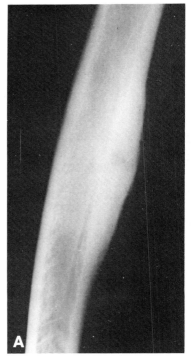

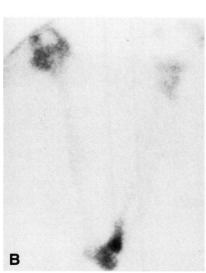

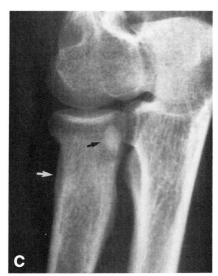

Figure 4–14. Osteoid osteoma. **(A)** Osteoid osteoma of the humerus. A small lucency within the anterior cortex is surrounded by a considerable amount of reactive bone, resulting in thickening of the cortex. **(B and C)** Osteoma of the proximal radius. Bone scan **(B)**. A focus of increased radioactivity is identified just distal to the elbow joint. A discrete, ovoid calcification (*black arrow*) **(C)** surrounded by a zone of radiolucency is identified. Note also the overlying periosteal new-bone formation (*white arrow*).

tense, and it may be sufficient to obscure the cavity. The central lucent area may contain a nidus of calcification (Fig. 4-14C). The periosteal reaction, the sclerotic wall, and normal cortex tend to merge into one another without sharp demarcation. Tomography or CT may be required to visualize the characteristic central lucency. In flat bones, such as the pelvis, a diffuse zone of sclerosis of variable width surrounds the cavity.

Osteoid osteomas arising within the intramedullary canal adjacent to joints are difficult to identify radiographically, since the nidus has no surrounding reactive bone.[11, 21, 32] The nidus may be identified as an intense focal uptake on bone scanning (Fig. 4-14B) and may be visualized by tomography or CT as a small, discrete lucency. Joint effusions, contractures, and periarticular osteoporosis may accompany an intra-articular osteoid osteoma.

Subperiosteal osteoid osteomas are small, round soft-tissue masses measuring approximately 1 to 2 cm in diameter and found immediately adjacent to bone.[32] They most commonly occur about the neck of the femur and in the hands and feet. The masses cause pressure atrophy of the adjacent cortex, which radiographically appears as a saucerization or deeper erosion bordered by a rim of sclerosis. These lesions may cause an effusion in the neighboring joint and periarticular osteoporosis similar to those of the intra-articular, intramedullary osteoid osteoma.

Osteoid osteomas may be located in the posterior elements of the spine, where they typically cause a painful scoliosis. The surrounding reactive bone may be minimal, but the nidus is often calcified when osteoid osteoma is in this location. Bone scanning and tomography or CT are helpful.

The essential part of the tumor lies within the central lucency. This must be removed completely at the time of surgical excision or the lesion will recur. It is not necessary to remove the surrounding reactive cortical bone, even though this may form the major part of the lesion. Bone scanning is helpful to identify the nidus and is particularly useful at the time of surgery to ensure that the nidus has been removed.

Osteoblastoma (Giant Osteoid Osteoma)

Giant osteoid osteoma or osteoblastoma is similar in histologic appearance to the nidus of an osteoid osteoma arbitrarily divided by size as described previously. This is a relatively rare tumor occurring chiefly between the ages of 10 and 20 years. It is most frequently found in the vertebral column, involving the neural arch and pedicles, occasionally in the femur and tibia and rarely in the ribs, hands, feet, facial bones, skull, patella, scapula, or ilium.[27] When the tumor occurs in the posterior elements of the spine, it is characteristically lytic and expansile, with minimal marginal sclerosis. Stippled calcification or plaques of osteoid ossification are often present within the lesion. In the long bones, the lytic areas tend to expand the overlying cortex and are bounded by a sclerotic rim. Osteoblastomas of the spine must be differentiated from giant cell tumors and aneurysmal bone cysts.

BENIGN FIBROUS TUMORS[22]

Nonossifying Fibromas and Benign Fibrous Cortical Defects

Fibrous cortical defects and nonossifying fibromas are not true neoplasms but represent a localized defect in bone growth. These lesions have been known in the past as xanthomas or fibroxanthomas or xanthofibromas. They are found in children and adolescents. It has been estimated that 30% to 40% of all children will develop one or more fibrous cortical defects. The lesions are rarely identified before the age of 2, are most frequently encountered around the age of 10 years, and begin to involute at age 14. The lesions are rarely encountered in mature adults.

The only difference between a nonossifying fibroma and benign cortical defect is size. The pathologic characteristics of the two are essentially the same. If a lesion is more than $1\frac{1}{2}$ to 2 cm in its greatest dimension, it is usually referred to as a nonossifying fibroma.

There are usually no symptoms referable to the lesions. They are found incidentally during examinations performed for other reasons, usually trauma. These lesions are encountered in the lower extremities and are usually metaphyseal in location. Frequent sites are the distal femur, proximal and distal tibia, and proximal and distal fibula. They may be single or multiple.

Roentgenographic Features. These tumors are so characteristic in their radiographic appearance that the majority can be diagnosed with absolute assurance on the basis of their radiographic features, without requiring biopsy or treatment.

The benign cortical defect is a small area of rarefaction, sharply marginated and bound by a thin rim of sclerosis (Fig. 4-15). It often has a scalloped border and may appear multiseptated. It is found in or directly beneath the cortex and may cause a slight localized bulging or thining of the overlying cortex.

Nonossifying fibroma is a larger lesion measuring more than 2 cm in its greatest dimension. It also appears as a sharply marginated area of radiolucency bound by a thin sclerotic shell (Fig. 4-16). There is often an expansion or bulging of the cortex, but no periosteal reaction occurs. The lesions are eccentric and rarely extend completely across the shaft but may

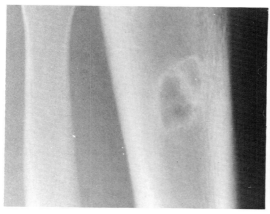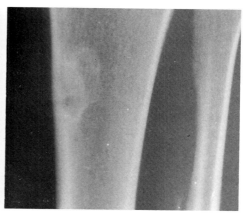

Figure 4–15. Benign fibrous cortical defect of the tibia. The lesion is radiolucent but is limited by a thin, slightly lobulated sclerotic margin of bone. This was an incidental finding on a radiograph obtained because of trauma.

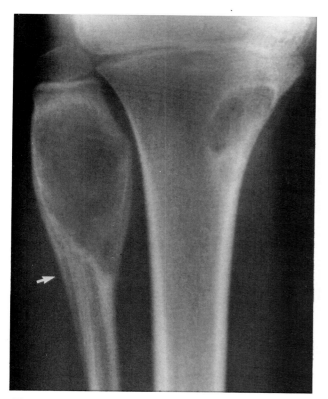

Figure 4–16. Two nonossifying fibromas in an 11-year-old boy. A typical nonossifying fibroma with eccentric location and a thin rim of sclerosis is present in the proximal tibia. The lesion of the proximal fibula has enlarged and expanded the cortex, but note that the cortex remains intact. There is a buttress of bone formed inferiorly and laterally (*arrow*). (Courtesy of Theodore Keats, M.D., Charlottesville, Virginia)

occupy the width of smaller bones such as the fibula and may expand them. Pathologic fractures may occur in larger lesions.

These lesions rarely persist into adult life, but occasionally in younger adults some remnant of an involuting fibrous lesion may be identified, often by an area of amorphous ossification on the endosteal aspect of the cortex within the metaphysis.

Desmoplastic Fibroma

Desmoplastic fibromas are rare benign tumors consisting of fibroblasts set in a matrix of collagen fibers, and they must be distinguished histologically from a low-grade fibrosarcoma.[22] They are locally aggressive lesions that tend to recur after resection. The average age at presentation is 25 years. Radiographically, they present as purely lytic, honeycomb, often expansile lesions of the metaphysis, usually surrounded by a sclerotic rim.

Ossifying Fibroma

Ossifying fibroma is an unusual tumor occurring in the diaphysis of the tibia and fibula, in the mandible, and in the facial bones. In the tibia and fibula, the lesion usually occurs in the first decade of life and is manifested by an enlargement and bowing of the shaft.[2] Characteristic radiographic features include an eccentric radiolucency that may be solitary or bubbly.[22] The external surface of the cortex is expanded and thin. Osteoid occurs within the lesion, resulting in a homogeneous amorphous opacification of the tumor.

In the mandible, the lesion is expansile and radiolucent; in the sinuses, it is also expansile but opacifies the sinus. The lesion often contains hazy, osteoid calcification and therefore may appear homogeneously dense.

CYSTIC TUMORS OF BONE

The lesions described as cystic tumors of bone do not have the same tissue of origin. Most are true, fluid-filled cystic lesions, but others are solid. They all have in common the radiographic appearance of a cyst, being more or less sharply outlined, radiolucent cavities in bone.

Unicameral Bone Cyst (Simple or Solitary Bone Cyst)

Unicameral or solitary bone cyst is a lesion of unknown origin arising in childhood and adolescence and found most commonly in the proximal humerus and proximal femur.[25] It may also occur in the tibia, fibula, or smaller bones such as the calcaneus and in flat bones, including the ribs and pelvis. It is twice as common in males. The lesions are usually asymptomatic and discovered incidentally on a radiograph obtained for another reason. Many present with a pathologic fracture. After fracture, some cysts heal by ossification. Most, however, do not and eventually require surgical intervention and packing with bone chips. More recently, unicameral cysts have been successfully treated by direct percutaneous injection of steroids into the cyst.[14]

Roentgenographic Features. A unicameral bone cyst is an expansile, radiolucent, centrally situated lesion with a well-defined, thin, sclerotic margin (Fig. 4-17). The lesion characteristically arises in the metaphysis and abuts against the physis or growth plate. In the most common location, the proximal humerus, it does abut against the growth plate (Fig. 4-17A), but in the proximal femur it is usually located in the intertrochanteric region and rarely extends into the femoral neck (Fig. 4-17B). It does not cross the growth plate to involve the epiphysis. The cortex is often thinned by

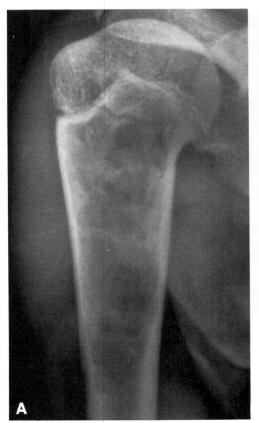
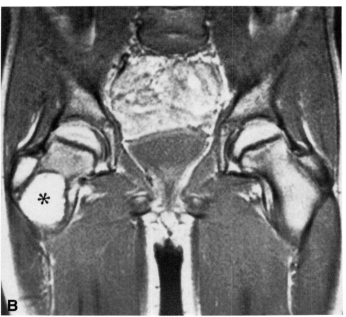

Figure 4–17. Unicameral bone cysts. (**A**) Simple bone cyst of the proximal humerus in a 13-year-old boy. The lesion is sharply defined, slightly expansile with endosteal erosion, and abuts the physis. (**B**) MRI of a unicameral bone cyst (*asterisk*) of the intertrochanteric region of the proximal femur in a 10-year-old boy. The lesion is sharply defined by a thin rim of cortical bone.

the expansion. Most cysts are not septated but composed of a single chamber, thus the term *unicameral*.[36] Some cysts have a multilocular appearance as though composed of multiple communicating cavities, but these result from ridging along the cortex rather than actual bone septa within the lesion.

Bone cysts presenting with a pathologic fracture may be noted to contain a spicule or fragment of bone in the dependent portion of the lesion. This is termed the *fallen fragment sign* and, although not common, is quite characteristic of a unicameral bone cyst.[36]

During its active phase, the cyst is located near or adjacent to the epiphyseal plate. When it becomes inactive, normal metaphyseal bone may form at the growth plate and the lesion appears to migrate toward the diaphysis and may be found some distance from the growth plate. These cysts have a thin sclerotic border and may be slightly expansile. It is uncommon for a simple cyst to be located in the diaphysis, and when faced with a lesion of this description, one would have to also consider a brown tumor of hyperparathyroidism and fibrous dysplasia.

Giant Cell Tumor

Giant cell tumor is an expansile, destructive lesion usually found in the end of long bones after epiphyseal closure and thus is rarely encountered in persons younger than 17 years of age.[7] It is essentially a lesion of early adult life and is uncommon after the age of 35. Its favorite locations are the distal femur, proximal tibia, and distal end of the radius (Fig. 4-18). It may arise in

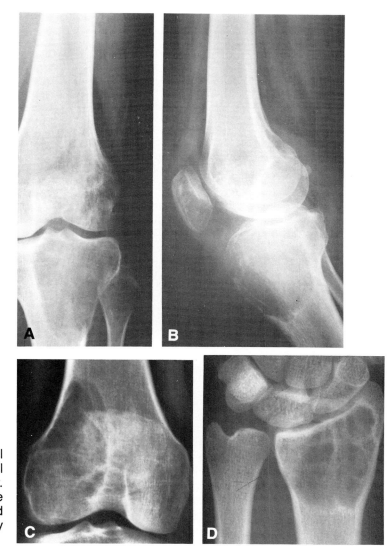

Figure 4–18. (**A** and **B**) AP and lateral views of a giant cell tumor of the proximal tibia. (**C**) Giant cell tumor of the distal femur. (**D**) Giant cell tumor of the distal radius. The lesions are radiolucent, eccentric, and sharply defined, and they characteristically extend to the joint surface.

the ilium and other pelvic bones and in the ribs, spine, clavicle, metacarpals, metatarsals, and tarsal bones.

Roentgenographic Features. The lesion is radiolucent and arises at the site of the epiphyseal scar, extending into both the metaphysis and the epiphysis. Initially the lesion is often eccentric, but as it enlarges may involve the entire width of the bone. In a smaller bone such as a metacarpal or fibula, giant cell tumors expand and balloon the bone. Characteristically the lesion extends to the subarticular bone or joint surface but does not involve the joint. The lesion usually has a sharp zone of transition and is fairly well demarcated from normal bone, but there is no sclerotic rim. At times, the zone of transition is wider and the medullary extent of the lesion is not as sharply defined (Fig. 4-19). The lesions may appear to contain thin septa of bone, but these are actually ridges on the inner surface of the cortex and are not true septations. There is no periosteal new-bone formation unless there has been a pathologic fracture. Large lesions may destroy portions of the cortex.

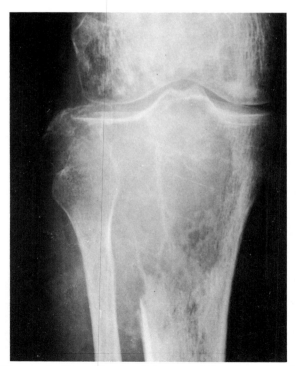

Figure 4–19.   Giant cell tumor of the tibia. A lytic tumor that has expanded and has apparently destroyed the lateral tibial cortex. The margin is less sharply defined than those in Figure 4-18, suggesting the possibility of a malignancy, although this lesion was benign.

Benign giant cell tumors have a malignant counterpart.[33] Recurrences following surgical therapy are suggestive of malignancy. Lesions that appear aggressive, with destruction of the cortex and a wider zone of transition, also suggest malignancy. Local recurrence following curettage is common. Pulmonary metastases are very rare and tend to be indolent.

Giant Cell Reparative Granuloma

Giant cell reparative granuloma is an uncommon lytic lesion that usually involves the mandible, but it more recently has been recognized to occur in the metacarpals, metatarsals, and phalanges.[15] Typically it presents as a markedly expansile and ballooned lesion in small bones.

Aneurysmal Bone Cyst

Aneurysmal bone cyst may arise de novo or in association with various benign lesions such as giant cell tumor, chondroblastoma, chondromyxoid fibroma, fibrous dysplasia, or malignant tumors, including osteosarcoma and chondrosarcoma.[8, 9] One must be aware of this possibility when the diagnosis of an aneurysmal bone cyst is made. Small biopsy specimens or biopsies of only one portion of such a tumor may be misleading. In general, an aneurysmal bone cyst occurring under 20 years of age is primary, whereas an increasing percentage of those occurring beyond this age are secondary and associated with other tumors.

Approximately half are found in the major long bones, and the remainder in the axial skeleton, particularly the spine,[3] sacrum, and pelvis.[25] The posterior elements of the vertebrae rather than the body are the usual sites of origin or maximal involvement.

The lesion may be difficult to distinguish from a giant cell tumor. The age of the patient is helpful. Eighty-five percent of giant cell tumors occur in patients over 20 years of age, whereas 78% of aneurysmal bone cysts occur in patients less than 20 years old.

Roentgenographic Features. Aneurysmal bone cysts often have a characteristic radiographic appearance (Figs. 4-20 and 4-21).[6] Typically, the lesion consists of an eccentric ballooned or aneurysmal, expanded radiolucency originating in the metaphysis. The margin is usually well circumscribed, with or without a sclerotic rim. Trabeculation is sometimes seen within the lesion, but there is no significant mineralization or calcification. Soft-tissue extension is produced by bulging of the periosteum, resulting in a thin layer of new bone outlining the periphery of the tumor, which may or may not be visible. The elevation of the periosteum may result in a buttress or Codman's triangle at the

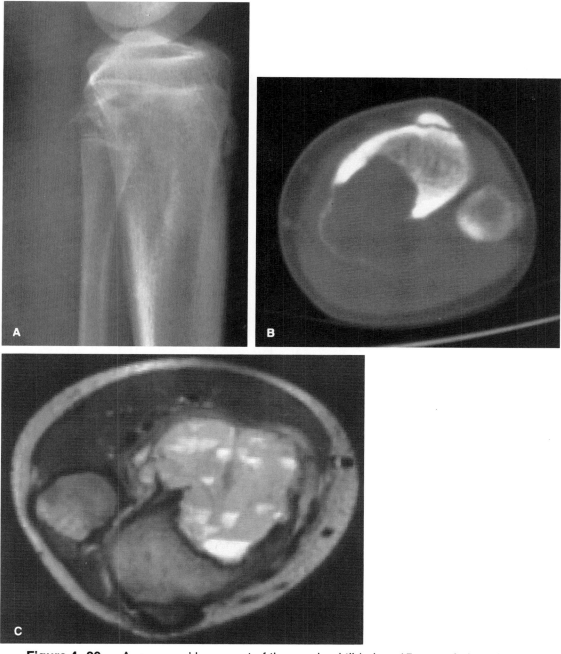

Figure 4–20.   Aneursymal bone cyst of the proximal tibia in a 15-year-old boy. (**A**) An eccentric, markedly expansile lesion of the distal tibial metaphysis is bordered posteriorly by a very thin rim of bone. There is no matrix within the lesion, which is poorly defined anteriorly and superiorly. (**B**) CT scan demonstrates the sharply defined thin rim of sclerosis and the eccentric nature of the lesion. There is a variation in the density within the lesion suggesting fluid–fluid levels. (**C**) T2-weighted axial image confirms the presence of fluid–fluid levels within the lesion. Examination was performed in the supine position. Note that the thin rim of sclerosis is not as well defined by MRI as it was by CT. (Case courtesy of W. Michael Hensley, M.D., Parkersburg, West Virginia)

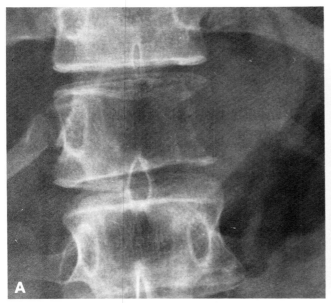

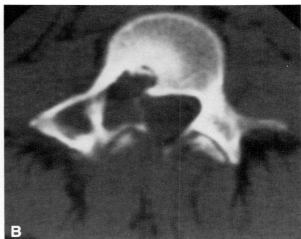

Figure 4–21.   Two cases of aneurysmal bone cyst of the spine. (**A**) This lesion involves the left side of the body and arch of T12 and the adjacent portion of the 12th rib. Note the absence of the left pedicle. The lesion is purely destructive. (**B**) CT of an aneurysmal bone cyst of L4 demonstrates an expansile lesion involving the pedicle, transverse process, and facet, with extension into the vertebral body. The lesion is obviously expansile and purely lytic.

periphery of the lesion. Aneurysmal bone cysts have been shown to demonstrate a fluid–blood level on CT and MRI (see Fig. 4-20C). Though highly suggestive of an aneurysmal bone cyst, fluid–blood levels have also been reported in cases of giant cell tumor, telangiectatic osteosarcoma, metastases, and chondroblastoma.

The typical spinal lesion[3] consists of a purely lytic process of the posterior elements and body or less commonly is limited to the posterior vertebral elements alone (Fig. 4-21). Involvement of the body alone is rare. An unusual feature of the aneurysmal bone cyst is its ability to cross the disc space and involve adjacent vertebrae. As in long bones, inability to visualize the thin outer cortical shell may suggest malignancy. The principal differential diagnostic consideration of such an expansile lesion of the spine is an osteoblastoma.

Intraosseous Ganglion

Intraosseous ganglion usually arises in the epiphysis or adjacent metaphysis, particularly in the region of the medial malleolus of the distal tibia and in the carpal and tarsal bones.[13] Radiographically it appears as a solitary, sharply defined lucency with a thin rim of sclerosis. The small, common, rounded cystlike lesion in the neck of the femur, although suggestive of an intra-

osseous ganglion, is actually a normal variant—the so-called herniation pit, described in Chapter 8.

Post-Traumatic Bone Cyst

Small cystic areas often found in the bones of the wrist and hand may be caused by trauma, possibly forming as a result of a localized hemorrhage within the bone. Multiple cysts of this type have been reported in workers using pneumatic air drills. Similar cystlike lesions also are found in persons without a history of previous injury. Some of these may be islands of cartilage that failed to ossify during the course of skeletal growth.

Synovial cysts are discussed in Chapter 3, Diseases of the Joints.

Brown tumor of hyperparathyroidism is discussed in Chapter 6, Metabolic, Endocrine, and Related Bone Diseases.

Epidermoid Cyst (Cholesteatoma)

A sharply marginated, cystic-appearing tumor is occasionally encountered in the cranial bones, usually in children or young adults. Pathologically, it is a squamous epithelium-lined cyst filled with mushy, pearl-colored material consisting of cholesterol and cellular debris. These tumors are known as cholesteatomas, epidermoidomas, or epidermoid cysts. When the cyst is as described previously, the term *epidermoid cyst* is used. When dermal structures (hair, teeth, and so on) are also included, the lesion is known as a *dermoid cyst*. The latter are usually midline structures found either within the occiput or anteriorly in the region of the nasion, whereas the epidermoid elements are found throughout the skull. Occasionally, primary cholesteatomas are encountered in the temporal bone.

In the skull, epidermoid cysts are of congenital origin, arising from epidermoid inclusions at the time of closure of the neural groove. The lesion arises in the diploic space and expands the inner and outer tables (Fig. 4-22). Viewed *en face*, it characteristically appears as a sharply outlined rounded or ovoid area of bone deficit with a thin surrounding zone of sclerosis. The edge of the defect is often slightly scalloped in places. Viewed tangentially, it will be seen that the tables have been expanded symmetrically. The tumor grows very slowly and may be asymptomatic except for the deformity caused by the mass.

Epidermoid Inclusion Cyst

A lesion pathologically similar to the epidermoid cyst is found in the terminal phalanx. These lesions are acquired by the implantation of epidermal cells occurring as the result of an injury such as a puncture wound by a sewing needle. Radiographically, the lesion presents as a sharply circumscribed round or oval destructive lesion, often with a very clearly defined, thin sclerotic rim marking the border between it and the adjacent bone.[11, 32] A glomus tumor may have a similar appearance in the distal phalanx.

Hemangioma of Bone

Hemangiomas of bone are uncommon tumors except in the cranial vault and vertebrae. Multiple lesions are common in the spine but not elsewhere. They are benign lesions corresponding histologically to the more frequent hemangiomas of the skin and subcutaneous tissues. Osseous hemangiomas are relatively common in adults but are infrequent in children. In the skull, the lesion presents as a small palpable mass but is usually found incidentally in a vertebra. Rarely, the tumor may cause collapse of a vertebral body and result in clinical signs and symptoms of vertebral compression. The rare tumors of the long tubular bones may cause symptoms because of growth of the tumor mass.

Roentgenographic Features. In the skull, the lesion is a round, lucent area about 1 to 2 cm in diameter, often in the frontal bone. When viewed *en face*, it has a fine granular appearance. When viewed in profile, the lesion is a smoothly convex bony mass protruding from the outer table containing characteristic and fine vertical, radiating sunburst-like striations (Fig. 4-23A, B). Rare hemangiomas arising in the cortex of tubular bones or in flat bones such as the scapula or pelvis are similar in appearance to cranial hemangiomas. In extracranial locations, this might possibly suggest an osteogenic sarcoma; however, the margin of a hemangioma is sharp and distinct without an accompanying soft-tissue mass. Clinical symptoms are minimal or nonexistent.

In the spine, hemangiomas produce coarse vertical

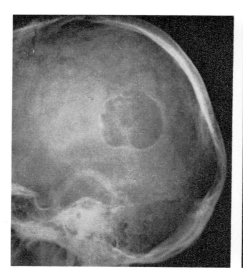
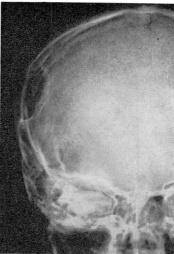

Figure 4–22. Epidermoid cyst of the skull. An area of radiolucency is surrounded by a thin rim of sclerosis. The lesion is scalloped.

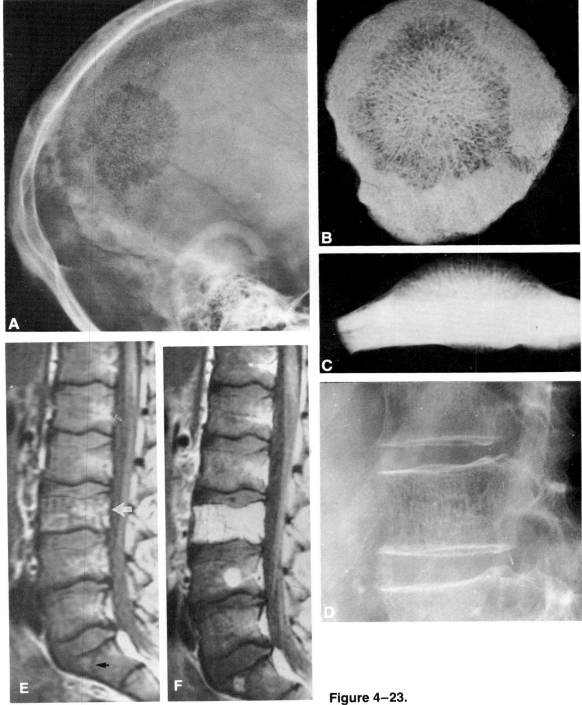

Figure 4–23.

striations within the vertebral body (Fig. 4-23C). The normal trabecular architecture is more or less completely replaced by these alternating vertical trabeculations and the clear spaces between them. Short horizontal striations may extend between two or more of the vertical trabeculations to produce a honeycomb appearance. In some persons, a large number of vertebral bodies will show some features of this pattern, perhaps to only a slight degree. In these, the changes represent hardly more than an anatomic variation. The vertebral processes are infrequently affected, and, rarely, the bone is eroded and soft-tissue extension produces a paravertebral soft-tissue mass.

Hemangiomas are commonly encountered as incidental findings when the spine is examined by MRI. They appear as areas of mixed signal intensity, both intermediate and high, within the vertebral body on T1-weighted images, which become bright, high signal on T2 (Fig. 4-23E, F). Hemangiomas within the vertebral body are interspersed with fat, accounting for foci of increased signal on T1-weighted images. The vascular component itself is of intermediate signal on T1. Foci of fat are commonly found within vertebral bodies by MRI. They are readily identified by high signal on T1 but reduced signal on T2, which distinguishes them from vertebral hemangioma.

Hemangiomas rarely occur in the intramedullary portion of long bones, and when they do so are expansile and trabeculated in a manner somewhat similar to that in the vertebral body.

Soft-tissue hemangiomas and arteriovenous malformations occasionally invade bone, producing erosions. Phleboliths are often present in the soft-tissue component and should suggest the diagnosis.

Diffuse Cystic Angiomatosis (Hemangiomatosis and Lymphangiomatosis)

Diffuse cystic angiomatosis, a rare condition, is a congenital malformation involving endothelium-lined vessels that may contain blood or lymph. Widespread skeletal involvement, including the skull, vertebrae, ribs, and long bones, produces numerous lucent lesions of varying sizes and shapes. The cortex may be eroded and expanded. The condition is usually discovered in an adolescent following a pathologic fracture. Individual lesions are clearly defined and many have a thin sclerotic margin. The prognosis is usually good unless the condition is associated with visceral involvement. Arteriography is useful in establishing the presence of visceral lesions. Malignancy is always a possibility, with hemangiosarcoma usually rapidly fatal.

Spontaneous Osteolysis (Disappearing Bone)

There are a number of syndromes associated with osteolysis that can be differentiated clinically and radiographically.[11, 32] They are as follows: (1) Idiopathic hereditary osteolysis. This is inherited as an autosomal dominant trait and manifested in early childhood by pain that may resemble arthritis. The carpal and tarsal bones are involved first, and the bone destruction may extend to involve adjacent long bones. There is no angiomatosis, no renal disease, and no threat to life. (2) Autosomal recessive carpal and tarsal osteolysis. Several syndromes have been described in which there is progressive and extensive destruction of carpals and tarsals. Elbows may also be involved. (3) Idiopathic osteolysis with nephropathy. This also involves the carpal, tarsal, and adjacent tubular bones of young children. These patients develop azotemia and usually die early in adult life. (4) Massive osteolysis of Gorham. This is a painless condition usually affecting the proximal skeleton; it is usually unifocal. There is complete destruction of all or part of involved bone by angiomatous tissue, which may spread to adjacent bones and soft tissues. This syndrome occurs in children and young adults and is not life threatening unless vital structures are encroached on. Some of these patients

◄ **Figure 4–23.** Hemangioma of bone. (**A**) Hemangioma of the skull. Note the somewhat granular appearance in the parietal bone. (**B**) Excised specimen of a benign hemangioma of the skull shown in two projections. Characteristic linear striation is noted in the tangential view. (Courtesy of Radiological Registry of the Armed Forces Institute of Pathology, Washington, DC) (**C**) Hemangioma of a vertebral body. Note the characteristic palisade-like vertical striations. (**E** and **F**) MRI examination of multiple vertebral hemangiomas in a 33-year-old man. T1-weighted image (**E**) demonstrates obvious vertical striations across the entire L3 vertebral body (*white arrow*). The signal within this vertebra is mixed, containing some foci of higher signal. There are smaller foci of signal within the midportion of the fourth lumbar vertebra and the first sacral segment (*black arrow*). T1-weighted image (**F**) following administration of gadolinium demonstrates an extremely bright signal from the entire third lumbar vertebral body and small, rounded similar foci within L4 and the first sacral segment. These findings are typical of hemangioma. T2-weighted images would give a similar though less intense bright signal.

recover spontaneously, often with some residual deformity. (5) Post-traumatic osteolysis. This is a relatively rare phenomenon occurring principally in the outer margin of the clavicle following repeated injury of the acromioclavicular joint. A similar process has also been reported following injuries of the distal ulna.

The radiographic features of these osteolytic syndromes are those of bone destruction without evidence of callus formation, sclerosis, or an associated soft-tissue mass.

Lipoma

Lipoma is an extremely rare lesion of bone usually reported within either the calcaneus or proximal femur.[28] It presents as a lucent lesion with a sclerotic rim that is characteristically thin in the calcaneus but wider in the proximal femur. Occasionally, calcification fills most of the

lesion. Lipomas commonly arise in the intertrochanteric region of the proximal femur (Fig. 4-24) or in the calcaneus. They are sharply defined, rarely expansile, and sufficiently characteristic to allow the diagnosis to be established with confidence by radiographic and CT criteria. This is important because practically all patients are asymptomatic and the lesion is only found incidentally on radiographs obtained for trauma or other reasons. Lipomas have no malignant potential and are rarely the focus of a pathologic fracture; therefore, once the true nature of the lesion is recognized, no surgical intervention is required. Lipomas represent another good example of a "leave me alone" lesion.

Synovioma

Synovioma is discussed in Chapter 3, Diseases of the Joints.

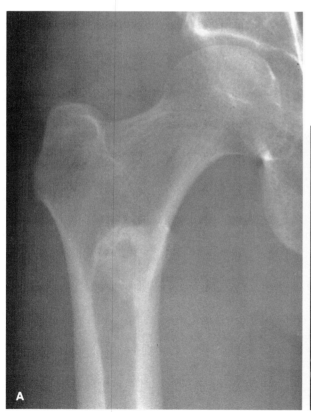
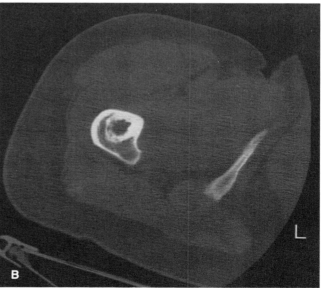

Figure 4–24.   Intramedullary lipoma in an asymptomatic 47-year-old woman. (**A**) Note the sharply marginated, slightly eccentric lesion with a heavily calcified, swirling thick margin of calcification at the level of the lesser trochanter. The overlying cortex is intact. (**B**) CT scan confirms the sharp definition of the lesion with a thick, irregular border contiguous with the cortex anteriorly and medially. The density of the center of the lesion is that of fat and confirms the diagnosis of lipoma.

Neurofibroma

Neurofibromatosis, or von Recklinghausen's disease, is discussed in Chapter 9. Neurofibroma occurring as a solitary lesion without the other stigmata of von Recklinghausen's disease is a moderately common lesion. A neurofibroma of an intercostal nerve causes an extrapleural soft-tissue mass, often associated with pressure erosion of the adjacent inferior cortex of the rib. If the mass is large, the rib interspace may be locally widened. Tumors arising from a spinal nerve root often are of the dumbbell type, with intra- and extraspinal extensions. They are best evaluated by CT. Erosion of vertebral pedicles and widening of the intervertebral foramen are common, and the intraspinal component may cause concave erosion of the posterior surface of the vertebral body (Fig. 4-25). The extraspinal component can be visualized as a rounded, soft-tissue mass adjacent to the spine in the thoracic area. In the lumbar spine, the extraspinal mass usually cannot be seen on a plain film unless very large, when it may cause a lateral bulge of the psoas muscle. Neurofibroma of a long tubular bone may cause a localized cystlike lucency in the shaft. Occasionally it is seen as a small excavation in the cortex of the bone, when it is described as a "pit" or "cave" defect. Neurofibromas of the cranial nerves often cause enlargement of the corresponding foramen. The acoustic nerve is the most frequent site of the tumor within the skull.

Teratoma

A teratoma is a tumor containing all of the germinal tissues—ectodermal, mesodermal, and entodermal. A malignant tumor, either carcinoma or sarcoma, may develop within a teratoma, and the lesion is then referred to as a malignant teratoma. External teratomatous malformations are most frequently encountered in the upper jaw and the sacrococcygeal area. Practically all teratomas contain bone or calcified cartilage. The normal structure, jaw or sacrum, to which the teratoma is attached often shows abnormal ossification and may be grossly distorted. The characteristic locations, the presence of the mass at birth, and the finding of bone or calcification within it are reliable diagnostic signs (Fig. 4-26).

Other sacrococcygeal masses include meningocele and myelomeningocele, chordoma, and neurofibroma.

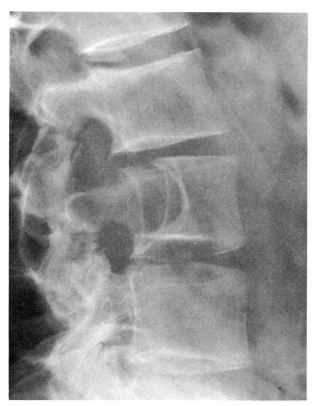

Figure 4–25. Neurofibroma. A large neurofibroma arising from a lumbar nerve root has resulted in pressure erosion of the posterior aspect of the vertebral body and adjacent posterior elements of the spine.

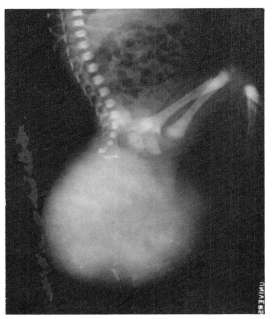

Figure 4–26. Sacrococcygeal teratoma. This large mass found in a newborn infant contains scattered areas of calcification and bone. The lower sacrum and coccyx are deformed.

MALIGNANT BONE TUMORS

SECONDARY MALIGNANCIES OF BONE (METASTATIC CARCINOMA)

Primary malignancies of bone are relatively rare. Secondary malignancies of bone are as common as primary bone tumors are rare. As a rule, when a bone lesion is observed in a patient over 45 years of age, the primary considerations must be metastatic carcinoma and multiple myeloma.

Cancer of the breast and prostate account for the majority of bone metastases, and the lungs, kidneys, and thyroid are relatively frequent sources. Metastatic disease to bone develops in two-thirds of carcinomas of the breast and in 50% of carcinomas of prostate. Twenty-five percent of tumors in the lungs and kidneys produce skeletal metastases, but skeletal metastases occur in only 10% or less of all other malignancies. Carcinomas of the gastrointestinal tract (esophagus, stomach, pancreas, and colon) and genital tract (ovaries, uterus, cervix, and testicles), though common, rarely metastasize to bone. Likewise, sarcomas rarely metastasize to bone.

The favorite sites of metastases are the axial skeleton (the spine, pelvis, ribs, and skull) and the appendicular skeleton in the proximal ends of the humerus and femur. All are sites of persistent red marrow. Metastases distal to the elbow and knees are infrequent but may occur.

Bone metastases sometimes present with a pathologic fracture, but most present with a history of pain at the site of the metastatic deposit. Some are occult and may be discovered incidentally on a routine radiologic examination or bone scan. Bone scanning is much more sensitive than radiography in the detection of bone destruction. Fifty percent of trabecular bone must be destroyed within an area such as the vertebral body before it is radiographically apparent. Neoplastic deposits may be detected by bone scanning when as little as 5% to 15% of trabecular bone is destroyed within a given area, well before they are evident on the radiograph.

^{99m}Tc-MDP is the most common nuclide used in bone scanning. Because of its sensitivity, a radionuclide bone scan should be the initial examination for the detection of metastatic disease to bone.[5, 20] Only 3% of all patients with x-ray documentation of metastases have no evidence of increased uptake on bone scan. All sites of activity suggesting metastatic disease can then be radiographed for further evaluation (Figs. 4-27 and 4-28). In symptomatic patients, the reverse order of examination is often used—that is, sites of pain are evaluated by radiographs, and, in those cases in which

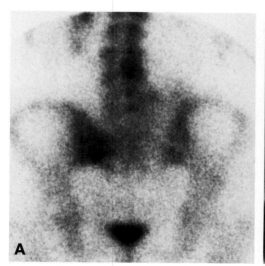
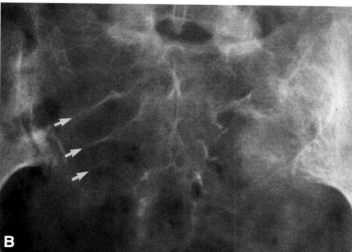

Figure 4–27. Metastatic carcinoma of the breast to the sacrum. **(A)** Posterior view of a bone scan demonstrates increased radioactivity in the left sacral ala. There is also a focus in the lower lumbar vertebra. **(B)** A subtle, lytic destructive lesion present in the left sacral ala is manifested by destruction of the sacral foraminal lines. The normal sacral foraminal lines on the right are identified by *arrows*. Note that the bone scan is actually a mirror image of the radiograph, since it was obtained and is displayed as though looking from the back, whereas the radiograph was obtained and displayed looking from the front of the individual.

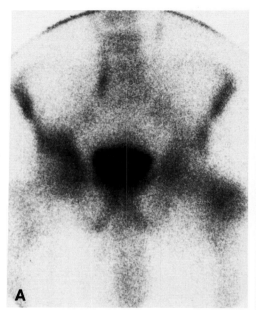

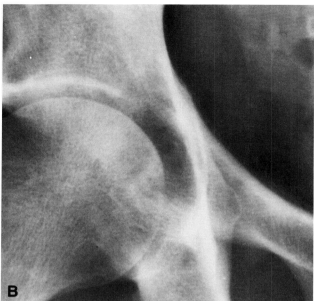

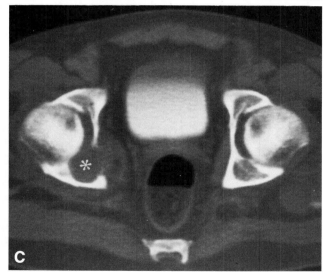

Figure 4–28. Metastasis to the right acetabulum from carcinoma of the lung. (**A**) Anterior view of a bone scan demonstrates increased radioactivity in the right acetabulum and left greater trochanter. (**B**) Closeup view of the right acetabulum demonstrates a vague radiolucency medially. (**C**) CT demonstrates bone destruction in the medial acetabulum posteriorly (*asterisk*), with an adjacent soft-tissue mass.

the radiograph is negative or equivocal, a bone scan is obtained.

CT and possibly MRI are more sensitive than radiography in the detection of metastases, particularly in the spine and pelvis. Therefore, in those cases with a positive bone scan in the spine and negative x-rays, consideration should be given to a CT[18] or MRI examination (see Figs. 4-28 and 4-32*B*).

MRI is a distinct advantage in those patients presenting with neurologic findings or significant collapse of vertebral bodies on plain film radiographs since it directly visualizes extension of disease from the ver-

tebra that abuts, surrounds, or compresses the spinal cord (Fig. 4–32*B*).

Roentgenographic Features. Most metastases are osteolytic and purely destructive; a smaller number are osteoblastic and produce well-defined areas of increased density. Still others are of a mixed variety, combining both osteolytic and osteoblastic types.

Osteolytic Type. The lesion begins in the medullary canal and is poorly marginated, often with a moderate to wide zone of transition. The margins are somewhat frayed and seldom sharp and smooth, and in almost all cases they lack a sclerotic rim (Fig. 4–29). As the lesion grows, it erodes and thins the cortex, possibly leading to a pathologic fracture. There is usually no periosteal new-bone formation. The most common sources for osteolytic metastases are the breast, lungs, kidney, and thyroid.

Tumors of the kidney and thyroid are prone to have a single metastatic focus, whereas metastases from breast or lung carcinoma are more often multiple when first encountered. Occasionally, metastatic foci from carcinomas of the kidney and thyroid are expansile and coarsely trabeculated, resulting in a soap-bubble appearance (Fig. 4–30). A solitary myeloma may have a similar appearance (see Fig. 4–41).

Metastases are occasionally found limited to the cortex[10] and usually arise from a primary bronchogenic carcinoma of the lung and rarely from other sources (see Fig. 4–29). These are probably due to unique characteristics of the cortical blood supply (see Cortical Bone Abscess in Chapter 5). When small, the lesions

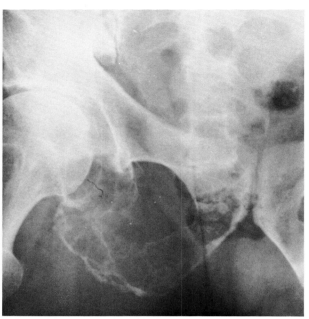

Figure 4–30. Osteolytic expansile metastasis from carcinoma of the thyroid. The metastasis destroys and expands the inferior ischiopubic ramus.

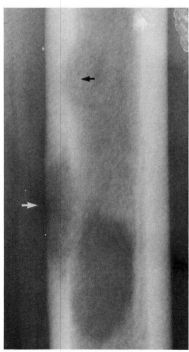

Figure 4–29. Metastasis of the femoral shaft from carcinoma of the breast. Distally there is a lytic, ill-defined lesion in the intramedullary canal. The *white arrow* demonstrates an ill-defined, lytic lesion within the cortex. The *black arrow* demonstrates a poorly defined intramedullary lesion, identified by the presence of endosteal erosion.

present as a well-defined radiolucency within the cortex. When they are larger, the overlying cortex is destroyed, leaving an elongated saucerlike defect on the outer margin of the cortex.

Osteolytic metastases within ribs are commonly identified on chest radiographs by the "extrapleural sign" (Fig. 4-31). This is created as a metastatic focus grows, destroys, and expands beyond the rib, lifting the underlying pleura and bulging into the lung. This sign is seen in profile on the chest radiograph as a moundlike protrusion arising from the chest wall, broader at its base than height, and having obtuse angles with the chest wall. The surface of the lesion is smooth and sharply defined against the underlying lung. Multiple myeloma (Fig. 4-31*B*) and benign tumors may present in a similar fashion. Fractures of the ribs can also be recognized by an extrapleural sign due to the surrounding hematoma.

The principal sign of spinal involvement is a vertebral body collapse with cortical destruction and often a small surrounding soft-tissue mass. The disease often extends into the pedicles and occasionally into the neural arches. Rarely, metastatic disease is limited to posterior elements. Involvement of the pedicles may be evidenced on anteroposterior radiographs of the spine by a destruction of some portion of its oval, cortical outline, the "pedicle sign" (Fig. 4-32*A*). In

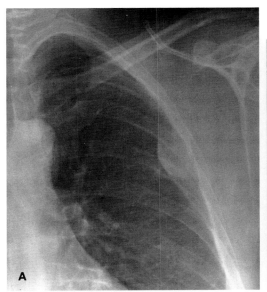

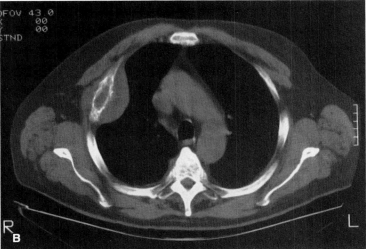

Figure 4–31.   Two cases of extrapleural sign. (**A**) Metastatic squamous cell carcinoma of the pharynx involving the anterolateral aspect of the third left rib. The lesion has a smooth, sharply defined interface with the lung and is broader at its base than its height. The angles formed with the chest wall are obtuse. Close inspection reveals destruction of the underlying rib. (**B**) Multiple myeloma in the anterolateral margin of the third right rib in a 66-year-old man. The rib is expanded and the cortex destroyed. The lesion has a sharp, smooth interface with the underlying lung. The lesion is characteristically broader at its base than its height.

actuality, destruction of any portion of cortical bone within the spine, not just the pedicle, is suggestive of metastatic disease. CT and MRI are more sensitive than standard film radiography in the detection of metastatic disease in the spine and elsewhere (Fig. 4-32*B*). In patients having a positive bone scan and a negative radiograph, a CT or MRI examination should be considered since either may demonstrate areas of cortical and trabecular destruction before they are evident on the radiograph. In the presence of a metastatic deposit, the normal high-intensity signal from the marrow fat found on a T1-weighted MR image is replaced by a lower-intensity signal from a metastatic deposit. Cortical destruction is better seen by CT than MRI.

The disease that must be considered in the differential diagnosis is multiple myeloma. In the spine, myeloma is less likely to involve a pedicle but more likely to have a large soft-tissue mass than metastatic carcinoma. In the skull and long bones, the myeloma deposits tend to be multiple and more sharply defined.

Osteoblastic Type (Sclerotic). Osteoblastic metastases are characterized by their pronounced density. About 10% of carcinomas of the breast and virtually 90% of carcinomas of the prostate are osteoblastic. They may occur as more or less isolated, rounded sclerotic densities or as a diffuse sclerosis involving a large area in the bone such as an entire vertebral body or multiple bones (Figs. 4-33 and 4-34). The density within the lesion is fairly uniform, amorphous, and homogeneous, similar to that of cortical bone. The normal trabecular architecture is lost. The involved intramedullary bone approaches cortical bone in density; thus, for instance, where the entire width of a rib is involved one cannot distinguish between the cortex and medullary portion of the bone.

The principal differential diagnostic task is to distinguish blastic metastases from Paget's disease. In Paget's disease, the cortex is thickened and the overall width of the bone increased, with coarsening of the trabecular pattern of intramedullary bone. In metastatic disease, the patches of density are amorphous but without coarsening of the trabecular pattern, and the width of the cortex and size of the bone remain normal. With diffuse involvement of the entire skeleton, as sometimes happens in prostatic carcinoma, there may be a superficial resemblance to osteopetrosis.

In males, the sclerotic metastases are usually sec-

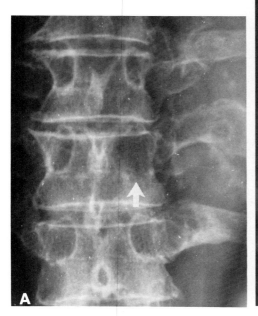

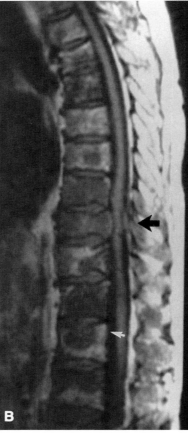

Figure 4-32. Two cases of metastases to the spine. (**A**) Metastases from carcinoma of the breast to the left pedicle (*arrow*) of a lower thoracic vertebra. Note the absence of a normal ovoid "ring" shadow of the pedicle. There are also destructive lesions in the ribs. (**B**) T1-weighted MRI. Metastases to the dorsal and lumbar vertebrae from carcinoma of the lung are identified by areas of low signal on T1-weighted image. Some vertebral bodies are almost completely filled by metastatic disease. A lower thoracic vertebra is compressed and the posterior wall protrudes into the spinal canal compressing the spinal cord (*black arrow*). In a mid-lumbar vertebra the end-plate has collapsed (*white arrow*) and the intervertebral disc protrudes into metastatic deposit located centrally within the subjacent vertebral body.

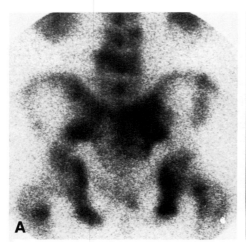

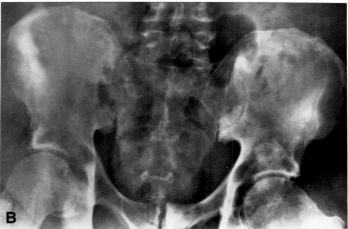

Figure 4-33. Blastic metastasis from carcinoma of the prostate. (**A**) Bone scan demonstrating multiple areas of increased uptake in the lower lumbar spine and pelvis. (**B**) AP view of the pelvis. Multiple sclerotic lesions correspond to positive areas on the bone scan.

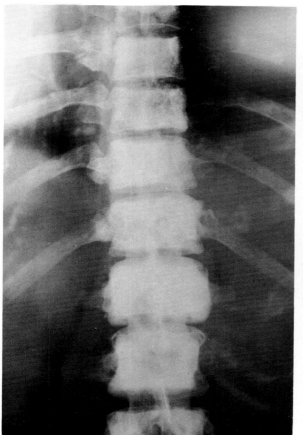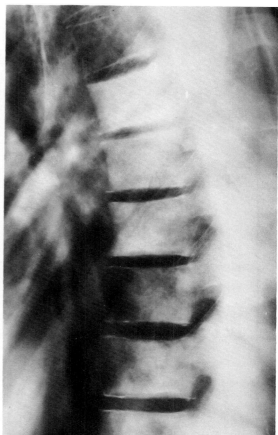

Figure 4–34. Blastic metastases in carcinoma of the prostate. The areas of involvement are manifested by dense sclerosis that tends to obliterate the normal architecture. All of the vertebrae show some degree of involvement.

ondary to carcinoma of the prostate, often associated with the increase in the serum acid phosphatase. In females, sclerotic metastases are usually secondary to carcinoma of the breast. Sclerotic metastases are also encountered from small cell carcinoma of the lung, uroepithelial tumors (transitional cell carcinoma), and less commonly gastrointestinal carcinomas (stomach, pancreas, and colon) and carcinoid tumors. Lymphoma and Hodgkin's disease also incite a sclerotic reaction in bone.

Metastatic carcinoma of the prostate sometimes causes a sunburst periosteal reaction, which gives the metastatic focus the appearance of primary osteogenic sarcoma. Lesions of this type are also rarely encountered from primary lesions of the rectum and colon.

Mixed Type. In the mixed type, there is a combination of destruction and sclerosis, usually with destruction predominating. The affected bone has a mottled appearance with intermixed areas of rarefaction and increased density. About 10% of carcinomas of the breast and a similar percentage of carcinomas of the prostate are of this variety.

Metastatic Neuroblastoma

Neuroblastoma is a highly malignant tumor encountered in infants and children. It arises from sympathetic nervous tissue, often within the adrenal gland. A palpable mass in the abdomen may be the first evidence of disease, or the tumor may present as a paraspinous mass in the thorax. Calcification is often visible within the primary tumor. The tumor shows a pronounced tendency to metastasize to the skeletal system.

Roentgenographic Features. In the skull, neuroblastoma produces rather characteristic changes (Fig.

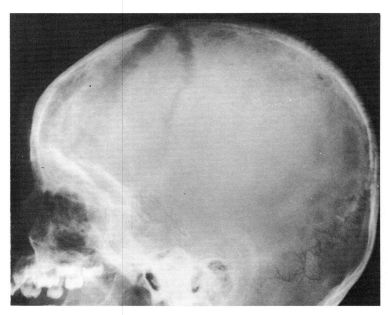

Figure 4–35. Neuroblastoma metastasis to the skull. An area of mixed sclerotic and lytic involvement is seen in the frontal bone. The coronal suture is widened, indicating increased intracranial pressure secondary to metastatic involvement of the meninges. Patches of bone destruction are also demonstrated in the parietal bone.

4-35). The cranial sutures are spread, owing to plaques of tumor tissue growing within the meninges over the surface of the brain. There are poorly defined areas of spotty rarefaction, creating a permeative destruction within the skull. Thin, whiskerlike calcifications frequently extend outward and inward from the tables of the skull. The combination of these findings is highly suggestive of metastatic neuroblastoma.

In the long tubular bones, the metastatic foci are most often permeative or moth-eaten, and the cortex often eroded (Fig. 4-36). Bilateral and symmetrical foci may occur. Periosteal new-bone formation may parallel the cortex or, as in the skull, form thin spiculations at right angles to the cortex.

All so-called round cell tumors of childhood, Ewing's tumor, neuroblastoma, and leukemia, may have a similar radiographic appearance, particularly in the long bones.

MYELOPOIETIC LESIONS OF BONE

Multiple Myeloma (Plasma Cell Myeloma)

Multiple myeloma is made up of plasma cells, which appear to arise from cells within the bone marrow, but the precise cell of origin is not clear. It is the most common primary tumor arising within bone, and it occasionally arises in extraskeletal tissues. It is associated with abnormal gamma globulins and an abnormal protein, the Bence Jones protein, in the urine. Multiple myeloma may be associated with amyloidosis.

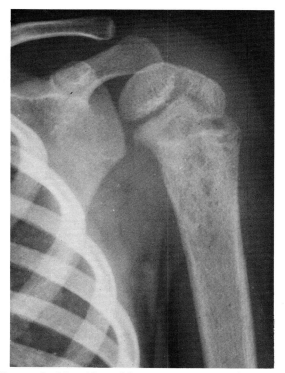

Figure 4–36. Neuroblastoma metastasis to the proximal humerus. Note the ill-defined permeative destructive process (compare with Figs. 4-51 and 4-52, Ewing's tumor). Round cell tumors of bone are very similar in radiographic appearance.

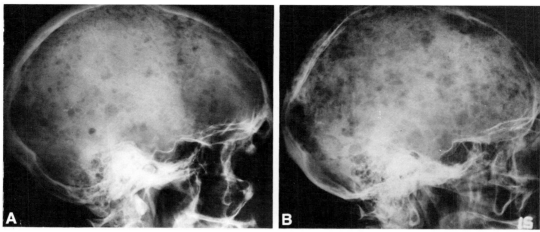

Figure 4–37. (**A** and **B**) Multiple myeloma in two patients. Multiple lytic areas are scattered throughout the calvarium. Note that the lesions tend to coalesce when widespread.

Myeloma is found chiefly in persons between 40 and 70 years of age and is somewhat more common in males than in females. The bones involved by myeloma are the same as those in metastatic carcinoma—the spine, ribs, pelvis, skull, and proximal ends of the humerus and femur.

Roentgenographic Features. The lesions of myeloma are typically multiple, round, punched-out, clean-cut areas of destruction with no surrounding sclerosis. In the flat bones, such as the pelvis and skull, the individual lesions can be seen to best advantage, appearing as numerous small, punched-out defects (Fig. 4-37). As a rule, the lytic lesions in the skull are smaller and better defined than those of metastatic carcinoma, but occasionally large and less well-defined lesions are observed. In some patients, the lesions in the skull may be very small and produce a porous, salt-and-pepper appearance somewhat similar to that observed in hyperparathyroidism.

In the long bones, lesions tend to appear as small or coalescing discrete areas of lytic destruction frequently associated with endosteal scalloping (Fig. 4-38). Lesions may enlarge or coalesce and lead to pathologic fractures. Pathologic fractures are particularly common in the ribs. On occasion, the lesions appear moth-eaten or even permeated. Occasionally myeloma may cause expansion of the cortex and appear trabeculated or honeycombed (see Fig. 4-41). Extension into the surrounding tissues is common. Soft-tissue masses are more common in myeloma than in metastatic carcinoma: Myeloma may occasionally cross joints to involve adjacent bones (Fig. 4-39). This is

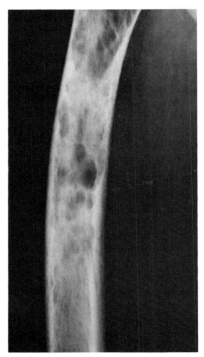

Figure 4–38. Multiple myeloma. The midfemoral shaft is involved by a number of lytic lesions. Note the endosteal erosion by several of the lesions.

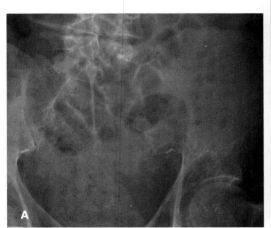
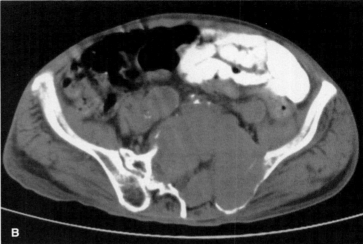

Figure 4–39. Plasmacytoma of the sacrum in a 72-year-old man. **(A)** AP view of the pelvis demonstrates a destructive lesion of the entire body of the sacrum that extends across the L5–S1 intervertebral disc to destroy the left inferior aspect of the fifth lumbar vertebral body and across the left sacroiliac joint to destroy the adjacent iliac bone. **(B)** CT scan confirms a large destructive mass arising from the sacrum and extending into the iliac bone. There is no matrix within the lesion. The anterior border of the lesion is slightly lobulated.

exceedingly rare in metastasis and other malignancies and might be considered characteristic of myeloma. In the ribs, these tumors may produce large extrapleural masses that protrude into the thorax (see Fig. 4-31*B*).

In perhaps one-fourth of cases, typical circumscribed defects are absent in the initial phases of the disease. In some patients, the bones may appear normal or simply osteoporotic. This is particularly true of spinal or rib involvement, in which the identification of discrete foci of disease is uncommon. Involvement of the pedicles in multiple myeloma is less common, and paraspinous soft-tissue masses tend to be larger than in metastatic carcinoma. Involvement of the spine leads to compression fractures of vertebral bodies similar to that seen in senile osteoporosis or metastatic disease (Fig. 4-40). The collapse of several discontiguous vertebral bodies should suggest the possibility of multiple myeloma.

Rare examples of myeloma have been reported in which the foci of disease were sclerotic rather than lytic. The sclerotic lesions may be solitary or diffuse, the latter simulating osteoblastic metastases observed in prostatic metastases. Also, occasionally osteolytic lesions may have thin sclerotic margins.

Bone scanning is not as sensitive to the presence of multiple myeloma as it is to metastatic carcinoma or other primary diseases of bone. Indeed, as many as 40% to 50% of patients with foci of multiple myeloma

may demonstrate no evidence of increased radionuclide activity. A negative bone scan does not rule out foci of myeloma, and a positive bone scan may miss a significant number of lesions in any given patient. Thus, the radionuclide bone scan takes a secondary role to plain film radiography in the evaluation of multiple myeloma.

As in metastatic disease, CT and MRI may be of value in demonstrating foci of disease that are inapparent on standard radiographic examinations.

Solitary Myeloma (Plasmacytoma)

Infrequently, myeloma occurs as an apparently solitary lesion, and some of these may pursue a relatively benign course, remaining as a single lesion for years. In the majority of cases, however, the tumor develops into typical multiple myeloma and eventually becomes widespread. The average age when first detected is 45 years. The tumor is more common in males than in females. The favorite sites are the spine, ribs, upper femur, pelvis (see Fig. 4-39), and upper humerus.

Roentgenographic Features. In long bones, solitary myeloma causes a central area of destruction, usually in the shaft; expansion and trabeculation are common, with little or no periosteal reaction. In the pelvis, scapula, and ribs, markedly expansile and trabeculated

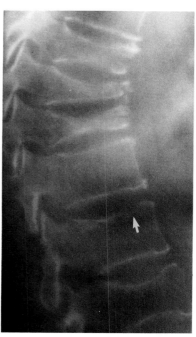

Figure 4–40. Multiple myeloma of the spine. There are multiple compression fractures of the lower dorsal vertebrae and a biconcave lumbar vertebra. Discrete foci of disease are rarely identified in the spine in multiple myeloma. Note that the tomogram does demonstrate one single area of destruction in a vertebral end-plate (*arrow*).

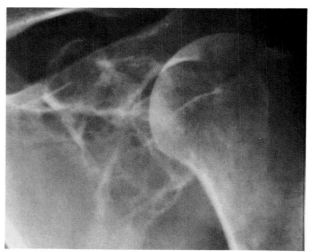

Figure 4–41. Plasmacytoma of the scapula. Note the soap-bubbly, slightly expansile process in the neck of the scapula.

tumors resembling soap bubbles may be encountered (Fig. 4-41). Expansile lesions are also common in the spine, whereas others are purely destructive and cause a collapse of the vertebral body. A soft-tissue mass surrounding the vertebra is common. Extension into the vertebral processes is sometimes encountered.

Acute Leukemia

Bone involvement with radiographic findings is quite common in acute leukemias of infants and children. Occasionally, bone lesions precede typical findings in the peripheral blood, and the radiographic examination may suggest the diagnosis. Early findings consist of a transverse zone of lucency crossing the width of the metaphyses of long bones. These findings are similar to the lucent zone seen in infantile scurvy. Fractures may occur through such a weakened area and should suggest the possibility of leukemia, particularly before the age of 2 years. In others, there are metaphyseal or diaphyseal patches of moth-eaten or permeative bone destruction and laminated periosteal new-bone formation (Fig. 4-42). These may be found in any bone and

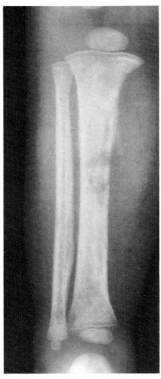

Figure 4–42. Leukemia involving the tibia. There are poorly defined areas of destruction as well as periosteal reaction forming a Codman's triangle on the medial aspect of the tibia. Note the thin, translucent band crossing the upper and lower metaphyses of the tibia and, to a lesser extent, of the fibula (compare with Figs. 4-51 and 4-52).

are often symmetrical. Larger areas of destruction may be encountered.

Chronic Myelogenous Leukemia

It is not to be expected that roentgenographic examination of the skeleton will yield any significant information in most patients having chronic myelogenous leukemia. Although involvement of bone marrow is common, the disease rarely causes distinct roentgenographic changes other than, perhaps, a nonspecific osteoporosis. Osteosclerosis has been described; however, it seems likely that most cases are actually examples of myelofibrosis that terminate with a leukemoid blood picture (see Chapter 7).

Lymphocytic Lymphoma

Involvement of bone by lymphocytic lymphoma is not common, but when it does occur, the lesions are usually destructive and osteolytic, resembling metastatic carcinoma (Fig. 4-43). Rarely the bone lesions are sclerotic, and occasionally of mixed density.

Hodgkin's Disease

Hodgkin's disease affects bone more frequently than does lymphosarcoma. In many instances, the lesions closely resemble those of metastatic carcinoma and the diagnosis of Hodgkin's disease cannot be made from the roentgenographic appearance. About two-thirds of cases are mixed lytic and sclerotic, a few are lytic, and the remainder (about 10% to 15%) are sclerotic lesions. In the pelvis, the lesions are of mixed osteolytic and osteoblastic type.

Sclerotic lesions tend to be confined to the vertebrae ("ivory vertebrae"), which are relatively common sites of the disease. In some cases, there is erosion of the anterior surfaces of one or several contiguous vertebral bodies, suggesting that the tumor invaded the bone by direct extension from adjacent lymph nodes. At times, there may be preservation of the cortex, suggesting a form of pressure atrophy from adjacent lymphadenopathy rather than invasion of the vertebra. As would be expected, the greatest incidence occurs in the upper lumbar and lower thoracic regions corresponding to the sites of paravertebral nodes.

PRIMARY MALIGNANCIES OF BONE

Osteosarcoma

Osteosarcoma is the most common primary malignant tumor of bone. It is more common in males than in females, with greatest incidence between the ages of 10 and 25 years. Less commonly, osteosarcoma occurs in patients older than 25 years. Some of these lesions originate in bone involved by Paget's disease, especially in individuals over the age of 50.[30]

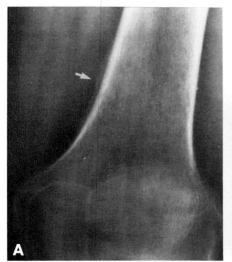
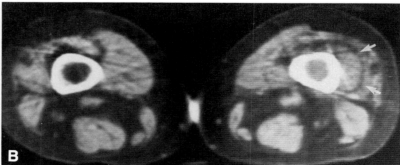

Figure 4–43. Primary lymphoma of bone. **(A)** An ill-defined permeative process is present in the distal femoral metaphysis and is overlaid by periosteal new-bone formation (*arrow*). **(B)** CT reveals the presence of increased absorption in the medullary cavity and the presence of a surrounding soft-tissue mass (*arrows*). The normal intramedullary canal has a fat density, whereas marrow infiltrated by infection or tumor has a soft-tissue density.

The most common sites of origin are the distal end of the femur and the proximal ends of the tibia and humerus. Less commonly, osteosarcoma appears in the pelvic bones, particularly in the iliac wings, the proximal femur, the mandible, the proximal fibula, and the distal tibia. Occasionally, osteosarcomas are encountered in almost any bone within the body. Pain and local swelling are the usual presenting symptoms. Bone formation may occur within the metastatic deposits and may be homogeneously dense.

There are four histologic types of osteosarcoma: osteoblastic (the most common), chondroblastic, fibroblastic, and telangiectatic.[12] For radiographic purposes, three forms of osteosarcoma may be recognized, depending on the presence or absence of tumor matrix ossification, or osteoid formation within the tumor. These are osteolytic, sclerosing or osteoblastic, and mixed.

Roentgenographic Features. The mixed form of osteosarcoma is the most common, and it is characterized by a mixture of bone destruction and osteoid production (Figs. 4-44 and 4-45).[12] One or the other may predominate, but in most, the destructive aspect overshadows the productive. Bone destruction is characteristically ragged, uneven, and poorly defined, with a broad zone of transition. The tumor disrupts the cortex and extends into the soft tissue. Codman's triangles are frequently seen at the edges of the tumor (Fig. 4-44A). Periosteal new-bone formation is either irregular, of sunburst appearance, or consisting of coarse radiating spiculations arranged in an arc about the mass. Patches of amorphous, homogeneously dense osteoid are scattered throughout the lesion and may occur within the soft-tissue component of the mass (Figs. 4-44 and 4-45).

The osteoblastic (sclerosing) form of osteosarcoma arises within the medullary canal and is manifested by an amorphous haze of mottled sclerosis indicative of osteoid formation (Fig. 4-45). The amount and density of bone formed by the tumor are characteristic of this type of osteosarcoma. As the cortex becomes involved,

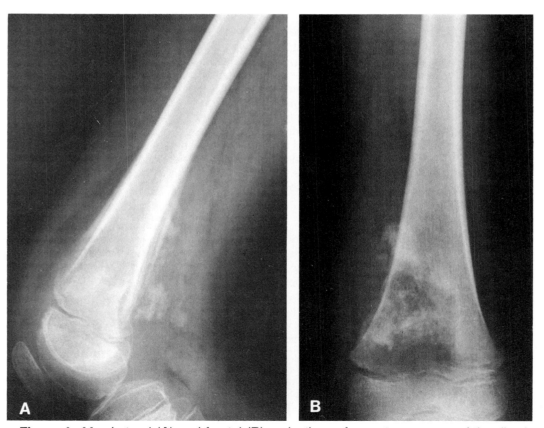

Figure 4–44. Lateral (**A**) and frontal (**B**) projections of an osteosarcoma of the distal femur. An area of irregular destruction is best seen on the frontal projection. Laminated or layered periosteal reaction is seen posteriorly, and tumor bone formation, osteoid, is noted within the medullary canal and extends into the soft tissues of the lower thigh.

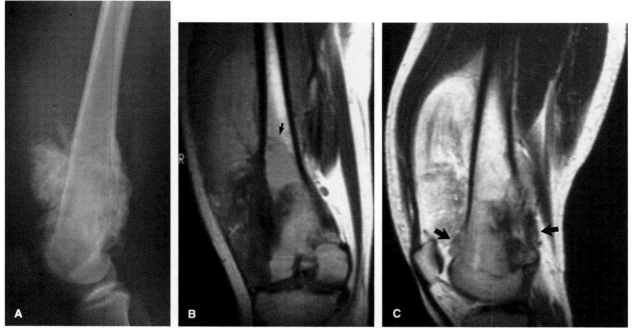

Figure 4–45. Osteosarcoma of the distal femur in a 19-year-old man. **(A)** Lateral view demonstrates sunburst pattern of dense periosteal new-bone formation anteriorly, dense osteoid in the medullary cavity, and cortical destruction with expansion of the lesion posteriorly. The lesion is poorly defined proximally. **(B)** T1-weighted coronal MRI demonstrates proximal medullary extension of the lesion (*arrow*). The entire distal medullary cavity is filled with tumor. The dense osteoid gives a low signal. The medial cortex is destroyed. Note that the associated soft-tissue mass is less well defined than on the T2-weighted image. **(C)** T2-weighted sagittal MRI clearly demonstrates the high-signal soft-tissue mass that bows the quadriceps muscle anteriorly. There is low signal within the lesion, representing areas of osteoid bone formation. The cortex of the femur is perforated by the tumor both anteriorly and posteriorly (*arrows*).

its outline is lost within the sclerotic tumor. The lesion soon disrupts the cortex and extends into the soft tissue, often forming dense spicules and irregular patches of bone. Although there is always a destructive aspect pathologically, it is largely obscured by the proliferative reaction and the dense osteoid. There is a tendency for this form to metastasize to other bones as well as to the lungs, forming dense masses of metastatic tumor.

The osteolytic form characteristically begins in the metaphyseal end of a long bone as a central area of poorly marginated destruction with little or no new-bone formation (Fig. 4-46*B*). Codman's triangles may be identified at the margins of the tumor. The margins of the lesion are poorly defined and ragged, and the cortex is involved early and destroyed. The tumor extends into the soft tissue, often with a rather large soft-tissue mass (Fig. 4-46*C*). It may be difficult, if not

impossible, to distinguish between the osteolytic form of osteosarcoma, fibrosarcoma, reticulum cell sarcoma, and malignant fibrous histiocytoma on the basis of their radiographic appearance. In general, osteosarcoma tends to occur in younger individuals than do the other tumors.

Osteosarcoma shows a great tendency to metastasize to the lungs. The pulmonary lesions are visualized as discrete, usually multiple round nodules of variable size, sometimes partially or completely ossified. Pulmonary metastases may develop early, and chest radiographs must be obtained to rule out metastases. CT is more sensitive than the chest radiograph in the disclosure of metastases.

Metastases may also occur to other sites in the skeletal system, including the skull, spine, and distal long bones, particularly in the osteoblastic form. Bone scanning is necessary to rule out this possibility. These

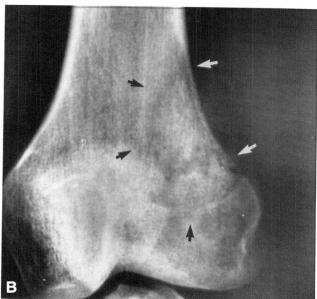

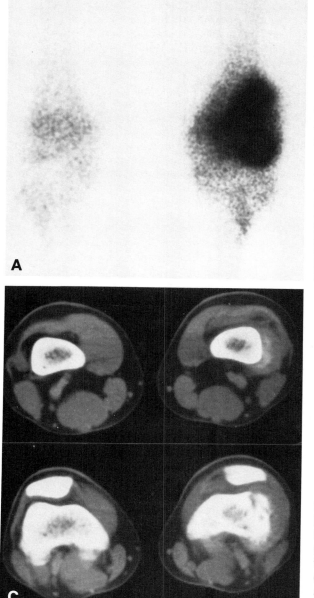

Figure 4–46. Osteolytic osteosarcoma of the distal femur. (**A**) Bone scan demonstrates a large area of increased radioactivity in the distal femur. (**B**) AP radiograph reveals an ill-defined area of destruction in the metaphysis involving both medullary bone and the overlying cortex (*arrows*). (**C**) CT shows cortical destruction, possibly osteoid formation, and a surrounding soft-tissue mass.

metastases may be identified at the initial presentation or may occur subsequently and have the same appearance as the primary tumor. In some cases, there is an extended delay between the appearance of the primary lesion and the second site of osteosarcoma. The question then arises about whether this represents a metastasis or the metachronous origin of a second primary tumor. This is debatable and not easily resolved.

Rarely, in young children, osteogenic sarcoma occurs in multiple sites in the metaphysis of long bones, all sites being similar in appearance, osteoblastic, and size, suggesting that they have originated synchronously or simultaneously. This condition is known as *osteosarcomatosis.*

Parosteal and Periosteal Osteosarcoma. Two additional distinct types of osteogenic sarcoma are recognized, parosteal and periosteal, each having a distinctive radiographic and pathologic appearance and prognosis allowing them to be distinguished from the more common osteogenic sarcoma arising in the medullary portion of bone.[8] Parosteal osteosarcoma accounts for 4% of all osteogenic sarcomas, and periosteal osteosarcoma is even less common, accounting for about 1%. The prognosis is more favorable in these two types than in the standard osteogenic sarcoma. Both can be treated successfully by wide local excision.

Parosteal Osteosarcoma (Juxtacortical Osteosarcoma). Parosteal osteosarcoma is an uncommon tumor that is found in a somewhat older age group than osteosarcoma, in a broad range of ages between 15 and 55 years, and it is more common in females than males. The classic location is the posterior distal metaphysis of the femur in the region of the popliteal space (Fig. 4-47). Less commonly it arises in the posterior metaphysis of the proximal tibia and the proximal metaphysis of the humerus and rarely elsewhere. It is slow growing but has a tendency to recur after inadequate excision, and it may metastasize.

Radiographically it is a broad-based, juxtacortical, densely ossified mass, the periphery somewhat less dense than the base.[23] The lesion often consists of three layers: At the cortical surface it is dense and compact, it has a middle layer of cloudlike amorphous dense bone, and in the outer layer there are dense compact spicules extending into the periphery of the mass. The mass is usually sharply demarcated from the soft tissue and is often lobulated. It is attached to the cortex at some portion of the base and tends to encircle the shaft,

leaving a narrow clear zone between the tumor and the cortex. The lesion may eventually progress to cortical destruction and medullary invasion. Cortical destruction and medullary invasion cannot usually be seen on the plain radiograph (Fig. 4-48). CT or MRI is required to determine the medullary extent of the lesion and the presence or absence of cortical disruption.

The lesion bears a superficial resemblance to myositis ossificans. However, myositis ossificans is more densely calcified at its periphery and usually does not involve the adjacent cortex. Osteochondroma is another diagnostic consideration, but the stalk of an exostosis is contiguous with the cortex of the bone from which it arises and the medullary bone within the stalk is also contiguous with that of the adjacent bone. Chondroid calcification within the cartilaginous cap may be present and is also distinctive.

Periosteal Osteosarcoma. Periosteal sarcomas occur in the second and third decades of life and characteristically arise in the mid-diaphysis of long bones, particularly the tibia, femur, and humerus.[1] They are characterized radiographically as an eccentric thickening of the cortex that has a central, saucer-shaped defect, out of which rise radiating spicules of periosteal reaction. The location and superficial cortical erosion are highly suggestive of periosteal osteosarcoma. The medullary cavity is usually not involved.

Chondrosarcoma

Chondrosarcoma is about half as common as osteogenic sarcoma, develops at a later age, grows more slowly, and metastasizes later. It is more common in males than females. The majority of patients are older than 40 years, and the peak incidence is between the ages of 50 and 60.

Chondrosarcoma may be either primary or secondary. In the primary form, it originates without a preexisting lesion, whereas the secondary type develops in a preexisting enchondroma or osteochondroma (exostosis). Chondrosarcoma is reported to occur in about 10% of patients with hereditary multiple exotosis. The incidence of chondrosarcoma in a solitary exostosis is less than 5%. The change from a benign to a malignant chondroma may be difficult to recognize. Any enchondroma or osteochondroma that becomes painful or begins to enlarge should be suspected of malignant degeneration.

Chondrosarcoma can also be classified as central or peripheral, depending on its location in the bone of origin. Chondrosarcomas occur most frequently around the hip, in the iliac bone or pubis, and proximal femur, and less commonly in the proximal humerus and around the knee. They also occur in the ribs and less commonly in the spine and sacrum. Despite the

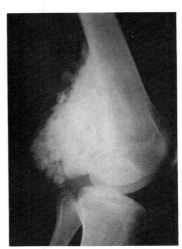

Figure 4–47. Parosteal osteosarcoma. A large, dense mass protrudes from the posterior aspect of the lower femur. There is no evidence of extension into the intramedullary canal. This is a typical location and appearance for this tumor.

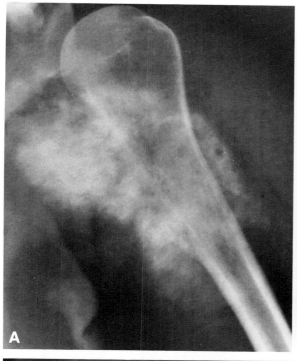

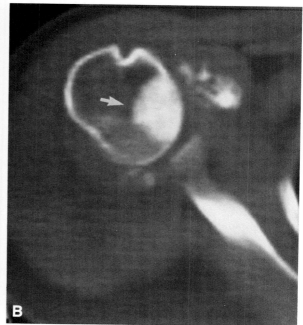

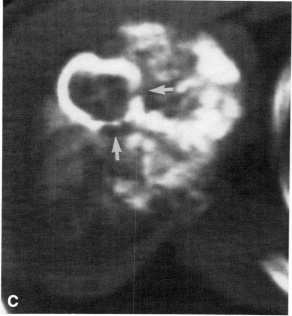

Figure 4–48. Parosteal osteosarcoma of the proximal humerus. **(A)** AP radiograph demonstrates an irregular cloudlike density typical of osteoid surrounding the proximal humerus. There is no obvious intramedullary extension, nor is there evidence of cortical destruction. **(B)** Proximal CT scan demonstrates extension of the disease process into the humeral head (*arrow*). **(C)** A more inferior CT scan demonstrates areas of cortical destruction (*arrows*).

frequency of benign chondromas in the small bones of the hands and feet, chondrosarcomas are exceedingly rare in these locations.

Central Chondrosarcoma. Solitary enchondromas may become malignant, the potential decreasing from

the hip or shoulder distally to the fingers or toes. Central chondrosarcoma of a tubular bone presents as a geographic radiolucent area of bone destruction within the cancellous bone of the diaphysis or metaphysis; it is poorly marginated. It is associated with endosteal erosion of the cortex and at times rather compact periosteal new-bone formation, giving an appearance of thickening and local expansion of the cortex (Fig. 4-49). The tumor usually contains characteristic chondroid calcification, nodules, or floccules of dense calcification, the same as those seen in benign tumors. In some cases these may be absent, but the cortical changes, age of the patient, and other aspects of the radiographic appearance of the tumor should suggest the diagnosis. Eventually the tumor erodes through the cortex and forms a soft-tissue mass adjacent to the lesion.

Benign enchondromas of long bones are usually manifested only by the presence of typical chondroid calcification (see Fig. 4-7B). Since the lesion is confined to the cancellous bone, it is usually poorly defined. Whenever endosteal erosion or cortical thickening is encountered in association with chondroid calcification, the possibility of chondrosarcoma must be considered. Under these circumstances, the lesion is more

likely to be a chondrosarcoma than a benign enchondroma. Benign enchondromas are not associated with pain; therefore, the presence of pain suggests chondrosarcoma. Similarly, any change in the radiographic appearance of a previously identified enchondroma must be viewed with suspicion.

Peripheral Chondrosarcoma. This type of chondrosarcoma arises within a preexisting osteochondroma or exostosis. The presence of pain or mass around a known or preexisting peripheral exostosis should suggest the possibility of malignant transformation.

Peripheral chondrosarcoma arises adjacent to the external surface of bone and is more common in the flat bones, particularly in the pelvis (Fig. 4-50). The lesions present as a soft-tissue mass adjacent to bone, are often large and bulky, and characteristically contain chondroid calcifications. Initially the underlying cortex may

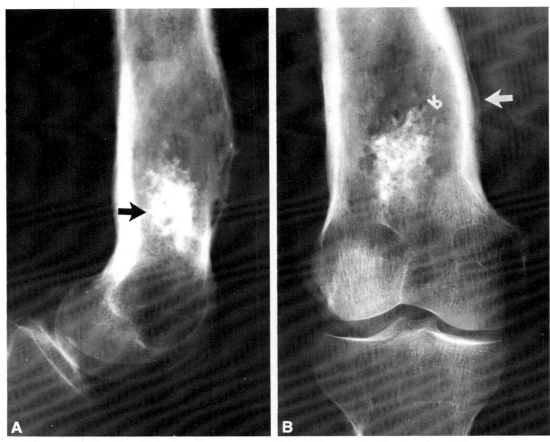

Figure 4–49. Central chondrosarcoma. This lesion probably developed from an enchondroma in the medullary canal, designated by the *arrow* in **A**. Note the expansion and thinning of the cortex, with overlying periosteal new-bone formation designated by the *white arrow* in **B** (compare with benign enchondroma in Fig. 4-7B).

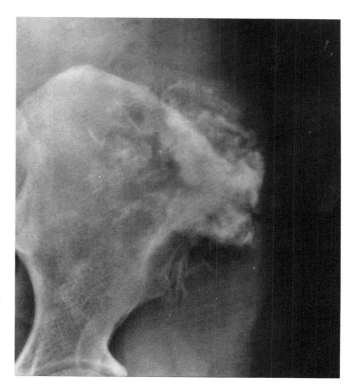

Figure 4–50. Peripheral chondrosarcoma. This chondrosarcoma is presumed to have arisen from an exostosis of the iliac bone. Note the chondroid calcification. Malignant degeneration is revealed by the presence of the discontiguous calcifications extending into the large soft-tissue mass.

be intact or may show erosion of its external surface. Eventually the cortex is destroyed, and the tumor invades the medullary cavity as well as the adjacent soft tissues.

Chondrosarcomas may also arise in parosteal chondromas. These are associated with saucerized erosion of the metaphysis of long bones, and they often contain chondroid calcification. The presence of an enlarging soft-tissue mass or poor definition of the adjacent bone should suggest the possibility of malignant degeneration.

Ewing's Tumor

Ewing's tumor is a primary malignant tumor arising in the red bone marrow and closely related histologically to reticulum cell sarcoma. It is found most frequently between the ages of 5 and 25 and rarely occurs in persons over 30 years old. Males are affected more frequently than females.

The most frequent sites of involvement are the long bones of the extremities, particularly the femur. Classically the lesion is said to occur in the diaphysis of long bones but, in fact, arises more often in the metaphysis. The tumor also occurs quite frequently in the flat bones of the pelvis, scapulae, and ribs. In patients over 20 years of age, the incidence is higher in flat bones than in long bones. The tumor may also occur in the ver-

tebrae and tarsal bones. This tumor shows a distinct tendency to metastasize to other bones, and multiple lesions may be present at the time of the initial study.

The clinical symptoms of pain and swelling are often accompanied by fever and leukocytosis, suggesting osteomyelitis. On some occasions, particularly when these lesions are located in the metaphysis, the radiographic distinction between the two is not easy.

Roentgenographic Features. In the long bones, the lesion usually involves a considerable length of shaft (Figs. 4-51 and 4-52). Although it is said to arise in the diaphysis, it is more often limited to the metaphysis or located in the metadiaphysis. Characteristically there is a permeative, poorly marginated, destructive lesion that perforates the cortex and is overlaid by a laminated, onionskin periosteal reaction. In other cases, Codman's triangles are present at the margins of the lesion and the periosteal reaction is disrupted. Fine, hair-on-end spicules are identified in other cases, and in still others the periosteal reaction is irregular and interrupted. Sometimes the lesion appears to originate parosteally, in which case there is characteristic saucerization of the diaphysis or metaphysis, with Codman's triangles at the margins of the lesion. In the long bones, differentiation of Ewing's tumor and osteomyelitis may be difficult. In a young

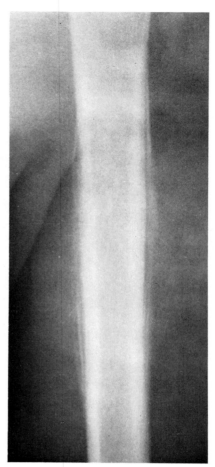

Figure 4–51. Ewing's tumor involving the diaphysis of the femur in a young adult. Laminated, onion-skin, periosteal new-bone formation extends over a considerable length of the shaft. The medullary destruction is permeative and poorly defined.

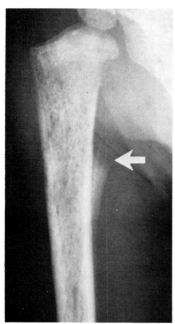

Figure 4–52. Ewing's tumor involving the metaphysis and proximal shaft of the humerus. There is a permeative destruction and a well-defined, laminated Codman's triangle (*arrow*) at its distal margin.

Reticulum Cell Sarcoma of Bone

Reticulum cell sarcoma is closely related to Ewing's tumor in its histology, distribution, and radiographic appearance. In contrast to Ewing's tumor, it occurs mainly in older persons, most commonly over the age of 50 years, but occasionally between the ages of 20 and 50. It is more common in males than females.

Reticulum cell sarcoma occurs at both ends and in the diaphysis of long bones in a manner similar to Ewing's tumor. In addition, it also appears in the flat bones such as the ilium, scapulae, and ribs, and occasionally in the vertebrae and sacrum.

The lesion is quite similar in its radiographic appearance to Ewing's tumor, causing a permeative, ill-defined, destruction of bone arising in the medullary cavity and soon involving the cortex. Periosteal new-bone formation is frequent, but absent in some cases. The tumor incites reactive bone formation in some cases, and therefore patches of sclerosis may be identified. It is often associated with large soft-tissue masses. Pathologic fracture occurs in as many as 25% of cases.

Because of the similarity in appearance, reticulum cell sarcoma can only be distinguished from Ewing's tumor by the age of the patient. In older individuals, it is similar in appearance to fibrosarcoma, malignant fibrous histiocytoma, and osteolytic osteosarcoma. The

patient, Ewing's tumor mimics the radiographic appearance of the other "round cell" tumors, leukemia, and metastatic neuroblastoma. Lesions occurring in the flat bones are also permeative and poorly defined; but in the flat bones, Ewing's tumor often stimulates osteoid formation and therefore there are patches of osteosclerosis (Fig. 4-53). Similar patches of sclerosis are much less common but are sometimes encountered in the long bones.

Vertebral involvement varies in appearance from pure lysis to sclerosis. Soft-tissue masses are usually present. The tumor has an extremely poor prognosis, which has been improved by the use of combined irradiation and chemotherapy. Pathologic fractures are common in the treated area.

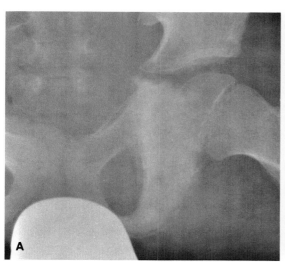
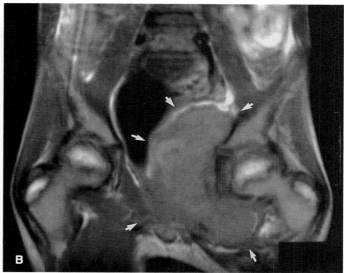

Figure 4–53.   Ewing's sarcoma of the ischium in a 10-year-old boy. (**A**) AP view demonstrates poorly defined sclerotic lesion of the ischium with cortical destruction and surrounding soft-tissue mass. There is periosteal new-bone formation at the margins of the lesion. (**B**) T1-weighted coronal MRI anterior to the inferior ramus demonstrates a large soft-tissue mass (*arrows*) poorly defined medially and inferiorly. The lesion has a homogeneous intermediate signal. (Case courtesy of Martin Gross, M.D., Detroit)

distinction between these tumors cannot be made with any degree of certainty on the basis of radiographic appearances.

Fibrosarcoma

Fibrosarcoma is a malignant lesion of bone arising from spindle-shaped cells that produce no osteoid, the malignant counterpart of the desmoplastic fibroma. It appears over a broad range of age, from the second to the eighth decades, and is generally more common after the age of 40 years. Males and females are affected equally often. It is most common at the distal ends of the bones around the knee but may be found in any long bone, and on occasion it arises in the midshaft. The lesion also occurs in the flat bones, sacrum, and occasionally the spine and ribs. Fibrosarcoma is a known complication of Paget's disease, and it may arise following previous irradiation for either benign bone lesions or nonosseous tumors.

There are no radiographic features that distinguish fibrosarcoma of bone from an osteolytic osteosarcoma. The lesion usually has poorly defined borders. At times it is somewhat geographic, but more often it appears moth-eaten or both moth-eaten and permeative. When the cortex is perforated, periosteal new-bone formation and soft-tissue masses are common. The dif-

ferential diagnosis must include reticulum cell sarcoma, malignant fibrous histiocytoma, osteosarcoma, and Ewing's sarcoma in an appropriate age group.

Malignant Fibrous Histiocytoma

Malignant fibrous histiocytoma is a recently recognized rare tumor of bone that is reported with increasing frequency. It most commonly arises around the distal and proximal ends of the femur, proximal tibia, and pelvis but has been found randomly throughout most long bones.[4] The age of occurrence is over a broad range, beginning at age 10 years. The lesion occurs with a slightly greater frequency in males than females. Here again, the radiographic features are those of an osteolytic lesion that may be geographic with poorly defined margins or on occasion frankly moth-eaten or permeative, with cortical destruction and a soft-tissue mass. On occasion, the lesion is expansile, particularly in the ribs. Periosteal reaction may occur following pathologic fracture.

Chordoma

Chordoma is an infrequent tumor arising from remnants of the fetal notochord. There are three common sites of origin. The most common is the sacrum, the second the region of the clivus, and the third the area of the upper cervical spine. The tumors are more common in males than females, and most occur after the age of 40 years. The tumors are rather slow growing and of a low order of malignancy, spreading by infiltration and metastasizing only in the late stages of the disease.

Radiographically, chordoma presents as a localized destruction of bone with an associated soft-tissue mass containing flocculent areas of calcification (Fig. 4-54). In the cervico-occipital lesions, destruction of the clivus, the margins of the foramen magnum, or portions of the upper cervical vertebrae are seen. The mass may project into the retropharyngeal space and cause a demonstrable thickening of the soft tissues. In the sacral region, the lesion usually causes a sharply marginated area of destruction, often involving a large part of the sacrum. The mass displaces the rectum forward. There is usually very little in the appearance of the lesions to establish the diagnosis from roentgenographic findings alone, but whenever localized bone destruction is found in either of these two characteristic regions—and particularly when associated with soft-tissue calcifications—one should consider the possibility of a chordoma.

Synovial Sarcoma

This disease is discussed in Chapter 3, Diseases of the Joints.

Adamantinoma

Adamantinoma of long bones is a peculiar neoplasm, based on its histologic appearance. The name *adamantinoma* was given to these tumors of long bone because of their histologic resemblance to the common adamantinoma (ameloblastoma) of the mandible. It is rare, and occurs equally in males and females after the age of 20 years. The classic site of the majority of these lesions is the midshaft of the tibia. On occasion the tumor arises in the fibula, and on rare occasions simultaneously in both the tibia and fibula. Radiographically the most typical appearance is multiple, sharply circumscribed lucent defects with sclerotic bone interspersed between, above, and below the lucent zones. Some lucent zones are entirely cortical. Typically, the lytic area in the midshaft is the largest and most destructive and appears to expand the overlying cortex.

Malignant Hemangioendothelioma of Bone (Angiosarcoma)

This is another rare tumor of bone that reveals itself mainly as a localized destructive lesion. A diagnosis based on roentgenographic evidence usually cannot be made. Multiple sites of involvement in a number of bones are common, as in the benign lesion cystic angiomatosis of bone. There is no tendency to produce sclerosis or calcification. The periphery of the individual areas of bone destruction produced by the tumor is

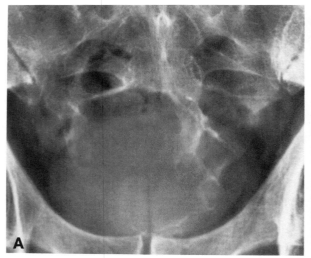
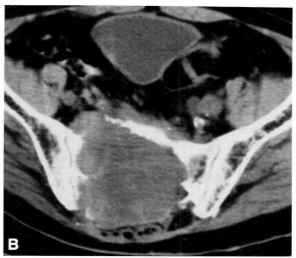

Figure 4–54. Two cases of chordoma of the sacrum. **(A)** AP view of the sacrum demonstrates destruction, with a soft-tissue mass containing calcification, findings typical of a chordoma. **(B)** CT demonstrates to excellent advantage the extensive destruction and soft-tissue mass.

poorly defined. Periosteal new-bone formation may occur when the lesion breaks through the cortex.

DIFFERENTIAL DIAGNOSIS OF SOLITARY BONE LESIONS

The most common solitary lesion is a cortical defect or a nonossifying fibroma. These characteristically occur in children prior to epiphyseal closure, arise in the metaphyses of long bones of the lower extremity, are radiolucent, and are characteristically sharply defined by a rim of sclerotic bone. The lesions are eccentric and tend to expand the overlying cortex. Osteochondromas arise at the end of long bones, projecting beyond the bone, and should present no diagnostic difficulties. Enchondromas are radiolucent lesions characteristically found in the phalanges. They may contain small areas of stippled calcification. Simple bone cysts are sharply defined lesions in children; they arise in the metaphysis, particularly proximal in the humerus and intertrochanteric region of the femur. They have a thin rim of sclerotic bone. Giant cell tumors arise after epiphyseal closure and extend to the joint surface. They are characteristically at the end of the bone, are slightly expansile and radiolucent, and lack a sclerotic rim, although they are usually sharply defined. Aneurysmal bone cysts also arise at the end of the bone but characteristically do not extend to the joint surface. They are markedly expansile and ballooned radiolucent lesions. The peripheral rim of the cortex may not be visible. Chondroblastomas arise in the epiphysis in children before the growth plate closes. They may contain small stippled areas of calcification, and periosteal reaction is occasionally noted. Chondromyxoid fibromas are eccentric lesions that arise in the metaphysis and usually are well marginated by a thin rim of sclerotic bone. They may extend through the cortex, and the peripheral margin of cortical bone may be so thin that it is invisible on the radiograph. Eosinophilic granulomas arise any place within the bone, including the diaphysis; they are radiolucent in the long bones and cause a thickening or expansion of the cortex, often with overlying periosteal reaction.

Malignant lesions are generally poorly defined, are associated with cortical destruction, and often have an accompanying soft-tissue mass. Metastatic lesions are by far the most common. Ewing's tumor occurs in childhood, classically in the diaphysis but probably more frequently in the metaphysis. It causes a motheaten or permeative destruction, with overlying periosteal new-bone formation that is classically onionskin in appearance. Other round cell lesions, metastatic neuroblastoma, and leukemia have the same appear-

ance. Metastases to long bones usually appear as geographic, somewhat poorly defined lesions in the medullary portion of bone. Osteosarcomas occur at the metaphysis or metadiaphysis of long bones and characteristically contain osteoid matrix calcification that is homogeneous, amorphous, and cloudlike. They may be purely blastic, lytic, and mixed (both blastic and lytic). Chondrosarcoma occurs in individuals over the age of 40 years and is characteristically found within the pelvis or proximal femur, but it may arise in any location, manifested by an ill-defined destructive lesion that contains nodules or floccules of chondroid calcification. In the long bones, it may be less aggressive and simply result in cortical thickening and endosteal scalloping. Multiple myeloma causes discrete, punched-out, lytic areas with endosteal scalloping in long bones and skull. Fibrosarcoma, malignant fibrous histiocytoma, reticulum cell sarcoma, and osteolytic osteosarcoma are similar, if not indistinguishable, in appearance. They are poorly defined geographic or moth-eaten destructive lesions with variable degrees of overlying periosteal reaction. Although it may be difficult if not impossible to distinguish one from the other, they all definitely appear malignant.

The most common tumor of the spine is a metastasis that usually involves the red marrow in the vertebral body and pedicle, resulting in cortical destruction and collapse of the vertebral body. Multiple myeloma is similar in appearance but may spare the cortex of the pedicles and at times is expansile. Osteoblastoma and aneurysmal bone cyst arise in the posterior elements of the spine and are characteristically expansile. Tumors can be differentiated from infections because they spare the intervertebral disc space, whereas infections characteristically result in narrowing of the disc space and the destruction of adjacent vertebral end-plates.

REFERENCES AND SELECTED READINGS

1. BERTONI F, BORIANTI S, LAUS M, ET AL: Periosteal chondrosarcoma and periosteal osteosarcoma. J Bone Joint Surg [Br] 64:370, 1982

2. CAMPANACCI M, LAUS M: Osteofibrous dysplasia of the tibia and fibula. J Bone Joint Surg [Am] 63:367, 1981

3. CAPANNA R, ALBISINNI U, PICCI P, ET AL: Aneurysmal bone cyst of the spine. J Bone Joint Surg [Am] 67:527, 1985

4. CAPANNA R, BERTONI F, BACCHINI P, ET AL: Malignant fibrous histiocytoma of bone. The experience at the Rizzoli Institute: Report of 90 cases. Cancer 54:177, 1984

5. CORCORAN RJ, THRALL JH, KYLE RW, ET AL: Solitary abnormalities in bone scans of patients with extraosseous malignancies. Radiology 121:663, 1976

6. CORY DA, FRITSCH SA, COHEN MD, ET AL: Aneurysmal bone cysts: Imaging findings and embolotherapy. Am J Roentgenol 153:369, 1989

7. DAHLIN DC: Giant cell tumor of bone: Highlights of 407 cases. Caldwell Lecture. Am J Roentgenol 144:955, 1985

8. DAHLIN DC: Bone Tumors. General Aspects and Data on 8,542 Cases, 4th ed. Springfield, IL, Charles C Thomas, 1986

9. DAHLIN DC, MCLEOD RA: Aneurysmal bone cyst and other nonneoplastic conditions. Skeletal Radiol 8:243, 1982

10. DEUTSCH A, RESNICK D: Eccentric cortical metastases to the skeleton from bronchogenic carcinoma. Radiology 137:49, 1980

11. EDEIKEN J, DALINKA M, KARASICK D: Roentgen Diagnosis of Diseases of Bone, Vol 1, 4th ed. Baltimore, Williams & Wilkins, 1991

12. EDEIKEN-MONROE B, EDEIKEN J, JACOBSON HG: Osteosarcoma. Semin Roentgenol 24:153, 1989

13. FELDMAN F, JOHNSTON A: Intra-osseous ganglion. Am J Roentgenol 118:328, 1973

14. FERNBACH SK, BLUMENTHAL DH, POZNANSKI AK, ET AL: Radiographic changes in unicameral bone cysts following direct injection of steroids: A report of 14 cases. Radiology 140:689, 1981

15. GLASS TA, MILLS SE, FECHNER RE, ET AL: Giant-cell reparative granuloma of the hands and feet. Radiology 149:65, 1983

16. GREENSPAN A, STEINER G, KNUTZON R: Bone island (enostosis): Clinical significance and radiologic and pathologic correlations. Skeletal Radiol 20:85, 1991

17. HALL FM, GOLDBERG RP, DAVIES JAK, ET AL: Scintigraphic assessment of bone island. Radiology 135:737, 1980

18. HARBIN WP: Metastatic disease and the nonspecific bone scan: Value of spinal computed tomography. Radiology 145:105, 1982

19. HUDSON TM: Radiologic-pathologic correlation of musculoskeletal lesions. Baltimore, Williams & Wilkins, 1987

20. JACOBSON AR, STOMPER PC, CRONIN EB, ET AL: Bone scans with one or two new abnormalities in cancer patients with no known metastases: Reliability of interpretation of initial correlative radiographs. Radiology 174:503, 1990

21. KATTAPURAM SV, KUSHNER DC, PHILLIPS WC, ET AL: Osteoid osteoma: An unusual cause of articular pain. Radiology 147:383, 1983

22. KUMAR R, MADEWELL JE, LINDELL MM, ET AL: Fibrous lesions of bones. Radiographics 10:237, 1990

23. LEVINE E, DESMET AA, HUNTRAKOON M: Juxtacortical osteosarcoma: A radiologic and histologic spectrum. Skeletal Radiol 14:38, 1985

24. MADEWELL JE, RAGSDALE BD, SWEET DE: Radiologic and pathologic analysis of solitary bone lesions. I. Internal Margins. Radiol Clin North Am 19:715, 1981

25. MARIO C, RODOLFO C, PIERO P: Unicameral and aneurysmal bone cysts. Clin Orthop 204:25, 1986

26. MCLEOD RA, BEABOUT JW: Roentgenographic features of chondroblastoma. Am J Roentgenol 118:464, 1973

27. MCLEOD RA, DAHLIN DC, BEABOUT JW: Spectrum of osteoblastoma. Am J Roentgenol 126:321, 1976

28. MILGRAM JW: Intraosseous lipomas with reactive ossification in the proximal femur. Report of eight cases. Skeletal Radiol 7:1, 1981

29. MILGRAM JW: The origins of osteochondromas and enchondromas. A histopathologic study. Clin Orthop 174:264, 1983

30. MOORE TE, KING AR, KATHOL MH, ET AL: Sarcoma in Paget disease of bone: Clinical, radiologic, and pathologic features in 22 cases. Am J Roentgenol 156:1199, 1991

31. MUNK PL: Recent advances in magnetic resonance imaging of musculoskeletal tumors. J Canad Assoc Radiol 42:39, 1991

32. MURRAY RO, JACOBSON HG: The Radiology of Skeletal Disorders. Vol 1, 2, 3. New York, Churchill-Livingstone, 1977

33. NASCIMENTO AG, HUVOS AG, MARCOVE RC: Primary malignant giant cell tumor of bone. Cancer 44:1393, 1979

34. PEAR BL: Epidermoid and dermoid sequestration cysts. Am J Roentgenol 110:148, 1970

35. RAGSDALE BD, MADEWELL JE, SWEET DE: Radiologic and pathologic analysis of solitary bone lesions. II. Periosteal reactions. Radiol Clin North Am 19:749, 1981

36. RESNICK D, NEMCEK AA JR, HAGHIGHI P: Spinal enostoses (bone islands). Radiology 147:373, 1983

37. REYNOLDS J: The "fallen fragment sign" in the diagnosis of unicameral bone cysts. Radiology 92:949, 1969

37. SEEGER LL, ECKARDT JJ, BASSETT LW: Cross-sectional imaging in the evaluation of osteogenic sarcoma: MRI and CT. Semin Roentgenol 24:174, 1989

38. SPRINGFIELD DS, CAPANNA R, GHERLINZONI F, ET AL: Chondroblastoma. J Bone Joint Surg [Am] 67:748, 1985

39. SWEET DE, MADEWELL JE, RAGSDALE BD: Radiologic and pathologic analysis of solitary bone lesions. III. Matrix patterns. Radiol Clin North Am 19:785, 1981

40. WILSON AJ, KYRIAKOS M, ACKERMAN LV: Chondromyxoid fibroma: Radiographic appearance in 38 cases and in a review of the literature. Radiology 179:513, 1991

Paul and Juhl's Essentials of Radiologic Imaging, Sixth Edition, edited by John H. Juhl and Andrew B. Crummy. J.B. Lippincott Company, Philadelphia, © 1993.

CHAPTER **5**

Infections and Inflammations of Bones

Lee F. Rogers

OSTEOMYELITIS

Osteomyelitis was once a common, devastating, often crippling, and much-feared disease. Since the advent of antibiotics, it has become manageable, less common, and much less serious. The general improvement in personal hygiene, greatly improved surgical antisepsis, and early antibiotic treatment of lesions that predispose to septicemia have resulted in an appreciable reduction in the incidence of osteomyelitis.

Infections of bone have been conveniently divided into three categories reflecting the source of the infection:[20, 30] (1) hematogenous osteomyelitis, (2) implantation osteomyelitis caused by bacteria implanted or introduced with an open fracture, penetrating wound, or surgical procedure, and (3) secondary osteomyelitis with the bone involvement secondary to a contiguous focus of soft-tissue infection related to peripheral vascular disease. In the series by Waldvogel and associates,[30] hematogenous osteomyelitis accounted for only 19% of all cases, implantation osteomyelitis 47%, and secondary osteomyelitis related to vascular insufficiency 34%. Osteomyelitis may also be divided into acute, subacute, and chronic forms, dependent on the virulence of the organism, the response of the host, and the effectiveness of antibiotic treatment.

Staphylococcus aureus is the most frequent offending organism. In children, in whom hematogenous infection is the rule, multiple foci of disease are relatively frequent, whereas in adults, the infection is usually limited to a single focus. The cause is usually established by obtaining a positive blood culture, a culture from an aspiration of the adjacent joint, or a direct aspiration of the involved bone or overlying soft tissues. Early recognition and treatment with antibiotics may minimize the radiographic findings of osteomyelitis.

PATHOGENESIS

Hematogenous Osteomyelitis

The source of bacteria in the hematogenous form is usually infections of the skin, boils or carbuncles, insect bites, infected abrasions, and less commonly infections of the respiratory tract. The offending organism is usually *S. aureus*, less commonly *Streptococcus*, *Haemophilus influenzae*, or pneumococcus. The organisms enter the bloodstream and become entrapped in the terminal vascular networks of long bones, the site and consequences dependent on the age of the patient (Fig. 5-1). In childhood, these networks are located in the metaphysis just beneath the physis, and thus the infections in childhood are most often located in and limited to the metaphyseal ends of long bones, particularly the femur and tibia[20, 28] (see Figs. 5-4 and 5-5). Involvement of adjacent joints is rare.[15] Terminal vascular networks are also located in the epiphysis, but isolated infections of the epiphysis are much less common than those in the metaphysis.[24] In contrast, in infants under the age of 1 year, the vascular network commonly crosses the growth plate from the meta-

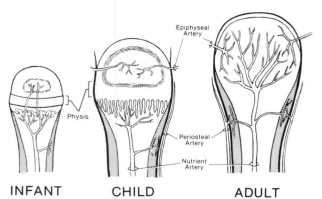

INFANT   CHILD   ADULT

Figure 5–1. Vascular supply of bone. The principal blood supply to the end of bone is from the nutrient artery in the medullary canal. In the infant and until 18 months of age, small vessels perforate the physis to enter the epiphysis. After 18 months of age, the vascular supply assumes the pattern of childhood and the perforating vessels involute. The epiphysis and metaphysis then have separate blood supplies. In the adult, following closure of the physis, the branches of the nutrient artery extend to the end of bone. Note the blood supply to the cortex. Branches of the periosteal artery supply the outer cortex, whereas branches of the nutrient artery supply the inner cortex.

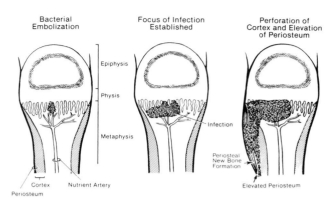

Figure 5–2. Pathomechanics of hematogenous osteomyelitis. Bacterial embolization occurs through the nutrient artery, and bacteria lodge in the terminal blood supply in the metaphysis. After the infection is established, it expands within the medullary canal toward the cortex and the diaphysis. The physis is an effective barrier. The infection then extends through the vascular channels in the cortex to elevate and strip the periosteum from the cortex. Periosteal new-bone formation occurs. Note that the bond between the periosteum and perichondrium at the physis prevents extension of the infection into the joint.

physis to the epiphysis; therefore, infections in infancy are more likely to originate within the epiphysis or extend quickly from the metaphysis into the epiphysis and then into the adjacent joint.[20, 28] Extension of the infection into the adjacent joint is much less likely after the age of 1½ years, except in the hip, where the metaphysis is located within the joint capsule. Following the closure of the epiphysis, the terminal blood supply is located in the end of the bone. Thus in adults, the hematogenous infections occur at the end of the bone and may extend into the adjacent joint space. However, primary hematogenous osteomyelitis of long bones is uncommon in adults. Adults are more likely to suffer vertebral osteomyelitis or suppurative spondylitis, often secondary to infection or manipulation of the urinary tract.

The infectious process begins in the intramedullary portion of the bone, eventually leading to the destruction of the trabeculae, penetration of the overlying cortex through vascular foramina, elevation of the periosteum, and extension into the overlying soft tissues (Fig. 5-2).

The periosteum is easily elevated by the extension of pus through the cortex. Because the periosteum is tightly bound to the perichondrium of the physis or growth plate, the periosteum is preferentially stripped

or elevated from the metaphysis toward the diaphysis, often well beyond the extent of involvement of the intramedullary bone or marrow. The tight bond between the periosteum and perichondrium at the physis prevents extension of pus into the epiphysis or adjacent joint except at the hip, where the metaphysis lies within the joint. In contrast to that in children, the periosteum of adults is tightly adherent to the cortex and much less easily stripped. Therefore, in adults, periosteal elevation is not as marked, the extent of periosteal stripping is more limited, and involucrum formation is uncommon.

Implantation Osteomyelitis

Implantation osteomyelitis is due to bacteria introduced into the soft tissues and bone by a penetrating wound, surgical procedure, or open fractures and dislocations (see Fig. 5-8). Blood clot, necrotic marrow, muscle, and other soft tissues provide an excellent culture medium for the localization and colonization of pathogenic bacteria. *S. aureus* is a common offending organism, but other gram-positive organisms like *Streptococcus* and gram-negative organisms such as *Pseudomonas*, *Proteus*, or *Escherichia coli* may be involved.

Secondary Osteomyelitis

Osteomyelitis associated with vascular insufficiency is almost always encountered in the diabetic patient and localized to the foot, affecting the phalanges and metatarsals (see Fig. 5-16). Infection of bone is always secondary to an overlying cellulitis or deep penetrating ulcer of the skin. The most common offending organism is *S. aureus* or *Streptococcus*, although gram-negative bacterial infections are also encountered.

Infections of bone are discussed in this chapter. Infections of joints and infectious spondylitis are detailed in Chapter 3.

RADIOGRAPHIC FINDINGS IN ACUTE OSTEOMYELITIS

In acute osteomyelitis there is a latent period of 10 to 12 days between the time of onset of clinical symptoms and the development of definite radiographic changes in bone.[20] Because it is essential that adequate therapy be instituted as early as possible, one should not wait for the development of radiographic evidence of disease before instituting appropriate treatment. Radioisotopic bone scan is very sensitive to the changes of osteomyelitis, revealing areas of increased radioactivity at sites of infection well before there is any plain film radiographic sign of disease (Fig. 5-3). A bone scan is warranted in every case of clinically suspected osteomyelitis in which the radiographs are unrevealing.

The first radiographic evidence of disease is the swelling of soft tissues, characteristically deep and adjacent to bone (Figs. 5-3A and 5-4).[4] The early swelling is recognized because of displacement or obliteration of the normal fat planes adjacent to and beneath the deep muscle bundles. At first the superficial fatty layer is unaffected. In contrast, with skin infection, soft-tissue swelling is superficial and does not involve the deeper tissues adjacent to the bone. The first evidence of disease in the bone is usually an area of indefinite rarefaction or destruction in the metaphysis (Figs. 5-5 and 5-6). The area of destruction is poorly defined and has a fine, granular, or slightly mottled appearance. Associated with this or even at times preceding it is a minimal amount of periosteal new-bone formation laid down parallel to the outer margin of the cortex. The limits of the bone destruction remain poorly defined throughout the acute stage. The actual disease process is usually much more extensive than demonstrated by the radiograph.

In a short time, bone destruction becomes more prominent, causing a ragged, moth-eaten appearance

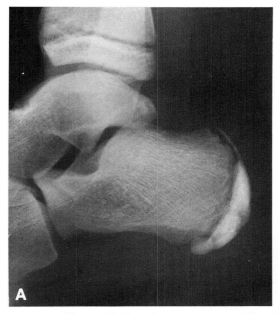
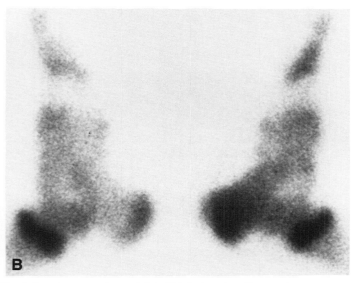

Figure 5–3. Acute osteomyelitis of the left calcaneus in a child. **(A)** Lateral radiograph demonstrates no bony abnormality. Deep soft-tissue swelling is present adjacent to the posterior and inferior surfaces of the calcaneus. **(B)** Technetium-99m bone scan reveals focus of increased activity in the left calcaneus. Bilateral increased activity at the distal tibial epiphysis is normal. (Courtesy of James Conway, M.D., Chicago)

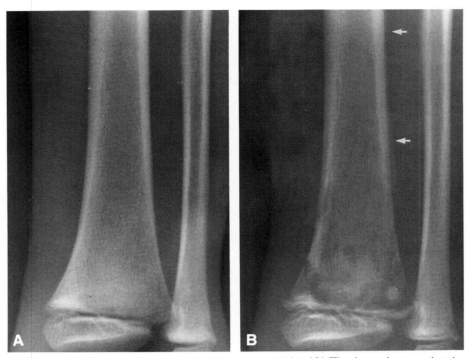

Figure 5–4. Acute osteomyelitis in the distal tibia. **(A)** The bone is completely normal; however, note the edema and soft-tissue swelling adjacent to the medial surface of the tibia, with obliteration of portions of the subcutaneous fat. This is the earliest radiographic sign of osteomyelitis. **(B)** Repeat examination obtained in 11 days demonstrates irregular permeative and mottled destruction within the metaphysis, with a perforation and destruction of the cortex in several areas. Periosteal elevation is identified proximally (*arrows*).

of the medullary bone, with foci of destruction intermingled with areas of apparently more or less normal bone. Periosteal new-bone formation is more pronounced, and both the periosteal reaction and intramedullary destruction extend into the diaphysis (see Fig. 5-6). In the neonate, the infection commonly extends to the overlying joint, forming a suppurative arthritis (Fig. 5-7, see also Figs. 3-5 and 3-6).

In the phalanges and other small bones there is little or no periosteal reaction. Bone is simply dissolved (see Fig. 5-16). At times this proceeds internally, hollowing or shelling out the bone by destroying intramedullary trabeculae, leaving only a thin rim of cortex (Fig. 5-8).

RADIOISOTOPIC BONE SCANNING

Technetium-99m radiophosphate (see Figs. 5-3 and 5-8), gallium-67 (^{67}Ga) citrate, and indium-111 leukocytes have been used to diagnose osteomyelitis and to differentiate osseous infections from those limited to the soft tissues (e.g., cellulitis).[3, 13, 22] To distinguish skeletal from soft-tissue infection, a triple-phase ^{99m}Tc radiophosphate scan is performed (see Fig. 5-17). The three phases are perfusion, blood pool, and delayed images. Acute osteomyelitis is characterized by enhanced activity in the blood pool and delayed bone images, whereas septic arthritis and cellulitis demonstrate increased activity in the blood pool phase but normal or only slightly increased uptake in the delayed image. Sequential radiophosphate and gallium scanning may also be used, since increased radiophosphate uptake is nonspecific, occurring in areas of high bone turnover from whatever cause—fracture, infection, metabolic, or tumor. Gallium-67 uptake is more specific for infection. Indium-111 leukocytes deposit wherever there is an active migration of white cells, and therefore this examination is also more specific for infection.[22]

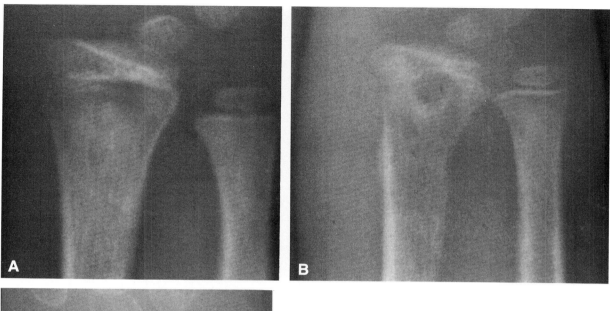

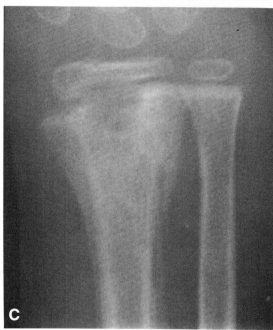

Figure 5–5. Acute osteomyelitis of the distal radius. **(A)** Initial examination demonstrates irregular lysis and destruction in the distal metaphysis. The epiphysis remains intact. **(B)** Repeat examination in 9 days demonstrates obvious destruction, which now extends proximally toward the diaphysis. Cortical destruction and considerable overlying soft-tissue swelling are present. Note the periosteal new-bone formation. **(C)** Eight-week follow-up examination. Healing is demonstrated by the compact periosteal reaction filling in a portion of previously destroyed bone. Note that the process did not extend into the epiphysis.

COMPUTED TOMOGRAPHY

Computed tomography (CT) is a useful adjunct in the evaluation of osteomyelitis.[10, 31] Increased attenuation occurs within the bone marrow early in the disease, prior to plain film changes and simultaneously with increased radioisotopic activity. The increased attenuation is due to the presence of edema and pus, which replaces the fat within the marrow. The attenuation of normal marrow fat is on the order of -80 to -100 Hounsfield units, increasing in the presence of an infection to -10 Hounsfield units or higher, well within the positive range. This is similar in appearance to infiltration by tumors (see Fig. 4-43). Small bubbles of intraosseous gas may be seen within the intramedullary canal as a result of infection by gas-forming organ-

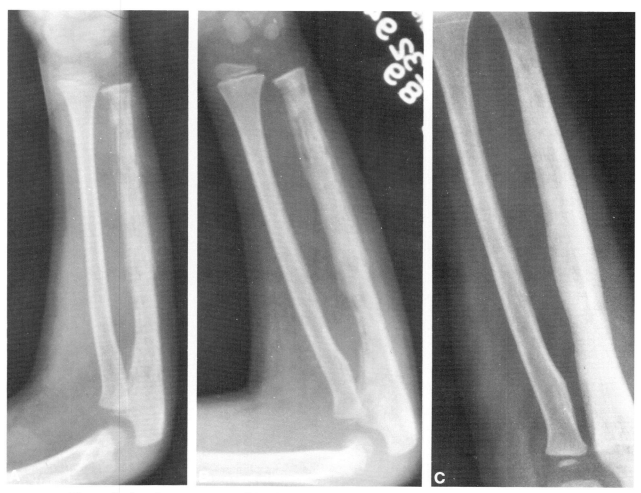

Figure 5–6. Acute osteomyelitis of the ulna. (**A**) Examination obtained 10 days after the onset of symptoms demonstrates permeative destruction of most of the ulna, with periosteal new-bone formation surrounding the distal shaft and metaphysis. (**B**) Repeat examination 1 week later shows an increase in the amount of subperiosteal new-bone formation. (**C**) Examination 6 months later shows residual cortical thickening but no definite areas of bone destruction.

isms. CT demonstrates to good advantage cortical destruction and associated soft-tissue changes (see Fig. 5-9B). Fat–fluid (pus) levels have been reported to occur within the medullary canal and adjacent bursae.[17] CT is also advantageous in the evaluation of chronic osteomyelitis,[10, 31] allowing the detection and localization of bony sequestra, the demonstration of cortical defects leading to subcutaneous sinus tracts, and the identification of adjacent soft-tissue abscesses. Abscesses appear as sharply defined areas of low density within surrounding muscle or subcutaneous tissue.

MAGNETIC RESONANCE IMAGING

Magnetic resonance imaging (MRI) has proved to be more sensitive than standard radiography, conventional tomography, or CT in the evaluation of osteomyelitis.[5, 8, 26, 29] MRI demonstrates changes in the marrow before they are evident on a radiograph. The initial manifestation of the disease is a reduction in the signal from the fat in the bone marrow, seen as a diminished signal on a T1-weighted image. On a T2-weighted image, the signal from the infected area is greater than

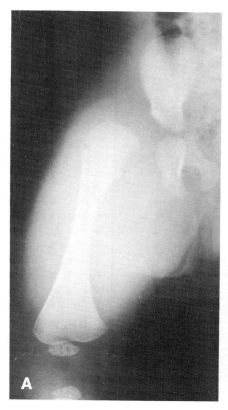
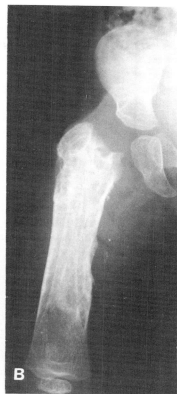

Figure 5–7. Acute osteomyelitis of the femur associated with suppurative arthritis of the hip in an infant. (**A**) Examination 7 days after the onset of fever and swelling of the thigh. Note the massive soft-tissue swelling and lateral dislocation of the femur, indicating an associated joint effusion. Minimal cortical destruction is evident in the medial aspect of the metaphysis. (**B**) Examination obtained 3 months later shows extensive new-bone formation surrounding much of the shaft. Remnants of the old shaft are visible. Several rounded or oval radiolucencies are seen in the proximal femur, possibly representing residual foci of infection. The hip joint is no longer dislocated.

that of the fat within the marrow, and the soft-tissue extent of the infectious process may also be demonstrated (see Figs. 5-14 and 5-15). MRI may distinguish between osteomyelitis and surrounding soft-tissue infection by demonstrating normal signals from the underlying intramedullary bone, clearly indicating the absence of osseous infection. Since there is essentially no signal from cortical bone, this method is not sensitive to changes within the cortex.

SUBACUTE AND CHRONIC OSTEOMYELITIS

Unless treated, osteomyelitis gradually progresses into subacute and chronic stages, with considerable variation in the time required for these developments. Among the factors involved are the virulence of the organism, the resistance of the host, and treatment with antibiotics. It has been suggested that the subacute form of osteomyelitis has become more prevalent, unrelated to the use of antibiotics[11], in the suppression of acute osteomyelitis.

BONE ABSCESS

The infection is gradually walled off by reactive bone formation, forming a bone abscess (Figs. 5-10 and 5-11). Chronic bone abscesses, often called *Brodie's abscess*,[25] are characterized by sharply outlined areas of rarefaction or lucency of variable size located in the metaphysis and surrounded by an irregular zone of dense sclerosis. The overlying cortex is usually thickened by periosteal new-bone formation.

In subacute osteomyelitis of childhood, abscesses are often elongated, serpiginous lucencies with a sclerotic border and oriented in the long axis of the bone (Fig. 5-10). They abut against the growth plate and may, on occasion, extend across the physis to involve the adjacent epiphysis.[2] When examined in the axial plane by CT or MRI, they may be found to have breached the overlying cortex and to be contiguous with a well-defined soft-tissue abscess.

Intraosseous abscesses examined by MRI are of low to intermediate signal on T1, brighter than normal marrow on T2 (Fig. 5-15), and surrounded by a low-intensity rim on both T1- and T2-weighted images.[26, 29]

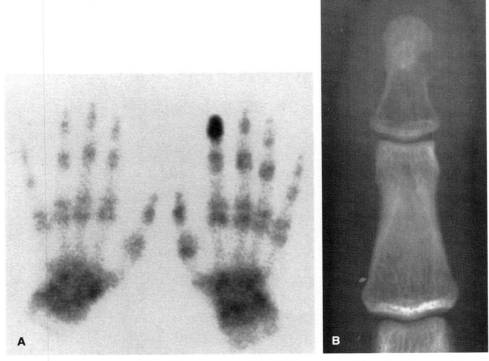

Figure 5–8.   Human bite with osteomyelitis. This man sustained a human bite on the tip of the index finger 2 weeks ago. He presented with obvious swelling and redness over the distal phalanx. The clinical question was to distinguish between cellulitis and osteomyelitis. (**A**) Technetium-99m bone scan, 2-hour delay, demonstrates increased activity in the distal phalanx. (**B**) AP radiograph demonstrates a breach in the lateral cortex just beneath the ungual tuft and a hollowing or shelling out of the trabeculae in the distal phalanx. There is no periosteal reaction. Findings are indicative of osteomyelitis.

INVOLUCRUM AND SEQUESTRUM FORMATION

Segments of cortical bone isolated in the midst of a chronic infection and devoid of blood supply are known as *sequestra*. Sequestra become avascular by losing the periosteal supply as the periosteum is stripped and elevated from the cortex and the intramedullary supply, because the infection of the marrow causes vascular thrombosis. Sequestra are evident on the radiograph as areas of dense bone surrounded by zones of rarefaction or lucency (Fig. 5-12). They remain as dense as normal bone, standing out clearly from the surrounding demineralized bone. An *involucrum* is a shell of bone formed by the periosteum that surrounds and encloaks a sequestrum. Involucrum and sequestrum formation are more common in osteomyelitis

in children than in adults, although sequestra often occur in secondary forms of osteomyelitis, particularly those associated with open fractures.

The end result of a chronic osteomyelitis, after the infection has subsided, is a thickened bone with a sclerotic cortex and a wavy outer margin interspersed with lucent areas where sequestra have been absorbed or surgically removed (Fig. 5-13). The cortex may become so dense and thickened that the medullary cavity is not apparent. Chronic osteomyelitis is subject to recurrent reactivation. Because of the irregular density and marked sclerosis, it is often impossible to determine with certainty whether or not an active infection is present. CT and MRI are used to visualize the interior of the bone (Fig. 5-14). If the infection becomes reactivated, it is usually

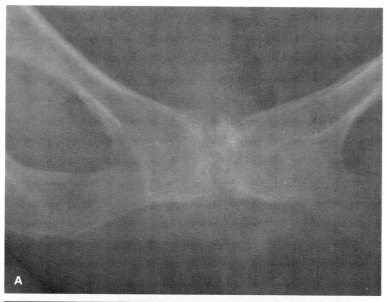

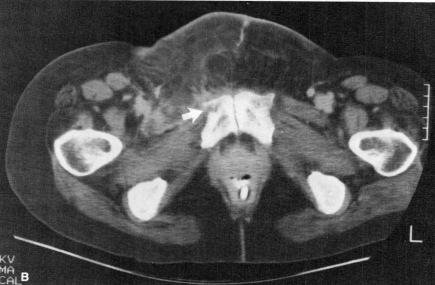

Figure 5–9. Osteomyelitis of the right pubic bone. (**A**) AP view. There is no definite abnormality. (**B**) CT scan. Extensive soft-tissue changes anterior to the pubis and a break in the cortex (*arrow*) consistent with osteomyelitis and overlying cellulitis.

manifested by soft-tissue swelling, by new areas of periosteal new-bone formation, and by the development of sharply defined radiolucent cavities within the bone. Comparison with previous examination is very helpful. The bone scan will usually remain positive throughout the entire course of the disease and therefore cannot be used to determine the presence or absence of reactivation.

MRI is useful in the evaluation of chronic osteomyelitis[5, 26] because of its ability to detect foci of persistent or recurrent infection. Scar and sinus tracts are of low to intermediate signal on both T1- and T2-weighted images, whereas a focus of active infection is similar to that of a bone abscess, low on T1, higher than marrow on T2, surrounded by a low-intensity rim on

(*text continues on page 198*)

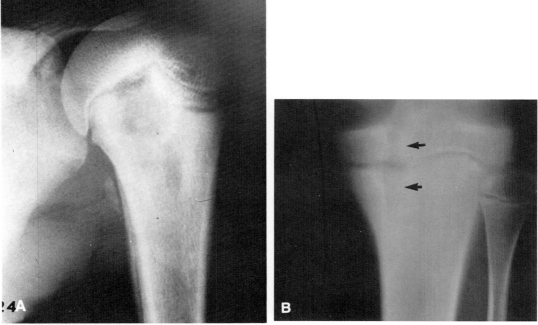

Figure 5–10. Two cases of subacute bone abscess in children. (**A**) An elongated radiolucency in the proximal humerus surrounded by sclerosis with overlying periosteal new-bone formation extends for some distance down the humeral shaft. Proximally, it abuts the growth plate. (**B**) Serpiginous lucency in the proximal metaphysis of the tibia extends across the growth plate into the epiphysis (*arrows*). Note that it is marginated by a fine sclerotic rim. (Case courtesy of Andrew K. Poznanski, M.D., Chicago)

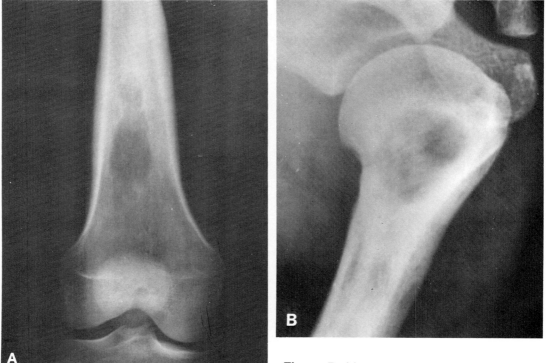

Figure 5–11.

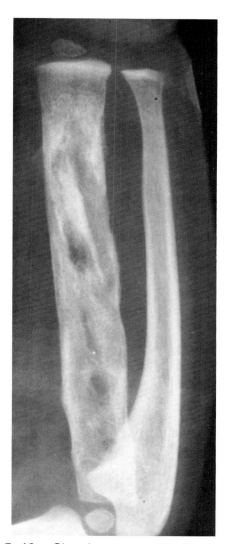

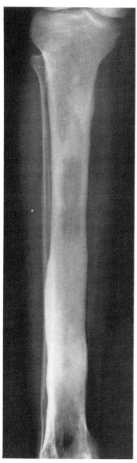

Figure 5–12.   Chronic osteomyelitis. The entire radius has been involved. There are irregular cavities representing chronic abscesses, and a large, dense sequestrum surrounded by involucrum is noted within the cavity in the distal end of the shaft. The original cortex has been completely replaced.

Figure 5–13.   Chronic osteomyelitis. Cortical thickening and sclerosis involve the entire shaft, particularly distally. Some ovoid radiolucencies can be seen within the thickening.

◀ **Figure 5–11.**   Chronic bone abscess, or Brodie's abscess. **(A)** The abscess cavity is seen as a well-demarcated area of radiolucency surrounded by sclerotic bone. The overlying cortex is thickened by compact periosteal new-bone formation. **(B)** Chronic bone abscess of the proximal humerus. A rounded radiolucency is surrounded by a relatively thickened wall of sclerosis. Periosteal new-bone formation is present in the metaphysis.

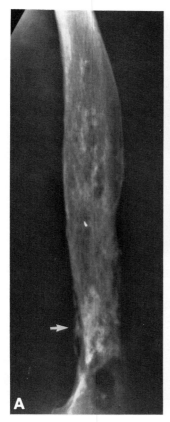

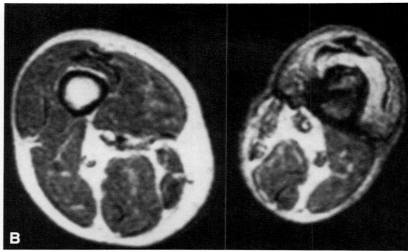

Figure 5–14. Chronic osteomyelitis of the femur, with intermittent drainage over a period of 40 years. (**A**) The cortex has expanded. Irregular patches of sclerosis and lucency are present throughout the diaphysis. A large radiolucency is present distally. Periosteal new-bone formation is present (*arrow*). (**B**) T1-weighted MRI. Note the obvious atrophy of the involved extremity. The cortex is poorly defined and is expanded and thin. The intramedullary cavity has a low signal compared with the opposite side, indicative of persistent infection.

both, and possibly containing a sequestrum of low signal by both techniques.

SPECIAL SITUATIONS

NEONATAL OSTEOMYELITIS

Osteomyelitis in the neonate, in the first month of life, is sufficiently distinctive to warrant consideration separate from osteomyelitis in older children.[12] The systemic manifestations of fever, malaise, and toxicity are much less pronounced or even absent in the neonate. Parents usually seek care for focal manifestations of disease—swelling, tenderness, and decreased motion of an extremity, a pseudoparalysis. This commonly occurs within the first 2 weeks of life and may affect either full-term or premature infants. The majority will have had an antecedent illness, frequently requiring umbilical catheterization or other potentially infective procedures or exposure to illness in family members or other close contacts. *S. aureus* is the most common causative organism. Multiple sites of involvement are common. The infection most frequently involves the ends of the femur (particularly the hip), tibia, and humerus, with septic arthritis of the adjacent hip, knee, and shoulder joints in as many as 50% of cases (see Figs. 5-7 and 3-5). Significant residual deficits are common.

Approximately 80% of affected neonates will have radiographic manifestations at the time of presentation. The most common finding is deep soft-tissue swelling, and half will have definite bone destruction or joint abnormalities. In a neonate, the radiographic findings of a joint dislocation associated with a surrounding soft-tissue mass are characteristic of septic arthritis (see Fig. 5-7). Technetium bone scanning will be helpful in questionable cases and may demonstrate other foci of disease in those with overt radiographic evidence of disease at a single site.[3]

CORTICAL BONE ABSCESS

Cortical bone has a dual blood supply, arising both externally from the periosteal blood vessels and centrally from the nutrient artery within the medullary canal. These two systems join in the middle of the cortex, forming an anastomotic network (see Fig. 5-1). Occasionally, foci of bacteria become entrapped and implant, giving rise to an infection manifested radiographically as eccentric, circular, ovoid, or elongated radiolucencies within the cortex of the diaphysis.[20] The outer cortex is usually either markedly thin or completely disrupted and the abscess surrounded by periosteal new bone (Fig. 5-15). At times the periosteal response is so marked that a tomogram or CT is required to demonstrate the lucency with certainty. CT and MRI will also demonstrate soft-tissue swelling and edema within the surrounding soft-tissues (Fig.

5-15*B*, *C*). The lesion may be difficult to distinguish from an osteoid osteoma on radiographic findings alone. However, clinical signs of infection or the characteristic nocturnal pain pattern relieved by aspirin, indicating an osteoid osteoma, will be helpful in establishing the correct diagnosis. A similar lesion may result from the cortical deposition of metastatic disease (see Fig. 4-29). However, the periosteal response is usually less prominent than that encountered with a cortical abscess. Intracortical metastatic disease is most commonly found in carcinoma of the lung but may be found occasionally with other primary carcinomas.

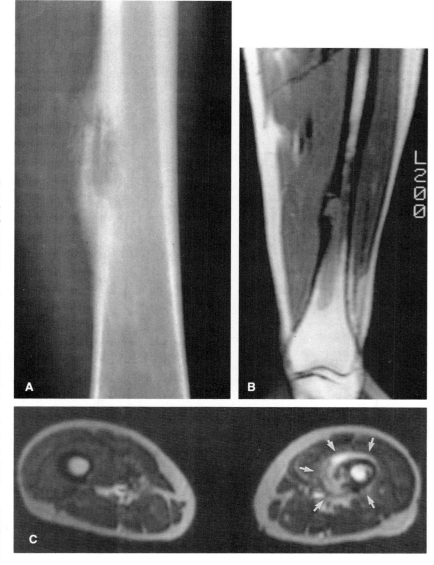

Figure 5–15. Cortical abscess of the midfemoral shaft in an intravenous drug abuser. (**A**) AP view demonstrates considerable linear and nodular (sometimes known as lamellonodular) periosteal reaction overlying a lucent lytic defect in the medial cortex. This type of periosteal reaction is usually indicative of infection. (**B**) Coronal T1-weighted MRI demonstrates low signal within the marrow surrounding the lesion in the medial cortex. The overlying soft-tissue mass is not sharply defined. (**C**) T2-weighted axial image. This image demonstrates a high signal from the surrounding soft-tissue mass surrounding the lesion and cortex (*arrows*). Note that the signal emanating from the intramedullary space is higher than the normal bone marrow on the opposite side. This is indicative of active infection. The cortical abnormality is well demonstrated. (Case courtesy of Alfred L. Horowitz, M.D., Chicago)

OSTEOMYELITIS IN FLAT BONES (SKULL, PELVIS)

Flat and irregular bones have anatomic subdivisions comparable to long bones. Apophyses, as encountered in the pelvis, are the equivalent of the metaphyses in long bones. Prior to skeletal maturation, metaphyseal-type vascular anatomy predisposes these sites to involvement by hematogenous osteomyelitis.[16] Hematogenous osteomyelitis is relatively frequent at these sites and often poses diagnostic problems. CT is useful in the evaluation of suspected lesions in the pelvis (see Fig. 5-9).

In children the most common presenting symptoms are a gait disturbance and pain about the hip with only mild limitation of motion.[6] The patients may not be febrile and leukocytosis is variable, although the erythrocyte sedimentation rate is almost uniformly elevated.[6, 19] Initial radiographs are usually normal. ^{99m}Tc and ^{67}Ga citrate scans are abnormal. The diagnosis can usually be substantiated by CT or MRI, demonstrating foci of bone destruction with surrounding soft-tissue changes. Similar problems and findings may be encountered with infections of the sacroiliac joint in children[19] and adults.

Osteomyelitis of flat bones is characterized by patchy destruction without sharp demarcation. In the skull, periosteal reaction is absent, but a certain amount of sclerosis may be present. In the pelvis, periostitis occurs but is not as prominent as in long bones.

OSTEOMYELITIS IN THE DIABETIC FOOT

Diabetic foot is a term used to describe the peculiar combination of circulatory, infective, neuropathic, and degenerative changes affecting persons with long-standing diabetes. The radiographic hallmark of the diabetic foot is the presence of calcification of the small arteries of the foot and ankle, particularly the metatarsal arteries. Neuropathic and degenerative changes are described in Diabetic Osteoarthropathy in Chapter 3. Cellulitis and ulcers of the skin and subcutaneous tissues of the toes and plantar surface, beneath the head of the metatarsals and over the calcaneus, are quite common (Fig. 5-16A). Such superficial infections may eventually involve the underlying phalanges, metatarsals, and calcaneus, resulting in secondary osteomyelitis. This is manifested initially by demineralization or rarefaction, and subsequently by destruction of trabecular bone and cortex associated with periosteal new-bone formation, often underlying or adjacent to an obvious, lucent soft-tissue ulcer (Fig. 5-16B).[14, 20] The problem is to determine whether or not osteomyelitis is present when radiographic findings are minimal or absent (Fig. 5-17), as is frequently the case. Somewhat

less frequent but equally difficult to distinguish are changes due to osteomyelitis from those due to diabetic neuropathic arthropathy. This is further complicated by the relatively frequent simultaneous occurrence of both processes. In general, osteomyelitis is more likely a lytic, destructive process involving the phalanges and distal metatarsals, whereas neuropathy is more likely to be sclerotic and involve the tarsal bones, tarsometatarsal joints, and proximal metatarsals. Soft-tissue swelling may occur in either and is often due to a concomitant cellulitis. Pathologic fractures may occur in both processes—in osteomyelitis, usually through lytic foci in the phalanges; in neuropathy, as fragmentation of sclerotic tarsal bones. The combination of the three-phase radiophosphate bone scan and ^{67}Ga-citrate scan is useful in this determination (see Fig. 5-17).[14] The three-phase radiophosphate scan is used to differentiate between cellulitis and osteomyelitis, as described earlier. Both neuropathy and infection may show an increased uptake on the radiophosphate scan; however, ^{67}Ga will be taken up avidly by osteomyelitis, whereas neuropathic bone either does not reveal any or at best reveals only modest uptake of ^{67}Ga.

OSTEOMYELITIS IN DRUG ADDICTS

Acute osteomyelitis and septic arthritis are common in drug addicts because of the intravenous injection of drugs using nonsterile paraphernalia. Drug addicts are particularly prone to vertebral osteomyelitis (suppurative spondylitis) and infections of unusual joints, such as the sacroiliac or sternoclavicular joint.[7, 9] The infection may be secondary to an adjacent soft-tissue abscess, but more often it is hematogenous. There may be multiple sites of osseous involvement.

OSTEOMYELITIS IN SICKLE CELL DISEASE

Sickle cell disease is frequently complicated by acute osteomyelitis. The infection is unusual in that it commonly involves the diaphysis instead of the metaphysis (Fig. 5-18), and the causative organism is *Salmonella* in approximately 80% of patients. Multiple, often symmetrical lesions are occasionally encountered. The lesions may be extensive, involving the entire shaft. Large sequestra and extensive involucrum formation and pathologic fractures may occur. Differentiation from bone infarction, also common in sickle cell disease, may be difficult (see Chapter 7).

ACQUIRED IMMUNE DEFICIENCY SYNDROME (AIDS)

Surprisingly, bone and joint infections are rare in patients with human immunodeficiency virus (HIV)

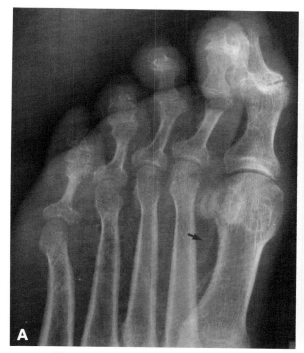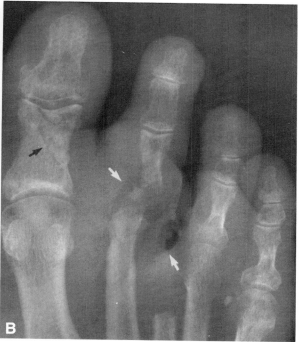

Figure 5–16. Infections in the diabetic foot. (**A**) Multiple small radiolucencies are present within the soft tissues of the foot underlying the metatarsals, identifying the site of a soft-tissue infection. No bony abnormalities are present, and thus there is no radiographic evidence of osteomyelitis. Note the arterial calcification (*arrow*) indicative of diabetes. (**B**) An amputation of the third toe was performed previously. A large collection of air (*white arrows*) identifies the site of ulcer on the plantar surface of the foot. Note the lytic destruction of the apposing surfaces of the second metatarsophalangeal joint, with associated subluxation indicative of osteomyelitis and suppurative arthritis. Closer examination will also reveal lytic destruction of the medial side of the head of the fourth metatarsal. There is also a fracture of the proximal phalanx of the great toe (*black arrow*) without a history of trauma, indicative of neurotrophic arthropathy.

infections. Bacillary angiomatosis is a recently recognized multisystem bacterial infectious disease that appears to represent an exception.[1] The disease consists of cutaneous vascular lesions that contain a bacterium similar to the bacillus of cat-scratch disease. Thirty-five percent of patients have multiple lytic lesions in bone.[1] The presence of bone lesions aids in differentiation of bacillary angiomatosis from Kaposi's sarcoma, which has similar cutaneous abnormalities but no associated bone lesions.[1]

CHRONIC GRANULOMATOUS DISEASE OF CHILDHOOD

Chronic granulomatous disease of childhood is characterized by infection, suppuration, and granuloma formation in the bones and lung.[32] The basic problem is a defect of the polymorphonuclear leukocytes in that they are able to ingest bacteria but cannot kill them. All other immune mechanisms, including plasma immunoglobulins, are normal. When the neutrophils die, live bacteria and their toxic products are released. Bone infection is very common and usually involves the small bones of the hands and feet. Initially it is similar to acute osteomyelitis, but it does not heal and proceeds to a chronic phase characterized by destructive, expansile, fairly well-marginated lesions that incite very little periosteal new-bone formation and usually do not break through the cortex or form sequestra. There may be a zone of rarefaction proximal to the growth plate similar to that observed in children with leukemia.

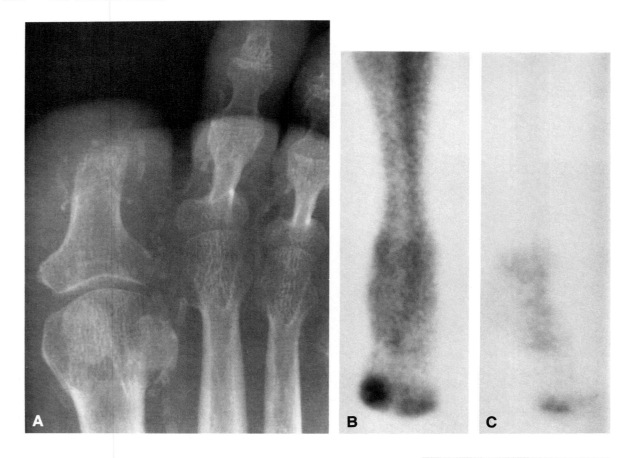

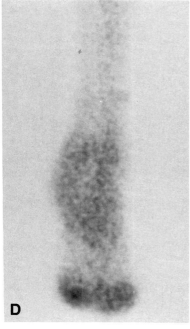

Figure 5–17.   Diabetic patient with soft-tissue infection. The ungual tuft of the great toe was previously amputated for osteomyelitis. There is now evidence of skin infection and a question of recurrent osteomyelitis. (**A**) Vascular calcification is present. The margin of the amputation of the distal phalanx of the great toe is poorly defined. (**B** and **C**) Two views from a three-phase ^{99m}Tc bone scan. The immediate static image (**B**) shows increased activity in the region of the great toe, and this diminished on the 2-hour delayed film (**C**). This suggests that the infection is a cellulitis without osteomyelitis. (**D**) A ^{67}Ga scan was obtained for confirmation. The activity is no greater than that on the delayed ^{99m}Tc scan and confirms the absence of osteomyelitis.

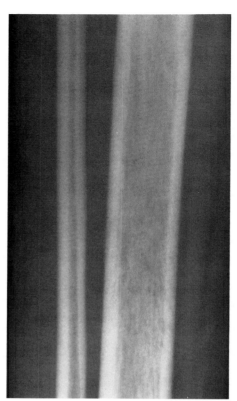

Figure 5–18. Osteomyelitis in sickle cell anemia. A permeative process is present throughout the mid-diaphysis, with tunneling in the cortex but no overlying periosteal reaction. Although the most common offending organism in such cases is *Salmonella*, *Escherichia coli* was present in this case.

CHRONIC SYMMETRICAL OSTEOMYELITIS

Chronic symmetrical osteomyelitis is a rare disease of childhood. It is a very indolent process, tending to involve the metaphyses, usually in the femur and tibia at the knee.[23] The lesions are osteolytic, rounded, or oval and surrounded by a thin sclerotic rim. Cortical breakthrough with resultant periosteal reaction occurs but is not common. The distal tibial metaphyses and distal ends of the clavicles may also be involved. Generalized symptoms are minimal, but there may be short, febrile episodes. The sedimentation rate is moderately elevated, and there is often an increase in leukocytes. Histologic features are those of chronic inflammation, but organisms often are not isolated. Some authors believe that this condition is of viral origin. The course is prolonged, and healing may not be complete for a number of years. There are usually no significant residua, however.

GARRÉ'S SCLEROSING OSTEITIS

As originally described by Garré, sclerosing osteitis was a peculiar type of osteomyelitis that, after an acute and virulent onset, subsided without drainage or the formation of sequestra, leaving only a thickened, sclerotic bone. The term *Garré's sclerosing osteitis* is now used infrequently. This is a rare condition, and many lesions so diagnosed initially turn out to be something else. If the possibility of other entities can be ruled out, the disease may be termed *chronic sclerosing osteitis*.

TUBERCULOSIS

Tuberculous osteomyelitis is infrequent when compared with tuberculosis of the spine or joints. It may occur as a localized bone abscess or less commonly as a diffuse disease. The clinical onset is insidious. The infection is of hematogenous origin, and simultaneous pulmonary disease is often demonstrated.

Disseminated tuberculous bone disease is not uncommon in heroin addicts and is usually associated with pulmonary tuberculosis. The ribs and spine are the most frequent sites of involvement. When draining sinuses are present, secondary infection may occur and the appearance may be similar to that of pyogenic osteomyelitis.

Tuberculous osteomyelitis may be difficult to distinguish from pyogenic osteomyelitis by radiographic examination. The lesion is largely destructive, and periosteal new-bone formation is minimal. The radiographic findings are those of chronic, nonvirulent infection.[20]

During infancy or childhood, tuberculous infection may involve one or more of the phalanges, tuberculous dactylitis (Fig. 5-19). It has a characteristic expanded cystic appearance, termed *spina ventosa*, with irregular destruction, expansion, and an absence of periosteal new-bone formation. In children and adults, there may be involvement of long tubular bones, characteristically a cystlike lesion located in the metaphysis, with marginal sclerosis and overlying periosteal reaction. In some cases they may be expansile. Ordinarily there is no sequestrum formation (Fig. 5-20).

Bone tuberculosis may occur in children as a complication of intradermal vaccination with BCG. The time interval between vaccination and appearance of detectable bone lesions ranges from 2 weeks to 2 months. The lesions are usually single and occur near the knee in the metaphysis of the femur or tibia. There is an eccentrically located area of destruction, often with cortical erosion and associated soft-tissue inflammation and swelling. Periosteal new-bone formation is slight or absent. There is very little tendency to diaphyseal

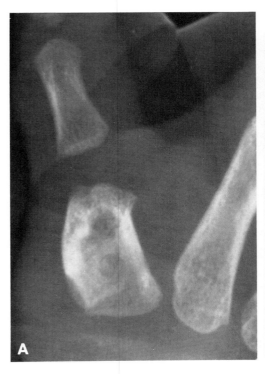

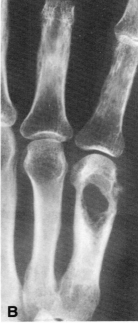

Figure 5–19. Tuberculous dactylitis in a child. (**A**) An expansile radiolucency with a slightly sclerotic rim involves the first metacarpal. The expansile nature of this process is characteristic of tuberculous dactylitis. Technically, the term should refer to an infection with similar changes in the phalanges. (**B**) Tuberculous abscess in the distal end of the fifth metacarpal in an adult. The cavity is clearly defined and slightly expanded and has a sclerotic margin and some sclerosis of bone proximal to the abscess.

spread, but about a third of patients develop involvement of the adjacent epiphysis.

Atypical mycobacteria may also produce osteomyelitis, and most of the reported cases have been in children. Manifestations vary from an indolent, chronic local bone lesion to a widespread dissemination with a fulminant course. The organism may be difficult to isolate. The osseous lesions usually respond satisfactorily to antituberculous therapy.

FUNGAL OSTEOMYELITIS

Fungal infections of bone are infrequent, the most common being blastomycosis and coccidioidomycosis. A lesion caused by a fungus is difficult to differentiate from other infections of bone. Fungal lesions are characteristically low-grade chronic infections with formation of a chronic bone abscess and possibly a draining sinus.[20] The appearance of the abscess resembles tuberculosis in that it is often found in cancellous bone, incites little periosteal new-bone formation, and characteristically has a relatively thin sclerotic margin. Findings suggestive of mycotic disease are (1) lesions arising at points of bony prominence such as the edges of the patella, the acromion or coracoid process of the scapula, the olecranon process, the styloid processes of the radius and ulna, the condyles of the humeri or

extremities of the clavicles, the malleoli, and the tuberosities of the tibias; (2) solitary marginal lesions of the ribs; (3) localized destructive lesions of the outer table of the skull; and (4) focal destructive lesions of the vertebra involving the neural arch or spinous and transverse processes.

COCCIDIOIDOMYCOSIS

Coccidioidomycosis is endemic to the San Joaquin Valley of California and arid zones of the Southwest. Hematogenous dissemination is uncommon in this disease, but when it occurs, the incidence of bone involvement is approximately 20%. The disease is more likely to be disseminated in blacks and Hispanics. A clue to dissemination is the presence of hilar adenopathy in association with pulmonary disease. Multiple bone lesions are the rule, and the spine is the most frequent site. The bony tuberosities and neural arch may be involved without involvement of the body of the vertebra.[20] The disc is often spared or involved late in the course of the disease. Epiphyseal involvement of long bones is common, but there is very little tendency to extend into the adjacent joint. The major roentgenographic finding is a focus of bone destruction with a moderate sclerotic margin (Fig. 5-21). Periosteal new-bone formation is uncommon. Paraspinal masses are common in vertebral disease and are often associated

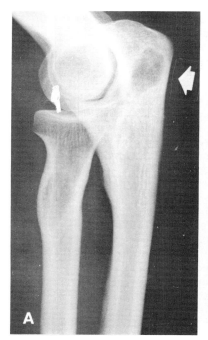
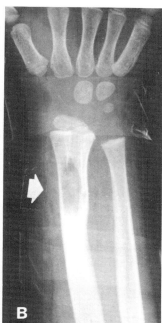

Figure 5–20. Tuberculous abscess. (**A**) Arrow indicates a radiolucent cavity in the olecranon process of the ulna, with very little surrounding reaction of bone. (**B**) Radiolucent focus in the distal radius (*arrow*) has slightly expanded the bone.

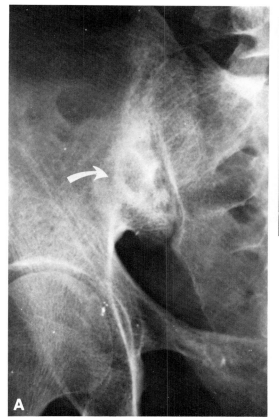

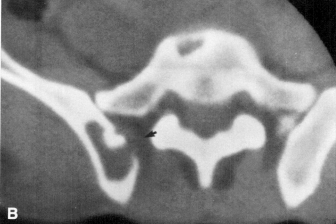

Figure 5–21. Two cases of coccidioidomycosis in the ilium. (**A**) Small, irregular radiolucencies are identified adjacent to the sacroiliac joint (*arrow*), with surrounding sclerosis of bone. (**B**) CT demonstrating radiolucency in the posterior aspect of the ilium, with perforation of the medial cortex (*arrow*). Note also a similar process within the body of the sacrum. Coccidioidomycosis characteristically involves bony projections and protuberances.

with involvement of the ribs, pedicles, and transverse processes. Recovery of the organism is necessary to confirm the diagnosis.

BLASTOMYCOSIS

Blastomycosis is endemic to the Eastern Mississippi River Valley, particularly Tennessee and Mississippi. Bones are involved in 25% to 50% of cases of the disseminated form of the disease. Blastomycosis commonly affects the skin and lungs, and this serves as an important clue to the skeletal disease process. Of patients with skeletal involvement, 75% have associated pulmonary disease. When an osseous lesion is encountered in association with disease of the skin or lung, the possibility of blastomycosis must be considered, particularly when the osseous process is distal to the knees or elbows. The most common sites affected are the long bones, ribs, short tubular bones of the hands and feet, and vertebrae. Facial bones may be involved, but the skull is rarely affected. In about one-third of the patients, bone lesions are multiple. Epiphyseal involvement is common, with rapid extension into the adjacent joint and formation of fistulous tracts. In the spine, the disease usually begins in the disc space and involves adjacent vertebrae and contiguous ribs in the formation of a paraspinal abscess. The bone lesions are usually indolent, expand slowly, and develop a sclerotic margin (Fig. 5-22). In the invasive form, bone destruction is rapid, inciting very little periosteal new-bone formation or sclerosis.

ACTINOMYCOSIS

Actinomycosis most commonly affects the mandible and forms sinus tracts. Involvement of the ribs is characteristically associated with underlying pneumonia and classically presents as marked periosteal new-bone formation along the margins of the rib. The bone involvement in actinomycosis most frequently occurs secondary to invasion from adjacent soft-tissue disease and results in a mixed osteolytic and sclerotic process.

CRYPTOCOCCOSIS

In cryptococcosis, osseous involvement is not common and usually occurs in patients with compromised defense mechanisms. The most frequent sites are the pelvis, ribs, and skull. The lesion tends to be lytic, with reasonably discrete margins and little or no periosteal reaction.

ASPERGILLOSIS

Aspergillosis of bone is also found in immunosuppressed patients. The organism is ordinarily a saprophyte but may cause osteomyelitis, with bone destruc-

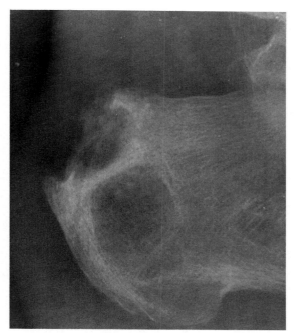

Figure 5–22. Blastomycosis. A lytic radiolucency with destruction of the overlying cortex is present on the posterior margin of the tuberosity of the calcaneus. This patient also had a lesion in the metacarpal that was quite similar in appearance to that in Figure 5-19B and had a right middle lobe abscess due to blastomycosis.

tion and a spread from an adjacent infection. This most commonly involves the ribs or spine secondary to pulmonary aspergillosis. Involvement of the spine is rather indolent and involves adjacent disc spaces, with minimal bone destruction or paraspinous mass.

MADURA FOOT

Madura foot is a chronic infection of the foot caused by a mixed group of fungi endemic to Mexico and Central and South America. It involves the soft tissue, causing sinus formation, and may result in an extensive destructive process of the small bones of the foot (Fig. 5-23).

ECHINOCOCCUS

Echinococcal disease is endemic to the Balkan states: Iceland, Australia, South Africa, and Argentina. Hydatid cysts are characteristically formed in the liver or lungs. Osseous lesions are located mainly in the spine and pelvis.[27] The typical lesion is a round or oval, often multiple and confluent osteolytic defect, with sharp,

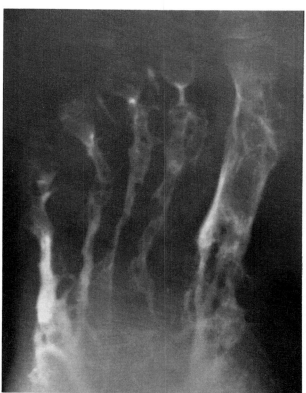

Figure 5–23. Madura foot. The metatarsals are all involved by a lytic process. The appearance is pathognomonic of this condition.

slightly sclerotic margins.[27] Occasionally there is rib involvement, which may extend into an adjacent vertebral body. Involvement of long bones is rare. The disease tends to destroy bone and may encroach on the spinal canal and cord when it involves the vertebral body.

SYPHILIS

There are three types of syphilis of bone: (1) congenital syphilis, present at birth or in early infancy, (2) late congenital syphilis, which appears later in childhood, in adolescence, or in early adult life and has the radiographic and pathologic characteristics of tertiary syphilis, and (3) acquired syphilis occurring in adults, the skeletal lesion appearing some time after the primary infection.

Congenital syphilis is characterized by symmetrical involvement of multiple long bones, whereas tertiary syphilis or gumma formation is characterized by a dramatic proliferation of new bone. Similar findings may occur in yaws.

CONGENITAL SYPHILIS

The principal radiographic features of congenital syphilis[18] are diffuse, linear, periosteal new-bone formation that symmetrically involves the shafts of multiple long bones and transverse bands of radiolucency of variable width within the metaphysis, located just beneath the zone of provisional calcification (Fig. 5-24). In the proximal tibia, these bands are associated with erosions of the cortex in the medial aspect of the metaphysis. The lesions of the tibia are characteristic of this disease and are known as Wimberger's sign. There may be similar lesions of the medial metaphysis of the distal femur. Pathologic fractures may occur through these foci of metaphyseal disease. When the disease is extensive, focal destruction may be demonstrated throughout the shaft. The epiphyses are characteristically spared.

Diffuse periosteal reaction must be differentiated from the periosteal growth of new-bone encountered in the premature infant. The periosteal new-bone formation may also suggest the diagnosis of Caffey's disease (infantile cortical hyperostosis). This disease characteristically involves the mandible, radius, ulna, or tibia and is asymmetrical and limited to a few long bones (see Figs. 5-30 and 5-31).

LATENT CONGENITAL SYPHILIS

Although the primary infection occurs in utero or at birth, in latent congenital syphilis the disease is not manifested until childhood, adolescence, or early adult life. The lesions of bone are manifestations of tertiary syphilis due to gumma formation. Bone is destroyed, but the destruction is overshadowed by extensive newbone formation. The disease characteristically involves the tibia. The affected bone becomes thickened as a result of chronic periostitis and new-bone formation. In the tibia, this is more intense on the anterior aspect and leads to a saber-shin deformity characteristic of latent congenital syphilis (Fig. 5-25). Gummas appears as small rarefactions within the dense and thickened shaft of the bone.

ACQUIRED (TERTIARY) SYPHILIS

Dense sclerosis of bone is a dominant feature of tertiary syphilis, involving the long bones and skull. In the long bones, the new bone is laid down on both the outer and inner aspects of the cortex, and the medullary cavity is narrowed (see Fig. 5-25). The affected segment is dense and spindle shaped, with a rough external surface. The lesion is characteristically elongated and may involve the entire circumference of the shaft or may be limited to just one portion of the cortex. There may be evidence of irregular destruction on the surface of the new-bone formation, giving a roughened or coarse

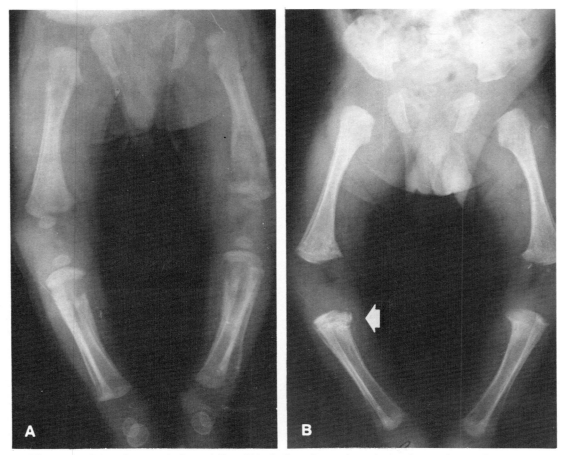

Figure 5–24. Congenital syphilis. **(A)** A fine line of periosteal new-bone formation parallels the diaphysis of the long bones, and focal areas of destruction are noted in the medial aspects of the metaphyses of the proximal tibia, distal femur, and distal tibia bilaterally—characteristic of congenital syphilis. **(B)** In this newborn infant, linear periosteal new-bone formation is seen to involve both femurs. A focal area of bone destruction at the medial margin of the proximal metaphysis of the tibia is present (*arrow*). A similar and less extensive focus is present in the distal femur.

appearance. Small foci of rarefaction or destruction may be identified within the thickened bone, representing areas of gumma formation. When the skull is affected, bone destruction is often seen but is usually limited to the outer table. Characteristically the destructive process is surrounded by a considerable proliferation of new bone to such an extent that the lesion mimics fibrous dysplasia.

Tabes dorsalis is another manifestation of tertiary syphilis. This may result in neurotrophic arthritis characterized radiographically by joint swelling and fragmentation, sclerosis, and resorption of bone (see Chapter 3).

LEPROSY

There are two principal forms of leprosy, the cutaneous (lepromatous or nodular) and the neural. The cutaneous form is not often associated with disease of the skeletal system, but bone changes are frequently found in neural leprosy.

The neurotropic changes of neural leprosy are found in the hands and feet.[20] The changes begin in the distal phalanges with a slowly progressive absorption of bone. The terminal tufts disappear, leading to a "collar-stud" appearance, followed by a gradual disappearance of the bone. The proximal phalanges are the last to

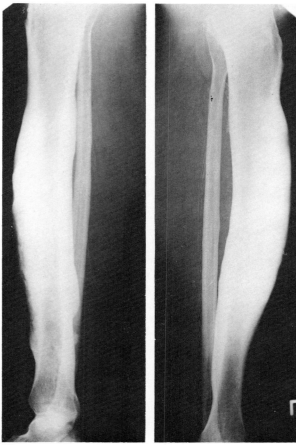

Figure 5–25. Chronic syphilitic osteoperiostitis of the tibia causing a bilateral saber-shin deformity characteristic of tertiary syphilis.

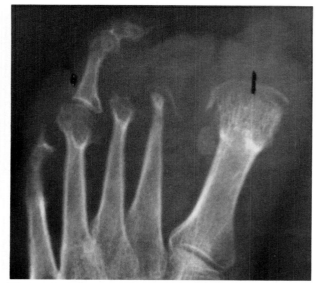

Figure 5–26. Leprosy. All of the phalanges of the feet have been resorbed, with the exception of the fourth toe and the base of the great toe. Tapered thinning of the distal ends of the metatarsals is evident.

disappear. Rarely, the metacarpals are affected, but the process does not ascend higher than this. In the feet, the absorption of bone begins in the metatarsal heads or in the proximal phalanges (Fig. 5-26). There is a gradual thinning of the shafts, and the ends become pointed. Eventually the involved bone may completely disappear. In some, a painless arthropathy resembling a Charcot joint develops, with gross disorganization of the articular ends of the bones. The lesions of neural leprosy are similar to those in a number of other diseases, including scleroderma, syringomyelia, tabes dorsalis, and the diabetic foot.

Granulomatous lesions occur in the hands and feet, producing focal areas of destruction and, when healed, they appear as small punched-out rarefied cysts with sclerotic margins ranging from 2 to 6 mm in diameter. They produce a honeycomb or cystlike appearance

associated with soft-tissue swelling. Periostitis may involve the tibia and fibula.

THE RUBELLA SYNDROME

During a virulent rubella epidemic in the United States in 1964, infants born of mothers who had the disease during the first trimester of pregnancy were found to have a syndrome of congenital heart disease, hepatosplenomegaly, and abnormalities of the skeletal system. The most frequent cardiac lesion is a patent ductus arteriosus, followed by pulmonary artery branch stenosis. Additional abnormalities include growth retardation, thrombocytopenic purpura, eye defects, and deafness.

Changes occur in the metaphyses of long bones, best demonstrated at the knees. The most striking characteristic is the presence of alternating lucent and sclerotic striations extending perpendicular to the epiphyseal plate and parallel to the long axis of the bone (Fig. 5-27) and fading into normal-appearing bone in the diaphysis. This has been termed *celery stalking*. The zones of provisional calcification are poorly defined and irregular. Transverse lucent metaphyseal bands are also seen. The bone changes improve rapidly in those infants who do well. In those infants who do poorly, the

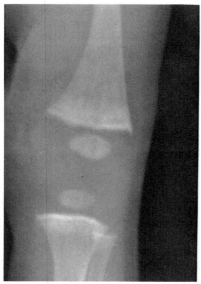

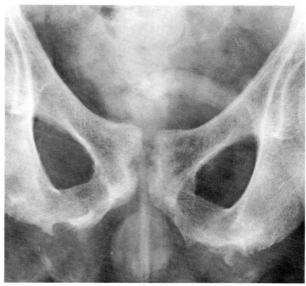

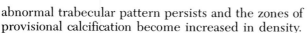

Figure 5–27.   Rubella syndrome. Note the vertical linear striations in the distal metaphysis of the femur and to a lesser extent in the proximal tibia. These marks are referred to as "celery stalking" and are characteristic of this disorder.

Figure 5–28.   Osteitis pubis following a suprapubic prostatic resection. The symphysis pubis is widened, and the margins are irregularly eroded.

abnormal trabecular pattern persists and the zones of provisional calcification become increased in density.

Similar skeletal changes have been reported in a patient having cytomegalic inclusion disease and other intrauterine-acquired infections; therefore, such changes may represent a nonspecific response to intrauterine viral infections. Lack of intracranial calcifications in the rubella syndrome tends to distinguish this syndrome from cytomegalic inclusion disease, but intracranial calcifications have recently also been reported in patients with the rubella syndrome.

OSTEITIS PUBIS

Osteitis pubis is the term given to an inflammatory condition that involves the pubic bones and that seems to develop chiefly after operations on the lower urinary tract, usually suprapubic or retropubic prostatectomies. The disease begins some weeks after the operation, with severe pain in the region of the pubis, aggravated by motion. A few weeks later, roentgenograms reveal rarefaction of the margins of the pubic bones. The affected bone has a washed-out appearance at first; later, complete dissolution occurs in the region of the symphysis (Fig. 5-28). The process may remain confined or may spread into the pubic rami. After a variable length of time, usually at least 3 or 4 months, there

is gradual reossification of the rarefied or destroyed bone. In patients with minimal involvement, the bone may eventually return to normal; in others, healing is shown by the development of sclerosis; and in the most severely involved, there will be a permanent loss of bone in the body of the pubis adjacent to the symphysis, the margin of the defect being bound by a zone of sclerosis (see Fig. 5-28). The cause of osteitis pubis is unknown, but the infectious theory has received considerable support.

Sclerotic lesions in the pubis with narrowing of the symphysis are fairly common in women who have borne children. Usually these women are asymptomatic and the lesions found by chance. Osteitis pubis is similar to osteitis condensans ilii, which also is seen in women who have borne children (see Chapter 3). Both the pubic and the iliac lesions may be seen in the same individual. The changes most likely represent a reaction of the bone to chronic stress.

SARCOIDOSIS

Sarcoidosis is a chronic, often widely disseminated disease, the cause of which remains unknown. Although originally considered to represent a form of tuberculosis of low virulence, the tuberculous nature of the disease has never been established.

The incidence of bone lesions in patients with cutaneous or visceral sarcoidosis is difficult to determine, but the lesions have been reported to occur in approximately 5% of cases.[20] Osseous lesions are usually associated with involvement of the skin, but this is not a prerequisite. Sarcoidosis is generally a more severe disease in the black race than in whites, and the incidence of osseous involvement in blacks is said to be higher.

Although the lesions have been found in practically all parts of the skeleton, the bones of the hands and feet are most frequently involved. The phalanges are commonly affected (Fig. 5-29). The lesions in the digits are usually asymptomatic and found on routine screening examinations or incidentally on radiographs obtained for the evaluation of trauma. Involvement varies from sharply defined, cystic radiolucencies to a lacelike or honeycomb pattern within the intramedullary canal. Destructive arthropathy and pathologic fractures are occasionally encountered.

Sclerotic lesions are occasionally encountered in the vertebral bodies and rarely elsewhere. No disc involvement appears to be present, but some of the destructive lesions may extend out to produce a soft-tissue mass in the paraspinal area. The posterior elements of the vertebrae are rarely involved.

INFANTILE CORTICAL HYPEROSTOSIS (CAFFEY'S DISEASE)

Infantile cortical hyperostosis is an uncommon disease of early infancy, and its cause is unknown. Although in many respects it behaves like an infection, with fever, irritability, and an increased erythrocyte sedimentation rate, there is no proof of an infectious etiology. The disease begins within the first few weeks of life, almost always before the age of 6 months but occasionally in older children up to the age of 4½ years. The disease presents with the sudden onset of an inflammatory process involving a few selected bones. The infant is febrile and irritable; hard, tender, soft-tissue swelling occurs around the affected bone. The favored sites are the mandible, clavicles, ulna, and less frequently the radius, ribs, tibia, and fibula. The mandible is almost always involved, representing the principal characteristic of the disease (Fig. 5-30). The diagnosis should be seriously questioned in the absence of mandibular involvement. The disease has been described in every bone except the phalanges and vertebral bodies. There may be extensive involvement of the ulna with no involvement of the adjacent radius. Scapular lesions may be misinterpreted for malignant tumors, but one should realize that malignancies of bone in this age

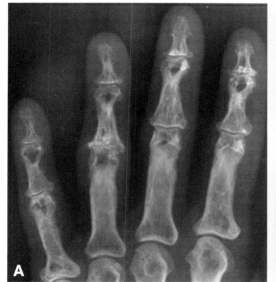 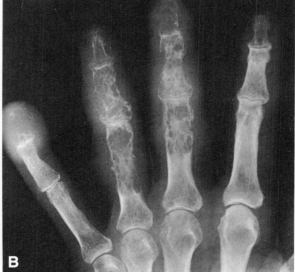

Figure 5–29. Sarcoidosis. (**A**) Characteristic punched-out, cystlike radiolucencies are seen in the ends of the phalanges. There is an erosive, destructive arthropathy involving the proximal interphalangeal joint of the ring finger. A lacelike trabecular pattern is present in the middle phalanges. (**B**) The disease is more advanced than shown in **A**. The cystic areas are larger, and the lacelike pattern of the trabeculae is more pronounced. The terminal phalanges of the third and fifth digits are almost completely destroyed.

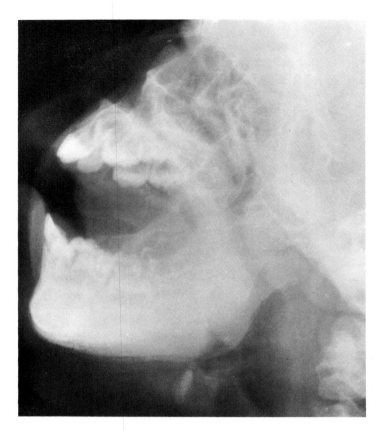

Figure 5–30. Infantile cortical hyperostosis (Caffey's disease). This 5-month-old male infant had symptoms for 3 months. The mandible is thick and dense, with a thin shell of periosteal new-bone formation along the inferior margin of the ramus, characteristic of Caffey's disease.

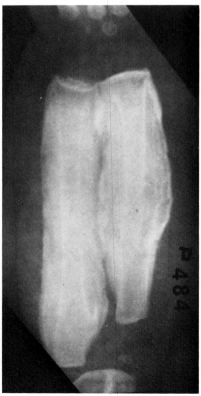

Figure 5–31. Infantile cortical hyperostosis (Caffey's disease) of the radius and ulna. There is extensive periosteal new-bone formation surrounding the shafts of both bones. The original cortex is barely visible.

group are exceedingly uncommon. The disease tends to show remissions and exacerbations, recovery taking place after a period of weeks to months. There is usually a prompt clinical response to corticosteroids; antibiotics have no effect.

The radiographic findings are a combination of soft-tissue swelling and extensive new-bone formation along the entire length of the involved bone (Fig. 5-31). Initial involvement may be limited to a short segment of the shaft, but eventually the process extends the entire length of the bone. The majority of the mandible is affected. Not all bones are affected simultaneously; some appear to be healing or improving while other cases become active or are reactivated. At first the subperiosteal new-bone formation is less dense than the cortex beneath it, but eventually the density increases. The outer margin may be rather irregular and wavy or smooth. As healing takes place, there is gradual resorption of the periosteal new-bone formation and the bone eventually returns to normal.

Infantile cortical hyperostosis must be differentiated from congenital syphilis and hypervitaminosis A. In congenital syphilis, the diffuse symmetrical involvement of multiple bones, the destructive process in the metaphysis, and the absence of soft-tissue swelling should allow the distinction (see Fig. 5-24). In hypervitaminosis A, the process is again more extensive and symmetrical, without overlying soft-tissue swelling, and affected children are generally older.

REFERENCES AND SELECTED READINGS

1. BARON AI, STEINBACH LS, LeBOIT PE, ET AL: Osteolytic lesions and bacillary angiomatosis in HIV infection: Radiologic differentiation from AIDS-related Kaposi sarcoma. Radiology 177:77, 1990
2. BOGOCH E, THOMPSON G, SALTER RB: Foci of chronic circumscribed osteomyelitis (Brodie's abscess) that traverse the epiphyseal plate. J Pediatr Orthop 4:162, 1984
3. BRESSLER EL, CONWAY JJ, WEISS SC: Neonatal osteomyelitis examined by bone scintigraphy. Radiology 152:685, 1984
4. CAPITANIO MA, KIRKPATRICK JA: Early roentgen observations in acute osteomyelitis. Am J Roentgenol 108:488, 1970
5. ERDMAN WA, TAMBURRO F, JAYSON HT, ET AL: Osteomyelitis: Characteristics and pitfalls of diagnosis with MR imaging. Radiology 180:533, 1991
6. FARLEY T, CONWAY J, SHULMAN ST: Hematogenous pelvic osteomyelitis in children: Clinical correlates of newer scanning methods. Am J Dis Child 139:945, 1985.
7. FIROOZNIA H, GOLIMBU C, RAFII M, ET AL: Radiology of musculoskeletal complications of drug addiction. Semin Roentgenol 18:198, 1983
8. FLETCHER BD, SCOLES PV, NELSON AD: Osteomyelitis in children: Detection by magnetic resonance. Radiology 150:57, 1984
9. GUYOT DR, MANOLI A II, KING GA: Pyogenic sacroiliitis in IV drug abusers. Am J Roentgenol 149:1209, 1987
10. HELMS CA, JEFFREY RB, WING VW: Computed tomography and plain film appearance of a bony sequestration: Significance and differential diagnosis. Skeletal Radiol 16:117, 1987
11. JONES NS, ANDERSON DJ, STILES PJ: Osteomyelitis in a general hospital. A five-year study showing an increase in subacute osteomyelitis. J Bone Joint Surg [Br] 69:779, 1987
12. KNUDSEN CJM, HOFFMAN EB: Neonatal osteomyelitis. J Bone Joint Surg [Br] 72:846, 1990
13. LEWIN JS, ROSENFIELD NS, HOFFER PB: Acute osteomyelitis in children: Combined Tc-99m and Ga-67 imaging. Radiology 158:795, 1986
14. MENDELSON EB, FISHER MR, DESCHLER TW, ET AL: Osteomyelitis in the diabetic foot: A difficult diagnostic challenge. Radiographics 3:248, 1983
15. NADE S: Acute septic arthritis in infancy and childhood. J Bone Joint Surg [Br] 65:234, 1983
16. NIXON GW: Hematogenous osteomyelitis of metaphyseal-equivalent locations. Am J Roentgenol 130:123, 1978
17. RAFII M, FIROOZNIA H, GOLIMBU C, ET AL: Hematogenous osteomyelitis with fat-fluid level shown by CT. Radiology 153:493, 1984
18. RASOOL MN, GOVENDER S: The skeletal manifestations of congenital syphilis: A review of 197 cases. J Bone Joint Surg [Br] 71:752, 1989
19. REILLY JP, GROSS RH, EMANS JB: Disorders of the sacroiliac joint in children. J Bone Joint Surg [Am] 70:31, 1988
20. RESNICK D, NIWAYAMA G: Diagnosis of Bone and Joint Disorders, 3rd ed. Philadelphia, WB Saunders, 1991
21. ROSEN RA, MOREHOUSE HT, KARP HJ: Intracortical fissuring in osteomyelitis. Radiology 141:17, 1981
22. SCHAUWECKER DS: Osteomyelitis: Diagnosis with In-111-labeled leukocytes. Radiology 171:141, 1989
23. SOLHEIM LF, PAUS B, LIVERUD K, ET AL: Chronic recurrent multifocal osteomyelitis. A new clinical-radiological syndrome. Acta Orthop Scand 51:37, 1980
24. SORENSEN TS, HEDEBOE J, CHRISTENSEN ER: Primary epiphyseal osteomyelitis in children. Report of three cases and review of the literature. J Bone Joint Surg [Br] 70:818, 1988
25. STEPHENS MM, MACAULEY P: Brodie's abscess: A long-term review. Clin Orthop 234:211, 1988
26. TANG JSH, GOLD RH, BASSETT LW, ET AL: Musculoskeletal infection of the extremities: Evaluation with MR imaging. Radiology 166:205, 1988
27. TORRICELLI P, MARTINELLI C, BIAGINI R, ET AL: Radiographic and computed tomographic findings in hydatid disease of bone. Skeletal Radiol 19:435, 1990

28. TRUETA J: The three types of acute haematogenous osteomyelitis: A clinical and vascular study. J Bone Joint Surg [Br] 41:671, 1959

29. UNGER E, MOLDOFSKY P, GATENBY R, ET AL: Diagnosis of osteomyelitis by MR imaging. Am J Roentgenol 150:605, 1988

30. WALDVOGEL FA, MEDOFF G, SWARTZ MN: Osteomyelitis: A review of clinical features, therapeutic considerations, and unusual aspects. N Engl J Med 282:198, 260, 316, 1970

31. WING UW, JEFFREY IB, FEDERLE WP, ET AL: Chronic osteomyelitis examined by CT. Radiology 154:171, 1985

32. WOLFSON JJ, KANE WJ, LAXDAL SD, ET AL: Bone findings in chronic granulomatous disease of childhood. A genetic abnormality of leukocyte function. J Bone Joint Surg [Am] 51:1573, 1969

Paul and Juhl's Essentials of Radiologic Imaging, Sixth Edition, edited by John H. Juhl and Andrew B. Crummy. J.B. Lippincott Company, Philadelphia, © 1993.

CHAPTER *6*

Metabolic, Endocrine, and Related Bone Diseases

Lee F. Rogers

The skeleton is the hard, bony framework of the body. It is difficult to imagine its mobility, mechanical properties, and vital role in metabolism and hematopoiesis when we study it in its dried state in the anatomy laboratory. A radiograph of bone is a static image chiefly of the inorganic salts it contains and therefore is an inadequate reflection of the living quality of the skeleton.

In its living state, bone is a blend of hard inorganic salts and resilient organic components. Bone tissue consists of a ground substance or matrix in which are embedded fibers impregnated with bone salts. The inorganic salts represent a mineral reservoir for the metabolic pathways of the body. In mature bone, approximately 20% of the weight of the matrix is water. Organic materials form one-third and mineral salts two-thirds of the dry weight of bone. The main organic component (90% to 95%) is collagen, a mucopolysaccharide, in combination with protein. Uncalcified organic matrix is known as osteoid matrix. Calcium and phosphorus are the principal mineral salts in the skeleton. Ninety-nine percent of body calcium is concentrated in bone.

Bone is living tissue, and old bone is constantly removed and replaced with new bone. Normally this exchange is in balance, and the mineral content remains relatively constant. This balance may be disturbed as a result of certain metabolic and endocrinologic disorders. The term *dystrophy*, referring to a disturbance of nutrition, is applied to metabolic and endocrine bone diseases and should be distinguished from the term *dysplasia*, referring to a disturbance of

bone growth. The two terms are easily confused but are not interchangeable. Metabolic bone disease is caused by endocrine imbalance, vitamin deficiency or excess, and other disturbances in bone metabolism leading to osteoporosis and osteomalacia.

The terms *osteomalacia* and *osteoporosis* describe specific bone dystrophies. Osteomalacia is a failure of deposition of calcium salts in bone matrix, whereas osteoporosis is a deficiency of the organic matrix of bone. However, the term *osteoporosis* is often used nonspecifically to describe a general loss of bone substance or bone atrophy.

A host of terms are used to describe a loss of bone mineral and decrease in radiographic density. These are deossification, demineralization, osteolysis, osteoporosis, rarefaction, and radiolucency. The terms are for the most part nonspecific and are used interchangeably. The loss of mineral salts causing bones to become more radiolucent than normal may be due to a lack of mineralization, lack of bony matrix, or an increased rate of bone removal.

Osteopenia is an acceptable and nonspecific descriptive term used to designate general or regional decrease in skeletal density. The term *osteopenia* is preferred to the term *osteoporosis* largely because it is difficult or even at times impossible to distinguish between the various causes of decreased radiographic bone density and the specific pathogenic implications attached to the term *osteoporosis*.

An increased radiopacity or increased density of bone is much less frequent. The increased radiopacity can result from either an increased formation of new bone, with the removal of bone remaining normal, or interference with normal removal of bone, with the rate of bone formation remaining normal.

MEASUREMENT OF BONE MINERAL

Bone minerals must be considered in two separate compartments, the compact cortical bone and the trabecular, intramedullary bone. The metabolic and turnover rates are not the same in both compartments, and diseases may affect each differently. Bone mineral loss occurs more rapidly in trabecular than in cortical bone. The surface area of trabecular bone is four times that of cortical bone, and the turnover rate of trabecular bone is eight times that of cortical bone.

The structural integrity of bone is in large measure dependent upon its trabecular content. Therefore, measurements of bone mineral content limited to or chiefly dependent upon the amount of cortical bone are either misleading or highly inaccurate in the determination of the clinical status of bone mineral. Bone mineral determinations have many research applications, but their most important clinical application is in the assessment of bone mineral in perimenopausal and postmenopausal females[13] to determine their susceptibility to fracture[14, 23] and need for estrogen therapy, dietary calcium supplements, and other means of treating osteoporosis. Measurement is also used to monitor the effect of treatment of osteoporosis[24] and to assess the impact of metabolic diseases known to affect the skeleton (e.g., chronic renal failure and Cushing's disease), and use of exogenous steroids.[4]

The estimation of bone mineral content on the basis of radiographic appearance is highly subjective and is greatly dependent upon exposure parameters. This precludes an accurate evaluation. In particular, overexposed radiographs give the false impression of decreased bone density. In general, 30% to 50% of bone mineral or bone must be removed before it is apparent on the radiograph. In the adult, it is important not only to evaluate the overall density of bone but to determine specific characteristics of both the cortex and trabecular bone. In children, metabolic abnormalities are most evident in the growing ends of the bone, resulting in specific changes within the metaphysis, growth plate, and epiphysis.

Because of the difficulties in the subjective assessment of bone mineral density on plain radiographs and the importance of determining bone mineral content, a number of in vivo methods have been devised to measure the mineral content of bone more accurately than by observation of radiographs. These noninvasive techniques include radiogrammetry, single- and dual-photon absorptiometry, and quantitative computed tomography.

RADIOGRAMMETRY

Radiogrammetry is the simplest method of quantitative bone mineral assessment. A conventional radiograph of the long bone is obtained, and the cortical thickness on either side of the medullary space is measured and expressed as a combined cortical thickness (CCT). This technique can be used at several skeletal sites, but the midshaft of the second metacarpal is most commonly measured (Fig. 6-1). In a normal individual with normal bone density, the combined cortical thickness of the second metacarpal is at least 50% of the width of the shaft at the point measured. In other words, the combined cortical width is equal to or greater than the width of intramedullary space in the plane of measurement. This ratio represents an excellent rule of thumb in the gross estimation of bone density in the everyday interpretation of radiographs but is too imprecise and insensitive to be used for clinical management.

SINGLE-ENERGY PHOTON ABSORPTIOMETRY

Single-energy photon absorptiometry requires a gamma-ray source, a detector, and intervening electronics to measure the beam attenuation through bone and to express the result in some convenient form. These devices measure the radial shaft using an ^{125}I source interfaced with a sodium iodide scintillation detector. The forearm is surrounded by a water bag or water bath. The gamma-ray source and detector are then translated across the forearm, and changes in the beam intensity are measured. Electronics calculate the average attenuation of the ^{125}I beam due to bone and then compare this result with a standard curve derived from potassium phosphate (K_2HPO_4). Two sites are commonly measured in the radius: the middiaphysis, composed of nearly 100% cortical bone, and the distal radial metaphysis, containing approximately 75% cortical and 25% trabecular bone. The accuracy is plus or minus 6%. Radiation exposure is low, less than 10 mrem. The gamma ray of ^{125}I is 26 and 37 keV. This is quite soft and of limited penetrance. Because of dosimetric and statistical considerations, the low-energy wide ^{125}I source cannot be used for body parts thicker than the forearm and is a major clinical limitation of this technique. It reflects the status of peripheral long bones and measures primarily the cortex. These measurements may not reflect the overall skeletal status in many metabolic diseases.

tons. The examination is performed on a rectilinear scanner. The spine and femoral neck may be examined with this method. Usually the lumbar spine is examined from L1 to L4 (Fig. 6-2*A*, *B*). This technique yields a measurement of the sum of all the minerals within the scan path, including not only the predominantly trabecular bone of the vertebral bodies but also the vertebral end-plates and posterior elements, which contain a greater percentage of compact bone. Vertebral compression fractures, scoliosis, bone hypertrophy, and extraosseous calcification such as in the aorta are also included in the measurement and may result in inaccuracies. All of these findings are common in elderly patients, but in healthy subjects under the age of 40, the precision is on the order of 2% to 3%. The radiation dose is about 15 to 20 mrem. When combined with radiography of the lumbar spine, this method allows accurate and clinically useful estimation of trabecular mineral bone content.

DUAL-ENERGY X-RAY ABSORPTIOMETRY (DXA)

DXA differs from DPA in that an x-ray tube replaces the isotopic source of photons. This greatly increases the speed and precision of DPX in comparison with DPA. It improves the accuracy of trabecular bone density assessment by facilitating scanning of the spine in the lateral projection, which limits evaluation to the vertebral body and eliminates the inclusion of the compact bone of the posterior spinal elements in the calculation of bone density.

QUANTITATIVE COMPUTED TOMOGRAPHY (QCT)

Quantitative bone measurements can be made on CT scanners with the addition of a K_2HPO_4 calibration phantom.[19, 24, 25] Single axial scans are obtained simultaneously through the phantom and the midplane of two to four lumbar vertebral bodies (Fig. 6-3). Quantitative readings are obtained from a region of interest over the trabecular bone encompassing 3 to 4 cc of each vertebral body and from four different reference solutions in the phantom. The readings are averaged and used to calculate the mineral density of trabecular bone in mineral equivalence of K_2HPO_4 (milligrams/cubic centimeter) (see Fig. 6-5). The precision is 1% to 3% for single-energy 80-kVp and 3% to 5% for dual-energy 80-kVp/140-kVp techniques. The accuracy of QCT as well as dual-photon absorptiometry decreases to 20% to 25% in the elderly osteoporotic population. The QCT inaccuracy is due to the presence of fatty yellow marrow in the spine in the elderly. This changes the spinal mineral equivalent. The inaccuracy can be reduced by the use of a dual-photon method using both

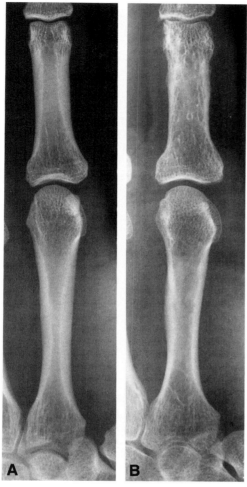

Figure 6–1. Comparison of the second metacarpal and proximal phalanx in a 19-year-old man (**A**) and an 82-year-old woman (**B**). Note the thickness of the cortex and the absence of identifiable bone trabeculae in the midshafts of the bones in **A** compared with the thinness of the cortices and coarse trabecular pattern in **B**. The combined cortical thickness (CCT) of the midshaft of the second metacarpal is 6 mm in **A** and 3 mm in **B**.

DUAL-ENERGY PHOTON ABSORPTIOMETRY (DPA)

The advantages of dual-energy scanning over single-energy scanning are higher gamma-ray energies, permitting larger body parts to be scanned and examined without the necessity of a water bath.[25] The usual source is ^{153}Gd, which emits 42-keV and 100-keV pho-

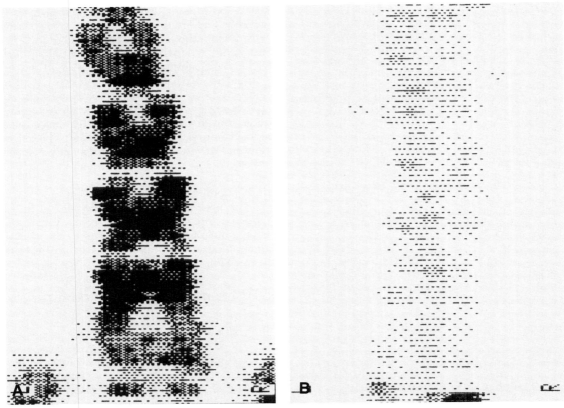

Figure 6–2. Dual-energy photon[153] Gd absorptiometry. (**A**) Normal 42-year-old woman with 94% of expected bone mineral content for this age. (**B**) Osteoporotic 79-year-old woman with 80% of expected bone mineral content for her age and 56% of that of normal young women.

80-kVp and 140-kVp techniques. This is the most accurate noninvasive means of measuring vertebral mineral content.

OSTEOPOROSIS

Skeletal disorders associated with osteoporosis may be conveniently subdivided into those associated with generalized osteoporosis of the entire skeleton and those associated with a regional osteoporosis usually limited to a single extremity or portion of an extremity (Table 6-1).

SENILE (POSTMENOPAUSAL) OSTEOPOROSIS

Senile osteoporosis is a state of increased porosity or rarefaction of bone caused by a loss of bone substance occurring in the elderly.[13, 14, 20] Women are much more severely affected than men, with an earlier onset and

more profound loss of bone. Osteoporosis is encountered in women as young as 45 years but is normally not identifiable in men until the age of 65 years. Undoubtedly the etiology is multifaceted, but the dominance of hormonal influence is beyond question. The disorder is dependent on the loss of stimulation by estrogen in women and therefore often described as postmenopausal. Osteoporosis is initiated prematurely by oophorectomy. The hormonal status in men is less clearly defined.

The changes are predominantly quantitative; qualitative changes are considered much less important and to date are poorly defined. Resorption of bone occurs in three locations (Fig. 6-4): the endosteal surface, resulting in thinning of the cortex; the haversian canals, giving rise to porosity of the cortex; and the trabeculae within intramedullary bone, significantly reducing internal structural support.

Osteoporosis is a disease mainly of white persons. Although the loss of bone occurs in all races, no evi-

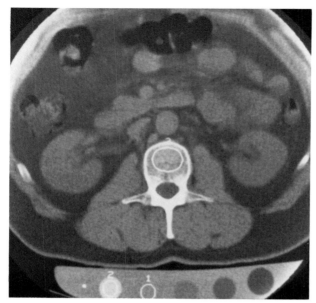

Figure 6–3. Quantitative computed tomography (QCT). A computer compares the density in a region of interest in trabecular bone with a K_2HPO_4-calibrated phantom. The phantom contains several tubes of varying concentration. The density of trabecular bone is calculated by comparing with densities of the phantom.

Table 6–1. Classification of Osteoporosis

Generalized
   Senile (postmenopausal)
   Idiopathic osteoporosis of males (alcoholism, cirrhosis)
   Idiopathic juvenile osteoporosis
   Cushing's disease and exogenous steroids
   Malnutrition (celiac disease)
   Scurvy (vitamin C deficiency)
   Osteogenesis imperfecta
   Homocystinuria
Others
   Hyperparathyroidism
   Hyperthyroidism
   Acromegaly
   Heparin-induced
   Multiple myeloma
Regional
   Disuse osteoporosis
   Reflex sympathetic dystrophy (Sudeck's atrophy)
   Transient osteoporosis of the hip
   Regional migratory osteoporosis
   Periarticular osteoporosis associated with arthritis

dence exists that the rate of loss is greater in one race than in another. The bone mass of black persons exceeds that of whites, and because blacks initially have a larger bone mass, their bones are not as weakened by the loss of bone occasioned by aging.

The principal effect of loss of bone in osteoporosis is an increase in the fragility of bone; as bone mass decreases, bones are more susceptible to fracture.[14, 20, 21, 23] Most fractures result from falls from a standing position by tripping or stumbling. The proximal end of the femur, the distal end of the radius, the proximal ends of the humerus, the thoracolumbar spine, and the pelvis are common sites of fracture in the elderly (see Chapter 2). The cumulative prevalence of all these fractures in women is about 7% by the age of 60 years and increases to about 25% by the age of 80 years. The female-to-male ratio of fractures in these locations varies from 2 to 1 in the spine and pelvis, 3 to 1 in the femur and humerus, and 6 to 1 in the distal forearm.

The mineral content of bone decreases progressively after the age of 45 years in women and 65 years in men. The cumulative loss of mineral from the vertebrae between young adulthood and extreme old age approaches 50% for women and approximately 15% for men. A bone mineral density below the threshold for fractures of vertebrae and hips is found in half of all women by age 65 years and in essentially all women by age 85. Men are at risk to a lesser extent and at a later age. The fracture threshold is slightly less than 1 mg of calcium per cubic centimeter of bone. Although it is possible to determine the fracture risk from a determination of bone mineral density at a given site (Fig. 6-5A), there is considerable difficulty in estimating the fracture risk at another site from a bone mineral density determination at the original site (Fig. 6-5B). In fact, it may not be possible. This implies that it may be necessary to examine each site separately to make accurate predictions of fracture risks. This is a continuing source of both research and controversy.[14, 23]

The extent of the loss of bone can be estimated grossly by the radiographic appearance of the skeleton. The cortex of the affected bone is thin and the trabecular pattern coarsened (see Fig. 6-1). The width of the cortical bone determined at specific sites, usually in the metacarpal as described previously, is found to achieve maximal cortical width by age 20 and begins to decline after 40 years of age. The rate of decline or decrease in the cortical width is greater in females than in males. Coarsening of the trabecular pattern is due to a selective resorption of smaller trabeculae; by removing smaller trabeculae, the larger trabeculae become more evident and more sharply defined.

The consequences of the loss of bone mineral are particularly well demonstrated in the spine by the presence of anterior wedging, "codfish" deformities, or overt fractures of the vertebral bodies (Fig. 6-6). The

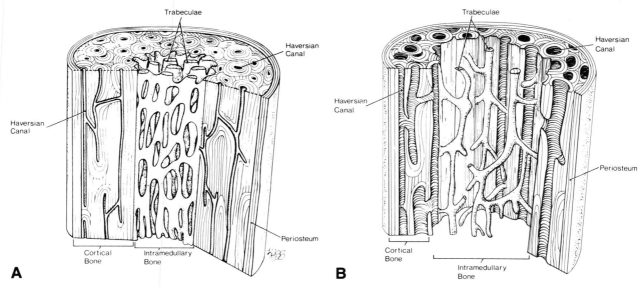

Figure 6–4. Cross section of normal bone (**A**) compared with osteoporotic bone (**B**). Note the thinning of the cortex caused by endosteal resorption, the widening of the haversian systems, and the reduction in the size and number of intramedullary trabeculae in osteoporotic bone.

presence and number of spinal fractures and deformities of the vertebral bodies correlate well with a decrease in bone mineral density; the more fractures, the greater the degree of bone mineral loss. The mid-thoracic, lower thoracic, and upper lumbar vertebral bodies are more severely affected. There is a gradual reduction in the height of the vertebral body, more marked anteriorly, that leads to an anterior wedged deformity and an overall reduction in height. The most characteristic abnormality is a codfish deformity of the vertebral body, so named because the end-plates be-come deeply concave, similar to the vertebral bodies of fish. This is caused by an expansion of the intervertebral disc or invagination of the disc into the vertebral body weakened by the loss of trabeculae. Elderly females may lose as much as 6 inches or more in height because of loss of vertebral height. Multiple wedging of the vertebral bodies leads to a kyphosis of the mid-dorsal spine. This deformity is obvious clinically and is known as a dowager's hump. Differentiation of the vertebral deformities from acute fractures is described in Chapter 2.

Figure 6–5. QCT determination of bone mineral density (BMD) of the spine in osteo- ➤ porotic women with vertebral fractures (**A**) and hip fractures (**B**). Center line within speckled areas depicts the mean spinal trabecular bone in 419 normal women at 90% confidence limits. (**A**) This diagram plots the bone mineral content (*dots*) in 74 osteoporotic women with vertebral fractures. The fracture threshold selected was the 5th percentile spinal BMD values in healthy premenopausal women 45 years old. Eighty-five percent of women with osteoporotic vertebral fractures had spinal BMC measurements below this value. Sixty-four percent of women with vertebral fractures had BMD values below the 5th percentile for age-matched control subjects. (**B**) BMD of the spine in 83 osteoporotic women with hip fractures. Only 38% of patients with hip fractures had spinal BMD values below the 5th percentile for healthy premenopausal women, and only 9% had BMD values below the 5th percentile for age-matched control subjects. (Firooznia H, Rafii M, Golimbu C et al: Trabecular mineral content of the spine in women with hip fracture: CT measurement. Radiology 159:737, 1986)

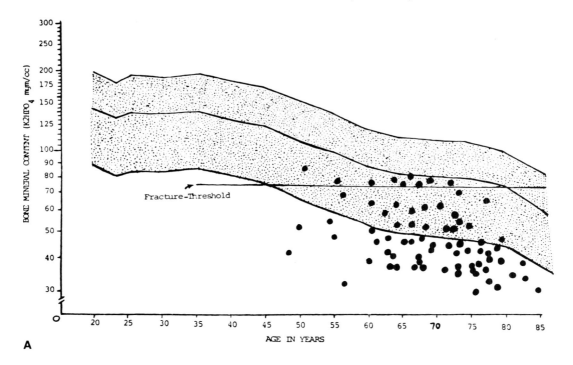

A

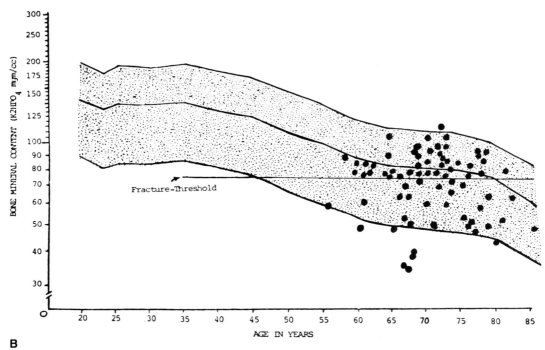

B

Figure 6–5.

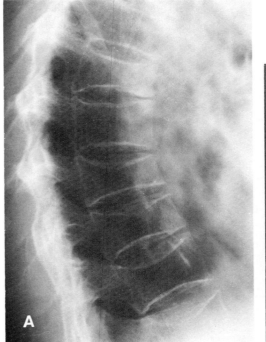
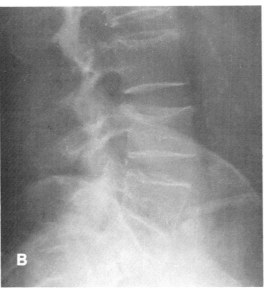

Figure 6–6. Postmenopausal osteoporosis. **(A)** There are multiple deformities of the thoracic vertebral bodies. The cortical margins are thin, the vertebral bodies are wedged anteriorly, and the end-plates are concave. The biconcave vertebral bodies are known as "codfish" vertebrae. **(B)** In the lumbar spine, there is no wedging of the vertebral bodies, but note the concave deformity of the superior end-plates.

IDIOPATHIC OSTEOPOROSIS OF MALES (ALCOHOLISM, CIRRHOSIS)

Persons with alcoholism and cirrhosis have a reduced bone mass compared with the controls and an increased bone fragility evidenced by an increased incidence of fractures of the vertebral bodies, hip, distal forearm, and proximal humerus similar to senile osteoporosis. Both males and females are affected. The early onset of osteoporosis in males is usually associated with alcoholism and cirrhosis. The cause of bone loss is unknown, but undoubtedly there is a relationship between bone mass, nutrition, and other variables such as physical activity and gastric surgery for peptic ulcer disease in alcoholic individuals. The disease is usually manifest radiographically by deformities of the thoracic and lumbar vertebral bodies typical of osteoporosis (see Fig. 6-6) and a generalized reduction of bone mass in the peripheral skeleton revealed by thinning of the cortex and coarsening of the trabecular pattern. Loss of bone can be verified and quantified by determination of bone mineral content.

IDIOPATHIC JUVENILE OSTEOPOROSIS

Idiopathic juvenile osteoporosis is an uncommon self-limited disease of childhood.[27] Afflicted children present about 2 years before puberty with spinal and extraspinal symptoms that may simulate those of arthritis; pain in the ankles, slowness in walking, and abnormal gait are characteristic. Radiographs show multiple compressed or biconcave vertebrae and often metaphyseal fractures of long bones. The serum calcium, phosphorus, and alkaline phosphatase are normal.

The differential diagnosis includes Cushing's syndrome, celiac disease, homocystinuria, and osteogenesis imperfecta. The main diagnostic problem is ruling out mild osteogenesis imperfecta and metastatic disease or leukemia. In idiopathic osteoporosis, the width of the long bones is normal, although the cortex is thin and metaphyseal fractures are common. In osteogenesis imperfecta, the width of the bones may be abnormally thin and most fractures occur in the diaphysis; metaphyseal fractures are rare. Osteogenesis imperfecta will also be associated with blue sclerae, progressive cranial, facial, and pelvic deformities, and a qualitative abnormality of bone on histologic examination. Biopsies in idiopathic juvenile osteoporosis reveal no qualitative changes in bone.

CUSHING'S SYNDROME AND ENDOGENOUS STEROIDS

Osteopenia is the principal skeletal manifestation of hypersteroidism, whether due to endogenous or exogenous sources. Excessive endogenous production of steroids resulting in Cushing's syndrome is usually due to bilateral adrenocortical hyperplasia and, less frequently, an adrenocortical adenoma or carcinoma.

Excessive steroids result in a demineralization of bone, particularly in the vertebrae, which are prone to collapse with multiple compression fractures manifested by anterior wedging and biconcave deformities of the vertebral bodies (Fig. 6-7). Marginal condensa-

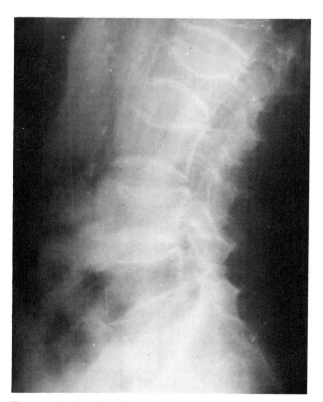

Figure 6–7. Cushing's syndrome. There is a "codfish" deformity of all the lumbar vertebral bodies. Expansion of the intervertebral discs into the softened vertebral bodies causes this characteristic biconcavity of the upper and lower end-plates.

tion of the end-plates of compressed vertebrae is seen more commonly than in vertebral compressions due to other causes. It has been suggested that this change is a manifestation of attempted repair with excess callus formation. Rib fractures are also common. Fractures of the pubic and ischial rami may also occur. The rib and pubic fractures often have exuberant callus formation.

Ischemic necrosis of the head of the femur (Fig. 6-8) and head of the humerus is another frequent complication of hypersteroidism.[18] The exact cause is not known. The characteristic radiographic manifestations of ischemic necrosis in the humeral and femoral heads are an increase in radiodensity or sclerosis, sometimes known as "snowcapping," collapse of bone with loss of volume, and linear subcortical radiolucencies, the "crescent sign" (see Chapter 7).

There is a generalized decrease in the skeletal density; this may be manifested in the skull as granular rarefaction. In children, there may be a delay in skeletal maturation.

Nonskeletal radiographic manifestations include excess subcutaneous and intra-abdominal fat and mediastinal widening from excess fat deposits. Extrapleural fat pads and epicardial fat accumulations may also be seen.

MALNUTRITION AND RELATED CAUSES

Severe malnutrition and protein deficiency or abnormal protein metabolism cause osteoporosis. Osteoporosis and osteomalacia may both occur after periods of starvation. Osteoporosis may develop in nephrosis or celiac disease as a result of loss of protein, in poorly controlled diabetes and in hyperthyroidism, probably owing to catabolic destruction of amino acids.

SCURVY

Vitamin C is necessary for normal osteoblastic activity. The organic matrix of bone cannot be laid down without it. Infantile scurvy is a form of osteoporosis caused by a deficiency of vitamin C. Scurvy is not a disease of the immediate postnatal period but is encountered in children between the ages of 6 months and 2 years. There are no authentic cases of symptomatic or radiographic scurvy in infants younger than 3 months. It is a rare disease in present-day America. Heating cow's milk for the purpose of pasteurization destroys vitamin C in sufficient amount to lead to clinical scurvy. In such circumstances, the addition of orange juice or ascorbic acid to the diet easily and effectively prevents scurvy.

The clinical manifestations are irritability, digestive disturbance, loss of appetite, and tenderness and swelling, particularly of the lower extremities. Swelling of

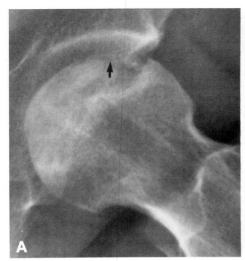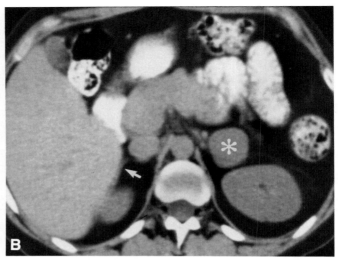

Figure 6–8.   Cushing's syndrome presenting with the chief complaint of hip pain. (**A**) Characteristic changes of avascular necrosis of the femoral head manifested by increased densities and lucencies and slight collapse of the femoral head. Note the subchondral fracture (*arrow*). (**B**) CT scan of the abdomen demonstrates presence of a left adrenal adenoma (*asterisk*). Note the normal thin, linear right adrenal gland (*arrow*).

the gums is also characteristic. In far advanced cases, hemorrhages occur in the skin, mucous membranes, and soft tissues because of the lack of intercellular substance in the capillaries.

Because of the lowered activity of the osteoblasts, the serum alkaline phosphatase is usually low or occasionally normal. The serum calcium and phosphorus are normal.

Radiographic Observations

The diagnosis or exclusion of scurvy is usually based on the roentgenographic changes in the long bones, especially at their distal ends. Changes, as a rule, are most marked in the knee (Fig. 6-9).

A diffuse demineralization of the entire skeleton gives rise to a ground-glass appearance. The trabecular structure is lost, and the cortices of the bone are thinned.

Characteristically there are two zones of increased density. The first forms at the margin of the epiphyseal centers. As the cancellous bone of the center becomes more translucent than normal, the dense outer rim has the appearance of a ring, sometimes known as the ring sign. The second zone develops in the zone of provisional calcification at the metaphysis of the long bones. This zone of density, known as the white line of scurvy, represents an abnormally wide zone of provisional calcification and is caused by a failure of normal proliferation of cartilage cells so that the change from cartilage to bone becomes arrested.

A small area of rarefaction involves the cortex and spongiosa just proximal to the metaphysis on one or both sides of the shaft. This is known as the corner sign of scurvy. It is an early and characteristic finding and represents the early development of the scurvy zone. The scurvy zone is a transverse band of rarefaction that crosses the shaft just beneath the white line of scurvy. This is an area where active bone formation would normally be taking place but in the presence of vitamin C deficiency cannot. It is a weakened portion of the bone, and fractures may occur with or without displacement of the shaft, giving the appearance of an epiphyseal separation (Fig. 6-10). The scurvy zone often disappears as the epiphysis, together with the zone of provisional calcification, becomes impacted into the shaft.

During the active phase of the disease, extensive hemorrhages may develop beneath the periosteum. During infancy and childhood, the periosteum is loosely attached to the cortex of the bone and is easily elevated by hemorrhage beneath it. However, it is firmly attached at the end of the shaft and hemorrhage is limited at this point and therefore does not extend over the epiphysis. It is the subperiosteal hemorrhage that accounts for the swelling of the extremities.

Healing is first shown by new-bone formation beneath the elevated periosteum (see Fig. 6-10). As a result of adequate treatment, bone is deposited throughout the area of hemorrhage surrounding the shaft, the scurvy zones recalcify, there is gradual remineralization of the skeleton, and cortices regain their normal thickness. As

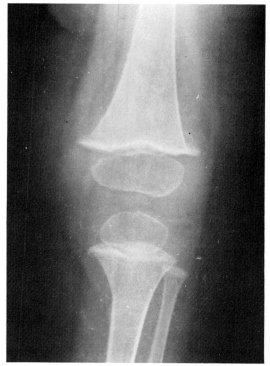

Figure 6–9. Infantile scurvy. The white line of scurvy is particularly distinct in the metaphysis of the femur. Note the spurlike projection at the zone of provisional calcification laterally. The translucent scurvy zone is not visible because of the impaction of the shaft into the zone of provisional calcification. Note the distinct ringlike contour of the epiphyses.

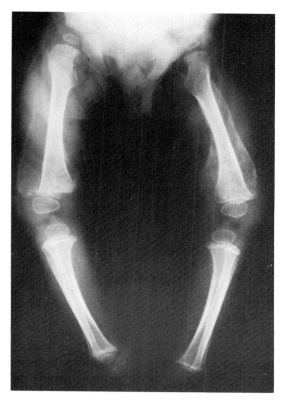

Figure 6–10. Infantile scurvy. Examination obtained shortly after the beginning of the patient's treatment. There has been epiphyseal fracture, with lateral displacement of the right lower femoral epiphysis. Large calcifying subperiosteal hematomas are present bilaterally about the femurs. Note the distinct ringlike contour of the epiphyses.

growth proceeds, the thickened zone of provisional calcification appears to migrate into the shaft, where it remains for a variable time as a thin, dense, white line (a growth-arrest line). In like manner, a ring of density may be visible within the epiphyseal center, as normal bone forms around the edge of the old center (ghost epiphysis, or bone within a bone). The calcified subperiosteal hemorrhages are gradually absorbed. If epiphyseal dislocation did occur, deformity is eventually corrected by growth and remodeling.

OSTEOGENESIS IMPERFECTA

Osteogenesis imperfecta is a congenital form of osteopenia due to a defect or deficiency of osteoblasts. It is discussed in Chapter 9.

OTHERS

Homocystinuria is an inborn error of metabolism resulting in osteopenia, and it may simulate Marfan's syndrome. It is transmitted as an autosomal recessive trait. Osteoporosis is present; arachnodactyly is found only occasionally.[18]

Osteopenia and osteoporosis are also found in a host of other diseases (e.g., hyperparathyroidism and occasionally acromegaly) and may be induced by large doses of heparin. In the elderly, multiple myeloma may cause diffuse osteopenia of the spine, with or without associated vertebral fractures, and must always be considered in the differential diagnosis of diffuse spinal osteoporosis.

REGIONAL OSTEOPOROSIS

DISUSE OSTEOPOROSIS

Disuse osteopenia or disuse osteoporosis is an acute form of osteopenia occurring in an extremity because of lack of use. This occurs following immobilization of a fracture and occasionally is secondary to other causes of forced inactivity. There is a generalized disuse atrophy of bone in astronauts because of the absence of gravity.

The process consists of a resorption of trabecular and cortical bone. It begins rather abruptly at or just proximal to a fracture and extends distally to involve all bones beyond the fracture site (Fig. 6-11). With resumption of activity, the process is reversed and the bone is restored. This acute form of osteopenia can be differentiated from senile osteoporosis. Disuse atrophy is a focal rather than a generalized phenomenon. There are two distinctive radiographic features,[8, 21] two findings peculiar to disuse atrophy: (1) a pronounced resorption of the endosteal surface of the cortical margins of the joints, resulting in a characteristic thin radiolucent line beneath the articular cortex, and (2) a tendency for a broad, transverse band of accentuated resorption in the metaphysis in the region of the epiphyseal scar in adults. The other characteristic radiographic findings are generalized osteoporosis, speckled or spotty osteoporosis, and changes within the cortex. The generalized osteoporosis consists of a loss of the finer trabeculae, resulting in a coarsened appearance of the intramedullary bone. Spotty or speckled osteoporosis consists of small oval or rounded translucencies found most commonly in the carpal and tarsal bones and in the bases of the metacarpals and metatarsals. The cortical changes consist of tunneling (thin linear longitudinal cortical radiolucencies due to enlargement of haversian canals) and scalloping of the outer margin of the cortex.

It is important to appreciate the similarities between the findings in this process and those associated with Sudeck's atrophy (Fig. 6-12). Radiographic evidence of disuse atrophy is usually present in all patients after 5 weeks of immobilization.

Chronic disuse osteoporosis may develop gradually when it results from partial limitation of activity, or it may be the continuation of an acute process, for instance in a paralyzed limb. The bones involved show uniform radiolucency, thinning of the cortex, and a poorly defined trabecular structure. The osteopenia is limited to the paralyzed extremity.

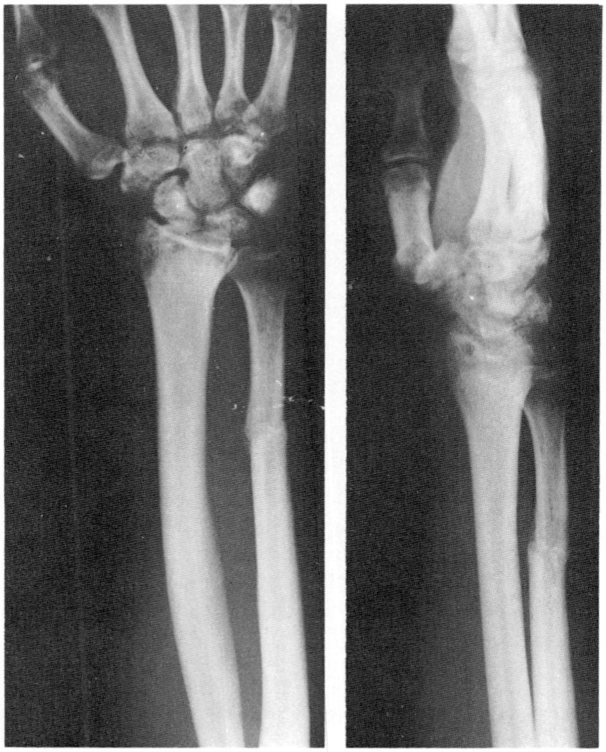

REFLEX SYMPATHETIC DYSTROPHY SYNDROME (SUDECK'S ATROPHY)

Sudeck's atrophy is a severe form of local osteopenia, usually following trauma with or without fracture. It may also follow infection, peripheral neuropathy, central nervous system abnormality, or cervical osteoarthritis. In about 25% of sufferers, no predisposing disorder is recognized. The cause is not clearly understood, but abnormal neural reflexes leading to muscle atrophy and sometimes marked hypervascularity are evidently the result of the stimulus of the inciting factor. Clinical manifestations consist of pain, often severe, resulting in far more disability than would be expected to follow a relatively minor injury. There are atrophic changes in the skin, making it smooth and glistening. The pain is often aggravated by immobilization, and the dystrophy tends to progress.

The radiologic hallmark of these syndromes is osteoporosis.[6] However, osteoporosis may be absent in as many as one-third of cases of nontraumatic cause, particularly during the early course or first stage of the disease process. The radiologic appearance of the osteoporosis has been characterized as spotty or patchy, but in reality it is little different from severe disuse osteoporosis discussed previously. It is manifested by thinning of the cortices, loss of finer trabeculae, and tunneling of the cortex due to widening of intracortical haversian canals (Fig. 6-12).[6] In reflex dystrophy, however, the osteoporosis is generally more rapid in progression. Periarticular swelling is noted. Juxta-articular and subchondral erosions are often present and are best demonstrated by fine-detail radiography.

Figure 6–11. Disuse osteoporosis. These radiographs were obtained 6 weeks following fracture of the distal ulna. Note the loss of bone density distal to the fracture site within the carpal and metacarpal bones, particularly prominent about the carpal joints.

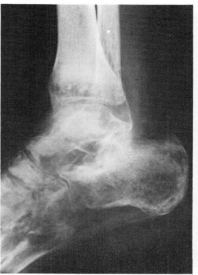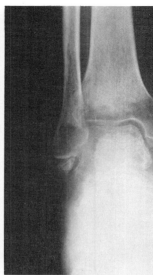

Figure 6–12. Reflex sympathetic dystrophy (Sudeck's atrophy). There is a severe osteopenia, which followed a fracture of the tip of the lateral malleolus. The osteoporosis involves all the tarsal bones, and a zone of radiolucency traverses the shafts of both the tibia and fibula. The cortical margins are thinned but intact. The patchy and mottled character of the loss of bone is characteristic. Note also the subchondral resorption, which leaves the articular cortices of the tarsal bones as fine, sharply defined lines of cortical bone.

Although the reflex dystrophy syndrome may exist in the absence of osteoporosis, the diagnosis of reflex dystrophy or Sudeck's atrophy cannot be made on the basis of radiographic appearance of the osteoporosis alone. The diagnosis requires that the osteoporosis be associated with pain or trophic changes or both.

The course of the disease may be prolonged or may revert at any stage, although the longer the process continues, the less likely there is to be a subsequent remission. There is no specific treatment.

TRANSIENT REGIONAL OSTEOPOROSIS

There are two general patterns of transient regional osteoporosis[18]—transient osteoporosis of the hip and regional migratory osteoporosis.

Transient osteoporosis of the hip is usually observed in young and middle-aged males. Either hip may be affected. However, the disease was originally recognized in pregnant females, the onset occurring in the third trimester and the process almost invariably involving the left hip.[2] Clinically there is gradual onset of hip pain, with no antecedent history of injury. There may be a joint effusion, and on biopsy, a mild, chronic synovitis may be observed. Recovery usually occurs spontaneously in 6 months or less. Radiographic findings consist of a severe loss of bone density in the femoral head and to a lesser extent in the femoral neck and acetabulum (Fig. 6-13). Characteristically there is no narrowing of the joint space.

Regional migratory osteoporosis is a transient, painful osteoporosis of the lower extremities in which the knee, ankle, and foot are involved more commonly than the hip. Females are affected more often than

males. There is gradual onset of regional pain and swelling accompanied by a rapid development of osteopenia, localized to the painful area. Pain often lasts as long as 9 months, and there may be subsequent involvement of other areas in the same or opposite extremity. Roentgenographic study reveals a decrease in bone density, with no evidence of local destruction similar to reflex osteodystrophy (see Fig. 6-12). The trabecular pattern is coarse and irregular and tends to change slowly, gradually returning to normal over a period of several years. There are no alterations in calcium, phosphorus, or alkaline phosphatase. The cause is unknown.

Isotopic bone scans demonstrate a diffuse increase in activity on both sides of the joint in either form of regional osteoporosis (Fig. 6-13A). MRI[1] (Fig. 6-13C, D) reveals a decreased signal in the marrow on T1-weighted images and an increase in signal on T2-weighted images. When the process involves the hip, the activity on bone scanning and signal intensity changes on MRI will be greater in the femoral head and neck than on the acetabular side of the joint.

PERIARTICULAR OSTEOPOROSIS

Periarticular osteoporosis refers to a pattern of focal osteoporosis at the apposing ends of bone at a joint, usually associated with some form of joint disease. It is particularly common and is characteristic of rheumatoid arthritis but is also encountered, to a lesser extent, in other noninfectious arthritides such as Reiter's syndrome. It also occurs in later stages of acute septic arthritis or chronic infectious arthritis (see Diseases of the Joints in Chapter 3).

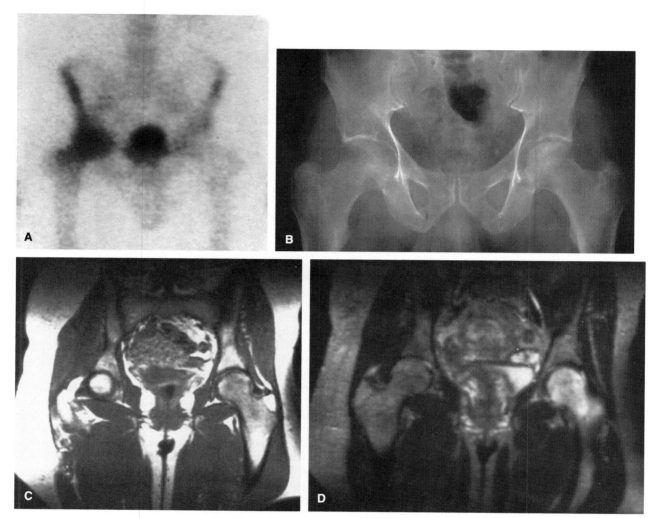

Figure 6–13.   Two cases of transient osteoporosis of the hip. (**A** and **B**) Case 1: Young man with involvement of the right hip. Technetium-99m bone scan (**A**). Increased activity is present in the femoral head and neck. AP view of the pelvis (**B**). Note the marked reduction in density of the right femoral head and neck and to a lesser extent in the acetabulum. The cortical margin of the femoral head is almost completely lost. The joint space is normal. (**C** and **D**) Case 2: MRI examination of a second case involving the left hip in a 38-year-old women. T1-weighted MR image (TR 500, TE 40) (**C**). Reduced signal in the intermedullary bone in the head, neck, and intertrochanteric region of the left femur. The cortical bone is intact. T2-weighted MR image (TR 2000, TE 120) (**D**) demonstrates increased signal from the same area. There is a small accompanying joint effusion identified by the linear bright signal at the lateral and inferior margins of the femoral head.

PRIMARY FORMS OF OSTEOMALACIA AND RICKETS

Normally the process of bone removal and formation is in balance. Unless adequate calcium and phosphorus are available, proper calcification of osteoid cannot oc-cur and the process of bone formation is arrested; removal of bone continues, and the balance is disturbed in favor of demineralization. When this happens in an adult, it results in a condition known as osteomalacia. During childhood, the effect is two pronged, affecting bone already formed in the same manner as in the adult and, in addition, new bone formed in the epiphyseal complex—the metaphysis, physis, and epiphysis. As a result, the process of growth is greatly altered and changes are seen in the epiphyseal complex that have no counterpart in the adult. This form of osteomalacia is known as rickets. Osteomalacia and rickets are therefore essentially the same disease. The roentgenographic findings differ only because of the presence of the epiphyseal complex and actively growing bone in childhood.

The causes of osteomalacia are varied and include an inadequate intake of vitamin D or failure of absorption of calcium and phosphorus singly or in combination. The importance of calcium and phosphorus in the proper mineralization of bone is well recognized. The major effect of vitamin D is to increase absorption of calcium and phosphorus from the intestinal tract. It may also have a direct effect on bone. Certain renal diseases in which there is tubular insufficiency and failure of phosphorus resorption may also cause osteomalacia.

VITAMIN D METABOLISM[18]

Vitamin D is in reality not a true vitamin. The metabolism of vitamin D is summarized in Figure 6-14. The chemical compound vitamin D_3 is produced from the interaction of ultraviolet light with a natural, endogenously produced cholesterol derivative, 7-dehydro-

cholesterol, in the deeper layers of the skin. Small amounts of exogenous vitamin D_3 may be derived in the diet from dairy products, fish, and liver oils. Vitamin D_2 is artificially prepared from yeast or fungi and is the compound used for food supplementation and pharmaceutical preparations. Vitamin D_2 and D_3 are quite similar in their chemical makeup and physiologic action. Both are hydroxylated at the carbon-25 position in the liver to form 25-(OH)-D_3 and 25-(OH)-D_2, respectively. Twenty-five hydroxy vitamin D_3 (and D_2) is further hydroxylated at the carbon-1 position to form 1,25-(OH)$_2$-D_3 (and D_2). Hydroxylation at this position occurs in the kidney and yields the most active form of vitamin D. The hormone acts at three main target organs: bone, kidney, and intestine. The effect on the intestine is to increase the absorption of calcium and phosphorus. In the skeleton, it has two actions: the mobilization of calcium and phosphorus from previously formed bone and the promotion of maturation and mineralization of organic matrix. The presence of vitamin D is essential for adequate deposition of bone mineral. Two hormonal roles are possible: the maintenance of adequate serum calcium and phosphorus levels and a direct effect on skeletal tissue. Vitamin D plays a lesser role in renal tubular resorption of phosphate and the regulation of parathormone excretion by the parathyroid gland. Vitamin D is excreted directly into the bile, where it facilitates the intestinal absorption of both calcium and phosphorus.

The serum calcium level and deposition of calcium in bone are very sensitive to the renal tubular excretion of phosphorus. When the renal tubular resorption of phosphorus is excessive, there is an associated loss of serum calcium and a mobilization of calcium from the bone. Therefore, renal tubular disorders are an important source of rickets and osteomalacia.

PATHOLOGIC CHANGES IN RICKETS AND OSTEOMALACIA

Rickets displays a disorganization of the growth plate and subjacent metaphysis. The resting or proliferative zones of the growth plate are not significantly altered; however, the zone of maturation or hypertrophy is grossly abnormal, with a disorganized increase in the number of cells and a loss of the normal columnar arrangement, resulting in an increase in the length and width of the growth plate. Vascular intrusion from the metaphysis and subsequent calcification of the intervening cartilage bars are decreased and grossly disordered. Defective mineralization occurs in the metaphysis, resulting in the failure of proper formation of bone lamellae and haversian systems.

Osteomalacia is characterized by abnormal quantities of osteoid, inadequately mineralized bone ma-

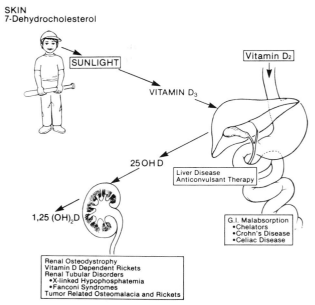

SKIN
7-Dehydrocholesterol

SUNLIGHT

Vitamin D_2

VITAMIN D_3

25 OH D

Liver Disease
Anticonvulsant Therapy

1,25 (OH)$_2$D

G.I. Malabsorption
•Chelators
•Crohn's Disease
•Celiac Disease

Renal Osteodystrophy
Vitamin D Dependent Rickets
Renal Tubular Disorders
•X-linked Hypophosphatemia
•Fanconi Syndromes
Tumor Related Osteomalacia and Rickets

Figure 6–14. Vitamin D metabolism. Deficiencies and diseases resulting in rickets and osteomalacia are identified in the enclosures.

Table 6–2. Clinical Syndromes of Rickets and Osteomalacia

Primary forms
　Adults
　　Osteomalacia in adults
　　Atypical axial osteomalacia
　Children
　　Vitamin D deficiencies
　　Neonatal rickets
　　Vitamin D-resistant rickets (renal tubular disorders)
　　Hereditary vitamin D-dependent rickets
　　Hypophosphatasia
　　Metaphyseal chondrodysplasia (Schmid type)
Secondary forms
　Gastrointestinal malabsorption
　Liver disease (primary biliary atresia)
　Anticonvulsant drug-related rickets and osteomalacia
　Tumor-associated rickets and osteomalacia

trix, coating the surfaces of trabeculae and lining the haversian canals in the cortex. Excessive accumulations of osteoid may also be deposited beneath the periosteum. Bone trabeculae become thin and decrease in number. In the cortex, the haversian systems become irregular and large. Osteoid seams, known as Looser's zones or pseudofractures, form in areas of high bone turnover within the cortex. These focal accumulations of osteoid are the radiographic hallmarks of osteomalacia in the adult.

The various clinical syndromes of rickets and osteomalacia are listed in Tables 6-2 and 6-3.

OSTEOMALACIA IN ADULTS

The disease osteomalacia is the same as infantile rickets, but it occurs after bone growth has ceased. In the United States, osteomalacia probably is most often

Table 6–3. Rickets: Age Versus Etiology

1. Onset less than 6 months of age
　　Biliary atresia
　　Vitamin D–dependent rickets
　　Hypophosphatasia
　　Neonatal rickets
2. Onset 6 to 18 months of age
　　Vitamin D deficiency
3. Late onset over 2 years of age
　　(Rickets resistant to usual doses of vitamin suggests)
　　a. Renal tubular disorders
　　b. Hypophosphatasia
　　c. Metaphyseal chondrodysplasia
　　d. Tumor-associated

caused by faulty absorption of fat-soluble vitamin D and other substances from the intestinal tract because of the steatorrhea in malabsorption syndromes, of which idiopathic sprue is the most common. Osteomalacia secondary to dysfunction of the proximal renal tubules (renal osteomalacia) is encountered less frequently, and dietary deficiency, the common cause of infantile rickets, is infrequent in the United States. Most cases identified in adults in the United States prove to be idiopathic. Some patients experience bone pain, and in others the condition is recognized incidentally on radiographs or at the time of the initial evaluation for a fracture.

Radiographic Diagnosis of Osteomalacia in Adults

Pseudofractures, or Looser's zones, are frequent in and characteristic of osteomalacia, although they may be found in a few other conditions. These are fissurelike defects or clefts extending transversely partly or completely through the cortex (Figs. 6-15 and 6-16). They are filled with uncalcified osteoid and fibrous tissue. Pseudofractures are commonly found along the axillary borders of the scapulae, the inner margins of the femoral necks, the ribs, the pubic and ischial rami, and the bones of the forearms. Pathologic fractures may occur through these weakened areas. The condition described by Milkman[12] and known as Milkman's syndrome is now considered to represent a mild form of osteomalacia in which pseudofractures are particularly numerous.

The basic roentgenographic abnormality is a generalized undermineralization of the skeleton. The texture of the bones is coarse and poorly defined. This is caused by an irregular absorption of trabeculae; the total trabecular structure of the bone is decreased, and the primary trabeculae that remain stand out more prominently. In contrast to osteoporosis, the cortical borders of the bones may not be very distinct. It is difficult to differentiate between osteoporosis and osteomalacia on the basis of the radiographic appearance. Because bone growth has ceased, the metaphyseal and epiphyseal changes that form a large part of the findings in infantile rickets are not observed.

Because osteomalacia causes softening of the bones, they may bend or give way as a result of weight-bearing. In the pelvis there may be an inward bending of the pelvis sidewalls, with deepening of the acetabular cavities (protrusio acetabuli). In the skull, softening of the bones may lead to a downward molding of the skull over the first and second cervical vertebrae. The basal angle of the skull is flattened; the condition is known as platybasia.

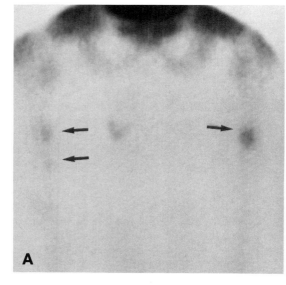 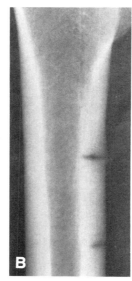

Figure 6–15. Osteomalacia. This 35-year-old male complained of diffuse bone pain. (**A**) Technetium bone scan demonstrates three small foci of increased uptake in the proximal shaft of the femurs (*arrows*). (**B**) AP radiograph of the proximal right femur demonstrates two short radiolucencies in the medial cortex, typical of pseudofractures.

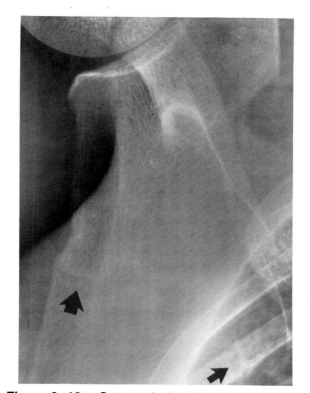

Figure 6–16. Osteomalacia in a 30-year-old female on long-term diphenylhydantoin sodium (Dilantin) therapy who complained of diffuse bone pain. A pseudofracture of the lateral border of the scapula and rib fracture (*arrows*) are identified.

ATYPICAL AXIAL OSTEOMALACIA

Atypical axial osteomalacia is a rare condition in which skeletal involvement is limited to the axial skeleton, sparing the extremities. A dense, coarse trabecular pattern primarily involves the cervical spine, but the lumbar spine, pelvis, and ribs are involved to a lesser extent. Looser's zones are not encountered. All reported patients have been adult men.

VITAMIN D–DEFICIENCY RICKETS

Classic vitamin D–deficiency rickets is uncommon in the United States because of the widespread addition of synthetic vitamin D to dairy products and bread and routine vitamin supplements administered to infants. Worldwide, however, rickets represents a significant health problem. In temperate northern climates, the most common cause is the lack of sufficient exposure to sunshine. This is more likely to occur during the winter months in crowded urban centers and occurs only in the absence of dietary supplementation. It also occurs in more tropical climates because of ethnic or cultural traditions. In some cultures, infants are wrapped and prevented from exposure to sunshine. Dietary staples, particularly grains, contain phytates, which act as chelators and bind calcium within the intestine, resulting in a fecal loss of calcium that is so great as to cause rickets and osteomalacia.

Dietary rickets is usually manifested between the ages of 4 and 18 months. The age of onset is an important clue to the cause of rickets (see Table 6-3). The earliest sign is craniotabes, manifested as a softening of the occiput and posterior parietal bones. In the thorax, there is both palpable and visible enlargement of the costochondral junctions, causing beading of the rib ends and forming a row of knobs, which constitute the "rachitic rosary." In the extremities, enlargement of the ends of the bones may be painful on palpation. The extremities may bow, more pronounced in the lower extremity than in the upper. The bending is produced by gravity and muscle pull on the softened bones. In severe cases, this results in a reduction in height—rachitic dwarfism.

Radiographic Diagnosis

Rachitic changes are more obvious in regions of active growth. Therefore, in order of decreasing sensitivity, the disease affects the costochondral junctions of middle ribs, the distal femur, the proximal femur, the proximal humerus, both ends of the tibia, and the distal radius and ulna (Fig. 6-17). The zone of provisional calcification marking the distal extent of the metaphysis disappears, and the metaphysis develops a very irregular coarse and frayed appearance. This is characteristic of rickets. Typically the metaphyses become concave, often referred to as cupping. The margins of the ossified epiphyseal centers become indistinct, and in severe cases the centers may be difficult to visualize or may even disappear because of pronounced demineralization. In severe rickets, thin, stripelike shadows frequently parallel the outer cortical margins of the long bones. These resemble periosteal new-bone formation but actually represent zones of poorly calcified osteoid laid down by the periosteum, which would normally result in transverse growth of bone.

Nonspecific radiographic features of rickets include general retardation in growth and osteopenia, a generalized demineralization of the skeleton, giving the bones a coarse texture. The smaller trabeculae are resorbed, and the larger and coarser trabeculae remain. Because of the weakening effects of the demineralization, bowing of the weight-bearing bones will develop if the infant has begun to stand or walk (Fig. 6-18).

Greenstick fractures may occur. These are more likely to develop in the older child than in the very young infant. Children with severe disease may develop pseudofractures or Looser's zones, similar to those in osteomalacia of adults. These are transverse, fissurelike clefts in the cortex of long bones, the axillary border of the scapulae, the pubic rami, and other areas.

Demineralization of the cranial bones occurs, and in the young infant the sutural margins become indistinct. The bones are soft, and the skull is readily molded by pressure. The tendency for piling up of poorly calcified bone leads to the formation of prominences or bosses in the skull, particularly in the frontal bone. These are especially noticeable after healing begins. The changes noted in the metaphysis of the long, tubular bones also develop in the sternal end of the ribs and lead to the clinical sign of beading, forming the rachitic rosary.

Healing of rickets is shown by recalcification of the zone of provisional calcification (see Fig. 6-18). At first, this is seen as a broad band of uniform density extending across the end of the shaft. Remineralization of the skeleton is a slow process and may take several months or even longer. The epiphyseal centers gradually regain normal density and sharpness of outline. The subperiosteal, poorly calcified osteoid is transformed into bone, and the periosteal stripes disappear. If the bones have become bowed or otherwise deformed during the active stage of disease, the deformities are likely to persist. Thus when rickets has completely healed, only the deformities from bowing or fracture will remain as evidence of the previous disease (see Fig. 6-18).

NEONATAL RICKETS

Neonatal rickets occur in premature infants with very low birth weight.[17] The requirements for calcium phosphate and vitamin D in premature infants are greater than those of infants born at term. Rickets may be manifested in those who have experienced necrotizing enterocolitis or neonatal respiratory distress syndrome. The radiographic diagnosis may be made on the basis of changes in the proximal humerus and ribs. The possibility of rickets in these newborns has been recognized and is successfully treated by oral administration of vitamin D. It is now rare to identify radiographic evidence of rickets in this population.

VITAMIN D–RESISTANT (REFRACTORY) RICKETS (RENAL TUBULAR DISORDERS)

Refractory rickets has also been called *rachitis tarda* or *late rickets* because it is found in older children (beyond the age of $2\frac{1}{2}$ years). It was formerly considered to be due to a high tissue threshold for the effects of vitamin D, since massive doses of the vitamin are necessary to effect a cure, thus the term *vitamin D–resistant rickets*. It is now known that this can result from a number of renal tubular disorders. The diseases may affect the proximal tubules, distal tubules, or both proximal and distal tubules. These result in renal loss of phosphorus and thus are known as hypophosphatemic

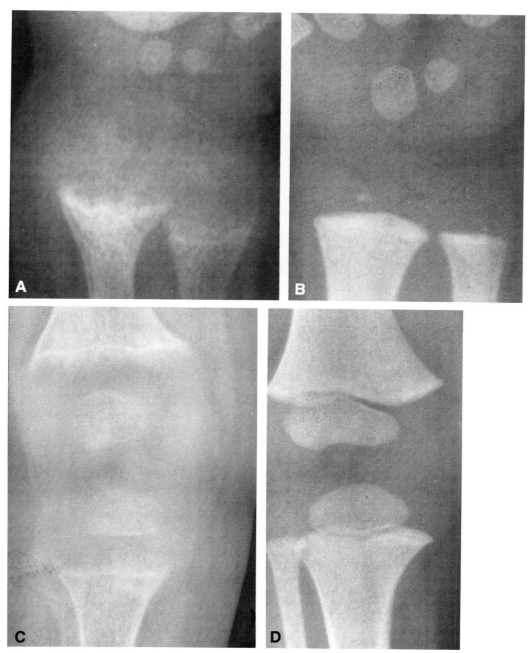

Figure 6–17.   Nutritional rickets in a 10-month-old girl. (**A**) Distal radius and ulna. The metaphyses are flared, with concave or cupping deformity. The zone of provisional calcification is decreased in density, broadened, and brushlike. (**B**) Normal wrist of a 10-month-old girl for comparison. (**C**) AP view of the knee demonstrated flaring of metaphysis with a broad, brushlike provisional zone of calcification. Note the widening of the growth plate and the poor definition of the epiphysis. (**D**) Knee of normal 10-month-old for comparison.

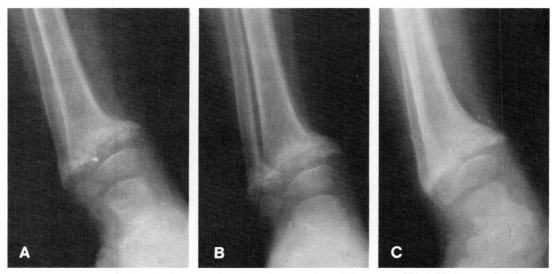

Figure 6–18. Infantile rickets showing the results of therapy. **(A)** Initial examination showing typical changes of rickets. Note the varus deformity at the ankle. **(B)** The same patient after 18 days of therapy. The metaphyses are beginning to recalcify. **(C)** Four weeks later, the healing is well advanced. There is bowing because the infant started to walk before therapy was initiated. Note that the growth plate has reduced considerably in width over the period of observation.

rickets. Four types have been reported: (1) Classic vitamin D–resistant (hypophosphatemic) rickets or phosphate diabetes is transmitted as an X-linked dominant trait. Most children having this type of rickets fall below the third percentile in height by the age of 2 years. Enlarged wrists and ankles, rachitic rosary, frontal bossing, and sometimes craniosynostosis are observed. (2) In vitamin D–resistant rickets with glycosuria, there is an abnormal resorptive mechanism for glucose and inorganic phosphate. (3) In the proximal tubular type (Fanconi's syndrome), there is defective resorption of phosphate, glucose, and several amino acids. The rachitic lesions are severe, but this type appears to be less refractory to vitamin D therapy than the others. (4) A rare type of hypophosphatemic syndrome does not become manifest until late adolescence or early adult life. It may be an acquired lesion and is probably of toxic origin.

There are several syndromes in which proximal and distal renal tubules are involved. The proximal and distal Fanconi's syndrome is transmitted as an autosomal recessive trait and is probably genetically unrelated to the proximal Fanconi's syndrome. In children with the combined proximal and distal Fanconi's syndrome, rickets is usually severe, with multiple fractures occurring in the first few months of life. There are several other very rare lesions in which both proximal and distal tubular abnormalities are found. The distal

renal tubules are involved in renal tubular acidosis. In one form, bicarbonate is excreted in excess amounts, with a reduced excretion of ammonia. In another, the acidosis results from loss of bicarbonate because of reduction in tubular resorption, and there is also increased excretion of sodium and potassium along with a decrease in water reabsorption, resulting in severe dehydration. More than 70% of patients with chronic renal tubular acidosis have nephrocalcinosis.

Radiographic Findings

Rachitic changes at the growth plate are usually only mild or moderate in degree, much less severe than those encountered in full-blown dietary rickets. Characteristically, metaphyseal changes persist unchanged even after prolonged treatment with high doses of vitamin D, thus the designation vitamin D–resistant rickets (Figs. 6-19 and 6-20). Bowing of the long bones of the lower extremity may occur, but the deformity is frequently minimal.

The trabecular pattern becomes coarsened as the patients become older, and by adulthood a generalized increase in bone density is characteristic, especially in the axial skeleton. Ectopic calcification in both the axial and appendicular skeleton occurs. The spinal changes may resemble ankylosing spondylitis. Calcification occurs in the paravertebral ligaments, annulus fibrosus,

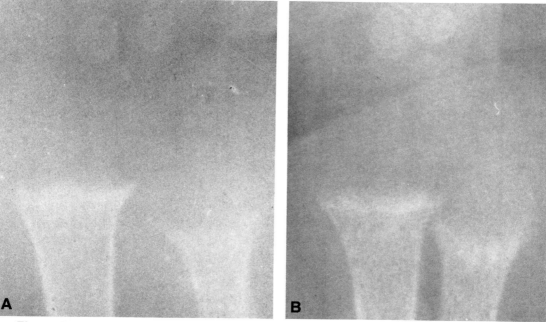

Figure 6–19. Fanconi's syndrome, with vitamin D–resistant rickets. Distal radius and ulna, with mild changes of rickets manifested by minimal flaring and slight cupping of the metaphysis. (**B**) Repeat examination following 10 months of high-dose vitamin D therapy demonstrates little change in the radiographic appearance of the rachitic changes.

and capsules of apophyseal joints. In the pelvis, calcification may involve the ligaments and joint capsules of the acetabulum and the sacroiliac ligaments, partially obscuring the sacroiliac joints. Entheses (bony spurs) form at muscle and ligamentous attachments. Separate small ossicles may develop around various joints, particularly the carpus.

HEREDITARY VITAMIN D–DEPENDENT RICKETS

Hereditary vitamin D–dependent rickets is due to an inborn error of vitamin D metabolism. The clinical and biochemical features resemble advanced nutritional rickets. Symptoms may be present as early as 3 months of age in contrast to nutritional rickets, and most patients are identified by 1 year of age. Rachitic bone changes may be severe and rapidly progressive, with pathologic fractures. In contrast to vitamin D–resistant rickets, large doses of vitamin D lead to complete healing.

HYPOPHOSPHATASIA

Hypophosphatasia is an inborn error of metabolism characterized by a low level of serum alkaline phosphatase and the presence of phosphoethanolamine in the urine and serum.

It is probably inherited as an autosomal recessive trait. The lack of adequate amounts of alkaline phosphatase causes failure of proper mineralization of osteoid and results in an appearance similar to that of rickets or osteomalacia. The disease may be present at birth. The earlier the disease is detected, the more severe it is likely to be, and infants born with it seldom survive more than a year or two. In these patients, there is severe undermineralization of the metaphyses, the ends of which have a coarse, frayed appearance somewhat similar to that of rickets. However, in contrast to rickets, the metaphyseal cupping is deep and irregular and often contains irregular linear streaks of calcification. The long bones in the newborn tend to be short and thin and have a coarse texture. The bones of the cranial vault are largely unossified, and there is bulging of the anterior fontanelle. Fractures of the long bones may occur. In older children, the changes are similar but less severe and resemble infantile rickets (Fig 6-21). If the patient survives and the cranial bones ossify, craniosynostosis often develops. Dwarfism also becomes a feature, and a genu valgum deformity is common. Anterior and lateral femoral bowing, early loss of teeth, pseudofracture, and fractures caused by minimal trauma are common. Many of these patients improve spontaneously. In its mildest form, hypo-

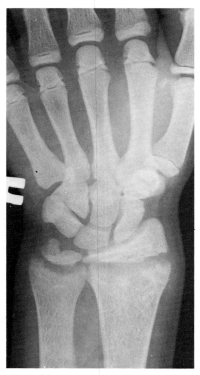

Figure 6–20.   Vitamin D–resistant rickets in an adolescent. The growth plate is widened, and the metaphysis is slightly flared and cupped.

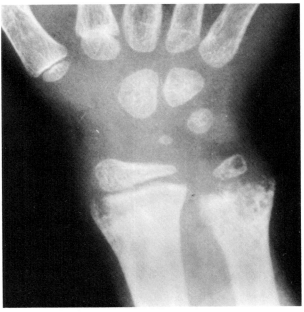

Figure 6–21.   Hypophosphatasia in a child. There is deficient ossification of the metaphysis of the ulna. Note the roughened, frayed appearance of the metaphyses, more marked in the ulna than in the radius. The changes are somewhat similar to those of rickets, but the depth of the cupping deformity and its irregularity are characteristic of hypophosphatasia.

phosphatasia manifests itself chiefly by an increased tendency of the bones to fracture and a low serum alkaline phosphatase. The disease is very rare in adults.

The essential histologic feature is the presence of abnormal amounts of osteoid.

METAPHYSEAL CHONDRODYSPLASIA (SCHMID TYPE)

Metaphyseal chondrodysplasias encompass a variety of disorders having in common a generalized symmetrical disturbance of endochondral bone formation, primarily at the metaphysis. The Schmid type is the most common and has radiologic features very similar to those of vitamin D–resistant rickets (see Fig. 9-12). Normal levels of serum phosphorus, alkaline phosphatase, and calcium differentiate these disorders from other rachitic syndromes. The disease is transmitted in an autosomal dominant pattern and presents in childhood with short stature and bowing of the long bones. In a child, the radiograph shows widening of the growth plates similar to rickets. In contrast to rickets, the metaphysis is well mineralized and may actually

show increased density. The skull is normal, and Looser's zones do not occur.

SECONDARY FORMS OF RICKETS AND OSTEOMALACIA

GASTROINTESTINAL MALABSORPTION

Rickets and osteomalacia may develop in small bowel malabsorption states, including sprue, celiac disease, regional enteritis, scleroderma, multiple jejunal diverticula, or stagnant loop syndromes. Decreased absorption in the small bowel and excessive fecal loss of vitamin D and calcium are contributory. Small intestinal bypass surgery and partial gastrectomy have also been associated with osteomalacia.

LIVER DISEASE

Metabolic bone disease is a complication of chronic hepatocellular and biliary disorders. Both osteoporosis and less commonly osteomalacia are found histologically. When present, radiologic changes are usually those of nonspecific osteopenia. Pseudofractures indicate the presence of osteomalacia.

Congenital biliary atresia is a rare anomaly that presents as progressive obstructive jaundice (beginning within the first 2 months of birth), hypercholesterolemia, and gradual liver deterioration.[9] The marked elevation of serum lipids leads to the formation of cutaneous xanthomata. The skeleton is normal at birth, but thereafter stress lines appear in the metaphyses and the bones become demineralized, associated with lack of tubulation of the diaphyses and sometimes expansion of the metaphyses. The cortex of long and short bones becomes quite thin. There are no changes in the calvarium. Soft-tissue masses appear over the extensor surfaces of the extremities. The epiphyses and growth plates are relatively normal except during periods of rapid growth, particularly during the end of the first year, when changes of rickets may be evident. The thinness of the bones leads to pathologic fractures in 50% of cases.

ANTICONVULSANT DRUG-RELATED RICKETS AND OSTEOMALACIA

Radiographic changes of rickets and osteomalacia associated with anticonvulsant drug therapy, particularly phenobarbital, and diphenylhydantoin (Dilantin) have been noted. The radiographic changes are nonspecific and cannot be differentiated from rickets or osteomalacia resulting from other causes. Changes of osteomalacia may be quite severe in nonambulatory, long-term, institutionalized patients.

TUMOR-ASSOCIATED RICKETS AND OSTEOMALACIA

Vitamin D–resistant rickets and osteomalacia have been associated with various neoplasms of soft tissue or bone occurring in both children and adults. Hypophosphatemia is the predominant biochemical feature and is secondary to a failure of renal tubular resorption, the cause of which remains unidentified. The most frequent soft-tissue tumor has been hemangiopericytoma. Bone lesions have included nonossifying fibroma, giant cell tumor, osteoblastoma, and a nonneoplastic disease, fibrous dysplasia. Patients present with generalized muscle weakness. Radiographic changes of rickets and osteomalacia may be advanced. A careful search for these lesions should be made in patients presenting with vitamin D–refractory rickets for which more common causes have not been identified. The removal of the responsible tumor is curative.

PARATHYROID DISORDERS

HYPERPARATHYROIDISM

Hyperparathyroidism is categorized into primary and secondary types.[18] In primary hyperparathyroidism, increased parathyroid hormone secretion is the result of a parathyroid tumor, usually a single adenoma, occasionally multiple adenomas, and rarely carcinoma. In 10% of cases, the excess secretion is due to diffuse hyperplasia of multiple glands. Secondary hyperparathyroidism is induced by alterations in renal function causing a hyperplasia of all parathyroid glands. The combination of renal failure and secondary hyperparathyroidism results in a spectrum of both soft-tissue and skeletal abnormalities commonly referred to as *renal osteodystrophy.*[29]

An excess of parathyroid hormone secretion produces excessive bone resorption, resulting in elevation of serum calcium and reduction of serum phosphorus. Parathyroid hormone acts to increase the number of osteoclasts, with resulting deossification of the skeleton. It may also diminish resorption of phosphate by the proximal renal tubules. When the renal threshold is exceeded, calcium is excreted in increased amounts. Eventually, renal stones are formed and calcification occurs in the kidney (nephrocalcinosis). These changes may lead to an impairment of renal function, further aggravating the retention of phosphate and the loss of calcium.

The initial clinical manifestations of hyperparathyroidism are often urinary tract calculi, peptic ulcer disease, or pancreatitis. A small percentage of patients complain of pain and tenderness of the peripheral joints or vertebral column. The diagnosis is substantiated by the characteristic biochemical findings of hypercalcemia, hypophosphatemia, increased urinary excretion of calcium and phosphorus, and elevated serum alkaline phosphatase. In fact, with the use of automated blood chemical analysis, the diagnosis is now often made on the basis of these biochemical abnormalities before the patient is symptomatic and, more to the point, before there are radiographic changes of disease. As many as 40% of cases are now diagnosed before there are radiographic manifestations of disease.

The parathyroid adenoma usually arises in the normal location of the gland but occasionally is ectopically located within the superior or anterior mediastinum. The radiographic localization of an adenoma can usually be accomplished by a barium swallow, chest radiograph, and CT scanning of the neck and mediastinum. Occasionally, mediastinal venous sampling for increased parahormone levels may be required to establish the location of smaller adenomas.

Radiographic Findings

The principal radiographic features of hyperparathyroidism are evidence of bone resorption (particularly subperiosteal bone resorption), diffuse osteopenia, cystlike lesions of bone, and chondrocalcinosis.[5]

Subperiosteal Resorption. Subperiosteal resorption of cortical bone is virtually diagnostic of hyperparathyroidism. It is most frequent along the radial aspect of the phalanges of the middle phalanx of the index and middle fingers (Figs. 6-22 and 6-23), although similar changes may be visualized in many skeletal locations. Normally the peripheral margins of the cortex are smooth. In the presence of subperiosteal resorption, there is a fine irregularity along the outer margins of the cortex. This roughened surface has been described as lacelike. Resorption of the terminal (ungual) tufts occurs in the distal phalanges (Fig. 6-23). These findings constitute the earliest and most sensitive radiographic findings of hyperparathyroidism. Similar changes occur in the medial, proximal metaphyseal surfaces of the tibia, humerus, and femur and the superior and inferior margins of the ribs. Resorption of the lamina dura, the fine line of increased density located about each tooth, is the equivalent of sub-

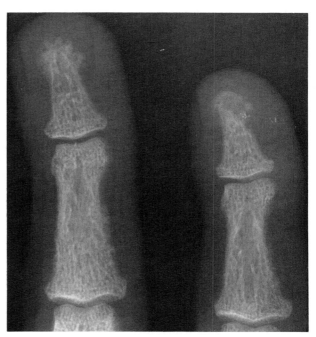

Figure 6–23. Hyperparathyroidism. Subperiosteal resorption is less pronounced than in Figure 6-22. Note also the resorption of the ungual tufts in this patient with secondary hyperparathyroidism.

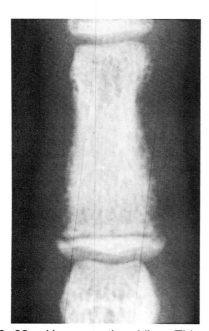

Figure 6–22. Hyperparathyroidism. This child with renal osteodystrophy demonstrates characteristic subperiosteal cortical resorption of the middle phalanx. Note the lacelike appearance of the peripheral margin of the cortex, typical of subperiosteal resorption.

periosteal resorption. However, this is nonspecific, as it may result from infections and a variety of other dental diseases.

Subchondral resorption of bone also occurs at the acromioclavicular, sternoclavicular, symphysis pubis, and sacroiliac joints (Figs. 6-24, 6-25). This causes irregularity and widening of these joints and a tapering or destruction of the outer end of the clavicle. Occasionally, subchondral resorption occurs about the margins of the smaller joints of the hand and feet in a manner somewhat suggestive of rheumatoid arthritis.[7, 18] However, the joint space is preserved. A destructive noninfective spondyloarthropathy is occasionally encountered in secondary hyperparathyroidism.[15]

Subligamentous bone resorption and erosions occur at the site of tendon and ligament attachment to bone. This is particularly frequent at the trochanters, the ischial and humeral tuberosities, the inferior surface of the calcaneus, and the inferior aspect of the distal clavicle. Additionally, intracortical bone resorption occurs within the haversian canals, and it may be radiographically detectable as intracortical linear lucencies. Endosteal bone resorption causes a scalloping of the endosteal surface. Trabecular resorption results in a granular appearance, with the loss of distinct trabecular detail. Fine-detail magnification radiography can

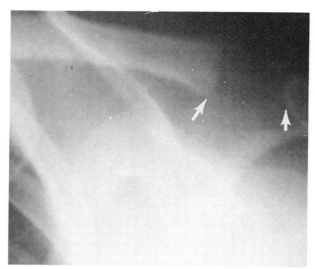

Figure 6–24. Hyperparathyroidism. There has been a loss of bone in the distal end of the clavicle. The *arrows* indicate the distal clavicle and the medial acromion. The resorption results in an apparent widening of the acromioclavicular joint.

detect these radiographic findings before they are visible on conventional radiographs.

Osteopenia. Generalized osteopenia frequently accompanies hyperparathyroidism. This is a subjective radiographic finding and is difficult to identify until 30% to 50% of bone mineral is lost. The degree of bone loss can be quantified by bone mineral density deter-

minations. The most characteristic manifestation of osteopenia is the "salt-and-pepper" appearance of the skull (Fig. 6-26), a pebbled pattern of reduced density due to endosteal resorption of the bony tables.

Brown Tumors. Localized destructive cystlike lesions of various sizes, referred to as *brown tumors*, are frequent in, and characteristic of, hyperparathyroidism. They contain fibrous tissue, giant cells, osteoclasts, and decomposing blood, which undergo necrosis and liquefaction. They appear as single or multiple well-defined lesions, frequently eccentric or cortical, commonly within the mandible, pelvis (Fig. 6-27), and femurs, but they may be found in any part of the skeleton. With removal of the offending parathyroid adenoma, brown tumors may heal, with increased radiodensity.

Chondrocalcinosis. Radiographic evidence of calcification in and around joints is identified in fewer than 50% of patients with primary hyperparathyroidism and is very infrequent in secondary hyperparathyroidism. This calcification is usually within the joint cartilage (chondrocalcinosis) and is similar in appearance to calcification associated with calcium pyrophosphate-dihydrate crystal deposition (CPPD), the pseudogout syndrome described in Chapter 3. Less commonly, calcification occurs in the joint capsule, ligaments, and tendons.

CPPD is a much more common cause of chondrocalcinosis than is hyperparathyroidism. The earliest radiographic finding of hyperparathyroidism is subperiosteal resorption, and therefore chondrocalcinosis in the absence of subperiosteal resorption is unlikely due to hyperparathyroidism and more likely indicative of CPPD or some other cause of chondrocalcinosis (see Chapter 3).

Osteosclerosis. Osteosclerosis is an infrequent finding in primary hyperparathyroidism but is a hallmark of secondary hyperparathyroidism or renal osteodystrophy. This is seen most often in the subchondral metaphyseal regions and is characteristically found in the superior and inferior margins of the vertebral bodies as poorly marginated broad bands of increased radiodensity resulting in the characteristic "ruggerjersey" spine (Fig. 6-28).

HYPERPARATHYROIDISM IN INFANTS AND CHILDREN

Primary hyperparathyroidism may occasionally be encountered in infants and children. Congenital primary hyperparathyroidism is a rare disorder occurring in infants demonstrating autosomal recessive inheri-

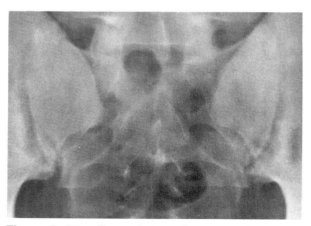

Figure 6–25. Secondary hyperparathyroidism, with erosion of the margins of the sacroiliac joint causing an apparent widening of the joint space.

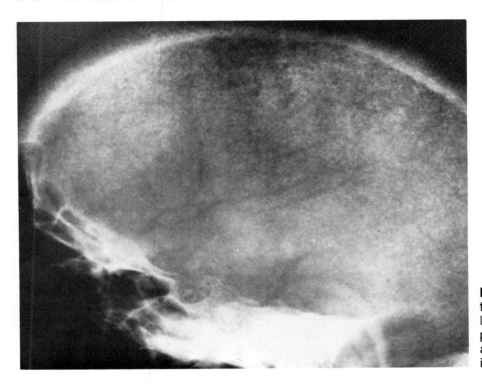

Figure 6–26. Hyperparathyroidism. Note the granular, "salt-and-pepper" appearance of the cranial vault associated with a decrease in overall bone density.

tance. In infants, radiographs reveal severe bone disease, with subperiosteal bone resorption, periosteal bone formation, trabecular reduction, extensive erosions of tubular bones, and pathologic fractures. The degree of periostitis may be so severe as to simulate congenital syphilis. In older children, hyperparathyroidism is characterized by osteopenia, genu valgum, cystic lesions of bone, and clubbing of the fingers.

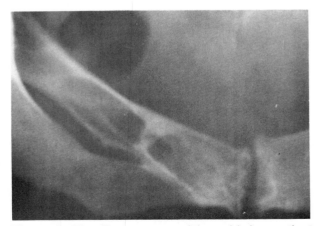

Figure 6–27. Brown tumor of the pubis in a patient with hyperparathyroidism. There is a lytic, slightly expansile lesion involving the superior pubic ramus.

Rickets-like changes of the metaphysis may be observed.

SECONDARY HYPERPARATHYROIDISM

Chronic renal insufficiency results in hyperplasia of the parathyroid glands, presumably due to phosphate retention and the consequent lowering of the serum calcium. The radiographic abnormalities associated with secondary hyperparathyroidism are very similar to those of primary hyperparathyroidism, differing only in degree. The hallmark of secondary hyperparathyroidism, as in primary hyperparathyroidism, is subperiosteal resorption of bone, particularly of the phalanges of the hand as previously described. Intracortical, endosteal, trabecular, subchondral,[7] and subligamentous bone resorption also occurs. The presence of osteosclerosis tends to separate secondary from primary hyperparathyroidism. Osteosclerosis is a prominent feature of secondary hyperparathyroidism encountered predominantly in the axial skeleton and more particularly in the superior and inferior margins of the vertebral bodies, forming the rugger-jersey spine (see Fig. 6-28). Osteosclerosis is much less common and much less severe when encountered in primary hyperparathyroidism. On the other hand, the incidence of brown tumors and chondrocalcinosis is much lower in secondary hyperparathyroidism than in

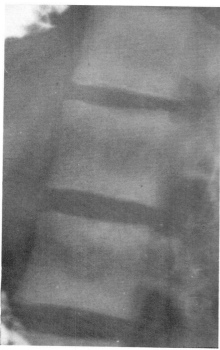

Figure 6–28. "Rugger-jersey" spine in secondary hyperparathyroidism. Osteosclerosis is present in both the superior and inferior portions of the vertebral bodies, giving rise to a striped or "rugger-jersey" appearance of the vertebral bodies that is characteristic of secondary hyperparathyroidism.

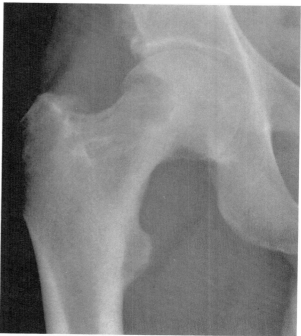

Figure 6–29. Beta$_2$-microglobulin deposition in the neck and head of the femur in a patient with chronic renal failure. The lytic deposit is well marginated superiorly and medially by a thin rim of sclerosis. Such depositions have served as the focus for pathologic fracture.

primary hyperparathyroidism. Lytic lesions of bone are found in patients with chronic renal failure on long-term dialysis.[22] They are single or multiple, often small, well-defined juxta-articular lytic lesions without matrix calcification (Fig. 6-29). Pathologic fractures may occur through such lesions particularly in the hip. When biopsied, they are found to contain beta$_2$-microglobulin, a type of amyloid, and a low-weight serum protein that is not filtered by standard dialysis membranes. Biopsy of spondyloarthropathies in hemodialysis patients has revealed the same substance.[15] Periosteal new-bone formation occurs in the metatarsals, femur, and pubic rami, although it may be visualized on any long bone. This is referred to as periosteal neostosis and presents as a thin layer of periosteal new-bone formation, paralleling the cortex from which it is frequently separated by a thin line of radiolucency.

Spontaneous ruptures of the infrapatellar tendon may occur, manifested clinically as an inability to extend the knee and radiographically by a high-riding patella and widening and poor definition of the tendon (Fig. 6-30).[10] Less commonly, rupture involves the

quadriceps tendon. The ruptures are depicted in exquisite detail by MRI (Fig. 6-30). Ruptures of these tendons have been observed in patients with renal failure, secondary hyperparathyroidism, systemic lupus erythematosus, and rarely primary hyperparathyroidism.

RENAL OSTEODYSTROPHY

The presence of chronic renal insufficiency has a profound effect on the skeletal system.[3, 29] In childhood or adolescence, the underlying renal disorder is related to some congenital structural abnormality of the urinary tract such as polycystic disease, hypogenesis, or congenital obstructions of the ureters, bladder outlet, or urethra. In adults, the underlying renal abnormality is usually a primary parenchymal disease such as glomerular nephritis or chronic pyelonephritis.

The radiographic findings are a combination of secondary hyperparathyroidism combined with rickets in the child and osteomalacia in the adult. In addition, there are characteristic soft-tissue calcifications: cal-

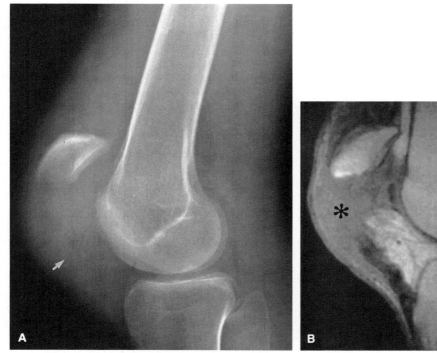

Figure 6–30.   Spontaneous rupture of the infrapatellar tendon in a patient with chronic renal failure. **(A)** Lateral radiograph demonstrates markedly elevated patella with poor definition of its inferior cortical margin. A few small irregular ossific densities are located inferiorly (*arrow*). These represent avulsions from the inferior pole of the patella. **(B)** T1-weighted sagittal MRI (TR616, TE 20) demonstrates elevated patella with hematoma (*asterisk*) anteriorly and inferiorly. The infrapatellar tendon is wrinkled and remains attached to the tibial tuberosity. Note the variation in signal intensity within the tendon.

cification of the smaller peripheral arteries and amorphous collections of calcifications, particularly about the joints. Additionally, avascular necrosis of the femoral head and, occasionally, of the ends of the other bones is frequently encountered. The latter may actually be due to the use of steroids and may not represent a manifestation of chronic renal insufficiency per se.

Rachitic changes are identified in the growth plates (Fig. 6-31). The radiographic features of rickets include osteopenia, irregular widening of the growth plate, and poor definition of the epiphysis.

Slipped epiphyses and spontaneous separations of the epiphysis are a frequent complication of renal osteodystrophy. The capital femoral epiphysis is most commonly affected (Fig. 6-32), followed by the proximal humerus, distal radius, distal ulna, distal femur, and rarely the small bones of the hands and feet. Bilateral involvement is frequent. Slippage of the capital femoral epiphysis may be preceded by evidence of subperiosteal erosion of the medial aspect of the femoral neck, an increase in the width of the cartilaginous growth plate, and bilateral coxa vara.

Osteomalacia is manifested by osteopenia and poor definition of trabeculae and cortex. Looser's zones are uncommon, in contrast to primary osteomalacia in adults.

Soft-Tissue and Vascular Calcification

Calcification in the soft tissues and vessels is frequently observed in patients with renal osteodystrophy. Periarticular deposits may reach considerable size, appearing as tumoral, radiodense masses about the hips, knees, shoulders, and ribs. Occasionally, there are bilateral symmetrical deposits. Arterial calcification is most commonly identified in the smaller arteries of the hand and foot as parallel linear radiodensities along the course of the artery (Fig. 6-33).

The bone changes of renal osteodystrophy will partially resolve in the majority of patients placed on

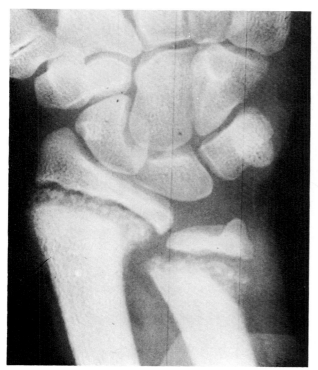

Figure 6–31. Renal osteodystrophy. There are severe changes in the metaphysis of the radius and ulna, with some medial epiphyseal subluxation.

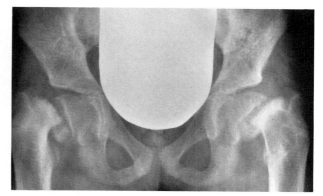

Figure 6–32. Renal osteodystrophy, with bilateral slippage of the capital femoral epiphyses. Note the widened growth plate and erosive or brushlike appearance of the metaphysis. A large brown tumor is present in the left femoral neck. (Courtesy of Sandra Fernbach, M.D., Chicago)

hemodialysis. Soft-tissue and vascular calcification is frequent in patients undergoing hemodialysis. Septicemia, osteomyelitis, and septic arthritis all are recognized complications of hemodialysis. The occurrence of osteonecrosis following renal transplantation is particularly common and may be in part due to the administration of steroids. The most common site of osteonecrosis is the femoral head. Radiographic changes are also frequently identified in the humeral head and to a lesser extent in the distal femur, talus, and elsewhere. The radiographic and pathologic manifestations of osteonecrosis are described in Chapter 7. The predominant changes are sclerosis, with varying degrees of lucency and ultimately collapse of the involved bone. A characteristic subchondral lucency beneath the articular cortex, the "crescent sign," often precedes the collapse of bone in the femoral head and elsewhere.

HYPOPARATHYROIDISM

Hypoparathyroidism usually results from injury or accidental removal of the glands during thyroidectomy. Spontaneous idiopathic hypoparathyroidism occurs but is uncommon. The clinical symptoms are those that result from the hypocalcemia (parathyroid tetany). The serum calcium is low and the phosphorus elevated. Roentgenographic changes are relatively few, and in some cases the skeletal system is normal. In others, the bones have shown increase in density, with widening of the cortices of the long bones, and the bones of the calvarium are thickened. In some patients, stippled areas of calcification occur within the brain. These tend to be symmetrically situated in the basal ganglia. Such calcification is also seen in pseudohypoparathyroidism, and occasionally it is idiopathic. In rare instances, paraspinal ossification is similar in appearance to that seen in diffuse idiopathic skeletal hyperostosis (DISH). Soft-tissue calcifications may be encountered.

PSEUDOHYPOPARATHYROIDISM AND PSEUDOPSEUDOHYPOPARATHYROIDISM

Pseudohypoparathyroidism (PH) is a congenital hereditary disorder characterized by a failure of normal response to parathyroid hormone. There is hypocalcemia and hyperphosphatemia as in hypoparathyroidism and little or no response to the administration of parathyroid hormone. Most patients are obese and of short stature, with a round facies, corneal or lenticular opacities, brachydactyly, and mental retardation. Usually all of the tubular bones of the hands and feet are short, but some, especially the fourth and fifth metacarpals (Fig. 6-34), are shorter than others. The shortening of the metacarpals may lead to a positive "metacarpal sign." Normally a line drawn tangential to the heads of the fourth and fifth metacarpals will not inter-

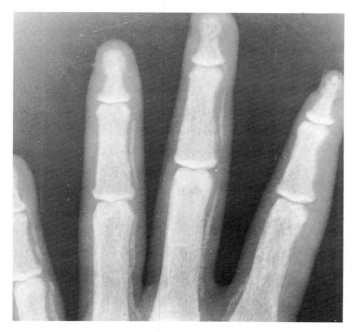

Figure 6–33. Secondary hyperparathyroidism (renal osteodystrophy) in a 21-year-old woman with chronic renal insufficiency. Subperiosteal resorption is noted, particularly along the radial aspects of the middle phalanges of the second and third digits. The bone texture is coarse, with prominent trabeculae. Calcification is present in the digital arteries.

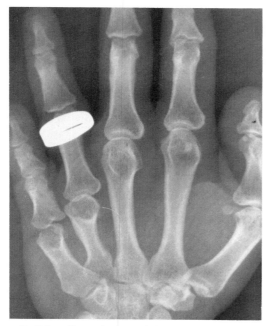

Figure 6–34. Pseudopseudohypoparathyroidism in a 33-year-old woman, manifested by shortening of both the fourth and fifth metacarpals. (Courtesy of Ronald Hendrix, M.D., Chicago)

sect the third metacarpal or will just contact its distal aspect. In PH and pseudopseudohypoparathyroidism (PPH), such a line may intersect the third metacarpal, indicating a disproportionate shortening of the fourth or fourth and fifth metacarpals. This sign is not specific since it is positive in other congenital syndromes such as basal cell nevus syndrome, Turner's syndrome, multiple epiphyseal dysplasia, and other conditions. It is also unreliable at times because the third metacarpal is also shortened. Short metacarpals and metatarsals also occur as isolated defects.

Calcified or ossified deposits may be found in the skin or subcutaneous tissues. Stippled calcification is often found in the basal ganglia or elsewhere in the brain, as in hypoparathyroidism. In some patients, the cranial bones are thickened and the skull has a brachycephalic shape. The interpediculate distances in the lumbar spine may decrease from above downward instead of showing the normal increase. The general skeletal density is decreased, apparently owing to osteoporosis, and the trabecular structure may be coarse. However, increased density has been reported in some patients. The changes of secondary hyperparathyroidism may develop because of the hypocalcemia. In some infants, the hands and feet are at first normal but become abnormal as the child grows older.

Dentition often is abnormal, including defective dentine, excessive caries, delayed eruption, and wide root canals. Other findings have been observed in some patients, including coxa vara or valga, bowing of long bones, and an occasional exostosis. The exostoses are frequently diaphyseal in location and project at a right angle to the bone, differing from those in multiple hereditary exostosis, which are usually at the metaphyseal end and directed away from joints.

The hereditary nature of PH has been established. It is possible for some members of the family to show roentgenographic findings characteristic of the disease but with normal blood chemistry studies and no evidence of tetany. This entity has been called PPH and is considered to be the partial expression of a disease of which PH is the complete syndrome.[18] Families showing only the characteristics of PPH have been reported, and in some members the bone changes have been very minimal, such as a shortening of one or more of the metacarpals. There also is a lower incidence of intracranial calcification in PPH than in PH.

Among the entities to be considered in the differential diagnosis are (1) peripheral dysostosis, (2) chondroectodermal dysplasia, (3) multiple hereditary exostosis, and (4) Turner's syndrome.[18] These as a rule have other roentgenographic, clinical, and genetic findings that aid in differentiation (see Chapter 9).

HYPERPHOSPHATASIA

Hyperphosphatasia is a hereditary familial disease transmitted by an autosomal recessive mode. It is a rare disease characterized by an elevation of the serum alkaline phosphatase and generalized bone thickening. Skeletal deformities include enlargement and bowing of the long bones and enlargement of the bones of the skull. The radiographic appearance is suggestive of Paget's disease, and therefore the disease is also known as *juvenile Paget's disease*, although the two diseases are not related.

The characteristic finding is marked thickening of the diaphyseal cortex of all tubular bones, both the short and long. The cortex is thickened, although decreased in density. There is a generalized deossification. Bowing of the long bones is a prominent feature. The bones of the cranial vault are thickened. Patches of sclerosis appear within the membranous bones, particularly within the skull and pelvis. The carpal and tarsal bones are normal, and the vertebrae show only minimal sclerosis.

Chronic Hyperphosphatasemia Tarda (Van Buchem's Disease)

Chronic hyperphosphatasemia tarda is most likely a distinct dysplasia and separate from familial hyperphosphatasia. The age of onset is later than in hyperphosphatasia, ranging from 23 to 52 years. The disease

is asymptomatic. The major roentgenographic finding is a symmetrical cortical thickening of the diaphysis of all the long tubular bones, chiefly on the internal surface. Short tubular bones are also involved in a similar fashion. The femurs are not bowed, and the epiphyses are spared. The cranial bones show marked thickening of both the vault and the base. The maxillary sinuses and the mastoids are densely sclerotic. The mandible and clavicle may be affected. There is diffuse sclerosis of the pelvic bones and ribs. The vertebrae are spared. Serum alkaline phosphatase is elevated, and calcium and phosphorus are normal.

CALCIUM OXALOSIS

Calcium oxalosis is a rare inherited metabolic disease[18] in which calcium oxalate crystals cause extensive renal damage leading to renal failure. Renal calculi and diffuse, extensive renal calcification are also observed. The skeletal changes resemble those of secondary hyperparathyroidism. There are destructive areas of subperiosteal resorption and sclerotic bands, producing rugger-jersey changes in the spine. Striking findings are noted in the hands and knees; these consist of irregular, transverse, sclerotic metaphyseal bands in the distal femur and proximal tibia and fibula as well as in the distal radius and ulna. There is a drumstick configuration of the metacarpals, evidently a combination of narrowing of the diaphysis plus widening of the metaphysis.

ENDOCRINE DISORDERS

HYPOFUNCTION OF THE THYROID GLAND

Cretinism

A congenital deficiency of thyroid secretion present at birth is known as cretinism. This results in characteristic radiographic findings. The time of appearance of ossification centers is greatly delayed, and their growth, once the centers appear, is slow. No other disorder causes as severe a delay in ossification as cretinism (Fig. 6-35). The centers that do ossify often are malformed and irregular in shape. Certain epiphyses, notably those of the proximal ends of the femurs, show a tendency to ossify from numerous small irregular centers rather than from a single one, as it normally should, the epiphysis does not grow properly, and the femoral head develops a flattened shape (Fig. 6-36). It may closely resemble the flattened and fragmented epiphysis occurring in Legg-Perthes disease (see Chapter 7), Morquio's disease, and dysplasia epiphysialis multiplex. The latter conditions are discussed in Chapter 9.

Stunting of growth may not be very obvious during

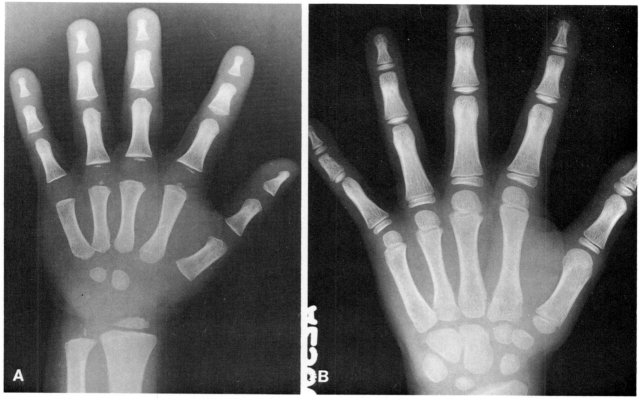

Figure 6–35. Cretinism. Hand of an 8-year-old cretin (**A**) shows delay in ossification compared with the hand of a normal 8-year-old child (**B**).

infancy, but as the child grows older, the thyroid deficiency will result in dwarfism. Roentgenographic examination is useful in the follow-up study of cretins who are undergoing treatment. The progress of skeletal development is a good index of the efficacy of therapy.

Dental defects, delay in the development and eruption of the teeth, tend to parallel the delay in ossification of the skeleton. The teeth that do erupt are structurally abnormal and are subject to caries. Other findings noted in cretinism include (1) increased thickness of the bones of the cranial vault, a narrow diploic space, and a brachycephalic shape; (2) wormian bones, which characteristically occur within the cranial sutures; (3) in severe involvement, some degree of flattening of the vertebral bodies (bullet shaped) and a thoracolumbar gibbus, with forward slipping of one vertebra on another, and wide disc spaces; and (4) slipping of a capital femoral epiphysis.

Wormian bones may be present in the skull early in skeletal development but usually disappear when the bone age reaches 5 years. Dense metaphyseal lines may be present very early in life, but they tend to

disappear at a bone age of approximately 6 months. Epiphyseal disturbances, particularly in the femoral head, persist beyond the bone age of 8 years. In many adult cretins, little or no residual skeletal deformity persists, even though insufficient or no treatment was given.

Juvenile Hypothyroidism

When the thyroid deficiency occurs after birth as an acquired disease, the process usually is less severe than in cretinism. The term *juvenile hypothyroidism* is used to designate this form of the disease. The roentgenographic signs will usually be limited to some degree of delay in ossification. In determining the significance of alterations in skeletal age, it must be remembered that there is a range of normal variation and a difference according to sex, females maturing more rapidly than males. It is good practice to allow a variation of 3 months, plus or minus, during the first year of life, and up to 1 year at the end of puberty before considering the skeletal age to be abnormal. This will prevent the

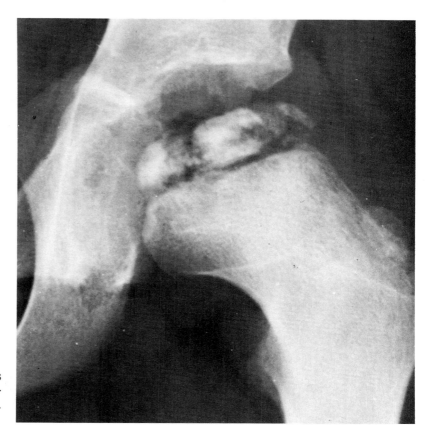

Figure 6–36. Epiphyseal changes in a cretin. The proximal femoral epiphysis arises from multiple centers. The femoral neck is broadened.

unnecessary use of potent preparations in treating children for supposed hormonal deficiency when none exists.

In chronic cases, the metaphyses may appear irregular, somewhat suggestive of rickets. Slipping of the capital femoral epiphyses has been observed. In more severe cases, the roentgenographic findings may be similar to those of cretinism.

HYPERFUNCTION OF THE THYROID GLAND

Hyperthyroidism occurring during childhood will cause some acceleration of skeletal development but is seldom marked, and frequently the skeletal age remains within or close to the normal range. In chronic cases, particularly in older children, there often is generalized demineralization of the skeleton. The loss of bone mineral is directly proportional to the duration of untreated hyperthyroidism.

Thyroid acropachy, a rare manifestation of hyperthyroidism, produces a peculiar periosteal reaction.[11] It usually occurs some years after partial thyroidectomy. The cause is unknown. Clinically there is swelling of the fingers and toes, exophthalmos, and pretibial myxedema. Radiographic examination reveals periosteal new-bone formation involving the metacarpals and phalanges (Fig. 6-37). It may be quite extensive and have a spiculated appearance. It is most intense in the area of greatest soft-tissue swelling.

HYPOFUNCTION OF THE PITUITARY GLAND

Since the pituitary is concerned with bone growth both directly and indirectly through the thyroid gland and the gonads, decreased function of the pituitary gland during childhood leads to generalized disturbance in bone growth and maturation. The epiphyseal centers are slow in appearing and delayed in uniting; at times union may never take place. Since epiphyseal closure is closely related to gonadal function, this is generally considered to be an indication of secondary hypogonadism. The bones do not grow normally in length or breadth so that affected persons are small in stature, usually well proportioned, of normal mentality, but sexually immature. In many patients, there is delay in eruption of the teeth, which tend to become impacted.

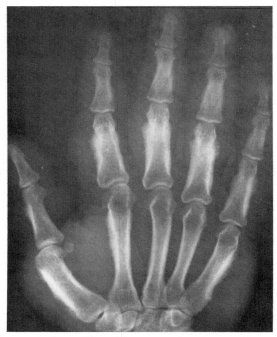

Figure 6–37. Thyroid acropachy, a peculiar periosteal reaction that is slightly lobulated and irregular on its outer margin. The findings are pathognomonic. (Courtesy of Col. Albert Hale, M.D., San Antonio, Texas)

This condition is known as the Lorain's type of pituitary dwarfism.

HYPERFUNCTION OF THE PITUITARY GLAND

Increased secretion by the eosinophilic cells of the anterior lobe of the pituitary gland, either as a result of an adenomatous tumor or from simple hyperplasia, leads to acceleration of bone growth. If this condition develops before growth has ceased, it will result in gigantism. If it begins after adulthood has been reached, it causes acromegaly.

Acromegaly

Increase in length of the bones does not occur in acromegaly if the disease develops after endochondral bone growth has ceased. Certain well-defined skeletal changes do appear, however, and these are characteristic of the disease.

Skull. The characteristic changes of acromegaly in the cranial bones are shown in Figure 6-38. In most patients, some enlargement of the sella turcica is noted, caused by pressure erosion from the eosinophilic adenoma. The increase in sellar size seldom is as pronounced as that caused by chromophobe adenoma of the pituitary. The cranial bones become thickened and of increased density. The diplöe may be obliterated, and the cranial bones have the density and appearance of cortical bone. Hyperostotic thickening, hyperostosis frontalis interna, may develop in the inner table, causing the internal surface of the vault to appear irregular. The nasal accessory sinuses become enlarged and the mastoids overpneumatized. The prognathic jaw, one of the obvious clinical features of acromegaly, can be demonstrated. There may be enlargement of the external occipital protuberance.

Long Bones. The terminal tufts of the distal phalanges enlarge, forming thick bony tufts with pointed lateral margins (Fig. 6-39). These curve proximally and may actually impinge against the phalangeal shafts. Hypertrophy of the soft tissues leading to the typical square, spade-shaped hand can be visualized. In some patients, there is widening of the joint spaces owing to hypertrophy of the articular cartilages. This is best demonstrated in the metacarpophalangeal joints. Degenerative changes in the joints manifested by marginal spurring and sclerosis of articular margins may be seen even in relatively young patients. Measurement of the heel-pad thickness has been used as an indicator of the increase in soft tissues. This distance is measured from the inferior surface of the os calcis to the nearest skin surface. In the normal person, this should not exceed 25 mm.

Spine. The vertebral bodies may actually increase in their anteroposterior diameters, particularly in the thoracic region (Fig. 6-40). "Scalloping" or increased concavity of the posterior aspect of the vertebral bodies occurs in a number of patients and is most prominent in the lumbar spine.

Gigantism

The roentgenographic features of gigantism are essentially those of an excessively large skeleton, because skeletal growth is accelerated; this happens before the epiphyses close. Additionally, there usually are the signs of acromegaly, and if the disease continues to be active after adult life is reached, the acromegalic aspects increase. The sella may or may not enlarge.

HYPOGONADISM

Deficiency of gonadal secretions occurring before skeletal growth has ceased results in delay of epiphyseal closure; therefore, the long bones become elongated and slender. The condition follows surgical removal of

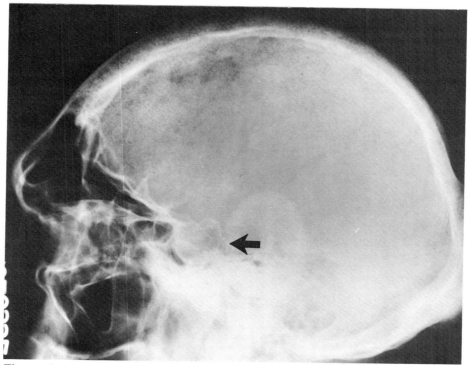

Figure 6–38. Acromegaly. The cranial bones are thickened, and the frontal sinuses are markedly enlarged. The sella turcica is moderately enlarged by an eosinophilic adenoma of the pituitary gland (*arrow*).

the gonads or atrophy from disease and is known as eunuchoidism. Fusion of the epiphyses is delayed.

CHEMICAL POISONING

LEAD POISONING

Lead deposited in the bones of adults produces no recognizable alteration in the roentgenographic appearance of the osseous system. If lead poisoning occurs before endochondral bone growth is completed, however, changes occur that may be of considerable value in arriving at the correct diagnosis. The significant finding is the appearance of dense, transverse bands, "lead lines," extending across the metaphyses of the long bones (Fig. 6-41) and along the margins of the flat bones, such as the iliac crest. The width of the lead line varies, depending upon the amount of lead ingested and the length of time it has been taken. The increased density is not caused by lead alone but also by increased calcium content as the result of a failure of resorption of calcium from the zones of provisional

calcification. Approximately 3 months after inhalation of lead and 6 months after ingestion of lead, the lead line can be observed in growing bone. Except for the development of these transverse zones of density, the bones and epiphyses remain normal. Because ingested lead shot may cause lead poisoning, abdominal films should be obtained as part of the investigation in persons suspected of having lead poisoning. When children have unexplained cerebral symptoms that may be caused by lead, a roentgenogram of the knee is indicated, since nearly all children with lead encephalopathy will demonstrate definite bony lead lines. After the intake of lead has been discontinued, normal bone forms on the epiphyseal side of the metaphysis and the lead line appears to migrate into the shaft, becoming wider and less dense, and gradually disappears. In normal infants, the zone of provisional calcification in the metaphyses of the long bones, particularly the distal femur, often shows an unusual whiteness and appears wider than one might expect. This should not be confused with lead poisoning. The incidence of lead poisoning in infants is low except in children living in the inner core of large cities.

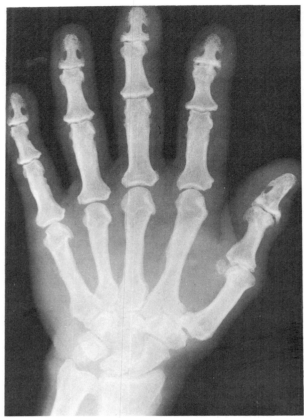

Figure 6–39. Acromegaly. The terminal tufts of the distal phalanges are spadelike, with spurlike bony projections. The soft tissues are thickened, and the joint spaces are slightly widened, best appreciated at the metacarpophalangeal joints.

Lead Arthropathy

Retained lead bullets are generally considered to be chemically inert and of no consequence, providing they are not adjacent to major vascular structures, through which they may erode and embolize to remote sites. However, retained intra-articular bullets are an exception. Bullets bathed in joint fluid gradually dissolve, and the lead is absorbed and initiates a proliferative painful destructive arthropathy.[26] The earliest radiographic finding is a fine punctate deposition of radiopaque lead on the articular cartilage and synovium. This becomes larger, coarser, and more confluent over time (Fig. 6-42). Resorption may be sufficient to cause systemic lead intoxication.[28] Bullets in joints should be removed.

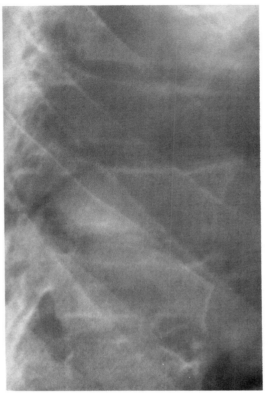

Figure 6–40. Acromegaly. Note the increase in the AP diameter of the vertebral bodies of the lower dorsal spine.

FLUORINE INTOXICATION

Fluorine poisoning is a rare cause of dense bones and is found mainly in adults, either as a result of an occupational exposure to high concentrations of fluorides or from drinking water containing a high concentration of this substance. In the United States, such concentrations occur in the drinking water only in certain parts of Texas. The mining and conversion of phosphate rock into fertilizer and the use of fluorides in the smelting of metals offer possible sources for poisoning. The major alteration in the skeleton is a diffuse increase in density. The trabecular architecture is accentuated, and the cortices become thickened. Coarse sclerosis of the spine and pelvis is usually present. Calcific spurs (entheses) may form at the sites of ligament attachments, and calcification may be observed in the interosseous membrane of the forearm. In spite of rather marked alteration in the bones, those affected are free of symptoms and surprisingly healthy.

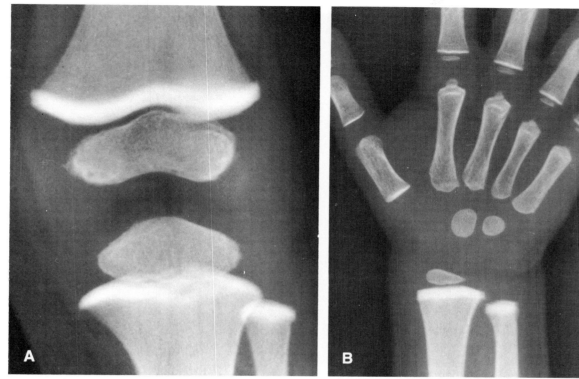

Figure 6–41. Lead poisoning. The dense transverse band of radiodensity within the metaphysis is characteristic of lead poisoning and often referred to as the "lead line." The line is usually more obvious in the knee, as shown in **A**. In **B**, similar densities are seen in the distal radius and ulna and to a lesser extent in the metaphyses of the phalanges.

HYPERVITAMINOSIS D

Excessive intake of vitamin D may lead to changes demonstrable by roentgenographic examination. In adults, hypervitaminosis D is encountered in patients with rheumatoid arthritis treated with large doses of vitamin D. The serum calcium is elevated, and the urine calcium is high. Roentgenographic examination of adults may reveal the following: (1) Deposition of calcium in the soft tissues, particularly around the joints. These deposits have an amorphous puttylike appearance. Calcification of the arteries may be noted, even in the young. Renal calcification often occurs. (2) Osteoporosis is frequent. Since many of these patients have rheumatoid arthritis usually accompanied by osteoporosis, this finding may be difficult to evaluate.

In infancy, hypervitaminosis D usually follows errors in dosage. It results in metastatic calcification in the media of the blood vessels, kidneys, heart, gastric wall, falx cerebri, tentorium, and adrenals. In the tubular bones, there is widening of the zones of provisional calcification, causing dense bands extending across the metaphyses similar to those noted in lead poisoning. Later there may be cortical thickening. Also, in the later stages there may be alternating bands of increased and decreased density crossing the ends of the shafts and an overall osteoporosis.

IDIOPATHIC HYPERCALCEMIA

In idiopathic hypercalcemia, a rare disorder, there is an elevated serum level of calcium, causing an osteosclerosis similar to that noted in some patients with osteopetrosis (marble bone disease) and in infants with hypervitaminosis D. The cause is obscure, but it has been suggested that the disease may represent an unusual sensitivity to vitamin D. The disease has been more prevalent in England than in the United States, and in the past, the amounts of vitamin D supplement in foods were not well regulated in Britain. It has been

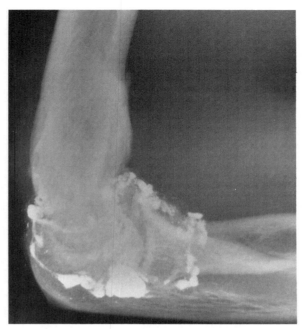

Figure 6–42. Lead arthropathy. This 41-year-old man sustained a gunshot wound to the elbow several years previously, resulting in a fracture of the distal humerus that has subsequently healed. The bullet was left within the joint and has partially dissolved. Coarse, irregular, dense particles of lead line the synovial surfaces of the joint. (Courtesy of Stephan I. Schabel, M.D., Charleston, South Carolina)

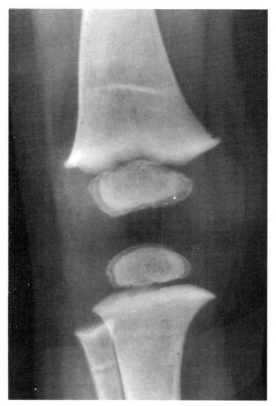

Figure 6–43. Idiopathic hypercalcemia. Note the poorly demarcated dense zones extending across the metaphyses and the "bone-in-bone" appearance of the epiphyses. The changes resemble those of heavy metal poisoning and are similar to those found in hypervitaminosis D.

suggested that some infants may have ingested excessive amounts of the vitamin in food and as a result developed vitamin D poisoning. More recently, stricter controls and limits have been put into effect and the incidence of the disease has decreased considerably. The clinical observations mirror the effects of the hypercalcemia and include muscle weakness and hypotonia, anorexia, vomiting, and failure of the infant to thrive and to develop properly. There is mental as well as physical retardation. The roentgenographic findings (Fig. 6-43) are essentially the same as those found in hypervitaminosis D. The most specific sign in both is the demonstration of calcium in the falx, tentorium, and gastric wall during infancy.

HYPERVITAMINOSIS A

Vitamin A poisoning from excessive administration is seen most frequently in young infants as a result of errors in dosage. Clinical manifestations include anorexia, failure to gain weight, pruritus, pain and swelling over the long bones, and hepatomegaly and spleno-

megaly. The serum alkaline phosphatase may be increased and the serum proteins lowered. The level of vitamin A in the blood serum is high. On roentgenographic examination, one may find linear periosteal new-bone formation, mainly involving the diaphysis of long bones (Fig. 6-44A). The bones most frequently affected are the ulna and clavicle; next in frequency are the femur and tibia. Split sutures may be identified in the skull (Fig. 6-44B).

Hypervitaminosis A must be distinguished chiefly from infantile cortical hyperostosis (see Chapter 5). In this latter disease, the mandible is almost always affected and is usually the first bone to be involved. Both diseases are accompanied by fever and the other signs of infection. Infantile cortical hyperostosis develops early in life, within the first few weeks or months; vitamin A poisoning usually occurs somewhat later, rarely before the child is 1 year old. The final diagnosis

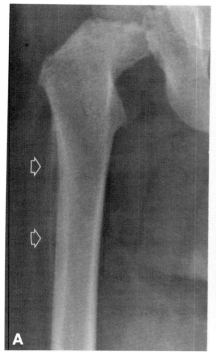

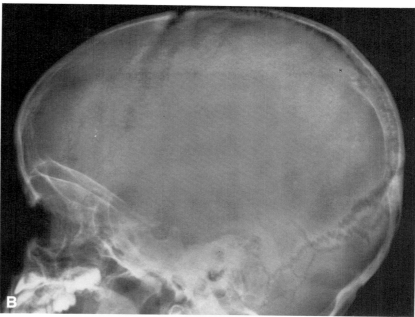

Figure 6–44. Hypervitaminosis A in a 2-year-old boy. (**A**) Periosteal new-bone formation is present along the lateral aspect of the shaft of the proximal femur (*arrows*). Similar findings were present on the opposite side. (**B**) Increased intracranial pressure has resulted in splitting or diastasis of the cranial sutures.

rests upon the history of the administration of excessive amounts of vitamin A and the determination of the level of vitamin A in the serum.

RETINOID HYPEROSTOSIS

Prolonged therapy with retinoid drugs (13-*cis*-retinoic acid, chemically similar to vitamin A) in the treatment of dermatologic disorders such as ichthyosis and cystic acne may result in a skeletal hyperostosis similar to that occurring in DISH.[16] The hyperostoses are often subtle, pointlike, or conical and tend to occur at the corners and promontories of bones, particularly on the anterior margin of the vertebral bodies of the cervical spine. Entheses (spurs) are also reported to occur on the calcaneus.[16]

REFERENCES AND SELECTED READINGS

1. ALARCON GS, SANDERS C, DANIEL WW: Transient osteoporosis of the hip: Magnetic resonance imaging. J Rheumatol 14:1184, 1987

2. BRODELL JD, BURNS JE JR, HEIPLE KG: Transient osteoporosis of the hip of pregnancy. J Bone Joint Surg [Am] 71:1252, 1989

3. ELMSTEDT E: Skeletal complications in the renal transplant recipient. A clinical study. Acta Orthop Scand 52:7, 1981

4. GENANT HK, BLOCK JE, STEIGER P, ET AL: Appropriate use of bone densitometry. Radiology 170:817, 1989

5. GENANT HK, HECK LL, LANZL LH, ET AL: Primary hyperparathyroidism. Radiology 109:513, 1973

6. GENANT HK, KOZIN F, BEKERMAN C, ET AL: The reflex sympathetic dystrophy syndrome: A comprehensive analysis using fine detail radiography, photon absorptiometry and bone and joint scintigraphy. Radiology 117:21, 1975

7. GRIFFIN CN JR: Severe erosive arthritis of large joints in chronic renal failure. Skeletal Radiol 12:29, 1984

8. JONES G: Radiological appearance of disuse osteoporosis. Clin Radiol 20:345, 1969

9. KATAYAMA H, SURUGA K, KURASHIGE T, ET AL: Bone changes in congenital biliary atresia. Radiologic observation of 8 cases. Am J Roentgenol 124:107, 1975

10. KRICUN R, KRICUN ME, ARANGIO GA, ET AL: Patellar tendon rupture with underlying systemic disease. Am J Roentgenol 135:803, 1980

11. McCarthy J, Twersky J, Lion M: Thyroid acropachy. J Can Assoc Radiol 26:199, 1975

12. Milkman LA: Pseudofractures (hunger osteopathy, late rickets, osteomalacia). Am J Roentgenol 24:29, 1930

13. Nilas L, Christiansen C: Bone mass and its relationship to age and the menopause. J Clin Endocrinol Metab 65:697, 1987

14. Nilas L, Podenphant J, Riis BJ, et al: Usefulness of regional bone measurements in patients with osteoporotic fractures of the spine and distal forearm. J Nucl Med 28:960, 1987

15. Orzincolo C, Bedani PL, Scutellari PN, et al: Destructive spondyloarthropathy and radiographic follow-up in hemodialysis patients. Skeletal Radiol 19:483, 1990

16. Pennes DR, Martel W, Ellis CN, et al: Evolution of skeletal hyperostoses caused by 13-cis-retinoic acid therapy. Am J Roentgenol 151:967, 1988

17. Poznanski AK, Kuhns LR, Guire KE: New standards of cortical mass in the humerus of neonates: A means of evaluating bone loss in the premature infant. Radiology 134:639, 1980

18. Resnick D, Niwayama G: (eds): Diagnosis of Bone and Joint Disorders, 3rd ed. Philadelphia, WB Saunders, 1991

19. Richardson ML, Genant HK, Cann CE, et al: Assessment of metabolic bone diseases by quantitative computed tomography. Clin Orthop 195:224, 1985

20. Rogers LF: Skeletal trauma in the elderly: Diagnostic and epidemiologic considerations. Arch Clin Imag 1:122, 1985

21. Rogers LF: Radiology of skeletal trauma, 2nd ed. New York, Churchill-Livingstone, 1992

22. Ross LV, Ross GJ, Mesgarzadeh M, et al: Hemodialysis-related amyloidomas of bone. Radiology 178:263, 1991

23. Ross PD, Davis JW, Vogel JM, et al: A critical review of bone mass and the risk of fractures in osteoporosis. Calcif Tissue Int 46:149, 1990

24. Ruegsegger P, Dambacher MA, Ruegsegger E, et al: Bone loss in premenopausal and postmenopausal women. J Bone Joint Surg [Am] 66:1015, 1984

25. Sambrook PN, Bartless C, Evans R, et al: Measurement of lumbar spine bone mineral: A comparison of dual photon absorptiometry and computed tomography. Br J Radiol 58:621, 1985

26. Sclafani SJA, Vuletin JC, Twersky J: Lead arthropathy: Arthritis caused by retained intra-articular bullets. Radiology 156:299, 1985

27. Smith R: Idiopathic osteoporosis in the young. J Bone Joint Surg [Br] 62:417, 1980

28. Stromberg BV: Symptomatic lead toxicity secondary to retained shotgun pellets: Case report. J Trauma 30:356, 1990

29. Sundaram M: Renal osteodystrophy. Skeletal Radiol 18:415, 1989

Paul and Juhl's Essentials of Radiologic Imaging, Sixth Edition, edited by John H. Juhl and Andrew B. Crummy. J.B. Lippincott Company, Philadelphia, © 1993.

CHAPTER 7

Miscellaneous Conditions

Lee F. Rogers

PAGET'S DISEASE (OSTEITIS DEFORMANS)

Paget's disease is predominantly a disease of Caucasians. It commonly occurs in England, Australia, New Zealand, Scandinavia, Canada, and northern United States but is relatively infrequent in the southern United States and rarely encountered in Asia.[11, 28] The average age of onset is between 50 and 55 years and rarely before the age of 40. It is twice as common in men as women. The cause is unknown.[11, 28]

Paget's disease may involve any bone in the body. It may affect a single bone and never extend to others; it may begin in one bone, with others becoming involved at a later date; and at times, it is widely distributed throughout the skeleton when first discovered. In order of frequency, the following bones are affected: pelvis, vertebrae, femur, skull, tibia, clavicle, humerus, ribs, and rarely the sternum, calcaneus, talus, phalanges, metastarsals, mandible, patella, and other sesamoid bones.[28]

Only 20% of patients are symptomatic, usually complaining of ill-defined pain at the site of involvement. Most cases are discovered incidentally at the time of a radiographic examination of the abdomen or a bone scan obtained to evaluate the possibility of metastatic disease. Characteristically there is elevation of the serum alkaline phosphatase, which may be elevated as much as 15 to 20 times normal. The serum calcium and phosphorus are usually normal; however, calcium may be markedly elevated in patients with Paget's disease who are immobilized. Renal calculi or nephrocalcinosis may develop from hypercalciuria under these conditions.

Pathologically, Paget's disease is characterized by destruction of bone (lysis) followed by attempts at repair. There is usually a combination of destruction and repair, but the destructive phase may predominate at some sites.

Roentgenographic Features. The radiographic appearance is dependent on the phase of the disease: lytic, reparative, or mixed. The principal radiographic findings are thickening of the cortex, coarsening of trabeculae, enlargement of bone, areas of lucency, patches of dense bone described as "cotton wool" or "cotton ball," and evidence of bone softening. In the long bone, the process almost always involves the end of the bone extending into the diaphysis. In the pelvis, it usually involves some portion of the acetabulum. Healing of the lytic phase has been described as a result of treatment with diphosphonates and calcitonin.[8, 10]

Pagetic bone takes up all radionuclide bone scanning agents avidly—in fact, more intensely than any other process. The diagnosis of Paget's disease can be made on the basis of a bone scan because of this intense activity and the pattern of bone involvement—involvement of the end of the bone with variable extension into the shaft and often evidence of softening manifested by bowing of long bones and flattening of vertebrae (Fig. 7-1).

Computed tomography (Figs. 7-3, 7-7B), mirrors the findings on plain film radiography in Paget's disease expansion; cortical thickening, coarsening of the trabeculae, and focal sclerotic densities in intramedullary bone, the equivalent of "cotton balls." The osteolytic phase demonstrates considerable thinning of the cortex of long bones and tables of the skull.[14]

MRI displays similar osseous changes as low signals

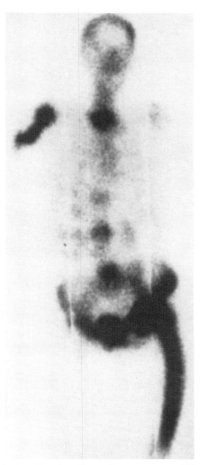

Figure 7–1. Technetium bone scan of Paget's disease involving the proximal right humerus, left femur, pelvis, several vertebral bodies, and skull. Note the intense activity, lateral bowing of the femur, and involvement of the ends of long bones, with variable extension into the shaft.

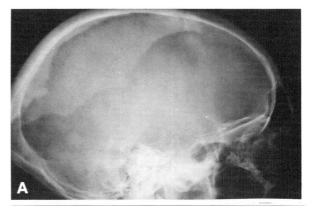

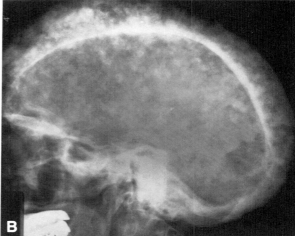

Figure 7–2. Paget's disease of the skull. (**A**) Osteoporosis circumscripta manifested by a large area of radiolucency sharply demarcated from the normal bone above it. (**B**) Far-advanced Paget's disease of the skull. Note the thickening of the skull and the interspersed areas of lucency and radiodensity, the cotton-wool or cotton-ball appearance. In this case, the process also involves the base of the skull and is associated with basilar impression. The base of the skull is flattened, platybasia, and the dens projects a well above both Chamberlain's and MacGregor's line. MacGregor's line is drawn from the posterior tip of the hard palate to the inferior cortex of the occipital bone. Chamberlain's line is drawn from the hard palate to the anterior margin of the foramen magnum.

on both T1- and T2-weighted images.[31] The marrow signal in the intramedullary and diploic spaces is variable with high signal foci of fat seen on T1 (Fig. 7-9) and high signal foci of fibrovascular marrow on T2-weighted images.

Both CT and MRI are useful in the analysis of the complications of Paget's disease; i.e., spinal cord or neural compression, basilar invagination, and sarcomatous degeneration. However, it is more likely that Paget's disease will be encountered unexpectedly as an incidental finding when these techniques are used to evaluate for other diseases. Plain film correlation is advisable to avoid confusion.

Skull. The classic expression of the lytic phase of Paget's disease in the skull is known as *osteoporosis circumscripta* (Fig. 7-2A). This is a sharply demarcated area of radiolucency within which the architecture of the bone is poorly defined. The lesion usually involves the frontal or parietal bones and may enlarge slowly.

Characteristically, the junction between the lucent and normal bone is very sharp. When repair begins, islands or patches of sclerosis appear, resembling cotton wool or cotton balls. The bones of the vault become thickened, usually only outward, and may measure 3 cm or more in thickness (Figs. 7-2*B* and 7-3). The outer edge of the lesion is better seen with a bright light. The base of the skull may be involved, and there may be basilar invagination (Fig. 7-2*B*) in which the cranium settles over the cervical spine and the craniovertebral junction protrudes into the base of the skull as a result of bone softening.

Long Bones. In long bones, Paget's disease almost invariably extends to and involves the subarticular bone immediately adjacent to the joint (Figs. 7-4 and 7-5). The length of involvement is variable, but in some cases the entire bone is involved. The cortex is thick-

ened, and the overall width of the bone is increased in diameter. The intramedullary cavity is maintained. The trabeculae are coarse and thickened and therefore radiographically prominent but remain in the same direction and relative position as they would in normal bone. Between the coarsened trabeculae, cystlike radiolucencies are often identified. The thickened cortex suggests increased strength, but actually the bone is

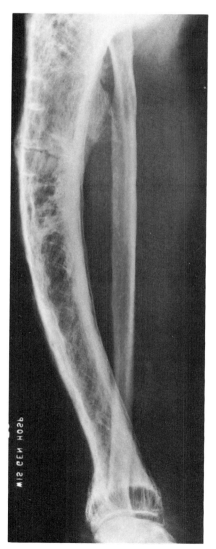

Figure 7–4. Paget's disease of the tibia showing anterior bowing, irregular thickening of the cortex, coarse trabecular pattern, and a number of linear horizontal radiolucencies in the anterior cortex, indicative of pseudofractures.

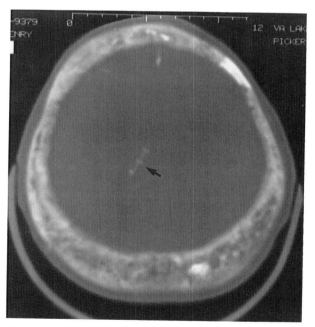

Figure 7–3. CT examination of Paget's disease of the skull in a case with plain films similar to Fig. 7-2*B*. The skull is markedly increased in thickness with a coarsened and thickened inner and outer table, and widened diploic space. A coarsened trabecular pattern in the diploic space and small foci of increased density (white arrow) give rise to the "cotton wool" appearance of the skull. The foci of sclerosis alternate with foci of lucency within the diploic space. A ventriculo-peritoneal shunt (*arrow*) was necessitated by platybasia leading to hydrocephalus.

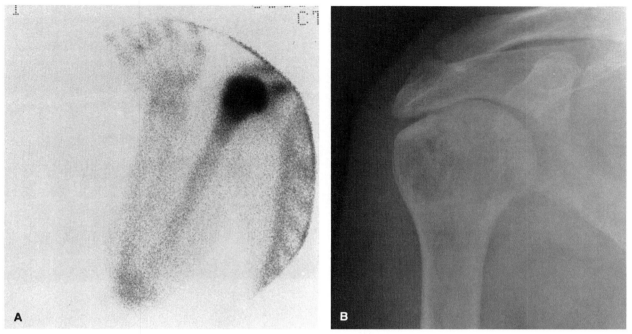

Figure 7–5. Paget's disease of the proximal humerus. **(A)** Technetium-99m bone scan demonstrates markedly increased homogeneous radioactivity in the humeral head and neck. The intense activity is indicative of Paget's disease. **(B)** AP view of the humerus confirms the presence of Paget's disease. Note the increased thickness of the articular cortex and coarsening of the trabecular pattern within the humeral head. A faint radiolucency extends beyond the humeral neck into the proximal shaft consistent with lytic phase of Paget's disease.

weakened as manifested by bowing of long bones, more pronounced in the lower than the upper extremities. Characteristically, the femur bows outward and the tibia anteriorly.

The osteolytic phase is less commonly encountered in long bones than is the mixed form described above. Inactivity such as bed rest or immobilization tends to accentuate bone destruction. The osteolytic phase is characterized by a clearly demarcated zone of radiolucency extending a variable distance into the diaphysis from the end of the bone. The process is often referred to as a "blade of grass" (Fig 7-6), because the lucency is elongated and involves only a segment of the cortex, the periphery of the lesion is clearly demarcated, and its distal margin is flame shaped or V-shaped and thus resembles a blade of grass.

Pathologic fractures are common and are characteristically transverse rather than oblique or spiral as in normal bone. These have been referred to as "banana fractures." Incomplete, transverse radiolucent fissures called pseudofractures are common in the cortex along the convex side of severely involved bowed bones (Fig. 7-4). They are often multiple. Pathologic fractures may be initiated at the site of a pseudofracture.

Pelvis. The most common expression of Paget's disease in the pelvis is thickening of the cortex, best appreciated in the pubic bones, and coarsening of the trabecular pattern, most easily recognized around the acetabulum and the margins of the sacroiliac joint (Fig. 7-7). Cystlike radiolucent spaces may be encountered. Larger areas of radiolucency are common in the central portion of the iliac bones. The sacrum may be the first or the only bone involved, manifested by a thickening of the cortex, best appreciated in the sacral foraminal lines. Coarse trabeculation causes a distinctive crosshatch pattern in the body of the sacrum. Less commonly, variable-sized patches of sclerosis may occur. These may resemble osteoblastic metastasis, but careful observation will usually reveal that they are associated with typical coarse trabeculation and thickening of the cortex not encountered in metastasis (Fig. 7-7).

When the pelvis and femur are both involved, there may be characteristic changes in the hip, manifested by concentric or medial narrowing of the hip joint unlike the superior narrowing commonly observed in osteoarthritis.[7] Hypertrophic spurring is common in Paget's disease of the hip.

Spine. The disease usually affects multiple vertebrae, occasionally is solitary, but rarely is universal. Involvement of the vertebral body is prominent, but closer examination will usually disclose involvement of the posterior elements, the laminae, pedicles, and transverse and spinous processes. The principal pattern of involvement is thickening of the cortex, which gives a broadened and somewhat smudged appearance. On the lateral view, due to the cortical thickening the vertebral bodies appear to be framed, the so-called "picture frame" vertebrae (Figs. 7-8 and 7-9). Similar changes can be seen within the pedicles and spinous process and occasionally the transverse process on the frontal view. The trabeculae within the vertebral body are coarsened. Occasionally the vertebrae are diffusely dense, with coarse trabeculae in a pattern similar to that seen in small bones of the hands and feet. The overall size of the vertebrae is increased, and softening results in compression. The vertebral bodies then appear flattened and slightly expanded. Expansion of pagetic bone may compromise the spinal canal, leading to spinal cord compression and neurologic symptoms.[2]

Flat Bones. In the ribs and clavicle, the bones are thickened and there is a general increase in density across their entire width. The trabecular pattern is typically coarsened. One or more ribs may be involved. The lesion will always extend to one or the other end of the bone.

Small Bones. Involvement of the small bones of the hands and feet is uncommon and almost invariably involves the entire bone. There are two principal patterns. In the calcaneus, prominent thickened trabeculae and thickening of the cortex occur, whereas in the phalanges, metacarpals, and metatarsals, the entire bone is enlarged and diffusely increased in density, and the trabecular pattern coarsened.

Complications. The most common complication is a fracture that is characteristically transverse and often initiated at the site of a pseudofracture (see Fig. 7-4).

Spinal cord compression may occur from expansion of the vertebral bodies.[2] Extramedullary hematopoiesis has been described, presenting as a mass adjacent to involved vertebral bodies and may lead to spinal cord compression.[29] Spinal epidural hematoma has also

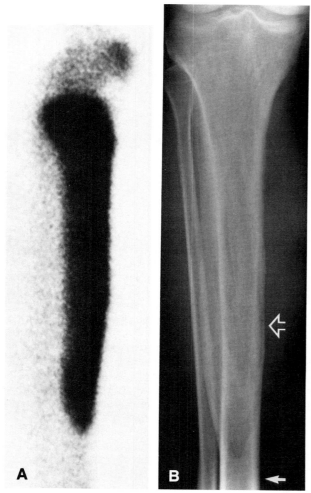

Figure 7–6. Lytic Paget's disease of the tibia. **(A)** Lateral view of bone scan demonstrates intense activity involving the entire proximal tibia with a flame-shaped distal margin. **(B)** An AP radiograph demonstrates expansion and lysis of the proximal tibia, with thinning of the cortex. The process ends distally with a characteristic flame shape beyond which there is a normal bone. Compare the character of the cortex of the normal bone (*closed arrow*) with that of the cortex in the lytic area (*open arrow*). This elongated lytic process with the characteristic pointed distal margin has led to the designation "blade-of-grass" appearance.

Often this can be done simply by comparison with the opposite side, but when both sides are involved, this is a greater problem. Because of bone softening, there may be intrapelvic protrusion of the acetabulum, termed *acetabuli protrusio.*

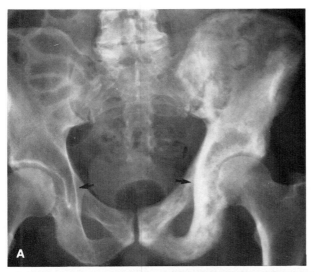

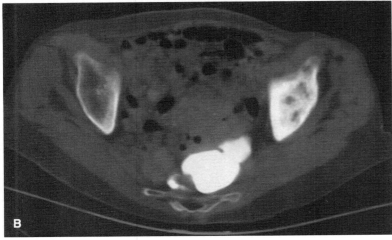

Figure 7–7. (**A**) Paget's disease of the left hemipelvis manifested by cortical thickening, coarse trabeculation, and expansion of bone. There are also several small radiolucencies, particularly within the pubic rami. The thickening of the cortex is best appreciated by comparing the cortex on the two sides—for instance, note the widening of the ilioischial line (*arrows*). (**B**) CT of the pelvis. Examination just above the acetabulum demonstrates the marked cortical thickening of the iliac bone with coarsening of the trabecular pattern and several lucent foci within the medullary cavity. Compare with the opposite side. The findings are typical of Paget's disease. Residual contrast is present within the rectum.

been reported in association with Paget's disease of the spine.[18]

Expansion of bone at the base of the skull may reduce the size of neural foramen and canals, leading to neurologic deficits such as deafness.

Heart failure is considered by many to be a complication and is thought to be caused by the arteriovenous fistulae within the involved bone. However, it is argued that most patients are older and their congestive heart failure is primarily related to concomitant arteriosclerosis. Arteriovenous shunting in pagetic bone is rarely responsible for cardiac failure.

Primary malignant tumors may develop in areas of pagetic bone.[12, 23] Sarcomatous degeneration leads to osteogenic sarcoma in most cases (Fig. 7-10) and less commonly to fibrosarcoma. The incidence is approx-

imately 1%. Nevertheless, Paget's disease accounts for most primary osteogenic sarcomas after the age of 50. Giant cell tumors have also been reported. Tumors are more frequent in the pelvis and long bones and occur rarely in the vertebrae. The most common manifestation is an area of poorly defined destruction, with destruction of the overlying cortex and an associated soft-tissue mass. Periosteal reaction is infrequent. Fibrosarcomas are lytic, and osteosarcomas will contain patches of sclerotic, blastic bone formation, particularly in the pelvis. Metastatic disease also occurs in the pagetic bone and cannot be differentiated from lytic primary tumors. Pathologic fractures are frequent complications of malignancy, and every pathologic fracture appearing in pagetic bone should be viewed suspiciously for evidence of an associated unsuspected malignancy.

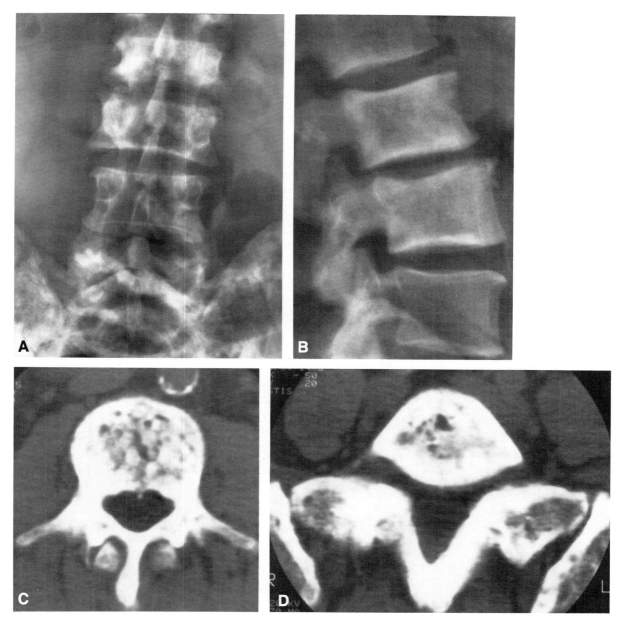

Figure 7–8. Paget's disease of the spine. (**A**) Anteroposterior view. (**B**) Lateral view. The fourth lumbar vertebra is normal. Note the cortical thickening and expansion of the involved vertebrae. Compare the thickness of the end-plates, cortical margins of the pedicles, and spinous process of the fourth lumbar vertebra with the corresponding portions of the involved vertebrae. (**C**) CT of the third lumbar vertebra. (**D**) CT of the fifth lumbar vertebral body and adjacent portions of the sacrum. Characteristic pattern of Paget's disease manifested by thickening of the cortex and coarse trabecular pattern interspersed with radiolucencies.

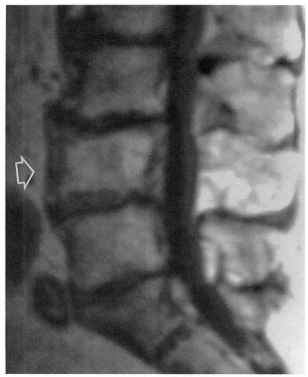

Figure 7–9. MRI of Paget's disease of the fourth lumbar vertebral body. The T1-weighted image demonstrates expansion of the fourth lumbar vertebral body (*arrow*). Note the intermediate signal of the thickened cortical bone that gives the "picture frame" appearance. The signal from the medullary bone is slightly increased, particularly posteriorly in keeping with the findings in Paget's disease.

HISTIOCYTOSIS X (RETICULOENDOTHELIOSIS)

The term *histiocytosis X* is the general designation for three conditions that range from the usually solitary, curable eosinophilic granuloma through the disseminated process of Hand–Schüller–Christian disease, to the fulminating and rapidly fatal variety known as Letterer–Siwe disease. The clinical presentations of the three syndromes are distinctive, but they share common microscopic features that cannot be distinguished histologically by pathologists.

In Letterer–Siwe disease, lesions are widely disseminated throughout the body. It is a disease of infants and young children, who present with splenomegaly, hepatomegaly, generalized lymphadenopathy, a tendency to hemorrhage, and a secondary anemia.

The course is rapid, and death occurs so early that radiographic changes often are not present, although the bone marrow may be extensively involved.

Hand–Schüller–Christian disease is a more benign process characterized by destructive lesions of the skull. It usually develops during childhood and may present with a classic triad of diabetes insipidus, exophthalmos, and lesions of the skull. However, presentation of the classic triad occurs in a distinct minority of cases, usually before the age of 5 years. The clinical course may extend over a period of years. The flat bones are most frequently involved—the skull, pelvis, scapula, ribs, and mandible—and less commonly, the long bones.

Eosinophilic granuloma is the most benign of these conditions, usually occurring as a solitary process in childhood or young adults. Lesions may respond well to curettage, steroid injection, or irradiation. Spontaneous regression may occur. It is widely distributed throughout the skeleton but is most frequent in the skull, pelvis, femur, and ribs. Lesions are infrequent below the knee and elbow.

Roentgenographic Features. Letterer–Siwe disease, although disseminated, rarely shows evidence of radiographic findings. The radiographic findings in Hand–Schüller–Christian disease and eosinophilic granuloma are essentially the same and differ only in the number of lesions. Eosinophilic granuloma is more likely to be solitary and occur in later childhood, adolescence, or early adult life. Hand–Schüller–Christian disease, on the other hand, occurs during childhood, and multiple lesions are usually present.

In general, bone scanning is not as sensitive as radiography in the evaluation of the histiocytosis.[24] Only 50% or less of lesions may be disclosed by scintigraphy, and therefore radiographic skeletal surveys must be performed for the discovery of additional lesions.

Skull. There are solitary or multiple areas of bone destruction. The edges of the individual lesions are sharply defined, punched-out areas that are slightly scalloped or irregular but have no boundary zone of sclerosis. The lack of a sclerotic boundary is characteristic (Fig. 7-11). Characteristically, the lesion originates in the diplöe and involves one or both tables, causing a sharply outlined and slightly irregular translucent defect. The lesion has a beveled edge, caused by unequal destruction of the inner and outer tables. Rarely, a small fragment of bone remains within the radiolucency, resembling a sequestrum. In Hand–Schüller–Christian disease, the lesions may become very large and maplike (Fig. 7-11A). The lesions of eosinophilic granuloma tend to be smaller, on the order of 1 cm to 2 cm.

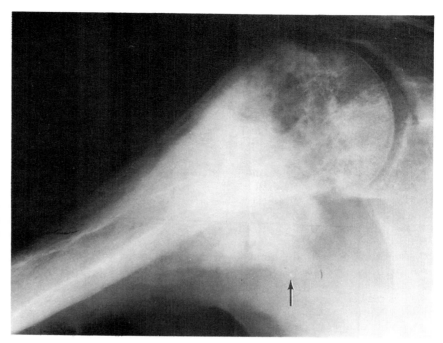

Figure 7–10. Osteosarcoma developing in a patient with Paget's disease of the humerus. Note the thickened cortex of the proximal humerus, indicative of Paget's disease. The tumor is largely sclerotic, with the tumor extending into the soft tissues (*arrow*). The homogeneous quality of the density indicates osteoid matrix.

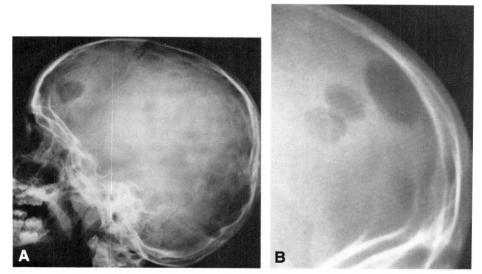

Figure 7–11. (**A**) Hand–Schüller–Christian disease. The lateral radiograph of the skull of a child reveals a large area of radiolucency in the posterior inferior parietal area. The margins of the lesion are scalloped and sharply defined without reactive sclerosis. (**B**) Three lytic foci are present in the frontal bone. They are sharply defined, with a beveled edge due to unequal involvement of the inner and outer table.

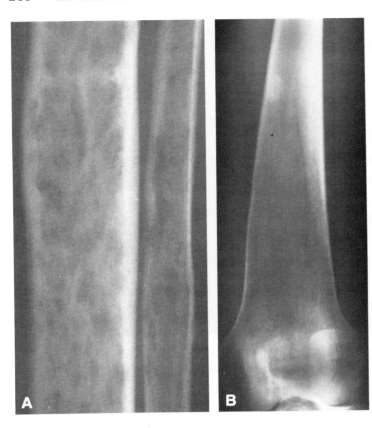

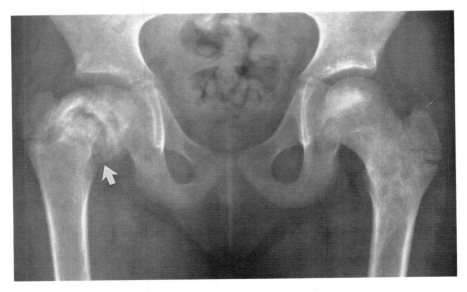

Figure 7–15. Gaucher's disease. (**A**) Patchy areas of bone destruction with endosteal scalloping are present in the midtibia and fibula. (**B**) A typical Erlenmeyer flask deformity of the distal femur. The deformity was caused by a lack of constriction of the metaphysis due to infiltration of the marrow by histiocytic cells of Gaucher's disease.

Figure 7–16. Gaucher's disease of the proximal femurs in an 8-year-old girl. Note the pathologic fracture of the right femoral neck (*arrow*). The medial portion of the proximal femoral epiphysis on the left is sclerotic in keeping with an avascular necrosis. There is a coarse swirled pattern of trabeculi in the intertrochanteric region of the left femur, consistent with the presence of Gaucher's deposits within the intramedullary space.

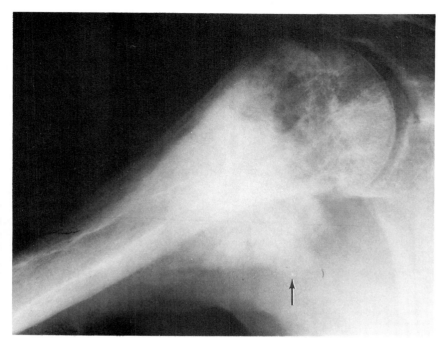

Figure 7–10. Osteosarcoma developing in a patient with Paget's disease of the humerus. Note the thickened cortex of the proximal humerus, indicative of Paget's disease. The tumor is largely sclerotic, with the tumor extending into the soft tissues (*arrow*). The homogeneous quality of the density indicates osteoid matrix.

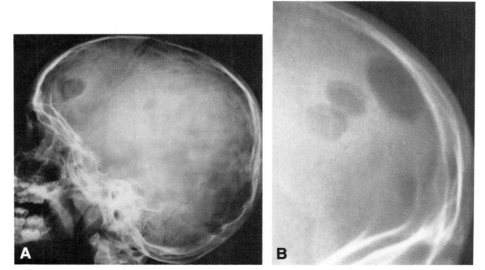

Figure 7–11. (**A**) Hand–Schüller–Christian disease. The lateral radiograph of the skull of a child reveals a large area of radiolucency in the posterior inferior parietal area. The margins of the lesion are scalloped and sharply defined without reactive sclerosis. (**B**) Three lytic foci are present in the frontal bone. They are sharply defined, with a beveled edge due to unequal involvement of the inner and outer table.

In the mandible, the lesions of histiocytosis cause destruction of bone without sclerotic reaction. The bone may completely disappear around one or more of the teeth, causing them to appear as if they were floating (Fig. 7-12). This is quite characteristic of histiocytosis.

Patients may present with draining ears secondary to histiocytosis within the mastoids. Radiographic examination will disclose a radiolucent focus of bone destruction within the temporal bone.

Flat Bones. In the pelvis and scapula, the lesions appear as radiolucent areas that may be bound by a rim of sclerosis. In the ribs, the lesions are often expansile and may have surrounding periosteal reaction.

Spine. Histiocytosis X causes extensive destruction of the vertebral body, leading to a uniform total collapse so that the body is thin and wafer like, often referred to as *vertebra plana* (Fig. 7-13). Perivertebral soft-tissue masses may be identified in association with vertebral lesions. Vertebra plana in an adult should suggest the possibility of multiple myeloma, Gaucher's disease, or Paget's disease.

Long Bones. In the long tubular bones, the appearance of histiocytosis is somewhat different from that

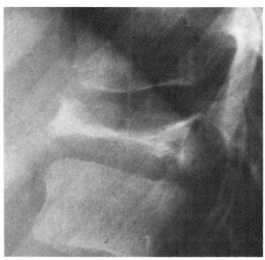

Figure 7–13. Eosinophilic granuloma of a vertebral body. The vertebra is markedly compressed and wafer like. This is termed *vertebra plana.*

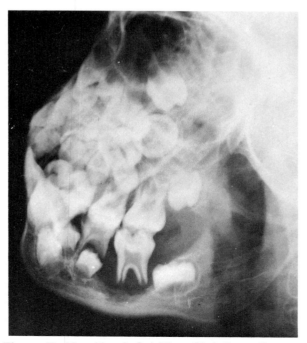

Figure 7–12. Hand–Schüller–Christian disease. A lytic lesion in the left mandible surrounds a tooth, the so-called "floating" tooth.

of the skull and is similar to that in flat bones. An area of bone destruction is noted any place along the length of the bone. It usually arises centrally but may be eccentric. The lesions may destroy or expand the cortex, and overlying periosteal new-bone formation is usually present (Fig. 7-14). The periosteal reaction is usually compact but may be laminated in younger children. At times, in young children, the lesion may have no visible outer or peripheral margin. Compact periosteal reaction is typical of histiocytosis X but is also noted in chronic infections. In younger children, the lesions may suggest Ewing's tumor, but the geographic area of bone destruction and the compact nature of the periosteal reaction are more in keeping with histiocytosis.

GAUCHER'S AND NIEMANN–PICK DISEASE

Gaucher's disease is not a tumor but a metabolic disorder characterized by the abnormal deposition of cerebrosides in the reticuloendothelial cells of the spleen, liver, and bone marrow. These develop a characteristic histologic appearance and are known as Gaucher's cells. A very large spleen and a moderately enlarged liver are clinical features of this disease, and roentgenographic evidence, particularly of the splenomegaly, will be present.

There is a wide spectrum of radiographic findings in Gaucher's disease.[25] Infiltration of the bone marrow

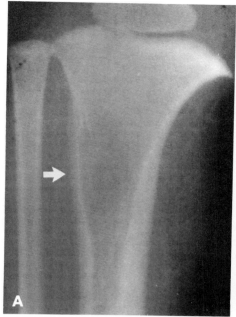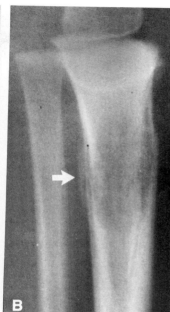

Figure 7–14. Histiocytosis X in the tibia. **(A)** Anteroposterior view. **(B)** Lateral view. A fairly well-defined radiolucent lesion is present in the medullary bone, with expansion of the overlying cortex (*arrow*). On the lateral view, periosteal new-bone formation is present posteriorly (*arrow*).

by these cells may lead to patchy areas of cortical destruction similar to myeloma. In some cases, there is only a rather generalized demineralization (Fig. 7-15A). If the disease has existed for some time, expansion of the lower end of the femur may occur, resulting in the "Erlenmeyer flask" appearance (Fig. 7-15B). This is suggestive but not diagnostic of Gaucher's disease.

Involvement of the vertebrae may lead to collapse of one or more vertebral bodies, which on occasion may be markedly compressed, thin, and waferlike as in vertebra plana. In the long bones, there may be numerous sharply circumscribed osteolytic defects resembling to some extent the lesions of metastatic carcinoma or multiple myeloma. The cortex is thinned and scalloped internally, and there may be periosteal new-bone formation over the involved area. Pathologic fractures of the femoral neck may occur (Fig. 7-16). Occasionally, sclerotic areas are present. The skull and bones of the hands and feet are rarely affected.

Infiltration of the bone marrow may compress and compromise the arterial supply to the end of a long bone, resulting in avascular necrosis. This is most commonly encountered in the head of the femur (Fig. 7-16) and humerus. The radiographic features of avascular necrosis are described below. The extent of bone marrow involvement may be assessed by technetium[99m] sulfur colloid (^{99m}Tc SC) bone marrow scanning.[13]

Niemann–Pick disease is apparently a very rare variant of Gaucher's disease occurring in families of whom about 50% are Jewish. It, too, is a form of lipid reticulosis, the lipid at fault being syringomyelin. The effect on the bones is similar to that of Gaucher's disease, but it occurs in infants (under 18 months of age) and is usually fatal within a year of onset.

HYPERLIPOPROTEINEMIAS

Primary familial hyperlipoproteinemias are a group of heritable diseases associated with an increase in plasma concentrations of cholesterol or triglycerides.[29] They are subdivided into five major types, I through V, according to the plasma lipoprotein pattern.

Xanthomas may be apparent in all five types. Localized deposits occur in the tendons of the palm and dorsum of the hand, patellar tendon, Achilles tendon, plantar aponeurosis, peroneal tendons, around the elbow, and the fascia and periosteum overlying the lower tibia. Tendinous xanthomas produce nodular masses in tendons (Fig. 7-17) that are characteristic of this disorder. They rarely calcify. Subperiosteal xanthomas are associated with scalloping of the external cortical surface. Intramedullary lipid depositions are well defined with sharp zones of transition between abnormal and normal bone. In the hands and feet, they may have a symmetric distribution.

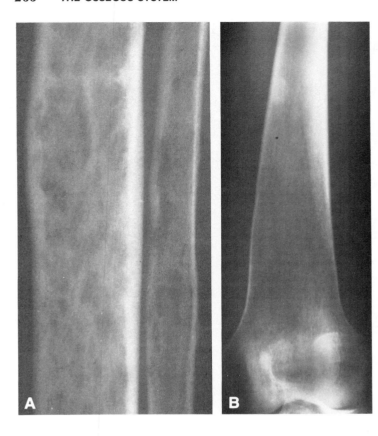

Figure 7–15. Gaucher's disease. (**A**) Patchy areas of bone destruction with endosteal scalloping are present in the midtibia and fibula. (**B**) A typical Erlenmeyer flask deformity of the distal femur. The deformity was caused by a lack of constriction of the metaphysis due to infiltration of the marrow by histiocytic cells of Gaucher's disease.

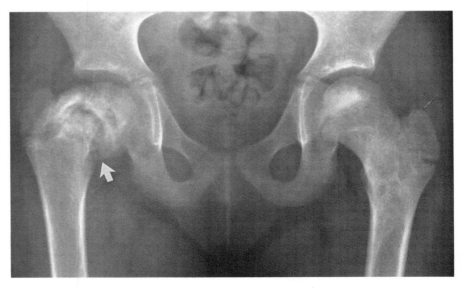

Figure 7–16. Gaucher's disease of the proximal femurs in an 8-year-old girl. Note the pathologic fracture of the right femoral neck (*arrow*). The medial portion of the proximal femoral epiphysis on the left is sclerotic in keeping with an avascular necrosis. There is a coarse swirled pattern of trabeculi in the intertrochanteric region of the left femur, consistent with the presence of Gaucher's deposits within the intramedullary space.

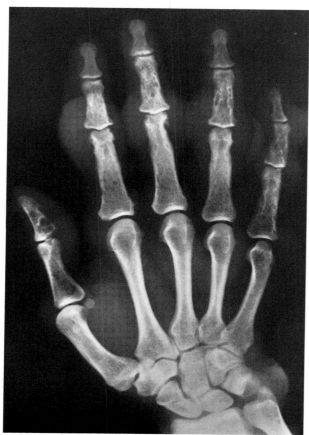

Figure 7–17. This is a Type II hyperlipoproteinemia. Note the multiple, asymmetrical, noncalcified soft tissue nodules of the digits. Within the phalanges are multiple small sharply defined radiolucencies. The intramedullary space of the middle phalanges is lacelike and slightly expanded. The opposite hand was similarly affected.

AMYLOIDOSIS

Bone lesions are occasionally found in primary amyloidosis. The upper part of the humerus and the proximal femur are the most frequent sites. Amyloid lesions may occur in two forms. In the first type, large deposits of amyloid may occur in and around the major joints; these are visualized roentgenographically as soft-tissue swellings. The masses may invade contiguous bones, causing multiple small erosions. In the second form, there is diffuse infiltration of the marrow, causing generalized demineralization with collapse of vertebral bodies, resembling multiple myeloma or other diseases causing diffuse demineralization, or there may be more localized areas of bone lysis.

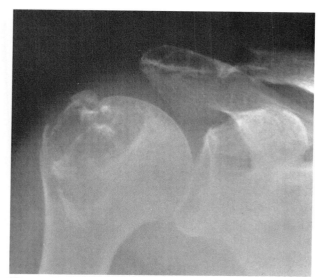

Figure 7–18. Amyloidosis of the shoulder. Note the large erosion on the lateral margin of the humeral head and greater tuberosity bordered medially by a coarse rim of sclerosis. (Case courtesy of Theodore E. Keats, M.D., Charlottesville, Virginia).

The most characteristic findings are soft-tissue masses around the shoulder and hip, with erosion of the adjacent bone (Fig. 7-18). The lesions are caused by replacement of bone by large deposits of amyloid, and they appear roentgenographically as well-demarcated areas of destruction.

AVASCULAR NECROSIS AND BONE INFARCTION

Trauma, several generalized diseases, and steroids are often associated with avascular necrosis of the ends of bone. Bone infarction involves the shafts, usually in areas of the metadiaphysis. Certain diseases such as caisson disease and sickle cell anemia are associated with both avascular necrosis and bone infarction. However, in most diseases the vascular disturbance is either avascular necrosis of the end of bone or bone infarction of the shaft.

AVASCULAR NECROSIS (ISCHEMIC NECROSIS OR OSTEONECROSIS)

Ischemic necrosis of the ends of bone in adults is relatively common. The heads of the femur and proximal humerus are most frequently involved. In trauma, ischemic necrosis is limited to one site, but multiple sites are frequently encountered as a result of systemic disease. The principal causes of ischemic necrosis are as follows:

1. Acute trauma (fracture or dislocation)
2. Steroid therapy
3. Alcoholism
4. Pancreatitis
5. Sickle cell anemia
6. Cushing's disease
7. Collagen vascular disease (particularly systemic lupus erythematosus)
8. Caisson disease
9. Gaucher's disease
10. Radiation therapy

The pathogenesis of ischemic necrosis involves a loss of blood supply.[29] Traumatic disruption occurs in association with the fracture or dislocation of the joint. In sickle cell anemia, thrombosis is considered to be the cause. In Gaucher's disease, the medullary spaces are filled with Gaucher's cells, leading to vascular compression and occlusion. In other entities, the mechanism of vascular compromise has not been clarified.

Roentgenographic Features. Pathologically, avascular necrosis consists of two principal stages, (1) vascular occlusion with cell death and (2) subsequent revascularization and repair of the involved bone. The radiographic findings reflect the pathologic changes. The earliest sign of avascular necrosis of the femoral head is the appearance of a thin, radiolucent line just beneath the articular cortex. This is called the "crescent sign" (see Figs. 7-21 and 7-25). In the femur, it is often best visualized in the frog-leg projection of the hip and may be seen in this projection when it is not apparent on the anteroposterior view. Following this, there is usually a collapse and loss of volume, with impaction of bone leading to an increased radiodensity (Figs. 7-19 and 7-20). The combination of repair and impaction causes bone sclerosis. These may be intermixed with smaller areas of radiolucency. Less commonly there may be a diffuse, homogeneous increase in density that represents deposition of reparative bone. This is seen without the crescent sign or collapse and is referred to as "snowcapping." Snowcapping is more commonly seen in the head of the humerus (see Figs. 7-21). The radiographic findings are similar, irrespective of the etiology.

The bone scan is more sensitive than the radiograph to the changes of ischemic necrosis and plays an important role in the evaluation of ischemic or avascular necrosis. Technetium-99m methyldiphosphonate (^{99m}Tc-MDP) is the agent of choice. In the initial stages of infarction, the area of involvement will be devoid of radioactivity (see Fig. 7-27). Later this area of decreased activity may be rimmed by a zone of increased activity as a result of the reparative process.

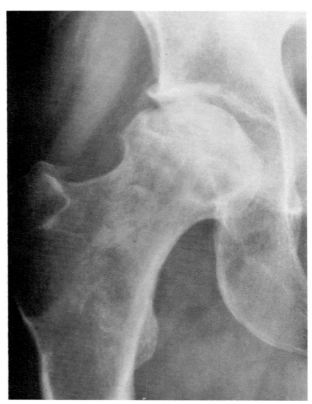

Figure 7–19. Ischemic necrosis of the femoral head in an adult. There is a loss of volume of the femoral head, with impaction of the articular surface. The head shows patches of increased density interspersed with areas of radiolucency. The distal margin of the lesion is demarcated by a zone of sclerotic bone.

MR imaging may even be more sensitive than the bone scan[3, 22] (Fig. 7-22). Infarction at the end of the bone causes changes in the fatty marrow, sharply reducing the normal T1 signal from the marrow. Thus, in T1-weighted images, the normal intense signal of the marrow fat is noticeably decreased and becomes gray to black on the image. The area of decreased signal tends to extend into the metaphysis. The border of the infarct is often sharply demarcated by a rim of low signal, the "ring sign," representing the margin of revascularization and new bone formation at the periphery of the infarction (Figs. 7-22B and 7-24B).[22]

Trauma

Following acute injury, there may be sufficient disruption of the blood supply to result in avascular necrosis of one or more of the fragments. This most commonly

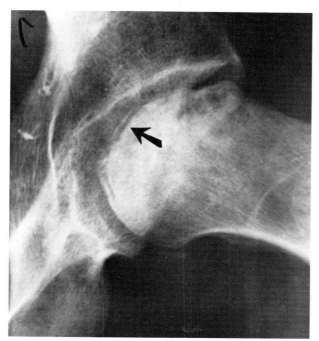

Figure 7–20. Ischemic necrosis of the femoral head of the femur after steroid therapy. Note the thin, lucent crescent separating the thin fragment of subchondral bone (*arrow*), the "crescent sign" of ischemic necrosis. The head is flattened and sclerotic and contains a few areas of radiolucency. The joint space and acetabulum are not involved.

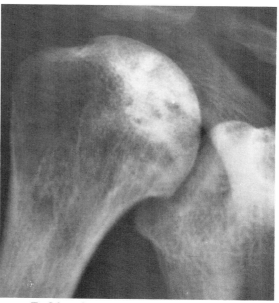

Figure 7–21. Avascular necrosis of the humeral head in sickle cell disease. The homogeneous increased density of the humeral head is sometimes referred to as "snowcapping."

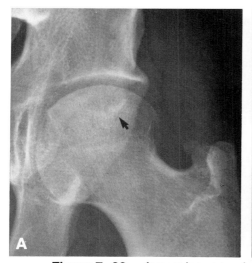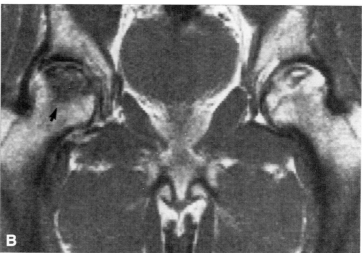

Figure 7–22. Avascular necrosis of the femoral head in sickle cell trait. (**A**) A fine-detail magnification view demonstrates no definite evidence of abnormality, with the exception of a suggestion of a short band of sclerosis (*arrow*). (**B**) MRI demonstrates bilateral avascular necrosis manifested on the right by a wedge-shaped area of decreased signal on this T1-weighted image (*arrow*). On the left there is a lesion in the femoral head bordered by a zone of decreased signal, which corresponds to the site of sclerosis in **A**.

occurs in the head of the femur following a fracture of the femoral neck or a dislocation or fracture-dislocation of the hip. These injuries may result in a disruption of the blood supply of the femoral head. Conversely, intertrochanteric fractures of the femur are rarely associated with avascular necrosis since the blood supply to the femoral head is left intact. Other common sites of ischemic necrosis following trauma are the proximal pole of the carpal scaphoid (navicular), the body of the talus as a result of a fracture of the neck of the talus (Fig. 7-23) and of the head of the second or third metatarsal (Freiberg's infraction) (Fig. 7-31), and of the entire lunate (Keinböck's disease) following injuries of the carpus.

During the early stage, the devitalized bone usually appears denser than the adjacent viable bone and may be separated from it by a thin lucent zone. The dead bone, being devascularized and having no blood supply, cannot change in density and thus maintains the appearance of normal bone, whereas the surrounding vascularized normal bone becomes osteoporotic and thus more radiolucent. Subsequently, the devascularized fragment undergoes compression, with a loss of volume and flattening of the articular surface. The

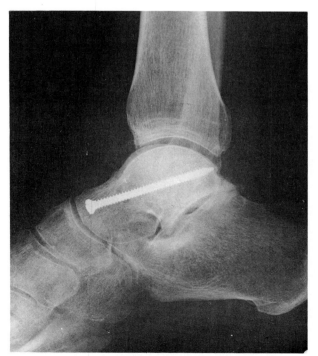

Figure 7–23. Ischemic necrosis of the body of the talus 4 weeks following open reduction of a fracture of the neck of the talus. The body of the talus is homogeneously dense and indicative of ischemia.

lucent zone separating the devascularized from the vascularized bone becomes more distinct, and a dense sclerotic reaction develops in the viable bone adjacent to the dead fragment (Figs. 7-19 and 7-20). The healing process is slow, with revascularization followed by removal of dead bone and the deposition of new bone and at least partial restoration of the involved bone. The larger the fragment, the less likely that this will be complete, but small fragments may be completely restored.

Exogenous Steroids

The potential musculoskeletal complications of corticosteroid therapy include osteoporosis, osteonecrosis, neuropathic-like articular destruction, osteomyelitis, septic arthritis, and rupture of tendons.[29]

The occurrence of a generalized osteoporosis is well recognized and is manifested by a collapse of single or multiple vertebral bodies and fractures of the ribs. There is often a peculiar condensation of bone or sclerosis of the affected vertebral body end-plate.

Osteonecrosis may follow oral, parenteral, topical, or intraarticular administration of steroids. The onset of symptoms and signs is usually delayed for two to three years following the administration of the drug, but on occasion symptoms may occur as early as six months. Single or multiple sites can be affected. The most common sites are the femoral head, the humeral head, the distal femoral condyles, and proximal tibia—in decreasing order of frequency. Approximately 30% to 50% of patients who have steroid-induced osteonecrosis of one femoral head will subsequently demonstrate changes on the contralateral side. The pathogenesis is unknown. The radiographic manifestations are the same as those of other etiologies and include patchy osteosclerosis, the crescent sign, osseous collapse, and fragmentation. Steroid-induced osteonecrosis is particularly common in association with systemic lupus erythematosus and renal transplants and is less common when administered for other conditions.

Neuropathic-like articular destruction is more likely to occur following intraarticular injection of the drug, but the pathogenesis of the process is not certain. The hip and knee are the most frequently involved, and the onset and progression of the disease are often rapid. The radiographic findings consist of fragmentation, sclerosis, joint-space narrowing, and an irregularity of the apposing margins of the joint.

Joint infections can complicate all types of steroid administration. Single or multiple joints may be involved.

Ruptures of the patellar and quadricep tendons are also encountered, particularly in association with systemic lupus erythematosus.

Alcoholism and Pancreatitis

The pathogenesis of ischemic necrosis developing in association with alcoholism and chronic pancreatitis is uncertain, although several theories have been proposed including that of fat embolism. However, the high incidence of trauma, often unremembered, in chronic alcoholics is well known. Many patients with chronic pancreatitis also suffer from chronic alcoholism, and the relationship may be significant. In acute pancreatitis, multiple lytic bone lesions have been reported; these progress rapidly (in a period of 10 days or so), destroying cortical and cancellous bone, with little if any periosteal reaction. This is thought to be caused by metastatic fat necrosis.

Caisson Disease

Caisson disease affects persons who have worked under increased atmospheric pressure and is caused by too rapid decompression. It is more familiarly known as "the bends." It is the result of liberation of bubbles of nitrogen from the blood after the body has absorbed an excess of the gas while under compression. In aviators, a rapid ascent to high altitudes may cause aeroembolism similar to that found in caisson disease. In this instance, the condition is due to a rapid reduction in atmospheric pressure. The bone and joint changes that may develop are the result of infarction. When infarcts involve the articular ends of the bone, ischemic necrosis results. The joints most frequently affected are those of the lower extremities and the shoulder. The radiographic appearance of these changes is similar to that seen from other etiologies. Bone infarcts also occur in this condition; therefore, the combination of avascular necrosis of the articular ends of bones and bone infarcts in the diaphysis should suggest the possibility of caisson disease. Similar changes may be seen in sickle-cell disease. Ischemic necrosis of bone will eventually lead to degenerative arthritis in the associated joint.

Other Areas

Spontaneous ischemic necrosis of the medial femoral condyle has been reported.[3, 21] This occurs in the elderly and is not associated with antecedent trauma. The pain precedes roentgenographic evidence of disease, often by months. Eventually, flattening and irregularity of the medial femoral condyle, followed by a semilunar break in the condylar margin surrounded by irregular sclerosis, is noted on the roentgenogram. The sequestrum formed is usually not detached, and the lesions tend to be larger than those in osteochondritis dissecans. Magnetic resonance imaging is more sensitive and may demonstrate conclusive findings of ischemic necrosis when the radiographic findings are questionable. On T-1 weighted images, a somewhat wedged-shaped area of low signal is found based upon the condylar joint surface. The area remains of low-to-intermediate signal on T-2 weighted images but may be surrounded by a corona of slightly increased signal on this sequence. Ischemic necrosis of the medial tibial plateau has also been described.[21]

Kümmell's Disease

Kümmell's disease has been considered to be an avascular necrosis of a vertebral body that develops after an injury, with no roentgenographic evidence of fracture immediately after the injury. The lesion, however, may very well be an unrecognized fracture with compression of the vertebral body occurring later because of continued weight-bearing. It occurs infrequently, and some authors have expressed doubt about its existence. Progressive collapse of obviously fractured vertebrae occurs with some frequency and leads to a progressive kyphosis at the fracture site. These changes are probably due to combination of avascular necrosis and continued weight-bearing.

BONE INFARCTION OF THE DIAPHYSIS

Infarction may occur in the shaft of bone, usually in the metadiaphysis, and has a distinctive roentgenographic appearance.[9] In some diseases, such as sickle cell anemia and caisson disease, infarction may occur in both areas. Also in sickle cell anemia, infarction of one or more of the short tubular bones may occur (i.e., the hand–foot syndrome). At other times, only shaft infarction is seen. Not infrequently, bone infarction is completely asymptomatic and roentgenographic changes are found by chance on examination for some other reason. The etiology of this infarction is unknown.

During the acute stage of an infarct of the diaphysis, there are no radiographic findings, and infarcted bone does not undergo a change in density. Not until revascularization does the density of the infarcted area change. The margin of the area of infarction is gradually and irregularly calcified. Usually there is a thin rim of sclerosis at the margin of the lesion (Fig. 7-24A), and this remains throughout the rest of life. This same rim is seen on MRI (Fig. 7-24B).

The principal differential diagnostic consideration is an enchondroma. Calcification in an enchondroma is typically chondroid, nodular or stippled, and more centrally located, and it lacks the rim of calcification typical of an infarct (Fig. 4-7B). Incomplete calcification of the rim of an infarct makes this distinction

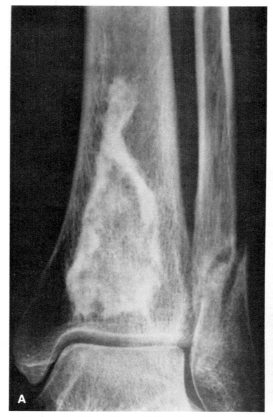
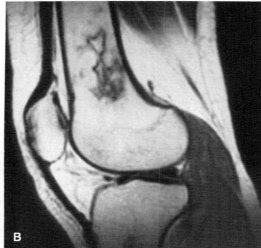

Figure 7–24. Bone infarcts of the shaft. **(A)** Bone infarct. The residual of the infarct remains as a triangular area of sclerosis bound by a sclerotic rim. This was an incidental finding on a radiograph performed to evaluate the fracture of the lateral malleolus. **(B)** T1-weighted MRI in a second case. Lesion in the metadiaphysis of the distal femur has a characteristic low-signal rim. Note smaller, similar lesion in proximal tibia. These were incidental findings on study to evaluate internal structures of knee.

difficult at times. Fortunately, this is rarely of importance. In asymptomatic individuals, an absolute diagnosis is not necessary because neither requires treatment.

In contrast, infarction of the shaft of long bones and the short tubular bones in the hands and feet in sickle cell anemia is usually symptomatic and has a different radiographic appearance, resembling osteomyelitis, with cortical destruction and periosteal new-bone formation. In some cases, both infarction and infection may occur simultaneously. The distinction is usually made on clinical grounds, but in severe cases infarctions may closely resemble osteomyelitis clinically and radiographically. The combination of ^{99m}Tc-MDP and gallium scintigraphy may be helpful in the differential diagnosis. In infarcts, the activity of ^{99m}Tc should be

greater than that of gallium, and the opposite is true of infection.

Osteosarcoma and malignant fibrous histiocytoma have been reported to arise in association with bone infarcts. This is rare.

OSTEOCHONDROSIS AND ISCHEMIC NECROSIS

Osteochondrosis and ischemic necrosis comprise two distinct groups of lesions, both involving an epiphyseal ossification center in one of the small bones of the hand or foot of a child or adolescent. The terms are not interchangeable. In ischemic necrosis, occlusion of blood vessels leads to death of bone. In the osteochondroses, the pathogenesis still is uncertain, and some may well represent nothing more than normal variations in normal ossification. Trauma is suspected as a causative factor in some, either an avulsion injury or chronic repetitive stress. At one time or another, practically every epiphyseal ossification center in the body has been described as the site of osteochondrosis or ischemic necrosis and has had an eponym attached to it. Some of the eponyms firmly established in the literature have proved difficult to eliminate.

CAPITAL FEMORAL EPIPHYSIS (PERTHES' DISEASE)

Ischemic necrosis of the proximal epiphysis of the femur is more commonly known as Perthes' disease or Legg–Calvé–Perthes disease. Other names applied to this lesion include *osteochondritis deformans* and *coxa plana*. The etiology of Perthes' disease has been debatable. Some authors have classified it as an idiopathic type of ischemic necrosis, even though occlusion of major arteries often cannot be demonstrated. Trauma or repeated microtrauma, with injury to the vessels supplying the epiphysis, has often been suggested as a cause.

Perthes' disease is a benign condition that runs a self-limited course and eventually heals. The pathology is one of degeneration and necrosis followed by eventual replacement of necrotic bone when revascularization occurs.[6, 26] It is a disease of childhood, with the greatest incidence at approximately 5 years of age. It is more frequent in boys than girls and is bilateral in about 10% of cases. Limpness and pain, sometimes referred to the knee, are the most common presenting complaints.

Roentgenographic Features. The early roentgenographic findings in Perthes' disease are largely in the soft tissues of the joint. The joint capsule is distended with fluid, and the joint space may be slightly widened, with a slight lateral displacement of the head of the femur. The joint effusion and displacement are due to hyperemia of the synovium and subsynovial tissues. These changes are often subtle and require comparison with the opposite normal side for detection. Similar changes are also seen in the entity known as transient synovitis of the hip. Only about 6% of such patients will progress to Perthes' disease. Because there is a relationship between these two diseases, patients with transient synovitis should be followed closely.

The first change in the femoral head is a thin, linear, arclike, radiolucent zone that develops in the subchondral bone just beneath the articular surface, along the anterosuperior aspect of the epiphyseal ossification center. This lucency is the crescent sign, and it is best seen in the frog-leg projection (Fig. 7-25). This is followed by a slight flattening and irregularity of the superior articular surface of the ossification center. During the early stages of Perthes' disease, the entire center may show a slight uniform increase in density (Fig. 7-26A). This is more apparent than real, owing to disuse osteoporosis in the viable bone immediately adjacent to the acetabulum and femoral neck. The head, having lost its blood supply, maintains the density of normal bone until revascularized.

The next well-defined stage is represented by crushing and fragmentation of the epiphysis (Fig. 7-26B and C). The extent of involvement varies; in some the entire center is affected, whereas in others the changes are limited to an area of subchondral bone along the superior aspect of the head. Once revascularization has taken place, dead bone can be removed. In some patients, this happens before much new bone has been formed, and large areas of the epiphysis will be absorbed. In others, reossification occurs before dead bone has been removed, the new bone being laid down on the scaffolding formed by the dead trabeculae. This is the major cause of increased density of the head or its fragments at this stage of the disease. Compression of the bone causes impaction of trabeculae and may add to the increased opacity. At this stage, the revascularization process is well advanced and reossification is taking place. Eventually the dead trabeculae are removed, and the center returns to a normal density. However, in some cases, old trabeculae may never be removed and the increased opacity of the head persists after healing is complete. Reossification begins adjacent to the epiphyseal plate, and the subchondral bone next to the articular surface is the last to ossify. Healing is a slow process and may require several years or longer.

During the active stage of the disease, there often is a slight widening of the epiphyseal line. (The epiphyseal cartilage derives its blood supply from the same vessels that supply the head.) The surface of the metaphysis becomes irregular, sometimes with small cystic areas, and the femoral neck is broadened and foreshortened (see Fig. 7-25B). The acetabulum is not involved in Perthes' disease.

Bone Scanning. Technetium radiophosphate bone scanning has been used to demonstrate epiphyseal ischemia (Fig. 7-27). High-resolution images with a pinhole or convergent collimator are essential in order to magnify hip structures for detailed assessment of the distribution of radioactivity. The diagnostic sensitivity approaches 100%. Bone scanning is much more sensitive than radiography to both the initial necrosis and healing stages of the disease.

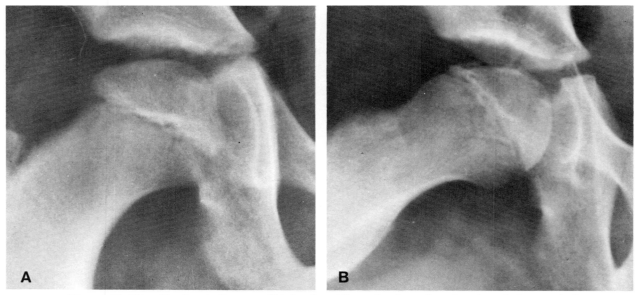

Figure 7–25. Perthes' disease (**A**) In the AP projection, the density of the capital femoral epiphysis is normal, although the head may be slightly flattened. (**B**) In the frogleg projection, a thin translucent zone is noted beneath the subchondral bone superiorly, the crescent sign. It represents a subchondral fracture through avascular bone. This is the earliest radiographic sign of Perthes' disease.

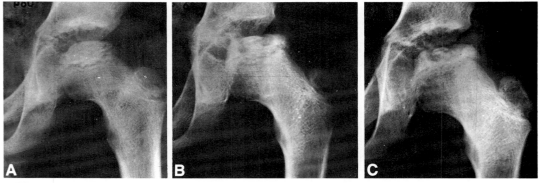

Figure 7–26. Perthes' disease (**A**) Initial film showing slight uniform increase in density of the femoral head and several fine radiolucent fissures within it. The joint space was widened when compared with the opposite normal hip. (**B**) Examination 10 months later shows increased flattening, sclerosis, and two lucent areas within the femoral head. (**C**) Five months later, the central fragment appears to lie within a cavity and is fragmented. The density has returned to normal, but flattening persists.

The initial finding is a photon-deficient area involving part or all the epiphysis (see Fig. 7-27). Healing is seen as a reactive zone of hyperconcentration or increased activity that surrounds the necrotic area. Eventually, with revascularization, radioactivity is demonstrated in the area of previous photon deficiency. In the early stages, photon deficiency may be demonstrated in the presence of a normal radiograph (Fig. 7-27). Similarly, scintigraphic evidence of healing manifested by activity in previously deficient areas is demonstrated before any radiographic evidence of repair.

The major late complication of ischemic necrosis is

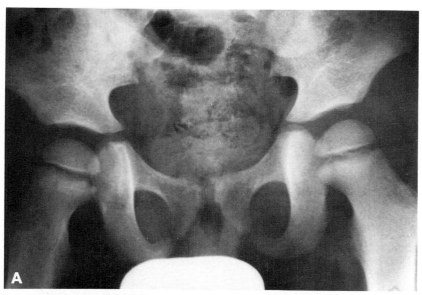

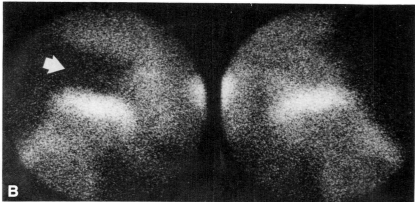

Figure 7–27. Perthes' disease in a 6-year-old boy with right hip pain. (**A**) Normal radiograph of the hips. (**B**) Bone scan reveals photo-deficient right femoral epiphysis (*arrow*) consistent with Perthes' disease. (Courtesy of James J. Conway, M.D., Chicago, IL)

premature degenerative disease of the hip joint, directly proportional to the amount of residual deformity of the femoral head. Another late complication is an increase in the incidence of osteochondritis dissecans of the femoral head. Discomfort in a hip previously affected by Perthes' disease should suggest this possibility. In one study, the average interval between the diagnosis of ischemic necrosis and the appearance of osteochondritis was found to be 8.8 years. The site is usually the superior lateral aspect of the femoral head. Separation of the bony fragment from its bed is uncommon.

OTHER OSTEOCHONDROSES

Some of the more common sites where osteochondrosis has been said to occur are described in the following paragraphs. As noted previously, some are now recog-

nized as being either avulsion fractures or chronic fatigue fractures instead of primary ischemic necrosis. Others may simply represent normal development.

Tarsal Navicular (Köhler's Disease)

Infrequently, the tarsal navicular may be involved by a process similar to Perthes' disease (Fig. 7-28). It occurs during childhood, and the roentgenographic findings consist of flattening, increased density, and a tendency for fragmentation of the bone. In some patients, the lesion has been asymptomatic.

Tibial Tuberosity (Osgood-Schlatter Disease)

The tibial tuberosity develops as a tonguelike extension on the anterior aspect of the proximal tibial epiphysis. Although the major part of this epiphysis begins to

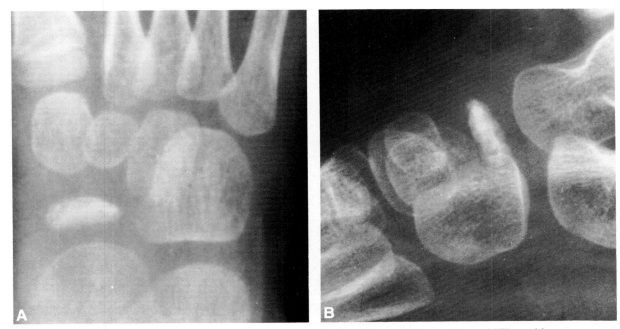

Figure 7–28.   Osteochondrosis of tarsal navicular in frontal (**A**) and lateral (**B**) positions. Note the dense, flat, and slightly irregular navicular characteristic of the lesion known as Köhler's disease.

ossify at or shortly before birth, the tuberosity remains cartilaginous until late childhood. When it begins to ossify it frequently does so from one or more centers; these fuse to the major part of the epiphysis within a relatively short time and subsequently the entire epiphysis fuses to the shaft. The tuberosity serves for the attachment of the patellar tendon and thus is readily subjected to injury.

Osgood-Schlatter disease is more frequent in boys than in girls and is more common during adolescence (i.e., 13 to 15 years). Most investigators believe this lesion represents a stress or fatigue fracture of the tuberosity rather than an ischemic necrosis.

The radiographic findings include irregularity, fragmentation, and an increase in density of the tibial tuberosity (Fig. 7-29). The inferior portion is often elevated slightly from its normal position. Localized swelling of the soft tissues over the tuberosity can be visualized, and indeed, in the absence of soft-tissue swelling the diagnosis is suspect.

The roentgenographic diagnosis of osteochondrosis of the tibial tuberosity should be made with caution and the findings correlated with clinical symptoms and signs, since there is considerable variation in the appearance of the normal tuberosity during the process of ossification. It may ossify from several centers, and its inferior portion may be elevated. The appearance may rather closely resemble that seen in osteochondrosis.

Visualization of soft-tissue swelling over the tuberosity plus the clinical signs of pain and local tenderness should be present before the diagnosis of Osgood-Schlatter disease is made. As a sequela to healing, some of the fragmented portions may not unite but remain as separate small, round or ovoid ossicles.

Vertebral Ring Epiphyses (Scheuermann's Disease)

At age 13 to 15 years, thin, ringlike ossification centers appear along the upper and lower margins of the vertebral bodies. These may be involved by an osteochondrosis clinically manifested by pain, particularly in the midthoracic spine. The epiphyseal plates lose their sharp outlines, become irregular and somewhat sclerotic, and often fragment. The involved vertebrae tend to be decreased in height and wedge shaped because the reduction is more pronounced anteriorly. This in turn leads to a dorsal kyphosis (Fig. 7-30). Although involvement of several or many vertebral bodies is the rule, occasionally the disease may be confined to only one or two. After the disease is healed, some irregularity of the disc surfaces, anterior wedging, and kyphotic deformity persist throughout life. Deficiency of the anterior portions of the apophyseal plates may cause a notchlike defect along the anterior corners of the bodies, as seen on the lateral view.

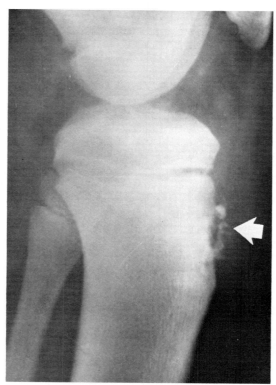

Figure 7–29. Osgood–Schlatter's disease of the tibial tuberosity. The apophysis is fragmented (*arrow*), and overlying soft-tissue swelling is present.

Schmorl's nodes are also common. These are small concave defects of the end-plates of one or more vertebrae, seen best on the lateral view. They are caused by a defect in ossification of the vertebral end-plate, allowing herniation or protrusion of the nucleus pulposus of the disc into the vertebral body. The protrusion is surrounded by a thin rim of sclerosis. When occurring in isolation or when scattered throughout several vertebrae, they are normal variants. In Scheuermann's disease, however, multiple Schmorl's nodes occur in the area affected by the disease process.

Metatarsal Head (Freiberg Infraction)

The Freiberg infraction is found in the head of the second metatarsal, less commonly in the third and the first. Although originally thought to be a form of aseptic necrosis, it is now generally considered to represent an infraction or a type of stress fracture involving the metatarsal head. It is found during late adolescence. The articular end of the bone becomes flattened, sometimes concave, and irregular. With healing, the neck of the metatarsal becomes thickened and sclerotic (Fig.

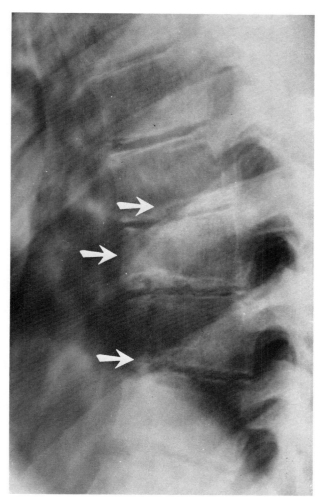

Figure 7–30. Scheuermann's disease of the thoracic spine. One of the vertebra (*central arrow*) is wedge shaped, and its endplate is irregular as a result of the fragmentation of the ring apophysis. There is lesser involvement with Schmorl's-node defects in several of the other vertebral bodies (*arrows*). The anterior wedging of several midthoracic vertebrae resulted in a kyphotic deformity.

7-31). Tiny fragments of bone may become separated from the articular surface and remain as small ossicles after healing is complete. Degenerative joint disease is commonly a late complication.

Apophysis of Os Calcis (Sever's Disease)

The apophysis of the os calcis is an epiphyseal plate that develops along the posterior border of the bone. It has been reported as the site of an osteochondrosis, the

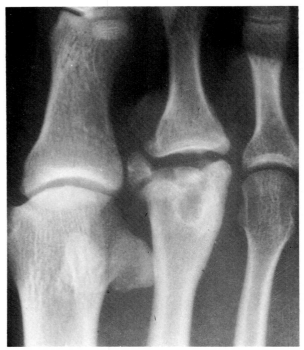

Figure 7–31. Freiberg's infraction of the head of the second metatarsal. The distal end of the metatarsal is irregular, the articular surface is concave, and the head and neck are thickened. The joint space appears slightly widened, and the base of the opposing proximal phalanx is normal.

apophysis becoming dense and sclerotic and undergoing fragmentation. This apophysis normally varies greatly in density. In many normal children, it has a uniform chalky white appearance and may ossify from several centers. The diagnosis of osteochondrosis involving the os calcis should be made with caution and is seldom justified on roentgenologic grounds alone.

In addition to the foregoing, many other epiphyseal centers have been reported as sites of osteochondrosis. Because of the possibility of normal irregular development of epiphyseal centers, we must emphasize the need for caution when the diagnosis of osteochondrosis is a clinical or radiographic consideration. An atlas of normal variants should be consulted.

Osteochondritis Dissecans

This lesion is a form of ischemic necrosis, but one that involves only a small portion of bone, usually the articular surface of the medial condyle of the femur. It occurs in young adults after epiphyseal closure, chiefly in males, and is characterized by the gradual separa-

tion of a button-shaped fragment of bone and cartilage from the condylar surface (Fig. 7-32A and B). It is bilateral in about 20% of cases. Why the disease involves this particular site is not clear. The fragment may separate completely from its bed and become a loose body within the joint, leaving a shallow defect in the articular surface of the femur. If it does not become completely separated, the button of bone may remain within its cavity, either becoming absorbed or eventually developing a new blood supply and becoming revitalized.

Osteochondritis dissecans must be differentiated from a normal irregular, flake-like ossification of the femoral condyles. This is characteristically seen between the ages of 10 and 13 and is situated on the posterior surface of the condyles, whereas osteochondritis dissecans occurs anteriorly and borders on the condylar notch.

Less frequently, osteochondritis dissecans is found in several other areas, particularly in the head of the femur, the medial or lateral edge of the dome of the talus (Fig. 7-32C), the capitellum of the elbow, the head of the radius, and the patella. Radiographic findings are similar to those seen in the femoral condyles, a shallow defect marginated by sclerosis usually with an overlying flake or button of articular bone. At times the articular fragment is displaced or has been completely resorbed, leaving only the defect.

Epiphysiolysis (Slipping of the Capital Femoral Epiphysis)

This lesion has been classified by some as an ischemic necrosis affecting the epiphyseal plate of the proximal end of the femur, but the head of the femur does not become avascular. However, many believe that the lesion is most likely caused by trauma, either in the form of an acute injury or chronic repetitive stress. The lesion develops during adolescence, ages 10 to 15 years, and is most frequent in overweight boys of the Fröhlich type. (There is an increased incidence of epiphysiolysis in renal osteodystrophy in the hip and elsewhere; see Chapter 6.)

The lesion is a gradual slipping of the femoral head on the neck or, more correctly, of the neck on the head. The head remains in the acetabulum. There is an upward displacement, external rotation, and adduction of the neck relative to the head. The head is displaced posteriorly, downward and medially. The initial displacement is seen to best advantage in a frog-leg view of the hip (Fig. 7-33) and may not be immediately obvious on the straight AP view. On the AP view, a line drawn along the superior cortex of the femoral neck should pass through the lateral margin of the femoral epiphysis. When the epiphysis is displaced medially,

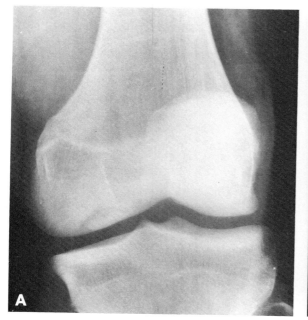

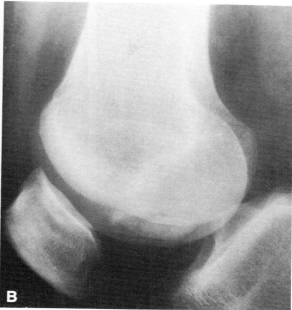

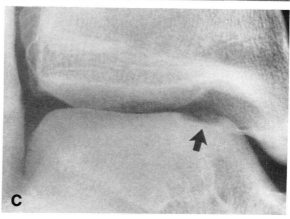

Figure 7–32. (**A** and **B**) Osteochondritis dissecans of the medial condyle of the femur. (**A**) The buttonlike, dense fragment of bone lies surrounded by an area of radiolucency. (**B**) In the lateral view, the fragment is quite clearly outlined along the surface of the medial femoral condyle. (**C**) Osteochondritis dissecans of the talus. Note the defect in the cortical surface of the medial dome of the talus (*arrow*). There are a few fine fragments of radiodensity lying within the defect.

the line will either pass tangential to or not transect any portion of the epiphysis. The displacement is accompanied by a widening of the physis or epiphyseal line and irregularity of the surface of the metaphysis. Treatment requires pinning of the hip using multiple threaded pins.

Both hips are affected in 20% to 40% of cases, so it is essential that the opposite hip be observed closely. Prophylactic pinning of the opposite side is occasionally performed.

When the epiphysis fuses, the lesion stops progressing, but any deformity that has occurred will be permanent. The neck of the femur is remodeled to some extent and develops a convex superior surface instead of the normal concavity; the characteristic appearance

is seen in straight AP views (Fig. 7-34). As with Perthes' disease, the early development of degenerative joint disease in the hip is a frequent complication.

ANEMIAS

The skeletal alterations of congenital hemolytic anemias are caused by erythroid hyperplasia of the bone marrow, which fills and expands the cancellous bone and disturbs the trabecular architecture. The three best-known anemias are (1) thalassemia, (2) sickle cell anemia, and (3) hereditary spherocytosis (familial hemolytic anemia). In addition, variants of these three and other rare hemolytic anemias can cause similar,

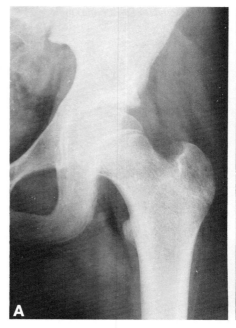
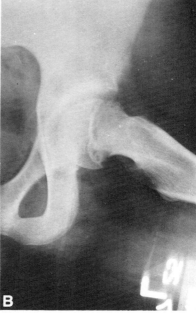

Figure 7–33. Epiphysiolysis. (**A**) No definite abnormality is observed on this anteroposterior projection. (**B**) A frog-leg oblique projection reveals characteristic medial displacement of the epiphysis and irregularity of the metaphysis, findings not apparent on the frontal projection. Frog-leg oblique projections are necessary to rule out this diagnosis.

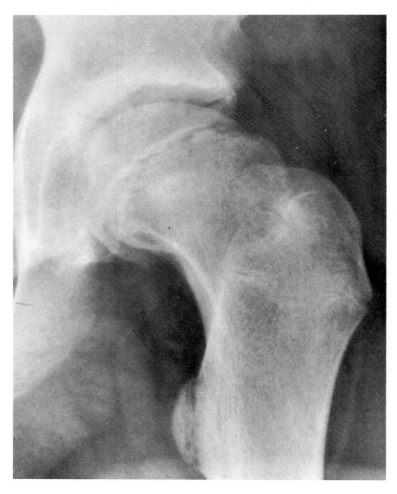

Figure 7–34. Epiphysiolysis. Postero-medial displacement of the capital femoral epiphysis and irregularity of the metaphysis are obvious in this case.

although usually much milder, changes. Also, changes in the skull similar to those of the congenital anemias have been found in chronic iron deficiency anemia, cyanotic congenital heart disease, and polycythemia vera in childhood.

THALASSEMIA (COOLEY'S ANEMIA)

Thalassemia, also known as Cooley's anemia or Mediterranean anemia, occurs predominately in Greeks and Italians and occasionally in persons of other nationalities. Cooley's anemia is the homozygous form of thalassemia inherited from both parents. The heterozygous form, thalassemia minor, is inherited from one parent. Persons with the heterozygous form usually have only a mild anemia and no skeletal stigmata. In adults, there may be some vertebral osteoporosis and minimal diploic widening in the skull.

The radiographic changes are seen in bones containing red marrow, and therefore the pattern of osseous changes is different in children and adults. In the young child, red marrow is present in all bones, including the small bones of the hand; in the mature adult, red marrow is replaced by yellow marrow in the majority of the peripheral skeleton. In the mature adult, red marrow is limited to the axial skeleton, the spine, pelvis, skull, and most proximal portion of femur and humerus.

In a child with Cooley's anemia, the peripheral skeleton is affected. The small bones such as the metacarpals, metatarsals, and phalanges have a rectangular appearance, the normal concavity of the shaft being lost, and the cortices are thinned. The medullary spaces have a spongy, mottled appearance. The trabecular pattern of the bone is coarsened (Fig. 7-35A). At times, thin transverse bands of increased density, or growth lines, can be seen crossing the shaft. In severe cases there is retardation of skeletal growth.

In the skull, the diploic space is characteristically widened, particularly in the frontal and parietal bones (Fig. 7-35B).[30] The occipital squamosa is usually not affected. The outer table is thinned and may become

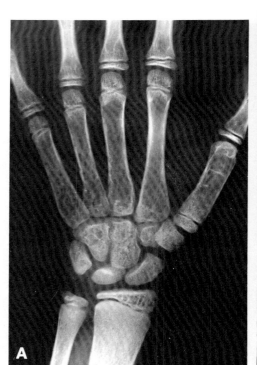
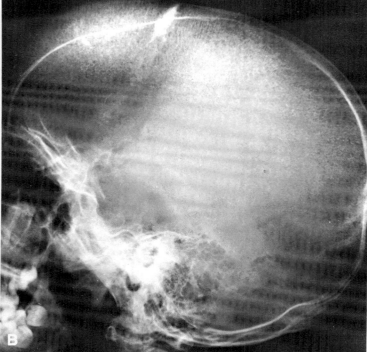

Figure 7–35. Cooley's anemia (thalassemia). (**A**) There is thinning of the cortex, with decrease in the normal constriction of the midshafts. Normal trabeculation is not observed in the area of mottled radiolucency. The phalanges are less involved than the metacarpals. (**B**) Lateral view of the skull illustrates marked thickening of bone in the frontal area, with characteristic vertical striations. (Courtesy of M. P. Neal, Jr., M.D. and T. R. Howell, M.D., Richmond, VA)

deficient in areas so that marrow can protrude into the subperiosteal space. There frequently are radiating trabeculae of bone extending at right angles to the inner table, giving a "hair-on-end" appearance.

The paranasal sinuses may be poorly developed, particularly the maxillary sinuses. Encroachment on the sinus air space is caused by a thickening of the bony walls due to marrow hyperplasia. Because of the absence of red marrow, the ethmoid cells are not affected. Enlargement of the maxilla may lead to malocclusion and overbite.

In older patients, the changes in the small bones of the hands and feet become less striking and may disappear completely by the time of puberty. Changes may become more pronounced after puberty in the skull, spine, and pelvis, where red marrow persists.

Occasionally, masses of extramedullary hematopoiesis are noted in the posterior mediastinum. These appear as multiple, bilateral, smoothly outlined soft-tissue masses projecting laterally in the posterior mediastinum. They apparently arise from bone marrow, extruded through the cortex of the ribs and vertebrae, following lysis of cortical bone by the expanding mass of hematopoietic tissue.[16, 17]

Pathologic fracture may occur through weakened bone, although it is not common. Gallstones also occur, often in young patients, as a complication of thalassemia.

SICKLE CELL ANEMIA

Sickle cell anemia is a hereditary disease transmitted as a dominant gene in the black race that results in an abnormal hemoglobin (hemoglobin S). Those who are heterozygous for the hemoglobin S gene have what is referred to as the sickle cell trait. Those who are homozygous, inheriting one such gene from each parent, develop sickle cell anemia. Sickle cell β-thalassemia is a doubly heterozygous condition in which the hemoglobin S gene is inherited from one parent and the β-thalassemia gene from the other. Bone changes are similar to those in sickle cell anemia (hemoglobin SC disease).

In general, the roentgenographic findings are similar to those in Cooley's anemia (Fig. 7-36). Loss of bone

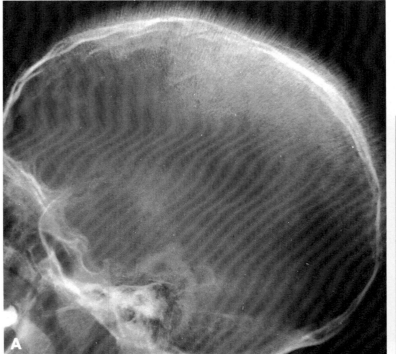
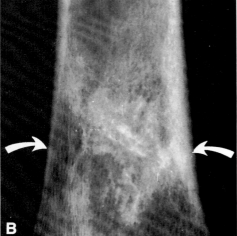

Figure 7–36.   Sickle-cell anemia. **(A)** Lateral view of the skull illustrates thickening of the bones of the cranial vault in the frontoparietal area containing perpendicular striations. The outer table is indistinct in some areas and absent in others. Note premature fusion of the sutures. **(B)** An infarct of the distal shaft of the femur is observed as an irregular patchy increase in radiodensity. There was a similar lesion in the opposite femur. (Courtesy of M. P. Neal, Jr., M.D. and T. R. Howell, M.D., Richmond, VA)

due to marrow hyperplasia, the most common finding, results in decreased bone density. The trabecular pattern is often sparse, with wide separation resulting in a wire-mesh pattern. In addition, bone infarction is common (Fig. 7-36*B*).[15] During infancy, the infarcts tend to involve the small bones of the hands and feet, producing a dactylitis (the hand-foot syndrome). This presents as an irregular, permeative, or moth-eaten destruction with overlying periosteal new-bone formation, and it very closely resembles an inflammatory process. Indeed, both infarction and infection may be present simultaneously, and the differentiation is extremely difficult because both cause rarefaction, periosteal new-bone formation, and occasionally sequestration. In older children, bone infarction is more common in the epiphyses and may cause an appearance quite similar to that of Perthes' disease.

Severe bone infarctions occasionally occur in the shafts of adults. Normally there is no radiographic sign of acute infarction, but in severe cases a moth-eaten or permeative destruction is evident, with perforation of the cortex and overlying thin lamellar or layered periosteal new-bone formation.[4] The incidence of infarcts in the long bone tends to increase with age. As a result of infarction, thin, strandlike bone densities appear within the intramedullary canal, paralleling the endosteal surface of the cortex. This gives the appearance of "bone within bone" (Fig. 7-37).

Hematopoietic marrow hyperplasia is a universal occurrence in sickle cell anemia. On MRI this results in a decreased signal from the marrow on both T-1 and T-2 weighted images.[27, 33] Acute and chronic infarction results in areas of further decreased signal on T-1. When infarction is acute, foci of increased signal are seen on T-2, but if infarction is chronic, decreased signal is maintained on T-2 as well.

Osteomyelitis is a frequent complication of sickle cell anemia and may develop in any bone.[4] It differs from the standard form of hematogenous osteomyelitis in that it frequently occurs within the diaphysis as opposed to the metaphysis and the organism is frequently *Salmonella* (see Fig. 5-18). The radiographic manifestations of osteomyelitis are an irregular rarefaction with a permeative pattern and lamellar or onionskin type of periosteal reaction (Fig. 7-38). The findings are identical to those of a severe infarction. The differentiation of infarction from osteomyelitis is difficult on the basis of radiographic findings alone. Differentiation of

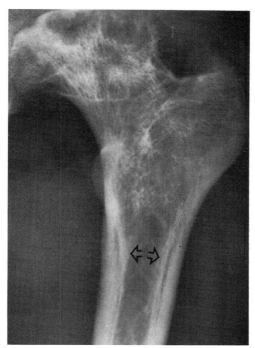

Figure 7–37. Sickle-cell anemia in an adult. Avascular necrosis of the femoral head is indicated by flattening, irregularity, and irregular areas of lucency and sclerosis. Infarction of the shaft has led to the characteristic "bone-in-bone" appearance of the proximal shaft (*arrows*).

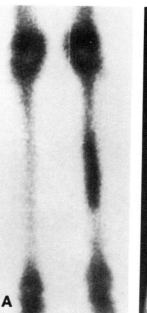 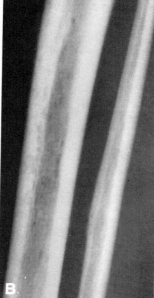

Figure 7–38. Salmonella osteomyelitis of the tibia in a 29-year-old black woman with sickle-cell anemia. **(A)** Technetium bone scan demonstrates an area of increased radioactivity in the diaphysis of the left tibia. **(B)** Permeative destruction of intramedullary bone is noted, associated with tunneling of the cortex and overlying soft-tissue swelling.

the two processes by combined technetium and gallium scanning may be possible.[1] Gallium has an avidity for infections, and in the presence of an infection will usually reveal a greater activity than technetium, whereas in infarction the activity of the technetium scan will be greater than that of gallium. Pathologic fractures may occur in bones thinned by both infarction and infection.

In the vertebrae, osteoporosis may be quite severe, leading to compression deformities. The vertebral end-plates become concave as the disc expands into the softened vertebrae. Reynolds has pointed out that the vertebral contour in sickle cell anemia is characteristic, consisting of a localized central depression of the end-plates and giving a "Lincoln log" or H-type vertebral pattern (Fig. 7-39).[30] This is in contrast to the biconcave or "codfish" vertebral contour seen in persons with osteoporosis and in those who use steroids. In adults, a diffuse sclerosis may be encountered resembling that seen in myelofibrosis. The vertebrae, in spite of a sclerotic appearance, are softer than normal and develop biconcave end-plates. This, combined with the sclerotic appearance, is distinctive for sickle cell anemia in the older child or adult. A hair-on-end appearance of the skull is infrequent, but there may be widening of the diploic space.[30]

When infarcts occur during childhood, growth disturbances may result. These consist of cupped metaphyses and triangular epiphyses, and there may be widening of the diaphysis near the metaphysis, usually in the lower femur, as a result of lack of modeling. A unilateral or bilateral tibiotalar slant may occur. This consists of a slant of the tibiotalar joint from above and laterally downward and medially, and it is probably a growth disturbance secondary to alteration in blood supply. Tibiotalar slant has also been reported in association with hemophilia, Still's disease, and epiphyseal dysplasia multiplex. In addition to bone changes, cardiomegaly, hepatomegaly, and splenomegaly are frequent. Cholelithiasis is fairly frequent and may be found in young individuals.

CHRONIC IRON DEFICIENCY ANEMIA

Iron deficiency anemia has been reported to cause widening of the diplöe of the skull and perpendicular trabeculation in the frontal and parietal areas, findings quite similar to those of Cooley's anemia. In other bones, changes are less striking however and they are usually essentially normal or, at most, slightly osteoporotic, even when well-marked skull changes are present.

MYELOFIBROSIS WITH OSTEOSCLEROSIS

Myelofibrosis runs a relatively benign course, and osteosclerosis will develop in approximately half of the patients. The disease is also known as nonleukemic myelosis, agnogenic myeloid metaplasia, osteosclerotic anemia, and leukoerythroblastic anemia, to mention only a few. It is usually idiopathic, but at times it may be secondary to some other disease such as polycythemia vera. It is estimated that from 10% to 20% of cases of polycythemia vera may ultimately have myelofibrosis. Clinical manifestations include the following: anemia; a normal, lowered, or moderately elevated white blood cell count; the constant presence of immature red and white cells in the peripheral blood; and significant enlargement of the spleen and the liver.

The osteosclerosis is often widely distributed throughout the bones of the trunk and some of the bones of the extremities, particularly the humerus and femur. In smaller bones such as the ribs, there may be a uniform increase in density, with loss of much of the trabecular architecture. In larger bones such as the femur, the sclerosis is more mottled and patchy in

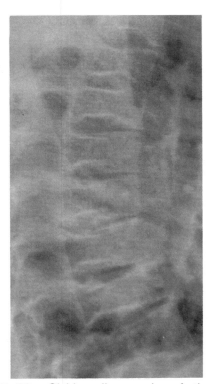

Figure 7–39. Sickle-cell anemia of the spine. Characteristic deformities of endplates of the vertebrae manifested by a central depression, sometimes referred to as the "H-type" or "Lincoln log" vertebra.

distribution (Fig. 7-40). In the femur, the earliest changes can often be recognized in the distal end.

When a diffuse increase in density of the skeleton is encountered in an adult, one should think first of the possibility of this disease. Osteoblastic metastases are rarely distributed as uniformly. Osteopetrosis (marble bones) is essentially a disease of the young.

SYSTEMIC MASTOCYTOSIS

Systemic mastocytosis is a rare cause of osteosclerosis. The osteosclerosis may consist of a generalized increase in density involving the skull, thorax, spine, and pelvis, and it closely resembles myelofibrosis. In other cases, the changes are scattered, well-defined foci of sclerosis. In still others, radiolucent zones have been found within areas of increased density, resembling mixed osteolytic and blastic metastases from which the systemic mastocytosis may be difficult to differentiate.

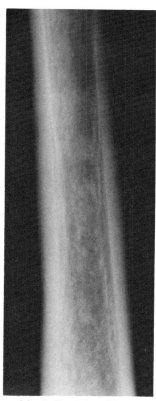

Figure 7–40. Myelofibrosis with osteosclerosis. An anteroposterior radiograph of a portion of the femoral diaphysis reveals a mottled sclerotic increase in density distributed throughout the medullary canal. The cortex is thickened, and there are linear stripelike areas of increased density along the endosteal cortical margins.

BONE CHANGES DUE TO PHYSICAL AGENTS

FROSTBITE

The initial radiographic manifestation of frostbite is soft-tissue swelling of the affected part, usually the distal portion of the foot and hand, particularly the toes and fingers. Superimposed infection is frequent, and amputation may be required. The first change in the bone is osteoporosis, which may be observed in 4 to 10 weeks following the incident and persisting for months. Other bone changes usually develop late, from six months to years after injury. Often there is soft-tissue atrophy followed by the appearance of small areas of increased density at the ends of the involved bones, usually more marked in the distal than in the proximal phalanges. These are presumed to represent small-bone infarcts.[34]

Periosteal new-bone formation may occur along the shaft of the involved bones. In some cases, small punched-out areas ultimately occur on the articular surfaces (Fig. 7-41). When the joint surfaces are severely involved, fusion may occur. This is more common in children than adults. Acro-osteolysis, a resorption of the ungual tufts and distal portions of the phalanges, may occur.

The more distinctive changes of frostbite occur in children. Freezing may lead to death of a portion or all of phalangeal epiphyseal growth plates, resulting in deformities and premature fusion of a portion or all of the affected growth plate (Fig. 7-42). This will usually be either more severe in or limited to the distal phalanges but may occur in the middle phalanges and less commonly in the proximal phalanges. The proximal growth plates will not be affected unless there is involvement more distally. The thumb is characteristically spared, because when subjected to severe cold, the thumbs are folded into the palms and covered by the fingers and therefore protected from frostbite.

THERMAL AND ELECTRICAL BURNS

Heat results in a necrosis of bone manifested initially by osteolysis and ultimately with bone resorption (Fig. 7-43), periosteal reaction, and possibly sequestrum formation.[32] Regional osteoporosis is common, and secondary osteomyelitis is frequent. Ultimately there may be soft-tissue calcification.[10] Periarticular calcification is particularly frequent around the elbow. Destruction of the articular surface and ultimately bony ankylosis may occur.

The changes of electrical burns may be limited to that portion of the body in immediate contact with the wire. For instance, if the patient stepped on a live wire, the changes may be limited to a narrow band across the

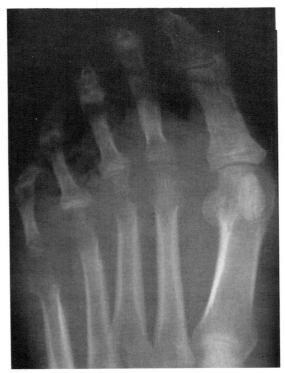

Figure 7–41. Frostbite. There is a loss of soft tissue distal to the metatarsal heads. The phalanges are osteopenic. Marginal erosions are present on the heads of the second through fifth metatarsals, and periosteal new-bone formation is identified along the margins of the metatarsals. The bone density is normal proximal to the heads of the metatarsals.

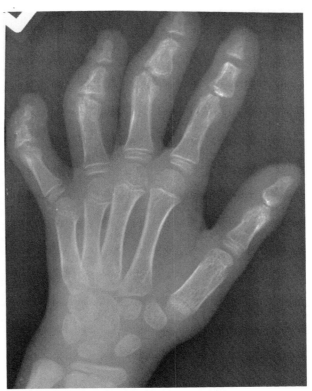

Figure 7–42. Residuals of frostbite in a young child. Note the epiphyses of the distal and proximal phalanges of all the digits have been destroyed. There is gross irregularity of the margins of both the proximal and distal interphalangeal joints. The epiphyses of the proximal phalanges, metacarpals, and distal radius are normal. The thumb is often spared, but not so in this case.

base of all of the metatarsals. Defects are characteristic in that they are in a line. Ultimately, the areas that undergo osteolysis heal and are marginated by a thin rim of sclerotic bone. Joint injury from electrical burns is essentially a destructive atrophy, and changes similar to those due to thermal injury may occur.

RADIATION INJURY OF BONE

The effect of irradiation on bone is often termed *radiation osteitis*, a term coined by Ewing in 1926. Radiation injury is limited to bone within the field of irradiation. The minimum dose is at least 1500 rad; the mean dose is in the range of 4000 to 5000 rad.[19] These doses are achieved in the treatment of carcinoma of the cervix and prostate, resulting in changes in the pelvis; carcinoma of the breast, affecting the pectoral girdle and ribs; orbital tumors, particularly retinoblastoma, affecting the skull and facial skeleton; and neuroblastoma

and Wilms' tumor, affecting the thoracolumbar spine and pelvis. The absorbed dose in bone with orthovoltage treatment techniques used in the past was probably twice as high as that received with current techniques using megavoltage. It is, therefore, quite likely the incidence of radiation injury of bone will decrease.

Pathologically, radiation leads to an inflammation and necrosis of the blood-forming elements within the medullary space, the osteoblasts, osteocytes, and osteoclasts, which recover slowly over a prolonged period. An obliterative endarteritis reduces the blood supply to the affected bone.

These changes are manifested radiographically one to two years after the irradiation by a minimal and subtle osteoporosis in the treatment area.[19] Within two

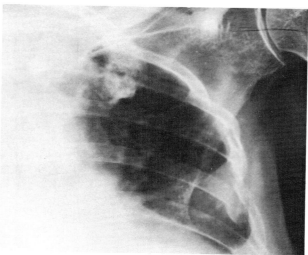

Figure 7–44. Radiation osteitis of the ribs. The patient received radiation therapy to the chest wall for carcinoma of the breast several years earlier. Note an area of absorption in the axillary margin of the fifth rib, with pathologic fractures of several ribs, some of which have healed.

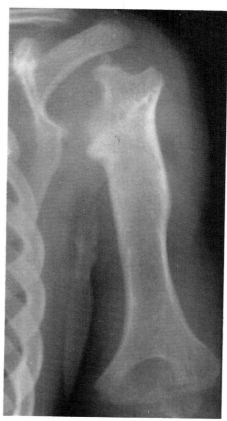

Figure 7–43. Effect of burns in a 6-year-old. Third-degree burns about the shoulder have destroyed the epiphysis of the proximal humerus, resulting in shortening and gross deformity.

years, new bone is laid down in the treatment area and is manifested as coarsening of the trabecular pattern and irregular small patches of sclerosis. These sclerotic patches are interspersed with small lytic areas, generally no larger than 5 mm.

Pathologic fractures occur particularly in the ribs and clavicle and are frequently asymptomatic (Fig. 7-44). These fractures can be differentiated from metastatic disease by the absence of symptoms and radiographically by the absence of a surrounding soft-tissue mass. In the past, fractures of the hip were noted following irradiation of the pelvis. This is now much less common, since the femoral heads and necks are rarely included in the treatment portals using modern equipment and techniques.

Radiation osteitis must be distinguished from invasive or metastatic bone destruction. Radiation osteitis occurs years rather than months after the completion of radiation therapy. The bone changes are localized to the radiation portal. The simultaneous presence of changes in several adjacent bones such as the humerus, scapula, clavicle, and ribs and nowhere else— as seen following radiation of carcinoma of the breast— strongly points to radiation change rather than metastatic disease. In most cases, radiation osteitis is only minimally symptomatic whereas metastatic disease is quite symptomatic.

The presence of multiple lytic areas or the presence of dystrophic calcification should always raise the possibility of radiation-induced sarcoma. Any alteration in stable radiation osteitis should also prompt consideration of the possibility of sarcomatous change. As a general rule, the absence of growth, destruction, or an associated soft-tissue mass favors radiation osteitis.

Radiation injury in children differs from that in adults because of the presence of growth centers.[5, 9] Radiation of growth centers may either destroy or severely disturb the growth plate, resulting in growth disturbances. In general, a minimum dose of 1000 rad and a mean dose between 3000 and 3500 rad is required before injury is evident. Injuries are most commonly encountered in the spine following treatment of Wilms' tumor and neuroblastoma. In general, several years elapse after the radiation before there is radiographic evidence of injury. In the spine, the radiographic evidence of injury consists of irregularity of the end-plates, an altered trabecular pattern, anterior beaking of the vertebral body, and asymmetry of vertebral body development, often with wedging of the lateral margin of the vertebrae toward the side of the original tumor. This ultimately results in a scoliosis.[5] If the iliac crest was included in the original treatment portal, a hypoplasia of the iliac bone may occur. If the acetabulum was in the treatment portal, it may be shallow and hypoplastic.

Radiation treatment of the extremities is not as frequent but is used in the treatment of Ewing's tumor. If the growth plate is included in the treatment portal, growth arrest with reduction in length and angular deformities at the joint may occur.

Radiation injury may ultimately induce neoplasia in bone.[5, 19] The resultant tumors are osteosarcoma, fibrosarcoma, and rarely chondrosarcoma. The average dose exceeds 4000 rad, and the tumor usually does not appear until eight or more years following irradiation. The majority of cases appear as lytic destruction within an area of radiation osteitis. A soft-tissue mass associated with evidence of destruction is frequently seen. Frank osteoid new-bone formation occurs within an area of rapidly destructive change within the irradiated field. Chondrosarcoma would produce cartilage matrix with chondroid calcification. Radiation-induced sarcoma should be considered when any change is noted in the region of stable radiation osteitis. This must be differentiated from metastatic disease. Recurrent tumors usually appear much sooner than radiation-induced sarcomas.

Osteochondromas (benign cartilaginous exostoses) have been noted to occur following radiation therapy in children.[20] These are similar in radiographic appearance to osteochondromas at other sites. They are usually incidental findings discovered on follow-up examinations and are rarely symptomatic. Osteochondromas are more likely to occur if the patient has been irradiated prior to the age of two years. They commonly arise from portions of the pelvis or posterior elements of the spinal column.

REFERENCES AND SELECTED READINGS

1. AMUNDSEN TR, SIEGEL MJ, SIEGEL BA: Osteomyelitis and infarction in sickle cell hemoglobinopathies: Differentiation by combined technetium and gallium scintigraphy. Radiology 153:807, 1984

2. AWWAD EE, SUNDARAM M: Vertebral Paget's disease causing paraparesis. Orthopedics 10:531, 1987

3. BJORKENGREN AG, AIROWAIH A, LINDSTRAND A ET AL: Spontaneous osteonecrosis of the knee: Value of MR imaging in determining prognosis. Am J Roentgenol 154:331, 1990

4. BOHRER SP: Bone changes in the extremities in sickle cell anemia. Semin Roentgen 22:176, 1987

5. BUTLER MS, ROBERTSON WW, RATE W ET AL: Skeletal sequelae of radiation therapy for malignant childhood tumors. Clin Orthop Related Research 251:235, 1990

6. CATTERALL A, PRINGLE J, BYERS PD ET AL: A review of the morphology of Perthes' disease. J Bone Joint Surg [Br] 64:269, 1982

7. DETENBECK LC, SIM FH, JOHNSON EW: Symptomatic Paget's disease of the hip. JAMA 224:213, 1973

8. DODD GW, IBBERTSON HK, FRASER TRC ET AL: Radiological assessment of Paget's disease of bone after treatment with the bisphosphonates EHDP and APD. Brit J Radiology 60:849, 1987

9. DESMET AA, KUHNS LR, FAYOS JV ET AL: Effects of radiation therapy on growing long bone. Am J Roentgenol 127:935, 1976

10. EVANS EB: Heterotopic bone formation in thermal burns. Clin Orthop 263:94, 1991

11. FREEMAN DA: Southwestern Internal Medicine Conference: Paget's disease of bone. Am J Med Sciences 31:144, 1988

12. GREDITZER HG, MCLEOD RA, UNNI KK ET AL: Bone sarcomas in Paget disease. Radiology 146:327, 1983

13. HERMANN G, GOLDBLATT J, LEVY RN ET AL: Gaucher's disease Type 1: Assessment of bone involvement by CT and scintigraphy. Am J Roentgenol 147:943, 1986

14. KELLY JK, DENIER JE, WILNER HI ET AL: MR imaging of lytic changes in Paget disease of the calvarium. J Comput Assist Tomogr 13:27, 1989

15. KEELEY K, BUCHANAN GR: Acute infarction of long bones in children with sickle cell anemia. J Pediatr 101:170, 1982

16. LAWSON JP, ABLOW RC, PEARSON HA: The ribs in thalassemia. I. The relationship to therapy. Radiology 140:663, 1981

17. LAWSON JP, ABLOW RC, PEARSON HA: The ribs in thalassemia. II. The pathogenesis of the changes. Radiology 140:673, 1981

18. LEE KS, MCWHORTER JM, ANGELO JN: Spinal epidural hematoma associated with Paget's disease. Surg Neurol 30:131, 1988

19. LIBSCHITZ HI (ED): Diagnostic Roentgenology of Radiotherapy Changes. Baltimore, Williams & Wilkins, 1979

20. LIBSHITZ HI, COHEN MA: Radiation-induced osteochondromas. Radiology 142:643, 1982

21. LOTKE PA, ECKER ML: Osteonecrosis of the knee. J Bone Joint Surg (Am) 70:470, 1988

22. MITCHELL DG, KRESSEL HY, ARGER PH ET AL: Avascular necrosis of the femoral head: Morphologic assessment by MR imaging, with CT correlation. Radiology 161:739, 1986

23. MOORE TE, KING AR, KATHOL MH: Sarcoma in Paget disease of bone: Clinical, radiologic, and pathologic features in 22 cases. Am J Roentgenol 156:1199, 1991

24. PARKER BR, PINCKNEY L, ETCUBANAS E: Relative efficacy of radiographic and radionuclide bone surveys in the

detection of the skeletal lesions of histiocytosis X. Radiology 134:377, 1980

25. PASTAKIA B, BROWER AC, CHANG VH: Skeletal manifestations of Gaucher's disease. Sem Roentgen 21:264, 1986

26. PONSETI IV, MAYNARD JA, WEINSTEIN SL ET AL: Legg-Calvé-Perthes disease. J Bone Joint Surg [Am] 65:797, 1983

27. RAO VM, FISHMAN M, MITCHELL DG: Painful sickle cell crisis: Bone marrow patterns observed with MR imaging. Radiology 161:211, 1986

28. RESNICK D: Paget disease of bone: Current status and a look back to 1943 and earlier. Am J Roentgenol 150:249, 1988

29. RESNICK D, NIWAYAMA G (EDS): Diagnosis of bone and joint disorders, 3rd ed., Philadelphia, WB Saunders, 1991

30. REYNOLDS J: The skull and spine. Sem Roentgen 22:168, 1987

31. ROBERTS MC, KRESSEL HY, FALLON MD ET AL: Paget disease: MR imaging findings. Radiology 173:341, 1989

32. SCHIELE HP, HUBBARD RB, BRUCK HM: Radiographic changes in burns of the upper extremity. Radiology 104:13, 1972

33. SMITH SR, WILLIAMS CE, DAVIES JM ET AL: Bone marrow disorders: Characterization with quantitative MR imaging. Radiology 172:805, 1989

34. TISHLER JM: Soft tissue and bone changes in frostbite injury. Radiology 102:511, 1972

*Paul and Juhl's Essentials of Radiologic Imaging,
Sixth Edition*, edited by John H. Juhl and
Andrew B. Crummy. J.B. Lippincott Company,
Philadelphia, © 1993.

CHAPTER *8*

Normal Anatomic Variants and Miscellaneous Skeletal Anomalies

Lee F. Rogers

Unlike the congenital and genetic disorders described in Chapter 9, the anatomic variants and miscellaneous skeletal anomalies described here are encountered daily in the practice of radiology. A general familiarity with these structures and their variants is necessary to lessen concern, decrease confusion, and increase the accuracy and confidence of radiographic interpretation. Their importance lies in the fact that they can easily be misinterpreted as pathologic by those unfamiliar with them, when in reality they are of little or no clinical significance. The texts by Keats[14] and by Kohler and Zimmer[16] are excellent, thorough references devoted to this subject. It is difficult to conceive of practicing radiology without one or both of them close at hand. In this chapter, only the most common variants of the peripheral skeleton will be described. Many are found in the skull and spine and are covered in Chapters 11 and 12, respectively.

Miscellaneous skeletal anomalies are isolated, anomalous developments. In most cases, they are sporadic and nonfamilial. They may be considered as (1) supernumerary development; (2) a failure to develop; and (3) segmentation defects.

Supernumerary development is usually seen in the hands and feet as the development of an extra digit, polydactyly on either side of the hand or foot (Fig. 8-1). These may be sporadic or genetically determined and, at times, associated with malformation syndromes.

Failure to develop is usually either hypoplasia of a structure or, less commonly, aplasia. Hypoplasia is most commonly identified in the middle phalanx of the fifth digit and is known as clinodactyly (Fig. 8-2). This may be sporadic, familial, or associated with a whole host of congenital disorders. Hypoplasia and aplasia are most commonly encountered in the posterior elements of the spine, particularly in the pedicle and transverse process.

Defects of segmentation are quite frequent. They may consist of a fusion of segments, commonly encountered in the vertebrae as a partial or complete fusion of two or more vertebral bodies, described in Chapter 12. Fusion occurs less commonly in the carpal (Fig. 8-3) and tarsal bones. The fusion of tarsal bones is often symptomatic (see Figs. 8-39 and 8-40).

The failure of segments to fuse is most commonly encountered in the spine, involving the laminae and spinous processes. This failure of fusion is known as spina bifida. When seen as an isolated radiographic abnormality it is known as spina bifida occulta, but it may be associated with other congenital abnormalities of the spine, as described in Chapter 12.

Bifid structures may also occur. These may develop from a natural growth, as in the bifid anterior margin of ribs (Fig. 8-4), or from a failure of fusion of structures that arise from more than one center, most commonly in the sesamoids of the great toe (see Fig. 8-36). Certain apophyses and epiphyses arise from multiple centers of ossification, which eventually fuse in most cases. Multiple centers of ossification are seen in the proximal humerus and elbow. The trochlear center of ossification

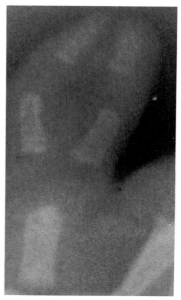

Figure 8–1. Duplication of the thumb in the newborn. Note the two separate and distinct distal and proximal phalanges, with fusion of the intervening soft tissues.

of the elbow itself may arise from separate centers, as may the epiphyses of the proximal phalanx of the great toe. Less commonly, individual carpal or tarsal bones arise from separate centers of ossification.

Accessory centers of ossification and accessory bones are found rather frequently in the skeleton (Figs. 8-6 and 8-7). An accessory bone represents either a supernumerary ossicle not ordinarily found in the skeleton or a secondary center of ossification that has failed to fuse and remains as a separate structure (Fig. 8-5). On occasion, they may predispose to injury or degenerative change and be responsible for symptoms.[18] This is often associated with a positive bone scan in the region of the abnormality. Sesamoid bones (Fig. 8-8) arise in tendons, particularly those of the feet, and are very similar in appearance to accessory centers of ossification. These small accessory bones and sesamoids may be mistaken for pathologic conditions, particularly fractures, and knowledge of their distribution and frequency is therefore important.

DIFFERENTIATION OF ANOMALOUS BONES FROM FRACTURES

A fracture line is ragged along its margin, irregular, and poorly defined. Anomalous ossification centers and sesamoids are characterized by smooth cortical mar-

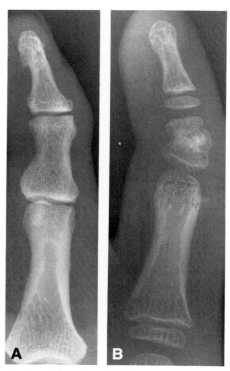

Figure 8–2. Clinodactyly in a 53-year-old father (**A**) and his 9-year-old son (**B**), an example of familial hypoplasia. The deformity was bilateral in both father and son. (**A**) The middle phalanx of the fifth digit is slightly shortened and curved inward. (**B**) The middle phalanx of the fifth digit is short and curved inward distally. The proximal epiphysis of the phalanx is already beginning to close. Compare with the epiphysis of the distal and proximal phalanx.

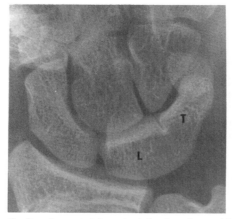

Figure 8–3. Lunatotriquetral fusion in a 13-year-old girl. The lunate (**L**) and triquetrum (**T**) are fused, with a small incomplete cleft between them distally.

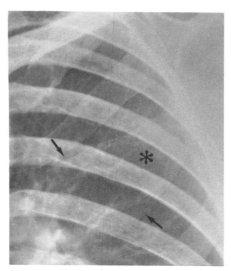

Figure 8–4. Bifid anterior third anterior left rib (*asterisk* and *arrows*).

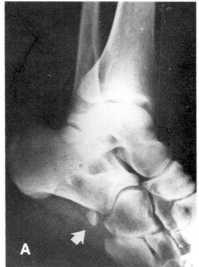

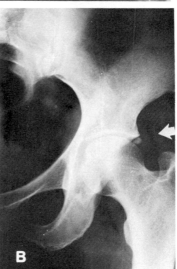

Figure 8–6. Two accessory ossicles. (**A**) Os peroneum. (**B**) Os acetabuli.

gins (Figs. 8-5, 8-6 and 8-8). An avulsion or small fracture will have an irregular, uncorticated surface at the line of fracture and a defect in the adjacent bone that corresponds to the avulsed fragment. Fresh fractures are accompanied by swelling of the contiguous soft tissue, which should not be present about an accessory center. Accessory centers and anomalous bones are commonly bilateral. Examination of the corresponding part of the opposite extremity is helpful in doubtful cases, but it is usually unnecessary. The precise diagnosis can usually be determined by reference to standard charts and diagrams (see Figs. 8-7 and 8-23).

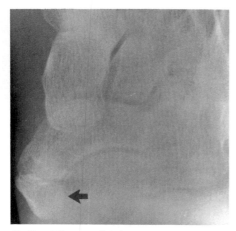

Figure 8–5. The os tibiale externum (*arrow*), adjacent to the proximal pole of the navicular.

NORMAL RADIOGRAPHIC FINDINGS CONFUSED WITH PATHOLOGY

Nutrient Canals and Foramina. Nutrient canals are present in all the long and short tubular bones. These are fine, sharply marginated radiolucencies that extend obliquely through the cortex, and they should not be mistaken for a fracture (Fig. 8-9). Nutrient canals are less radiolucent than a fracture and have a characteristic course. Nutrient foramina generally occur at the end of bones, presenting as a small circular radiolucency, and are seen most commonly at the intercondylar notch of the knee.

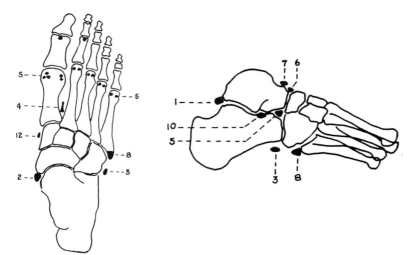

Figure 8–7. Common accessory ossicles in the foot: (**1**) os trigonum; (**2**) os tibiale externum; (**3**) os peroneum; (**4**) os intermetatarseum; (**5**) calcaneus secondarius; (**6**) supranavicular; (**7**) secondary astragalus; (**8**) os vesalianum; (**10**) os sustentaculi; (**12**) sesamoid tibiale anterius; (**S**) sesamoid bones (the small black dots over the metatarsal heads and proximal phalanges of first and second toes represent the most frequent sites of the sesamoid bones, but they may occur in other locations). There are no numbers **9** or **11** in this diagram.

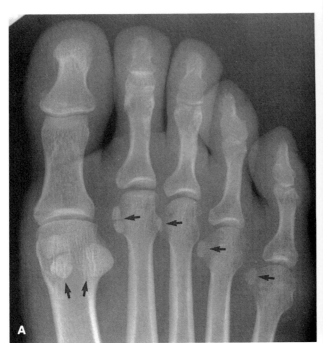
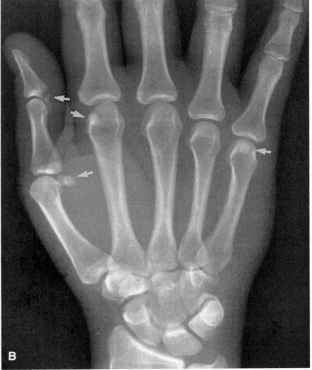

Figure 8–8. Sesamoid bones. (**A**) Feet. Sesamoid bones underlie the head of each metatarsal (*arrows*). There are two sesamoids on the great toe, a medial (tibial) sesamoid, and a lateral (fibular) sesamoid. The tibial sesamoid of the great toe and that of the second metatarsal are bifid, a common normal variant. Sesamoid bones are always present on the great toe and less commonly on the fifth. They are rarely encountered on the second, third, and fourth. Though unusual, the findings in this case are of no clinical significance. (**B**) Hands. Sesamoid bones are found in relation to the heads of the first, second, and fifth metacarpals (*arrows*). There is also a sesamoid at the base of the distal phalanx of the thumb (*arrow*). There are two sesamoids at the head of the first metacarpal. Sesamoid bones of the hand and feet lie within the anterior joint capsule.

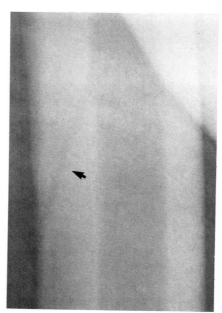

Figure 8–9. Lateral view of the proximal femur demonstrating a vascular groove in the posterior cortex (*arrow*). Note the slightly roughened but normal posterior surface of the cortex. This is known as the linea aspera and represents the site of the insertion of the adductor muscles.

Interosseous Ridges. Ossification of interosseous membranes occurs between the tibia and fibula and the radius and ulna. These are generally thin, slightly undulant, and smooth flanges of bone that may be mistaken for periostitis or periosteal new-bone formation (see Fig. 8-34). They are characteristically located on the apposing margins of the bones, although they may be more pronounced on one bone than the other. Ossification is more common on the diaphysis of the ulna and fibula and the proximal metaphysis of the tibia.

There are numerous osseous ridges and grooves at the site of muscular and ligamentous attachments. Many of these bony prominences are commonly encountered daily and dismissed without equivocation, such as the deltoid eminence of the humerus and linea aspera of the femur (see Fig. 8-29).

Irregular and Bifid Epiphyses. Certain ossification centers are often irregular in outline at some point during the course of development. This is particularly true of the distal femoral epiphysis (see Fig. 1-4B) in the child younger than 5 years of age. The trochlear ossification center at the elbow is similarly irregular.

Clefts may be seen in the epiphysis.[12] The basal epiphysis of the proximal phalanx of the great toe is the most frequent site, but clefts may occasionally be seen elsewhere and should not be mistaken for a fracture. Characteristically they are well margined, undisplaced, and have no surrounding soft-tissue swelling, allowing the distinction to be made with confidence.

Metaphyseal Spurs. Small spur-like projections are often encountered at the periphery of the metaphyses of both long and short bones in infants.[15] These are normal but might be mistaken for subtle evidence of injury or even child abuse by the unwary.

Epiphyseal Scars. For variable periods after closure of a physis, a fine radiodense line is present at the site, referred to as an epiphyseal scar. This is eventually resorbed and is usually no longer evident after the age of 40 years. Just after closure of a physis, there might be a slight irregular margin at the peripheral edge of the epiphysis, possibly suggesting a fracture. This is most commonly encountered at the lateral edge of the distal radius.

Bone Bars. In older individuals, after the onset of osteoporosis and on occasion earlier, groups of horizontally oriented large bone trabeculae may be encountered. When seen on edge, usually in the AP view, they present as a collection of punctate or increased densities; but when seen in profile on the lateral view, they are noted to represent elongated, horizontal bone trabeculae (Fig. 8-10). These are encountered in the phalanges, distal humerus, femoral shaft, proximal tibia, and occasionally elsewhere.[17] They are referred to as bone bars. Their significance is unknown.

SPECIFIC ANOMALIES AND NORMAL VARIANTS

RIBS

Bifid Ribs. The sternal end of a rib may be bifid or forked. The third and fourth ribs are most frequently affected (see Fig. 8-4).

Fenestrated First Rib. Fenestration of the first rib consists of a smooth, rounded opening in the anterior end of the rib. The significance of this deformity lies in the fact that it may be mistaken for a cavity in the lung in roentgenograms of the chest.

"Student's Tumor." The anterior chondral margin of the first rib is frequently irregularly calcified and easily mistaken by the unwary for a nodule or tumor mass within the lung (Fig. 8-11). An apical lordotic radio-

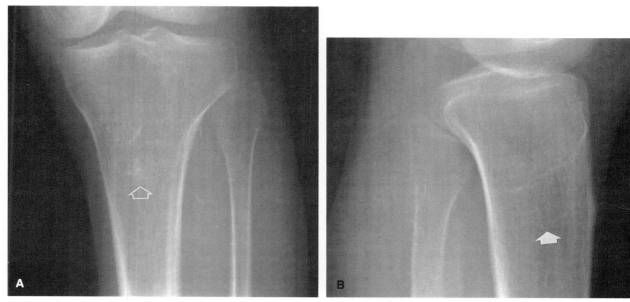

Figure 8–10.   Bone bars. (**A**) Anteroposterior (AP) view. The bright dots (*arrow*) of trabecular bone are even more dense than the cortex. This is a normal finding and should not be mistaken for evidence of bone infarction or chondroid calcification associated with an endochondroma. (**B**) Lateral view. The bright dots on the AP view are these elongated, horizontal, coarse trabeculae (*arrow*) seen on end. These are more commonly found in the osteopenic elderly at this site, the distal humerus and elsewhere.

graph of the chest should be obtained in doubtful cases to rule out the possibility of a true lung tumor. The irony is that underlying small lung cancers are sometimes obscured by calcification of the first rib.

Cervical Ribs. A small rib occasionally arises from the seventh cervical vertebra and is called a cervical rib (Fig. 8-12). It may occasionally give rise to a thoracic outlet syndrome and therefore may be of importance.

Hypoplastic Ribs. Hypoplasia of an entire length of a rib is sometimes encountered (Fig. 8-13). Hypoplasia most commonly involves the first or 12th rib but may be encountered elsewhere.

Fused Ribs. Occasionally the first and second ribs are fused anteriorly (Fig. 8-14). This is rarely of clinical significance.

Ununited Apophysis Transverse Process First Lumbar Vertebra

Occasionally the apophysis of the transverse process of first lumbar vertebra fails to unite (Fig. 8-15). This may occur unilaterally or bilaterally and rarely, if ever, occurs at other levels. It might easily be mistaken for a fracture or an abortive rib.

SHOULDER

Sprengel's Deformity. Sprengel's deformity also is known as congenital high scapula or congenital elevation of the scapula. The scapula is small, high in position, and rotated so that the inferior edge points toward the spine. The deformity may be unilateral or bilateral.

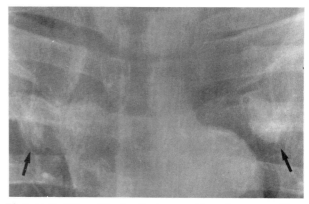

Figure 8–11.   Student's tumor. Prominent ossification in the cartilaginous ends of the first ribs (*arrow*). These are easily misconstrued as tumors in the underlying lung.

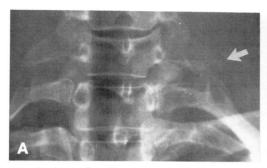
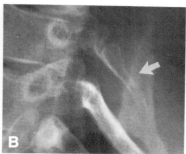

Figure 8–12. Cervical rib. (**A**) The transverse process of C7 is usually prominent, as seen on this case on the right. The cervical rib extends from this transverse process in a manner similar to the thoracic ribs, as seen on the left (*arrow*). (**B**) The cervical rib is better seen in the oblique view (*arrow*).

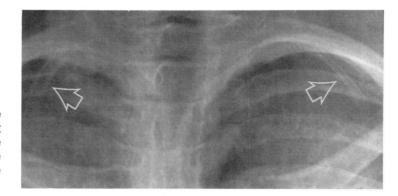

Figure 8–13. Hypoplastic first ribs. The first rib is hypoplastic bilaterally (*arrows*). It is often difficult to determine whether there is a hypoplastic first rib or a cervical rib. The distinction is made by simply counting the ribs on both sides.

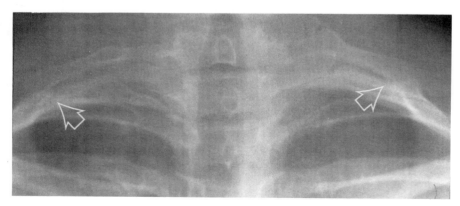

Figure 8–14. Fusion of the first and second ribs bilaterally (*arrows*).

A fusion of the cervical and upper thoracic vertebrae, the Klippel-Feil syndrome, is present in practically all cases (Fig. 8-16). This fusion anomaly may exist, however, without elevation of the scapula. In some cases there is a bony connection between the elevated scapula and either the fifth or sixth cervical vertebra. This bony connection is known as the omovertebral bone. It may join the scapula and the vertebrae by either bony or fibrous union (Fig. 8-17).

Pseudocyst of the Humeral Head. A normal area of rarefaction or lucency may be located in the lateral aspect of the proximal humerus, within the greater tuberosity (Fig. 8-18).[25] This may be prominent, on

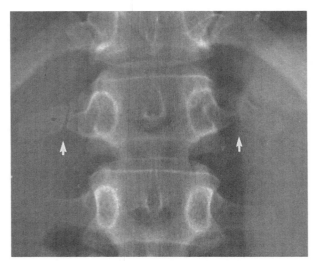

Figure 8–15. Ununited apophyses of the transverse processes of L–1. The transverse processes are not united with the main body of the vertebra (*arrows*). Note that the medial borders of the transverse processes are slightly rounded and faintly sclerotic as are the opposing margins of the base of the transverse processes. The sclerotic margin distinguishes this from a fracture. These may be either unilateral or bilateral.

occasion, and can be mistaken for a site of metastatic disease or other abnormality.

Deltoid Tubercle. The insertion of the deltoid muscle on the lateral surface of the proximal humerus normally projects as a flat cortical elevation.

Humeral Epiphyseal Line. The proximal humeral epiphysis arises from two centers, which usually fuse by 6 years of age. When viewed in the frontal projection with the shoulder in external rotation, the anterior aspect of the growth plate is chevron shaped, whereas the posterior portion of the line is transverse and may be mistaken for a fracture (Fig. 8-19).

Apophyses of the Coracoid and Acromion. In early adolescence, a flake-like ossification center appears at the superior aspect of the coracoid and the lateral margin of the acromion. These are normal ossification centers, which might be mistaken for fractures.

Rhomboid Fossa. The pectoralis insertion on the medial inferior margin of the clavicle is sometimes associated with a shallow, occasionally irregular marginal defect known as the rhomboid fossa (Fig. 8-20). This is often bilateral.

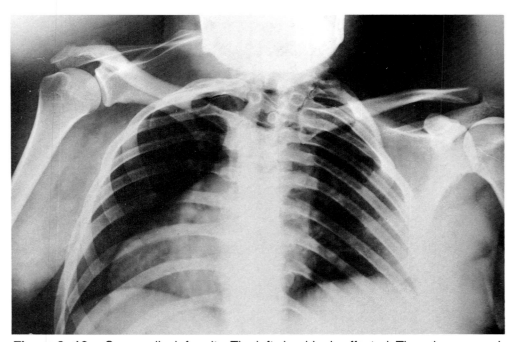

Figure 8–16. Sprengel's deformity. The left shoulder is affected. There is an associated abnormality of ossification of the cervical and upper thoracic vertebrae, with irregular segments fused together (Klippel–Feil deformity). These deformities frequently coexist.

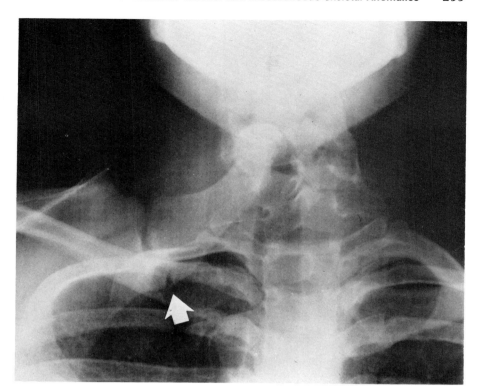

Figure 8–17. The omovertebral bone in association with Sprengel's deformity. The bone forms an articulation with the scapula (*arrow*) and the arch of one of the cervical vertebrae.

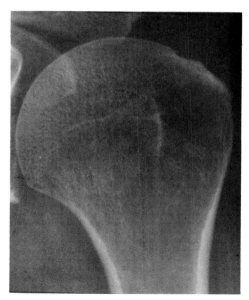

Figure 8–18. Pseudocyst of the humeral head. A radiolucency is present within the greater tuberosity because of the relative absence of bone trabeculae. This is a frequent normal finding that is easily mistaken for evidence of metastatic disease or other abnormalities (see Fig. 8-34).

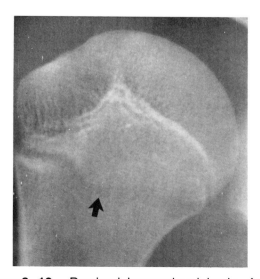

Figure 8–19. Proximal humeral epiphysis. Anteriorly the growth plate is chevron shaped, whereas posteriorly it is transverse (*arrow*) and could be misconstrued as a fracture.

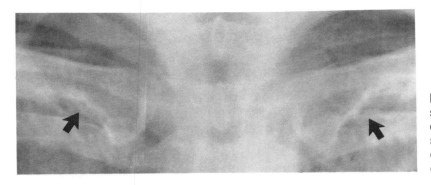

Figure 8–20. Rhomboid fossa. The scalloped inferior margin of the medial clavicle (*arrows*) represents the site of insertion of the pectoralis muscles. It is present bilaterally in this case but may be seen unilaterally.

Foramen for the Supraclavicular Nerve. A small radiolucency is sometimes seen in the superior cortex of the midclavicle (Fig. 8-21).

ELBOW

Supracondylar Process of the Humerus. A hook-like bony projection may arise from the metaphysis of the medial surface of the distal humerus, curving inferiorly (Fig. 8-22). The projection may be mistaken for an osteochondroma. It is presumed to represent an atavistic trait and is said to be found in 2% of Scandinavians.

HAND AND WRIST

Accessory Centers of Ossification. There are several reported accessory centers of ossification in the wrist and hand, but they are much less common than those in the foot. The most important ones are shown in Figure 8-23.

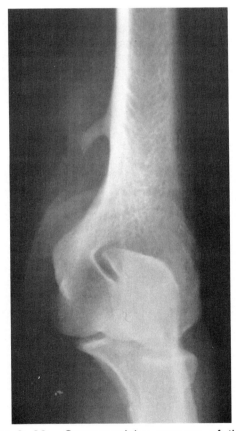

Figure 8–22. Supracondylar process of the humerus. There is a hook-like projection of cortical bone arising from the medial surface of the distal shaft of the humerus. This is the characteristic location and position of the supracondylar process, which should not be mistaken for an exostosis.

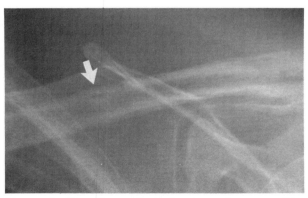

Figure 8–21. Supraclavicular nerve foramen. The small lucency in the superior cortex of the middle third of the clavicle (*arrow*) represents a foramen for the supraclavicular nerve.

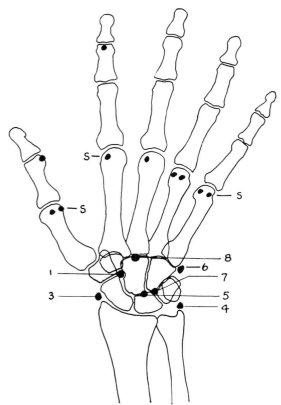

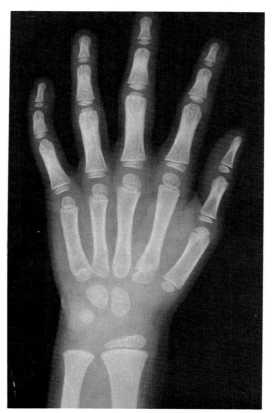

Figure 8–23. The most frequent accessory ossicles in the hand and wrist: (**1**) os centrale, (**3**) os radiale externum, (**4**) os triangulare, (**5**) epilunatum, (**6**) os vesalianum manus, (**7**) epipyramis, (**8**) os styloideum, (**S**) the most frequent sites for sesamoid bones in the hand. Number **2** is not included.

Figure 8–24. Pseudoepiphyses and supernumerary epiphyses. The former are represented by incomplete clefts in the distal ends of proximal phalanges and proximal end of the fifth metacarpal. The latter are present at the proximal end of the second and fifth metacarpals and the distal end of the first metacarpal.

Divided Scaphoid (Navicular). The carpal scaphoid may be found in two parts with a transverse fissure through the center. It is difficult to determine whether this is an anomaly or an old ununited fracture since fractures of this bone are notorious for their failure to unite. Eburnation of edges, roughness, and cystlike areas along the line of the fissure favor the diagnosis of an ununited fracture. When the fissure is the result of an anomaly, the bone is otherwise normal.

Pseudoepiphyses for the Metacarpals and Metatarsals. Partial cartilaginous clefts may appear in the proximal ends of one or more of the lateral four metacarpals or the distal end of the first metacarpal or metatarsal where normally no epiphyses are found.[23] Less frequently the clefts are complete, in which case they are termed supernumerary epiphyses (Fig. 8-24).

Clinodactyly. Clinodactyly refers to curvature of a finger in the plane of the hand. It may involve any finger, but the usual pattern is radial deviation of the fifth finger at the distal interphalangeal joint associated with a short middle phalanx, shorter on its radial than on its ulnar side (see Fig. 8-2). Most persons are otherwise normal; however, clinodactyly is also found in a wide variety of disorders, including Down's syndrome.[23]

Madelung's Deformity. Madelung's deformity is a chondrodysplasia of the distal radial epiphysis. Some investigators believe that this deformity is a minimal form of the dysplasia known as dyschondrosteosis (see Chap. 9); others believe that it can occur as an isolated deformity without other osseous stigmata.[9] It causes a curvature of the shaft of the radius, resulting in a deformity of the hand at the wrist and giving the appearance of an anterior dislocation of the hand. The reverse type also is seen but is very rare. The lesion is usually bilateral and is first noticed at about the beginning of adolescence.

The characteristic roentgenographic findings include shortening of the radius in comparison to the length of the ulna and a lateral and dorsal curvature of the radius (Fig. 8-25). There is early fusion of the radial epiphysis on the internal or ulnar side. This results in a tilting of the radial articular surface internally and anteriorly. The epiphysis develops a triangular shape. Because the radius fails to grow properly in length, the distal radioulnar articulation is disrupted and the lower end of the ulna projects posterior to the radius. The deformity of the radial articular surface leads to a derangement in the alignment of the carpal bones. The carpus assumes a triangular configuration, with the apex pointing toward the radius and ulna and the base formed by the carpometacarpal articulations.

Lunatotriquetral Fusion. Fusion of the lunate and triquetrum is encountered in approximately 2% of Africans and less commonly in Caucasians (see Fig. 8-3).[23] It is the most common carpal fusion and, when isolated, is of no clinical significance.

Os Styloideum. The os styloideum is an accessory center of ossification arising at the base of the second metacarpal and is visualized on the lateral view (see Fig. 8-20). Occasionally, an unmovable bony protuberance is located on the dorsum of the wrist at the base of the second and third metacarpals, adjacent to the capitate and trapezoid bones. This has been referred to as a "carpal boss."[6] It may represent either degenerative osteophyte formation at the metacarpal joint or the presence of an os styloideum (Fig. 8-26). Patients may complain of pain and limitation of motion of the hand.

PELVIS AND HIP

Os Acetabuli. The os acetabuli is a round or oval ossicle lying along the upper rim of the acetabulum (see Fig. 8-6B). There is normally an apophyseal center or centers for the upper rim of the acetabulum that appear at about the age of 13 and fuse with the acetabulum within a very short time. Failure to unite results in the formation of an os acetabuli. In other instances, a small sesamoid may be found in this area, usually situated more laterally than the apophysis but called by the same name.

Diastasis of Pubic Bones. Diastasis of pubic bones is ordinarily found in association with exstrophy of the bladder, epispadius, and other lower urinary tract anomalies. It may also be associated with cleidocranial dysostosis (see Chap 9). However, it has also been reported in a family with no other anomalies.[26]

Pubic Synchondrosis. The pubic synchondrosis is the site of fusion of the inferior ramus of the pubis and ischium and is located medially on the obturator fora-

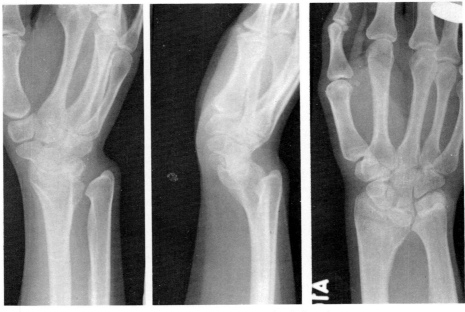

Figure 8–25. Madelung's deformity.

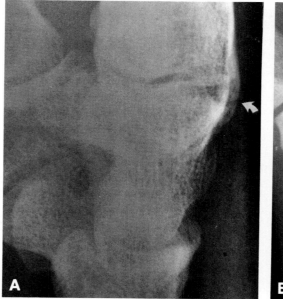
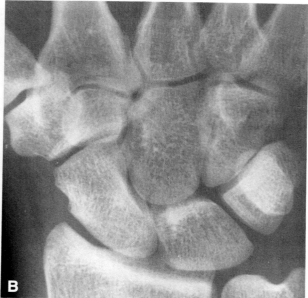

Figure 8–26. Carpal boss with os styloideum (*arrow*). (**A**) Lateral view. (**B**) Posteroanterior (PA) view. Bony prominence dorsally at the base of the second metacarpal as seen on the dorsum of the wrist (*arrow*) is not easily identified on the PA view. It is often difficult to determine on the plain films whether this is simply a bony protuberance or a separate ossicle, the os styloideum.

men (Fig. 8-27). The synchondrosis is often expansile and may be confused for a pathologic condition. It is usually most prominent about the age of 10 years.

Herniation Pit of the Femoral Neck. A round or oval radiolucency surrounded by a thin rim of sclerosis is often identified in the proximal, superior aspect of the femoral neck in adults (Fig. 8-28).[22] The radiolucency represents a cortical depression or cavity formed by the herniation of capsular soft tissues through defects in the cortex. This "herniation pit" is a normal finding.

Femoral Linea Aspera-Pilaster Complex. Frontal radiographs of the femur commonly demonstrate two longitudinally oriented, thin, parallel lines projected over the middle third of the shaft (Fig. 8-29).[21] These lines, called the "track sign," represent the site of insertion of the strong adductor and extensor muscles of the thigh. When seen in the lateral view, the surface of the linea aspera is often rough, undulant, and irregular. This may suggest periosteal reaction but is, in fact, a normal finding.

THE KNEE

Bipartite Patella. The patella may be divided into two or even more segments (see Fig. 2-60C and D). The smaller segment or segments are usually located

along the upper outer quadrant of the patella. These may be mistaken for fractures. In approximately 80% of the cases, the anomaly is bilateral. Flake-like ossification centers also appear on the anterior and occasionally on the inferior surface of the patella. These are likewise normal.

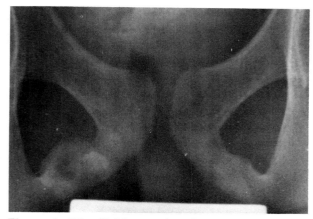

Figure 8–27. Pubic synchondrosis in a 12-year-old. This represents the junction of the inferior ischial and pubic rami. The pattern of ossification is highly variable, often asymmetrical, and easily misinterpreted.

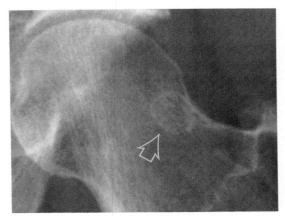

Figure 8–28. Herniation pit of the femoral neck. Note the circular sclerotic radiodensity on the lateral margin of the femoral neck (*arrow*). In some cases, the pit may be smaller and the rim of sclerosis thicker.

Fabella. The fabella is a small sesamoid bone that is very frequently found in the tendon of the lateral head of the gastrocnemius muscle at the level of the knee joint (see Fig. 8-29B). It may become enlarged and roughened in the presence of degenerative disease of the knee joint.

Physiologic Bowlegs of Infancy. During early infancy, a mild degree of bowleg deformity is physiologic.[27] It has been suggested that this bowing is the result of the normal internal tibial torsion that occurs during intrauterine life. This type of bowleg deformity tends to correct itself, and usually the legs have become perfectly straight by the time the child has reached the age of 4 to 5 years.

Occasionally the bowing is accentuated to the point where it may be considered abnormal (Fig. 8-30) and the result of disease, particularly rickets or Blount's tibia vara. Differentiation from rickets can be made with assurance in most cases because the metaphyses are well ossified and none of the other findings seen in active rickets are present. It may not be possible to rule out the possibility of rickets that has healed, but, since this type of bowing usually comes to the attention of the physician during the first months or year of life, there seldom will have been time for rickets to have been present and to have undergone complete healing. Differentiation from Blount's tibia vara may be more difficult.

Tibia Vara, Blount's Disease (Osteochondrosis Deformans Tibiae). Blount's disease is an infrequent cause of bowlegs during infancy and childhood. Its cause is uncertain, but it often is classified with the

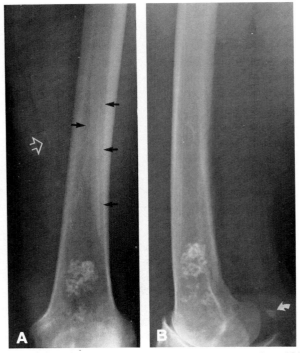

Figure 8–29. Linea aspera—pilaster complex. **(A)** The two long roughly parallel lines (*arrows*) represent the margins of the pilaster complex on the posterior surface of the femur. This represents the site of insertion of the adductor muscles of the thigh. Calcification is present in the femoral artery (*open arrow*), and distally there is the conglomeration of calcium representing either an enchondroma or the residuals of previous bone infarct. **(B)** Lateral view. Note the roughened surface of the posterior femoral cortex. This is the appearance of the pilaster complex or linea aspera when seen in profile. It is normal but might be misconstrued as evidence of periosteal new-bone formation. Note the fabella (*arrow*).

osseous dysplasias. The possibility of ischemic necrosis as a causative factor has been considered by some investigators. A progressive, nonrachitic outward bowing of the legs is the characteristic clinical finding. The medial aspect of the upper tibial metaphysis is evidently the site of partial growth arrest, resulting in medial flangelike broadening of the metaphysis in addition to shortening. This causes a rather sharp posteromedial slope of the medial tibial plateau. The amount of varus deformity depends on the angle of this slope.

The deformity actually is an angular one rather than a curved bowing, and is centered at the junction of the proximal tibial epiphysis and metaphysis (Fig. 8-31).

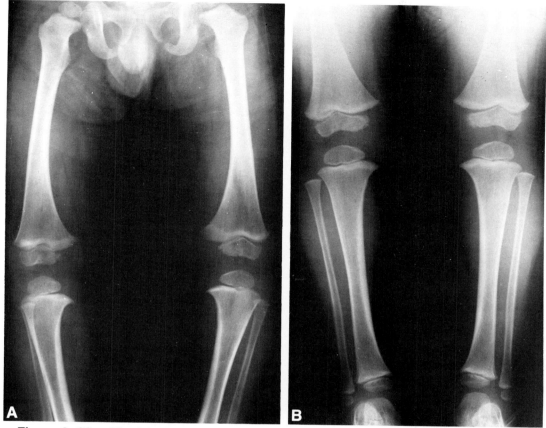

Figure 8–30. Physiologic bowlegs. (**A**) Initial views demonstrate moderate bowleg deformity. (**B**) Approximately one year later, the bowing has largely disappeared. Note that the bowing involves both femur and tibia.

Tibia vara must be differentiated from physiologic bowlegs. In tibia vara, the angular deformity is centered at the junction of the proximal metaphysis and epiphysis of the tibia. There is a broad, beak-like projection of the inner side of the metaphysis within which are small islands of cartilage, and the tibial epiphysis tends to be triangular with the apex pointing medially. In physiologic bowing, both the tibia and femur are affected, the femur often showing more deformity than the tibia.

Irregular Ossification Distal Femoral Epiphyses. Before age 5, the distal femoral ossification center is often irregular in outline (see Fig. 1-4B). This is a normal variant. In later adolescence, an irregular center of ossification often appears in the posterior margin of both condyles. This is likewise normal but is readily mistaken for osteochondritis dissecans. However, the latter occurs on the lateral margin of the medial femoral condyle anteriorly.

Pelligrini-Stieda Disease. Pelligrini-Stieda disease is an irregular calcification that appears on the superior margin of the medial femoral condyle. It is most likely related to previous injury of the medial collateral ligament (Fig. 8-32).

Cortical Desmoid. The adductor magnus and medial head of the gastrocnemius insert on the posterior superior junction of the condyles and metaphysis of the distal femur, often accompanied by radiographic evidence of cortical irregularity (Fig. 8-33).[24] This is a normal variant that may easily be misinterpreted as something sinister, such as a malignancy or infection.

The Soleal Line. A prominent ridge of bone along the origin of the soleus muscle in the proximal tibia as seen on the lateral projection may mimic periosteal reaction along the posterior margin of the proximal tibial shaft.[20] The underlying cortical bone is normal.

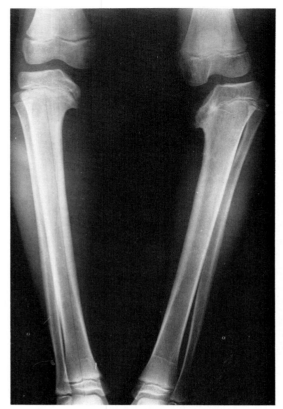

Figure 8–31. Blount's disease. There is bilateral involvement, with an angular deformity at the physis. The tibial shafts are straight and the femurs uninvolved.

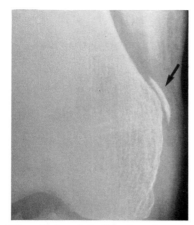

Figure 8–32. Pellegrini–Stieda disease. A thin, shell-like calcification at the superior margin of the medial femoral condyle (*arrow*).

to which the talofibular ligament is attached. Its shape varies from a small triangular fragment to one more rounded or oval. The division from the talus may be incomplete. A fracture of the posterior process of the talus may resemble an os trigonum.

Os Tibiale Externum. The unfused tuberosity on the medial proximal side of the tarsal navicular (scaphoid) is called the os tibiale externum (see Fig. 8-5). It is sometimes called the divided scaphoid or an accessory scaphoid. It is a common variation and is usually bilateral.

On the frontal projection, it is seen as a thin, obliquely oriented vertical band of sclerosis traversing the upper tibia (Fig. 8-34).

Tibial Tubercle. On the proximal medial metaphysis of the tibia, there is often a thin, smoothly defined flange of bone projecting into the interosseous space (Fig. 8-34A). This might be mistaken for periosteal new-bone formation, but it actually represents ossification at the base of the interosseous membrane.

ANKLE AND FOOT

The foot is a common site for accessory bones and sesamoids (see Fig. 8-7). The most frequent of these are described in the paragraphs that follow.

Os Trigonum. The accessory ossicle known as the os trigonum occurs in about 10% of individuals. It is a separate center for the posterior process of the talus,

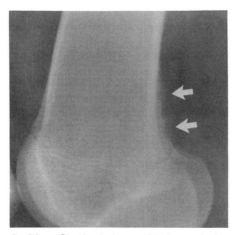

Figure 8–33. Cortical desmoid. Irregularity of the surface of the cortex of the distal femur (*arrows*) at the site of the insertion of the adductor magnus and gastrocnemius muscles.

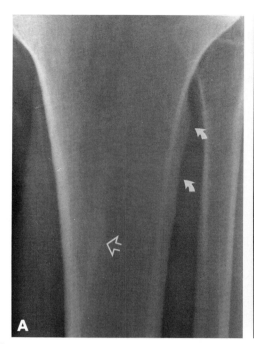
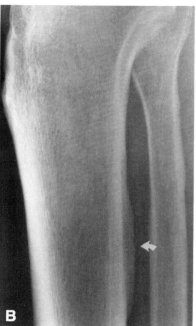

Figure 8–34.   Tibial tubercle and soleal line. (**A**) Anteroposterior view. Prominent ossification of the interosseous membrane on the lateral surface of the tibia (*arrows*) is known as the tibial tubercle. This is commonly present but is of variable size. A similar ossification is present on the apposing margin of the fibula. The soleal line is seen on edge as an oblique line projecting in the medullary canal (*open arrow*). (**B**) Lateral view. The soleal line is seen on the posterior surface of the tibial cortex (*arrow*). This might be misconstrued as evidence of periosteal new-bone formation associated with infection or stress fracture. The tibial tubercle cannot be seen on the lateral projection.

Os Peroneum (Peroneal Sesamoid). The os peroneum is a small ossicle found in or adjacent to the tendon of the peroneus longus, just lateral to and below the os calcis and cuboid (see Fig. 8-6*A*). It occurs in about 8% of persons. Occasionally there may be two or even three separate ossicles representing a bipartite or tripartite sesamoid.

Os Intermetatarseum. The os intermetatarseum is a small bone that has the form of a tiny rudimentary metatarsal and is found between the proximal ends of the first and second metatarsals. Its frequency is about 10%.

Calcaneus Secondarius. The secondary os calcis is a small, irregular bony mass found at the tip of the anterior process of the os calcis, where it articulates with the navicular. It is seen to best advantage in oblique roentgenograms of the foot. Its frequency is about 2%.

Supranavicular. The supranavicular is a small, triangular bone occurring at the proximal superior edge of the navicular and articulating with the talus and navicular. It is relatively common and can easily be mistaken for a fracture.

Secondary Astragalus. A small, rounded bone found just above the head of the talus, seen only in lateral views of the foot, is the secondary astragalus. It should not be confused with the supranavicular, which lies between the talus and navicular.

Os Vesalianum. A rare accessory bone found just proximal to the head of the fifth metatarsal is the os vesalianum. It should not be mistaken for the lateral apophysis of the metatarsal head, which is a normal finding (see below).

Apophysis at the Base of the Fifth Metatarsal. An apophysis that appears in individuals at about the age of 13 years and unites shortly thereafter is a flat bony center found along the lateral side of the proximal end of the fifth metatarsal (Fig. 8-35). It often is irregular in shape, but its long axis parallels the long axis of the metatarsal. A fracture in this location is also common (Fig. 8-35), but the line of fracture invariably extends transversely across the long axis of the shaft. The fracture surfaces are irregular, the soft tissues overlying the area are swollen, and the proximal fragment often is displaced or rotated.

Os Subtibiale. The os subtibiale is a separate ossification center for the tip of the medial malleolus.

Os Subfibulare. Corresponding to the subtibiale, the os subfibulare is a separate center for the tip of the lateral malleolus. It varies from a tiny, rounded ossicle to a fairly large triangular fragment. It is best seen in anteroposterior views of the ankle joint.

Some of these apparent accessory ossicles around the ankle joint may be old chip fracture fragments that have smoothed off and have united with fibrous rather than bony union. Others may be foci of ossification that have formed as a result of soft-tissue injury. It often is impossible to determine their precise origin from a single roentgenographic examination.

Bifid Sesamoids. The sesamoids of the great toe are commonly bipartite, particularly the tibial or medial sesamoid, which is bifid in 10% of cases. The fibular or lateral sesamoid is bifid in approximately 3% (Fig. 8-36).

Pseudocyst of the Calcaneus. A lucency is frequently encountered in the body of the calcaneus just beneath the tuber angle on lateral radiographs of the foot (Fig. 8-37). It is simply an area relatively devoid of trabeculae and of no clinical significance. Rarely, a lipoma, a simple bone cyst, or other tumor arises in this region. However, in contrast to a normal pseudocyst, they are usually sharply defined by a rim of sclerotic bone.

CONGENITAL SYNOSTOSIS

A congenital synostosis consists of a fusion of two or more bones. It is a frequent anomaly in the thorax, where there may be a partial fusion of several of the

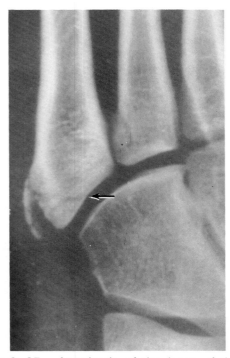

Figure 8–35. Apophysis of the base of the fifth metatarsal. The secondary ossification center parallels the lateral aspect of the proximal end of the metatarsal. In this case, there is also an undisplaced transverse fracture (*arrow*) at the base of the fifth metacarpal.

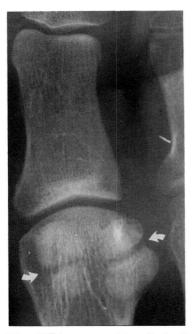

Figure 8–36. Bifid sesamoids. Both the medial and lateral sesamoids of the great toe are bifid (*arrows*).

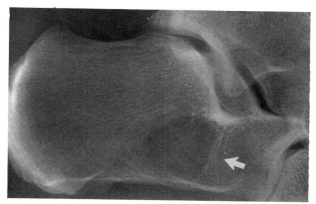

Figure 8–37. Pseudocyst of the calcaneus. The relative radiolucency beneath the tuber angle (*arrow*) represents an area devoid of trabeculae. This is a normal finding and is similar to the pseudocyst of the humeral head seen in Figure 8-18.

ribs. This may affect any part of the rib, but it is more frequent in the lateral portions and at the vertebral ends (see Fig. 8-14).

The proximal ends of the tibia and fibula occasionally are fused. Another uncommon site of fusion is at the proximal ends of the radius and ulna, resulting in an inability to supinate the forearm. In some cases, there is an associated dislocation of the head of the radius (Fig. 8-38).

Carpal and Tarsal Fusions. Fusions have been found in almost every combination in the carpal and metacarpal regions and in the corresponding portion of the foot. The fusions can be fibrous, cartilaginous, or osseous.

Carpal fusions may be sporadic or hereditary. Lunatotriquetral fusion is the most common (see Fig. 8-3). In general, fusions between bones in the same carpal row are of less significance than those that occur between the carpal rows, the latter being frequently associated with other, often clinically significant, congenital abnormalities and encountered in congenital malformation syndromes.[23]

Congenital fusion of tarsal bones is commonly referred to as a tarsal coalition. The unusual rigidity of the fused joints may cause pain. The condition is often referred to as "peroneal spastic flatfoot" or "rigid flatfoot." The latter term is preferred, since the rigidity of the tarsus is the result of a bony fixation and not spasm. In many cases, the clinical presentation suggests the correct diagnosis. Fusion may occur at any point between two bones but is most frequent between the calcaneus and navicular.

Radiographic verification is important. Calcaneonavicular coalition can often be recognized in conven-

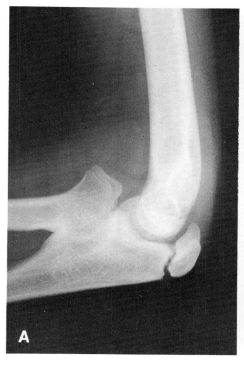
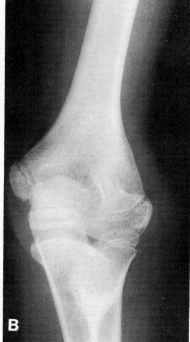

Figure 8–38. Congenital radioulnar synostosis with congenital dislocation of the head of the radius. There is bony fusion between the proximal radius and the ulna.

A

B

tional radiographs of the foot (Fig. 8-39). However, talocalcaneal coalition is frequently difficult to demonstrate radiographically, and special views supplemented by bone scintigraphy, tomography, and CT may be necessary to demonstrate the site of coalition (Fig. 8-40*B*).[5, 7, 10, 19]

Talocalcaneal fusion is often associated with a prominent beak on the anterior, superior margin of the head of the talus (Fig. 8-40*A*). Irregularity and a lack of definition of the posterior subtalar joint are indirect signs of talocalcaneal coalition. The coalition almost invariably occurs at the medial facet, between the talus and sustentaculum tali of the calcaneus, a joint not easily demonstrated by routine radiography. Individuals who have clinical signs and radiographic findings suggestive of coalition should have a CT scan performed. Bone scanning may demonstrate a focal increase in radionuclide activity in the region of the coalition or in the talar beak and posterior facet of the subtalar joint. Coronal CT in the axial plane demonstrates the site and nature of the fusion quite satisfactorily and at the same time allows comparison with the opposite side (Figs. 8-40*C* and 8-40*D*).

CONGENITAL DISLOCATION OF THE HIP

The hip is the most frequent site of congenital dislocation. It is six to ten times more common in girls than in boys, the left hip is involved more often than the right in the ratio of 3 to 2, and it is much more frequent in whites than in blacks. It is unusual for dislocation to be present at birth, displacement occurring gradually during the first year of life. It was formerly believed that faulty development of the hip joint and associated structures was responsible for the dislocation, referred to as "acetabular dysplasia." Most investigators now consider the fault to be in the supporting soft tissues of the hip joint, with the primary abnormality being a relaxation of the joint capsule.[3] Others consider shortening or tightening of the muscles that cross the joint to be the primary cause.

The diagnosis of the predislocation stage during the newborn period is important, since early treatment prevents the ultimate dislocation and results in a normal hip joint. The Ortolani maneuver of 45° of abduction and internal rotation of the leg is useful in detecting hips that are susceptible to dislocation. With this maneuver, the examiner feels a "click" as the hip dislocates.

Roentgenographic Features. Roentgenographic examination of the hips for a suspected hip joint dislocation should include an anteroposterior roentgenogram of the pelvis (Fig. 8-41) obtained with the patient's legs straight or slightly flexed at the knee and with the toes pointing forward. A so-called "frog" view is also included (Fig. 8-42). In this position, the thighs are flexed, externally rotated and maximally abducted, with the feet brought together in the midline. Careful positioning is necessary to make certain that the hips are symmetrically placed so that one side can be compared with the other.

Increased Acetabular Angle. The acetabular angle is a measurement of the slope of the upper half of the acetabular wall. The method of measurement is shown in Figure 8-41. Observations of Caffey and his associates, based on the measurement of a large number of infants, indicate that the normal angles vary widely and that the upper limit of normal should be close to 40°.[3] They also found that the acetabular angle for the left hip is usually slightly larger than for the right. The normal angle decreases considerably between birth and the age of 6 months and to a lesser degree between the ages of 6 months and 1 year. These observations indicate that considerable caution should be exercised in the diagnosis of hip joint dysplasia based only on the finding of an acetabular angle that measures more than 30°. When one hip is affected, the acetabular angle is a more useful indicator than when both are involved, and a definite discrepancy in the angles on the two sides is an important finding.

Lateral Displacement of the Femur. Lateral displacement of the femur in relation to the acetabulum is

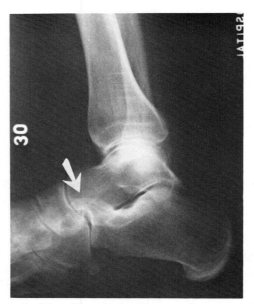

Figure 8–39. Tarsal coalition, calcaneonavicular bar (*arrow*).

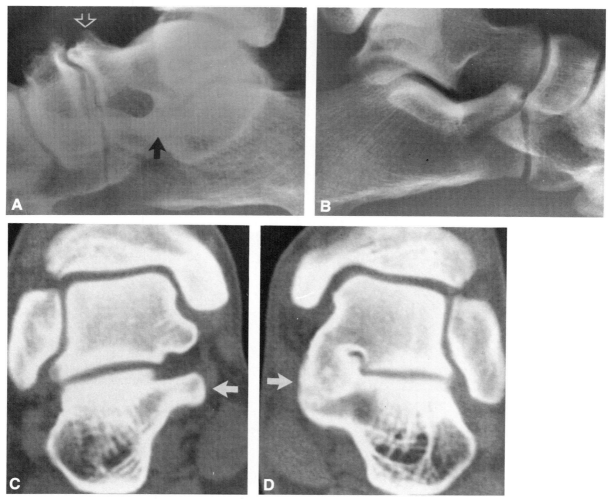

Figure 8–40. Tarsal coalition, talocalcaneal fusion. (**A**) Lateral view of the foot demonstrates pes planus, a prominent anterior beak of the talus (*open arrow*), and poor definition of the posterior facet of the talocalcaneal joint. There is a suggestion of fusion of the medial facet in the region of the sustentaculum tali (*arrow*). (**B**) Normal side for comparison. (**C** and **D**) Computed axial tomograms. (**C**) Normal side demonstrating normal appearance of sustentaculum tali (*arrow*). (**D**) Fusion of the medial facet of the talocalcaneal joint (*arrow*).

an important finding. Because the ossification center for the head of the femur is not present at birth and does not appear normally until the age of 3 to 6 months, the neck of the femur must be used for this determination in the newborn. Perkin's line, as shown in Figure 8-41, is useful when either one or both hips are involved. This consists of a vertical line drawn from the upper outer edge of the iliac portion of the acetabulum to intersect at a right angle the transverse line drawn through the centers of both acetabula. Caffey found that the beak of the femoral neck normally fell medial

to this line in practically every case, whereas in the majority of abnormal hips (60%) the femoral neck was situated lateral to this line.[3]

Disruption of Shenton's Line. Shenton's line is a smooth, curved imaginary line formed by the inner margin of the femoral neck and the inner surface of the obturator foramen, as shown in Figure 8-41. Lateral displacement of the femur disrupts the smooth curve. Some degree of upward displacement is usually required before a significant break in the curve is seen.

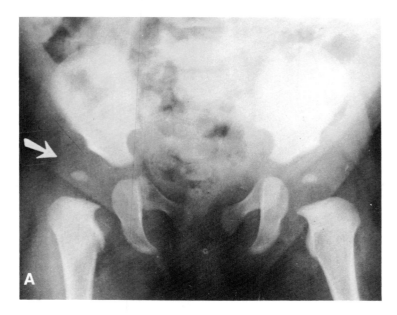

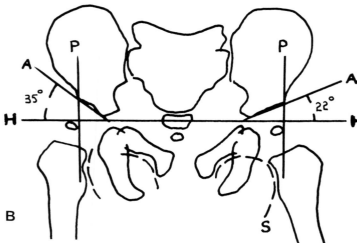

Figure 8–41. Congenital dislocation of the right hip in an infant. (**A**) Roentgenogram of the pelvis. (**B**) Tracing illustrating the method for determining the acetabular angle. Line **A** drawn along the upper margin of the acetabulum represents the bony roof of the fossa, although in an infant the acetabulum is composed largely of cartilage. Line **H** is drawn through the centers of the triradiate cartilages of the acetabular fossae. The vertical lines **P** are drawn through the outer limits of the bony margin of the acetabular roof of either side, perpendicular to the **H** line. The acetabular angle is larger on the right than on the left; however, this difference is not entirely diagnostic. The right capital femoral epiphysis is displaced laterally and very slightly superiorly. The curved broken line **S,** or Shenton's line, is disrupted on the right and normal on the left.

Delayed Ossification of the Femoral Epiphysis. The ossification center for the head of the femur normally appears between the ages of 3 to 6 months. In the presence of hip joint subluxation or dislocation, the center may be delayed in appearance, and, when it does appear, its growth lags behind normal (Fig. 8-42).

Later Stages. In older children and in adults, gross displacement is usually present and the diagnosis is made without difficulty (Fig. 8-43). In untreated subjects, the head and neck of the femur do not develop properly, remaining small and hypoplastic. The ace-

tabular fossa is very shallow, never having accommodated the femoral head. The head often impinges against the outer pelvic wall above and behind the shallow acetabulum and forms a shallow pseudoacetabular cavity.

Recognition in the Newborn. Diagnosis of congenital dislocation of the hip is principally based on clinical findings. In the newborn, the standard radiographic features described above in the older infant are not applicable. At this stage, it would be necessary to obtain an AP examination of the pelvis and hips with the legs in the Ortolani position—that is, abducted 45°

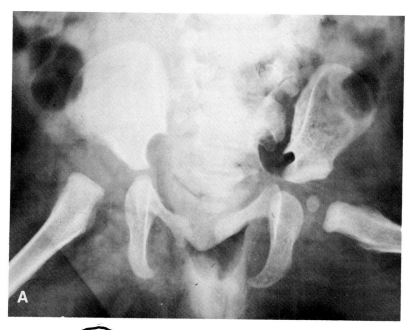

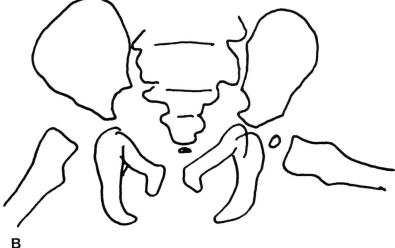

Figure 8–42. Congenital dislocation of the hip illustrated in the frog-leg position, with the thighs abducted and externally rotated. Note the absence of an ossified center for the right capital epiphysis, the poorly developed acetabular roof on this side, and an increased acetabular angle. The position of the femoral neck indicates the subluxation, even though the femoral head is not visible. The patient also had an extensive spina bifida in the lower lumbar and sacral spine. (**A**) Roentgenogram of the pelvis. (**B**) Tracing of the roentgenogram.

and internally rotated.[8] In this position, a line bisecting the femoral shaft should pass through the acetabulum and the lumbosacral articulation. In the presence of a dislocation, the line will pass laterally to both structures. Care should be taken that the line bisects the shaft and not the femoral neck, as this would give a false reading.

Computed Tomography. CT is a useful technique in the study of congenital dislocation of the hip, particularly in those cases in which there has been a failure to

obtain or maintain a reduction of the dislocated hip.[2, 13] In such cases, the iliopsoas tendon can interpose between the femoral head and the acetabulum, producing an infolding of the capsule and labrum. In other cases, there may be a hypertrophy of the pulvinar: a collection of fibrofatty tissue in the center of the acetabulum that decreases the capacity of the acetabulum and prevents relocation of the femoral head. The CT examination may be combined with hip arthrography to better visualize the unossified femoral epiphysis.

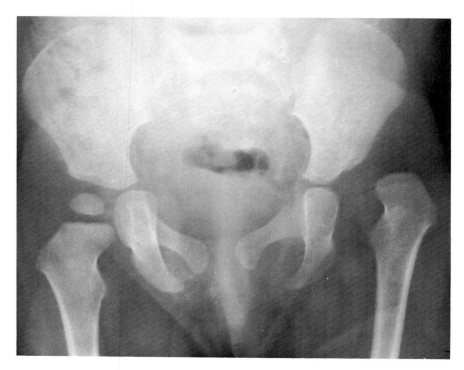

Figure 8–43. Congenital dislocation of the left hip in an older child. The capital epiphysis has not developed an ossification center. The left acetabulum is hypoplastic, with marked increase in the acetabular angle.

Ultrasonography. Ultrasonography has a distinct advantage in that it uses no ionizing radiation. Real-time examination from the lateral projection allows visualization of the unossified cartilaginous portion of the acetabulum and the cartilaginous femoral head to determine the presence or absence of a dislocation.[4, 29] US is of particular value in the screening of newborns and young infants for congenital dislocation of the hip.

Magnetic Resonance Imaging. MRI has proven to be a valuable adjunct in the assessment of congenital dislocation of the hip because of its superior visualization of cartilage and soft tissues.[11] It is of particular value in the demonstration of hip position and source of obstruction to relocation.

OTHER CONGENITAL DISLOCATIONS

Congenital dislocations affecting joints other than the hip are infrequent. Dislocation of the radial head is seen occasionally in the elbow joint. In these cases, the radial head is displaced forward on the humerus. In some cases there is an associated congenital fusion of the dislocated radius with the proximal part of the ulna, the latter bone maintaining a normal relationship with the humerus (see Fig. 8-38). This lesion may be uni-

lateral but more often is bilateral. With the passage of time, it will be noted that the head of the radius fails to develop properly and the proximal end of the bone is smaller than normal.

Traumatic dislocations due to birth trauma are decidedly rare. Most prove to be separations of the epiphyses. These are more likely to occur in high-weight babies of diabetic mothers during the course of a difficult delivery. The proximal femur and proximal and distal humerus are the most common sites of injury.

CLUBFOOT (TALIPES EQUINOVARUS)

Clubfoot is one of the more common birth defects. It may be sporadic and possibly is due to intrauterine abnormalities including severe oligohydramnios, a constriction in the uterus, and the amniotic band syndrome. There is also an increased incidence in some families, and it may be associated with other congenital abnormalities, including cleft palate and congenital heart disease. Clubfoot is also a feature of certain malformation syndromes (e.g., Gordon and Pierre Robin syndromes).

The three principal components of clubfoot are adduction of the forefoot, inversion, and cavus foot. In many cases the condition is bilateral. Everything dem-

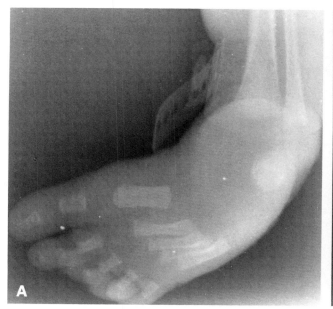
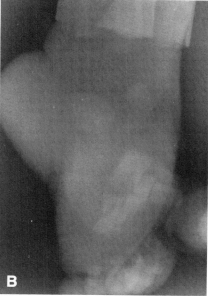

Figure 8–44. Clubfoot, talipes equinovarus in a newborn. (**A**) Anteroposterior view of the foot demonstrates inversion of the foot. The varus deformity of the foot is obvious. Inversion has displaced the calcaneus beneath the talus in this projection. (**B**) Lateral view demonstrates the associated equinus deformity with severe plantar flexion of the foot.

onstrated radiographically is better seen and evaluated by clinical methods. The radiographic findings are confirmatory and secondary. Elaborate radiographic procedures are unnecessary.

On the radiograph, there is medial angulation of the forefoot, revealed by medial displacement of the navicular and cuboid in relation to the talus and calcaneus (Fig. 8-44).[28] The inversion deformity is shown by an inward rotation of the calcaneus under the talus. Cavus foot is associated with posterior displacement of the calcaneus. The superior surface of the posterior segment of the calcaneus lies near the tibia. The talus overhangs the calcaneus, projecting well beyond it anteriorly. Regional hypoplasia of the tarsal bone and soft tissues of the foot often accompanies the deformity.

The diagnosis has been made in utero by ultrasonography.[1] When diagnosed in utero, it should suggest the possibility of other related abnormalities and syndromes, as listed above.

The diagnosis should be made clinically in the newborn. It is imperative to differentiate the rigid clubfoot from the flexible clubfoot, which needs minimal or no treatment. This differentiation can be made by clinical evaluation of the foot. The radiographic demonstration of spina bifida, dislocation of the hip, and amyotonia congenita (arthrogryposis) indicates a poor prognosis.

REFERENCES AND SELECTED READINGS

1. BENACERRAF BR, FRIGOLETTO FD: Prenatal ultrasound diagnosis of clubfoot. Radiology 155:213, 1985

2. BROWNING WH, ROSENKRANTZ H, TARQUINIO T: Computed tomography in congenital hip dislocation. J Bone Joint Surg [Am] 64:27, 1982

3. CAFFEY J, AMES R, SILVERMAN WA, ET AL: Contradiction of the congenital dysplasia predislocation hypothesis of congenital dislocation of the hip through a study of the normal variations in acetabular angles at successive periods in infancy. Pediatrics 17:632, 1956

4. CLARKE NMP, HARCKE HT, McHUGH P, ET AL: Real-time ultrasound in the diagnosis of congenital dislocation and dysplasia of the hip. J Bone Joint Surg (Br) 67:406, 1985.

5. CONWAY JJ, COWELL HR: Tarsal coalition: Clinical significance and roentgenographic demonstration. Radiology 92:799, 1969

6. CONWAY WF, DESTOUET JM, GILULA LA, ET AL: The carpal boss: An overview of radiographic evaluation. Radiology 156:29, 1985

7. DEUTSCH AL, RESNICK D, CAMPBELL G: Computed tomography and bone scintigraphy in the evaluation of tarsal coalition. Radiology 144:137, 1982

8. DOBERTI A, MANHOD J: A new radiologic sign for the early diagnosis of congenital hip dysplasia. Ann Radiol 11:276, 1968

9. FELMAN AH, KIRKPATRICK JA: Madelung's deformity. Observations in 17 patients. Radiology 93:1037, 1969

10. GOLDMAN AB, PAVLOV H, SCHNEIDER R: Radionuclide bone scanning in subtalar coalitions: Differential considerations. Am J Roentgenol 138:427, 1982

11. GUIDERA KJ, EINBECKER ME, BERMAN CG, ET AL: Magnetic resonance imaging evaluation of congenital dislocation of the hips. Clin Orthop 261:96, 1990.

12. HARRISON RB, KEATS TE: Epiphyseal clefts. Skeletal Radiology 5:23, 1980

13. HERNANDEZ RJ, TACHDJIAN MO, DIAS LS: Hip CT in congenital dislocation: Appearance of tight iliopsoas tendon and pulvinar hypertrophy. Am J Roentgenol 139:335, 1982

14. KEATS T: Atlas of Normal Roentgen Variants That May Simulate Disease, 3rd ed. Chicago, Year Book Medical Publishers, 1984

15. KLEINMAN PK, BELANGER PL, KARELLAS A, ET AL: Normal metaphyseal radiologic variants not be confused with findings of infant abuse. Am J Roentgenol 156:781, 1991

16. KOHLER A, ZIMMER EA: Borderlands of the Normal and Early Pathologic in Skeletal Roentgenology, 11th ed. New York, Grune & Stratton, 1968

17. KURSUNOGLU S, PATE D, RESNICK D, ET AL: Bone reinforcement lines in chronic adult osteopenia: A hypothesis. Radiology 158:409, 1986

18. LAWSON JP: Symptomatic radiographic variants in extremities. Radiology 157:625, 1985

19. LEE MS, HARCKE HT, KUMAR SJ, ET AL: Subtalar joint coalition in children: New observations. Radiology 172:635, 1989.

20. LEVINE AH, PALS J, BERINSON H, ET AL: The soleal line: A cause of tibial pseudoperiostitis. Radiology 119:79, 1976

21. PITT MJ: Radiology of the femoral linea aspera-pilaster complex: The track sign. Radiology 142:66, 1982

22. PITT MJ, GRAHAM AR, SHIPMAN JH, ET AL: Herniation pit of the femoral neck. Am J Roentgenol 138:1115, 1982

23. POZNANSKI A: The Hand in Radiologic Diagnosis With Gamuts. Philadelphia, WB Saunders, 1984

24. RESNICK D, GREENWAY G: Distal femoral cortical defects, irregularities, and excavations. Radiology 143:345, 1982

25. RESNICK D, CONE RO III: The nature of humeral pseudocysts. Radiology 150:27, 1984

26. SCHEY WL, LEVIN B: Familial pubic bone maldevelopment. Radiology 101:147, 1971

27. SHOFFNER CE, COIN CG: Genu varus and valgus in children. Radiology 92:723, 1969

28. SIMONS GW: A standardized method for the radiographic evaluation of clubfeet. Clin Orthop 135:107, 1978

29. TERJESEN T, RUNDEN TO, JOHNSEN HM: Ultrasound in the diagnosis of congenital dysplasia and dislocation of the hip joints in children older than two years. Clin Ortho 262:159, 1991

Paul and Juhl's Essentials of Radiologic Imaging,
Sixth Edition, edited by John H. Juhl and
Andrew B. Crummy. J.B. Lippincott Company,
Philadelphia, © 1993.

CHAPTER *9*

The Congenital Malformation Syndromes: Osteochondrodysplasias, Dysostoses, and Chromosomal Disorders

Lee F. Rogers

Congenital abnormalities of bone are relatively common. It has been estimated that approximately 3% of newborns have malformations and 1% have multiple malformations.[14, 22] Some are so common they may be considered as variations of normal. These and minor congenital anomalies are covered in Chapter 8. In this chapter, the congenital malformation syndromes are described. The term *malformation syndrome* refers to a constellation of abnormalities that frequently occur together.[31] The syndromes are often referred to by an eponym, named for those who originally described the abnormality, such as Hurler's syndrome. Alternatively, they are designated by a series of Latin or Greek phrases that include the principal sites of abnormalities, such as the acrocephalosyndactyly syndrome (Apert's syndrome), consisting of craniofacial, hand, and foot abnormalities. Many are known by both, as in the previous case.

The precise cause of most malformation syndromes is unknown.[14, 28, 29, 31] A few are known to be due to

The author gratefully acknowledges the insight, contribution, and assistance of Andrew K. Poznanski, M.D., in the development of this chapter.

specific abnormalities in metabolism, such as the mucopolysaccharidoses (i.e., Hurler's syndrome), and a small number have been related to chromosomal abnormalities such as trisomy 21 or Down's syndrome. Advances in genetic science have disclosed a number of chromosomal abnormalities and more are anticipated.

Osteochondrodysplasias are characterized by generalized abnormality of cartilage or bone growth.[30] Dysostoses are malformations of individual bones that may occur singly or in combination, differing from the osteochondrodysplasias in that they are focal and not generalized.

Although it is true that the malformation syndromes present a complex, complicated, rather bewildering array of seemingly endless variation, it is possible to develop a systematic approach that will, under most circumstances, lead to the correct diagnosis. There is a common misconception that most can be diagnosed by chemical analysis of enzymes or by chromosomal studies. In fact, most are based on their morphology—that is, the clinical appearance of the individual—or on the basis of the radiographic appearance of the skeletal system. In many cases, the radiographic examination of the skeleton is essential for accurate diagnosis.

A precise diagnosis is necessary to determine the prognosis, to offer genetic counseling, and to alert the physician to the presence of associated visceral abnormalities. Certain abnormalities are lethal either in the newborn or shortly thereafter. Many are associated with dwarfism or mental retardation. Several skeletal malformation syndromes are associated with congenital abnormalities of the heart, usually septal defects, and some with lenticular or retinal abnormalities affecting sight. Genetic counseling is necessary for those parents who have given birth to a child with a malformation syndrome or who have a family history of malformation syndromes.

In general, evaluation of congenital malformation syndromes requires a thorough evaluation of the clinical history and clinical findings, as well as a total skeletal survey.[28] This examination should include AP and lateral films of the skull and entire spine, as well as an AP of the trunk, including the pelvis and both extremities, and a separate AP examination of the hands and feet. This allows evaluation of the length of bones and other important characteristics. It is important to realize that not all of the findings are present in each case.

By the same token, if one is attempting to confirm the clinical diagnosis of a certain syndrome and significant radiographic findings are identified that are not included in the description of the disorder being considered, it is very likely that the clinical diagnosis is incorrect and that one is dealing with a different syndrome.

RADIOGRAPHIC FEATURES OF MALFORMATION SYNDROMES

The following is a list of important considerations in the radiographic evaluation of malformation syndromes:

1. *The relative length of various bones.* Are the bones too short or too long? Is there some form of dwarfism? In some forms of dwarfism, the trunk is normal and the extremities are affected or vice versa. When the extremities are affected, the distal bones may be affected more than the proximal bones or vice versa. Dwarfism may be identified in utero by ultrasonographic detection of short limbs (Fig. 9–1).[10, 12, 27, 32]

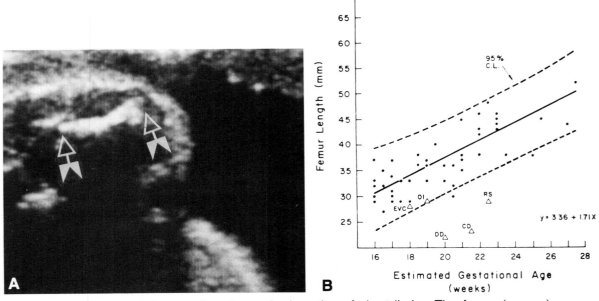

Figure 9–1. (**A**) Intrauterine ultrasonic detection of short limbs. The femur (*arrows*) measured two standard deviations below the expected length for the age. The fetus proved to have thanatophoric dysplasia. (**B**) Femur length of normal fetuses in utero measured by ultrasonography. Values from fetuses with skeletal dysplasia plotted on normal curve: **EVC,** chondroectodermal dysplasia, or Ellis–van Creveld syndrome; **OI,** osteogenesis imperfecta; **DD,** diastrophic dysplasia; **CD,** camptomelic dysplasia; **RS,** Robert's syndrome. (Hobbins JC, Bracken MB, Mahoney MJ: Am J Obstet Gynecol 142:306, 1982, with permission).

2. *Is the spine involved?* There is a major group of anomalies associated with abnormalities of the vertebrae.

3. *The age of onset.* Those abnormalities seen in early infancy can be separated from those in later life.

4. *Fusion of bones.* Fusion of various bones may be diagnostic in certain conditions. Fusion of carpal or tarsal bones may occur as a sporadic anomaly or may be associated with various syndromes. Normal persons may have fusions in the hand, usually involving carpals in the same proximal (see Fig. 8-3) or distal row, whereas fusion of carpal bones between rows is usually associated with a malformation syndrome. Fusions in congenital malformation syndromes may also involve carpals in the same row, however. In the foot, the syndrome-associated fusions usually involve the distal portions of the forefoot, which may be fused to each other or to the metatarsals. This type of fusion almost never occurs as an isolated anomaly. Fusion of proximal tarsals, such as the calcaneus and navicular (see Fig. 8-40), is often isolated and not syndrome associated, but it may be seen in syndromes as well.

5. *The appearance of the epiphyseal complex; the epiphysis, physis, and metaphysis.* Alterations in the epiphyseal complex are extremely important in the characterization of various abnormalities. When studied in adult life, many of these findings disappear and the diagnosis is often more difficult. Similarly, in the neonate, diagnosis of disorders affecting the epiphyses may be difficult since very few are ossified.

6. *The diaphysis.* Is the diaphysis thick or thin? Is the cortex abnormal? Is there bowing?

7. *Abnormalities in the number of digits.* Polydactyly or decreased number of digits is seen in a variety of conditions and may be a clue to the diagnosis.

8. *Symmetry of abnormalities.* Generally, symmetrical anomalies, such as polydactyly or absence of digits, are associated with a familial inheritance, whereas unilateral changes are more likely to be sporadic and not part of a major syndrome.

9. *Abnormalities of density.* Are the bones too dense or too lucent?

10. *Skeletal maturation.* In the majority of syndromes, skeletal maturation is delayed so that it is per se, of little diagnostic value. However, advanced skeletal maturation can be an important clue to diagnosis.

11. *Pattern of anomalies.* Many of the individual malformations are nonspecific. However, when associated with other anomalies, they suggest a diagnosis. Triangulation is important in establishing the diagnosis. For instance, a child is noted to have multiple carpal bones and a dislocated hip. By examining a listing of syndromes associated with multiple carpal bones and a separate listing of multiple dislocations, it is noted that multiple carpal bones are found in several disorders, as are multiple dislocations, but the combination of both is only found in Larsen's syndrome. Such listings are available in the texts by Poznanski and Taybi.[23, 31] Several texts include full descriptions of the malformation syndromes and serve as excellent references, such as Spranger, Langer, and Wiedemann's book on the bone dysplasias,[29] Taybi's book on radiology syndromes and metabolic disorders,[31] and Poznanski's book *The Hand in Radiologic Diagnosis.*[23]

NOMENCLATURE OF THE CONGENITAL MALFORMATION SYNDROMES

The designations of the congenital malformation syndromes will be those adopted by the Committee for the International Nomenclature of Constitutional Diseases of Bone (1991), in Table 9-1.[2] The nomenclature was adopted to minimize the problem presented by the many syndromes that were described under various names, and it is periodically revised to unify the terminology used in different parts of the world. It is not intended to be a classification of skeletal disorders. The term *gross dwarfism* was eliminated in 1977 because it was offensive to the patients or their families. Thus, the previous term, *diastrophic dwarfism,* is now *diastrophic dysplasia.* Since dwarfism is such an important characteristic, the author has marked with an asterisk those conditions associated with dwarfism. Otherwise, the nomenclature is as published. At first glance the list is rather foreboding, arcane, and mystic because of the combination of lexicon and eponyms; the use of Latin, Greek, and proper names—a seemingly incomprehensible nosology—a lexicographer's nightmare. Closer inspection reveals a considerable attempt to bring order out of chaos. The logic of the listing will be appreciated if a few minutes are spent in consideration of the major categories and subdivisions.

OSTEOCHONDRODYSPLASIAS

Osteochondrodysplasias are generalized abnormalities of growth and development of cartilage or bone. They are subdivided into those identifiable at birth and

(text continues on page 323)

Table 9–1. International Nomenclature of Constitutional Diseases of Bone (1983)[2]

OSTEOCHONDRODYSPLASIAS
Abnormalities of cartilage or bone growth and development

	TRANSMISSION			TRANSMISSION
A. Defects of growth of tubular bones or spine			**25.** Other multiple dislocation syndromes (Desbuquois)	AR
a. Identifiable at birth			**b.** Identifiable in later life	
α. Usually lethal before or shortly after birth			**1.** Hypochondroplasia	AD
*1. Achondrogenesis type I (Parenti-Fraccaro)	AR		*2. Dyschondrosteosis	AD
*2. Achondrogenesis type II (Langer-Saldino)			*3. Metaphyseal chondrodysplasia type Jansen	AD
*3. Hypochondrogenesis			*4. Metaphyseal chondrodysplasia type Schmid	AD
*4. Fibrinochondrogenesis	AR		*5. Metaphyseal chondrodysplasia type McKusick	AR
*5. Thanatophoric dysplasia			*6. Metaphyseal chondrodysplasia with exocrine pancreatic insufficiency and cyclic neutropenia	AR
*6. Thanatophoric dysplasia with cloverleaf skull			*7. Spondylometaphyseal dysplasia	
*7. Atelosteogenesis			**a.** type Kozlowski	AD
*8. Short rib syndrome (with or without polydactyly)			**b.** other forms	
a. type I (Saldino-Noonan)	AR		*8. Multiple epiphyseal dysplasia	
b. type II (Majewski)	AR		**a.** type Fairbanks	AD
c. type III (lethal thoracic dysplasia)	AR		**b.** Other forms	
β. Usually nonlethal dysplasia			**9.** Multiple epiphyseal dysplasia wih early diabetes (Wolcott–Rallison)	AR
*9. Chondrodysplasia punctata			**10.** Arthro-ophthalmopathy (Stickler)	AD
a. rhizomelic form autosomal recessive	AR		*11. Pseudoachondroplasia	
b. dominant X-linked form	XLD		**a.** dominant	AD
c. common mild form (type Sheffield)			**b.** recessive	AR
Exclude: symptomatic stippling (Warfarin, chromosomal abberation)			**12.** Spondylo-epiphyseal dysplasia tarda (X-linked recessive)	XLR
*10. Campomelic dysplasia			*13. Progressive pseudorheumatoid chondrodysplasia	AR
*11. Kyphomelic dysplasia	AR		**14.** Spondylo-epiphyseal dysplasia (other forms)	
*12. Achondroplasia	AD		**15.** Brachyolmia	
*13. Diastrophic dysplasia	AR		**a.** autosomal recessive	AR
*14. Metatrophic dysplasia (several forms)	AR, AD		**b.** autosomal dominant	AD
*15. Chondroectodermal dysplasia (Ellis–van Creveld)	AR		*16. Dyggve–Melchior–Clausen dysplasia	AR
*16. Asphyxiating thoracic dysplasia (Jeune)	AR		*17. Spondylo-epimetaphyseal dysplasia (several forms)	
*17. Spondyloepiphyseal dysplasia congenita			*18. Spondylo-epimetaphyseal dysplasia with joint laxity	AR
a. autosomal dominant form	AD		**19.** Otospondylomegaepiphyseal dysplasia (OSMED)	AR
b. autosomal recessive form	AR		**20.** Myotonic chondrodysplasia (Catel–Schwartz–Jampel)	AR
*18. Kniest dysplasia	AD		*21. Parastremmatic dysplasia	AD
*19. Dyssegmental dysplasia	AR		**22.** Trichorhinophalangeal dysplasia	AD
*20. Mesomelic dysplasia			**23.** Acrodysplasia with retinitis pigmentosa and neophropathy (Saldino–Mainzer)	AR
a. type Nievergelt	AD		**B.** Disorganized development of cartilage and fibrous components of skeleton	
b. type Langer (probable homozygous dyschondrosteosis)	AR		**1.** Dysplasia epiphysealis hemimelica	
c. type Robinow			**2.** Multiple cartilaginous exostoses	AD
d. type Rheinardt	AD		**3.** Acrodysplasia with exostoses (Giedion–Langer)	
e. others				
*21. Acromesomelic dysplasia	AR			
22. Cleidocranial dysplasia	AD			
23. Otopalatodigital syndrome				
a. type I (Langer)	XLSD			
b. type II (André)	XLR			
24. Larsen syndrome	AR, AD			

* Associated with dwarfism
(A, autosomal; D, dominant; R, recessive; S, sporadic; XL, X-linked)

Table 9–1.   (continued)

OSTEOCHONDRODYSPLASIAS
Abnormalities of cartilage or bone growth and development

	TRANSMISSION		TRANSMISSION
4. Enchondromastosis (Ollier)		a. type Apert	AD
5. Enchondromatosis with hemangioma (Maffucci)		b. type Chotzen	AD
6. Metachondromatosis	AD	c. type Pfeiffer	AD
7. Spondyloenchondroplasia	AR	d. other types	
8. Osteoglophonic dysplasia		4. Acroencephalopolysyndactyly (Carpenter) and others	AR
9. Fibrous dysplasia (Jaffe–Lichtenstein)		5. Cephalopolysyndactyly (Greig)	AD
10. Fibrous dysplasia with skin pigmentation and precocious puberty (McCune–Albright)		6. First and second branchial arch syndromes	
11. Cherubism (familial fibrous dysplasia of the jaws)	AD	a. mandibulofacial dysostosis (Treacher–Collins)	AD
C. Abnormalities of density of cortical diaphyseal structure and/or metaphyseal modeling		b. acrofacial dysostosis (Nager)	
1. Osteogenesis imperfecta (several forms)	AR, AD	c. oculoauriculovertebral dysostosis (Goldenhar)	
2. Juvenile idiopathic osteoporosis		d. hemifacial microsomia	
3. Osteoporosis with pseudoglioma	AR	e. others (probably parts of a large spectrum)	
4. Osteopetrosis		7. Oculomandibulofacial syndrome (Hallermann–Streiff–François)	
a. autosomal recessive lethal	AR	B. Dysostoses with predominant axial involvement	
b. intermediate recessive	AR	1. Vertebral segmentation defects (including Klippel–Feil)	
c. autosomal dominant	AD	2. Cervico-oculoacoustic syndrome (Wilderwanck)	
d. recessive with tubular acidosis	AR	3. Sprengel's anomaly	
5. Pyknodysostosis	AR	4. Spondylocostal dysostosis	
6. Dominant osteosclerosis type Stanescu	AD	a. dominant form	AD
7. Osteomesopyknosis	AD	b. recessive forms	AR
8. Osteopoikilosis	AD	5. Oculovertebral syndrome (Weyers)	
9. Osteopathia striata	AD	6. Osteo-onychodysostosis	AD
10. Osteopathia striata with cranial sclerosis	AD	7. Cerebrocostomandibular syndrome	AR
11. Melorheostosis	AD	C. Dysostoses with predominant involvement of extremities	
12. Diaphyseal dysplasia (Camurati–Engelmann)	AD	1. Acheiria	
13. Craniodiaphyseal dysplasia		2. Apodia	
14. Endosteal hyperostosis		3. Tetraphocomelia syndrome (Roberts) (SC pseudothalidomide syndrome)	AR
a. autosomal dominant (Worth)	AD	4. Ectrodactyly	
b. autosomal recessive (Van Buchem)	AR	a. isolated	
c. autosomal recessive (sclerosteosis)	AR	b. ectrodactyly–ectodermal dysplasia cleft palate syndrome	AD
15. Tubular stenosis (Kenny–Caffey)	AD	c. ectrodactyly with scalp defects	AD
16. Pachydermoperiostosis	AD	5. Oroacral syndrome (aglossia syndrome, Hanhart syndrome)	
17. Osteodysplasty (Melnick–Needles)	AD	6. Familial radioulnar synostosis	
18. Frontometaphyseal dysplasia	XLR	7. Brachydactyly (Bell's classification)	
*19. Craniometaphyseal dysplasia (several forms)	AD	a. type A	AD
20. Metaphyseal dysplasia (Pyle)	AR or AD	b. type B	AD
21. Dysosteosclerosis	AR or XLR	c. type C	AD
22. Osteoectasia with hyperphosphatasia	AR	d. type D	AD
23. Oculodentoosseous dysplasia		e. type E	AD
a. mild type	AD	8. Symphalangism	AD
b. severe type	AR	9. Polydactyly (several forms)	
24. Infantile cortical hyperostosis (Caffey disease familial type)	AD	10. Syndactyly (several forms)	
		11. Polysyndactyly (several forms)	
		12. Camptodactyly	
		13. Manzke syndrome	

DYSOSTOSES
Malformation of individual bones, singly or in combination
A. Dysostoses with cranial and facial involvement

1. Craniosynostosis (several forms)		14. Poland syndrome	
2. Craniofacial dysostosis (Crouzon)		15. Rubinstein–Taybi syndrome	
3. Acrocephalosyndactyly		16. Coffin–Siris syndrome	

(continued)

Table 9–1. (continued)

OSTEOCHONDRODYSPLASIAS
Abnormalities of cartilage or bone growth and development

	TRANSMISSION			TRANSMISSION
17. Pancytopenia–dysmelia syndrome (Fanconi)	AR		in 25-hydroxyvitamin D, alpha-hydroxylase	
18. Blackfan–Diamond anemia with thumb anomalies (Aase-S.)	AR		b. type II with target-organ resistance	AR
19. Thrombocytopenia–radial-aplasia syndrome	AR		3. Late rickets (McCance)	
20. Orodigitofacial syndrome			4. Idiopathic hypercalciuria	
a. type Papillon–Leage	XLD Lethal in male		5. Hypophosphatasia (several forms)	AR
b. type Mohr	AR		6. Pseudohypoparathyroidism (normo- and hypocalcemic forms, including acrodysostosis)	AD
21. Cardiomelic syndrome (Holt–Oram and others)	AD		B. Complex carbohydrates	
22. Femoral focal deficiency (with or without facial anomalies)			1. Mucopolysaccharidosis type I (alpha-L-iduronidase deficiency)	
23. Multiple synostoses (includes some forms of symphalangism)	AD		a. Hurler form	AR
			b. Scheie form	AR
24. Scapuloiliac dysostosis (Kosenow–Sinios)	AD		c. other forms	AR
25. Hand–foot–genital syndrome	AD		2. Mucopolysaccharidosis type II—Hunter (sulfoiduronate sulfatase deficiency)	XLR
26. Focal dermal hypoplasia (Goltz)	XLD Lethal in male		3. Mucopolysaccharidosis type III—San Filippo	
			a. type III A (heparin sulfamidase deficiency)	AR
IDIOPATHIC OSTEOLYSES			b. type III B (N-acetyl-alpha-glucosaminidase deficiency)	AR
1. Phalangeal (several forms)			c. type III C (alpha-glucosaminide-N-acetyl transferase)	AR
2. Tarsocarpal			d. type III D (N-acetyl-glucosamine-6 sulfate sulfatase)	AR
a. including François form and others	AR		4. Mucopolysaccharidosis type IV	
b. with nephropathy	AD		a. type IV A—Morquio (N-acetyl-galactosamine-6 sulfate sulfatase deficiency)	AR
3. Multicentric				
a. Hajdu–Cheney form	AD			
b. Winchester form	AR?		b. type IV B (beta-galactosidase deficiency)	AR
c. Torg form	AR			
d. other forms			5. Mucopolysaccharidosis type VI—Maroteaux–Lamy (aryl-sulfatase B deficiency)	AR
			6. Mucopolysaccharidosis type VII (beta-glucuronidase deficiency)	AR
MISCELLANEOUS DISORDERS WITH OSSEOUS INVOLVEMENT			7. Aspartylglucosaminuria (Aspartyl-glucosaminidase deficiency)	AR
1. Early acceleration of skeletal maturation			8. Mannosidosis (alpha-mannosidase deficiency)	AR
a. Marshall–Smith syndrome			9. Fucosidosis (alpha-fucosidase deficiency)	AR
b. Weaver syndrome			10. GM1-Gangliosidosis (beta-galactosidase deficiency) (several forms)	AR
c. other types				
2. Marfan syndrome	AD		11. Multiple sulfatases deficiency (Austin–Theiffry)	AR
3. Congenital contractural arachnodactyly	AD		12. Isolated neuraminidase deficiency (several forms included)	
4. Cerebrohepatorenal syndrome (Zellweger)			a. mucolipidosis I	AR
5. Coffin–Lowry syndrome	SLR		b. nephrosialidosis	AR
6. Cockayne syndrome	AR		c. cherry red spot myoclonia syndrome	AR
7. Fibrodysplasia ossificans congenita	AD		13. Phosphotransferase deficiency (several forms included)	
8. Epidermal nevus syndrome (Solomon)			a. mucolipidosis II (I cell disease)	AR
9. Nevoid basal cell carcinoma syndrome			b. mucolipidosis II (pseudo-polydystrophy)	AR
10. Multiple hereditary fibromatosis	AD		14. Combined neuraminidase galacto-sidase deficiency	AR
11. Neurofibromatosis	AD			

CHROMOSOMAL ABERRATIONS
PRIMARY METABOLIC ABNORMALITIES
A. Calcium or phosphorus
    1. Hypophosphatemic rickets   XLD
    2. Vitamin D dependency or pseudodeficiency rickets
       a. type I with probable deficiency   AR

Table 9–1. (continued)

OSTEOCHONDRODYSPLASIAS
Abnormalities of cartilage or bone growth and development

	TRANSMISSION			TRANSMISSION
15. Salla disease	AR		**D.** Nucleic Acids	
C. Lipids			**1.** Adenosine-deaminase deficiency and others	AR
1. Niemann-Pick disease (sphingomyelinase deficiency) (several forms)	AR		**E.** Amino acids	
2. Gaucher's disease (beta-glucosidase deficiency) (several types)	AR		**1.** Homocystinuria and others	AR
3. Farber's disease (ceraminidase deficiency)	AR		**F.** Metals	
			1. Menkes' kinky-hair syndrome and others	AR

those identifiable in later life. The other two principal categories are (1) disorders with disorganized development of cartilage and fibrous components of the skeleton and (2) abnormalities of density of cortical or diaphyseal bone structure.

DEFECTS OF GROWTH OF TUBULAR BONES OR SPINE IDENTIFIABLE AT BIRTH

Achondroplasia

Achondroplasia is the most common form of dwarfism. It has been recognized since antiquity, commonly identified in the past with court jesters and today with clowns in circuses. It is a hereditary congenital disturbance transmitted as an autosomal dominant trait, causing inadequate endochondral bone formation and resulting in dwarfism. Membranous bone formation is not affected. The mental status is normal.

Characteristically, the short limb bones contrast with the normal length of the trunk. The facies is characterized by prominent frontal bossing of the skull, saddle nose, and prognathic jaw. All achondroplastic persons bear a strong anatomical resemblance to each other. The following paragraphs describe the most typical changes in the skeleton.[26, 29]

Roentgenographic Findings.[17] *Long Tubular Bones.* Shortening of the long bones is responsible for dwarfism (Figs. 9-2 and 9-3). The humerus and femur tend to be relatively more affected than the distal bones of the extremities. The diameter is usually normal, but the bones appear thick because they are short. The ends of the shafts are flared. The zone of provisional calcification may be smooth or irregular. At times there is a sizable V-shaped notch in the metaphyses, and the epiphyseal centers may be partially buried in the metaphyses, the ball-and-socket epiphyses (Fig. 9-3). The fibula often is longer than the tibia, causing an inversion of the foot (Fig. 9-2). Bowing of the long bones is common.

Short Tubular Bones. These bones show changes similar to those in the long bones. They are short and

appear thick, and the fingers tend to be of similar lengths, the so-called "trident hand" (Fig. 9-3).

Pelvis. Characteristic changes occur in the pelvis. The ilia are short and square, and the sacrosciatic notch

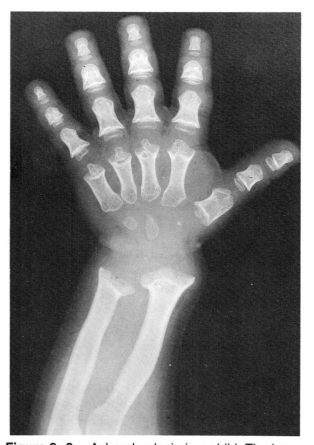

Figure 9–2. Achondroplasia in a child. The bones of the hand are short and broad; there are ball socket epiphyses at the distal ends of the metacarpals. Note the flaring of the metaphyses, particularly of the radius and ulna.

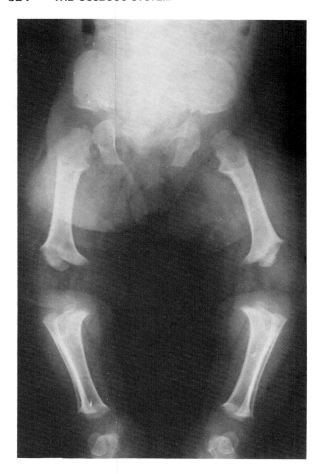

Figure 9–3. Achondroplasia in an infant. The shortening of the femurs is more pronounced than that of the tibia. Note that the length of the fibula is proportionally greater than that of the tibia. The distal femoral metaphyses are tilted upward and laterally, with laterally placed epiphyses. Typical changes are present in the pelvis.

is small. The ischial and pubic bones are also short and broad. The acetabular angles are decreased in infancy. The sacrum articulates low on the ilia (Fig. 9-4).

Spine. The length of the spinal column may be normal or nearly so, but vertebral development is affected. One or several vertebrae at the thoracolumbar junction (T12 to L3) may be rounded or wedged anteriorly. In the lumbar area, the interpedicular distances characteristically narrow progressively from above downward (see Fig. 9-4), the reverse of the normal, in which it increases from above downward. The pedicles are short and thick, and the posterior surfaces of the bodies are concave (Fig. 9-5). The net effect is a stenotic spinal canal, which in the adult may lead to severe neurologic symptoms, especially if a herniated disc or degenerative joint disease or kyphosis develops. The lumbar lordosis is increased, and the lumbosacral angle becomes more acute than is normal (Fig. 9-5). The long axis of the sacrum tends to be horizontal.

Skull. The skull is brachycephalic because the base of the skull is preformed in cartilage and therefore hypoplastic. The vault is relatively large, with bulging of the frontal bones. It is of membranous origin and thus is not affected. The growth of the mandible is relatively normal and thus appears prognathic.

Other Bones. The carpal and tarsal bones are normal. The scapula is short, and the sternum may be thick and short. The ribs are short, causing a decrease in the anteroposterior diameter of the thorax.

Hypochondroplasia

Hypochrondroplasia is similar to achondroplasia but with milder involvement. The skull in these patients may be normal or nearly so, but the interpedicular distance may decrease slightly from L1 to L5. The pelvis is small, and lordosis may be present. Shortening of the tubular bones is less than in achondroplasia. These bones are proportionately shortened, in contrast to disproportionate shortening in achondroplasia.

Thanatophoric Dysplasia

Thanatophoric dysplasia was previously mistaken for a severe type of achondroplasia because of its many similar features including dwarfing of the long tubular bones with a relatively long trunk, a prominent forehead with a short skull base and depression of the nasal root, small square iliac wings with horizontal acetabular roofs, a narrow thorax with short ribs, and a decrease from above downward of the interpedicular distances in the lumbar spine. Distinguishing features include extremely thin, wafer-like ossification of vertebral bodies with thick intervertebral spaces, very short limb bones with bowing, especially in the lower extremities (Fig. 9-6), and no history of a similar disorder in other members of the family.

Affected infants have been stillborn or have died shortly after birth, possibly from respiratory failure owing to the short ribs and narrow thorax.

Short ribs with a narrow thorax occurs in three principal dysplasias—thanatophoric dysplasia, asphyxiating thoracic dystrophy, and achondroplasia—and other changes common to achondroplasia may be seen in the other two abnormalities. A small chest is also a feature of the short rib polydactyly syndromes.[31]

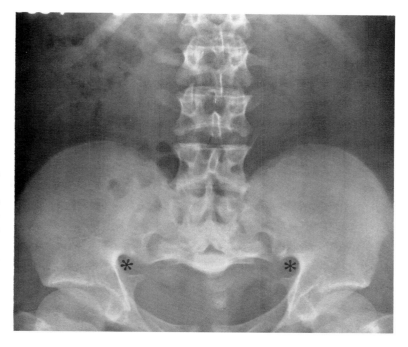

Figure 9–4. Achondroplasia in an adolescent. The ilia are short and square, and the acetabular angles are flat. The pelvis is foreshortened in the anteroposterior direction, and there are characteristic deformities of the sacrosciatic notches (*asterisk*). The sacrum is horizontal and projected on end. The interpediculate distance narrows progressively, proceeding from the upper to the lower lumbar spine, the reverse of normal.

Asphyxiating Thoracic Dystrophy

Asphyxiating thoracic dystrophy was first reported by Jeune in 1955 in two infant siblings who died of respiratory distress associated with small and relatively immobile thoraces. The major abnormalities identifiable on roentgenography consist of very short ribs and a variable degree of shortening of the long tubular bones with metaphyseal notching.

The ribs project horizontally and may be so short as to barely reach the anterior axillary line (Fig. 9-7). The shortened ribs reduce the volume of the thorax and are responsible for the respiratory distress. The cardiac silhouette often appears large, but this is probably an illusion because of the smallness of the thorax. In the pelvis, the ilium is shortened in its inferosuperior diameter, the acetabular roof is broad, and there may be a deep V-shaped notch in it. The disease may be fatal, with the infant dying from respiratory complications. Associated renal disease has also been reported. Renal failure may be the cause of death in patients with less severe skeletal changes.

Achondrogenesis

Achondrogenesis is a fatal form of neonatal dwarfism. The head is very large, the extremities small, and the trunk is short. There is almost complete absence of ossification of the vertebral bodies. The most characteristic finding distinguishing achondrogenesis from both thanatophoric and asphyxiating thoracic dysplasia is the absence of sacral ossification. The iliac bones are very small.

Diastrophic Dysplasia

Diastrophic dysplasia is inherited as an autosomal recessive trait. The syndrome is characterized by the combination of scoliosis and clubfeet. There is also a delay in appearance of the epiphyseal centers and subluxation of various joints (especially the hips).

The long bones are short and thick, with widened metaphyses, simulating achondroplasia. In the hands, the bones are short, especially the thumb, which may project at a right angle to the other digits, the "hitchhiker's thumb." The metacarpal of the thumb also may have an ovoid shape. The bones of the feet show changes similar to those in the hands. In addition, there is a bilateral clubfoot deformity.

The epiphyseal centers are late in appearing and, when they do appear, are apt to be flat and abnormal in shape. In the hand, the epiphyseal centers may be oriented parallel rather than perpendicular to the long axis of the phalanges. That is, the height is longer than the width, the reverse of the normal proportion. In most patients, laxity of ligaments and tendons causes subluxation of the joints. The subluxations are not present at birth but develop after the child begins to walk. Scoliosis and kyphosis also appear at about the same time. A severe kyphosis in the cervical region may be fatal in infancy. Other bones, including the vertebrae, skull, and pelvis, are normal. The tarsal

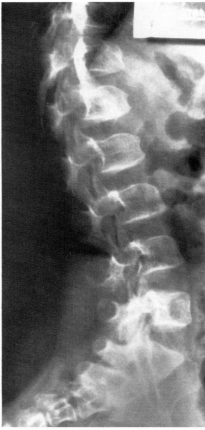

Figure 9–5. Achondroplasia in a 6-year-old. The vertebrae at the thoracolumbar junction are rounded and are wedged anteriorly and concave posteriorly. The pedicles are short. The lumbosacral angle is accentuated by the horizontal orientation of the long axis of the sacrum.

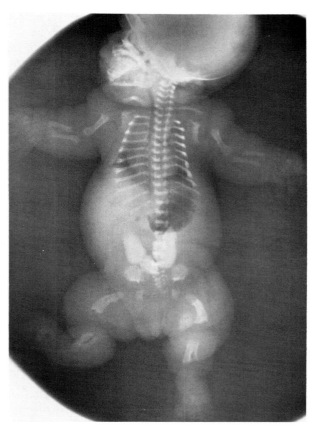

Figure 9–6. Thanatophoric dysplasia. This limb shortening is more pronounced proximally than distally. Note the narrow thorax with short ribs and characteristic flattening of the vertebral bodies. The pelvis is deformed in the characteristic pattern. The presence of sacral ossification centers distinguishes thanatophoric dysplasia from achondrogenesis.

bones may be distorted because of the equinovarus deformity, but otherwise are normal.

The differentiation from achondroplasia, in the average patient, is not difficult if all findings are taken into consideration. The normal appearance of the skull, vertebrae, and pelvis and the presence of clubfeet are helpful in this regard.

Chondrodysplasia Punctata (Stippled Epiphyses)

Infants affected with chondrodysplasia punctata are frequently stillborn or die within the first year of life of associated abnormalities or intercurrent disease. The disease is genetically transmitted with both dominant and recessive forms.

The characteristic roentgenographic finding is the presence of numerous small, round opacities in the unossified epiphyseal cartilages (Fig. 9-8). In some patients, the opacities appear to extend into the adjacent soft tissues. They also have been found in other cartilages such as the nasal septum, larynx, and trachea. Stippling of the vertebral cartilages is common in the more severe cases. The extremities may be dwarfed, and flexion deformities may also be present. The femur and humerus are most likely to be shortened. In many patients, there have been congenital cataracts, saddle nose, hyperkeratotic dermatoses, and failure of proper mental and physical development. If the infant survives, in some cases the foci may ossify and then merge to form a fairly normal epiphyseal center. The fingers and toes may be short and stubby.

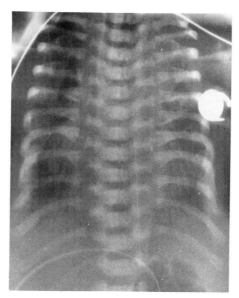

Figure 9–7.   Asphyxiating thoracic dystrophy. The thorax is extremely small and the ribs quite short. The cardiac silhouette appears large because of the smallness of the thorax. The vertebral bodies are larger and the intervertebral disc space is narrower than that encountered in thanatophoric dysplasia and achondrogenesis. The limbs are also relatively normal in length.

The carpal and tarsal bones may be normal or show some irregularity in shape.

Stippled calcification has also been noted in the cerebrohepatorenal syndrome, except that the calcified foci are most marked and may be limited to the patellae. Other findings include (1) marked flaccidity, (2) abnormal facies, (3) cataracts, (4) flexion contractures of the extremities, (5) small cortical renal cysts, (6) fibrosis of the liver, with increased deposits of hemosiderin, and (7) abnormality of the cerebrum including lissencephaly and sudanophilic leukodystrophy.

Chondroectodermal Dysplasia (Ellis–van Creveld)

Chondroectodermal dysplasia was first described among the Old Order Amish People of Pennsylvania. The disease is transmitted as an autosomal recessive trait. Cardiac anomalies (atrial septal defects being the most frequent) have been found in about 60%. The ectodermal component of the syndrome is manifested by small, friable nails; defective dentition; and, in a few cases, alopecia.

The changes in the skeleton are usually characteris-

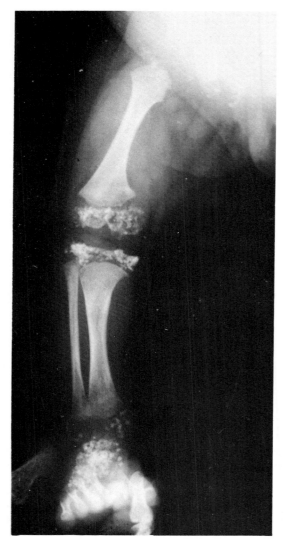

Figure 9–8.   Stippled epiphyses. Numerous tiny, dense foci were noted throughout the cartilages of the skeleton. They were most numerous in the right lower extremity. The bones are shorter than normal. (Paul LW: Am J Roentgenol 71:941, 1954. Copyright 1954 American Roentgen Ray Society. Reproduced with permission.)

tic. Polydactyly and syndactyly are almost universal. A partially or completely formed sixth metacarpal may be fused to the fifth (Fig. 9-9). Fusion of the hamate and capitate bones in the wrist is often present. Cone epiphyses are common during childhood (see the following section entitled "Peripheral Dysostosis"). Shortening of the long tubular bones characteristically becomes more severe distalward, the opposite of that

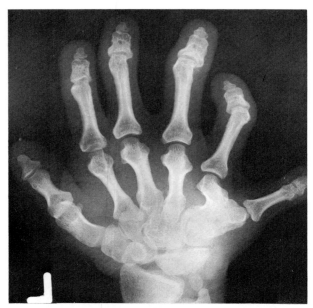

Figure 9–9. Ellis–van Creveld disease in a woman. There is progressive shortening of the bones distally from the wrist, with polydactyly, syndactyly, and carpal fusions. (Courtesy of M. Pinson Neal, Jr., M.D., Richmond, Virginia)

encountered in achondroplasia. The tibia and fibula thus are much shorter than the femur, and the distal phalanges more dwarfed than the proximal. The distal end of the radius and proximal end of the ulna are somewhat enlarged. Also, the radial head may be flared and frequently is dislocated. The proximal end of the tibia also is widened, and the epiphysis offset medially. A small exostosis is frequently present on the upper inner cortex of the tibia. The intercondylar notch of the femur is shallow, and the tibial spine is small. A severe cervical kyphosis with spinal cord compression may occur.

The iliac crest tends to be flared, but the pelvis of many of these patients is normal, as are the vertebrae, ribs, and skull.

Peripheral Dysostosis

The characteristic roentgenographic changes of peripheral dysostosis are limited to the short tubular bones of the hands and feet, which are short and broad and have cone-shaped or ball-and-socket epiphyses. The term *cone epiphysis* refers to an epiphyseal center that is partially or completely buried in the metaphysis and that usually has the shape of a cone. The terms are

often used interchangeably, however. Supernumerary epiphyses and pseudoepiphyses are often present.

Cone-shaped epiphyses also have been found in a number of other conditions, including[23] (1) cleidocranial dysostosis, (2) Ellis–van Creveld disease, (3) trichorhinophalangeal syndrome, (4) Apert's syndrome, (5) pseudohypoparathyroidism, (6) achondroplasia, (7) multiple hereditary exostoses, and (8) those due to no recognizable cause.

Spondyloepiphyseal Dysplasia Congenita

The roentgenographic signs of spondyloepiphyseal dysplasia vary with the age of the patient. Dwarfism is one of the major features. There is a general delay in ossification with particular delay in pubic ossification. Ossification centers for the distal femurs, proximal tibias, and the calcanei and tali are less delayed. Flattening of the vertebral bodies, platyspondyly, is present. The acetabular angles are small. There may be flaring of the anterior ends of the ribs, and the thorax is broad and bell shaped. Lateral bowing of the femurs is frequent. The long tubular bones are shortened and have various epiphyseal and metaphyseal abnormalities. In later infancy and early childhood, delay in ossification of the pubis and femoral head and neck persists. When ossification centers appear in the femoral heads, they may be multiple. The vertebral bodies remain flattened and have an ovoid shape in lateral views. Anterior hypoplasia of one or more vertebral segments often is pronounced at the thoracolumbar junction. In the pelvis there is a lack of normal iliac flare, and the ilia appear small in their cephalocaudal dimensions. There is little or no acetabular slant.

In later childhood there is accentuation of the dorsal kyphosis, and lumbar lordosis and scoliosis may develop. There is hypoplasia of the odontoid process, and platyspondyly persists into adult life. In adults, the dysplasia of the proximal femurs leads to a varus deformity. The hands and feet remain relatively normal. The degree of dwarfism varies from patient to patient and results from both vertebral and long-bone changes.

Spondyloepiphyseal dyplasia congenita was previously confused with Morquio's disease. Differentiation is based upon its mode of inheritance—that is, as a dominant trait, its manifestation at birth, the different roentgenographic changes (particularly coxa vara rather than coxa valga), the lack of corneal clouding, and the absence of keratosulfaturia.

Spondyloepiphyseal Dysplasia Tarda

Spondyloepiphyseal dysplasia tarda is an entirely different disease than spondyloepiphyseal dysplasia congenita.

The disease often is not recognized until adulthood, when precocious degenerative joint disease occurs. It may be impossible to determine the cause of the joint disease. Other epiphyseal dysplasias may lead to similar premature degenerative changes.

Metatrophic Dysplasia

Metatrophic dysplasia is another form of dwarfism that may be confused with achondroplasia.[17] Roentgenographic changes are apparent at birth, with shortening of the long tubular bones and hyperplastic, and greatly flared metaphyses. There is overconstriction of the midshafts, so that the bones have a dumbbell shape. Epiphyseal ossification centers are delayed in appearance, and when they do appear are deformed. The ribs tend to be short, with a narrow chest. Kyphoscoliosis is present, and there is platyspondyly (i.e., flattening of the vertebrae). In the pelvis, the iliac wings are short, the sacroiliac notches are short and deep, and the acetabula are horizontal. As the child grows older, there is lengthening of the long bones, more than is seen in achondroplasia. However, the platyspondyly and the kyphoscoliotic curvature worsen, and the child changes clinically from what appears to be achondroplasia to an appearance resembling spondyloepiphyseal dysplasia. The base of the skull is not fore-shortened, and the interpedicular distances in the lumbar spine usually remain normal, findings that aid in differentiating this dysplasia from achondroplasia during infancy.

Spondylocostal Dysostosis

Spondylocostal dysostosis[25] is a form of truncal dwarfism due to segmental abnormalities of the entire spine (Fig. 9-10). The extremities are normal. When severe, it may lead to death in the newborn. The spinal canal is normal, but the segmentation of the vertebral bodies is entirely abnormal. The ribs are thin and often fused medially, giving a fan-like appearance. It occurs in both autosomal dominant and autosomal recessive forms. The disease is common in Puerto Ricans.

DEFECTS OF GROWTH OF TUBULAR BONES OR SPINE IDENTIFIABLE LATER IN LIFE

Multiple Epiphyseal Dysplasia

The characteristic finding in multiple epiphyseal dysplasia is the presence of multiple ossification centers for the affected epiphyses, giving them a fragmented appearance. It is considered to be transmitted as an autosomal dominant trait with complete penetrance but variable expression. The epiphyses are usually flat, and the ends of the long bones may be somewhat

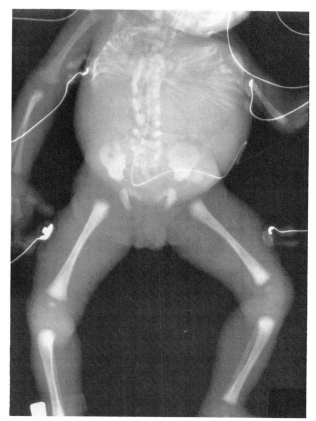

Figure 9–10. Spondylocostal dysostosis. The trunk is shortened because of segmentation defects throughout the entire spine. The limbs are normal. Note the thin ribs with multiple interosseous fusions.

flared. The involvement may be limited to a pair of epiphyses, or all epiphyses throughout the body. Symmetrical involvement of the capital femoral epiphyses is common. Knock-knee or bowleg deformity may be present, and flexion deformities at the knee joint may be seen. The tibias are usually curved. A coronal cleft in the patellas (i.e., "double-layered patella") has been described as a fairly consistent and characteristic finding in the tarda form.

The vertebrae may be flattened in the thoracic spine, with irregular end-plates. The skull is normal. The long bones appear to be short and thick. The thickness is an illusion because of the shortening. The carpal and tarsal bones are often irregular and the digits stubby. In many patients, however, the hands are normal.

Affected children usually are brought to the attention of a physician after they begin to walk, because of a peculiar waddling gait. Eventually the multiple centers merge and unite to the shaft. Irregularity of the articular plates frequently persists (Fig. 9-11) and leads to the early development of degenerative joint disease, particularly in the hips. At this stage it usually is impossible to determine what the primary disorder was, since the other epiphyseal dysplasias may also result in early degenerative joint disease.

In differential diagnosis, the presence of epiphyseal abnormalities serves to rule out achondroplasia. The normal vertebrae are significant in excluding Morquio's disease. When the heads of the femurs alone are involved, bilateral Perthes' disease and the epiphyseal dysgenesis of cretinism must be considered.

Metaphyseal Chondrodysplasia

McKusick Type (Cartilage-Hair Dysplasia). A characteristic type of dysplasia exists among the Old Order Amish of Eastern Pennsylvania and Canada.[28] Dwarfism is noted at birth owing to shortening of the tubular bones of the extremities, and it is said that adults seldom exceed 4 feet in height. The epiphyses and the skull are normal, an important point in differentiating this dysplasia from achondroplasia. The hair is fine,

sparse, short, and brittle and is said to be characteristic of this dysplasia. Other findings include flexion deformities at the elbows, and hyperextensibility of the wrists and fingers. The fingers are greatly shortened. The intelligence is not affected. The disorder is autosomal recessive.

Jansen Type. In 1934, Jansen reported a case of dwarfism that resembled achondroplasia except that the metaphyses were abnormal, being cup shaped with irregular mineralization consisting of radiolucent non-ossified cartilage mixed with scattered islands of bone and calcification.[32] The disorder is characterized roentgenographically by a rachitic rosary of the ribs, coxa vara, genu valgum, and anterior bowing of the femurs. The growth plates of the tubular bones are thickened and irregular owing to extensions of cartilage into the metaphyses.

Schmid Type. In 1949, Schmid reported a mild form of metaphyseal dysplasia. The Schmid type is relatively common.[20] The spine and skull are not affected. Dwarfism is of the rhizomelic type, as seen in achondroplasia. The skeletal changes are not present at birth

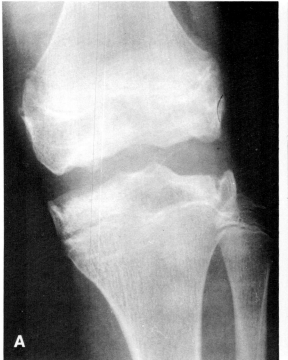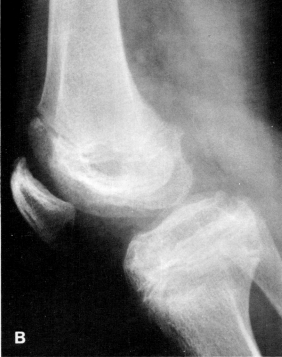

Figure 9–11. Multiple epiphyseal dysplasia in an adolescent. The articular surfaces are irregular as seen in both the frontal (**A**) and lateral (**B**) projections. The joint abnormality often leads to the early development of degenerative joint disease.

but appear between 3 and 5 years of age. Dwarfism is relatively mild compared with the Jansen type. Bowing of the legs is marked, and patients have a waddling gait. Mild to moderate inhibition of growth of all cylindrical bones is present. There is bilateral coxa vara. It is transmitted as an autosomal dominant trait. Irregularity of the zones of provisional calcification resembles rickets and is caused by extension of cartilage into the metaphyses (Fig. 9-12).

The appearance may be similar to Vitamin-D-resistant rickets. Differentiation may depend on biochemical analysis of blood and urine.

Cleidocranial Dysostosis

Cleidocranial dysostosis is transmitted as an autosomal dominant trait. In most patients, the clavicles and skull are involved, but other structures may be affected as well. The major and most obvious abnormality is a deficiency or absence of the clavicles (Fig. 9-13). There

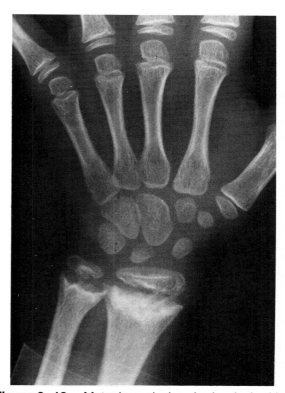

Figure 9–12. Metaphyseal chondrodysplasia (dysostosis) of the Schmid type. The metaphyses of the radius and ulna are concave and irregular. Similar changes were present in the metaphyses of the other long tubular bones. The epiphyses are normal. The bones of the hand are not affected.

are many variations in the appearance because the clavicle ossifies from three centers and any part may be absent. Clinically, the deficiency of the clavicles allows the individual to approximate the shoulders anteriorly, a significant feature of the disease. The cranial sutures remain open, and numerous wormian bones are present in the skull. Permanent patency of fontanelles is usually encountered. Often the anterior fontanelle is particularly large and extends forward between the frontal bones, with the metopic suture failing to close (Fig. 9-14). The mandible is prognathic as a result of hypoplasia of the maxilla and other facial bones.

In the pelvis, the bones are often underdeveloped and the symphysis pubis may be unusually wide. The sacrum and coccyx may be malformed or the coccyx may be absent.

MALFORMATION SYNDROMES ASSOCIATED WITH DISORGANIZED DEVELOPMENT OF CARTILAGE AND FIBROUS COMPONENTS OF THE SKELETON

Hereditary Multiple Exostoses (Osteochondromatosis; Hereditary Deforming Chondrodysplasia)

The anomaly known as hereditary multiple exostoses is characterized by the presence of numerous osteochondromas at the end of the shafts of the tubular bones and other bones preformed in cartilage. Lesions also occur in the pelvic bones, ribs, scapulae, vertebrae, and, very rarely, base of the skull. The disorder is inherited as an autosomal dominant trait with complete penetrance in males and reduced penetrance in females, so it usually passes from the father to his children. Males are affected more often than females, in a ratio of about three to one. The lesions are not present at birth but usually are first discovered during childhood and, as a rule, are asymptomatic unless they cause pressure on other structures. They are most common at the sites of greatest growth (i.e., the knee, shoulder, and wrist). Their number may vary from a few to hundreds, but they are usually bilaterally symmetrical. Small lesions in the hands and feet are noted in some patients, and the metacarpals and metatarsals may be shortened; in others, the hands and feet are normal.

The characteristic lesion is a broad-based, bony outgrowth with the apex pointing away from the nearest joint (Fig. 9-15). It consists of a cortical shell surrounding a core of cancellous bone. The cortex of the lesion merges smoothly with the normal cortex of the bone, and the growth is covered by a layer of cartilage that acts as an epiphyseal plate. This is not visible in roentgenograms. Occasionally, the lesion is more pedunculated, with a narrow base and a bulbous outer

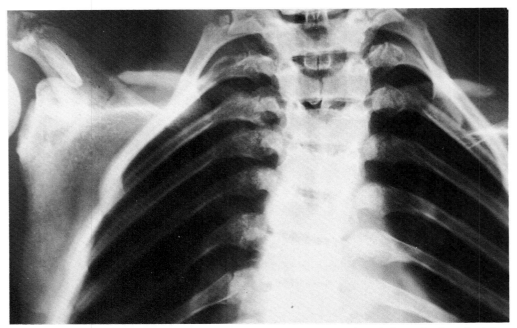

Figure 9–13. Cleidocranial dysostosis. Note the ossification defects in the clavicles and the midline spina bifida occulta involving the upper third thoracic vertebrae.

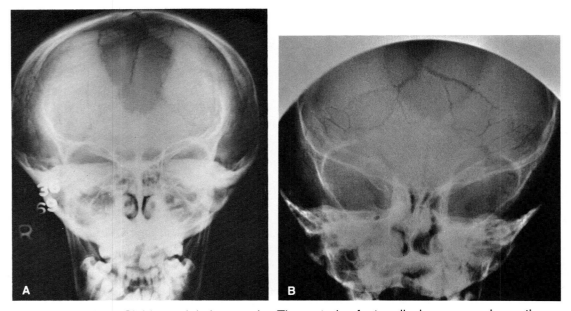

Figure 9–14. Cleidocranial dysostosis. The anterior fontanelle is open and greatly enlarged. There are numerous wormian bones adjacent to the lambdoidal suture.

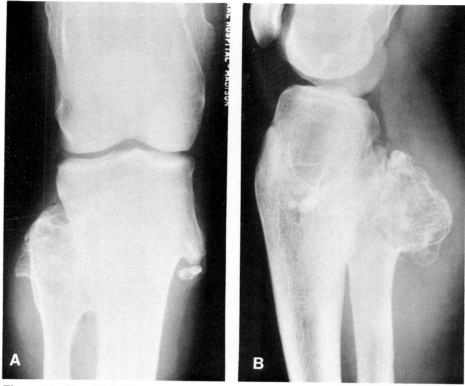

Figure 9–15. Multiple exostoses. (**A**) Note the characteristic deformity of all long bones, with a broad-based outgrowth with the apex pointing away from the nearest joint. (**B**) The cortex of the lesions is contiguous with the adjacent cortex of bone.

extremity containing lucent areas of cartilage and stippled areas of calcification, similar to the solitary osteochondroma. The osteochondromas originate in the metaphyseal region of the long tubular bones and cause the end of the shaft to be thickened and club shaped.

In about one third of affected persons, there is a characteristic deformity of the forearm due to shortening and bowing of the ulna, which does not extend far enough distally to take part in formation of the wrist joint. Another characteristic deformity occurs in the necks of the femurs. The neck is grossly thickened, particularly on the undersurface, caused by irregular, bony overgrowth sometimes likened to candle gutterings (Fig. 9-16), but also described as looking like the profile of the head and neck of a Brahma bull. The fibula may be shortened, and stunting of growth of other bones is seen in the more severe cases.

Growth of the osteochondromas continues throughout childhood and usually ceases when the nearest epiphysis fuses. Malignant degeneration is said to have

an incidence of about 1%. When an osteochondroma in an adult begins to enlarge or becomes painful, sarcomatous degeneration should be suspected.

Enchondromatosis (Ollier's Disease)

The basic lesion in enchondromatosis is the enchondroma, a proliferation of masses of cartilage within bone occurring in the ends of the shafts and causing an irregular, club-shaped enlargement. These lesions are radiolucent and contain characteristic spotty areas of calcification. In some cases, the lesions are limited to one extremity or to the extremities on one side of the body. The name Ollier's disease has been applied to the disseminated form. Even when widely disseminated, the involvement may be more severe on one side of the body than on the other. The femur and tibia are most often or most severely involved. Stunting of growth of the affected member is common, and at times a unilateral shortening of one leg has brought the patient to the physician. The epiphyses are not involved. The

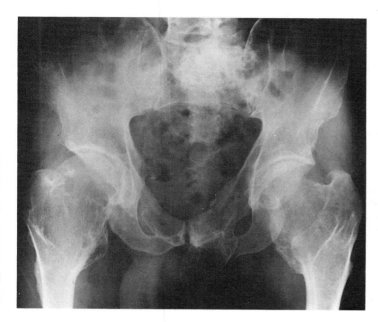

Figure 9–16.   Multiple exostoses in an adult illustrating the characteristic appearance of the upper ends of the femurs in this disease. The broad neck with the irregular bony overgrowths along the inferior surface is typical. There is also a large osteochondroma overlying the upper sacrum manifested by chondroid calcifications, and another is arising from the left pubis.

spine and skull usually are normal. The iliac crest and the vertebral border of the scapula have been affected in persons with more severe involvement.

In the long bones, the lesions may appear as elongated, radiolucent streaks extending in the direction of the long axis of bones and involving the metaphysis and adjacent diaphysis. In the hands and feet, the lesions tend to be globular and cause considerable expansion of the bone (Fig. 9-17). At other times, the lesion will involve the entire shaft of one of these short tubular bones. With growth, the lesions appear to migrate into the shaft. Eventually they may ossify, but residual deformity persists. Malignant transformation of an enchondroma into a chondrosarcoma can occur, particularly in the lesions in the long tubular bones.

Maffucci's Syndrome.   A combination of enchondromatosis and multiple cavernous hemangiomas that may be widely distributed throughout the body is known as Maffucci's syndrome. The presence of calcified thrombi (phleboliths) may allow roentgenographic recognition of the vascular lesions. The disease is rare but the potential of malignant degeneration of cartilage tumor is much higher than in other enchondromas.

Fibrous Dysplasia

Fibrous dysplasia usually begins during childhood and is characterized, pathologically, by replacement of normal bone by an abnormal proliferation of fibrous tissue. The disease may involve a single bone (monostotic) or the bones of one extremity or be widely distributed throughout the skeleton (polyostotic). There is some

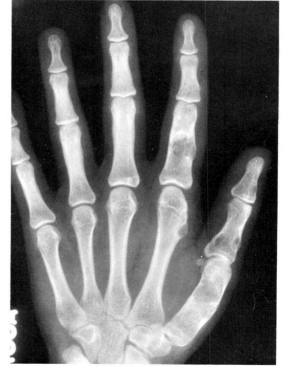

Figure 9–17.   Multiple enchondromatosis involving the hand. Note the lucent lesions with expansion of the shafts of the first and second proximal phalanges and metacarpals.

predilection for the long bones of the extremities, but any bone may be involved.

In the monostotic form, the femur, tibia, and ribs are the most common sites. The lesions are usually diaphyseal but may extend into the metaphysis. Most are discovered coincidentally on a radiographic examination obtained for trauma or some other reason. Occasionally, there is a pathologic fracture.

The polyostotic form is much less common than the monostotic and is usually associated with café-au-lait spots of the skin. Sexual precocity (Albright's syndrome) occurs in about one third of females with the polyostotic form but is rare in males. Other endocrine abnormalities are present in some of the patients. Acceleration of skeletal growth and maturation is fairly common, and thyroid enlargement, toxic and nontoxic, is found in about one fourth of the patients. Acromegaly and parathyroid hyperplasia are rare associated conditions.

Roentgenographic Findings.[16] The individual lesions vary, and some appear as that of a well-defined lucent area or "cyst." The cavity is filled with fibrous tissue rather than fluid so that it does not represent a true cyst. The margins often are ill defined, but in the cystic variety a thin sclerotic rim may bound the lesion (Fig. 9-18). The affected bone may have a milky or ground-glass appearance and may lack normal trabeculation (Fig. 9-19). The cortex may be eroded from within and the bone locally expanded, predisposing to fracture. Fractures heal with ample periosteal callus. A sequestrum may be found within an apparent cavity in a long bone.

Rib lesions have a ground-glass appearance, are usually well marginated, and occasionally are markedly expansile (Fig. 9-20). A markedly expanded lesion in a rib in a young individual should suggest fibrous dysplasia, whereas in an older patient a plasmacytoma is the most likely consideration.

In severe and long-standing disease, the bones may be bowed or misshapen. Some of the deformity may be the result of a previous fracture. The upper end of the femur characteristically has a "shepherd's crook" deformity and coxa vara, with lateral and anterior bowing of the shaft (Fig. 9-21).

In the skull, the lesion appears as a somewhat multilocular, cystlike area involving the diploic space and expanding the tables (Fig. 9-22). The margins are somewhat sclerotic but not sharply defined.

When fibrous dysplasia involves the base of the skull and the facial bones, the appearance is different. It causes a marked sclerosis and thickening. Thickening of the superior orbital wall giving rise to the "winking eye" sign on AP views of the skull and face is characteristic of fibrous dysplasia (Fig. 9-23). The sinuses may be obliterated. Computed tomography is helpful in diffi-

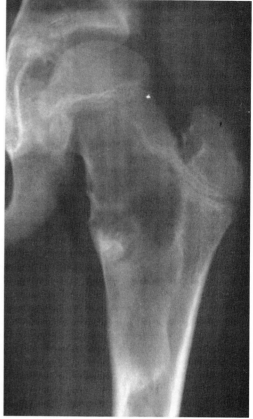

Figure 9–18. Fibrosis dysplasia monostotic form. There is a lucent, cystic lesion bordered by a rim of sclerosis in the neck of the femur extending into the trochanteric region and proximal shaft of the femur. (With permission from the Archives of the AFIP).

cult cases.[5] Involvement of the facial bones is similar to that of the base of the skull, with thickening and sclerosis. This appearance is known as *leontiasis ossea.*

In the base of the skull there is a striking similarity of the sclerosis to that associated with meningioma, and this may cause difficulty in diagnosis. Arteriography or CT scan may be necessary. The principal difference is that fibrous dysplasia is often encountered in the young, well before meningioma should be a consideration. Of great importance is the lack of involvement of the inner table in fibrous dysplasia and its occurrence in meningioma. There may also be involvement in the face or mandible in fibrous dysplasia, distinguishing it from a meningioma. In the differentiation from meningioma, the lack of dilated vascular grooves leading to the area of the bone lesion has been considered a significant finding. However, a few patients with fibrous dysplasia have been reported to have enlarged,

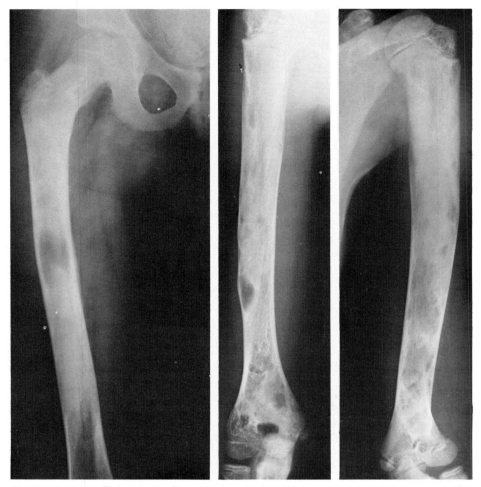

Figure 9–19. Polyostotic fibrous dysplasia. Widespread involvement of the skeleton is manifested by expansion of bone, with areas of ground-glass appearance interspersed with cystlike lesions.

tortuous vascular grooves, and this finding therefore cannot be considered specific for meningioma.

When skeletal involvement is extensive, there may be severe crippling and deformity. Solitary lesions or disease of lesser magnitude may cease to progress when skeletal growth is complete and may cause little or no permanent disability or deformity. Sarcomatous degeneration has been reported as a complication of fibrous dysplasia but appears to be very uncommon.

Hereditary Fibrous Dysplasia of the Jaws (Cherubism)

A multilocular, radiolucent lesion expands the jaw, causing a rounding of the facial features—hence the term *cherubism*. The lesions involve the mandible bi-laterally. The entire mandible, except the condyles, may be involved. Maxillary involvement is less frequent and less severe than mandibular disease and probably does not occur without lesions in the lower jaw. Although the exact cause is unknown, it has been suggested that the disease represents a hereditary form of fibrous dysplasia.

Dysplasia Epiphysealis Hemimelica (Trevor's Disease)

Dysplasia epiphysealis hemimelica is essentially an eccentric, usually intraarticular, overgrowth of an epiphysis of a long bone or a small bone of the foot, forming an irregular bony mass along one side of the affected epiphysis. Only a single epiphysis is involved; in the

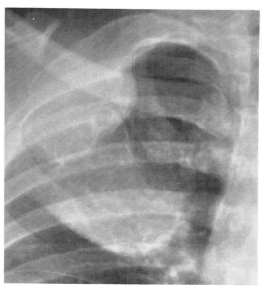

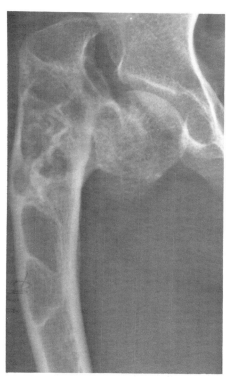

Figure 9–20. Fibrous dysplasia of a rib. The second rib is markedly expanded, but the cortex remains intact. The bone has a ground-glass appearance. (Courtesy of Harold Jacobson, M.D., Bronx, New York)

Figure 9–21. Fibrous dysplasia of the proximal femur. Shepherd's crook deformity of the femur, with considerable proximal migration of the shaft associated with an expansile lytic lesion that extends from the greater trochanter into the proximal femoral shaft. The femur is also bowed.

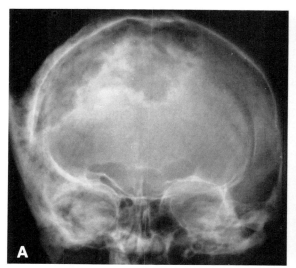

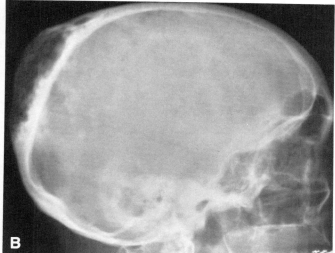

Figure 9–22. Fibrous dysplasia of the skull. (**A**) PA view. (**B**) Lateral view of the skull. Irregular expansile lesion involves the parietal bone and extends across the midline. The margin of the lesion is slightly irregular and sclerotic. The process extends anteriorly to involve the frontal bone. The inner and outer tables are intact, as demonstrated on the lateral projection.

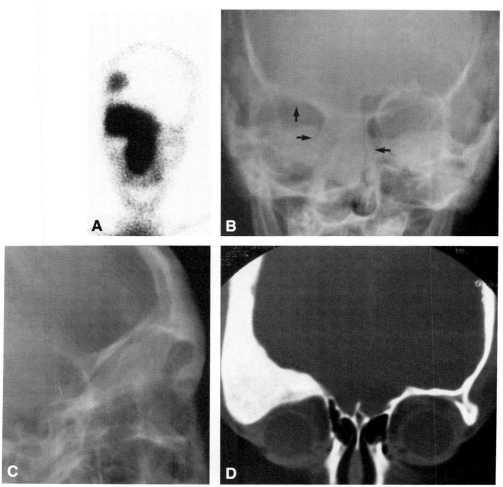

Figure 9–23.   Fibrous dysplasia of the frontal, sphenoid and ethmoid bones in a 15-year-old girl. **(A)** Bone scan demonstrates markedly increased uptake in the region of the right orbit and nasal fossa, with a separate focus in the right frontal bone. **(B)** AP view of skull reveals homogeneous sclerotic density involving the nasal fossa and ethmoid region, with the process extending to involve the upper rim of the orbit (*arrows*) giving rise to the "winking eye" appearance. **(C)** Lateral view of the face demonstrates homogeneous thickening of the roof of orbit extending into the base of the frontal bone. (Courtesy of John Ralsten, M.D., Parkersburg, West Virginia). **(D)** CT scan in the coronal projection in an 11-year-old girl demonstrates a characteristic mottled appearance of fibrous dysplasia involving the sphenoid and frontal bones. Note the characteristic mottled sclerotic appearance of the involved bone. Though expanded, the cortex remains intact; there are small foci of lucency interspersed within the sclerotic bone. (Courtesy of Thomas Naidich, M.D., Miami, Florida)

great majority of patients it is the talus, followed in frequency by the distal femur and distal tibia. Other areas less frequently affected include the upper tibia, upper fibula, lesser trochanter of the femur, and the tarsal navicular and first cuneiform. The bony mass may be attached to the adjacent epiphysis or may exist separately. It is usually first noticed during childhood and is asymptomatic until the mass interferes with joint function. Pathologically, the lesion is said to be identical with an exostosis or osteochondroma.

SYNDROMES ASSOCIATED WITH ABNORMALITIES OF DENSITY OF CORTICAL BONE OR DIAPHYSEAL STRUCTURE OR METAPHYSEAL MODELING

Osteogenesis Imperfecta (Fragilitas Ossium Congenita: Brittle Bones)

Osteogenesis imperfecta is a rare hereditary disorder characterized by an unusual fragility of bone, leading to multiple fractures often from a trivial cause. The underlying abnormality is a disorder of collagen. This results in fragile bones, thin skin, blue sclerae, poor teeth, and hypermobility of the joints.

There are several forms of the disease. The two principal forms are (1) osteogenesis imperfecta congenita and (2) osteogenesis imperfecta tarda. The inheritance is variable from type to type; some are autosomal dominant, others are recessive.

In the congenital form, the disorder develops in utero and the infant is born with multiple fractures (Fig. 9-24). The diagnosis has been established in utero using ultrasonography by recognizing angular defor-mities of long bones.[7, 10] Mortality is high, resulting from intracranial hemorrhage at birth or from recurrent respiratory infections in the first two years of life.

The tarda form of disease is first noted during childhood because of the unusual tendency for fractures. The joints are lax, dislocations are frequent, deafness caused by otosclerosis becomes apparent, and the teeth are discolored, fragile, and easily broken. Blue sclerae also become more apparent, evidently owing to the intraocular pigment, which shows through the thin sclerae.

Roentgenographic Findings. *Skull.* In the congenital type, the cranial bones are largely membranous at birth. If the infant survives, ossification progresses slowly, leaving wide sutures and multiple wormian bones (mosaic skull). Later the sutures become of normal width.

Tubular Bones. In the congenital form, the infant usually is born with multiple fractures of the long bones

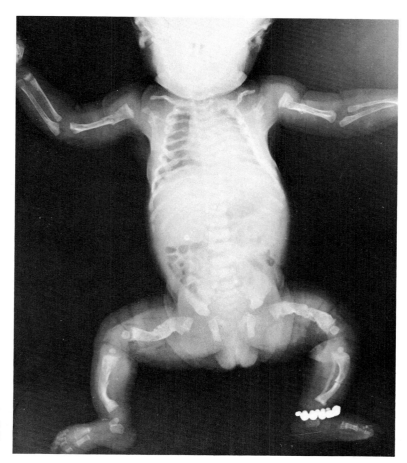

Figure 9–24. Osteogenesis imperfecta in a newborn. Note the multiple fractures and deformities of all bones of the skeleton.

(Fig. 9-24). The shafts are wide and appear short owing to the multiple fractures and the width of the bones. The fractures heal readily, occasionally with exuberant callus so extensive that a malignant tumor may be suspected (Fig. 9-25). The cortices are characteristically thin. In the tarda type, the long bones appear thin and gracile (Fig. 9-26). The ends appear wide, and the zones of provisional calcification may be denser than normal. Trabeculae are diminished. There often is extensive deformity owing to recent fractures and to previous fractures that healed. The epiphyses are normal. Fractures involving short bones are less frequent, but otherwise they show similar changes.

Spine. Growth of the vertebrae is normal, but they are osteoporotic and have thin cortical margins. Compression fractures are frequent, and multiple bodies may show biconcave disc surfaces (codfish vertebrae).

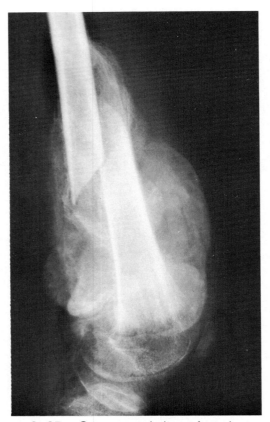

Figure 9–25. Osteogenesis imperfecta in an adolescent. Exuberant callus is present about the spiral fracture, forming a huge mass around and below the fracture site. This type of callus may be mistaken for a malignant tumor.

The intervertebral disc spaces may be widened. Scoliosis is frequent.

Flat Bones. The pelvis may show changes in shape secondary to the osteoporosis, and protrusio acetabuli is common. Fractures of the ribs also are common.

Osteopetrosis (Albers–Schönberg Disease; Osteosclerosis Fragilis; Marble Bones)

Osteopetrosis is characterized by an unusual density or radiopacity of the bones. Although dense, the bones are brittle and fracture readily. The disease may be discovered at birth, shortly thereafter, or not until adulthood. As with most of the other dysplasias, the earlier the disease is found the more severe it is likely to be.

Growth is often stunted in the infantile form; myelophthisic anemia may become severe and lead to death. Jaundice, hepatosplenomegaly, and cranial nerve palsies are common. Death often occurs within the first year of life. This form of the disease has been treated successfully by bone-marrow transplantation. In the infantile (congenita) form, the disease has been found in utero and the baby may be stillborn. This form is transmitted as an autosomal recessive trait, whereas the adult form may be either autosomal dominant (majority) or recessive.

In the adult form, the disease may first come to the attention of a physician because of a fracture of a long bone. Characteristically, these fractures are of a transverse type. There may be a history of repeated fractures during childhood. Another presenting symptom may be an unexplained anemia. These patients often suffer from carious teeth and dental or jaw infections.

Roentgenographic Findings. *Tubular Bones.* In the infant, all of the bones may be affected, having a uniform, dense, structureless appearance and complete obliteration of normal trabecular architecture (Fig. 9-27). The medullary canal is obliterated by dense sclerosis and merges with the cortex. The density of the bones is thought to be the result of failure of normal removal of old bone while new bone continues to be formed. The sclerosis is usually uniform in the infantile form. Occasionally there may be alternating bands of sclerotic and normal bone at the ends of the shafts. The trabecular pattern is completely obliterated. The length of the bones is usually normal but is occasionally decreased. Characteristically the bones are club shaped owing to failure of normal modeling. The epiphyseal ossification centers are dense, but they mature normally. In the adult, the increased density is limited to bands of sclerosis at the bone ends, sometimes alternating with bands of normal den-

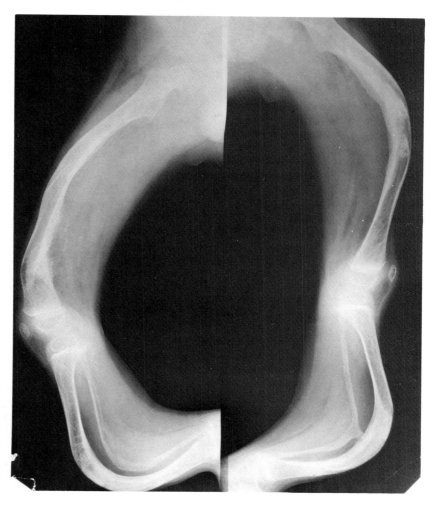

Figure 9–26. Osteogenesis imperfecta tarda. The misshapen bones are caused by multiple healed fractures and abnormal softness of the bone. Note the thin cortex and relative thinness of the bone sometimes described as gracile.

sity. The bones of the hands and feet are involved in the same way as the long tubular bones. The sternal ends of the clavicles may be widened.

Spine. The vertebrae are uniformly involved by the sclerosis, and there may be impingement on the spinal nerves. In the adult type, the sclerosis may be limited to the upper and lower margins of the vertebrae, creating a "sandwich" or "rugger-jersey" vertebra (Fig. 9-28) similar in appearance to that seen in renal osteodystrophy or secondary hyperparathyroidism, but the sclerosis in osteopetrosis is much more sharply defined than in secondary hyperparathyroidism. Other cases have a dense "bone-in-bone" appearance.

Skull. The base of the skull shows the most marked sclerosis, but all of the cranial bones may be involved.

The sinuses and mastoids may show complete lack of pneumatization. The cranial foramina are encroached upon, leading to various cranial nerve palsies such as blindness and deafness. The teeth are late in erupting and develop caries early. Dental infection may lead to osteomyelitis of the jaw. The lamina dura, the cortical margin of the tooth socket, may be unusually thick and dense, and the disease may be suspected from dental roentgenograms.

Pyknodysostosis

Pyknodysostosis is easily confused with osteopetrosis because of the generalized dense sclerotic appearance of the bones; however, it is separate and distinct and has characteristic and distinctive radiographic features that allow differentiation from the more common osteopetrosis.

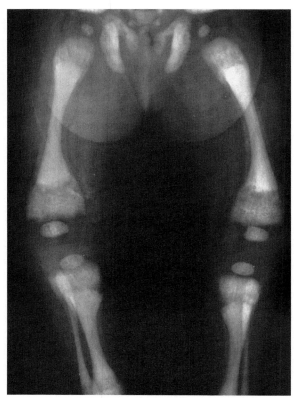

Figure 9–27. Osteopetrosis in an infant. The bones throughout the skeleton are chalky white, and no trabecular architecture is visible. Radiolucent bands cross the ends of the shaft, representing periods of normal ossification. The metaphyses are large and club shaped, owing to a failure of modeling as the bones increased in length.

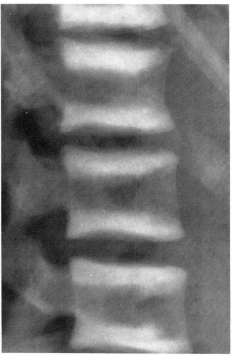

Figure 9–28. Osteopetrosis of the spine in a 34-year-old man. Note the characteristic sandwich or "rugger jersey" appearance of the vertebrae caused by sclerosis of the vertebral end plates.

In the skull, there is a failure of closure of the cranial sutures and fontanelles and numerous wormian bones are present (Fig. 9-29A). The mandibular rami are hypoplastic, with a characteristic loss of the normal mandibular angle. Sclerosis and thickening of the cranial and facial bones may be severe. The sinuses may fail to develop, particularly the frontals, and the mastoids often are not pneumatized. The hands are short and stubby, with acro-osteolysis of the terminal phalanges (Fig. 9-29B). The vertebrae are sclerotic, and there is a lack of fusion of the neural arches in some. Fractures are extremely common and often are of the transverse type. The stature is reduced, and deformity from old fractures may lead to further shortening of the long tubular bones. Henri Toulouse-Lautrec, the late 19th-century French lithographer and painter, very likely was afflicted with pyknodysostosis.

Osteopoikilosis (Spotted Bones)

Osteopoikilosis is an asymptomatic disorder characterized by the appearance of numerous small, round or oval densities in the ends of the long bones (Fig. 9-30), in the small bones of the hands and feet, and around the acetabulum. The lesions are composed of dense, compact bone. They are discovered by chance on roentgenographic examination obtained for trauma or some other condition. The disorder is transmitted as an autosomal dominant trait and has been discovered in newborns as well as in the fetus in utero. The lesions may increase or decrease in size and number during the period of active bone growth and have been noted to disappear altogether.

Solitary sclerotic foci of the same nature are common throughout the appendicular skeleton and pelvis and are known as bone islands (see Chap. 4).

Osteopathia Striata

Osteopathia striata is similar in many ways to osteopoikilosis, but, instead of rounded foci, striae of dense

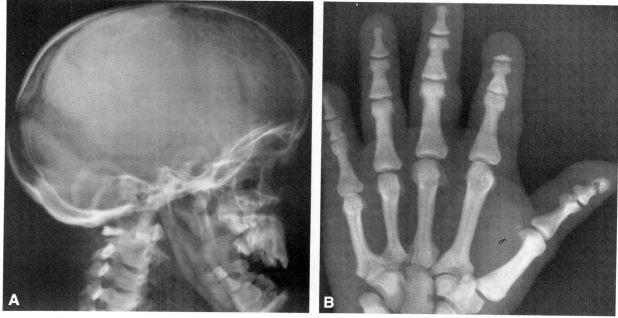

Figure 9–29. Pyknodysostosis. **(A)** Skull. The cranial sutures have failed to close. Note the markedly widened lambdoid suture. The skull is foreshortened. There is a characteristic deformity of the mandible caused by a hypoplasia of the mandibular rami. Note the loss of the normal mandibular angle characteristic of this disorder. **(B)** Hand. The bones are quite dense, and the hand is short with stubby fingers. The terminal phalanges are hypoplastic. Note acro-osteolysis of the terminal phalanges.

bone extending toward the nearest joint are encountered. In children, the striae begin at the epiphyseal line and extend for a short distance into the diaphysis. In the acetabulum, the striae have a "sunburst" appearance, fanning outward toward the iliac crest. Any or all of the long bones and the pelvis may be involved. The lesions are asymptomatic and are discovered by chance.

Tuberous Sclerosis

Tuberous sclerosis is a rare familial disease manifested by a classic triad of adenoma sebaceum of the face, epilepsy, and mental deficiency. Hamartomas are identified in the kidney (angiomyolipomas) and in the subependymal tissues of the brain (see Chap. 11).

The characteristic finding in the skeletal system is punctate osteosclerosis (Fig. 9-31). These lesions may be round, oval, or irregular in outline and vary in size from a few millimeters to several centimeters. Sclerosis may also occur in the ribs and spine. Periosteal new-bone formation along the shafts of the large and small tubular bones may be seen. Small cystlike lesions occur in the small bones of the hands and feet.

In addition, there may be a reticular or honeycomb pattern in the lung and diffuse intracerebral calcifications.

Melorheostosis

Melorheostosis presents as an irregular thickening of the cortex along one side of a bone or bones of one extremity.[3] The thickening may be external, internal, or both (Fig. 9-32). The appearance has been likened to molten wax flowing down the side of a candle. If an extremity is involved, the pelvis (or shoulder girdle) on the affected side is likely to show similar thickening. Fibrolipomatous masses occasionally containing amorphous calcification are sometimes encountered adjacent to the bony lesions.[9]

The onset may be in infancy or not until late adolescence, up until age 20. The presenting symptom is pain, which may be severe. The disease does not appear to be hereditary. If it begins early in life, the epiphyses may fuse prematurely, causing shortening of the involved extremity. The lesions usually cease progressing when skeletal growth is complete. Regression has not been noted.

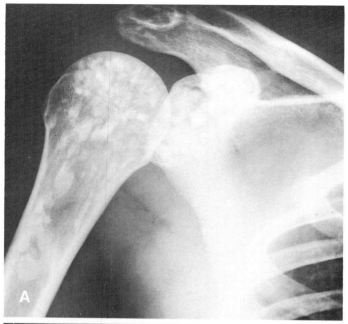

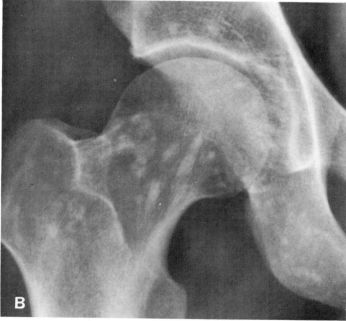

Figure 9–30. Osteopoikilosis. (**A**) Shoulder. There are dense, rounded, and slightly elongated foci on both sides of the joint, but they are best visualized in the head and proximal shaft of the humerus. (**B**) The hip in another patient. The sclerotic foci in this film are not quite as dense nor large as those in *A* but are seen on both sides of the joint.

Endosteal Hyperostosis (Van Buchem's Syndrome)

Endosteal hyperostosis, transmitted as an autosomal recessive trait, is characterized by symmetrical sclerosis of the skull, mandible, and clavicle. In the diaphyses of the bones of the extremities, endosteal thickening tends to thicken the cortex but does not increase the diameter of the bone. The medial aspects of the clavicles tend to be increased in diameter, however.

Engelmann's Disease (Diaphyseal Dysplasia, Progressive Diaphyseal Sclerosis)

The major manifestations of Engelmann's disease consist of symmetrical cortical thickening in the mid-diaphyses, particularly of the femur and the tibia.[13]

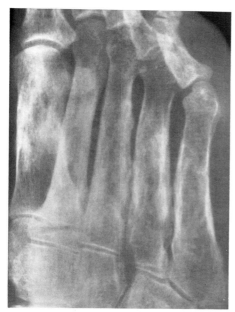

Figure 9–31. Tuberous sclerosis. Note the irregular patches of sclerosis and periosteal reaction. (Courtesy of James C. Reed, M.D., New Bern, North Carolina)

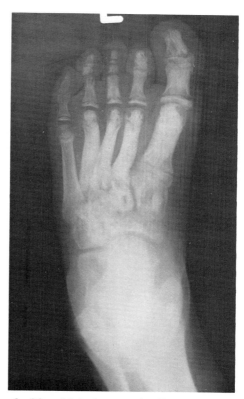

Figure 9–32. Melorheostosis. Dense sclerosis of the first to fourth metatarsals and phalanges of the great toe of the left foot is evident. Similar changes were present along the inner cortex of the long bones of the left leg and the left hemipelvis.

The lesion tends to progress and eventually involves most of the diaphysis. The epiphyses and metaphyses are spared. The disorder may begin in early childhood, with difficulty in walking and a shuffling or waddling gait. The cortical thickening begins subperiosteally, but, with failure of resorption, the medullary canal may be encroached upon, leading to anemia and hepatosplenomegaly (Fig. 9-33). The disease also progresses to involve other bones and, in some, may involve the short bones of the hands and feet as well as the bones of the trunk, skull, and face. The base of the skull may become thick and dense, with subsequent impingement on the cranial nerves. The vault is seldom involved except for frontal and occipital bossing. Muscles tend to be flabby and weak. Dental caries are often present. Mentality is not affected.

Metaphyseal Dysplasia (Pyle's Disease, Craniometaphyseal Dysplasia)

The basic disturbance in metaphyseal dysplasia appears to be a failure of modeling of cylindrical bones. The changes are often most noticeable at the lower ends of the femurs and upper ends of the tibias and humeri, leading to a club-shaped enlargement often referred to as an "Erlenmeyer flask" appearance. The cortices at the ends of the bones are thin, and thus the bone is subject to fracture.

In the hand, there is distal flaring of the metacarpals and proximal flaring of the phalanges. Marked thickening of the ribs, clavicles, and ischial and pubic bones is present, and there may be minimal vertebral flattening. Skull findings include a distinct supra-orbital bulge, and sometimes there is mild hyperostosis of the cranial vault. Minimal prognathism and a rounded, obtuse mandibular angle may also be present.

The disease is transmitted as an autosomal recessive trait, and consanguinity has been noted in many cases. Some authors separate craniometaphyseal dysplasia from Pyle's disease. Clinically, there is hypertelorism and broadening of the root of the nose in craniometaphyseal dysplasia. The bone sclerosis at the root of the nose leads to nasal obstruction. Temporal bone changes often lead to deafness and sometimes to facial paralysis. Frontal, paranasal, and occipital sclerosis or hyperostosis is present, and diaphyseal sclerosis is a common feature. There is no thickening of ribs, clavicles, or ischial and pubic bones. Metaphyseal flaring is less than in metaphyseal dysplasia.

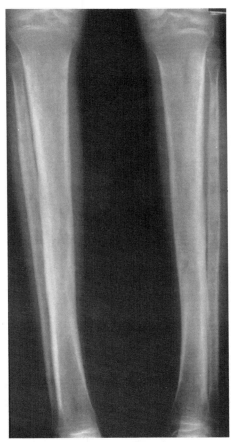

Figure 9–33. Diaphyseal dysplasia (Engelmann's disease). There is diffuse cortical thickening involving the shafts of both tibias and fibulas. The process extends into the metaphysis but does not involve the bone adjacent to the growth plates.

DYSOSTOSES

Dysostoses are malformations of individual bones, either singly or in combination. Some of these are associated with craniofacial involvement, whereas others predominantly involve the spine, and still others the extremities.

DYSOSTOSES WITH CRANIAL AND FACIAL INVOLVEMENT

Acrocephalosyndactyly (Apert's Syndrome)

Persons with Apert's syndrome have characteristic facial deformities that include a flat face, shallow orbits, hypertelorism, and osseous and cutaneous syndactyly

with hands and feet that appear as if they were in mittens and socks. The thumbs are usually broad and often short. Affected persons are often mentally retarded. The condition is inherited as an autosomal dominant trait, and most cases represent new mutations.

The most important radiographic findings are in the skull, hands, and feet. In the skull there is premature fusion of the coronal suture, which results in a decreased AP diameter of the skull, or brachycephaly. In the hand there are osseous and cutaneous syndactyly, symphalangia, and a very broad thumb (Fig. 9-34). In some forms, the changes are milder in the hand, with no syndactyly but with characteristic changes in the thumb.

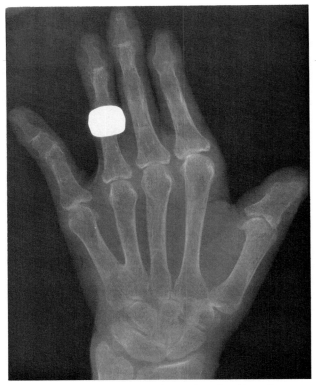

Figure 9–34. Acrocephalosyndactyly (Apert's syndrome) in a 60-year-old woman whose daughters had similar manifestations. Note symphalangism or fusion of the proximal interphalangeal joints of the second, third, and fourth digits; osseous syndactyly at the base of the fourth and fifth metacarpals; and cutaneous and soft-tissue syndactyly at the base of the third and fourth digits. (Note the position of the wedding ring). The thumb is characteristically short and broad. There is also a lunatotriquetral fusion.

Mandibulofacial Dysostosis (Crouzon's Disease) (See Chapter 11)

DYSOSTOSES WITH SPINAL INVOLVEMENT

1. Klippel-Feil (see Chap. 12)
2. Sprengel's anomaly (see Chap. 8)
3. Spondylocostal dysostosis (see previous description of conditions identifiable at birth; see also Fig. 9-10)

DYSOSTOSES WITH PREDOMINANT INVOLVEMENT OF EXTREMITIES

Brachydactyly

A variety of syndromes associated with shortening of various bones within the hand have been identified. These are generally characterized by the phalanges involved (Fig. 9-35A). The most commonly used classification of brachydactyly is that of Bell.[23] Most of the brachydactyly conditions are inherited as autosomal dominant traits.

There are also a variety of syndromes associated with polydactyly and clinodactyly, or curvature of the fingers. These may occur as sporadic abnormalities or may be associated with familial disorders.

Symphalangism

Symphalangism is characterized by fusion of one phalanx to another within the same digit. Most are inherited as an autosomal dominant trait. Some are related to syndromes, such as Apert's syndrome. The incidence of involvement decreases from the fifth to the second digit (Fig. 9-35B). The thumb is usually

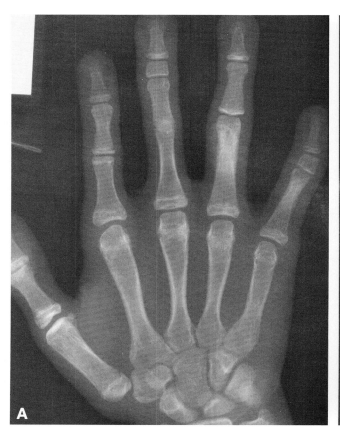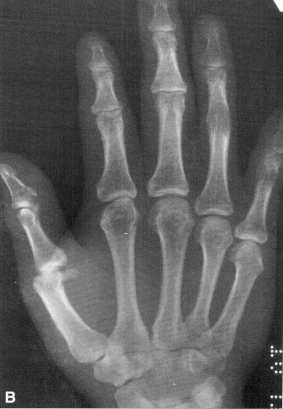

Figure 9–35. (**A**) Brachydactyly (Bell type C). In this form, the middle phalanges are predominantly involved, and there may be peculiar epiphyseal centers or segmentation defects as seen in the proximal phalanx of the third digit. The ring finger is characteristically spared, as in this case. (**B**) Symphalangism. There is congenital fusion of the proximal interphalangeal joints of the fourth and fifth digits and relative shortening of the phalanges. There is also a fusion of the capitate and hamate bones.

not affected. Associated carpal and tarsal fusions are common.[31]

Cardiomelic (Holt—Oram) Syndrome

Holt–Oram syndrome is an autosomal dominant inherited disorder consisting of characteristic abnormalities of the upper limbs and associated with congenital heart disease, usually a septal defect. The most characteristic radiographic findings are in the hand, where there may be a triphalangeal thumb having a finger-like configuration (Fig. 9-36). This anomaly is uncommon in other disorders and should suggest Holt–Oram syndrome when associated with congenital heart disease. In some cases, however, there may be hyperplasia or absence of the thumb. Accessory carpals and carpal fusions may occur.

MISCELLANEOUS CONGENITAL DISORDERS WITH OSSEOUS INVOLVEMENT

Marfan's Syndrome (Arachnodactyly)

Marfan's syndrome is a disease of connective tissue caused by abnormal collagen formation[24]. It involves the heart and aorta, and one of its common manifestations is aneurysm formation, usually of the ascending aorta and often complicated by dissection. Afflicted persons are tall and slender, usually over 6 feet in height. The muscles are poorly developed and have poor tone. Thus the joints may be hypermobile, there may be dislocation of the hips, genu recurvatum, dislocation of the patella, and pes planus. Ectopia lentis is common.

The bones are of normal density but long and gracile. Their thickness is normal, but the increased length gives an illusion of thinness. In the hands, elongation of the bones leads to a characteristic appearance, arachnodactyly, described as "spider-like" (Fig. 9-37). Scoliosis is frequent. The skull often has a dolichocephalic shape owing to increased length of the base. There is a decrease in subcutaneous fat, so that affected persons appear emaciated. There often is pectus excavatum. The disease is transmitted as an autosomal dominant trait.

Basal Cell Nevus Syndrome (Gorlin's Syndrome)

The basal cell nevus syndrome consists of a combination of multiple basal cell epitheliomas, rib anomalies (bifid, fused, etc.), odontogenic cysts of the maxilla and mandible, cystic lesions in long and short bones (Fig. 9-38A), and extensive calcification of the falx cerebri (Fig. 9-38B).[9, 19]

Neurofibromatosis (Von Recklinghausen's Disease)

Neurofibromatosis was first described by von Recklinghausen in 1882. It is a disease of the supporting tissues of the nervous system. Although skin tumors

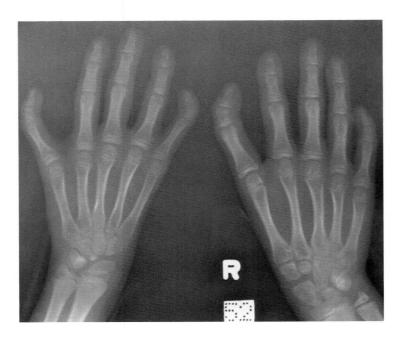

Figure 9–36. Holt–Oram Syndrome. Note characteristic bilateral triphalangeal thumb. At first glance the patient appears to have no thumbs. Carpal anomalies are also present. (Case courtesy of Andrew K. Poznanski, Chicago).

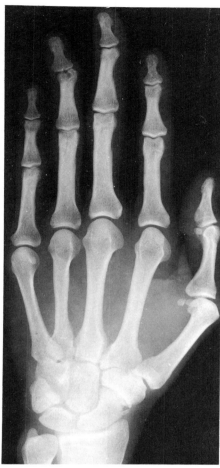

Figure 9–37. Arachnodactyly (Marfan's syndrome). The bones are elongated and slender, characteristic of this disorder. The deformity of the fourth finger is secondary to old trauma.

are the most prominent feature, the disorder may involve other systems, including endocrine, gastrointestinal, and skeletal. The present discussion chiefly centers on the latter. Brownish pigmented areas (café-au-lait spots) occur frequently on the skin. The extent of the disease may vary considerably. There is a tendency for the progression to slow or stop when skeletal growth is completed. A small percentage of the lesions may become malignant, indicating neurofibrosarcoma. There is an increased frequency of meningiomas.

Kyphoscoliosis is common in the spine.[4] The scoliosis is usually sharp and angular, and its cause often is obscure since associated neurofibromas are not found (Fig. 9-39). The vertebrae often are wedge shaped at the height of curvature.

The ribs often are thin and have been likened to a twisted ribbon (Fig. 9-39). In the long bones, pressure from an adjacent tumor may cause a small local excavation in the cortex, the "pit" or "cave" defect. A neurofibroma may arise within bone, causing a sharply outlined area of radiolucency.

A peculiar manifestation of the disease is localized enlargement of a part such as a finger or one extremity (focal gigantism). The bone, except for its greater size, appears normal.

In the skull, absence of part of the orbital wall may cause unilateral exophthalmos, often pulsating. The clinoid processes of the sella may be absent on the affected side. As with some of the other bone changes, an associated tumor need not be present, and the loss of bone is not caused by pressure erosion. Localized widening of the lambdoid suture has been reported. A neurofibroma may affect a cranial nerve, particularly the acoustic, causing enlargement of the corresponding foramen. Bilateral acoustic neuromas are characteristic of neurofibromatosis.

Lateral intrathoracic meningocele is found with some frequency in neurofibromatosis. It presents as a rounded, paraspinous mass projecting into the thoracic cavity and is usually associated with deformity of the contiguous vertebrae, including kyphosis, scoliosis, and erosions of the vertebral bodies, arches, and ribs. Scalloping of the posterior surfaces of one or more vertebral bodies is common. It has been shown that posterior scalloping of the vertebral body can occur in neurofibromatosis in the absence of any associated tumor.

A neurofibroma of a spinal nerve root often is of a dumbbell shape, having both intra- and extraspinal components. This type of tumor is prone to erode the contiguous vertebral pedicles, and, in the thoracic area, a paraspinous mass may be seen. A neurofibroma of an intercostal nerve causes a mass density along the thoracic wall, and often there is pressure erosion of adjacent ribs and localized widening of the rib interspace. It should be noted that a solitary neurofibroma may occur in many different areas of the body without the other stigmata of von Recklinghausen's disease.

Pseudarthrosis. During the newborn period (and occasionally noted at birth), a pathologic fracture may occur through a long bone, usually the distal one third of the tibia. The fracture fails to heal, the ends of the fragments become pointed or smoothly rounded, and pseudarthrosis results (Fig. 9-40).[4] Stigmata of neurofibromatosis, such as café-au-lait spots, are present in about one half of these patients. When observed early, the lesion appears as a gradual local lysis of bone. In some cases, the fracture heals temporarily but refractures when weight-bearing is attempted. The condition is very difficult to treat. Some authorities contend

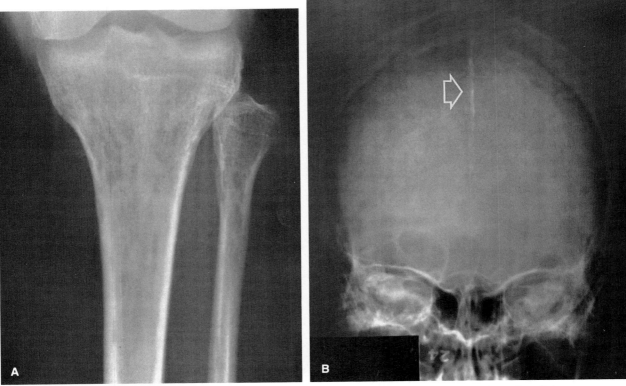

Figure 9–38.   Basal cell nevus syndrome. (**A**) A poorly defined, elongated, oval radiolucent pattern appears in the metaphysis of both the tibia and fibula. Similar findings were evident in the metaphysis of all long bones and lucencies were present in the phalanges of both hands. (**B**) Heavy calcification of the falx cerebri (*arrow*) is characteristic of this disorder. (Case courtesy of Martin Gross, M.D., Detroit)

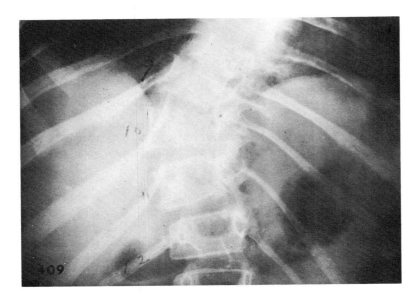

Figure 9–39.   Neurofibromatosis. There is a sharp scoliosis in the lower thoracic spine, the vertebrae are malformed, and the lower ribs are thin, particularly on the left side.

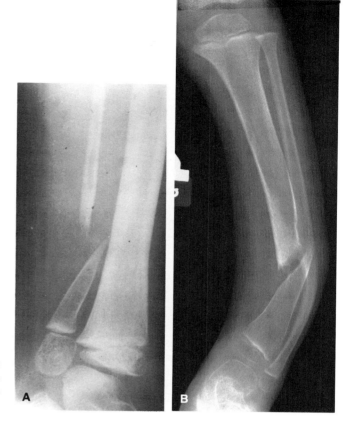

Figure 9–40. **(A)** Pseudoarthrosis of the fibula in a patient with neurofibromatosis. **(B)** Pseudoarthrosis of the tibia in a 5-year-old without evidence of neurofibromatosis.

that intraosseous neurilemoma is responsible for the lesion, but most investigators believe that it represents a mesenchymal defect or is perhaps related to the abnormal periosteum sometimes present in neurofibromatosis.

Congenital Fibromatosis

Congenital fibromatosis is an entity characterized by progressive benign fibrous tumors noted at or shortly after birth; these may involve the subcutaneous tissues, viscera, and bone.[1] The tumors are peculiar in that they grow for a limited time and then gradually regress over a period of two years. Skeletal lesions are lytic or cystic, with smooth, well-defined margins and occasional disruption of the overlying cortex (Fig. 9-41). Pathologic fractures can occur. Before regressing, the lesions enlarge and expand bone. Residual abnormalities after regression are minimal. In a small percentage of cases, the vital organs and viscera may be involved and the patients may not survive. However, patients survive if the lesions are found predominantly

within the skeletal system and there is little or no involvement of the viscera.

Progeria

Progeria is essentially premature senility developing in a child. Affected infants appear normal at birth, but the typical features become evident within the first few years of life. The appearance has been likened to that of a wizened old person. There is loss of subcutaneous fat, alopecia, and atrophy of the muscles and the skin. The facies show a receding chin, beaked nose, and exophthalmos. There is premature arteriosclerosis in the coronary arteries and other vessels, leading to death during late childhood or early adolescence. Afflicted persons are dwarfed. Roentgenographic findings include hypoplastic facial bones, open cranial sutures and fontanelles, and dwarfism. The long bones are apt to be short, thin, and osteoporotic, and there is coxa valga, which may be marked. A significant feature is acro-osteolysis of the terminal digits of the fingers and toes.

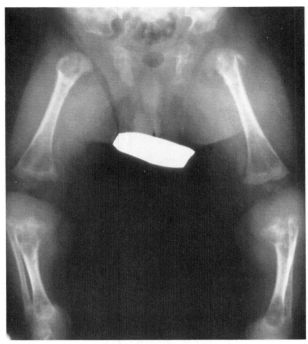

Figure 9–41. Congenital fibromatosis. There are lucent lesions in the metaphyses of all the long bones and within the pelvis. The overlying cortex is eroded in the proximal tibia. The lesions characteristically regress in time. (Courtesy of Leonard O. Langer, M.D., Minneapolis, Minnesota)

THE MUCOPOLYSACCHARIDOSES

The mucopolysaccharidoses are a group of metabolic diseases characterized by the excretion of abnormal amounts of one or more mucopolysaccharides in the urine and an abnormality in elaboration and storage of these substances. The following types have been defined according to the mucopolysaccharide involved, their mode of genetic transmission, and clinical and roentgenographic features.[18, 31]

Type I-H: Hurler's syndrome
Type I-S: Scheie's syndrome
Type II: Hunter's syndrome
Type III: Sanfilippo's syndrome
Type IV: Morquio's syndrome
Type V: Vacant
Type VI: Maroteaux–Lamy syndrome
Type VII: Glucuronidase deficiency

From the radiographic standpoint, Hurler's disease (gargoylism), Morquio's disease, and the Maroteaux–Lamy syndrome are the most important. The others differ chiefly in their nonroentgenographic manifestations.

Morquio's Disease (Type IV)

Morquio's disease is due to an abnormality in the elaboration and storage of the mucopolysaccharide keratan sulfate. The disease is rare and is characterized by dwarfism, kyphosis, and severe disability. The dwarfism is caused primarily by shortness of the spine, although some degree of shortening of the long tubular bones is common. Both sexes are affected with the same frequency. It is hereditary and familial, the genetic transmission being autosomal recessive. Consanguinity has been noted in some. The first symptoms usually occur when the child begins to sit, stand, or walk.

Roentgenographic Findings.[5, 18] *Spine.* The most characteristic change is universal platyspondyly, a flattening of the vertebral bodies. The disc margins are irregular and roughened, and an anterior, central, tonguelike projection is seen in the thoracolumbar region (Fig. 9-42). A sharp angular kyphosis at the thoracolumbar junction is one of the significant clinical observations. The intervertebral discs may be thick early in life but later are reduced in height.

Long Tubular Bones. Epiphyseal ossification centers may be multiple and are often irregular. They are late in appearing but mature normally. The degree of shortening of the long bones is variable. The zones of provisional calcification are irregular, and the metaphyses are broad. The proximal femur is often the most severely affected. Delay in appearance of the capital epiphysis, fragmentation, flaring, and irregularity of the metaphysis and subluxation of the hip are common (Fig. 9-43). The presence of coxa valga helps to distinguish Morquio's disease from most of the spondyloepiphyseal dysplasias in which coxa vara is more common.

Flat Bones. The ilia flare laterally, and the acetabular cavities are enlarged and have rough margins (Fig. 9-43). Rubin describes the ribs as canoe paddles, the vertebral end being narrow and the remainder broad.[26]

Short Tubular Bones. These bones often are short and have irregular epiphyseal ossification centers. The second, third, fourth, and fifth metacarpals often taper at their proximal ends. The metatarsals are similarly affected (Fig. 9-44).

Other Findings. The skull and facial bones are normal, significant in the differentiation from achondroplasia. A hypoplastic or absent odontoid process is noted in many patients. The carpal and tarsal bones are late in appearing and, when developed, have irregular or angular shapes.

The head appears large in relation to the size of the

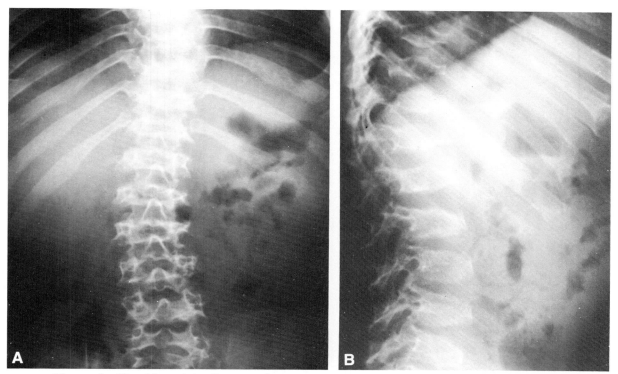

Figure 9–42. Morquio's disease. Anteroposterior (**A**) and lateral (**B**) views of lower thoracic and lumbar spine. The vertebrae are flattened and irregular. The anterior central beaking is best demonstrated in the lower thoracic vertebrae on the lateral projection. The ribs are broad peripherally but narrow at their vertebral ends.

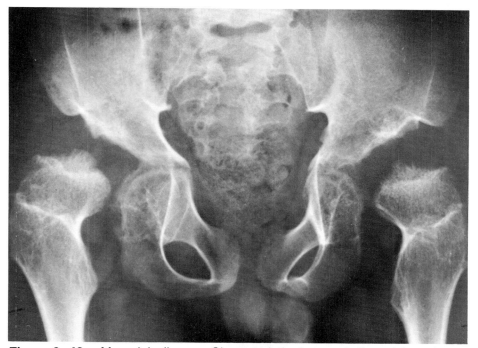

Figure 9–43. Morquio's disease. Characteristic changes in the pelvis and proximal femurs include the "wine glass" contour of the pelvis, the large irregular acetabulae, and the small, poorly formed femoral epiphyses and broad femoral necks. Ilia are flared, and the hip joint is partially subluxed.

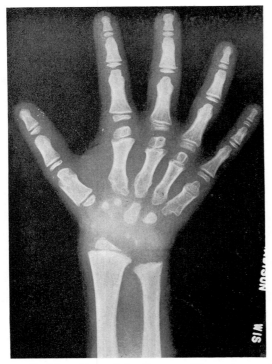

Figure 9–44. Morquio's disease. There is moderate tapering of the proximal ends of the second, third, fourth, and fifth metacarpals.

trunk. The lower extremities are more underdeveloped than the trunk, and the trunk more so than the head and the upper extremities. The joints appear widened, and some large joints are hypermobile owing to laxity of muscles and tendons. However, flexion deformities also occur in the elbows, hips, and knees, caused by the epiphyseal distortions. The hands are held in ulnar deviation.

Hurler's Disease (Gargoylism)

Hurler's disease is usually first noted after the first year of life. Clinical characteristics include a large, bulging head, hypertelorism, and corneal opacities leading to blindness. The lips are thick and the tongue large. The teeth are poorly formed. The facial appearance has been likened to that of a gargoyle, hence the designation gargoylism. Hepatosplenomegaly is present, often of considerable degree. The stature is dwarfed. The genetic transmission is autosomal recessive. There is excessive urinary excretion of dermatan sulfate and heparan sulfate.

Roentgenographic Findings. *Skull.* The skull often is scaphocephalic (elongated), owing to premature closure of the sagittal and metopic sutures. The anteroposterior diameter of the sella is lengthened and has an anterior depression, described as J shaped (Fig. 9-45). The sinuses and mastoids are poorly pneumatized. The mandible is short and thick, and the noted in many patients. The carpal and tarsal bones are

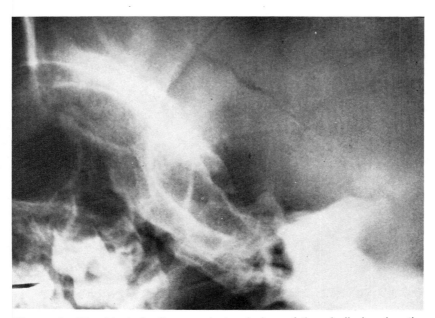

Figure 9–45. Hurler's disease. Lateral view of the skull showing the anterior depression of the tuberculum giving rise to the J-shaped sella.

late in appearing and, when developed, have irregular or angular shapes.

The head appears large in relation to the size of the trunk. The lower extremities are more underdeveloped than the trunk, and the trunk more so than the articular surfaces of the condyles are often concave, one of the characteristic findings. Hyperostotic thickening of the frontal and occipital area may develop, but the base does not become sclerotic.

Ribs. The ribs, especially the lower ribs, are broad and flat.

Long Tubular Bones. The upper extremities are more involved than the lower, which may be normal. The humerus is short and the shaft widened, and a constriction with a varus deformity of the humeral neck

may be seen (Fig. 9-46). The radius and ulna show similar changes, and the distal metaphyseal surfaces tend to be tilted toward one another (Fig. 9-47). The femoral neck is constricted, and there is a coxa valga deformity at the hips (Fig. 9-46). The epiphyseal ossification centers are often flattened and irregular.

Short Tubular Bones. The appearance of the hands usually is characteristic. The bones have a coarse texture and wide shafts, and the metacarpals in particular have conical or pointed proximal ends (Fig. 9-47). Similar changes may be seen in the feet.

Flat Bones. The pelvis may resemble achondroplasia during early infancy, but in persons who survive, its appearance comes to resemble that of Morquio's disease (Fig. 9-48).

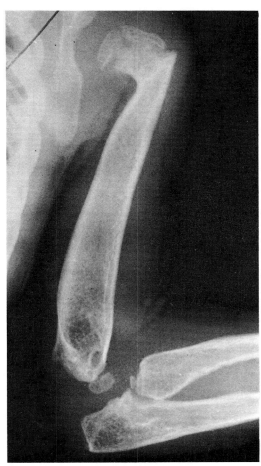

Figure 9–46. Hurler's disease. The proximal humeral metaphysis has a characteristic constriction and a varus deformity. There is expansion of the mid- and distal shaft.

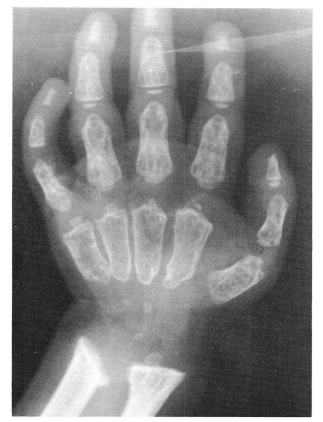

Figure 9–47. Hurler's disease. The hand and wrist show characteristic changes. The distal metaphyses of the radius and ulna are tilted toward each other. The bones of the hand are broadened, the cortices are thin, the trabecular pattern is coarsened, and there is a characteristic conical deformity of the proximal ends of the metacarpals.

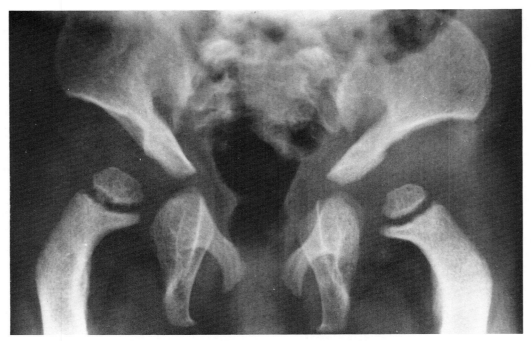

Figure 9–48. Hurler's disease. The contour of the pelvis resembles that in Morquio's disease (see Fig. 9-41). In Hurler's, the femoral epiphyses are better developed, the acetabulum is shallow, and there is moderate constriction of the femoral necks.

Spine. There is an angular kyphosis or gibbus at the thoracolumbar junction; one or several of the bodies are hypoplastic and have an anteroinferior beak (Fig. 9-49). Posterior displacement of one vertebra on the one above or below is often present at the level of T12 or L1. The intervertebral disc spaces are intact.

Other Bones. The carpal and tarsal bones may be late in appearing and then may show irregular or angular contours. The clavicle may be thickened. The teeth are poorly developed.

CHROMOSOMAL ABERRATIONS

Trisomy Syndromes

The normal human cell contains 22 pairs of somatic chromosomes, called autosomes and numbered from one through 22, and two sex chromosomes, XX in the female and XY in the male, for a total of 46. The addition of a chromosome to one of the autosomal groups leads to one of the trisomy syndromes, the most common locations being the 13, the 18, and 21 groups.

Many of the radiologic signs of the chromosomal disorders may also occur as isolated anatomical variants in otherwise normal individuals. However, the frequency in normal individuals is considerably less than that in the chromosomal disorders. When several of them are present together, the diagnosis of a chromosomal disorder can be suggested.[23, 31]

Trisomy 21 Syndrome (Mongolism, Down's Syndrome).

Mongolism is the result of an autosomal trisomy of chromosome 21 and is by far the most common chromosomal disorder, occurring in 1 of every 660 births. A number of skeletal stigmata have been described, some of which are fairly specific and aid in recognition of the disease when clinical findings are equivocal during the early months of life.

In the pelvis, during infancy the acetabular angles are flattened, the iliac bones large and flared, and the ischia elongated and tapering (Fig. 9-50). The iliac index is decreased. The iliac index is said to be more significant than the acetabular angle in the diagnosis of mongolism. This index consists of the sum of the acetabular and iliac angles on both sides, divided by two. The method for determining the index is shown in Figures 9-51 and 9-52. In the newborn, the normal iliac index has a mean value of 81° with a range of 68 to 97°. In mongolism, the index has a mean value of 62°

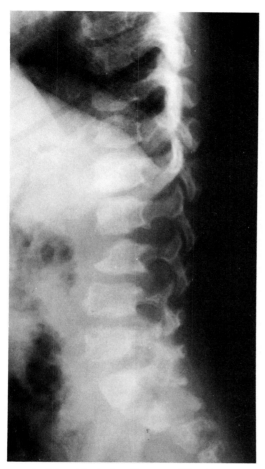

Figure 9–49. Hurler's disease. The lumbar spine shows anteroinferior beaking of L3, a moderate angular kyphosis, and malalignment of L2 on L3. The vertebrae are slightly flattened. Compare with Morquio's disease, Figure 9-40.

and a range from 49 to 87°. If the index is less than 60°, mongolism is very probable; if it is greater than 78°, the child is probably normal. These changes are most significant during the first 6 to 12 months of life.

Shortening of the middle phalanx (clinodactyly) of the fifth finger occurs. The manubrium sterni may ossify from two or three centers instead of one, as is normal, as identified on a lateral view of the chest. The lumbar vertebrae may be small in the anteroposterior diameter and increased in height.

Skull changes include (1) atlantoaxial subluxation, (2) hypoplastic nasal sinuses, and (3) decreased interorbital distance (hypotelorism).[8]

Visceral anomalies include congenital heart dis-ease—usually an atrioventricular canal, and increased frequency of an aberrant right subclavian artery—and duodenal obstruction (duodenal atresia or annular pancreas).

Trisomy 18 Syndrome. Trisomy 18 syndrome is one of the most frequent. The abnormalities result from an extra chromosome for number 18. The clinical and roentgenographic findings include (1) low-set, malformed ears and recession of the chin (mandibular and maxillary hypoplasia), (2) ulnar deviation of the fingers with the hand held as a clenched fist, (3) retarded bone age, (4) short, hypoplastic first metacarpals, (5) pseudoepiphysis for the metacarpals, (6) equinovarus and rocker-bottom feet with hammertoe deformities, short first toe, and hypoplastic distal phalanges, (7) thin ribs and short, undersegmented sternum and an increase in the anteroposterior diameter of the chest, (8) narrow transverse diameter of the pelvis due to anterior rotation of the ilia (antimongoloid pelvis), (9) hypoplasia or absence of the medial third of the clavicle, (10) hypoplastic, dislocated femoral heads with increased acetabular angles, and (11) thin cranial bones with a prominent elongated posterior fossa and a shallow, J-shaped sella.[11] Of these, the combination of thin ribs and antimongoloid pelvis are particularly characteristic of this disorder.[23]

In addition, congenital cardiac abnormalities are frequently present, usually a ventricular septal defect or patent ductus arteriosus. Eventration of the diaphragm and malformation of the kidneys are relatively common. The latter defects include double ureters, multicystic kidneys, horseshoe kidneys, and hydronephrosis.

Trisomy 13 Syndrome. Trisomy 13 syndrome is less common than trisomy 18. Affected infants are usually small and do not thrive, often dying during the first year of life. The ears are malformed and set low, and there is micrognathia. Major anomalies include cleft palate, microcephaly midline cleft defects in the brain, polydactyly, and syndactyly, together with various anomalies of the viscera. Other skeletal anomalies include malformed ribs with asymmetry of the thorax, increased interpediculate distance in the cervical spine and prominent heels.

The visceral anomalies include (1) congenital heart disease, particularly ventricular septal defect, patent ductus arteriosus, and dextroposition, (2) diaphragmatic, umbilical, or inguinal hernias, (3) genitourinary tract anomalies as seen in trisomy 18, (4) malrotation of the colon, (5) undescended testes, and (6) mental and motor retardation.

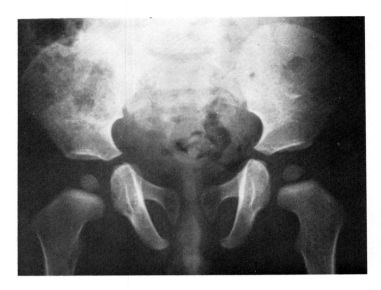

Figure 9–50. Down's syndrome (trisomy 21). There is flaring of the ilia and elongation and tapering of the ischia, with flattening of the acetabular angles giving rise to the "Mickey Mouse ears" deformity of the pelvis.

Turner's Syndrome

Of the syndromes associated with abnormal gonadal development, the one that may show significant roentgenographic findings is Turner's syndrome, or gonadal aplasia. Most common is a relative shortening of the fourth metacarpal in relation to the third and fifth, the metacarpal sign (Fig. 9-53). This is determined by drawing a straight line tangential to the distal ends of the heads of the fourth and fifth metacarpals. If this line passes through the head of the third metacarpal, the sign is said to be positive. Normally, the line will pass distal to the head of the third metacarpal. However, a positive sign occurs in some normal persons and in

persons with other disturbances such as pseudo-pseudohypoparathyroidism, and it therefore is not pathognomonic (see Chap. 6).

The time of appearance of epiphyseal ossification centers on normal, but fusion is occasionally delayed. The proximal row of carpal bones assumes an angular configuration somewhat similar to Madelung's deformity, with the apex pointing proximally. Various other abnormalities of the bones of the hands also have been described. At the knee, the medial femoral condyle is enlarged and the apposing tibial plateau is flattened or

Figure 9–51. Method for determining the acetabular and iliac angles and the iliac index. This index is the sum of the acetabular angles (**b** and **c**) and the iliac angles (**a** and **d**), divided by 2. The diagram illustrates the proper placement of the lines necessary for determining the various angles. (Tong ECK: The iliac index angle: a simplified method for measuring the iliac index. Radiology 91:376, 1968)

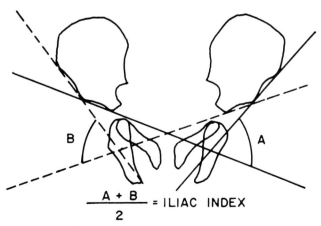

Figure 9–52. Tong's method for determining the iliac index (**A** and **B** divided by 2). The measurement of the larger angles gives less chance for error than the method shown in Figure 9-49. (Tong ECK: The iliac index angle: a simplified method for measuring the iliac index. Radiology 91:376, 1968)

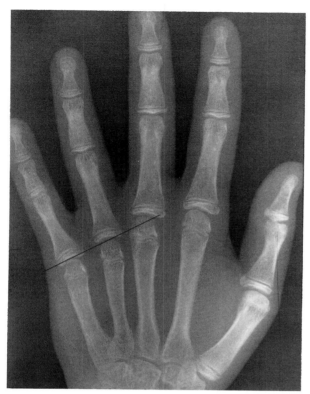

Figure 9–53. Turner's syndrome. Characteristic shortening of the fourth metacarpal gives the positive metacarpal sign. A line drawn tangential to the heads of the fourth and fifth metacarpal passes through the head of the third metacarpal. Normally it should be tangential or distal to the head of the third metacarpal. (Courtesy of Andrew Poznanski, M.D., Chicago, Illinois)

depressed. The medial part of the proximal tibial epiphysis may overhang the metaphysis, and in some cases an appearance rather similar to Blount's disease has been noted. There may be scoliosis and hypoplasia of the posterior arch of C1. An irregularity of the vertebral bodies similar to Scheuermann's disease also has been described. An increased carrying angle at the elbow, cubitus valgus, one of the significant clinical signs, also can be demonstrated radiographically.

REFERENCES AND SELECTED READINGS

1. BAER JW, RADKOWSKI MA: Congenital multiple fibromatosis. A case report with review of the world literature. Am J Roentgenol 118:200, 1973

2. BEIGHTON P, CREMIN B, FAURE C, ET AL: International nomenclature of constitutional disease of bone: Revision, May, 1983. Ann Radiol (Paris) 26:457, 1983

3. CAMPBELL CJ, PADEMETRIOU T, BONFIGLIO M: Melorheostosis. A report of the clinical roentgenographic and pathological findings in 14 cases. J Bone Joint Surg [Am] 50:1281, 1968

4. CRAWFORD AH JR, BAGAMERY N: Osseous manifestations of neurofibromatosis in childhood. J Pediat Orthop 6:72, 1986.

5. DAFFNER RH, KIRKS DR, GEHWEILER JA JR, ET AL: Computed tomography of fibrous dysplasia. Am J Roentgenol 139:943, 1982

6. DUNNICK NR, HEAD GL, PECK GL, YODER FW: Nevoid basal cell carcinoma syndrome: radiographic manifestations including cystlike lesions of the phalangens. Radiology 127:331, 1978.

7. FILLY RA, GOLBUS MS: Ultrasonography of the normal and pathologic fetal skeleton. Radiol Clin North Am 20:311, 1982

8. GABRIEL KR, MASON D, CARANGO P: Occipito-atlantal translation in Down's syndrome. Spine 15:997, 1990.

9. GARVER P, RESNICK D, HAGHIGHI P, GUERRA J: Melorheostosis of the axial skeleton with associated fibrolipomatous lesions. Skel Radiol 9:41, 1982.

10. HOBBINS JC, BRACKEN MB, MAHONEY MJ: Diagnosis of fetal skeletal dysplasias with ultrasound. Am J Obstet Gynecol 142:306, 1982

11. JAMES AE JR, BELCORT CL, ATKINS L, ET AL: Trisomy 18-syndrome. Radiology 92:37, 1969

12. JEANTY P, ROMERO R: Fetal limbs: Normal anatomy and congenital malformations. Semin Ultrasound CT MR 5:253, 1984

13. KAFTORI JK, KLEINHAUS U, NAVEH Y: Progressive diaphyseal dysplasia (Camurati–Engelmann): Radiographic follow-up and CT findings. Radiology 164:777, 1987.

14. KALTER H, WARKANY J: Congenital malformations. Etiologic factors and their role in prevention. N Engl J Med 308:424, 491, 1983

15. KAPLAN FS, AUGUST CS, FALLON MD, DALINKA M, AXEL L, HADDAD JG: Successful treatment of infantile malignant osteopetrosis by bone-marrow transplantation. A case report. J Bone Joint Surg [Am] 76:617, 1988.

16. KRANSDORF KJ, MOSER RP JR, GILKEY FW: From the archives of the AFIP: Fibrous dysplasia. Radiographics 10:519, 1990.

17. LANGER LO JR, BAUMANN FA, GORLIN RJ: Achondroplasia. Am J Roentgenol 100:12, 1967

18. LANGER LO JR, CAREY LS: The roentgenographic features of the K.S. mucopolysaccharidosis of Morquio (Morquio–Brailsford disease). Am J Roentgenol 97:1, 1966

19. LILE HA, ROGERS JF, GERALD B: The basal cell nevus syndrome. Am J Roentgenol 103:214, 1968

20. MILLER SM, PAUL LW: Roentgen observations in familial metaphyseal dysotosis. Radiology 83:665, 1964

21. MILGRAM JW, JASTY M: Osteopetrosis. A morphological

study of twenty-one cases. J Bone Joint Surg [Am] 64: 912, 1982

22. POZNANSKI AK: Bone dysplasias: Not so rare, definitely important. Am J Roentgenol 142:427, 1984

23. POZNANSKI AK: The Hand in Radiologic Diagnosis, 2nd ed. Philadelphia, WB Saunders, 1984

24. PYERITZ RE, MCKUSICK VA: The Marfan syndrome: diagnosis and management. N Engl J Med 300:772, 1979.

25. ROBERTS AP, CONNER AN, TOLMIE JL, CONNOR JM: Spondylothoracic and spondylocostal dysostosis: Hereditary forms of spinal deformity. J Bone Joint Surg [Br] 70:126, 1988.

26. RUBIN P: Dynamic Classification of Bone Dysplasias. Chicago, Year Book Medical Publishers, 1964

27. SANDERS RC, BLAKEMORE K: Lethal fetal anomalies: Sonographic demonstration. Radiology 172:1, 1989.

28. SCOTT CI JR: Dwarfism. Clinical symposia (CIBA-Geigy). 40: 1988.

29. SPRANGER JW, LANGER LO JR, WIEDEMANN HR: Bone Dysplasias. An Atlas of Constitutional Disorders of Skeletal Development. Philadelphia, WB Saunders, 1974

30. STANESCU V, STANESCU R, MAROTEAUX P: Pathogenic mechanisms in osteochondrodysplasias. J Bone Joint Surg [Am] 66:817, 1984

31. TAYBI H, LACHMAN RS: Radiology of Syndromes and Metabolic Disorders 3rd Ed. Chicago, Year Book Medical Publishers, 1990

32. SPIRT BA, OLIPHANT M, GOTTLIEB RH, GORDON LP: Prenatal sonographic evaluation of shortlimbed dwarfism: An algorithmic approach. Radiographics 10:217, 1990

Paul and Juhl's Essentials of Radiologic Imaging, Sixth Edition, edited by John H. Juhl and Andrew B. Crummy. J.B. Lippincott Company, Philadelphia, © 1993.

CHAPTER **10**

The Superficial Soft Tissues

Lee F. Rogers
Andrew B. Crummy
Mary Ellen Peters

THE SUPERFICIAL SOFT TISSUES—GENERAL CONSIDERATIONS

Lee F. Rogers

The soft tissues can be seen in every roentgenogram, even those that have been heavily exposed, by viewing the film with a strong beam of light (in addition to the usual illuminators). Some type of spotlight should always be available for the scrutiny of overexposed roentgenograms and particularly for the study of the soft tissues.

Although the density of the soft tissues as a whole is close to that of water, there is enough difference between fat and other tissues to make subcutaneous fat distinctly visible on roentgenograms as a more translucent area beneath the skin (Fig. 10-1). The fat also makes the outer surface of the muscles stand out clearly. Localized accumulations of fat near the joints aid in the recognition of joint effusion because of their displacement when the joint capsule is distended. When there has been wasting from disease with consequent loss of fat, the soft parts have a very homogeneous density.

When specifically indicated, a suitable selection of exposure factors ranging from 26 kV to 40 kV with relatively low filtration (e.g., 0.5 mm Al) will produce a roentgenogram of high quality in which the soft-tissue

outlines are preserved and good differentiation of the soft-tissue densities is obtained. This type of roentgenogram is useful when the examination is made primarily for soft-tissue evaluation. These factors have been used in mammography (see Fig. 10-36).

A small, localized soft-tissue enlargement such as a wart or a mole in close contact with the film cassette or tabletop can cause a sharply marginated increase in density that may be mistaken for a pathologic process within the tissues. It can be seen because it is contrasted by the surrounding air. When a similar mass is placed within the abdomen it cannot be visualized separately from the surrounding soft tissues of similar density. For example, a mole on the surface of the chest wall may produce a round density that can be mistaken for a nodule within the lung, and a similar lesion of the soft tissues of the lower back may suggest a renal or gallbladder calculus (Fig. 10-2). The nipples are a common source of difficulty in the interpretation of chest roentgenograms. If one breast is pressed more firmly against the film cassette than the other, the nipple on one side may form a sharply outlined round density but the other may be invisible. Absence of one breast following a radical mastectomy causes one lung to be more translucent than the other.

Contrast between soft tissue can be achieved by the injection of contrast material (i.e., angiography) (see Fig. 10-7), which allows visualization of the lumen of arteries and subsequently visualizes solid organs by perfusion. Computed tomography (Fig. 10-3*A*) demonstrates the soft tissues with greater clarity than plain

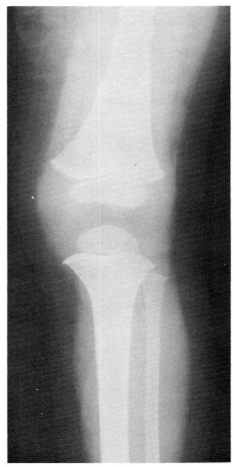

Figure 10–1. Normal soft tissues. This film demonstrates the difference in density of muscles and fat. The more radiolucent subcutaneous fat causes the muscles to stand out clearly.

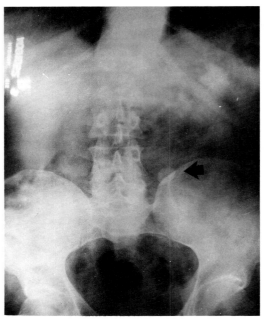

Figure 10–2. A mole on the skin of the back was responsible for the round density (*arrow*) seen in this film of the abdomen.

film radiography by clearly depicting the fat in fascial planes surrounding muscles and vascular structures; however, the density of these structures is similar, requiring contrast for the identification of vascular structures. Magnetic resonance imaging (Fig. 10-26) distinguishes between various soft tissue structures by a difference in signal intensity. This can be varied by changing the parameters of the examination to exploit or modify the relative signal intensity from differing tissues. Vascular structures are directly identified by signal voids or variations created by the flow of blood. Thus, the soft tissues have been freed from their murky lair in the radiographic shadows by the light of newer technologies.

THE DISORDERS OF MUSCLE

MYOSITIS OSSIFICANS

Calcification with subsequent ossification often follows trauma to the deep tissues of the extremities and is called traumatic myositis ossificans. So-called calcified hematomas involving the muscles of the thigh are observed frequently in athletes, particularly football players, but they may follow any local injury sufficient to cause bruising of the muscle or a frank hemorrhage within it. An injury of this nature that is severe enough to cause a deep muscle bruise often traumatizes the periosteum as well, and there may be hemorrhage beneath it; this also frequently undergoes calcification.

The calcified hematoma may become visible as a hazy shadow of increased density within a few weeks after the initiating trauma. Over a period of several weeks, this gradually becomes more dense and finally develops the appearance of actual bone. The mass has a laminated character (Fig. 10-4). The exact appearance of the lesion is closely related to its age and parallels the stage of maturation. The first finding is that of soft-tissue swelling. Calcification subsequently develops in a centrifugal pattern, which is flocculent at first.

Thus, the lesion is characteristically more densely calcified on its periphery than centrally. The active

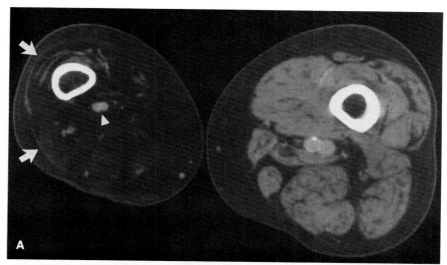

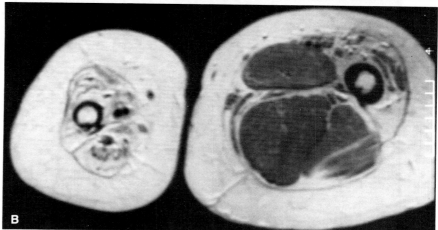

Figure 10–3. Two cases of muscle atrophy secondary to long-standing poliomyelitis. (**A**) CT of Case 1. There is a complete atrophy of muscles on the right. They are replaced by fat. The fascia remains intact at the periphery (*arrows*). The femoral artery and vein are central (*arrowhead*). The overall size and cortical width of the femur is reduced when compared with the opposite normal side. (**B**) MRI of Case 2. There is complete atrophy on the right similar to 3*A*. On the left the adductors and medial head of the gastrocnemius are not affected. However, the hamstrings (*open arrow*) and lateral head of the gastrocnemius (*arrow*) are severely affected.

nature of the processes results in the uptake of radioactive bone-seeking agents. In general, plain films are sufficient for diagnosis, especially if there is a history of trauma. CT scanning may be useful when the lesions are atypical.[80] Usually, after a period of time, the ossification gradually decreases in size; smaller masses may disappear completely.

MYOSITIS OSSIFICANS PROGRESSIVA

Myositis ossificans progressiva is a rare disorder of unknown cause. It appears to be a congenital dysplasia. It begins in early childhood with the development of doughy and often painful swellings, chiefly in the muscles of the neck and back. As these swellings subside, a diffuse fibrosis is left, and this in turn is followed by the development of platelike masses of bone (Fig. 10-5).

There is a slow progression. The abnormal ossifications are often observed first in the muscles of the neck and back. Initially, these ossifications are relatively hazy and somewhat difficult to identify. In time, irregular, elongated bony plates are observed extending along the long axis of the involved muscle. In later stages, numerous muscles become extensively ossified and the joints become virtually immobile. Associated anomalies of the small bones of the hand and feet are found in almost all patients.

MUSCULAR DYSTROPHIES

The replacement of muscle by fat in muscular dystrophies results in a fairly characteristic appearance in roentgenograms of the extremities. The muscles do not shrink appreciably in size, but the extensive accumula-

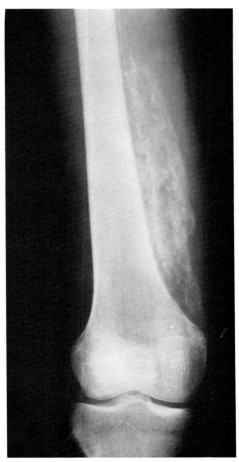

Figure 10–4. Traumatic myositis ossificans. There is calcification in a large hematoma on the inner aspect of the thigh. Note that the lesion is more calcified at its periphery than centrally. Centripetal calcification is characteristic of myositis ossificans.

tion of fat within the remaining muscle bundles gives them a finely striated or striped appearance. In later stages, most of the muscle tissue is replaced by fat, and the fascial sheath bounding the muscle will stand out as a thin line of increased density as it is visualized on edge (Fig. 10-6). One of the clinical subgroups is known as pseudohypertrophic muscular dystrophy (Duchenne's syndrome). It is characterized by the enlargement of certain muscle groups, usually those of the calves and shoulder girdles. The appearance clinically is that of a very muscular individual, but strength actually is markedly decreased. In addition to the extensive replacement by fat in this type of dystrophy, the muscles are enlarged. This is the only condition in which there is the combination of large muscles interlaced with fat (Fig. 10-6).

MUSCLE ATROPHY

In patients with long-standing paralysis of one or more extremities—including such conditions as poliomyelitis (see Fig. 10-3), spinal cord injuries, and cerebral vascular accidents—muscles may contain stripes of fat, but the affected muscle groups are decreased in size whereas the subcutaneous fat layer may be thick. When complete paralysis of an extremity has existed for a long time, the muscle bundles may be almost completely absent and subcutaneous fat makes up most of the soft tissues that surround the bones.

CALCIFICATION IN THE SOFT TISSUES

Calcification in the soft tissues may be of several etiologies. It may be *dystrophic*, occurring in necrotic tissues as found in infections or tumors; it may be *metabolic*, occurring as the result of deposition due to abnormal concentrations of calcium salts as in chronic renal failure or calcium deposition disease; or, it may represent *ossification*, which occurs in certain chondral tumors of soft tissues.

ARTERIAL CALCIFICATION

Calcification in the walls of the larger arteries of the abdomen and of the extremities is a frequent observation in roentgenograms of individuals of middle age or older. Intimal arteriosclerosis is characterized pathologically by the formation of atheromatous plaques in the thickened intima of the arteries. The atheromatous plaques may not be calcified. When they are calcified, they are seen as irregular plaques of variable size, from small flecks to larger areas a centimeter or more in length. They may be elongated or somewhat triangular, with a considerable variation in shape. They seldom completely encircle the lumen of the vessel and are distributed irregularly along the course without any specific arrangement (Fig. 10-7). The amount of visible calcification bears no relationship to the severity of the vascular occlusion; complete obstruction may exist with no visible calcification.

Mönckeberg's medial arteriosclerosis is characterized by the deposition of calcium in the media of the vessel. These deposits do not narrow the vessel lumen, nor do they interfere with flow. Müonckeberg's arteriosclerosis is an almost constant finding in elderly individuals, and it is frequently seen in persons 35 to 50 years old, particularly in diabetics. The vessels most often affected are the femoral, popliteal, and radial arteries. The calcification occurs in the form of closely spaced, fine concentric rings. These may be complete or incomplete, but the process generally is diffuse,

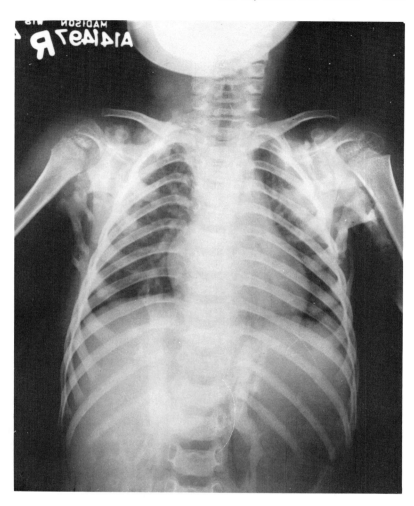

Figure 10–5. Myositis ossificans. Progressive extensive ossificans of back and shoulder muscles are evident in this child. Irregular bony plaques can be seen along the lower thoracic and upper lumbar spine, as well as around the shoulders.

involving long segments of multiple vessels (Fig. 10-7C).

Calcification of small arteries of the feet is characteristic of diabetes (see Figs. 5-16, 5-17). Small vessel calcification in both the hands and feet occurs in chronic renal failure (see Fig. 6-33).

CALCIFICATION OF VEINS

Phleboliths

A phlebolith is a calcified thrombus within a vein. Phleboliths are found very frequently in the pelvic veins, and most adults have a few of them. They occur in the form of small, round, or slightly ovoid calcified shadows of variable size, from very tiny ones up to those that measure on the order of 0.5 cm in diameter (Fig. 10-8). They may be of homogeneous density, may be laminated, or may have a ringlike appearance. Phleboliths are common in varicose veins of the lower ex-

tremities. They frequently form in the dilated venous spaces of a cavernous hemangioma and result in one of the characteristic roentgenographic signs of the lesion. When a number of small, rounded calcifications are seen in a localized area of the superficial soft tissues, one should consider the possibility of a cavernous hemangioma (Fig. 10-9). The phleboliths in a hemangioma very often have a ringlike appearance.

Calcification Associated With Venous Stasis

In the presence of venous stasis of long duration, usually secondary to varicosities and thrombosis, thin stripelike shadows of calcification may be seen in the subcutaneous tissues. These usually present as double parallel stripes or with distinctly tubular and branching characteristics. Additionally, there often are plaquelike calcifications in the subcutaneous tissues throughout the legs (Fig. 10-10A) or as a more localized process in

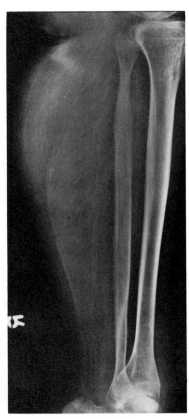

Figure 10–6. Pseudohypertrophic muscular dystrophy. The muscle of the calf is very large but contains fat, producing streaks of radiolucency. Note the wide fibular shaft.

the neighborhood of a varicose ulcer. The calcification in some of these patients resembles very closely that seen in patients with diffuse scleroderma or dermatomyositis, except that it is localized to the leg. Phleboliths are often seen in association with the plaques. Smooth, wavy periosteal reaction along the tibial and fibular shafts is common (Fig. 10-10B). The stasis ulcers that are often present may be seen as defects in the soft tissues when the film is viewed with a high-intensity light.

CALCIFICATION OF LYMPH NODES

After being involved by infection, usually tuberculosis or histoplasmosis, the peripheral lymph nodes may calcify. The most frequent site is the cervical chain (Fig. 10-11), with the axillary nodes second in frequency. Calcification of other peripheral nodes is very infrequent. The calcifications are visualized as mottled areas of calcific density, often multiple, and distributed along the course of the cervical lymph node chains or in the axilla.

PARASITIC CALCIFICATION

Cysticerosis. The larvae of the pork tapeworm *(Taenia solium)*, known as *Cysticerus cellulosae*, may lodge in the brain, meninges, muscles, and other structures and become encysted. Normally, the pig is the intermediate host of *C. cellulosae*, and human infestation occurs from eating improperly cooked pork. The eggs may be swallowed as the result of self-infection, and the larvae may enter various tissues and become encysted. Thus, humans would act as the intermediate host. The encysted parasites may become sufficiently calcified to be visualized roentgenographically as small or slightly elongated masses of one to several millimeters in diameter or length. The small size of the calcifications and their wide dissemination, particularly in the brain, meninges, and muscles, is very suggestive of the diagnosis (Fig. 10-12).

Trichinosis. The encysted embryos of *Trichinella spiralis* are said to undergo calcification very frequently, but the parasite is so small that it cannot be seen readily on roentgenograms so the diagnosis of trichinosis usually cannot be made from roentgenographic examination.

Hydatid Disease. Hydatid disease is due to infestation with hydatid cysts, the larval forms of an ecchinococcal tapeworm. The cysts are usually found in visceral organs of the thorax and abdomen. Rarely, they occur in the soft tissues of the extremities, where they tend to be small and fragmented in contrast to large visceral cysts. Therefore, the appearance is not characteristic, and the calcifications may present a variety of bizarre patterns.

Dracunculiasis (Guinea Worm Infestation). Guinea worm infestation may be manifested on roentgenograms when fibrositis or myositis develops around a dead female guinea worm that migrates in the subcutaneous tissues before discharging eggs. The worm may calcify, particularly if it remains deep in the tissues. It appears as a long, stringlike calcification, up to 10 cm to 12 cm, usually in the lower limbs.

ARTICULAR AND PERIARTICULAR CALCIFICATION

Any bursa adjacent to a joint may become distended with fluid and may present as a cystic mass. This is particularly common in the prepatellar bursa of the knee and the olecranon bursa overlying the olecranon

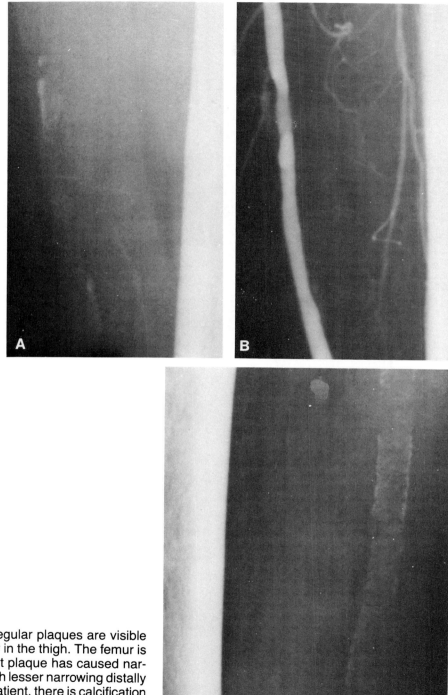

Figure 10–7. (**A**) Several irregular plaques are visible in the superficial femoral artery in the thigh. The femur is at the right. (**B**) The uppermost plaque has caused narrowing of the arterial lumen, with lesser narrowing distally in this arteriogram. (**C**) In this patient, there is calcification of the femoral artery of the type usually found in association with involvement of the media.

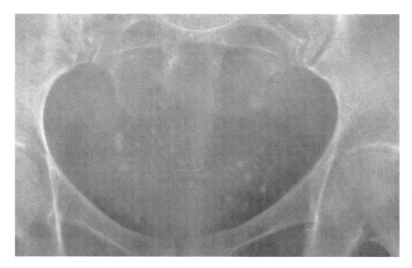

Figure 10–8. Phleboliths in pelvis. Numerous rounded calcific densities in the pelvis are typical of phleboliths. Note that many are slightly more dense on their periphery than centrally.

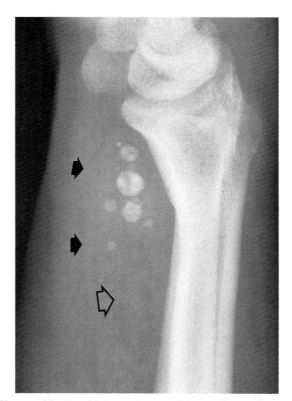

Figure 10–9. Hemangioma of the volar surface of the distal forearm arising in the pronator quadratus muscle. Note the bulging of the fascial plane (*arrows*). In addition to the phleboliths distally there is a mottled lucency proximally (*open arrow*) indicative of fat that is often found in hemangiomas. The volar surface of the underlying radius is eroded.

process of the ulna. Trauma may result in hemorrhage into these bursae. Olecranon bursitis is a frequent complication of gout. Extensive distension of the iliopsoas bursa associated with the hip joint has been found in rheumatoid arthritis. The distended bursa bulges into the pelvis and presents as a mass that displaces both the rectum and bladder. Similar large, fluid-distended bursae may be found near other large joints in rheumatoid arthritis. Such distended bursae rarely show evidence of calcification.

CALCIFIC BURSITIS AND TENDINITIS

Inflammatory changes in tendons and bursae are common, particularly in the shoulder. This results in pain and limitation of motion, and it is the most frequent cause of shoulder disability. It is referred to variously as bursitis, tendinitis, calcific tendinitis, or, more obscurely, as peritendinitis calcarea. Radiographically, calcium deposits may be identified in the tendons of the rotator cuff. These usually occur in the tendon of the supraspinatus and are found directly above the greater tuberosity of the humerus (Fig. 10-13). Similar deposits in the tendons of the subscapularis, infraspinatus, and teres minor components of the cuff are less common. These deposits in the tendons are often associated with inflammation of an overlying bursa, and hence the clinical designation of bursitis or subacromial bursitis. Rupture of the mass of calcium into the bursa may occur. The calcium may be spontaneously resorbed.

It is not at all infrequent to find calcium deposits around the shoulder in patients who have no complaints, or at least none at the time of the examination.

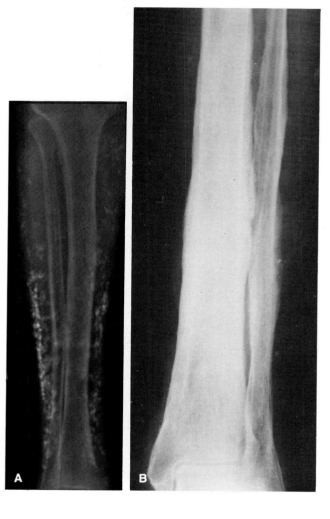

Figure 10–10. (**A**) Subcutaneous calcification in a patient with long-standing venous stasis. (**B**) Periosteal reaction associated with chronic venous stasis. Note the characteristic, irregular, wavy periosteal formation along the tibial and fibular shafts.

Thus, the mere presence of demonstrable calcium does not indicate the existence of an acute inflammatory process.

In addition to their presence in the shoulder, calcifications of a similar nature are at times found in the trochanteric bursa that overlies the greater trochanter of the femur. They are also encountered in the periarticular tissues around the elbow, hand (Fig. 10-14), wrist, around the prepatellar bursa of the knee, and in the retropharyngeal tissues of the upper cervical spine.[35] Bursal calcification should be sought in any patient complaining of acute pain around a joint.

Calcium Hydroxyapatite Deposition Disease

Calcium hydroxyapatite has been identified as the crystal most commonly responsible for calcium deposits in tendons and bursae. This and other related calcium phosphate crystals may occur in association with both interarticular and periarticular changes involving one or many joints. This constellation of findings is known as Calcium Hydroxyapatite Deposition Disease.[37, 72] Calcium hydroxyapatite crystals are so small (75 to 250 nm) they are not individually visible by light microscopy, and are seen only in the aggregate. Therefore, the diagnosis is usually presumptive and based on the radiographic findings.

Calcium Pyrophosphate Deposition Disease

The principal finding in this disease is chondrocalcinosis, calcium salts deposited in the joint cartilage and less commonly in the periarticular tissues. This entity and the differential diagnosis of chondrocalcinosis are described in Chapter 3, Diseases of Joints.

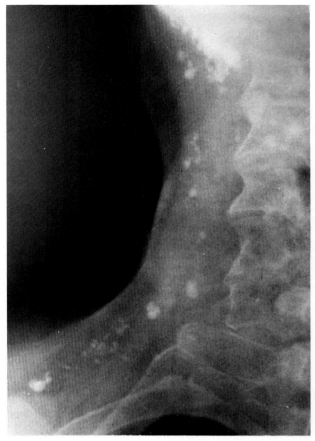

Figure 10–11. Calcified cervical lymph nodes. Multiple calcifications showing a variety of sizes and shapes are observed in the cervical nodes.

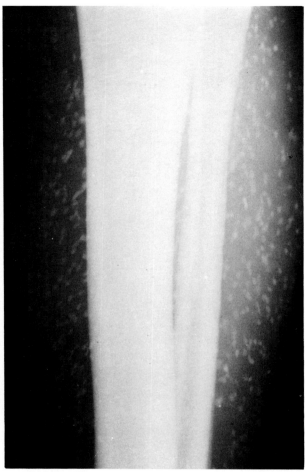

Figure 10–12. Cysticercosis. Numerous tiny round and oval calcifications in the muscles of the leg. The patient had eaten a considerable amount of raw pork while he was a prisoner of the Japanese during World War II. (Courtesy of Dr. Margaret Winston)

INTERSTITIAL CALCINOSIS

Interstitial calcinosis is an uncommon condition in which there is either a localized or a widely disseminated deposition of calcium in the skin, subcutaneous tissues, muscles, and tendons. Calcinosis is often associated with collagen diseases, scleroderma, and dermatomyositis. However, it can exist in a relatively asymptomatic form with no signs of any associated disorder.

Calcinosis Universalis (Diffuse Calcinosis)

Calcinosis universalis is characterized by the wide dissemination of thin calcific plaques of various sizes throughout the soft tissues, chiefly in the subcutaneous layer, and occasionally within the muscles and tendons. From a clinical point of view, there are several types of diffuse calcinosis:

1. Asymptomatic. This has been reported, but is rare.
2. Diffuse calcinosis associated with generalized scleroderma (Fig. 10-15). This includes the CREST syndrome (calcinosis, Raynaud's phenomenon, esophageal hypomobility, sclerodactyly, and telangiectasia) and the Thibierge–Weissenbach syndrome (calcinosis and acrosclerosis).
3. Diffuse calcinosis associated with dermatomyositis (Fig. 10-16).

In scleroderma and dermatomyositis, the calcification occurs in the form of thin plaques. In scleroderma, they are limited to the skin and immediate subcutaneous tissues; in dermatomyositis, calcification

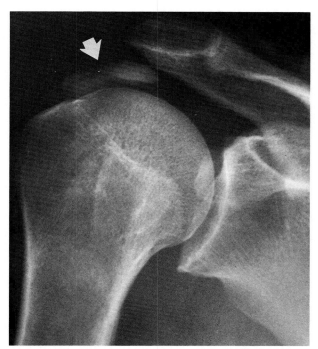

Figure 10–13. Calcific tendinitis supraspinatus muscle. There is an elongated ovoid homogeneous cloud-like collection of calcification projected (*arrow*) between the humeral head and the acromion typical of calcific tendinitis.

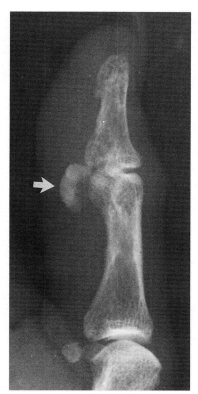

Figure 10–14. Calcific tendinitis involving the flexor tendons of the thumb. Note the crescentic homogeneous calcification (*arrow*). The smaller underlying ossific densities represent sesamoid bones.

also occurs in the muscles. The calcification appears in four distinct patterns: superficial masses, deep masses, deep linear deposits, and a lacy reticular subcutaneous deposition that encases the torso. This last pattern is of particular importance because it is associated with a steadily progressive deterioration and is therefore of prognostic significance. In addition to the plaques, there is a general loss of soft-tissue differentiation, with the subcutaneous fat layer becoming very scanty or disappearing altogether.

Calcinosis Circumscripta

In the localized type of calcinosis, the calcifications occur in the form of small rounded foci having an amorphous appearance. These foci are found chiefly in the tips of the fingers and along the margins of the joints in the hands and feet. The changes are noted more frequently in the hands than in the feet and, when present in both areas, are usually more intensive in the hands. As is true with the diffuse form of calcinosis, the localized type occurs in several different clinical manifestations:

Without Associated Skin or Vasopastic Phenomena. The lesions appear most frequently in elderly persons and are more common in women than in men. There may be some aching in the joints of the affected areas. The foci may be numerous, and some may be sufficiently large to cause visible swellings. In some of these patients, ulceration of the skin occurs over the larger lumps, followed by extrusion of cheesy, whitish material and subsequent healing.

With Associated Scleroderma. Calcinosis is of frequent occurrence when scleroderma affects the fingers and hands. The calcification may be in the form of a few tiny rounded subcutaneous nodules or may occur as larger masses. These are commonly found in the terminal phalanges or along the margins of the joints. Other roentgenographic signs of scleroderma often are present, including (1) diminution in the amount of soft tissues in the tips of the fingers so that these digits develop a tapered or almost pointed appearance, (2) absorption of bone. The latter begins in the terminal

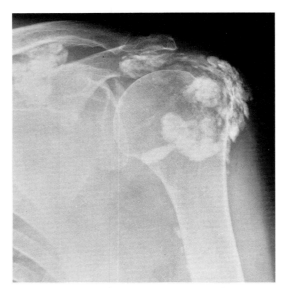

Figure 10–15. Extensive calcification about the shoulder in a patient with scleroderma. Much of the calcification is located within and about the rotator cuff. (Case courtesy of Harry Genant, M.D., San Francisco, CA)

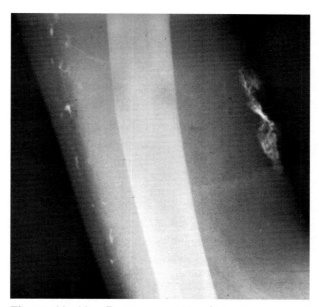

Figure 10–16. Dermatomyositis. Subcutaneous calcification of the arm is in two distinct patterns; anteriorly a plaque and posteriorly a weblike, reticular pattern. Calcification in dermatomyositis is characteristically located at the subcutaneous tissues.

tufts of the distal phalanges of the affected fingers, so that the tufts disappear and the shaft of the phalanx becomes pointed. The absorption may extend to involve the shaft and can be sufficiently severe so that most of the bone disappears or fragments (Fig. 10-17).

Tumoral Calcinosis

Tumoral calcinosis is a rare entity characterized by the occurrence of a large calcified mass, usually near one of the larger joints, particularly the hip.[19, 54] The hallmark is the presence of large, multiglobular, paraarticular calcific masses (Fig. 10-18) usually related to the extensor surface of the involved joints. In order of decreasing frequency the hips (Fig. 10-19), elbows, shoulders,

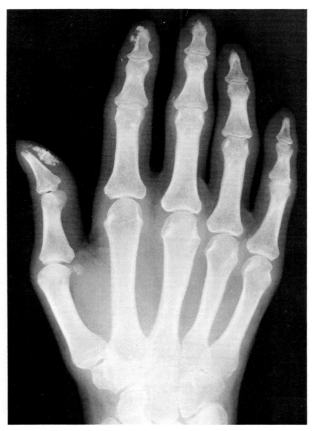

Figure 10–17. Scleroderma with associated interstitial calcinosis. Note the punctate calcifications in the soft tissues of the thumb and index finger. There is absorption of the terminal tufts, giving the phalanges a pointed shape. There is also some decrease in the amount of soft tissue at the fingertips. The latter two findings are particularly evident in the fourth and fifth digits.

and feet are affected. Multiple masses may be present. Generally the adjacent bone is not involved. Clinically there is pain and localized swelling. The condition is benign but often recurs following surgical removal. Roentgenographic findings are a round or oval, well-circumscribed mass of calcium, which may be lobulated. It appears in periarticular soft tissues and consists of multiple smaller opacities separated by radiolucent lines representing fibrous tissue septa (Figs. 10-18

and 10-19A). Occasionally, fluid levels may be observed in upright films (Fig. 10-18). Fluid levels are also demonstrated by CT, which also shows that the calcific collections arise in the fascial planes between muscles (Fig. 10-19B). CT demonstrates this phenomenon quite nicely with dependent layering of the calcium, and, less commonly, calcium lining a cystlike structure (Fig. 10-19B).[4]

Deposits of calcium pyrophosphate within the med-

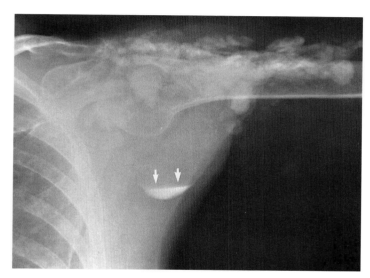

Figure 10–18. Tumoral calcinosis. There are multiple globular calcifications that are contiguous but separated by septae. This radiograph was obtained in the upright position. Note the fluid level (*arrows*) outlining a large cystic collection. (Case courtesy of Theodore Keats, M.D., Charlottesville, VA)

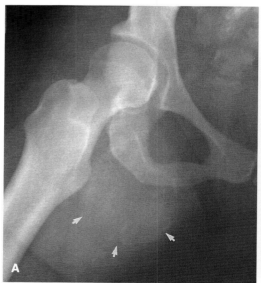

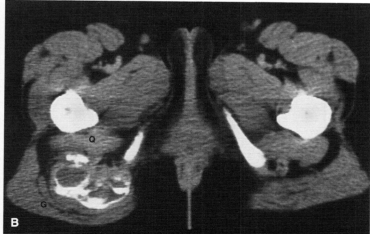

Figure 10–19. Tumoral calcinosis. **(A)** A vague, large radiodensity occurs within the soft tissues of the upper thigh (*arrows*). The bone is intact. **(B)** CT scan demonstrates multilocular cystic collections containing several fluid levels. Note that the collection lies between the gluteus maximus (G) and quadratus femoris (Q) muscles. (Case courtesy of Ginteras E. Degesys, M.D., St. Petersburg, FL)

ullary space of long bones in this condition have resulted in a painful, inflammatory response, a diaphysitis, manifested by surrounding periosteal reaction and changes in the marrow signal on MRI.[54]

Specific biochemical abnormalities have been identified in tumoral calcinosis, establishing it as a metabolic disease. These are hyperphosphatemia, elevated serum 1,25- dihydroxy-vitamin D, and elevation of renal phosphate reabsorption threshold. The serum calcium, parathyroid hormone, renal function, and alkaline phosphatase are normal.

Similar masses of calcium have been found in association with pseudoxanthoma elasticum, a rare hereditary disorder characterized by degeneration of elastic tissue. The most common findings are xanthoma-like lesions of the skin. Arterial calcification is common. Multiglobular masses of calcium, indistinguishable from those of tumoral calcinosis, may be encountered in chronic renal failure patients undergoing hemodialysis (Fig. 10-20).

MISCELLANEOUS FORMS OF SOFT-TISSUE CALCIFICATION

Burns. Heterotopic soft-tissue calcifications occur in about one fourth of patients with severe burns. They tend to be flocculent and occur more commonly in children than in adults. Some spontaneous regression is the rule unless tissues adjacent to and surrounding a joint are involved. In the latter instance, a bony bridge may form, resulting in immobilization of the joint involved.

Spinal Cord Injury. Heterotopic periarticular ossification occurs about the joints in the injured spinal cord, most frequently about the hip, although it may occur about any joint (Fig. 10-21). The process begins as early as three to four weeks after injury and continues actively for two to three years. The activity may be determined by skeletal scintigraphy. The radiographic evidence consist of irregular sheets, bands, and plaques of bone when mature. Early in the process the calcification is more filamentous. Surgery is occasionally required to excise a segment of the ossification to free a completely immobilized joint. This may recur if performed while the process is active, therefore bone scanning is performed before contemplated surgery.

Head Injury. Patients who are comatose from head injury may experience heterotopic ossification similar to the injured spinal cord.

Subcutaneous and Intramuscular Calcification in Calcium Gluconate Therapy

When calcium gluconate is administered intramuscularly to infants or when it extravasates during intravenous injection, a tissue reaction occurs. This results in hazy amorphous calcification in muscle and sub-

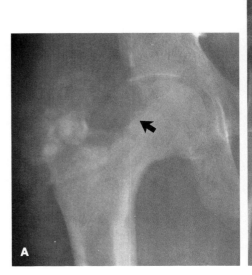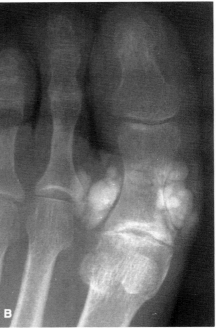

Figure 10–20. Tumoral calcinosis in two patients with chronic renal failure. **(A)** Amorphous, large collection of calcification within the trochanteric bursa in a 30-year-old. Note the subperiosteal erosion of the superior cortex of the femoral neck (*arrow*) consistent with secondary hyperparathyroidism. **(B)** Tumoral calcification about the great toe in a second patient. Note also the degenerative arthritis of the metatarsophalangeal joint.

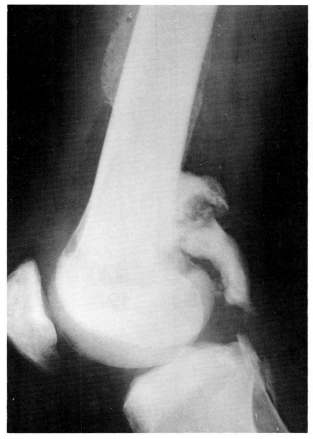

Figure 10–21. Heterotopic paraarticular ossification in a paraplegic patient. Large masses of calcium have formed in the popliteal area, and there is some subperiosteal calcification along the shaft of the femur.

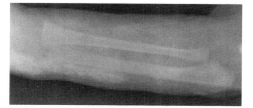

Figure 10–22. Calcium gluconate infusion occurred approximately six days before this radiograph. Following the infusion there was swelling and erythema. Note the sheets of calcification in the soft tissues of the forearm and wrist. Clinical findings had suggested osteomyelitis.

cutaneous tissues that is not produced by the administered calcium, since no roentgenographic findings are present initially. Erythema and induration develop, causing a hard mass that begins to calcify in a few days and thus becomes visible radiographically (Fig. 10-22). The mass may continue to increase in size for about two weeks. There is then a gradual decrease in size followed by eventual disappearance of the calcium. If large subcutaneous doses are administered, ulceration and extrusion of the calcium may occur. Calcification may also be observed in vessels in the area of extravasation.

THE EHLERS-DANLOS SYNDROME

The Ehlers-Danlos syndrome, a congenital dystrophy with hereditary and familial aspects, is a rare cause of disseminated subcutaneous calcifications. It is charac-

terized by an unusual hyperelasticity and fragility of the skin and blood vessels, hypermobility of the joints, pseudotumors over the bony prominences, and disseminated movable subcutaneous nodules. The subcutaneous nodules may calcify. They appear as round discrete densities, usually ringlike with a central zone of translucency ranging from 2 mm to 10 mm in diameter. They occur most frequently over the bony prominences of the forearms and legs. Additional findings include a variety of thoracic deformities, among which are scoliosis, kyphosis, pectus excavatum, and subluxation of the sternoclavicular joints.

CALCIFICATION IN TUMORS

Calcification is not a specific finding for any single type of tumor of the soft tissues, with the exception of hemangioma. Calcification in the form of phleboliths is a frequent finding in cavernous hemangioma and is often diagnostic (see Fig. 10-9). In other tumors, calcification results usually because of a deficient blood supply, with subsequent necrosis within a solid, slowly growing neoplasm. Deposits of calcium may be seen most commonly in lipomas; liposarcomas, fibrosarcomas, and synovial sarcomas (see Fig. 3-50). Chondral calcification is seen in parosteal chondromas (see Chapter 4, Tumors of Bone) and in the less common cartilage tumors of soft tissues. Rarely, *osteosarcoma* has been found arising in the soft tissues, apparently as a result of cellular metaplasia.

GAS IN THE SOFT TISSUES

Accumulations of gas in the soft tissues can be easily recognized in roentgenograms because of the extreme radiolucency of gas compared with the opacity of the surrounding soft tissues. Occasionally, a localized deposition of fat, such as is present in a lipoma, may appear sufficiently lucent in roentgenograms with very high contrast to suggest the presence of a local pocket of gas. An accumulation of air or other gas of a size similar to that of a deposit of fat, however, would appear considerably darker, and it usually requires little experience to differentiate the two. Two major types of gas can be found in the soft tissues. One is air that may have gained entrance through a wound or following a surgical procedure. The other is gas that has been formed as a result of anaerobic bacterial action. Occasionally, in patients with massive pneumomediastinum, gas will dissect into the peritoneum and into superficial soft tissues of the face, neck, thorax, and abdomen. The presence of any appreciable amount of subcutaneous air is termed *subcutaneous emphysema.*

SUBCUTANEOUS EMPHYSEMA

Small bubbles or streaks of air are frequently seen in the region of soft-tissue wounds of penetrating nature. The air shadows may persist for several hours or longer following the injury, but they usually disappear after a day or two. Subcutaneous emphysema may follow injuries to the thorax; usually rib fracture (Fig. 10-23).

There may or may not be an associated pneumothorax. Occasionally, after this type of an injury the subcutaneous emphysema becomes very extensive and the air extends widely through the fascial planes of the body. After surgical procedures on the thorax, fairly large amounts of subcutaneous emphysema may be seen for several days. Traumatic rupture of the trachea, larynx, or esophagus may also result in subcutaneous emphysema. Because of the free communication of the fascial spaces of the body, air may extend far from its point of origin. The recognition of subcutaneous emphysema is not difficult unless the amount of gas is small.

GAS GANGRENE

Infection with gas-forming organisms may result in the roentgenographic visualization of bubbles or streaks of gas in the subcutaneous or deeper tissues. This may follow penetrating or crushing injuries as well as surgical procedures. The organisms most frequently found are *Bacillus welchii (Clostridium perfringens).* It is not possible to distinguish gas formed by anaerobic bacteria from air that has been introduced from without, and

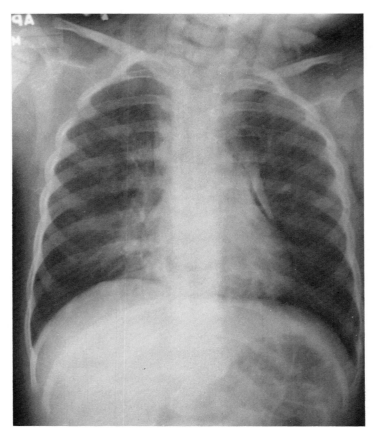

Figure 10–23. Subcutaneous and mediastinal emphysema. There is air in the soft tissues of the neck, left axilla, and left side of the mediastinum, noted as linear radiolucent streaks in these areas. This condition followed an injury to the upper thorax.

therefore the diagnosis of gas gangrene cannot be made from roentgenographic evidence during its very early stage. If the gas shadows extend for a considerable distance from the known site of the soft-tissue wound, one can suspect the possibility of infection. If serial examinations over a period of hours or several days show definite evidence of increasing amounts of gas and spread of the gas shadows, the evidence for gas bacillus infection is more conclusive (Fig. 10-24).

In diabetic gangrene involving the foot, it is common to find small bubbles of gas in the region of the gangrenous tissue and occasionally even more extensively throughout the soft tissues of the foot or in the distal part of the leg (see Fig. 3-43).

TUMORS OF SOFT TISSUES

Many tumors that involve the peripheral soft tissues of the body cause no roentgenographic signs other than a diffuse increase in density. Diagnosis of tumor type may be difficult or impossible, but differentiation between tumor and inflammation and between benign and malignant tumor should be the goal in the study of soft-tissue masses. Such features as relative density, homogeneity, the presence of calcification or ossification, the interface between tumor and adjacent tissues, alterations in adjacent bone or soft tissues, and rapidity of growth may help in the differential diagnosis. Plain films are of limited value except in lipomas (Fig. 10-25A) and hemangiomas (see Fig. 10-9). CT is of greater value, particularly in lipomas (Fig. 10-25B and C), but the ultimate examination is MRI (Figs. 10-26 and 10-27) which can identify the presence and extent of soft tissue masses with certainty. But it is still difficult to determine the precise histologic diagnosis by MRI. The latter remains elusive.

LIPOMA AND LIPOSARCOMA[8]

Larger, deep-seated lipomas can usually be identified without difficulty because of the translucency of fat as compared with that of the muscles. Only when the lipoma is small and located superficially is there an absence of this finding. The margin of the tumor is usually sharply defined. The lesions are clearly visualized by CT. Fibrous tissue septa are occasionally seen within the lipoma and cause a certain amount of striation of the fat shadow (Fig. 10-25). Calcium deposits are sometimes found within a lipoma. Calcification follows ischemic necrosis within the central part of the tumor mass. Liposarcoma causes roentgenographic findings similar to those of its benign counterpart, except for the fact that the boundary of the mass may be poorly defined and there may be irregular extensions of fat into the adjacent muscles. However, in many instances, very little fat can be recognized radiographically in liposarcoma, it may also erode the adjacent bone. Liposarcoma tends to be in deep intermuscular or periarticular planes in contrast to the more superficial benign lipoma. Calcification within the tumor is somewhat more common than in lipoma. The demonstration of fat within a lesion does not establish the diagnosis of a lipoma. Fat is also found in several other tumors including lipoblastoma, hibernoma, hemangioma (see Fig. 10-9), and neural fibrolipoma.[16] MRI of lipoma and liposarcoma is discussed below.

FIBROMA AND FIBROMATOSIS

Benign fibroma is a superficial tumor of little radiographic significance. *Juvenile fascial or aponeurotic fibroma* arises from the aponeurotic tissues of the forearm, hand, leg, or foot. Calcification often occurs within the mass, which is also termed *fascial fibromatosis*. This mass may be very large and cause pres-

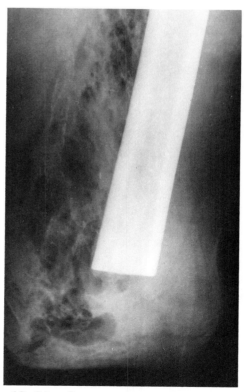

Figure 10–24. Gas gangrene of the thigh following amputation. The gas forms irregular streaks and rounded translucent areas in the soft tissue of the thigh.

(text continues on page 380)

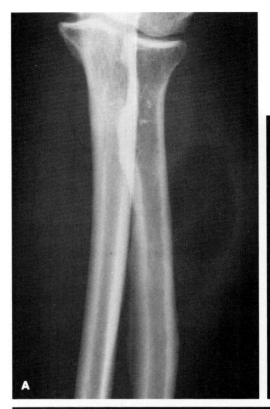

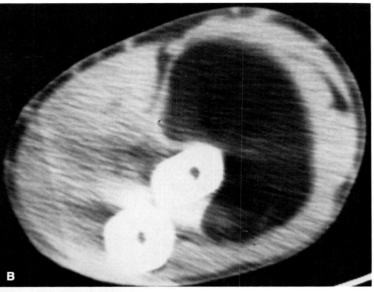

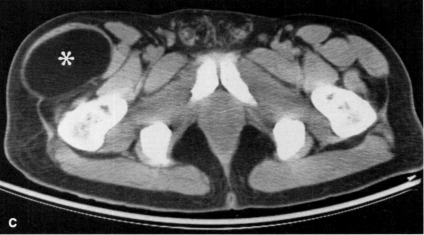

Figure 10–25. Two lipomas in a 59-year-old man. (**A** and **B**) Lipoma of forearm. (**A**) Radiolucency is present within the lateral soft tissues of the proximal left forearm. The lucency is well defined and contains a few septations. (**B**) CT scan demonstrates conclusively that this is a benign lipoma. The lesion is sharply defined, homogeneous, and of characteristic low-fat density. (**C**) CT scan of a second lipoma arising within the tensor fasciae latae muscle(*). This is likewise typical in density, sharply defined and smooth, and indicates a benign lipoma.

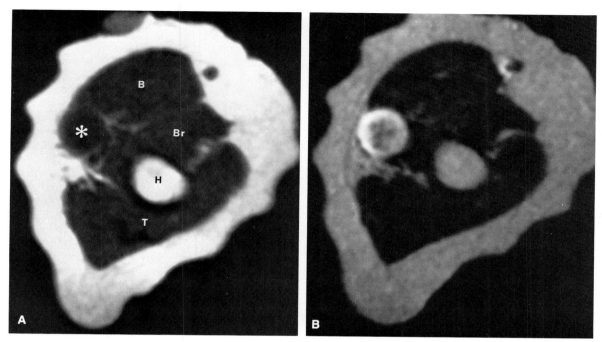

Figure 10–26. MRI of neuroma of upper arm. (**A**) T1-weighted image shows mass(*) is isointense with adjacent muscle. (**B**) T2-weighted image. High signal and sharp definition are consistent with benign lesion. H—humerus; B—biceps brachii muscle; Br—biceps brachialis muscle; and T—triceps brachii muscle.

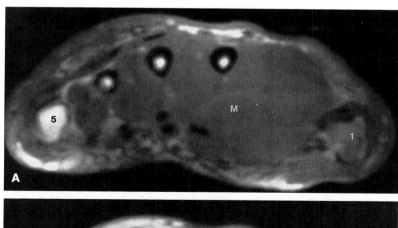

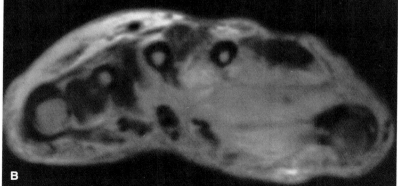

Figure 10–27. MRI of poorly differentiated sarcoma of the hand. (**A**) T1-weighted image reveals poorly defined mass of the palm and thenar eminence that is isointense with surrounding muscle. It is impossible to separate mass from adductor pollicis muscles. 1—first metacarpal; 5—fifth metacarpal; and M—mass. (**B**) T2-weighted image shows mass of variable high-signal intensity with poor marginal definition.

sure changes in the shafts of adjacent bones. *Nodular fasciitis* tends to develop in the superficial soft tissues of the upper extremities. It presents as an oval or round subcutaneous mass that is clearly defined. There may be some difficulty in histologic differentiation between it and sarcoma.

NEUROFIBROMATOSIS AND NEUROFIBROMA

In von Recklinghausen's neurofibromatosis, nodules over the body (widely disseminated cutaneous) are seen as rounded shadows of increased density. In roentgenograms of the chest, these tumor nodules may cause round shadows overlying the lungs. On casual inspection, these may simulate nodules within the lung. If the examination consists of more than one view, the superficial location of the soft-tissue nodules may be apparent. Nodular shadows along the margins of the chest wall may clearly indicate that the lesions are extrapulmonary and suggest the nature of the disease.

Solitary neurofibroma and schwannoma can be identified on MRI by noting the tumor is the axis of, and intimately related to, the course of a nerve.

OTHER TUMORS

Numerous other mesenchymal tumors arise in the soft tissues: arteriovenous malformations, lymphangioma, intramuscular myxoma, desmoid tumors, fibrosarcoma hemangiopericytoma, malignant fibrous histiocytoma, and rhabdomyosarcoma to list a few. Synovial cyst and synovial sarcoma arise around joints. Cysts can be identified as such by various techniques including ultrasound. Otherwise, a specific diagnosis, even the distinction between benign and malignant, is often difficult if not impossible.

MRI of Soft-Tissue Tumors

MRI is the technique of choice for the evaluation of soft-tissue neoplasms because of its superior soft-tissue contrast, ability to image in multiple planes, and lack of beam-hardening artifacts as encountered in CT.[10, 25, 48, 67, 80] However, even then it may be difficult to distinguish between benign and malignant processes.

Benign tumors are homogeneous in signal intensity, sharply defined, do not invade bone or encase neurovascular bundles, and lack surrounding edema (Fig. 10-26). Malignant lesions are generally the opposite (Fig. 10-27). Unfortunately, the exceptions to this generalization are numerous. The T-1 and T-2 relaxation times of benign and malignant lesions overlap considerably and are, therefore, not useful in establishing a distinction between the two.

Most benign tumors are low-signal intensity on T-1

weighted images but have a high signal on T-2 (Fig. 10-26). *Lipomas* are an exception. The signal intensity is the same as subcutaneous fat, high on both T-1 and T-2. Low-signal fibrous septation is frequently noted. *Liposarcoma* should be considered when a fatty lesion is either inhomogeneous or has poorly defined irregular margins. Desmoid tumors, although benign, are often both of inhomogenous signal intensity and irregularly margined. *Hemangiomas* and *vascular malformations* are often irregular and of mixed or variable signal intensity. Feeding vessels may be obvious.

Most malignant soft-tissue neoplasms are inhomogeneous in signal intensity on both T-1 and T-2 sequences, usually most obvious on T-2 weighted images (Fig. 10-27). The margin of most malignant lesions is irregular, although some are well marginated. Irregular margins may be due to inflammation rather than malignant extension. Increased signal intensity surrounding masses on T-2 weighted images is commonly encountered with malignancies but may also be seen in infection or hemorrhage. Neurovascular encasement and invasion of adjacent bone are more common in malignant lesions.

Recent surgery or needle biopsy makes MRI evaluation more difficult. Hemorrhage and inflammation occasioned by this intervention result in an inhomogeneous signal intensity within the lesion in question.

ANGIOGRAPHY
Andrew B. Crummy

VENOGRAPHY

Venography is the radiographic study of the venous system following the injection of a water-soluble radiopaque contrast agent. During the study multiple exposures are made in various projections as the contrast flows through the venous structures. Venography had its widest application in examination of veins in the lower extremities for the detection of thrombosis, particularly of the deep venous system (Fig. 10-28). Venography is also useful in identifying incompetent perforators in patients who have varicose veins. In the upper extremity venography is used to study obstructions of the axillary and subclavian veins as well as the superior vena cava. This application is increasing because of the widespread use of long-term indwelling catheters for hyperalimentation as well as for the infu-

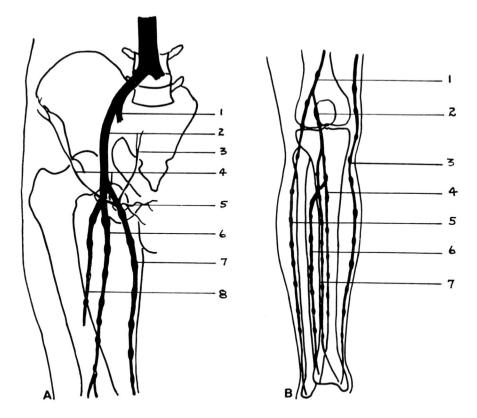

Figure 10–28. Diagram of veins of lower extremity. **(A)** Veins of the thigh: **(1)** hypogastric, **(2)** external iliac, **(3)** superficial epigastric, **(4)** superficial circumflex dendal, **(5)** superficial external pudendal, **(6)** femoral, **(7)** greater saphenous, and **(8)** deep femoral. **(B)** Veins of the leg: **(1)** femoral, **(2)** popliteal, **(3)** greater saphenous, **(4)** posterior tibial, **(5)** lesser saphenous, **(6)** peroneal, and **(7)** anterior tibial.

sion of immunosuppressive and chemotherapeutic agents. This has resulted in an increase in the thrombosis of these veins.

The value of venography for the determination of deep venous thrombosis in lower extremities has been disputed. This is primarily because in the face of extensive obstruction, the deep veins may not fill, and one can only infer that they are thrombosed. Nevertheless, in a properly performed study, the deep veins should fill, and failure to fill should allow one to infer with a high degree of confidence that obstruction is present. Ideally, the thrombus will be outlined by the contrast agent and then the final diagnosis can be made.

Many techniques have been described for the performance of lower extremity venography, but basically we use the following technique. The examination is performed with the patient semi-upright (30° to 45°) from a horizontal position. The patient stands with one foot on a box so that the extremity being examined is nonweight-bearing and completely relaxed. A superficial vein on the dorsum of the foot, preferably the dorsal metatarsal vein of the great toe, is punctured with a 22- or 23-gauge needle. The small needle is easier to place and causes the patient less discomfort. Nevertheless, its lumen is sufficient for the slow injection of dilute contrast agent. Any of the currently approved water soluble contrast agents of 30% concentration are satisfactory. Higher concentrations are unnecessary, they are more difficult to inject, and they produce a greater incidence of undesirable side effects, particularly thrombophlebitis. The injection is performed by hand, and fill of the venous system is monitored fluoroscopically. The total amount of contrast material necessary for complete opacification is determined by direct observation, and the injection site can be monitored to detect any extravasation. One can then take views of the various areas of the venous system as they fill. AP views are supplemented with lateral and oblique projections as necessary.

Use of a remote control fluoroscope with large spot film views has proved to be eminently satisfactory. Upon completion of filming of the vessels of the calf and distal thigh, the tilt table can be lowered so that the contrast agent will be displaced cephalad. Elevation of the extremity will also aid in the displacement of the contrast agent and optimize filling of the common femoral and iliac venous systems.

In instances when the deep venous system does not fill or there is preferential filling of the saphenous veins, application of a tourniquet may tend to force the contrast agent into the deep system. Following the completion of the study, a small amount of saline is infused to aid in the complete clearing of the contrast agent from the venous system. This decrease in contact time diminishes any adverse effects on the venous endothelium.

ROENTGENOGRAPHIC OBSERVATIONS

Deviation of the venous system from its normal anatomic path, fill of incompetent perforating veins, and varicosities are readily recognized, and present no particular diagnostic problems. While observing the incompetent perforators fluoroscopically, it is useful to mark on the skin their exact location to aid the surgeon in locating them.

The recognition of the clots as intraluminal filling defects is a pathognomonic sign (Fig. 10-29). Failure to visualize portions of a given vein or venous system presents more of a problem, and the question always arises, "Is this due to a technical shortcoming?" Injection into a vein of the foot should preferentially fill the deep system, and failure to do this may be the result of

obstruction of the deep system or preferential flow into the saphenous vein. Under these circumstances one should apply a tourniquet to the distal portion of the extremity and repeat the injection with the superficial system occluded. If the deep system does not fill, one may conclude that it is obstructed. Confirmatory signs under these circumstances are the presence of collateral vessels around the nonopacified veins.

Visualization of one of the deep veins to a certain point with failure of the contrast to outline any higher segment, as well as the presence of tortuous vessels in the region with filling of other deep veins more centrally, is positive evidence of obstruction. In instances of doubt, it is helpful to repeat the examination, concentrating on the areas of interest.

Most venograms of the upper extremity are performed to study obstructions of the axillary and subclavian veins as well as the superior vena cava. Under these circumstances, the contrast agent is preferably injected into a branch of the basilic vein at the elbow. Multiple serial films can be made with the use of a film changer or rapid spot filming. Fluoroscopic observation of the initial small bolus is generally helpful to outline the area of interest. Late films should be taken to follow the flow of the contrast agent through collaterals and to see how far centrally the thrombus may extend.

The use of digital subtraction recording techniques has proved to be useful in some circumstances. When injecting through an indwelling catheter that may be partially thrombosed, it may be difficult to inject a quantity sufficient for satisfactory opacification. In these circumstances, a small amount of contrast may prove to be satisfactory because of the increased contrast detection of the electronic technique. Similarly, one may inject through a very small vein with a small needle and use the Digital Subtraction Angiography (DSA) to provide satisfactory delineation of the vessels.

ARTERIOGRAPHY

Arteriography is the study of arteries by the injection of a water-soluble radiopaque contrast agent. Generally, access to the arterial system is achieved through the percutaneous route as described by Seldinger, and the position of the catheter tip for the injection is dictated by the clinical problem. As a rule, the closer the injection is made to the area of interest, the more satisfactory the opacification will be. For study of both the upper and lower extremities the percutaneous transfemoral route is most commonly employed. In instances of severe iliac artery disease, the aorta may be entered either through the translumbar route, or using the Seldinger approach to the axillary or brachial artery

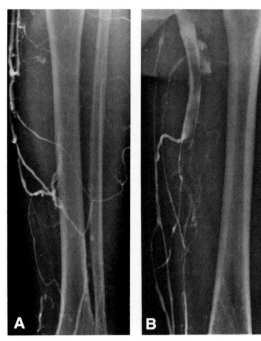

Figure 10–29. **(A)** This lower-extremity venogram shows lack of opacification of the deep system of the leg secondary to thrombosis. **(B)** Only a portion of the superficial femoral vein of the thigh has filled, and radiolucent filling defects are noted within it, indicating the presence of thrombosis.

with retrograde passage of the catheter into the aorta. Injection into the abdominal aorta allows filming of both iliac vessels simultaneously, as well as study of both lower extremities (Fig. 10-30). Study of the abdominal aorta is discussed in Chapter 20.

The most common indication for extremity arteriography is the evaluation of occlusive disease, generally atherosclerotic. However, aneurysms and arteriovenous fistulae are readily evaluated. The study of the vascularity of neoplasms and their extent has decreased in recent years as the use of CT scanning and ultrasound have become more widespread.

The contrast material used is similar to that used for venography, CT scanning, or intravenous pyelography. Because the blood flow is fast, it is necessary that a film changer be employed so that multiple films can be obtained as the contrast courses through the vascular tree. When the area of pathology is known, it is centered over the film changer. In cases of obstructive disease it may be necessary to film large segments of the vascular systems, and under these circumstances the use of a moving tabletop to follow the contrast agent distally through the vascular system is of considerable help.

More recently, the use of digital subtraction arteriography (DSA) has allowed considerable modification in the study of peripheral vascular problems. In some instances, such as abdominal aortic aneurysm or iliac artery disease, venous injection of the contrast agent will provide sufficient detail for clinical management. The use of digital subtraction arteriography in conjunction with intraarterial injections has considerably reduced the volume of contrast agent required. This results in marked reduction in patient discomfort, as well as a decrease in the nephrotoxicity imposed by a large volume of contrast agent. Because many patients with peripheral vascular disease have renal insufficiency secondary to longstanding hypertension and arteriolar nephrosclerosis, this is a very important consideration.

ROENTGENOGRAPHIC OBSERVATIONS

The recognition of an aneurysm is usually accomplished without difficulty. The appearance of the dilated portion of the vessel is characteristic. Occasionally, an aneurysm may be almost completely filled with thrombus and the remaining channel may simulate a relatively normal artery. Under such circumstances, one may be alerted to the presence of an aneurysm by the separation of calcification in the wall of the vessel from the lumen. In addition, failure to fill

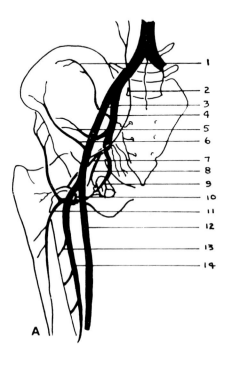
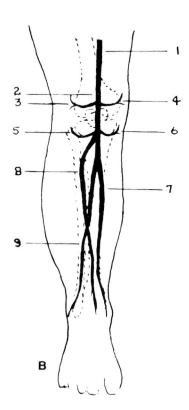

Figure 10–30. Diagram of the arteries of the pelvis, thigh, and leg. (**A**) Arteries of the pelvis and thigh: (**1**) iliolumbar, (**2**) inferior epigastric, (**3**) external iliac, (**4**) hypogastric, (**5**) superior gluteal, (**6**) deep circumflex iliac, (**7**) inferior gluteal, (**8**) internal pudendal, (**9**) obturator, (**10**) medial femoral circumflex, (**11**) lateral femoral circumflex, (**12**) femoral, (**13**) perforating branch, and (**14**) deep femoral (profunda). (**B**) Arteries of the lower thigh and leg: (**1**) femoral, (**2**) popliteal, (**3**) lateral superior genicular, (**4**) medial superior genicular, (**5**) lateral inferior genicular, (**6**) medial inferior genicular, (**7**) posterior tibial, (**8**) anterior tibial, and (**9**) peroneal (Morton S, Byrne R: Radiology 69:63, 1957)

the lumbar arteries that may be thrombosed, or their ostia occluded by the thrombus, may indicate the true nature of what is present.

Arteriovenous fistulae may be congenital, but more frequently are caused by penetrating wounds, and give unequivocal arteriographic signs. The vessels leading to the fistula, as well as the exiting veins, will be increased in size and there will be rapid flow through the area of communication. Usually the diagnosis is made clinically and arteriography demonstrates the exact site and extent of the fistula. This will aid in the management of the fistula which may be performed surgically, or radiologically with the use of intravascular occluding materials such as autologous clots, coils, glue, or detachable balloons.

The most frequent indication for arteriography of peripheral vessels is the study of occlusive disease. Because in most patients the clinical manifestations are diagnostic, the arteriogram delineates the site and extent of the disease and determines whether lesions suitable for bypass or transluminal angioplasty are present. Intimal atherosclerotic plaques cause areas of irregular narrowing of the vessel or, if severe, complete occlusion (Figs. 10-31 and 10-32). Areas of involvement

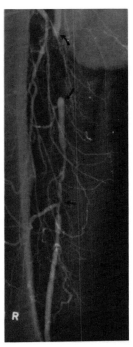

Figure 10–32. Femoral arteriogram. The proximal portion of the superficial femoral artery has a complete obstruction approximately 4 cm in length (*curved arrows*). Further distally, the vessel is involved with high-grade but incomplete obstruction secondary to atherosclerosis (*straight arrow*). Note the collaterals from the profunda femoral artery communicating with muscular branches of the superficial femoral.

may be focal, but in most instances are diffuse with the degree of severity of involvement being quite variable. It is important that the vessels proximal and distal to the areas of hemodynamically significant obstruction or stenosis be identified. If there is insufficient inflow to the area of involvement, any local treatment will fail because of inadequate perfusion. Likewise, for a vessel that has been dilated or a graft to stay patent, there must be sufficient outflow to prevent stagnation of flow and thrombosis.

LYMPHANGIOGRAPHY

Until the advent of ultrasound and CT scanning, lymph nodes could not be visualized except by lymphangiography. Lymphangiography is performed by injecting oily contrast material directly into lymph vessels, nodes, or, rarely, lymphocytes. In clinical practice the injection sites are the lymph vessels of the lower extremity

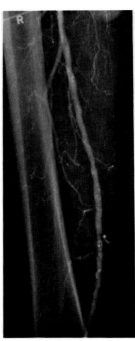

Figure 10–31. Femoral arteriogram. The artery is diffusely involved with atherosclerotic plaques throughout its course; however, none of the plaques has resulted in a hemodynamically significant obstruction.

or the spermatic cord. Lymphangiography is used as a method for opacifying the lymphatic channels and lymph nodes (Figs. 10-33 and 10-34).

TECHNIQUE

Staining of lymphatic channels in the feet is performed by intradermal injection of a mixture of 1% xylocaine (1 cc) and 4% direct sky blue (3 to 4 cc) or similar dye between the first three toes of each foot. In 15 to 30 minutes the subcutaneous lymphatic vessels are stained and can be seen through the skin. Under local anesthesia a small skin incision is then made over a lymph channel on the dorsum of each foot. The vessel is freed from its fibrous sheath for 1½ to 2 cm on each side. It is then stabilized with a small clip. A 30-gauge cannula especially designed for the purpose is then inserted. Generally this is accomplished with the aid of magnifying lens or glasses. Once the cannula is seated, 6 to 8 cc of ethiodol are injected in each foot. Films of the upper thighs and abdomen are obtained to monitor the progression of the contrast material, and when it

reaches the level of L3 or L4, the injection is discontinued. Films of the upper femurs, pelvis, and abdomen demonstrate the vascular phase. A second set of films if obtained at 24 hours and sometimes 48 hours to demonstrate nodal filling.

Lymphography is indicated to (1) evaluate extremity edema of unknown cause; (2) assess the extent of adenopathy to stage lymphoma; (3) localize nodes for treatment planning; (4) evaluate the nature of intraabdominal mass; (5) localize abnormal nodes for percutaneous biopsy.

Contraindications include known iodine hypersensitivity, severe pulmonary insufficiency, cardiac disease, and advanced renal or hepatic disease.

Complications in the main are related to embolization of the contrast material into the lungs. The thoracic duct empties into the venous system, so there will always be some pulmonary embolization, which temporarily diminishes pulmonary function. Thus, lymphography may be hazardous in patients with diminished pulmonary reserve. Rarely, a patient may develop a lipid pneumonia. Extravasation is a compli-

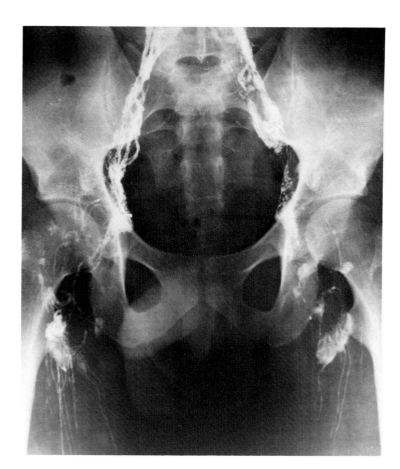

Figure 10–33. Normal lymphangiogram. Vascular phase showing filling of lymphatic vessels in the upper thighs and pelvis. A few nodes are opacified.

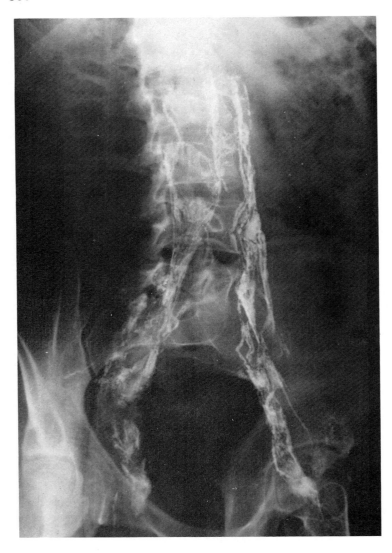

Figure 10–34. Lymphangiogram. The vascular phase shows displacement of channels by large nodes that are not opacified.

cation that usually does not cause any clinically significant changes.

Normally the initial films show filling of the lymphatic channels in the thigh, pelvis, and abdomen. Some of the nodes may be filled at this time (Fig. 10-33). On the 24-hour film, the lymph channels are no longer visible in the normal person and the lymph nodes are filled (Fig. 10-34). Interpretation of lymphangiograms is difficult, and there are limitations: nodes completely replaced by neoplasm may not take up contrast material, while nodes involved by inflammatory disease may have alteration of the lymph nodes architecture which may simulate primary or secondary neoplasm (Fig. 10-35). The details of lymphangiographic interpretation are discussed elsewhere.

The wide use of ultrasound and particularly CT scanning have markedly reduced the use of lymphangiography. However, ultrasound and CT scanning will only allow the identification of masses, while lymphangiography permits characterization of nodal architecture. If lymphatic channels are completely blocked or masses of nodes totally replaced by tumor, they will not be opacified by the contrast agent and will remain undetected. Masses identified by ultrasound and CT scanning as well as lymphography can be biopsied percutaneously so that a histologic diagnosis can be made. Ultrasound and CT scanning have reduced the need for lymphangiography. The application of the various modalities in the detection of lymph node disease, however, remains unsettled.

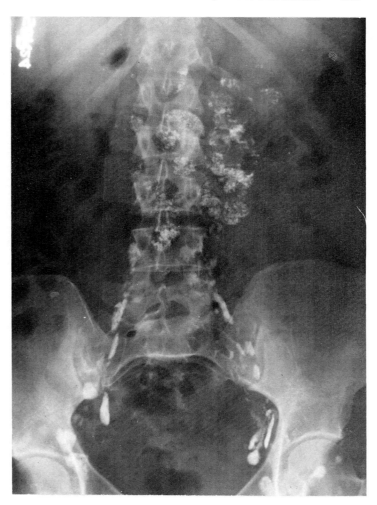

Figure 10–35. Lymphangiogram of a patient with Hodgkin's Disease. This 24-hour film shows a number of midabdominal para-aortic nodes that are enlarged and appear foamy. Pelvic and iliac nodes are normal.

MAMMOGRAPHY

Mary Ellen Peters

MAMMOGRAPHY

The goal of mammography is to detect small, curable carcinomas. In order to accomplish this, the radiologist and the surgeon must be willing to accept a low positive biopsy rate. A 15% to 30% positive rate is considered acceptable.[43] The radiologist must be as discriminating as possible, however, in the recommendation for biopsy, and, therefore, must know the signs of benign processes as well as those of malignancy.

A fundamental knowledge of breast anatomy is essential in understanding mammographic findings. The breast is divided into 15 to 20 lobes. Each lobe is drained by a collecting duct with multiple branches that end in a terminal ductal lobular unit (TDLU). The TDLU consists of an extralobular terminal duct and the lobule, the smallest structural unit. The lobule consists of an intralobular terminal duct, ductules that have a sac-like appearance, and the surrounding connective tissue.[84] It is in the TDLU that most carcinomas arise. It is also the site of benign proliferative and epithelial changes and the area in which cysts develop.

The basic screening mammographic views are the craniocaudal and mediolateral oblique. Additional views may be necessary for further evaluation of suspected pathology. The lateromedial, exaggerated medial craniocaudal, and valley (which is performed with the medial aspects of both breasts on the film) views are useful for delineation of medial masses. An exaggerated lateral craniocaudal view (Cleopatra view) is used for accessing lesions located far laterally. The 90° lateral view is useful in evaluating for fluid levels and meniscus signs. The tangential view can aid in differentiation of an intradermal lesion from a parenchymal lesion. The coned compression and 90° lateral views can help confirm if the area in question is a mass or superimposed glandular tissue. The magnification view is often helpful in defining masses and calcifications.

The craniocaudal views should be placed on the viewbox adjacent to one another, and likewise for the mediolateral views. In this manner, it is easier to perceive masses or areas of asymmetry that could represent a carcinoma. A magnifying glass is mandatory to detect calcifications. It is also necessary to have a bright light, because often in the properly exposed screen–film study the skin cannot be visualized using the viewbox. If the patient has had previous mammograms, they must be carefully compared to the current study.

There is a wide variation of normal parenchymal patterns. The glandular tissue is usually symmetric although asymmetry can be seen as a normal variant. The glandular tissue may extend far into the axillae and often this is asymmetric.[5] The density of the breasts is variable. The breasts are usually dense in the young patient. As patients grow older, fatty replacement commonly occurs, with the parenchyma in the superolateral quadrant being the last to be replaced. (It also in this quadrant that most carcinomas arise.) The breasts have more fatty replacement after pregnancy and lactation, as well as in obese patients. Estrogen and progesterone therapy frequently produce an increase in the glandular tissues.[9, 78] During lactation, the breasts are extremely dense.

MALIGNANCY

Primary signs of ductal and infiltrating ductal carcinoma (not otherwise specified) are as follows:

I. Calcifications—usually have some or all of the following characteristics (Figs. 10-36 and 10-37):
   A. Location: In a cluster measuring 1 to 2 cm. More than one cluster may be present.
   B. Size: Variable within a cluster, measuring from less than 1 to 2 mm. Intermixed larger calcifications can be seen. Classification of a cluster into a benign or malignant category should be determined by the smallest calcification, not the largest.[47]
   C. Shape: Pleomorphic within a cluster. Configurations can be Y or V shaped, rod-like, angular, granular, lacy, or round.
   D. Contour: Irregular.
   E. Number: Usually 15 to 20 or more; occasionally only four or five. Most mammographers do not recommend biopsy for a group of calcifications numbering less than four or five except for unusual compelling reasons. If there are two or three calcifications that are questionable, they can be monitored with followup studies and biopsied if they increase in number.[43]
II. Mass—may contain calcifications. Malignant

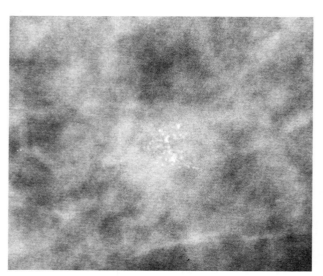

Figure 10–36. Malignant calcifications. Innumerable calcifications of varying size, shape, and density. Magnified.

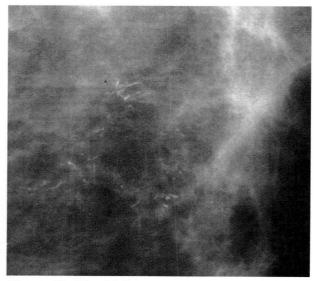

Figure 10–37. Malignant calcifications. Linear, branching, and punctate calcifications. Magnified.

masses usually are dense, but this is not always true.[44] More than one malignant mass may be present. The masses may be characterized as follows:

A. Stellate: Spicules radiating in straight lines from a central mass (Figs. 10-38 and 10-39*A* and *B*).

B. Nodular: A mass with an irregular or "knobby" border. Commonly, a portion of the border is ill defined (Fig. 10-40).

C. Lobulated: A minimal and rather smooth lobulation, often with only a small, poorly defined local irregularity or indistinct border.

D. Well defined: Can be round or oval. A halo sign, which is a fine rim of radiolucency partially or entirely surrounding a mass, can be associated with malignant masses. However, it is more commonly seen with benign masses.[53, 62, 81]

III. Neodensity—a new appearing density as compared with previous studies.

IV. Density that increases in size or opacity.

V. Focal asymmetric density is a mass, the margins of which are ill defined or obliterated by the surrounding glandular tissue. It is dense centrally and may be associated with architectural distortion, microcalcifications, or a palpable mass. It can be identified as a mass density in two planes (Figs. 10-41*A* through *D*). This needs to be differentiated from normal asymmetrical glandular tissue, which is not associated with a palpable mass, architectural distortion, or microcalcifications, and is not volumetric.[45, 47] (Asymmetry can also be the result of a previous biopsy).

VI. Architectural distortion. History is important since a previous biopsy, infection or trauma can cause distortion of the parenchyma as well as a carcinoma.

Secondary signs are as follows:

I. Skin thickening over the site of a malignancy may be helpful in calling attention to a mass (Fig. 10-38).

II. Skin retraction resulting in straightening or concavity of the normal contour (Fig. 10-38). Spicules extending to the skin may be observed (Fig. 10-38).

III. Nipple retraction—may be normal, but when associated with increased retroareolar density, mass, malignant calcifications or enlarged duct or ducts retraction is an important sign.

IV. Abnormal lymph nodes.

V. Vascularity—an increase in size or in number of veins is often of little help since this may be seen as a normal variant.

VI. Duct pattern—asymmetrically enlarged duct or ducts. It is rare for asymmetry of ducts to herald the presence of a carcinoma unless associated with nipple retraction, discharge, eczema, malignant calcifications, or a mass that is palpable or seen on the mammogram.

Lesions that are questionable but are thought most likely to be benign can be monitored with followup mammograms. Depending on the degree of suspicion, the initial followup examination of a lesion should be obtained at three to six months. If the lesion is unchanged, this is usually followed by either a six-month study or yearly studies for two to three years. If there is no change, routine screening can resume.[4, 13, 42, 74]

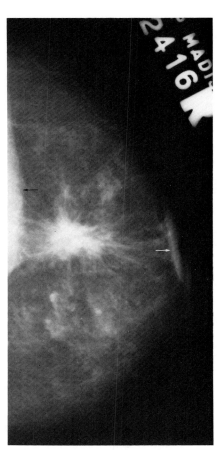

Figure 10–38. Stellate, mass-infiltrating ductal carcinoma. Craniocaudal view. Spicules extending out from dense central mass. Associated skin thickening and retraction (*white arrow*). Black arrow points to pectoralis muscle.

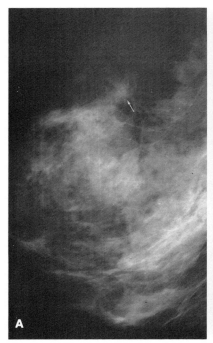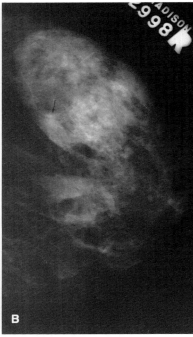

Figure 10–39. Stellate, mass-infiltrating ductal carcinoma. Mediolateral oblique (**A**) and craniocaudal (**B**) views. Small spiculated mass (*arrow*).

OTHER BREAST MALIGNANCIES

Comedocarcinoma is primarily an intraductal carcinoma, although areas of invasion may be present. Dilated ducts are filled with malignant cells that undergo necrosis and calcification. Mammographically,

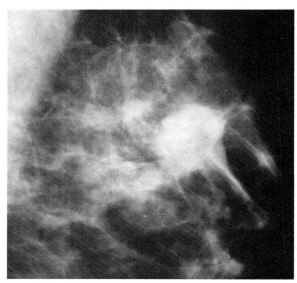

Figure 10–40. Ill-defined mass containing malignant calcifications—infiltrating ductal carcinoma.

malignant calcifications are usually seen along the course of the ducts. The extent of involvement is variable. It may involve a single duct, several ducts in a segment of a breast, or have multiple foci.[43, 68]

Inflammatory breast carcinoma is the result of dermal lymphatic carcinomatosis.[59] It causes the breast to appear dense and the skin thickened. If the internal architecture is not obscured by the generalized increase in density, the trabeculae will often appear thickened. No specific masses can be visualized. Axillary adenopathy is common (Figs. 10-42A and B).

Medullary and mucoid (colloid) carcinomas are frequently peripheral in location. Both appear as round or lobulated masses that are well circumscribed and may have an associated halo sign. Alternatively, a segment of the margin may be ill defined (Fig. 10-43). Medullary carcinomas are of high density while mucoid carcinomas tend to be of low density.[68]

Papillary carcinomas occur as intraductal, intracystic, and invasive lesions. They are usually of low density, and present as round, lobulated, dumbbell-shaped or bilobed masses. Margination may be sharp and a halo sign may be seen. However, the borders may be ill defined secondary to invasion or an associated usual ductal carcinoma. The wall of an intracystic papillary carcinoma may calcify.[61, 73]

Tubular and lobular carcinomas are indistinguishable from the usual invasive ductal carcinoma mammographically.[56] *Lobular carcinoma in situ* is found

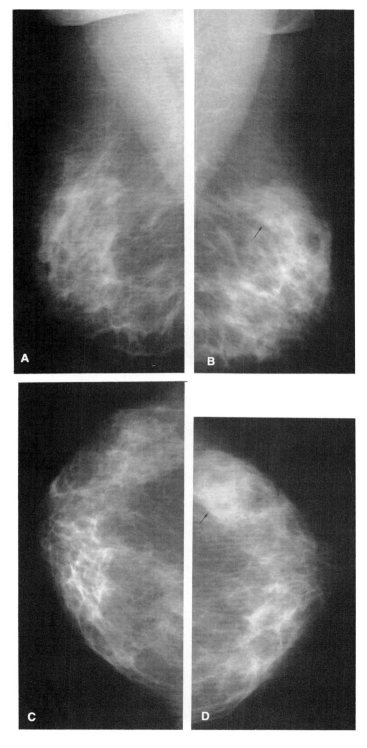

Figure 10–41 (A through **D).** Infiltrating carcinoma of the left breast presenting as an asymmetrical density. Mediolateral oblique left **(A)** and right **(B)**, and craniocaudal left **(C)** and right **(D)**. Asymmetrical density (*arrow*) in the superolateral quadrant of the left breast. The abnormality can be recognized in two planes.

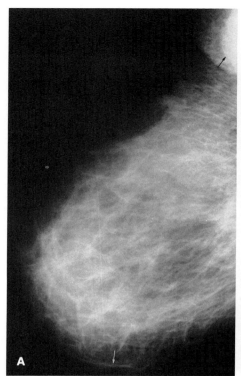

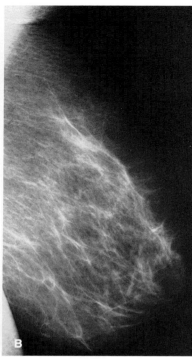

Figure 10–42. Inflammatory carcinoma. Left (**A**) and right (**B**) mediolateral obliques. Increased density and trabecular thickening of left breast. Enlarged axillary lymph node (*black arrow*). Only a small area of skin thickening is reproducible on print (*white arrow*).

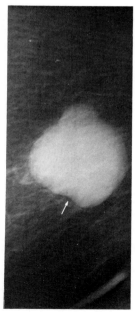

Figure 10–43. Mucoid carcinoma. Large, lobulated, low-density mass. The white arrow indicates a halo sign.

incidentally on biopsy specimens, and does not produce mammographic findings.

Paget's disease presents clinically as an eczematoid lesion of the nipple. It may be secondary to an intraductal or an infiltrating ductal carcinoma. Rarely, it is the result of a lobular carcinoma. Neoplastic cells (Paget cells) are found in the epidermis.[6, 59] Findings of a retroareolar carcinoma are usually present on the mammogram, but the carcinoma may occur anywhere in the breast. Malignant calcifications may be seen extending into the nipple.

Sarcomas: Cystosarcoma Phyllodes and Stromal Sarcoma. Breast sarcomas are divided into two types: those with epithelial elements, cystosarcoma phyllodes, and those without epithelial elements, stromal sarcomas. Only 20% of cystosarcoma phyllodes tumors are malignant.[59] However, the benign form can recur after surgery because of its tentacle-like projections. Both types of sarcomas are classified into fibrosarcoma, liposarcoma, chondrosarcoma, osteosarcoma, and leiomyosarcoma. Angiosarcoma is another type of stromal sarcoma. It may present with bluish discoloration of the skin. The stromal sarcomas are rapidly growing tumors. Mammographically, the cystosarcoma phyllodes tumors and the stromal sarcomas present as round or multilobulated masses, the borders of which may be well defined, although a segment is often obscured.[20, 27, 33, 79] Calcifications may be observed within the mass if chondroid or osteogenic elements are present.[2, 83] Liposarcomas may contain areas of lucency. Axillary adenopathy, if present, is the result of necrosis and inflammation since sarcomas metastasize by a hematogenous route.

Lymphoma. Primary and secondary lymphoma can involve the breast. In both types, masses that are round, ovoid, or lobulated with well-defined or spiculated borders measuring 2 to 3 cm can be seen. Multiple and bilateral masses can be observed in the secondary form, but this is unusual in primary lymphoma. Findings similar to those of inflammatory breast carcinoma also may occur more commonly in secondary lymphoma.[23, 49, 58, 60, 65] Axillary adenopathy is seen in both forms.

Leukemic involvement, which is usually bilateral, may present as multiple masses or generalized increased density and skin thickening. All types of leukemia may occur in the breast.[60, 68]

Metastases. The most common metastasis is from a contralateral breast carcinoma. The findings may be similar to inflammatory breast carcinoma, or the presentation may be that of a mass. Malignant melanoma is the second most common metastasis, followed by lung carcinoma, sarcoma, and ovarian carcinoma.[55] Any type of neoplasm, however, may metastasize to the breast. The metastases usually present as solitary, well-demarcated masses, but the borders can be ill defined.[12] They can be multiple and bilateral. Frequently, they occur in the superolateral quadrant and often are superficial.[23, 82] Metastatic ovarian carcinoma may contain calcifications.[63] A less common presentation of extramammary metastatic disease is skin thickening, which may be diffuse or focal.[55]

BENIGN BREAST MASSES

Fibroadenomas are comprised of fibrous stroma and glandular tissue. It is theorized that they are a form of lobular hyperplasia.[59] They can occur at any age, but are more common before the age of 30. Fibroadenomas are generally solitary, but can be multiple and bilateral. Their radiographic characteristics are those of an ovoid, round, or lobulated mass with sharp borders that may be associated with a halo sign. The margins can be ill defined secondary to overlying glandular tissue (Fig. 10-44). Fibroadenomas frequently calcify as the result of myxomatous degeneration, particularly in the postmenopausal age group. The calcifications may entirely

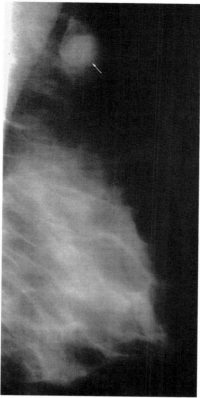

Figure 10–44. A mediolateral oblique view of a fibroadenoma. Note the round, homogenous mass (*arrow*) in accessory axillary glandular tissue. The borders are ill-defined secondary to surrounding parenchyma.

replace the soft-tissue component. Typically, the calcifications are large. They may be solitary or multiple, and have a round, "popcorn," comma, shell, or rim-like appearance (Figs. 10-45 and 10-46). Because fibroadenomas can appear as new masses, increase in size, or contain malignant-appearing calcifications, they may be mistaken for carcinomas.

Giant or *juvenile fibroadenoma* is the most common mass in the teenager. It is similar to the fibroadenoma seen in adults except that it can grow rapidly and become very large. *Tubular adenomas (pure mammary adenomas)* are rare tumors that are composed of epithelially lined tubular structures.[6] *Lactating adenomas* occur before or during lactation. Some theorize that they are the result of the hormonal effects on an ordinary fibroadenoma, but others believe them to be a variant of the tubular adenoma.[6] They can grow rapidly and attain a large size. When lactation stops, they usually decrease in size.

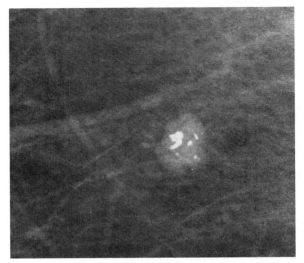

Figure 10–45.   Fibroadenoma. Lobulated mass with large, smooth calcifications.

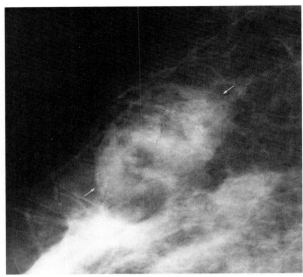

Figure 10–47.   Lipofibroadenoma.   Inhomogeneous mass (*arrows*) with areas of lucency.

Lipofibroadenomas (hamartomas) contain fatty, glandular, and fibrous elements. Characteristically, they present as masses with a center of mixed radiolucency–radiodensity and a lucent periphery. Often they appear to have a capsule that anatomically represents the normal trabeculae that have been displaced. Lipofibroadenomas may also appear as homogenous masses with ill-defined borders. They can measure up to 10 cm, but more commonly measure 2 to 3 cm (Fig. 10–47).[22, 23, 38]

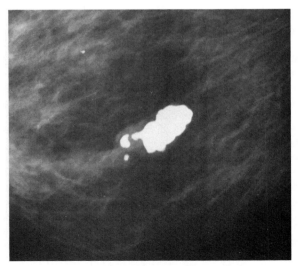

Figure 10–46.   Fibroadenoma. The soft tissue component has been largely replaced by calcification.

Cysts most commonly occur between the ages of 30 and 50 years. It is unusual for a cyst to develop in the postmenopausal age group unless the individual is on hormonal replacement. If a cyst is seen in these women, one must carefully search for signs of an associated carcinoma that may be obstructing the duct. Radiographically, cysts appear as round, ovoid, or lobulated homogeneous masses that may be of low or high density (Fig. 10–48). Usually the margins are distinct and an associated halo sign may be seen. However, they may be indistinct secondary to overlying glandular tissue or inflammatory reaction as the result of cyst contents leaking into the parenchyma. They can change in size relatively rapidly, becoming either very large or disappearing. Usually they are multiple but can be single as well as unilateral or bilateral. The wall of a cyst can calcify. Occasionally, calcium particles can be identified within a cyst layering against the dependent wall.

Intraductal papillomas are villous lesions that have a fibrovascular core and are covered by an epithelium.[59] They are the most common cause of serous or bloody nipple discharge, but are usually too small to be identified mammographically. Solitary papillomas usually occur in the retroareolar area, and can present as a mass or as a dilated duct. Multiple papillomas tend to occur peripherally, and can present as a cluster of small round densities. Small calcifications can develop within them or the calcification may have a rosette or raspberry appearance. Solitary papillomas have no potential for developing malignancy.[6] Multiple papillomas,

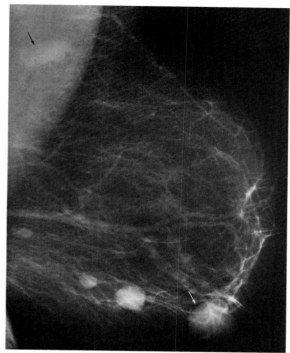

Figure 10–48. Cysts. Mediolateral oblique view. Four round-to-ovoid well-defined densities. Halo sign (*white arrow*). Cysts proven with ultrasound. Normal, fatty replaced axillary lymph node (*black arrow*).

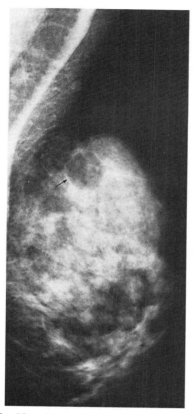

Figure 10–49. Lipoma. Mediolateral oblique view. Round, well-defined lucency with surrounding capsule (*arrow*).

however, are associated with an increased incidence of carcinoma.[6]

Lipomas are seen more commonly in older women, and are of no clinical consequence unless they grow so large that they cause a cosmetic problem. Radiographically, they present as an area of lucency with a surrounding capsule (Fig. 10-49). Calcification secondary to fat necrosis may develop within them. Lipomas should not be confused with fatty lobules that are partially surrounded by trabeculae and Cooper's ligaments.

Galactoceles are cysts that contain a milky fluid, and are the result of inspissated milk obstructing a duct. They develop during or shortly after cessation of lactation. Because the diagnosis is often evident clinically, no mammogram is needed. If radiographed, they may appear entirely radiolucent or radiodense depending upon the fat content. A 90° lateral view may demonstrate a fat–fluid level or a fat–calcium level. Inspissation of the contents of a galactocele produces a varied appearance of radiolucency–radiodensity.[31]

Fibromatosis (extraabdominal desmoid tumor) is an infiltrative fibroblastic proliferation. It usually originates in the pectoralis fascia and involves the breast secondarily. Rarely, it originates in the breast. It simulates a breast carcinoma clinically and mammographically.[18, 34] Associated calcification has not been reported.

Radial scar (elastosis, indurative mastopathy, benign sclerosing ductal proliferation) is composed of ductal elements, elastic tissue, and hyalinizing fibrosis.[59] The mammographic presentation is difficult or impossible to distinguish from a stellate carcinoma. Unlike the stellate carcinoma, it does not have a central mass nor does it appear the same in all projections. In addition, fat can be seen traversing through it.[3] However, fat can become incorporated into a carcinoma. These lesions warrant biopsy.

BENIGN MISCELLANEOUS

The response of the glandular tissues to the fluctuations in hormonal levels leads to what has been collectively termed "*fibrocystic changes.*" Various entities, including adenosis, cystic lobular hyperplasia, fibrosis, cysts, fibroadenomas, radial scar, epitheliosis, apocrine and squamous metaplasia, atypical hyperplasia, ductal ectasia, and sterile mastitis have been classified under this heading.[21, 68] It is better to consider each entity and understand its histopathology rather than to use the term "fibrocystic change."[47] Atypical hyperplasia, which is associated with an increased risk for developing carcinoma, and the metaplasias have no specific radiographic findings.

Adenosis is a form of benign epithelial hypertrophy and hyperplasia. There is an increase in the number of lobules and a hypertrophy of the myoepithelium and epithelium, which may be diffuse or localized. As a result, an increase in density of the breasts is seen.[47, 59, 68] If it is diffuse, a "snowflake pattern" may be observed. In *sclerosing adenosis*, proliferation of the connective tissues is also present.[59] When the proliferation is localized, a mass that is indistinguishable from malignancy may be present. Inspissated secretion within the ductules may calcify in all forms of adenosis. The calcifications can be clustered or diffuse. Classically, the calcifications within a cluster are tightly grouped, smoothly rounded, and homogenous in size and density (Fig. 10-50). However, the characteristics of the cluster can simulate malignancy. Multiple groups are commonly present, and usually they are bilateral. In the diffuse form, numerous calcifications are seen scattered throughout both breasts, which tend to appear dense. The calcifications are relatively the same size and are rounded. The borders of the calcifications can be indistinct. Biopsy is recommended if the calcifications are unilateral.[43] Homer recommends followup mammograms on patients with diffuse calcifications because of the possibility of a hidden carcinoma.[43]

Cystic lobular hyperplasia is a form of adenosis in which the ductules are dilated and are referred to as microcysts. Milk of calcium can form in the dilated ductules. Since the milk of calcium layers out in the dependent portion of the microcyst, a meniscus is seen with a horizontal beam and often it can be identified on the standard mediolateral oblique view. This meniscus is called a teacup calcification (Fig. 10-51). En face it appears as a small, round, ill-defined, calcific density.[68]

Fibrosis (chronic indurative mastopathy, fibrous mastopathy) consists of fibrous tissue without glandular elements. It is questioned whether this represents a true pathologic entity or is simply the result of normal atrophy of the glandular elements. It occurs most commonly in the superolateral quadrant, and often cannot be clinically or radiographically differentiated from a malignant mass.[59]

Secretory disease occurs in older women, and is the result of accumulations of secretions within ducts. The secretions can inspissate and calcify, producing large, smooth, rod-shaped or branching calcifications that are oriented toward the nipple (Fig. 10-52). Occasionally,

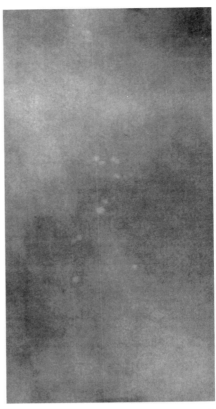

Figure 10–50. Adenosis. Note the smooth, round calcifications, some of which are tightly grouped. Magnified.

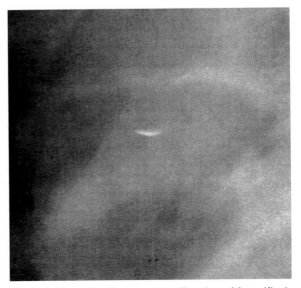

Figure 10–51. Teacup calcification. Magnified.

the calcifications are small and are difficult to differentiate from malignant calcifications. Enlargement of retroareolar ducts (*ductal ectasia*), which generally is bilateral and symmetrical, can also be observed.[47, 68]

Plasma Cell Mastitis. Ductal secretions may extravasate causing a chemical mastitis and plasma cell infiltration. As a result, periductal calcifications develop. These calcifications have a relatively lucent center and can be round, ovoid, rod shaped, or branching (Fig. 10-52). The spherical calcifications are likely the result of fat necrosis. The inflammatory reaction can secondarily cause fibrosis, which usually develops in the retroareolar area and may be palpable. The nipple is frequently retracted, and there may be nipple discharge. Mammography reveals a homogenous subareolar mass with indistinct margins that tends to be bilaterally symmetrical. Plasma cell mastitis occasionally occurs deeper in the breast.[47, 68]

Fat necrosis can be the result of surgery, trauma, radiation therapy, and inflammation. The three major radiographic findings of fat necrosis are oil cyst, stellate mass, and calcifications. The oil cyst is composed of a fibrous capsule surrounding a lipid material. It can measure from a few millimeters to several centimeters.

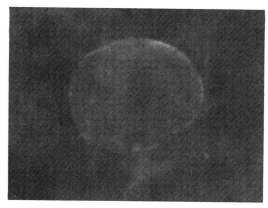

Figure 10–53.   Oil cyst with calcification in the wall.

The center may be entirely radiolucent or may be radiolucent–radiodense. A fat fluid level may be seen with a horizontal beam. The capsule may calcify producing a rim or shell-like appearance (Fig. 10-53). Calcification of the contents may also occur causing coarse or small malignant-like calcifications.[28] As the result of the fibrotic response associated with fat necrosis, stellate masses can be seen that may be associated with skin retraction and thickening (Fig. 10-54).[7, 75]

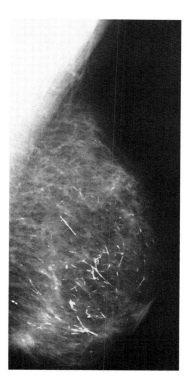

Figure 10–52.   Secretory and plasma cell mastitis calcifications. Mediolateral oblique view. Linear, branching, ovoid calcifications.

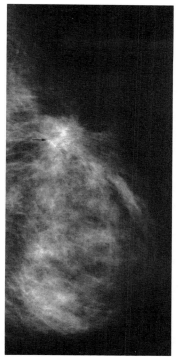

Figure 10–54.   Stellate mass secondary to fat necrosis (*arrow*). Mediolateral oblique view.

These masses usually decrease in size, but they may remain unchanged.[76] Benign or malignant-appearing calcifications can also develop. These may be seen in isolation or be associated with a mass. History is important in evaluating these findings. Followup mammograms or biopsy may be needed, depending on the circumstances.

Most *hematomas* are seen after surgical procedures although they can be the result of trauma. The mammographic presentation may be either that of a sharply or poorly marginated mass or a vague area of increased density. Skin thickening may be an accompanying finding. Hematomas usually resolve in four to six weeks. However, those presenting as a mass may have residual architectural distortion or persist as a mass-like lesion secondary to organization of the hematoma (Fig. 10-55).

Mastitis and Abscess. Acute generalized mastitis cannot be distinguished mammographically from an inflammatory breast carcinoma. Usually it develops during lactation, and the diagnosis is clinically evident. In the older woman, acute mastitis and abscess are often superficial as the result of an infected sebaceous gland. Acute inflammation produces a localized increase in density, the area of which depends on the size of the inflammatory reaction. An abscess presents as a poorly defined mass. Both are frequently associated with skin thickening. The history and clinical findings are important in differentiation from a carcinoma.[68]

The characteristic "tram track" sign of *arterial calcifications* does not cause a diagnostic dilemma. Occasionally, however, the calcifications assume a dot–dash or irregular configuration, which can be mistaken for malignancy. Magnification and oblique views are helpful for further evaluation.

MALE BREAST

Gynecomastia is the most common abnormality of the male breast. Radiographically, it presents in the retroareolar area as prominent ducts extending posteriorly or as a homogeneous density (Fig. 10-56). Gynecomastia is often asymmetric.

Carcinoma of the breast is uncommon in males. The mammographic manifestations are similar to those seen in women.

LYMPH NODES

Lymph nodes are bean shaped, ovoid, or round. Often an associated central or umbilicated lucency can be seen secondary to fat within the hilum. Almost without exception, *intramammary lymph nodes* are located in the superolateral quadrant (Fig. 10-57). They can be

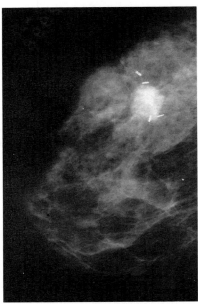

Figure 10–55. Organized hematoma. Craniocaudal view. Round mass present at surgical site six months after resection of carcinoma. Proven with ultrasound and aspiration.

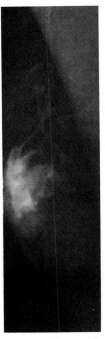

Figure 10–56. Gynecomastia. Mediolateral oblique view. Homogenous density in the retroareolar area.

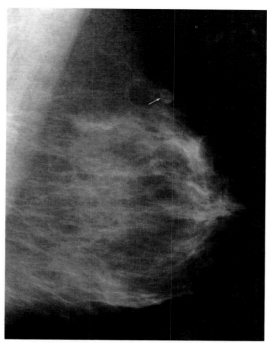

Figure 10–57. Normal intramammary lymph node (*arrow*). Mediolateral oblique view. Smooth, ovoid density with central lucency.

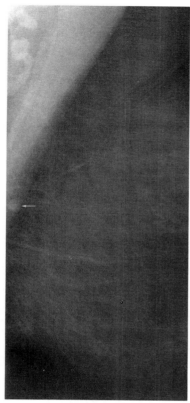

Figure 10–58. Normal axillary and lateral thoracic (*arrow*) lymph nodes. Mediolateral oblique view. Fat (lucency) can be seen with the axillary lymph nodes.

multiple and bilateral.[57] An intramammary lymph node that measures 1 cm or greater and does not have an identifiable fatty hilum is abnormal. A carcinoma or an inflammatory process in the ipsilateral breast are the most likely etiologies.[51] *Lateral thoracic lymph nodes* can measure up to 1 cm. Frequently they are solitary and unilateral, and often do not have a fatty hilum (Fig. 10-58).

Axillary lymph nodes measure 1 to 1.5 cm, although in the presence of a large, fatty hilum they can measure up to 2 to 3 cm (Fig. 10-58). In the younger patient, they may measure up to 2 cm and appear solid. Metastatic lymph nodes appear dense, lack a fatty hilum, and may be matted together. They need not be enlarged. In advanced disease, the borders may become ill defined.[11] Microcalcifications can be seen in metastatic breast carcinoma and secondary to gold therapy for rheumatoid arthritis.[15, 39] Enlargement of axillary lymph nodes can be the result of lymphoma, leukemia, infectious processes, rheumatoid arthritis, sarcoid, and dermatitis, as well as metastatic carcinoma.

SKIN

Skin is normally not more than 2 to 3 mm thick. It is thicker inferomedially.[70, 85] Causes for *bilateral skin thickening* include central venous and lymphatic ob-

struction and anasarca, which can be more pronounced in one breast as the result of positioning (Fig. 10-59). Etiologies for *unilateral skin thickening* are inflammatory breast carcinoma, acute mastitis, radiation therapy, surgery, cellulitis, lymphoma, leukemia, unilateral venous and lymphatic obstruction, extramammary metastatic carcinoma, Mandor's disease (thrombophlebitis), and contralateral spread of a breast carcinoma, which is usually more pronounced medially. *Localized skin thickening* can be secondary to a primary carcinoma, plasma cell mastitis, fat necrosis, surgery, trauma, abscess, extramammary metastatic carcinoma, Mandor's disease, and intradermal masses.[30, 41]

Retraction of the skin is almost always associated with skin thickening. It can be seen as the result of carcinoma, fat necrosis and postsurgical and inflammatory changes. *Nipple retraction* is a common normal variant. However, it can be secondary to plasma cell mastitis, carcinoma, and surgery.

Sebaceous cysts are the most common intradermal lesions and are usually located in the periareolar region or in the lower quadrants. Viewed en face, their mar-

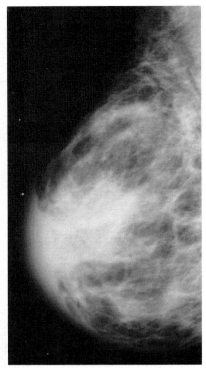

Figure 10–59. Skin thickening. Mediolateral oblique view. Thickening is most pronounced in periareolar area. Secondary to central venous obstruction. Both breasts were involved.

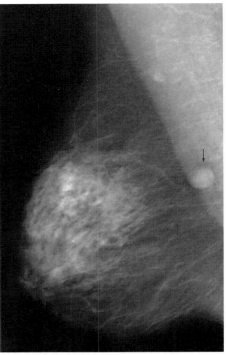

Figure 10–60. Skin lesion. Mediolateral oblique view. A broad rim of lucency surrounds a mole (*arrow*).

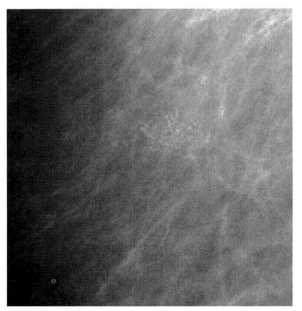

Figure 10–61. Calcification in a wart. Small, irregular calcifications. Beware of skin calcifications mimicking a carcinoma.

gins are distinct unless infected. In tangent, they appear as a localized area of skin thickening.

Skin Lesions. Moles and warts present as sharply defined masses viewed en face. Commonly, a wide rim of radiolucency surrounds them (Fig. 10-60). Warts have a variegated appearance, and may contain calcium (Fig. 10-61). Accessory nipples are less well defined since they have sloping margins. They are more easily diagnosed when viewed in tangent. Placement of a BB on a skin lesion is often helpful in the clarification of its etiology on the mammogram.

Skin Calcifications. Closely approximated, small, round, or ovoid lucencies are frequently seen on the mammogram. These represent normal skin pores (sebaceous glands) (Fig. 10-62). Calcifications associated with sebaceous glands are also commonly seen. Viewed en face, the calcifications appear round, ovoid, or dumbbell shaped. In tangent, they have a discoid configuration. They measure 1 to 1.5 mm, and a lucent center is often identifiable. Their occurrence may be multiple and diffuse or grouped, or they may appear as

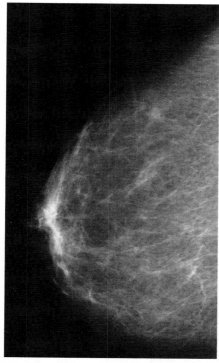

Figure 10–62. Skin pores (sebaceous glands). Craniocaudal view. Scattered small lucencies.

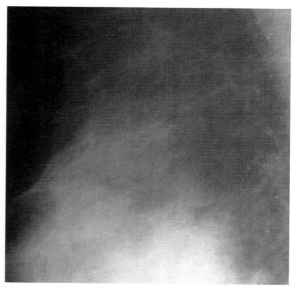

Figure 10–63. Calcified sebaceous glands. Small, round-to-ovoid calcifications with central lucency.

an isolated calcification (Fig. 10-63). Postsurgical changes are another etiology for skin calcifications. These are plaquelike or punctate in appearance. The mammographer must be aware that skin calcifications can masquerade as malignant calcifications (Fig. 10-61).[46] If this possibility is questioned, tangential views should be obtained for clarification. Since deodorants, skin creams, and tattoos all contain metallic salts, they can simulate skin calcifications.[14]

POSTSURGICAL AND IRRADIATED BREAST

Breast conservation is limited by two factors: the presence of only one dominant carcinoma and a satisfactory postoperative cosmetic result. The preoperative mammogram is used to determine the size of the carcinoma, to detect the presence of multifocal carcinoma, and to assess the contralateral breast.[66] A postlumpectomy mammogram should be obtained approximately two weeks after surgery, allowing time for healing of the incision and for a decrease in edema. This mammogram is used as a baseline for future mammograms and to help detect residual tumor. However, the sensitivity in detecting residual tumor is very low.[40] Early postoperative changes include edema of the fibroglandular

tissues and skin. The edema is usually localized to the area of the incision, but may involve the entire breast. Usually it resolves within four weeks; however, the thickening of the skin in the area of the incision may never entirely resolve. Hematomas may be seen in the surgical bed. In addition, lymphoceles can develop as the result of axillary dissection. These usually present as well-defined masses.

The first postradiation mammogram should be obtained at six months, followed by a second six-month study if there are no suspicious findings. Subsequent yearly studies are then obtained unless an earlier mammogram or biopsy is warranted. Radiation therapy causes edema of the entire breast. This is manifested by a generalized increase in density with trabecular and skin thickening.[17, 50] The edema caused by radiation therapy is more extensive and dramatic than that produced by surgery. The changes are greatest at six months after initiation of therapy. Usually most of the changes will have resolved within one year, although findings can persist (Fig. 10-64A and B).

Calcifications are commonly seen in the postsurgical irradiated breast. These include surgical or radiation-induced calcified oil cysts, large linear incisional calcifications, and sutural calcifications that may be linear or knotlike in appearance.[8, 24, 69] Smooth, round calcifications, malignant-appearing calcifications and dermal calcifications that may be punctuate or plaque-like may also develop at the lumpectomy site. Secretory-like calcifications may occur as the result of radiation therapy, but this is uncommon.

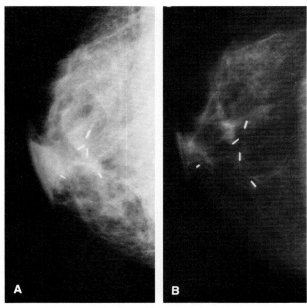

Figure 10–64. Postradiation mammogram. Craniocaudal view at six months (**A**) demonstrates increased density of the parenchyma and thickening of the trabeculae and skin. Surgical clips at surgical site. (**B**) Marked resolution on the craniocaudal view at one year.

The greatest challenge to the radiologist in evaluating the postsurgical and irradiated breast is deciding if the mammographic changes are the result of fat necrosis, architectural distortion, a hematoma, or edema secondary to surgery or radiation therapy, or if they are the result of a recurrent or residual carcinoma.

The mammographic manifestations of a recurrence include the development of malignant-appearing calcifications or a new density, increase in size of a pre-existing density, an inappropriate increase in edema, and an increase in skin thickening.[26, 36, 69, 71, 77] The recurrence rate in the conservatively treated breast is 2%/year for the first 14 years, and it is higher in premenopausal women.[71] Approximately 35% of these carcinomas are only detected by mammography.[77] Also, it should be remembered that the conservatively treated breast and the contralateral breast are at a higher risk for developing another primary carcinoma.

PROCEDURES

Needle localization is performed by the radiologist before surgical biopsy of a nonpalpable lesion. This is accomplished by using a needle through which a spring-hooked wire is inserted and left in place to be used as a guide by the surgeon or by using a straight needle through which methylene blue is injected. To assist the radiologist in localizing the lesion, specialized grid compression paddles have been devised for mammographic units. Mammograms are performed to document the localization. It is important that the biopsy specimens be radiographed to assure that the lesion has been removed. If calcifications are present in the lesion, usually there is no difficulty in determining if the surgeon has resected the area in question. If there are no calcifications associated with the lesion, however, it may not be possible to make this determination. Compression and magnification views may prove helpful in these instances.

Mammographic guided *fine-needle aspiration and large-core biopsy* using stereotaxic techniques are also used in obtaining tissues for histopathology. A 77% sensitivity for fine-needle aspiration has been reported.[29] However, in one series insufficient tissue on fine-needle aspiration occurred in 26% of the cases.[52] Parker and coworkers found large-core biopsy an acceptable option to surgical biopsy.[64]

Galactography is used to evaluate abnormal nipple discharge. The suspected duct is cannulated and a water-soluble agent is injected. Mammograms are then performed. If positive, they may demonstrate a mass or masses within the duct, ductal dilatation, or irregularity of the wall of the duct. It cannot be determined from the galactogram if the findings represent a benign or malignant process. Galactography is not performed in most instances of pathologic nipple discharge since the surgeon is usually able to resect the abnormal duct.

Ultrasound can be used to prove the presence of a cyst if puncture and aspirations are not feasible. Some mammographers rely on ultrasound to evaluate for the presence of an intraluminal mass, but others prefer to inject an aqueous contrast medium and air for a *double contrast study*. Ultrasound cannot reliably differentiate malignant and benign solid masses.

REFERENCES AND SELECTED READINGS

1. ABRAMS HL, ED: Vascular and Interventional Radiology, Volume 1, 3rd ed. Little Brown and Company, Boston, 1983

2. ACHRAM M, ISSA S, RIZK G: Osteogenic sarcoma of the breast: Some radiological aspects. Br J Radiol 58:264, 1985

3. ADLER DD, HELVIE MA, OBERMAN, ET AL: Radial scle-

rosing lesion of the breast: Mammographic features. Radiology 176:737, 1990

4. ADLER DD, HELVIE MA, IKEDA DM: Perspective, nonpalpable, probably benign breast lesions: Follow-up strategies after initial detection on mammography. Am J Roentgenol 155:1195, 1990

5. ADLER DD, REBNER M, PENNES DR: Accessory breast tissue in the axilla: Mammographic appearance. Radiology 163:709, 1987

6. AZZOPARDI JG: Problems in Breast Pathology. Philadelphia, W. B. Saunders, 1979

7. BASSETT LW, GOLD RH, CORE HC: Mammographic spectrum of traumatic fat necrosis: The fallibility of "pathognomonic" signs of carcinoma. Am J Roentgenol 130:119, 1978

8. BASSETT LW, GOLD RH, MIRRA JM: Non-neoplastic breast calcifications in lipid cysts: Development after excision and primary irradiation. Am J Roentgenol 138:335, 1982

9. BERKOWITZ JE, GATEWOOD OMB, GOLDBLUM LE, ET AL: Hormonal replacement therapy: Mammographic manifestations. Radiology 174:199, 1990

10. BERQUIST TH: MRI of the Musculoskeletal System, 2nd ed. New York, Raven Press, 1990

11. BJURSTAM N: The radiographic appearance of normal and metastatic axillary lymph nodes. Recent Results Cancer Res 90:49, 1984

12. BOHMAN LG, BASSETT LW, GOLD RH, ET AL: Breast metastases from extramammary malignancies. Radiology 144:309, 1982

13. BRENNER RJ, SICKLES EA: Acceptability of periodic follow-up as an alternative to biopsy for mammographically detected lesions interpreted as probably benign. Radiology 171:645, 1989

14. BROWN RC, ZUEHLKE RL, EHRHARDT JC, ET AL: Tattoos simulating calcifications on xerographs of the breast. Radiology 138:583, 1981

15. BRUWER A, NELSON GW, SPARK RP: Punctate intranodal gold deposits simulating microcalcifications on mammograms. Radiology 163:87, 1987

16. BUCK JL: Fat-containing soft-tissue masses of the extremities. From the Archives of the AFIP. Radiographics 11:81, 1991

17. BUCKLEY JH, ROEBUCK EJ: Mammographic changes following radiotherapy. Br J Radiol 59:337, 1986

18. CEDERLUND CG, GUSTAVSSON S, LINELL F, ET AL: Fibromatosis of breast mimicking carcinoma at mammography. Br J Radiol 57:98, 1984

19. CLARKE E, SWISCHUK LE, HAYDEN CK: Tumoral calcinosis, diaphysitis, and hyperphosphatemia. Radiology 151:643, 1984

20. COLE-BEUGLET C, SARIANO R, KUTZ AB, ET AL: Ultrasound, x-ray mammography, and histopathology of cystosarcoma phylloides. Radiology 146:481, 1983

21. CONSENSUS MEETING (CONVENED BY THE CANCER COMMITTEE OF THE COLLEGE OF AMERICAN PATHOLOGISTS): Is

"Fibrocystic disease" of the breast precancerous? Arch Pathol Lab Med 110:171, 1986

22. CROTHERS JG, BUTLER NF, FORTT RW, ET AL: Fibroadenolipoma of the breast. Br J Radiol 58:191, 1985

23. D'ORSI CJ, FELDHAUS L, SONNENFELD M: Unusual lesions of the breast. Radiologic Clinics of North American 21:67, 1983

24. DAVIS SP, STOMPER PC, WEIDNER N, ET AL: Suture calcification mimicking recurrence in the irradiated breast: A potential pitfall in mammographic evaluation. Radiology 172:247, 1989

25. DEMAS BE, HEELAN RT, LANE J, ET AL: Soft tissue sarcomas of the extremities: Comparison of MR and CT in determining the extent of disease. Am J Roentgenol 150:615, 1988

26. DERSHAW DD, MCCORMICK B, COX L, ET AL: Differentiation of benign and malignant local tumor recurrence after lumpectomy. Am J Roentgenol 155:35, 1990

27. EPSTEIN EE: Fibrosarcoma of the breast: A case report. South Afr Med J 57:288, 1980

28. EVERS K, TROUPIN RH: Pictorial essay. Lipid cyst: classic and atypical appearances. Am J Roentgenol 157:271, 1991

29. FAJARDO LL, DAVIS JR, WIENS JL, ET AL: Mammography-guided sterotactic fine-needle aspiration cytology of nonpalpable breast lesions: Prospective comparison with surgical biopsy results. Am J Roentgenol 155:977, 1990

30. GOLD RH, MONTGOMERY CK, MINAGI H, ET AL: The significance of mammary skin thickening in disorders other than primary carcinoma: A roentgenologic-pathologic correlation. Am J Roentgenol 112:613, 1971

31. GOMEZ A, MATA JM, DONOSO L, ET AL: Galactocele: Three distinctive radiographic appearances. Radiology 158:43, 1986

32. GORDON LF, ARGER PH, DALINKA MK, ET AL: Computed tomography in soft tissue calcification layering. J Comput Assist Tomogr 8:71, 1984

33. GRANT EG, HOLT RW, CHUN B, ET AL: Angiosarcoma of the breast: Sonographic, xeromammographic and pathologic appearance. Am J Roentgenol 141:691, 1983

34. GUMP FE, STERSCHEIN MJ, WOLFF M: Fibromatosis of the breast. Surg Gynecol Obstet 153:57, 1981

35. HALL FM, COCKEN WP, HAYES CW: Calcific tendinitis of the longus coli: Diagnosis by CT. Am J Roentgenol 147:742, 1986

36. HASSELL PR, OLIVOLTO IA, MUELLER HA, ET AL: Early breast cancer: Detection of recurrence after conservative and radiation therapy. Radiology 176:731, 1990

37. HAYES CW, CONWAY WF: Calcium hydroxyapatite deposition disease. Radiographics 10:1031, 1990

38. HELVIE MA, ADLER DD, REBNER M, ET AL: Breast hamartomas: Variable mammographic appearance. Radiology 170:417, 1989

39. HELVIE MA, REBNER M, SICKLES EA, ET AL: Calcifications in metastatic breast carcinoma in axillary lymph nodes. Am J Roentgenol 151:921, 1988

40. HOMER MJ, SCHMIDT-ULLRICH R, SAFAII H, ET AL: Residual breast carcinoma after biopsy: Role of mammography in evaluation. Radiology 170:75, 1989

41. HOMER MJ: Mammary skin thickening. Contemp Diagn Radiol 4:1, 1981

42. HOMER MJ: Nonpalpable mammographic abnormalities: Timing the follow-up studies. Am J Roentgenol 136:923, 1981

43. HOMER MJ: Mammographic Interpretation: A Practical Approach. New York, McGraw-Hill, Inc., 1991

44. JACKSON VP, DINES KA, BASSETT LW, ET AL: Diagnostic importance of the radiographic density of noncalcified breast masses: Analysis of 91 lesions. Am J Roentgenol 157:25, 1991

45. KOPANS DB, SWANN CA, WHITE G, ET AL: Asymmetric breast tissue. Radiology 171:639, 1989

46. KOPANS DB, MEYER JE, HOMER MJ, ET AL: Dermal deposits mistaken for breast calcifications. Radiology 149:592, 1983

47. KOPANS DB: Breast Imaging. Philadelphia, J.B. Lippincott Company, 1989

48. KRANSDORF MJ, JELINEK JS, MOSER RP, JR, ET AL: Soft-tissue masses: Diagnosis using MR imaging. Am J Roentgenol 153:541, 1989

49. KUSHNER LN: Hodgkin's disease simulating inflammatory breast carcinoma on mammography. Radiology 92:350, 1969

50. LIBSHITZ HI, MONTAGUE ED, PAULUS DD: Skin thickness in the therapeutically irradiated breast. Am J Roentgenol 130:345, 1978

51. LINDFORS KK, KOPANS DB, McCARTHY KA, ET AL: Breast cancer metastasis to intramammary lymph nodes. Am J Roentgenol 146:133, 1986

52. LOFGREN M, ANDERSSON I, LINDHOLM K: Sterotactic fine-needle aspiration for cytologic diagnosis of nonpalpable breast lesions. Am J Roentgenol 154:1191, 1990

53. MARSTELLER LP, dePAREDES ES: Well defined masses in the breast. RadioGraphics 9:13, 1989

54. MARTINEZ S, VOGLER JB III, HARRELSON JM, LYLES KW: Imaging of tumoral calcinosis: New observations. Radiology 174:215, 1990

55. McCREA ES, JOHNSTON C, HANEY PJ: Metastases to the breast. Am J Roentgenol 141:685, 1983

56. MENDELSON EB, HARRIS KM, DOSHI N, ET AL: Infiltrating lobular carcinoma: Mammographic patterns with pathologic correlation. Am J Roentgenol 153:265, 1989

57. MEYER JE, KOPANS DB, LAWRENCE WD: Normal intramammary lymph nodes presenting as occult breast masses. Breast 40:30, 1982

58. MEYER JE, KOPANS DB, LONG JC: Mammographic appearance of lymphoma of the breast. Radiology 135:31, 1974

59. MILLIS RR: Atlas of Breast Pathology. Lancaster, England, MTP Press Limited, 1984

60. MILLIS RR, ATKINSON MK, TONGE KA: The xerographic appearances of some uncommon malignant mammary neoplasms. Clin Radiol 27:463, 1976

61. MITNICK JS, VAZQUEZ MF, HARRIS NM, ET AL: Invasive papillary carcinoma of the breast: Mammographic appearance. Radiology 177:803, 1990

62. MITNICK JS, ROSES DF, HARRIS MN, ET AL: Circumscribed intraductal carcinoma of the breast. Radiology 170:423, 1989

63. MONCADO R, COOPER RA, GARCES M, ET AL: Calcified metastases from malignant ovarian neoplasm. Radiology 113:31, 1974

64. PARKER SH, LOVIN JD, JOBE WE, ET AL: Nonpalpable breast lesions: Sterotactic automated large-core biopsies. Radiology 180:403, 1991

65. PAULUS DD: Lymphoma of the breast. Radiologic Clinics of North America 28:833, 1990

66. PAULUS DD: Conservative treatment of breast cancer: Mammography in patient selection and follow-up. Am J Roentgenol 143:483, 1984

67. PETASNICK JP, TURNER DA, CHARTERS RJ, ET AL: Soft-tissue masses of the locomotor system: Comparison of MR imaging with CT. Radiology 160:125, 1986

68. PETERS ME, VOEGELI DR, SCANLAN KA, (EDS.) Breast Imaging. New York, Churchill Livingstone, 1989

69. PETERS ME, FAGERHOLM MI, SCANLAN KA, ET AL: Mammographic evaluation of the postsurgical and irradiated breast. RadioGraphics 8:873, 1988

70. POPE TL, READ ME, MEDSKER T, ET AL: Breast skin thickness: Normal range and causes of thickening shown on film-screen mammography. J Can Assoc Radiol 35:365, 1984

71. REBNER M, PENNES DR, ADLER DD, ET AL: Breast microcalcifications after lumpectomy and radiation therapy. Radiology 170:691, 1989

72. RESNICK D: Calcium hydroxyapatite crystal deposition disease. In: Resnick D, Niawayama G, eds. Diagnosis of bone and joint disorders, 2nd ed. Philadelphia, W.B. Saunders, 1988

73. SCHEIDER JA: Invasive papillary breast carcinoma: Mammographic and sonographic appearance. Radiology 171:377–379, 1989

74. SICKLES EA: Periodic mammographic follow-up of probably benign lesions: Results in 3,184 consecutive cases. Radiology 179:463, 1991

75. SICKLES EA, HERZOG KA: Intramammary scar tissue: A mimic of the mammographic appearance of a carcinoma. Am J Roentgenol 135:349, 1980

76. SICKLES EA, HERZOG KA: Mammography of the postsurgical breast. Am J Roentgenol 136:585, 1981

77. STOMPER PC, RECHT A, BERENBERG AL, ET AL: Mammographic detection of recurrent cancer in the irradiated breast. Am J Roentgenol 148:39, 1987

78. STOMPER PC, VanVOORHIS BJ, RAVNIKER VA, ET AL: Mammographic changes associated with postmenopausal hormone replacement therapy: A longitudinal study. Radiology 174:487, 1990

79. STRASSER W, HEIM K, MULLER E, ET AL: Phylloides tumor: Findings on mammography, sonography and aspiration cytology in 10 cases. Am J Roentgenol 157:715, 1991

80. SUNDARAM M, MCGUIRE MH, HERBOID DR: Magnetic resonance imaging of soft tissue masses: An evaluation of fifty-three histologically proven tumors. Magn Reson Imaging 6:237, 1988

81. SWANN CA, KOPANS DB, KOERNER FC, ET AL: The halo sign and malignant breast lesions. Am J Roentgenol 149:1145, 1987

82. TOOMBS BD, KALISHER L: Metastatic disease to the breast: Clinical, pathologic, and radiographic features. Am J Roentgenol 129:679, 1977

83. WATT AC, HAGGAR AM, KRASICKY GA: Extraosseous osteogenic sarcoma of the breast: Mammographic and pathologic findings. Radiology 150:34, 1984

84. WELLINGS SR, WOLFE JN: Correlative studies of the histological and radiographic appearance of the breast parenchyma. Radiology 129:299, 1978

85. WILLSON SA, ADAM EJ, TUCKER AK: Patterns of breast skin thickness in normal mammograms. Clin Radiol 33:691, 1982

The Brain
and Spinal Cord

Paul and Juhl's Essentials of Radiologic Imaging,
Sixth Edition, edited by John H. Juhl and
Andrew B. Crummy. J.B. Lippincott Company,
Philadelphia, © 1993.

CHAPTER *11*

Intracranial Diseases

Charles M. Strother

INTRODUCTION

Over the past five years, advances in magnetic resonance imaging (MRI) have revolutionized the ability to visualize the brain and its coverings. Exceptional contrast resolution, multiplanar capability, and the lack of known harmful effects combine to make MRI, in the majority of circumstances, the preferred technique for the initial diagnostic evaluation of patients with neurologic disease. Ongoing developments in magnetic resonance techniques that link the acquisition of physiologic and biochemical information to the display of morphology will soon further enhance the value of this technique as a diagnostic method. In spite of these advantages, however, computed tomography (CT) will continue to be the most widely applied tool for diagnostic imaging of the brain because of its widespread availability, accuracy, speed, and the easy ability to evaluate uncooperative or critically ill patients.

Skull radiography no longer has any meaningful role in the diagnostic evaluation of patients suspected of having neurologic disease. The technique is insensitive and nonspecific. It is also redundant, because even when abnormalities are seen on skull radiographs it is rare that the findings provide sufficient information on which to base patient management.[70] Even though skull radiography no longer plays a role in clinical practice, knowledge of skull anatomy is essential for proper interpretation of CT and magnetic resonance scans of the brain. This knowledge may be facilitated through the study of multiple projections of skull radiographs, which provides a means for correlating the spatial relationships of structures seen on cross-sectional images. For a complete discussion of the changes that occur in

the skull as a result of intracranial disease, see Yock[75] and Newton and Potts.[53]

THE CHOICE OF A DIAGNOSTIC TECHNIQUE

When available, MRI is the technique of choice for the initial diagnostic evaluation of the great majority of patients with neurologic disease. Important exceptions where CT remains the technique of choice for initial examination are 1) evaluation of patients after acute trauma; 2) evaluation of patients suspected of having an acute subarachnoid or parenchymal hemorrhage; and, 3) evaluation of patients with diseases affecting primarily the skull base or calvarium.

The array of techniques available with which to perform an MRI examination of the brain is too large and complex for discussion in this chapter. If one is to achieve optimal results from the examination, however, each scan should be tailored to maximize information that can be brought to bear on a particular case. Careful consideration must be given to the choice of pulse sequences and timing parameters used for each study, because depending on factors such as the age of the patient and the type of pathology suspected greatly influences the appearance of the images obtained. One of the great advantages of MRI over other imaging techniques is its ability to depict changes in chemical makeup of tissue. To maximize information obtained from a particular examination, one must not only have some understanding of the changes occurring with various disease states but also understand how images obtained from these altered tissues are affected by variation in MRI pulse sequences.[2] Generally, every initial examination of the brain should include as a minimum one set of T1, proton density, and T2-weighted images.

With modern devices there are also many different ways to perform a CT scan, and as with MRI, each scan should be tailored to optimize information that may influence a particular case. Proper evaluation of some lesions, for example, requires the use of thin sections and special reconstruction algorithms and variation in the plane of section in which the scan is taken.

INTRACRANIAL CALCIFICATION

Certain structures within the skull are found with considerable frequency to contain calcium or other mineral deposits. Calcification of the dura and choroid plexus and mineralization of basal ganglia structures in the elderly are without known clinical significance. In other instances the presence of these deposits provides a valuable clue to the presence of an abnormality and its etiology. CT is the most sensitive technique for the recognition of intracranial calcifications. MRI is not a sensitive technique for the detection of calcification, nor does it allow calcifications to be distinguished from air, rapidly flowing blood, or hemosiderin. An outline listing the major causes of normal and abnormal intracranial calcification is found in Table 11-1.

The Pineal Gland

The pineal gland, also known as the pineal body, contains sufficient calcium to be visible radiographically on from 33% to 76% of adult skull x-rays. Calcification in the gland is seen even more frequently on CT scans. The location of the pineal gland adjacent to the Great Vein of Galen and the similarity of signal intensities caused by most pineal calcifications and flowing blood make recognition of pineal calcifications difficult with MRI. Because, however, MRI provides a means to view the gland directly in multiple planes, this poses no limitation for the technique.

Visualization of calcification in the pineal on CT scans is rare in individuals younger than 6 years of age, in which case its presence suggests a neoplasm.[76] Pineal calcification is usually in the form of a cluster of amorphous, irregular densities, but may be solitary. The size of the calcification ranges from 10 or 12 mm in the greatest diameter, but usually is between 3 and 5 mm. When calcifications greater than 1 cm in diameter are observed, the question of an abnormality such as a pinealoma or arteriovenous malformation should be raised.

Table 11–1. Causes of Intracranial Calcification and Mineralization

I. Physiologic sites
  A. Pineal gland
  B. Habenular commissure
  C. Choroid plexus
  D. Dura
  E. Pacchionian bodies
  F. Basal ganglia and dentate nucleus
II. Abnormal causes
  A. Traumatic lesions
    1. Subdural hematoma
    2. Epidural hematoma
    3. Intracerebral hematoma
  B. Parasitic lesions
    1. Cysticercosis
    2. Trichinosis
    3. Toxoplasmosis
    4. Echinococcosis
  C. Vascular lesions
    1. Arteriosclerosis
    2. Aneurysms
    3. Arteriovenous malformations
    4. Capillary and venous angiomas (Sturge-Weber syndrome)
  D. Tuberous sclerosis
  E. Inflammatory and other lesions
    1. Tuberculosis
    2. Viral (cytomegalic inclusion disease)
    3. Other infections
      a. Old abscesses
      b. Nontuberculous granulomas
      c. Torulosis
  F. Degenerative and atrophic lesions
    1. Congenital atrophy or hypoplasia (lissencephaly)
  G. Symmetric calcification of basal ganglia
    1. Hypoparathyroidism
    2. Pseudohypoparathyroidism
  H. Neoplasms
    1. Glioma
    2. Craniopharyngioma
    3. Dermoid, teratoma, and epidermoid
    4. Meningioma
    5. Lipoma
    6. Pituitary adenoma (rarely)
    7. Metastic tumors (rarely except for primary osseous tumors)
  I. Toxicosis
    1. Hypervitaminosis D
    2. Idiopathic hypercalcemia
  J. Other causes
    1. Lead poisoning
    2. Fahr's disease
    3. Cockayne's disease (progeria)

The Choroid Plexus

The choroid plexus is formed as the result of invagination of the ependyma into the cavities of the ventricular system. Its major function is the elaboration of cerebrospinal fluid. The choroid plexus of the two lateral ventricles and third ventricle is continuous; that of the fourth ventricle is separate. In the lateral ventricles the choroid plexus extends posteriorly from the interventricular foramen along the ventricular floor, passing around the atrium to reach the temporal horn. The choroid plexus of each lateral ventricle is continuous at the interventricular foramen with that of the third ventricle. Choroid plexus in the third ventricle extends posteriorly from the interventricular foramen along the roof of the ventricle to reach the suprapineal recess. In the fourth ventricle the choroid plexus has the shape of a "T"; the vertical limb extends from near Magendie's foramen to the fastigium, and the two horizontal segments pass laterally along each lateral recess, where they reach Luschka's foramina and project into the subarachnoid space of the cerebello-pontine angle cisterns. The glomus of the choroid plexus is a localized enlargement found along the posterior part of the floor of the ventricle at or in front of the atrium. Calcification of portions of the choroid plexus sufficient to allow visualization on CT scans occurs in a high percentage of individuals and is frequently present in children. Calcification is most frequently seen at the glomera, but may be present at any site.

The importance of choroid plexus calcification is only that one be aware of the normal distribution of the choroid plexus so that physiologic calcification is not mistaken for an abnormality. The choroid plexus is usually enhanced, sometimes quite markedly, on both CT scans and MRI scans performed after administration of intravenous contrast medium. Like calcification, this enhancement should not be mistaken for an abnormality. Most calcifications on MRI are seen as a signal void. Not uncommonly, however, the combinations of calcium salts that occur in the choroid plexus result in a hyperintense signal intensity.[12] The position of the choroid plexus within the lateral ventricles is essentially symmetrical; thus, asymmetry should alert one to the possibility of a mass lesion.

Calcifications of the Dura

Plaque like areas of calcification are common in the dura, particularly in the falx, along the margins of the superior sagittal sinus, and along both the free and attached edges of the tentorium. These calcifications are often quite prominent. They tend to be larger and occur more frequently anteriorly in the falx than elsewhere. Heavy calcification of the falx, and less fre-

quently of the tentorium, is reported as a component of the basal cell nevus syndrome. Otherwise, no significance can be attached to the finding of these plaques.

Because calcification is an important sign of many lesions that occur in the juxtasellar area, it is particularly important that one be aware of the relationships of the dura in this region so that physiologic calcification is not interpreted as a sign of pathology. Calcification is frequent in the free edges of the tentorium, posterior to the sella in the so-called petroclinoid ligaments. These are formed by the margins of the tentorium as it extends from the petrous ridges of the temporal bones to the posterior clinoid processes of the dorsum sellae. The calcifications are seen as spur-like projections extending posteriorly and downward from the dorsum. In older individuals, calcification is often seen in the cavernous segments of the internal carotid arteries.

The Sella Turcica

In the past, careful scrutiny of the sella turcica on plain films of the skull often provided direct evidence of the presence of an abnormality of the pituitary gland or indirect evidence of a more remote abnormality. It has been demonstrated that the size and shape of the sella turcica have no consistent relationship to abnormalities of the pituitary gland.[71] The pituitary gland as well as those remote abnormalities (i.e., aneurysms or tumors), that affect the size or shape of the sella turcica are seen more directly on CT or MRI scans. Plain radiographs of the sella turcica are thus no longer indicated.

Hyperostosis Frontalis Interna

Hyperostosis frontalis interna is a peculiar overgrowth of bone developing on the inner table of the frontal bone. The hyperostosis usually is bilateral and symmetrical and is found chiefly in females over the age of five. The bony proliferation is confined to the internal surface of the inner table; the diploe and external table are not affected. The overgrowth of bone forms a dense, irregular thickening that surrounds the venous sinuses but does not obliterate them. The extent of the thickening varies considerably, but the hyperostosis may measure 1 cm or more in thickness. The process spreads upward and laterally from the midline of the frontal area for a variable distance. The external limits may be abrupt, or the process may fade gradually into bone of normal thickness. While usually limited to the frontal area, occasionally a process of this nature extends into the parietal bones and over the orbital roofs. Hyperostosis calvariae diffusa, a variant of hyperostosis frontalis interna may manifest a more diffuse thickening of the vault, involving both tables with a poorly defined or absent diploe.

The etiology of hyperostosis frontalis interna is not known. Generally, especially in females, it is not thought to be of clinical significance. Some, however, have considered it part of an endocrine dysfunction and have variously called it metabolic craniopathy, Morgagni's syndrome, and Stewart–Morel syndrome. On both CT and MRI, it appears as irregular cortical thickening in the frontal area, sparing the areas occupied by the superior sagittal sinus and venous channels. It is important to distinguish the changes of hyperostosis frontalis interna from the bony hypertrophy that results from meningioma and fibrous dysplasia or from the generalized calvarial thickening that can be seen in the presence of atrophic lesions or chronic dilantin ingestion. Except for the rare *en plaque* meningioma, there is generally little problem in making this distinction.

Intracranial Tumors

Calcification occurs commonly in many intracranial diseases and its presence is often an important indication of underlying pathology. There is, however, with few exceptions, little diagnostic specificity in the type of calcification occurring as the result of intracranial pathology. In general, one obtains much more indication of the etiology of abnormal calcification from a careful analysis of its location and the characteristics of adjacent parenchyma (i.e. CT density or MRI signal intensities, the presence or absence of mass effect, or enhancement), than from attempting to characterize the features of the calcifications. Calcifications may mimic enhancement or hemorrhage on CT scans and air or rapidly flowing blood on MRI examinations; however, a careful analysis of CT density levels, anatomic location, and a comparison of enhanced and non-enhanced scans usually allows accurate recognition of most calcifications.

SPECIAL PROCEDURES

Computed Tomography and Magnetic Resonance Imaging

Since the last edition of this book, improvements in the capabilities of MRI coupled with widespread dissemination of MRI devices have made MRI, in most instances, the technique of choice for the initial diagnostic imaging evaluation of the brain and its coverings. Recent advances in MRI angiography now also permit this technique to be, in many instances, a substitute for the traditional angiographic examination. CT, however, because of its speed, availability, and accuracy, remains an important and extremely useful diagnostic

tool. CT will continue to be a mainstay for the diagnostic imaging of the brain.

With both CT and MRI, there are many different ways to perform an examination of the brain, and, for best results, each study should be tailored to optimize the information necessary to solve a particular diagnostic problem. Proper evaluation of some lesions requires the use of thin sections and special reconstruction algorithms or pulse and timing sequences; evaluation of others requires performance of examinations both with and without intravenous contrast medium. Finally, the ideal plane of section in which to view the area of concern varies considerably depending on the suspected location of the abnormality. While a complete discussion of factors such as these is beyond the scope of this text, a few general comments are appropriate.

The characteristics of the MR image depend upon multiple variables involving both the tissue being imaged and the pulse/timing sequence used to obtain the image. Continued innovations and improvements in available techniques and applications make it unrealistic in this discussion to report systematically these aspects of MRI. For a good and thorough discussion of these variables, their effect on MR images, and ways in which they may be manipulated so as to optimize information obtained, refer to Chapter 2 and Atlas.[2] In general, the use of a short TR/short TE sequence and long TR/short and long TE pulse sequence provides a set of images that displays adequately the T1, proton density, and T2 characteristics of the tissue being imaged (Fig. 11-1).

The rationale for the use of intravenous contrast medium in CT scanning of the brain is two-fold. First, administration of intravenous contrast medium increases the sensitivity of the technique for detection of active areas of abnormality in the blood–brain barrier (BBB). Second, CT scans done after administration of intravenous contrast medium allow improved definition of both vascular and dural structures (Fig. 11-2). The use of paramagnetic intravenous contrast medium in conjunction with MR examinations also increases the sensitivity of the technique for detection of some disease processes. Like intravenous iodine-containing contrast media, the paramagnetic contrast medium used in MRI accumulates in areas of BBB disruption, and, because of its T-1 shortening effect, results in the appearance of enhancement (i.e., increased signal intensity). Unlike CT, widespread dural enhancement is not a normal feature of contrast enhanced MR examinations (Fig. 11-3).

While many lesions are seen "better" following infusion of intravenous contrast medium, the added information is often trivial while the added cost may be quite significant. Frequently, the added cost of enhanced scans outweighs their advantages. In general,

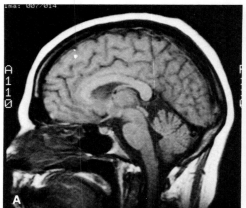
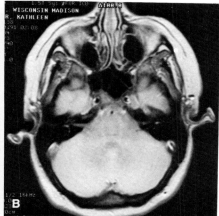
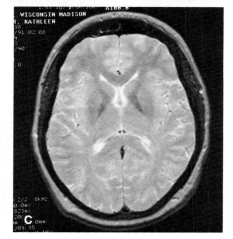

Figure 11–1. Normal MRI. (**A**) Short TR/TE (T1-weighted) sequence. (**B**) Long TR/short TE (proton-density weighted) sequence and (**C**) long TR/long TE (T2-weighted) sequence. These images illustrate well the differences in signal intensities of cerebrospinal fluid, gray matter, and white matter as seen on these commonly used pulse sequences.

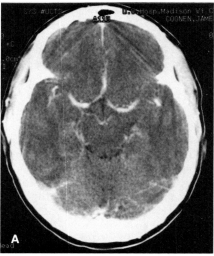
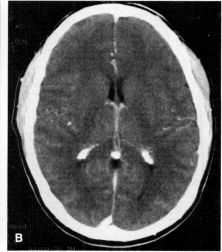

Figure 11–2. Normal CT scan performed (**A** and **B**) following the intravenous administration of iodinated contrast medium. Arterial and venous structures at the base of the brain are prominent in these images. There is also enhancement of the falx cerebri and choroid plexus of the lateral ventricles.

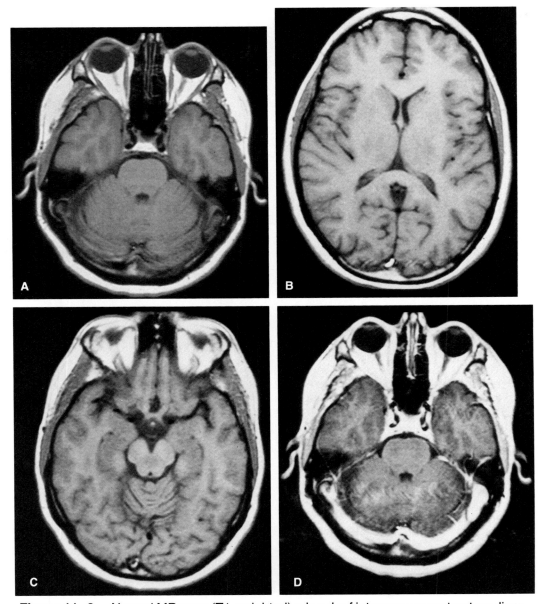

Figure 11–3. Normal MR scan (T1-weighted) a,b,c,d,e,f intravenous contrast medium.

intravenous contrast media should not be used in association with either CT or MRI scans done for evaluation of congenital malformations, dementia, trauma, hydrocephalus, or suspected brain infarction. Contrast administration is indicated in evaluation of many but not all patients with other vascular abnormalities such as suspected aneurysm or arteriovenous malformations, as well as for studies performed because of suspected neoplasms, and infectious or inflammatory disorders. The routine use of a precontrast or nonenhanced CT

scans before an enhanced scan has, in my experience, not been useful and is recommended only for the evaluation of lesions thought to have hemorrhagic or calcified components.

The usual dosage for intravenous contrast medium results in the administration of 42 grams of iodine, which can be given as an intravenous (IV) drip or as an IV bolus depending on the clinical situation.[37]

Intrathecal contrast media, either air or an appropriate water-soluble medium, can also be used to advan-

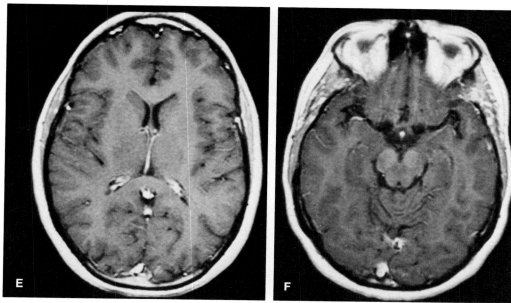

Figure 11–3. *(Continued)*

tage in association with CT scanning. Scans performed shortly after the injection of low doses of water-soluble contrast medium (up to 5 cc of a 190 mg I/cc concentration) into the lumbar subarachnoid space provide excellent depiction of the cisternal spaces about the brain. This technique is only indicated in circumstances when an MR examination cannot be performed or when information about (CSF) flow patterns and the presence or absence of communication between various CSF-containing spaces is required (Fig. 11-4).[14] Small volumes of subarachnoid air may also be used effectively as a contrast medium in conjunction with CT scans (Fig. 11-5).[58] It is noteworthy, however, that with very few exceptions the natural contrast provided by the CSF on MRI examinations has eliminated the need for both air and positive subarachnoid contrast medium in conjunction with CT scans.

ANGIOGRAPHY

Angiography remains an important tool in neuroradiology; however, as is the case with plain skull films and more recently with CT, many of the indications for cerebral angiography have been eliminated because of the information provided by MRI and MR angiography. Over the last decade, cerebral angiography has evolved from a technique used largely to detect the presence of structural lesions to one that is performed primarily only to add specificity to ambiguous CT findings or to assist in the planning of neurosurgical or interventional radiologic procedures. In the future,

many of these indications will be further reduced because of the capabilities of MR angiography.

The primary indication for cerebral angiography is for the evaluation of patients with vascular disease of all types (atherosclerosis, aneurysms, arteriovenous malformations and fistulas, arteritis and posttraumatic vascular lesions), either intra- or extracranial. Only occasionally is angiography required as part of the diagnostic assessment of neoplasms or other neurologic diseases. Current capabilities of MRI angiography make it quite suitable in many instances as a screening examination for both intracranial and extracranial diseases that involve primarily the large vascular structures of the neck, skull base, or dural coverings.

Conventional film–screen angiography is performed by rapidly injecting an iodine-containing contrast medium into one of the arteries supplying the brain or its coverings and then obtaining a series of roentgenograms in rapid sequence. The site of injection, the volume of contrast medium used, and the filming sequence employed all depend on the specific problem under evaluation. Almost all conventional cerebral angiography is now performed with the Seldinger technique, in which a catheter is inserted percutaneously into one of the femoral arteries and then under fluoroscopic control is positioned at an appropriate site. Direct carotid puncture or brachial artery injections are rarely required or indicated. Biplane filming, magnification, and subtraction techniques are considered routine parts of conventional angiography. The risks of conventional angiography conducted by experienced

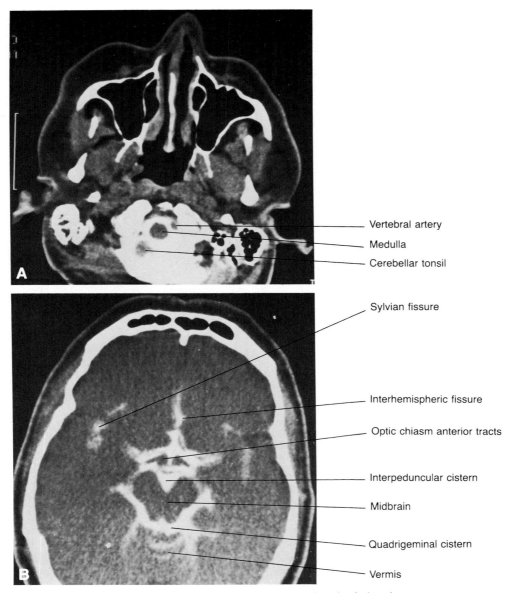

Figure 11–4. (**A**) Axial computed tomogram at level of the foramen magnum. Water-soluble contrast medium in the subarachnoid space outlines the margins of the vertebral arteries, cerebellar tonsils, and the medulla. (**B**) Axial computed tomogram at midbrain level. Water-soluble contrast medium opacifies the subarachnoid space and allows clear definition of the midbrain and adjacent structures.

personnel are small but significant in that they include stroke and damage to the site of arterial puncture. The age and general medical condition of the patient are important factors that influence the magnitude of these risks.

The application of digital electronic techniques to

angiographic equipment has eliminated much of the need for film–screen techniques in neuroangiography. Digital subtraction techniques allow one to perform angiography following either an intravenous or an intraarterial injection of contrast medium at a smaller volume and concentration than would be possible if

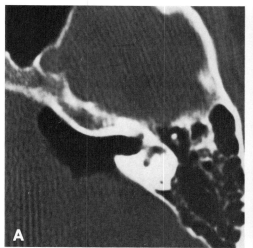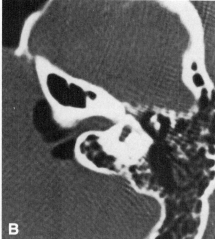

Figure 11–5. **(A)** Axial air-contrast computed tomogram at level of the internal auditory canal. Air fills both the cerebellopontine angle cistern and the internal auditory canal. **(B)** Axial air-contrast computed tomogram at level of the internal canal. The neurovascular bundle of the seventh and eight cranial nerves is seen crossing the cerebellopontine angle cistern. Air entered and almost filled the canal at a slightly higher level.

film–screen techniques were employed. Intraarterial digital subtraction angiography allows procedures to be carried out in less time and at less expense than with conventional methods, with, generally, an insignificant loss of spatial resolution.

SPECIFIC DISEASE STATES

In this discussion of specific disease states the findings on CT and MRI examinations are emphasized. When pertinent, angiographic findings are also presented.

NEOPLASMS

The term "brain tumor," as used here, includes those neoplasms that occur within the brain parenchyma, those that arise from the meninges or cranial nerves, and those that originate from adjacent structures such as the skull or pituitary gland. These lesions have been classified by a variety of methods, their anatomic location and cell origin being the basis of the most common classification. Precise anatomic localization of an intracranial neoplasm is of fundamental importance in that through use of this information, one has the best hope of being specific about the diagnosis, and, thus, the prognosis of the lesion. The wide availability of CT has made this technique the procedure of choice for the initial evaluation of patients suspected of having a brain

tumor. Because of its increased contrast sensitivity and multiplanar capabilities, MRI is rapidly eroding the role of CT in this regard.

There is no routine CT method that optimizes the capabilities of the technique for detection of all brain tumors. If properly used CT is, however, quite sensitive and can detect the great majority of these lesions; it can also provide information that in many instances allows accurate prediction of the tumor's origin. MRI is more sensitive than CT for the detection of neoplasms and also allows more precise localization of their anatomic extent. When available, MRI is the technique of choice for initial diagnostic evaluation of such patients. Unless contraindicated, the administration of intravenous contrast medium is indicated for both CT and MR scans performed for study of suspected brain tumor. Noncontrast CT scans are not routinely required. MRI examinations are best performed both with and without intravenous contrast administration.

Some tumors of the central nervous system (CNS) tend to have a predilection for certain anatomic sites while others occur throughout the intracranial space. It is thus useful to identify a lesion's location and to define whether it is within (intraaxial) or outside (extraaxial) the brain. Nearly 70% of tumors in adults are supratentorial, while the reverse is the case in children. The most common primary tumors of the adult are astrocytomas and glioblastomas; in children, at least half of all such lesions are astrocytomas of the cerebellum or brain stem. In general an extraaxial location of a neoplasm implies a more favorable prognosis than does an intraparenchymal location.[63] The incidence of various intracranial tumors as listed by Potts is as follows: gliomas, 43%; meningiomas, 15%; pituitary adenomas, 13%; acoustic neuromas, 6.5%; congenital tumors, 4%; blood vessel tumors, 3%; and miscellaneous, 9%. These figures vary somewhat depending upon the source (i.e., surgical versus autopsy series).

SUPRATENTORIAL TUMORS

Gliomas

Glioblastoma Multiforme. Glioblastoma multiforme is an invasive, malignant tumor of astrocytic origin; it is the most common of the gliomas occurring above the tentorium, forming about 40% of all such tumors. The tumor occurs most frequently between the ages of 40 and 60 years. The duration of symptoms usually is short, the time between onset and the initial examination averaging about six months. Glioblastoma may occur anywhere in the brain; it is characterized by its infiltrative nature and its ability to spread rapidly. Involvement of both cerebral hemispheres through spread across the corpus callosum is common. The tumor also may spread through the ventricular system

or subarachnoid space. True multicentric tumors of this nature are rare.

Unenhanced CT scans classically show the tumor margin to be of slightly higher density than the surrounding brain, with fingerlike projections of low attenuation tissue, representing edema, extending along white-matter pathways. The great majority of these tumors show marked enhancement following administration of intravenous contrast medium. This enhancement occurs because of the tumor's neovascularity plus disruption of the adjacent BBB. On contrast-enhanced scans, the margins of the tumor are usually irregular and the pattern of the enhancement is inhomogeneous. Evidence of mass effect is usually present in these lesions, and some displacement of the ventricular system away from the lesion is usual. Temporal lobe tumors displace or compress the temporal horn of the lateral ventricle. Often there is gross distortion of the ventricle on the side of the lesion. When the tumor involves a frontal lobe, it is prone to extend across the midline beneath the falx by way of involvement of the corpus callosum so that some deformity of the opposite ventricle may be visualized. Low-density regions in the central areas of these tumors often represent regions of tumor necrosis. Gross cystic areas sometimes occur but are relatively rare in untreated tumors (Fig. 11-6).[73]

MR scans of glioblastomas more closely reflect the

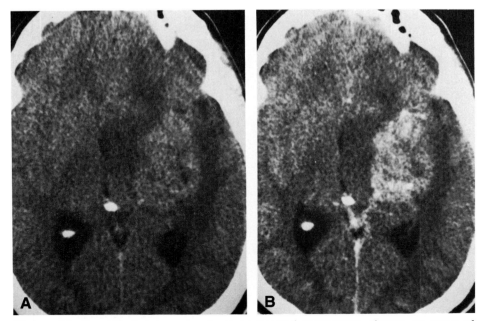

Figure 11–6. **(A)** Axial noncontrast computed tomogram shows an area of slightly increased density in the basal ganglia and thalamus surrounded by low-density areas of edema on the left. **(B)** Axial computed tomogram following administration of intravenous contrast medium. There is diffuse nonhomogeneous enhancement of the tumor.

pathologic changes of hypercellularity, hemorrhage, necrosis, and hypervascularity than do CT scans. Thus, on these examinations, areas of cystic change, hemorrhage, and neurovascularity are more commonly demonstrated than on CT scans. MRI also allows more precise recognition of the tumor mass than does CT. It has been shown to be impossible, however, to differentiate accurately the margin of these tumors from adjacent normal brain tissue. The tumors are usually hypointense on T1-weighted scans and hyperintense on proton density and T2-weighted images. Inhomogeneity of signal intensity is characteristic of these lesions. Enhancement following administration of intravenous contrast medium is almost always present to some degree; it is usually inhomogeneous also (Fig. 11-7).

The angiographic findings in glioblastomas vary somewhat, but typically the tumor is very vascular and a bizarre pattern of neurovascularity with irregularly dilated arteries and early filling of dilated veins is seen. On angiography these tumors may appear to be well circumscribed, and the extent of neurovascularity may vary greatly from one area to another. Avascular areas within a glioblastoma are usually the result of necrosis or cyst formation. Vascular displacements away from the area of the lesion with stretching and straightening of branches is a common observation. In some cases a diffuse stain or blush is seen during the late arterial or capillary phase. Angiography is now seldom required for either the diagnosis or management of tumors of this type.

MRI is now the primary method for investigating suspected supratentorial tumors. It should be noted that while MR images show the extent and characteristics of these lesions to better advantage than does CT, it is still to be demonstrated that this advantage has a positive impact on either the treatment or earlier diagnosis of these tumors.

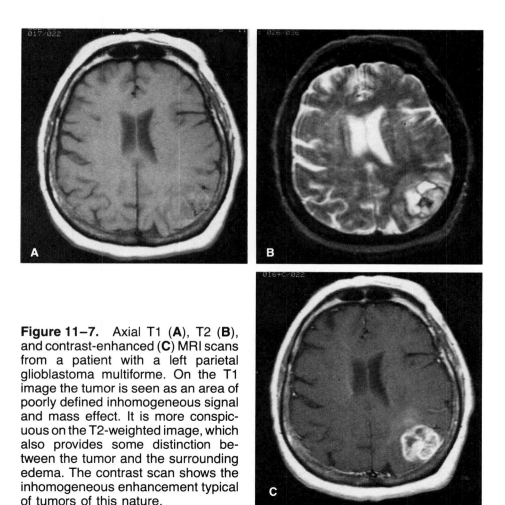

Figure 11–7. Axial T1 (**A**), T2 (**B**), and contrast-enhanced (**C**) MRI scans from a patient with a left parietal glioblastoma multiforme. On the T1 image the tumor is seen as an area of poorly defined inhomogeneous signal and mass effect. It is more conspicuous on the T2-weighted image, which also provides some distinction between the tumor and the surrounding edema. The contrast scan shows the inhomogeneous enhancement typical of tumors of this nature.

Astrocytoma

The second most common glioma occurring above the tentorium, astrocytoma represents approximately 32% of all such tumors. Formerly these neoplasms were graded on a numeric scale, from 1 through 4, a higher number indicating a more malignant tumor histology. This classification is now less frequently employed, because it is realized that in many instances variations of grades occur throughout any particular tumor; therefore biopsy samples are subject to considerable error. Classification of these tumors by predominant cell line (i.e., fibrillary or pilocystic), and also by site of origin (i.e., supra- or infratentorial), also provides some idea about their biologic behavior and, thus, about prognosis. As was the case with the numeric grading scale, these classifications are not without fault because these lesions are seldom of a pure histologic type. Except for the juvenile pilocystic astrocytoma, which almost uniformly has an excellent prognosis, it is difficult to offer guidelines about the biologic behavior of these tumors based on imaging studies.

The duration of symptoms at the time of diagnosis averages three years. Like glioblastoma, astrocytoma may involve any part of the brain; depending upon their topography and biologic behavior, the radiographic features of these tumors are quite diverse. This discussion is limited to those astrocytomas occurring above the tentorium; others will be discussed in a subsequent section. Large cysts commonly form in astrocytomas, particularly in those of a pilocystic nature, and the cystic element may predominate in both the pathologic and radiographic appearance of the lesion. Calcification occurs in as many as 15% of these tumors.

Depending upon the size of the lesion, unenhanced CT scans may show only mass effect, with displacement, distortion, or compression of the ventricular system. In some small or low-grade lesions, there is very little mass effect and the tumor may be difficult or impossible to detect on CT scans. The degree of contrast enhancement seen varies depending both on the degree of BBB disruption and the cellular makeup of the tumor. It is important to recognize that in these tumors as well as in other neoplasms of the CNS the degree of enhancement tends to be more intense and more frequently present in malignant than in benign tumors, although this feature does not correlate in a reliable manner with the malignancy of any particular tumor.

Because of its increased contrast sensitivity, MRI is more accurate than CT in demonstrating the *gross borders* of these tumors which typically are seen as regions of abnormal signal intensity on both T1- and T2-weighted sequences. Most astrocytomas are slightly hypointense on T1 and hyperintense on T2 images.

The degree of homogeneity varies, with the more benign lesions tending to be homogeneous while the more malignant ones are heterogeneous. The degree of adjacent edema also varies, with more malignant tumors being associated with considerable edema. As with CT, the degree of contrast enhancement is variable; with both modalities, enhancement is not rare in the more benign tumors, and it is usually present in the high-grade or malignant tumors.

The juvenile pilocystic astrocytoma, a variety of tumor that occurs predominantly in children, has features that usually allow accurate diagnosis on both CT and MRI. The great majority of these tumors occur either in or adjacent to the visual pathways or cerebellar vermis, they are well defined, and they enhance markedly both on CT and MRI. Cyst formation is common. Regardless of their location, these tumors are low grade and only occasionally recur after resection.[44] These will be discussed further in the sections on juxtasellar tumors and posterior fossa tumors.

The angiographic features of astrocytomas depend on the histologic nature of the tumor; lesions with predominant malignant features show abnormalities quite similar to those described for glioblastomas; tumors with mixed benign and malignant features show intermediate changes; lesions of a benign nature show only evidence of avascular mass effect or no changes at all. In the capillary phase of the arteriogram a tumor stain may be present, at times either in a nodular component of the lesion or if the entire mass is solid, throughout the tumor. Only rarely is angiography required for either the diagnosis or management of these tumors.

Oligodendroglioma

Oligodendrogliomas make up about 7% of the supratentorial gliomas. Most of them are found in adults, the average age at the time of diagnosis being 45 years. Oligodendrogliomas usually grow slowly, and the duration of symptoms before diagnosis averages 11 years. These tumors occur almost exclusively in the cerebral hemispheres, and there is a definite predilection for the frontal lobes. Because of its slow growth, calcification within the tumor occurs very frequently; the calcium usually is distributed in the form of coarse, irregular strands. As in astrocytoma, other types of calcification may also occur and the pattern of calcification does not allow one to make a specific histologic diagnosis.

The findings on CT scans are similar to those seen with low-grade astrocytomas. Because of a lack of neurovascularity and little disruption of the BBB, the enhancement following administration of intravenous contrast medium is usually only slight. The presence of

heavy calcification may provide a clue about the nature of the lesion, but as already mentioned is a nonspecific sign. Cystic or necrotic changes are rare unless the lesion has undergone malignant degeneration.[73]

These tumors have no specific or distinguishing features on MRI. The calcifications in these tumors are seen on spin echo sequences as areas of inhomogeneity of signal intensity. These may be confused with signal void in abnormal vascular structures.[45]

Arteriography shows displacement of vessels away from the mass, with stretching of small adjacent branches. Seldom is there significant neurovascularity; the interior of the tumor usually does not develop a tumor stain during the capillary phase of the angiogram.

Ependymoma

Ependymomas comprise about 5% of all supratentorial gliomas. The duration of symptoms at the time of diagnosis is usually relatively short, being less than one year in many cases. The average age at the time of diagnosis in supratentorial ependymomas is reported to be 30 years. Infratentorial ependymomas occur most frequently in children and adolescents and are much more common than are the supratentorial variety.

Many supratentorial ependymomas probably arise from ependymal cell rests situated about the margins of the lateral ventricles; they frequently occur near the atrium of one of the lateral ventricles. Ependymomas often contain small, scattered, punctate, calcified deposits, which may be visible on unenhanced CT scans. On these scans, ependymomas most often are isodense or slightly hyperdense as compared with the adjacent normal brain. Cystic changes frequently occur and at times the lesion may appear to be almost entirely cystic. Most ependymomas are enhanced to some degree following administration of intravenous contrast medium. These neoplasms show no specific signal characteristics on MRI. Nonetheless, the multiplanar capabilities of MRI are advantageous in demonstrating the location and pathway of spread of these tumors.[66]

Meningiomas

Meningiomas are extraaxial tumors that arise from the arachnoid; the great majority of them are benign. The common locations of meningiomas include sites along the superior sagittal sinus, particularly in the posterior frontal and parietal areas and adjacent to the convexities of the cerebral hemispheres a short distance away from the midline. Other frequent sites for development of these tumors are in the region of the tuberculum sellae or just anterior to the tuberculum along the olfactory groove, along the edges of the sphenoidal ridge, and somewhat less frequently, along the margins of the falx cerebri and the tentorium. Grossly, meningiomas vary in shape from a globular configuration to a flat type of growth, the so-called meningioma en plaque.

Meningiomas usually receive a major portion of their blood supply from the arteries that supply the normal dura at the site from which they arise. Aggressive or malignant types of this tumor may also parasitize the vasculature of the adjacent brain. Meningiomas that arise from or adjacent to the dural sinuses may invade and obstruct these structures. Most meningiomas that arise near bone exhibit some type of osseous response, most often hyperostosis (i.e., hypertrophy). They may invade the bone and occasionally will extend through it to form a hyperostotic density along the outer table of the skull. In other instances, extensive bone destruction is apparent; rarely, the bone overlying a meningioma is completely destroyed with a soft-tissue mass bulging externally.

Tumors that cause a pure hyperostotic type of bone reaction tend to recur infrequently, while those that cause a destructive or mixed bone reaction recur much more often. In 60% to 65% of patients with meningiomas, changes seen on plain films of the skull will strongly suggest both the diagnosis and location of the tumor; nevertheless, these studies are not indicated because they do not allow assessment of the tumor's size and thus are not of value in deciding on management. Likewise, angiography provides typical findings but is now rarely used for diagnostic purposes. Depending upon the size, location, and likely vascularity of the tumor, angiography may be indicated to decide whether removal will be facilitated by preoperative embolization. Initial assessment of all these features is best performed with CT or MRI. Although CT is accurate in the diagnosis of meningiomas, having a specific diagnostic rate of 86% and an overall accuracy rate of 96% in one series, the superior contrast sensitivity and multiplanar capabilities of MRI have now made this method the preferable technique for evaluation of patients with these tumors.[9, 28] MRI allows more precise assessment of the extent, location, and vascularity of these tumors than does CT.

Calcification within meningiomas is found in 15% to 20% of cases. The calcium deposits typically are in the form of small punctate densities that are rather uniformly distributed throughout the tumor mass. These sandlike deposits are known as psammoma bodies and are in part responsible for the homogeneous increase in attenuation values that are typical of the unenhanced CT appearance of these lesions. Some very slow-growing meningiomas form densely calcified masses, which may have little if any soft-tissue component.

On unenhanced CT scans, most meningiomas are homogeneous and have slightly increased attenuation values. The degree of edema surrounding them varies

greatly; some lesions cause marked edema of the adjacent brain and others do not. This feature depends in part on their rate of growth. Scans usually show a relationship of the tumor to an adjacent dural structure, and often some reaction of the overlying bone can be seen. Following intravenous contrast administration, the typical meningioma is enhanced in a homogeneous manner and has very well-defined margins (Fig. 11-8). Slow-growing, heavily calcified lesions may not show any enhancement; aggressive or malignant lesions often show inhomogeneous enhancement. Primary lymphomas of the CNS may closely simulate the CT appearance of meningiomas.[32,64]

On MRI studies, meningiomas are typically isointense to slightly hypointense with the adjacent brain on T1-weighted images, and slightly to markedly hyperintense on proton density and T2-weighted images. Most of these tumors have sharply defined margins and heterogeneous signal intensities. Early reports of a superiority of CT over MRI for detection of some of these tumors have not proven to be accurate.[81] The ability to do brain imaging in multiple projections without the presence of artifact created by bone in the calvarium greatly improves the ability to define the full extent of these lesions, especially when they involve the skull base (Fig. 11-9). Most meningiomas enhance significantly following administration of paramagnetic contrast medium. Enhancement of the meninges adja-

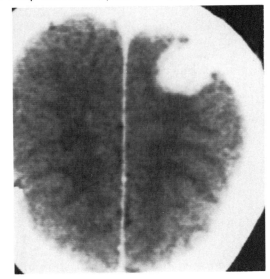

Figure 11-8. Axial computed tomogram done after administration of intravenous contrast medium. A right parietal meningioma is enhanced in a homogeneous manner. Its margins are sharply defined and there is some edema in the adjacent white matter.

cent to the bulk of the tumor mass is a useful diagnostic sign (Fig. 11-10).

The angiographic findings of the typical meningioma are quite characteristic: the major arterial supply is from dural arteries; tumor vessels are usually uniform so that opacification is relatively constant throughout the tumor; and the arterial branches surround the tumor in an archlike manner, sending small tributaries toward the center of the mass. Nonetheless, angiography is not required in the diagnostic evaluation of meningiomas unless there is concern about the ability at surgery to control the arterial supply because of the location of the lesion. In these instances, a preoperative embolization procedure may be required.

JUXTASELLAR TUMORS

Pituitary Adenoma

Historically, the classification of pituitary adenomas was based on their predominant staining characteristics, and on this basis three primary tumor types were recognized: eosinophilic adenomas (associated with acromegaly), basophilic adenomas (associated with Cushing's disease), and chromophobe adenomas (associated with hypopituitarism). A more meaningful classification divides these lesions into two major groups, those that are hormonally active and those that are hormonally inactive. The active ones are then further divided according to the hormones they secrete. Depending on their size, pituitary adenomas are designated as either macroadenomas (> 1 cm) or microadenomas (< 1 cm). Macroadenomas are the majority of hormonally inactive tumors and typically become clinically manifest as a result of their size, causing compression of adjacent neural structures. Patients with microadenomas usually seek medical attention because of abnormal hormone secretion. Specific types of pituitary adenomas include prolactin, growth hormone, and ACTH-secreting adenomas. Prolactinomas in women are associated with galactorrhea and amenorrhea; in men, they most often cause hypogonadism. Growth-hormone-secreting adenomas that occur before bone growth has ceased cause giantism, while those that occur later result in acromegaly. ACTH-secreting tumors are associated with Cushing's disease. Most pituitary adenomas occur in adults.

There is no longer any place for plain film or complex motion tomographic evaluation of the bony contours of the sella turcica as part of the diagnostic workup of patients suspected of having a pituitary tumor. Several studies have provided clear evidence of the lack of correlation between the configuration and size of the sella turcica and the presence or absence of a pituitary tumor.[72] MRI has replaced CT as the technique of choice for

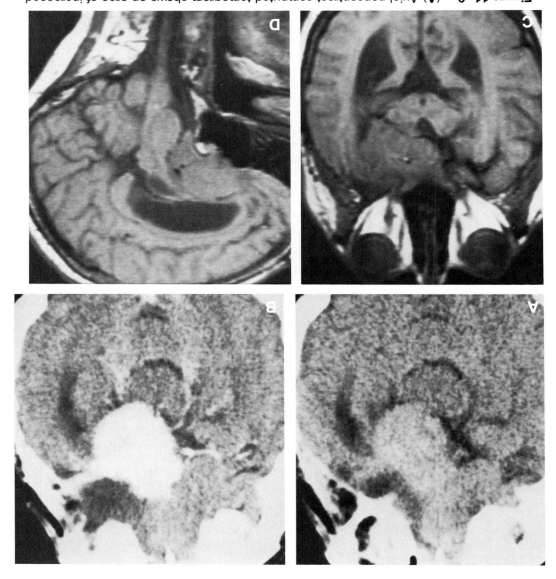

Figure 11–9. (**A**) Axial noncontrast computed tomogram shows an area of increased density extending from the suprasellar cistern into the interpeduncular and left sylvian fissure. This is a recurrent sphenoid wing meningioma. (**B**) Following administration of intravenous contrast medium there is homogeneous enhancement of the tumor. (**C**) Axial MR image. The meningioma is isointense with the adjacent brain. Nonetheless, its extension along the paths of the optic nerves and its effect on the adjacent midbrain are more clearly seen than on the computed tomogram. (**D**) Sagittal MR image. The extension of the tumor into the interpeduncular cistern and prepontine cistern is clearly demonstrated.

evaluation of the juxtasellar area. This has occurred because although CT is in many instances satisfactory for evaluation of pituitary tumors, its optimal use depends upon the routine use of intravenous contrast medium, the absence of dental or postsurgical metallic elements, and the ability to obtain direct coronal scans. On CT scans performed immediately following administration of intravenous contrast medium, most pituitary microadenomas are seen as an area of reduced attenuation within the enhancing pituitary gland. This pattern is variable, however, with exceptions occurring both as a result of differences in the tumor histology and as a function of the time occurring between administration of the contrast and performance of the scan. Other CT findings seen with microadenomas are an increase in the height of the gland (normally < 10 mm), alteration in the contour of the upper margin of the gland from concave or straight to convex, erosion of the floor of the sella turcica adjacent to an area of hypodensity, and displacement of the normally midline pituitary stalk away from an area of hypodensity in the gland (Fig. 11-11). Considerable variation occurs in the size and configuration of the normal pituitary gland, especially in women of childbearing age; great care must be exercised in the diagnosis of pituitary microadenomas on the basis of CT scans performed without associated evidence of a hormonal abnormality.[61, 69]

Depending on their size and pattern of growth, pituitary macroadenomas have a variable appearance on CT scans. Most of them are isodense or slightly hyperdense on unenhanced CT scans; following administra-

tion of an intravenous contrast medium, a pattern of marked homogeneous enhancement is typical (Fig. 11-12). Cystic or necrotic areas occur frequently in very large pituitary adenomas, and, on CT scan, appear as areas of reduced attenuation. Pituitary macroadenomas must be distinguished from other mass lesions that occur in the juxtasellar area, such as giant

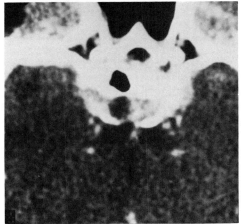

Figure 11-11. Coronal computed tomogram done after administration of intravenous contrast medium. An area of hypodensity is seen in the left side of the pituitary fossa. The infundibular stalk is displaced to the right.

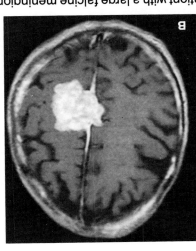

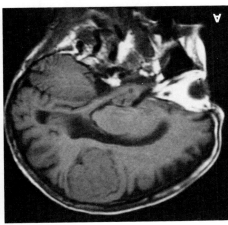

Figure 11-10. (A) Parasagittal MRI from patient with a large falcine meningioma. On this T1-weighted image the tumor appears as a well-defined mass having slightly hypointense signal. (B) Axial T1-weighted image performed following intravenous administration of paramagnetic contrast medium. The tumor enhances in a homogeneous manner. Well demonstrated on this image is the extension of enhancement from the tumor mass along adjacent dural margins, typical of this kind of tumor.

aneurysms, meningiomas, and optic gliomas. In most instances, the use of direct coronal scans and intravenous contrast medium allows this to be determined without difficulty because the relationship of the mass to adjacent vascular and neural structures as well as the presence or absence of any associated bony abnormality can be well assessed with this technique. Only occasionally is angiography required as part of the diagnostic evaluation of a suspected pituitary macroadenoma.

On MRI, microadenomas are most often seen as areas of hypointensity on T1-weighted scans and hy-perintensity on T2-weighted scans. Many micro-adenomas have some areas of high signal intensity on the T1-weighted images; this reflects the presence of prior hemorrhage. The superior contrast resolution of MRI has made it unnecessary to use intravenous contrast medium in MR examinations done for evaluation of pituitary tumors in most instances (Fig. 11-13). In circumstances in which a noncontrast scan is negative and a functioning tumor is highly suspected, the use of intravenous contrast medium has, however, been shown to be of use in detecting very small tumors. When it is used, the pattern of enhancement is similar

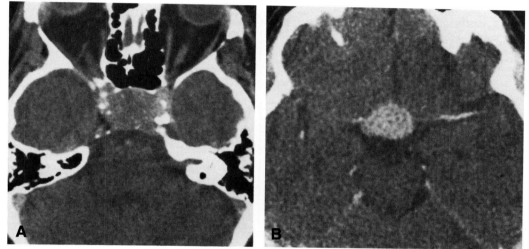

Figure 11–12. **(A)** Axial computed tomogram performed after administration of intravenous contrast medium. The pituitary fossa is enlarged because of a macroadenoma. **(B)** Axial computed tomogram of the same patient taken at a higher level shows a homogeneously enhancing mass extending into the suprasellar cistern.

Figure 11–13. Coronal T1 images without (**A** and **B**) and with (**C** and **D**) intravenous contrast medium. This small pituitary adenoma is clearly seen on the non-contrast scans as an area of low-signal intensity. Extension into the cavernous sinus on the right is also evident. On the contrast-enhanced scans the tumor is still hypo-intense compared with the adjacent normal pituitary gland.

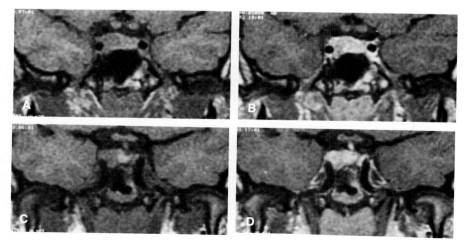

to that described for contrast-enhanced CT scans. Macroadenomas are best imaged with MRI because this technique provides the best means for visualizing the relationship of these tumors to adjacent neural and vascular structures. The extent of a suprasellar tumor is easily demonstrated in both coronal and sagittal images. It is more difficult to be sure about lateral extension of these tumors. Displacement of the cavernous segments of the internal carotid arteries may occur without tumor invasion of the cavernous sinus. Abnormal signal intensity lateral to this segment of the artery, however, usually indicates extension of the tumor into the cavernous sinus. Cystic and hemorrhagic changes within these tumors are common (Fig. 11-14).

Craniopharyngioma

This congenital tumor arises from remnants of Rathke's pouch. Craniopharyngioma is largely a tumor of childhood and adolescence; however, occurrence in older adults is by no means rare. In younger children the presenting complaint is often related to increased intracranial pressure; in older children and adults, symptoms are most often of a visual or endocrine nature. Delayed growth is the most common endocrine-related symptom associated with craniopharyngioma.

Calcification occurs very frequently in craniopharyngiomas and has been reported in as many as 80% of children with this tumor; it is much less common in adults. Most craniopharyngiomas are suprasellar in location, but at least 10% to 15% are confined solely to the pituitary fossa. Cystic changes of either a unilocular or a multilocular nature occur very frequently in these tumors.

As is the case in evaluation of pituitary adenomas, MRI has replaced CT as the technique of choice for evaluation of craniopharyngiomas. Thin-section coronal projections performed without the use of intravenous contrast medium are usually sufficient for the diagnosis. Craniopharyngiomas have a variable appearance on MRI, depending upon their degree of calcification as well as the extent of cystic changes in the tumor. Solid portions of craniopharyngiomas are usually heterogeneous with calcifications appearing as low intensity on both T1- and T2-weighted images, while noncalcified portions are isointense or hypointense on T1 images and hyperintense on T2 images. Cystic portions of this tumor are often filled with a machine-oil-type fluid that is of high-signal intensity on both T1- and T2-weighted images.

The CT scan appearance of these tumors is also variable depending on the amount of calcification and cystic change present with the tumor.[20] Tumors that have extensive cystic change most often appear as well-defined areas of decreased attenuation with areas of calcification about their periphery (Fig. 11-15). Tumors that are mostly solid are usually of increased attenuation on noncontrast scans.

Following intravenous contrast medium administration, the capsule of cystic tumors shows enhancement both on CT and MRI. Solid portions of these tumors often enhance in a homogeneous manner on contrast-enhanced scans.

Optic Gliomas

These gliomas, which involve the optic pathways, are slow-growing tumors that occur most often in children with neurofibromatosis Type 1. They may involve one or both optic nerves, the optic chiasm, optic tracts or

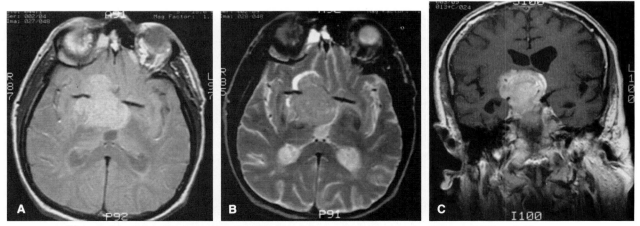

Figure 11–14.   Proton-density (**A**), T2- (**B**), and T1-contrast enhanced (**C**) axial images from the scan of a patient with a pituitary macroadenoma. The extent of these large tumors both into the suprasellar cisterns and into the cavernous sinuses and sphenoid sinus is most clearly defined with MRI.

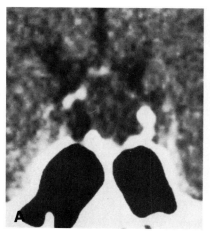 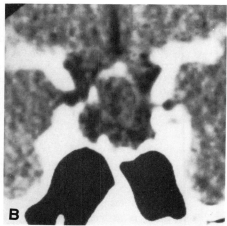

Figure 11–15. (A) Noncontrast coronal computed tomogram shows an isodense mass within the suprasellar cistern. Its upper margin is calcified. **(B)** Computed tomogram at the same level performed after administration of intravenous contrast medium. There is no enhancement of the tumor. Adjacent normal vascular structures are clearly seen.

optic radiations. Because of their early occurrence and slow rate of growth, optic gliomas frequently are associated with enlargement of the optic foramen and alteration in the configuration of the pituitary fossa. It is often impossible to distinguish these tumors either by their behavior or their location from a primary glioma of the hypothalamus.[65]

MRI is the technique of choice for evaluation of the patient suspected of having an optic glioma (Fig. 11-16). These tumors are usually hypointense on T1-weighted images and hyperintense on T2-weighted scans. They usually enhance homogeneously following intravenous contrast medium administration.

The Empty Sella Syndrome

The term "empty sella" is used when there is extension of the subarachnoid space into the pituitary fossa, a situation that may occur as a result of either a congenital or acquired defect in the diaphragma sellae. Pulsations of the cerebrospinal fluid and the anterior recesses of the third ventricle may enlarge this defect and, when their extension into the sella is significant, can cause enlargement of the pituitary fossa and compression of the pituitary gland. Rarely is the empty sella syndrome of clinical significance; this discussion illustrates that this condition is recognized and will not be confused with either a low-density or low-signal intensity pituitary tumor on CT or MRI. When cerebrospinal fluid density or intensity is seen within the pituitary fossa, one should try to identify the infundibular stalk and then trace this structure to its junction with the pituitary gland, which usually will be found in the posterior inferior aspect of the pituitary fossa.[36] Rarely, a largely cystic pituitary microadenoma may simulate closely the findings of an empty sella. Microadenomas may also occur in association with a partially empty sella.

OTHER SUPRATENTORIAL TUMORS

Tumors of the Pineal Gland

Tumors of the pineal gland are rare, contributing approximately 0.5% or 1% of all intracranial tumors. They are usually manifested during the first three decades and originate either from pineal parenchymal cells (pinealoblastoma and pinealocytoma), from germ cells (germinomas, teratomas, embryonal carcinoma, choriocarcinoma), or from glial cells. Germ cell tumors are the most common type and occur much more often in males than in females. Tumors arising from the pineal parenchymal cells occur in equal numbers in males and females. Teratomas contain multiple tissues including fat, the characteristic CT and MRI appearance of which often provides a clue to the nature of the lesion. A variety of glial tumors also occur in the pineal region, which is also a common site for lipomas. Because many of these tumors tend to infiltrate diffusely, it is often impossible to determine from imaging studies whether a lesion has its origin within the pineal gland or the adjacent neural parenchyma. The so-called ectopic pinealoma is actually a teratoma that usually arises in the region of the infundibulum and presents as a suprasellar mass.

Teratomas and most pineal parenchymal tumors (i.e., pinealocytomas and pinealoblastomas), show some degree of calcification. The observation of calcification in the region of the pineal gland in a child under the age of 7 years is thus somewhat suggestive of a neoplasm because the normal pineal gland usually does not calcify at this age. In one study, fewer than 11% of children between the ages of 11 and 14 had pineal calcification present on CT scans.[77]

The various types of pineal and pineal region tumors cannot be distinguished accurately on the basis of CT scan findings alone. All may have calcifications and all usually show significant enhancement following the

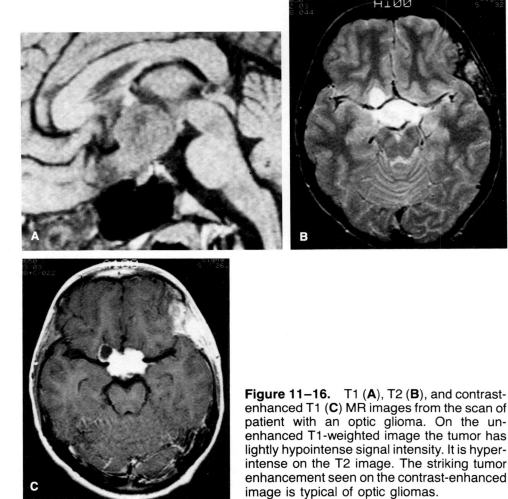

Figure 11–16. T1 (**A**), T2 (**B**), and contrast-enhanced T1 (**C**) MR images from the scan of patient with an optic glioma. On the unenhanced T1-weighted image the tumor has lightly hypointense signal intensity. It is hyperintense on the T2 image. The striking tumor enhancement seen on the contrast-enhanced image is typical of optic gliomas.

administration of intravenous contrast medium. The pattern of enhancement that these tumors show varies; some are homogeneous while others are not, some have well-defined margins while the margins of others are indistinct. Edema of the brain adjacent to a pineal tumor is unusual. Because of their relationship to the aqueduct of Sylvius, many of these tumors are associated with hydrocephalus.[23]

Aside from its other advantages, the ability of MRI to provide high-quality coronal and sagittal images has made it superior to CT for evaluating patients with pineal region tumors. Multiplanar images greatly assist in the location of the epicenter of a mass and, therefore, are useful in judging the nature of its origin. Except for teratomas, which are almost always partially cystic and are markedly heterogeneous in signal intensity because of the presence of fat, hair, and bone, there are no

specific MRI features of these lesions. Germinomas and pinealoblastomas often are isointense with gray matter on both T1 and T2-weighted images. Most pineal gland region tumors enhance following administration of intravenous contrast medium.

Colloid Cyst

Colloid cysts develop in the anterior portion of the third ventricle, usually arising from the roof. Because of its location, the lesion may block either one or, as is more often the case, both of the interventricular foramina, thereby causing hydrocephalus. In some instances obstruction is intermittent. This tumor shows no predilection for either sex and usually becomes manifest during adult life.

As seen on unenhanced CT scans, colloid cysts characteristically appear as well-demarcated, symmetrical, midline masses of increased density, located at the level of the interventricular foramina. On contrast scans, the mass, particularly its outer margins, may become enhanced slightly (Fig. 11-17).[22]

Tumors that obstruct the interventricular foramen cause enlargement of the lateral ventricles, the third ventricle remaining normal in size. An occasional colloid cyst that is isodense with the adjacent brain has been reported; these may be difficult to visualize without the use of CT scans performed following injection of water-soluble contrast medium into the ventricular system. Astrocytomas that originate from the tissue around the interventricular foramen can usually be distinguished from colloid cysts because they typically are poorly defined, have indistinct margins, and are either isodense or hypodense or unenhanced CT scans.

Because the diagnosis of a colloid cyst depends primarily upon the recognition of its location and the ability to discern that the adjacent brain is normal, the multiplanar nature of MRI alone makes it the technique of choice for evaluation of these lesions (Fig. 11-1). The contents of colloid cysts are variable; therefore, their signal characteristics on MRI are not specific.

Because colloid cysts are benign lesions that cause symptoms only as a result of the hydrocephalus they produce, it is important that they be recognized so that appropriate treatment may be attempted. Treatment may either be removal of the cyst or decompression of the hydrocephalus without cyst removal.

Epidermoid Tumor

Epidermoids are congenital lesions derived from ectoderm. They are found more frequently as intradiploic lesions in the bones of the skull than as intracranial lesions; both are uncommon. There is no age or sex predilection. Desquamation of cholesterol-containing debris from the lining of this tumor accounts for its slow growth. Symptoms usually occur as the result of compression of adjacent neural structures. The most common location for an epidermoid is the cerebellopontine angle cistern. Other sites of occurrence are the juxtasellar area, in one of the lateral ventricles or the fourth ventricle.

The CT density of an epidermoid is the same as or slightly lower than that of cerebrospinal fluid. Calcification of the tumor's margins is uncommon but when it occurs it is one feature that helps in distinguishing epidermoids from arachnoid cysts which on CT scan may otherwise closely resemble each other. Characteristically, the surface of an epidermoid is rough and nodular, and some are cauliflower like with deep clefts. Arachnoid cysts are smooth. Epidermoids do not enhance after administration of intravenous contrast medium. On MRI, epidermoids tend to have signal intensities that are slightly hyperintense to CSF on all pulse sequences. The signal intensities from epidermoids are often heterogeneous.

Dermoid Tumor

Dermoids are rare congenital tumors derived from ectoderm and mesoderm. Almost all dermoids occur in the midline and, like epidermoids, most of these tu-

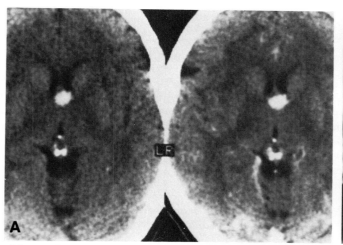
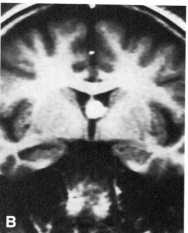

Figure 11–17. **(A)** Noncontrast and contrast computed tomograms taken through the level of the interventricular foramen. A well-circumscribed high-density mass is located in the midline at this level. It does not enhance on the contrast scan. **(B)** Coronal MRI allows better definition of the relationship of this colloid cyst to the septum pellucidum and the interventricular foramen (partial saturation TR 600; TE 25).

mors cause symptoms because of compression of adjacent neural structures. Occasionally, a dermoid may rupture spontaneously either into the ventricular system or into the subarachnoid cisterns, causing an intense meningitis or ventriculitis. The lining of these lesions contains hair follicles and glandular elements as well as squamous epithelium. On CT scan the density of dermoids is variable but typically is similar to that of fat. Dense calcification representing partially formed dental elements is seen within some dermoids, and calcification of a portion of the outer margin is commonly observed.

The characteristic fat-like signal intensities from the secretions of these tumors often allow an accurate diagnosis to be made with MRI. On both CT and MRI, fat fluid levels are sometimes seen within some dermoids; their presence within the ventricular system indicates rupture.[11] Dermoids do not enhance following administration of intravenous contrast medium.

Lipoma

Lipomas, lesions derived from mesoderm, occur infrequently. Like dermoids, they usually occur in the midline, the most common locations being the corpus callosum, the vermis, and the quadrigeminal cistern. The majority of lipomas are incidental findings. When they occur in the corpus callosum they are often associated with callosal agenesis. The fat density of these lesions gives them a characteristic appearance on both CT scans and MRI (Fig. 11-18). Calcification is frequent in their periphery, especially in lipomas that occur in the corpus callosum.

INFRATENTORIAL TUMORS

GLIOMAS

Astrocytoma

Astrocytoma is the most common primary infratentorial tumor. Astrocytomas of the brain stem and cerebellum account for as many as 50% of childhood tumors in some series. These tumors range in their biologic behavior from very slow-growing, diffusely infiltrating lesions to rapidly spreading malignant lesions that result in death within a few months after symptoms become apparent. Their radiographic appearance depends primarily on their histologic nature but also is influenced by their location.

Astrocytomas of the brain stem occur most frequently in children but are not unusual in adults. They account for about one third of all infratentorial tumors. They may originate at any level of the brain stem, but are most common in the pons. Rapidly growing, dif-

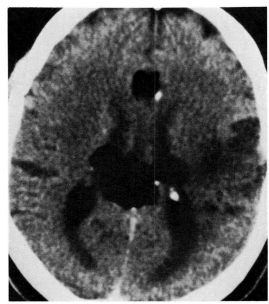

Figure 11–18.   Axial noncontrast computed tomogram through the level of the body of the corpus callosum. The low attenuation values of fat are characteristic of a lipoma. The flecks of calcification about the margins of the lipoma are also typical.

fusely infiltrating tumors (fibrillary astrocytomas) are more common than the slow-growing varieties. Because of diffuse infiltration of these tumors, large segments of the brain stem are often found to be abnormal. At the time of diagnosis, the clinical signs and symptoms produced by brain-stem astrocytomas are often mild when compared with the large size of the tumor. It is not uncommon to observe a low-grade astrocytoma involving the entire brain stem and even extending into both the cervical portion of the spinal cord and the cerebellum. Astrocytomas commonly form exophytic extensions along the surface of the brain stem, and, occasionally, can simulate an extraaxial mass lesion. In very low-grade lesions, the only indication of the presence of an abnormality may be distortion of the shape and increase in the size of the involved brain stem segment. The use of low-dose, intrathecal, water-soluble contrast medium in conjunction with CT scanning has been of great value in the early detection of such tumors. Because of improvements in the capability of CT scanning and the development of MRI, this technique is now seldom if ever needed (Fig. 11-19). Calcification in brain-stem astrocytomas is not observed as frequently as in the case of similar supratentorial tumors. Following the administration of intravenous contrast medium, there is a variable pattern;

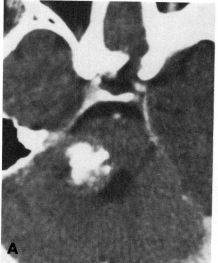

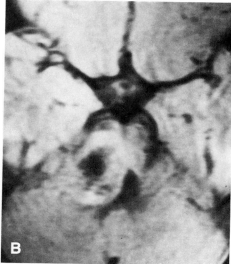

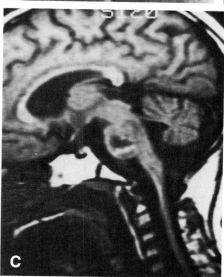

Figure 11–19. (**A**) Axial computed tomogram performed after administration of intravenous contrast medium. An area of dense calcification surrounded by some edema is seen in the right side of the pons and cerebellum. (**B**) Axial MR image at the same level (SE Tr 2000; TE 30). The calcification is seen as an area of signal void. The extent of the tumor into the pons and cerebellar hemisphere is more clearly seen on this image than on the computed tomogram. (**C**) Sagittal MR image (partial saturation TR 800; TE 25). The enlargement of the pons and the rostral and caudal extent of the tumor are clearly seen on this projection.

higher-grade or malignant tumors tend to enhance intensely while those that are less aggressive enhance slightly or not at all.[3]

MRI is more sensitive than CT for detection of both the presence and the extent of these tumors. On T1-weighted images, most of these lesions are hypointense: on T2 images they are hyperintense. Small cystic changes are not uncommon. As is the case with CT scanning, enhancement following intravenous contrast administration is variable.

Astrocytomas arising in the cerebellum are a common CNS tumor of childhood. Two major types of cerebellar astrocytoma exist. The most frequent is the pilocystic variety, which is well demarcated, benign,

and often cystic. Less common is the diffusely infiltrative (fibrillary) variety that is poorly defined and often malignant. Calcification is unusual in either the solid or the cystic variety of this tumor.[50] Most of the lesions of either type arise in the cerebellar hemispheres.

On CT scans the cystic pilocystic astrocytoma is seen as a well-circumscribed mass with attenuation values that are similar to those of cerebrospinal fluid. On MRI, signal intensities from the cystic portion of the tumor are similar to those of cerebrospinal fluid. Often there is a mural nodule that enhances after administration of intravenous contrast medium. Solid varieties of these tumors are isodense on CT scans performed without intravenous contrast medium; on MRI they are hypointense on T1-weighted images and hyper-intense on T2-weighted scans (Fig. 11-20).

The infiltrating variety of cerebellar astrocytoma (fibrillary astrocytoma) has an appearance on both CT and MRI that is similar to that of its brain-stem counterpart.

Hemangioblastoma

These benign tumors, found mostly in adults, occur most often in the cerebellum. They also occur regularly, however, in the brain stem and spinal cord; supratentorial occurrences are rare. These neoplasms are sometimes associated with the von Hipple–Lindau disease, and, in this setting, the chance of their being multiple increases significantly. As many as half of all hemangioblastomas are mostly cystic; the remainder are divided between those that are partially cystic and solid and those that are entirely solid. Regardless of whether they are cystic or solid, hemangioblastomas have extensive vascularity. The cystic variety typically has a well-defined mural nodule that receives its blood supply from adjacent pial vessels. At times the vascularity of these tumors is so extensive that they may simulate arteriovenous malformations. Calcification is usually not seen.

As seen on unenhanced CT scans, these tumors vary in appearance depending primarily upon whether they are cystic or solid. Lesions that are largely cystic appear as well-defined masses, the attenuation values of which are similar to those of cerebrospinal fluid. Careful observation will usually reveal an area along the margin of the mass that is isodense as compared with the adjacent brain; this represents the mural nodule. Solid hemangioblastomas are most often isodense. Likewise, on MRI, the cystic portion of a hemangioblastoma typically has signal characteristics that are the same as those of cerebrospinal fluid. Solid portions of these tumors are usually hypointense to adjacent brain on T1-weighted scans and hyperintense on T2-weighted

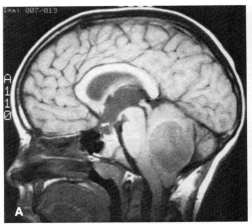
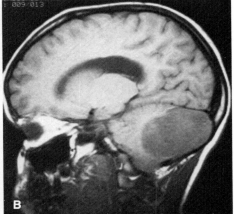
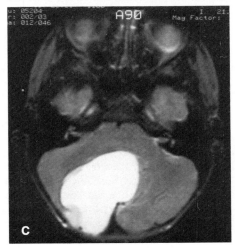

Figure 11–20.   (**A** and **B**) Sagittal T1- and (**C**) axial T2-weighted images from a patient with a pilocystic cerebellar astrocytoma. The sharp demarcation from adjacent normal brain, the large cyst, and the mural nodule are characteristic features of this kind of tumor.

images. Following administration of intravenous contrast medium, the solid portion of a hemangioblastoma enhances intensely both on CT and MRI. On the basis of CT findings alone it may be difficult or even impossible to distinguish a cystic cerebellar hemangioblastoma from a cystic cerebellar astrocytoma (Fig. 11-21). Angiography usually allows this differential to be made, since the mural nodule of a cystic hemangioblastoma typically has enlarged feeding arteries and draining veins, a feature not common in astrocytomas of this nature.[67] Because of its ability to portray vascular structures, MRI is probably more sensitive than is CT in allowing this distinction to be made without the use of angiography.

Medulloblastoma

These malignant tumors, which originate solely in the cerebellum, are the most common posterior fossa tumors of childhood and are unusual in adults. They spread both by direct extension and by dissemination of tumor cells throughout the subarachnoid space. The great majority of childhood medulloblastomas occur in the vermis along the roof of the fourth ventricle. Most medulloblastomas in adults originate more laterally in one of the cerebellar hemispheres. It is unusual for a medulloblastoma to have a significant cystic component, the majority of them being composed of densely cellular tissue; likewise, calcification within these tumors is atypical. With increasing length of survival of patients with these as well as some other malignant tumors of the CNS, there are increasing reports of extraneural metastases particularly to lymph nodes

and bone. Osseous metastases from medulloblastomas occur chiefly in the axial skeleton and may be osteolytic, osteoblastic, or of mixed type.[56] Because most medulloblastomas originate in the cerebellar vermis and grow into the fourth ventricle, obstructive hydrocephalus is common and is frequently the cause of the initial complaint.

On unenhanced CT scans the most typical appearance of a medulloblastoma is a midline vermian mass with attenuation values that are slightly higher than those of the adjacent brain. Except for their location, tumors that originate in the cerebellar hemispheres have a similar appearance. On enhanced CT scans medulloblastomas show an intense increase in their density and are seen to have sharply defined margins. Both the subarachnoid and subependymal metastases of these tumors enhance following administration of intravenous contrast medium (Fig. 11-22).[50, 80]

As with other posterior fossa tumors, MRI is superior to CT for depicting the origin and full extent of these lesions. Probably because of their dense cellularity and scant cytoplasm, most medulloblastomas are of somewhat lower signal intensity on T2-weighted images than are most other primary brain tumors. Both the primary lesion and its parenchymal and subarachnoid metastases enhance markedly after administration of paramagnetic contrast medium.

Ependymoma

From 60% to 75% of ependymomas occur in the posterior fossa and usually have their origin along the floor of the fourth ventricle. Except for location, they are simi-

Figure 11–21. **(A)** Axial noncontrast computed tomogram shows a large, well-circumscribed area of reduced density in the right cerebellar hemisphere. The fourth ventricle is displaced forward and to the left. **(B)** Axial computed tomogram at the same level performed after administration of intravenous contrast medium. A crescent-shaped peripheral area of enhancement is seen on the posterolateral margin of the tumor.

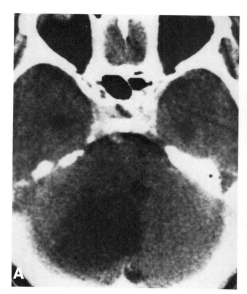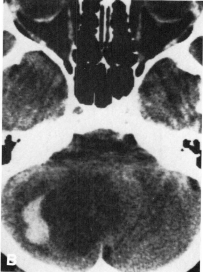

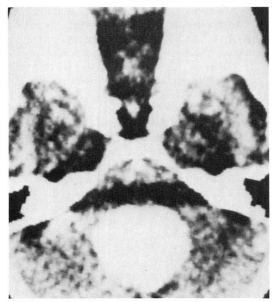

Figure 11–22. Axial computed tomogram performed after administration of intravenous contrast medium. A large, homogeneously enhancing mass fills the fourth ventricle.

lar in appearance to supratentorial ependymomas, which have already been described. Their tendency to spread along the outlets of the fourth ventricle and into the upper cervical spinal canal, along with the frequent occurrence of prominent calcifications, helps in differentiating them from medulloblastomas. As an additional differential point, on both CT and MRI the enhancement seen in these tumors tends to be considerably more heterogeneous than that which occurs in medulloblastomas.

Schwannoma

Schwannomas are benign tumors that occur along the course of cranial, spinal, and peripheral nerves. The previous designation of these tumors as neuromas or neurilemmomas is misleading and should not be used. The discussion that follows is limited to those tumors that involve the cranial nerves.

Schwannomas are primarily tumors of adults and occur considerably more often in females than in males, a 2:1 ratio being reported in some series. The eighth cranial nerve is most frequently involved; most of the other tumors occur on the fifth nerve. There is no explanation for the tendency of these tumors to occur in sensory nerves almost exclusively. Of those schwannomas that originate from the eighth cranial nerve approximately 75% involve the vestibular division, usually its intracanalicular portion. Because of their

location, eighth-nerve schwannomas often produce signs and symptoms when they are quite small. These include a characteristic hearing loss, tinnitus, vertigo, and dizziness. Large eighth-nerve lesions may also cause dysfunction of the fifth and seventh cranial nerves. Schwannomas account for the great majority of tumors that occur in the cerebellopontine angle.

The appearance of an acoustic schwannoma on an unenhanced CT scan depends primarily on its size. Large lesions are visible because of obliteration of the ipsilateral cerebellopontine angle cistern, displacement of the brain stem and fourth ventricle, and widening of the contralateral cerebellopontine angle cistern (Fig. 11-23). Small lesions may be occult or may manifest themselves only by enlargement of the ipsilateral internal auditory canal. Following administration of intravenous contrast medium, schwannomas enhance significantly. Very small tumors that are confined to the internal auditory canal may not, however, be visualized on even the best routine CT scans. MRI is, therefore, recommended over CT as the technique of choice for the evaluation of patients suspected of having a cerebellopontine angle lesion. Except when MRI or modern CT devices are not available, there is now no longer a place for complex motion tomography or CT following placement of air in the subarachnoid space in the evaluation of acoustic schwannomas.

Most schwannomas are well seen on thin-section (3 mm), T1-weighted scans performed in either an axial or coronal projection (Fig. 11-23). On T2-weighted images, these tumors have signal characteristics similar to those of cerebrospinal fluid and may thus be obscured. Because of almost constant, dense enhancement after administration of contrast medium, this technique allows visualization of very small tumors within both the cerebellopontine angle cistern and the internal auditory canal itself.

Except for location, schwannomas of the other cranial nerves appear similar on MRI and CT scan to those of the eighth nerve. MRI is also the technique of choice for evaluation of these lesions.

Neurofibromas are pathologically distinct from schwannomas; however, on the basis of imaging features, differentiation is not possible. Almost all neurofibromas occur in association with von Recklinghausen's disease; bilateral eighth nerve tumors as well as multiple tumors of other cranial nerves are common.

OTHER TUMORS

Choroid Plexus Papilloma

This rare, benign tumor, which usually occurs in children, may originate anywhere that choroid plexus occurs but is most often found within either the fourth ventricle or one of the lateral ventricles. It is often pedunculated, giving it some mobility. It is frequently

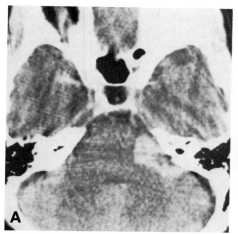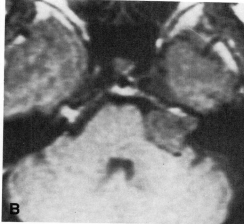

Figure 11–23. **(A)** Axial computed tomogram performed after administration of intravenous contrast medium. There is a homogeneously enhancing mass in the left cerebellopontine angle cistern. The mass is centered at the level of the internal auditory canal. **(B)** Axial MR image taken at the same level as the computed tomogram shown in A. A mass having reduced signal as compared with adjacent normal brain is seen filling the left cerebellopontine angle cistern and extending into the internal auditory canal.

associated with hydrocephalus, the cause of which may be both obstruction of cerebrospinal fluid circulation and overproduction of cerebrospinal fluid. On CT scans performed with the use of intravenous contrast medium, a choroid plexus papilloma is often visible as a mass within a ventricle. Because these tumors are within the choroid and thus outside the BBB, contrast enhancement is marked.[78]

Choroid plexus papillomas typically have multiple areas of calcification and cystic changes. Their vascularity is usually prominent and areas of hemorrhage are common. The MRI appearance of these lesions reflects these characteristics so that typically these tumors have heterogeneous signal intensities on both T-1 and T-2-weighted images. In many instances, prominent areas of hypointensity due either to calcification or vascularity are present. Contrast enhancement is prominent. Angiography is usually required before operative removal of these tumors. It demonstrates the lesion and outlines the extensive blood supply, which is derived from the choroidal arteries.

Chordoma

Chordomas are benign but locally invasive tumors that arise from intraosseous remnants of the notochord. Their most common locations are at either end of the spinal column—the body of the sphenoid bone and clivus and the sacrocoxygeal area. They grow slowly but cause extensive local bone destruction. Neurologic

signs and symptoms are produced as the result of the compression of local neural structures. On unenhanced CT scans, chordomas of the clivus and sphenoid bone appear as areas of bone destruction associated with an irregular soft tissue mass, which may extend into both the basilar cisterns and the nasopharynx. Calcification is usually present within the soft-tissue component of the tumor. Most chordomas are somewhat enhanced following administration of intravenous contrast medium. On occasion these tumors may invaginate the adjacent brain stem, and on the basis of axial CT scan findings alone may be difficult to distinguish from an intraaxial mass. They may also resemble a clivus meningioma, because a clivus meningioma usually does not contain large areas of calcification and does not typically produce florid bone destruction; however, this differential is usually not difficult with careful study.

Although MRI is inferior to CT for demonstrating the bone destruction associated with these tumors it is superior in defining the extent of the lesion and usually allows an accurate diagnosis to be made. Typically these lesions are hypointense on T1 images and are hyperintense on T2-weighted scans.

METASTATIC TUMORS

Metastasis of a remote primary tumor to the brain, its coverings, and the skull is common. Most metastatic tumors arise as the result of hematogenous spread; the initial tumor implants thus tend to occur in the distribution of end arteries, that is, at the gray–white matter junction and in the distribution of deep perforating arteries. Common primary sources are tumors of the lung, breast, colon, kidney, skin, and paranasal sinuses. Carcinomas of the breast and lung account for over half of all metastatic brain tumors. There is wide variability in the CT and MR appearance of metastatic brain tumors. Among factors that influence this variation are the primary source of the tumor (i.e., its cellularity); vascularity and biologic behavior; the number and location of the tumor(s) within the brain; and whether previous treatment has been directed to the area of the tumor.

On unenhanced CT scans, metastatic tumors most often are seen as multiple (solitary metastases also occur commonly, 0% to 40%), fairly discrete areas of isodensity or slight hyperdensity surrounded by low density that extends along and through the white matter. The low density abnormality is believed to be a reflection of edema, and in the majority of metastatic tumors it is substantial. For reasons that are not clear, however, some metastases produce almost no edema, and, when isodense with the adjacent brain, may be occult on scans performed without the use of intravenous contrast. Except for metastases from primary osseous tumors, especially osteogenic sarcomas, calcification is unusual in untreated metastatic brain tumors. Some metastatic tumors show a tendency to hemorrhage spontaneously; these include melanoma, renal cell carcinoma, and choriocarcinoma.

As is the case on unenhanced CT scans, the appearance of metastatic brain tumors on scans performed following the use of intravenous contrast medium varies. Most metastases will be enhanced to some degree, but the pattern that they exhibit shows great variability; enhancement may be ringlike, diffuse (either homogeneous or inhomogeneous), or only in scattered areas with no apparent particular distribution (Fig. 11-24). Tumors in individuals being treated with corticosteroids may not become enhanced because of the medication's stabilizing effect on the BBB. Metastases to the brain may involve the subarachnoid space because of meningeal involvement. This may occur either as an isolated phenomenon or may be seen in association with parenchymal tumors. These meningeal implants appear on contrast-enhanced CT as either areas of nodular high density or as generalized enhancement occurring along the subarachnoid cisterns, fissures, and sulci. Melanoma is one tumor that is particularly prone to this type of involvement.[60]

MRI is more sensitive than CT for the detection of CNS metastatic tumors and is thus the technique of choice for evaluating patients suspected of having such disease. While many metastatic tumors can be recognized on noncontrast-enhanced scans, the use of intravenous contrast medium increases detection of small

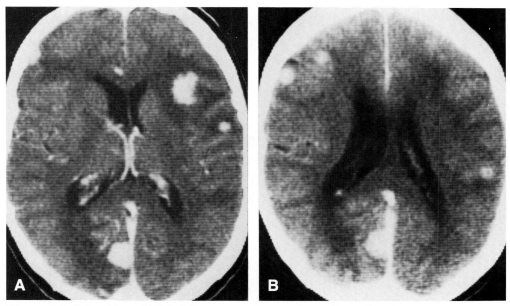

Figure 11–24. (**A** and **B**) Axial computed tomograms done after the administration of intravenous contrast medium. Both cerebral hemispheres show numerous areas of abnormal enhancement. They were metastases from carcinoma of the breast.

and peripheral tumor deposits.[36] As is the case on CT scans, the appearance of metastatic tumors on MRI is variable. Typically, however, the tumor is seen as an area of hypointensity on T1-weighted images and heterogeneous hyperintensity on T2-weighted images. Surrounding most metastatic tumors is edema, which has less signal variation (i.e., it is more homogeneous than the tumor itself). Hemorrhage, cystic change, and necrosis are all common in metastatic tumors and account for the variable signal intensities of these lesions. Most metastases enhance following administration of intravenous contrast medium; as with CT, the pattern of enhancement is variable.

On the basis of CT or MRI scan findings alone it is impossible to predict with accuracy the primary source of a metastatic tumor. Likewise, a solitary metastasis cannot reliably be distinguished from a primary neoplasm of the brain.

Lymphoma

In the absence of systemic disease, involvement of the CNS by non-Hodgkin's lymphoma is designated primary CNS lymphoma. This previously unusual lesion, representing less than 2% of all brain tumors, is now occurring with increasing frequency because of the AIDS epidemic. Patients who are immunosuppressed are at increased risk for the occurrence of primary CNS lymphoma. A significant number of these tumors are multicentric at the time of their diagnosis. While some primary CNS lymphomas are responsive to treatment, the overall prognosis is worse than for tumors with similar histology occurring outside the CNS.

Non-Hodgkin's lymphoma that occurs in the CNS as the result of spread of systemic disease is also uncommon. This type of involvement occurs most often with tumors of diffuse histology and in patients with advanced disease. Hodgkin's disease rarely involves either the brain or the meninges but is more frequent in the latter site.

All types of lymphoma are found most frequently in the cerebral hemispheres, with the basal ganglia, corpus callosum, and periventricular white matter being the areas that are especially likely to be involved. On CT scans performed without contrast medium, these tumors are most often isodense or slightly hyperdense. Following the administration of intravenous contrast medium they typically are enhanced significantly (Fig. 11-25). The pattern of enhancement varies considerably, some tumors being homogeneous with distinct borders and others having areas of irregular enhancement and poorly defined margins. On CT scan some primary lymphomas may closely mimic a meningioma.[10, 49]

On MRI, lymphomas tend to show hypointensity on T1-weighted images and to be hyperintense on T2-weighted scans. Almost all lymphomas enhance following administration of intravenous paramagnetic con-

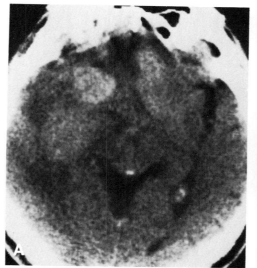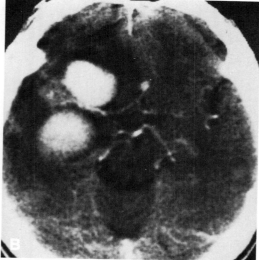

Figure 11–25. (A) Axial noncontrast computed tomogram shows an area of increased density and mass effect in the right frontal and temporal lobes. (B) Axial computed tomogram through the same area performed after administration of intravenous contrast medium shows two well-circumscribed areas of homogeneous enhancement. This was a non-Hodgkin's lymphoma that originated outside the central nervous system.

trast medium. There are no specific signs that allow differentiation of CNS lymphomas from other neoplasms of the brain.

Leukemia

With increasing survival of patients with many types of leukemia, CNS complications are of increasing incidence and significance. The major CNS complications of leukemia are infections, hemorrhages, parenchymal or subarachnoid leukemic infiltrations, and abnormalities related to therapy. CT scans are effective in demonstrating most of these, and the technique plays an important role in the management of such patients.[33, 55] MRI is superior to CT for demonstration of parenchymal or subarachnoid infiltrations. It is less efficient in detection of small recent hemorrhages.

DEMENTIA

Alzheimer's Disease

Brain atrophy is a pathologic description, and therefore, its presence cannot be diagnosed accurately using currently available imaging techniques. Loss of brain substance is a normal function of aging. Studies done using CT scanning have demonstrated that with aging there is both an increase in size of the ventricular system and an increase in the prominence of the cortical sulci; these alterations, however, do not correlate either with changes in the metabolism of the brain as measured with Positron Emission Tomography (PET) techniques or with the presence or absence of cognitive impairment. A strong relationship between the degree of prominence of cortical sulci and age, however, has been demonstrated using CT scans.[27] Alzheimer's disease is the most common cause of both presenile (onset before the age of 60) and senile (onset after the age of 60) dementia. Clinically, it is characterized by the gradual and relentless progression of cognitive impairment; with time, multiple neurologic deficits appear, so that by the terminal phase of the disease patients are totally dependent. Pathologically, it may be impossible in individual cases to distinguish the changes of both presenile and senile dementia of the Alzheimer's type from those that occur with normal aging; neurofibrillary tangles and senile plaque formation are seen in all three conditions.

The CT and MRI scans of patients with Alzheimer's disease show enlargement of the lateral and third ventricles and prominence of cortical sulci (Fig. 11-26). The severity of these changes varies greatly, and they

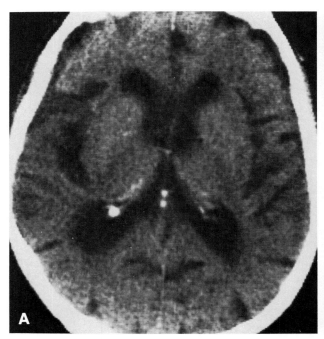
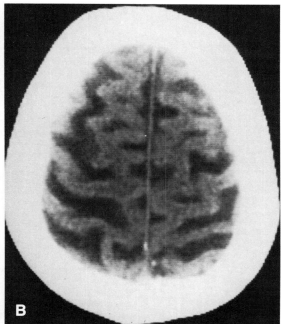

Figure 11–26. (**A** and **B**) Axial noncontrast computed tomograms of a patient with Alzheimer's disease and severe dementia. The ventricular system is dilated, and the sulci over the cerebral hemispheres are enlarged. Identical changes may be seen in some elderly patients who have normal cognitive function.

overlap with those that occur with aging to a degree that makes it impossible to base the diagnosis of Alzheimer's disease on CT or MRI findings alone. Recent studies indicate that structural (i.e., atrophic) changes in the temporal lobe, particularly the hippocampus, are most likely to occur in Alzheimer's disease. The multiplanar capability of MRI combined with the lack of artifact from the bony boundaries of the middle cranial fossa make this technique ideal for assessment of the temporal lobes. MRI is, therefore, the technique of choice for the imaging assessment of patients with dementia of unknown etiology.

Other Causes of Dementia

There are many other causes of loss of intellectual function. Some, such as Huntington's chorea, Parkinson's disease, and a large variety of metabolic disorders, typically produce only nonspecific morphologic changes and cannot be diagnosed using currently available imaging techniques. Others such as severe head trauma and cerebrovascular disease result in changes in the brain that are recognizable on routine CT and MRI scans.

Atherosclerotic cerebrovascular disease, particularly when associated with chronic hypertension, is a common etiologic factor in dementia. Loss of intellec-

tual capacity is frequently noted in patients who suffer large bilateral infarcts; the location of infarction, however, does not correlate well with either the degree or presence of cognitive dysfunction. Binswanger's disease is a particular form of multiinfarct dementia in which multiple, small subcortical infarcts, often of a subclinical nature, result in white-matter ischemic changes and a slowly progressive dementing illness (Fig. 11-27).[47] On CT scan, patients with either multiinfarct dementia or with Binswanger's disease are seen to have multiple areas of low density throughout their cerebral hemispheres. In multiinfarct dementia, these areas of infarction may involve both large and small areas of vascular distribution in the cortex, white matter, and basal ganglia. In Binswanger's disease, the areas of ischemic change tend to be more confined to the distribution of perforating vascular territories (i.e., the basal ganglia and deep white matter with sparing of the immediate subcortical tissue). On MRI these areas of ischemia appear as hypointensities on T1-weighted images and as hyperintensities on T2-weighted sequences. It should be emphasized that there is marked overlap in findings seen on imaging studies of many patients with Alzheimer's disease, multiinfarct dementia and Binswanger's disease, and it is seldom that an accurate diagnosis can be made on the basis of imaging studies alone.[6]

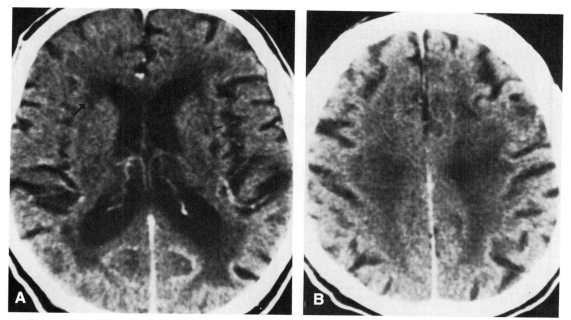

Figure 11–27. **(A)** Axial noncontrast computed tomogram through the level of the basal ganglia shows multiple areas of infarction. **(B)** Computed tomographic section at a higher level shows diffuse abnormality in the white matter of both cerebral hemispheres. The patient had severe dementia.

WHITE-MATTER DISEASE

Multiple Sclerosis

Multiple sclerosis is the most common demyelinating disease. The age of clinical onset of symptoms is most often after the age of 20 and before the age of 50; females are more often affected than are males. The disease is characterized clinically by exacerbations and remissions, and pathologically by multiple plaques representing areas of demyelination of varying activity. While the distribution of demyelination seen in multiple sclerosis is rather random, there is a tendency toward involvement of certain areas. These include the periventricular area, the corpus callosum, and the visual system, from optic nerves to the occipital lobes. The spinal cord is also frequently a site of involvement. The lesions of multiple sclerosis tend to be symmetrical.

Until the development of MRI, imaging techniques had little place in the diagnostic evaluation of patients suspected to have multiple sclerosis. Although on occasion CT scans were of use in excluding other diseases that might simulate multiple sclerosis, several studies have shown this method to be markedly deficient as a tool for detecting areas of demyelination. Other radiologic techniques play no role at all in the diagnosis of this disease. MRI has proved to be a sensitive method for demonstration of multiple sclerosis plaques; in the opinion of some it is the best diagnostic method for use in patients suspected of having multiple sclerosis who have inconclusive or atypical clinical manifestations of the disease.

Plaques of multiple sclerosis are best seen on long TR/TE or long TR, short TE images, and appear as areas of hyperintensity (Fig. 11-28). Currently, it is not possible to distinguish accurately acute from chronic areas of demyelination using MRI techniques. Acute (i.e., active areas of demyelination), often enhance following administration of intravenous contrast medium. The number and distribution of areas of demyelination do not accurately correlate with the clinical severity of the disease. On occasion, solitary plaques of multiple sclerosis may present as a large mass lesion. It is emphasized that there are no specific MRI findings of multiple sclerosis, and numerous other white-matter diseases may simulate this condition.[24]

Progressive Multifocal Leukoencephalopathy (PML)

This progressive, fatal demyelinating disease occurs in patients who are immunosuppressed. It is now commonly seen in patients with AIDS. The myelin destruction is thought to result from invasion and alteration of oligodendroglia by a virus of the papova group.

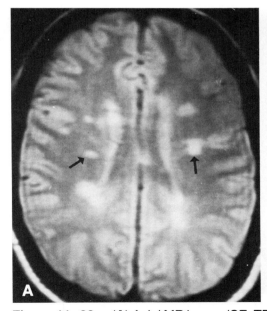 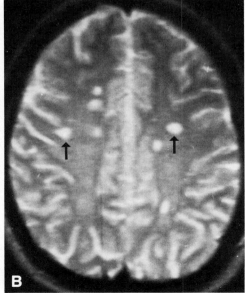

Figure 11–28. (**A**) Axial MR image (SE, TR 2000; TE 30) at the level of the body of the lateral ventricles. Multiple areas of signal abnormality are seen in the white matter of both cerebral hemispheres. (**B**) Axial MR image (SE TR 2000; TE 90) at a slightly higher level shows additional areas of myelin destruction in both cerebral hemispheres.

On unenhanced CT scans, the lesions of PML are seen as areas of white-matter hypodensity that tend to be symmetrical and are most often parietooccipital in location. They do not respect vascular territories and may or may not have some mass effect.[4] Following administration of intravenous contrast medium, enhancement may occur in a few instances.

Necrotizing Leukoencephalopathy

Necrotizing leukoencephalopathy is a disease of unproven cause that occurs primarily in children who have leukemia. It is seen most often in those who have been treated with a combination of cranial radiation and methotrexate. The outcome of the disease is variable. On CT scan necrotizing leukoencephalopathy is characterized by diffuse areas of hypodensity in the white matter; as the disease progresses, white matter calcifications are common. During the active phase of the disease, contrast enhancement is typical but the pattern is variable.[33, 43] As is true for other white matter diseases, MRI is more sensitive than CT for detection of necrotizing leukoencephalopathy. Early lesions are seen best on T2-weighted scans where they appear as areas of high-signal intensity.

Other White Matter Diseases

A host of other diseases involves the white matter either because of myelin destruction (myelinoclastic diseases) or because of inadequate myelin formation or maintenance (dysmyelinating diseases). All of these are uncommon and a discussion of them is beyond the scope of a general text. Radiographic manifestations is discussed elsewhere.[15, 74]

TRAUMA

Until recently, CT had supplanted all other radiographic techniques as a method for the diagnostic evaluation of patients with head trauma, whether acute or chronic. This role is now gradually being supplanted by MRI. In spite of the demonstrated superiority of MRI over CT for detection of posttraumatic injuries, CT remains the technique of choice for the initial assessment of patients with severe head injury. This is true both because a CT examination is faster than an MR scan, and it also allows accurate recognition of those patients who require acute neurosurgical intervention (i.e., hematoma evacuation). Following stabilization, patients who have had significant head injury or who have unexplained neurologic deficits may benefit from an MRI examination because this technique has been shown to depict more clearly the full extent of injury to the brain more effectively than CT.[26]

With currently available CT and MRI techniques it is now possible to visualize clearly both the direct and the indirect effects of trauma on the brain. Subarachnoid, parenchymal, and extraaxial hemorrhages (i.e., subdural and epidural hematomas), occur commonly as the result of both closed head injury or following penetrating trauma; these types of injuries are usually best evaluated with CT scanning. Contusions, shearing injuries, and diffuse swelling of the brain also often occur both separately and together after significant trauma; these types of injuries are often more clearly and more completely demonstrated with MRI than with CT scans.

On CT scans, traumatic parenchymal hematomas appear as clearly defined areas of increased density. If acute, their margins may be irregular but are distinct, and there is little adjacent edema. Unless there is an impairment of the clotting mechanism, hematomas of this nature are homogeneous in character. Traumatic hematomas occur most frequently in the frontal and temporal lobes and in the basal ganglia. As they resolve, these injuries as well as all other significant head injuries may be associated with the development of secondary obstructive hydrocephalus because of associated arachnoid scarring, which causes blockage of the cerebrospinal fluid absorptive pathways.

Shearing injuries are thought to result from severe stresses placed on both the small penetrating arteries and brain parenchyma as the result of the action of sudden rotational forces associated with high-velocity trauma. The result of this type of injury is multiple, small, well-defined hematomas that tend to occur in the subcortical areas, the basal ganglia, corpus callosum, and brain stem. Shearing injuries often reflect severe and extensive damage to the brain and are frequently associated with severe neurologic deficit (Fig. 11-29).

Contusions of the brain are often noted in patients who have experienced significant head trauma. Unless these lesions are very large or are associated with significant hemorrhage, they may not be seen well on CT scans performed shortly after an injury. Later, they become more apparent as areas of mixed low and high density, findings that represent small hemorrhages and surrounding edema. These injuries tend to be superficial, occurring adjacent to bony prominences; they are especially frequent in the portions of the frontal and temporal lobes that lie next to the calvarium (Fig. 11-29). Enlargement of a hematoma in an area of contusion occurring 24 to 72 hours following an initial injury is one of the complications associated with closed head trauma.

CT allows excellent detection and evaluation of intracranial foreign bodies and depressed skull fractures, making other radiographic techniques seldom needed in these conditions.

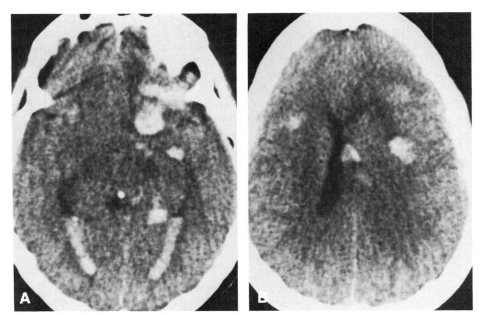

Figure 11–29. (**A**) Axial noncontrast computed tomogram of a patient with severe head trauma. A hemorrhagic contusion is present in the left frontal lobe adjacent to the orbital roof. Two small hematomas are present in the left temporal lobe; there is blood in the posterior portions of both lateral ventricles. (**B**) Computed tomographic section at a higher level shows multiple white matter hemorrhages.

Subdural Hematoma

Bleeding into the subdural space is a frequent complication of head injury; when it occurs, the result is the formation of a subdural hematoma. These lesions are most common over the convexity of the cerebral hemisphere, but may develop at any site over the surface of the brain. They occur infrequently, however, in the posterior fossa. Bilateral subdural hematomas are not uncommon, occurring in approximately 20% of patients. The early use of CT scanning in patients suffering acute head trauma has significantly reduced the previously high mortality rate associated with acute subdural hematomas.

The appearance of a subdural hematoma on CT scan depends on several important factors: the age of the lesion, whether repeated episodes of bleeding have occurred, whether the lesion is unilateral or bilateral, and the level of the patient's hematocrit at the time of the injury. It is most useful to divide subdural hematomas into those that are hyperdense, isodense, and hypodense in relation to the adjacent area of the brain.[30] In general, blood within the subdural space in the early stages of its presence is hyperdense; over a period of two to six weeks it becomes isodense, and after six weeks hypodense, as compared with the CT values present in a healthy brain. Extensive variation in this sequence occurs as the result of rebleeding into a subdural collection, a frequent occurrence, as well as because of differences in the attenuation values of blood caused by variations in the hematocrit levels.

Using CT scan criteria it is thus impossible to accurately classify subdural hematoma as acute, subacute, or chronic. In the majority of instances, however, hyperdense subdural collections have occurred recently, isodense lesions will have been present for at least several days, and hypodense lesions are likely to be of a chronic nature.

With the exception of those instances in which the patient has a very low hematocrit, subdural hematomas studied with CT soon after their occurrence appear as hyperdense collections having a crescentic configuration. The degree of mass effect present in association with these lesions is almost always greater than that which can be accounted for on the basis of the size of the hematoma, a reflection of the underlying brain injury that accompanies most such injuries. The medial margin of very large lesions may be straight or even convex, thus somewhat simulating an epidural collection. If scans are performed soon after the injury or if there are disorders of the coagulation system, the subdural collection may be inhomogeneous, a phenomenon thought to be due to the presence of incomplete clotting within the hematoma (Fig. 11-30).

Although they are encountered infrequently, it is important to be aware of the existence of the isodense subdural hematomas because they may be occult on even high quality CT scans. Unilateral effacement of cortical sulci, asymmetries in the gray–white-matter junction, ventricular asymmetries, and unilateral mass effect are all signs that usually serve to alert one to the presence of a unilateral, isodense, subdural hematoma[29] (Fig. 11-31). Bilateral lesions of this nature may be more difficult to recognize. In older adults, the presence of a "super normal" appearing scan (i.e., one in which the cortical sulci and ventricular system appear like those of a much younger person), is one clue that such lesions may be present. The administration of intravenous contrast medium is valuable in that it results in opacification of dural margins and cortical vessels, thereby allowing good definition of the margins of the brain.

Chronic subdural hematomas usually appear on CT scans as well-defined crescentic collections, the attenuation values of which are hypodense as compared with those of the adjacent area of the brain. As is the case with acute lesions, a very large chronic subdural hematoma may have a straight or even concave medial margin. Episodes of rebleeding may be indicated by inhomogeneous densities within the hematoma. Occasionally, sedimentation levels are seen in dependent portions of such lesions. Calcification of the margins of these lesions occurs frequently.

On MRI, subdural hematomas that appear hypodense on CT will have high-signal intensity on T-1-weighted images because of the hemoglobin that they contain. Because of its sensitivity in detecting blood degradation products of different ages, MRI is more sensitive than CT for identification of subdural hematomas that have undergone multiple episodes of bleeding. These lesions are seen as having multiple collections with signal intensities characteristic of hemoglobin breakdown products of different ages. The membranes separating these areas have low-signal intensities on images made with all pulse sequences.

Subdural Hygroma

A subdural hygroma represents the accumulation of clear fluid in the subdural space. It may be observed following head trauma, in which case it represents either the residual of an old subdural hematoma, or an injury of the arachnoid membrane that has allowed accumulation of cerebrospinal fluid in the subdural space. The mechanisms causing those that are noted in the absence of trauma are poorly understood. Subdural hygromas are usually not symptomatic, and with time they resolve spontaneously. Except for their size, subdural hygromas appear similar on CT scan to the description given for chronic subdural hematomas. These lesions should not be confused with atrophic changes, because the CT scan appearance of the two conditions is quite different (Fig. 11-32). Atrophy produces widening of the cortical sulci, and the involved gyri are not significantly displaced away from the margin of the calvarium. Subdural hygromas represent mass lesions and as such displace the brain away from the skull margin; the adjacent gyri and sulci are effaced and obliterated.

Epidural Hematoma

Epidural hematomas occur as a result of injury to meningeal vessels, and are most often the result of arterial rather than venous disruptions. The most common location of an epidural hematoma is over the lateral surface of one of the cerebral hemispheres; however, like subdural hematomas, they may occur in other places as well.

Except for the rare instances in which they occur in

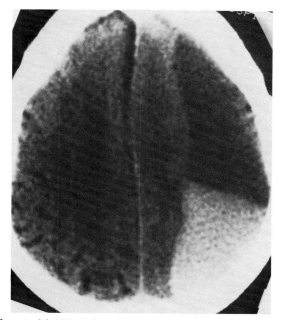

Figure 11–30. Axial noncontrast computed tomogram shows a large subdural hematoma extending over the entire lateral surface of the left cerebral hemisphere. A sedimentation level is seen in this acute subdural hematoma of a patient whose clotting function was impaired.

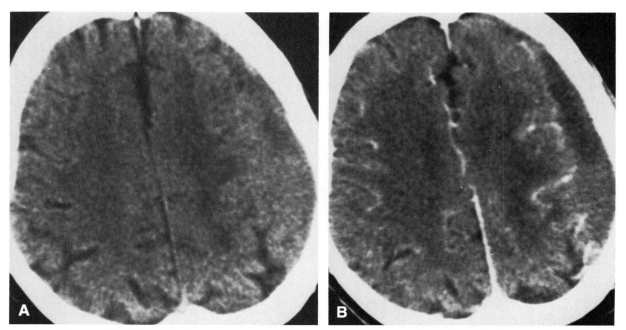

Figure 11–31. (**A**) Axial noncontrast computed tomogram shows inward displacement of the gray white matter junction of the left cerebral hemisphere. Although most of this chronic subdural hematoma is isodense, a small sedimentation level is apparent in its posterior portion. (**B**) Computed tomographic section at the same level as *A* performed after administration of intravenous contrast medium. There is now good visualization of the lateral margin of the left cerebral hemisphere, which is marked by opacified cortical veins.

the presence of severe anemia or severe recent blood loss, epidural hematomas are hyperdense on CT scans. Because they occur peripheral to the dura, which is the periosteum of the inner table of the calvarium, they are more restrained than subdural collections. This is the explanation for their typical biconvex configuration; it also accounts for the observation that they sometimes cross the midline, not being limited as are subdural hematomas by dural attachments. On CT scans, as is the case in subdural hematoma, areas of inhomogeneity within an epidural hematoma indicate either incomplete clotting or active bleeding (Fig. 11-33). Angiography is no longer performed in the evaluation of patients with either subdural or epidural hematomas.

Carotid Cavernous Fistula

As it passes from its bony canal, through the cavernous sinus and into the intracranial cavity, the internal carotid artery is situated so that a laceration can easily result in development of a fistula between the artery and the cavernous sinus and its multiple tributaries. Patients presenting with internal carotid artery cav-

ernous sinus fistulas have usually suffered severe head trauma. Abnormal communications may also occur between the meningeal branches of the external carotid arteries and the cavernous sinus; these fistulae are, however, usually unrelated to trauma. Fistulae between the internal carotid artery and the cavernous sinus are usually high-flow lesions that produce striking ocular signs and symptoms.[13] Endovascular techniques are the treatment of choice for treating carotid cavernous sinus fistula (Fig. 11-34).

The CT and MRI findings of a high-flow internal carotid artery cavernous sinus fistula are enlargement of the cavernous sinus and the ipsilateral superior ophthalmic vein; proptosis may also be present. Depending on their size, dural or indirect fistulas may show similar findings or may be occult on both CT and MRI scans. Angiography provides the definitive diagnosis in both of these conditions.

Porencephaly

The term porencephaly originally indicated a congenital defect consisting of a cavity extending from the surface of one cerebral hemisphere into the adjacent

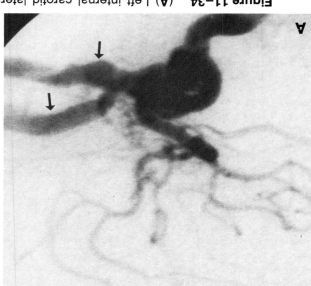

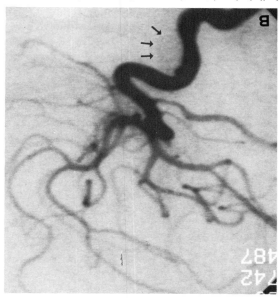

Figure 11–34. **(A)** Left internal carotid lateral digital subtraction arteriogram shows rapid opacification of the cavernous sinus and both the superior and inferior ophthalmic veins (*arrows*). There is a tear in the cavernous segment of the internal carotid artery. **(B)** Left internal carotid lateral digital subtraction arteriogram performed following detachment of a balloon within the cavernous sinus. The fistula is occluded and the internal carotid artery now appears normal. The margins of the balloon are faintly seen (*arrows*).

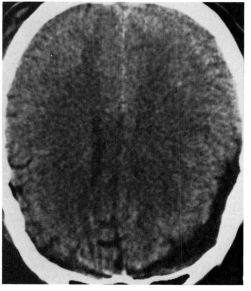

Figure 11–32. Axial noncontrast computed tomogram shows a small, low-density, extra axial collection over the right frontal lobe. There is slight mass effect and the adjacent sulci are compressed. Contrast the appearance of this scan with that of Figure 30B.

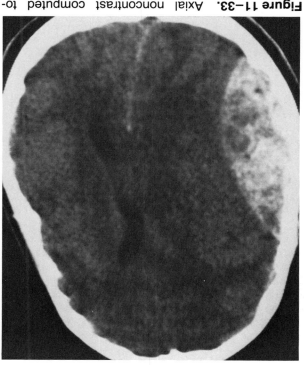

Figure 11–33. Axial noncontrast computed tomogram shows an acute epidural hematoma over the lateral surface of the right cerebral hemisphere. The nonhomogeneous attenuation levels within it are the result of incomplete clotting.

lateral ventricle. It is now used without precise mean-ing, however, and indicates a variety of either single or multiple defects in the parenchyma of the brain of various etiologies. As defined by this usage, poren-cephalic cavities may communicate with either the subarachnoid space, the ventricular system, or with neither; they may be of congenital, posttraumatic, postischemic or postinflammatory etiology.

On CT and MRI scans areas of porencephaly appear most often as cerebrospinal fluid density/intensity col-lections extending from one of the superficial margins of a lateral ventricle. A small porencephaly is seen as an area of focal ventricular dilatation with no apparent abnormality in the adjacent brain. Large areas of por-encephaly are seen as round, cystlike lesions extending from the side or top of a lateral ventricle, often reaching the surface of the cerebral hemisphere. The sulci im-mediately adjacent to a porencephalic cyst are usually dilated, a feature that helps distinguish this lesion from an arachnoid cyst. When major destruction of brain tissue, leading to the development of an extensive area of porencephaly, occurs either in utero or in early postnatal life, there is often compensatory thickening of the calvarium and overexpansion of the frontal and ethmoid sinuses and mastoid cells. Large porencepha-lic cysts may act as mass lesions and thereby have the potential to cause a variety of neurologic signs and symptoms; they may also cause secondary hydro-cephalus because of blockage of the interventricular foramen or aqueduct of Sylvius.

ARACHNOID CYSTS

Intracranial arachnoid cysts are found in various loca-tions, with the most common being within the sylvian fissure. Other sites of involvement are the cerebello-pontine angle cisterns, the suprasellar region, the paracollicular area, and the interhemispheric fissure. The majority of arachnoid cysts are congenital. The symptoms they produce depend on both their size and location; it is by compression of the adjacent neural structures that they cause neurologic dysfunction. On CT scan they appear as well-demarcated, thin-walled masses with attenuation values the same as those of cerebrospinal fluid. They do not contain calcium or fat, and their margins are not enhanced following adminis-tration of intravenous contrast medium. Large arach-noid cysts may cause deformity of the adjacent cal-varium. Some arachnoid cysts communicate freely with the subarachnoid space and ventricular system, while others are at least partially isolated. CT scans performed with low doses of water-soluble contrast medium in the intracranial subarachnoid space are valuable in determining the cerebrospinal fluid dy-namics associated with these lesions.[25,46] Largely be-

cause of its multiplanar nature, arachnoid cysts are demonstrated more clearly on MRI than on CT; their signal characteristics match those of CSF on all pulse sequences (Fig. 11-35).

INFECTIOUS DISEASES OF THE BRAIN

The role of imaging studies in evaluation of patients suspected of having infectious disease of the brain or its coverings has increased greatly with recent advances in the capabilities of CT, MRI, and intracranial ultra-sound. In large part because of the increased numbers of immunosuppressed patients, there has been an in-crease in the variety of agents that cause infections of the CNS. Because the pathologic and, thus, by neces-sity, the imaging manifestations of CNS infections are limited, the information provided by the diagnostic methods of CT, MRI, and ultrasound can be optimized only if the clinical setting in which an infectious illness occurs is known. The role of imaging techniques in the diagnosis and management of patients with CNS infec-tions is discussed elsewhere.[16,38]

Brain Abscess

Brain abscesses occur most frequently because of he-matogenous dissemination of infectious agents from a distant site (most often the lung). They may also result, however, from the direct spread of an infection from a location such as a paranasal sinus or the middle ear. Abscesses that develop from the hematogenous spread of microorganisms occur most frequently in the cere-bral hemispheres, along the corticomedullary junction and in the basal ganglia. A wide variety of organisms has been associated with brain abscesses; none of these produce totally characteristic radiographic findings. Immunosuppression, cyanotic heart disease, and pul-monary arteriovenous fistulae predispose patients to the development of brain abscess. The ability to define the extent and characteristics of a brain abscess with CT, MRI, and ultrasound, as well as the use of these methods as guides for the surgical treatment of ab-scesses that do not respond to medical therapy have greatly reduced the high morbidity and mortality pre-viously associated with these lesions.

During the course of its development, a brain ab-scess evolves through a number of stages.[7] Initially, it is a poorly defined area consisting of small, scattered foci of inflammation (i.e., cerebritis); when mature, it is a well-demarcated, encapsulated lesion, the central por-tion of which consists of suppurative material and tis-sue debris. The appearance of a brain abscess on CT, MRI, or ultrasound depends primarily on the stage in its development during which the study is performed.[17] On CT scans, early lesions may be seen only as areas

of hypodensity, with little, if any, enhancement occurring after administration of intravenous contrast medium. Over time, as neovascularity and a collagen capsule develop, however, a pattern of ring enhancement will become apparent. The ring or margin of an incompletely encapsulated abscess becomes thicker and shows increased intensity of enhancement on scans performed 30 to 45 minutes following intravenous contrast administration. The margin of a mature abscess does not show this pattern and often may even decrease in intensity on delayed scans. Except in immunocompromised patients who are taking corticosteroids, studies done before the onset of treatment usually show extensive vasogenic edema surrounding the area of a brain abscess (Fig 11-36). Except in the immunocompromised patient, multiple abscesses are unusual. On ultrasound examination, an

abscess appears as a hypoechoic area surrounded by an echogenic rim.

MRI is superior to CT for evaluation of patients with brain abscesses because of its increased contrast sensitivity (i.e., better detection of edema and characterization of the various elements of an abscess), the lack of associated artifact from bone at the skull base, and, because of its multiplanar capability, its superior ability to detect subtle mass effect.[32] The abscess capsule is its hallmark and this is best characterized on either contrast-enhanced or T2-weighted MRI scans. The thin, relatively smooth capsule enhances uniformly. On T2-weighted scans it is hypointense as compared with gray matter. Often, adjacent, smaller, so-called satellite capsules are present, particularly along the margin of an abscess that faces one of the lateral ventricles. Healing of an abscess is indicated by a decrease in its size; it is

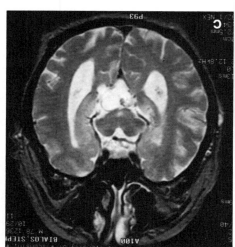

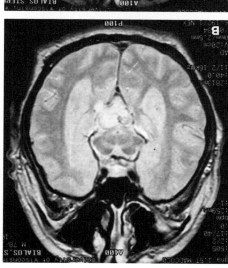

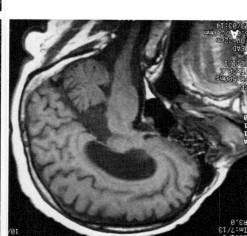

Figure 11-35. (A) Sagittal T1- (B) axial proton density, and (C) axial T2-weighted images from a patient with a quadrigeminal cistern arachnoid cyst. The signal characteristics of the lesion follow those of cerebrospinal fluid. Signal from adjacent vascular and dural structures accounts for the low-signal intensity areas seen around the anterior margin of the lesion on the axial images.

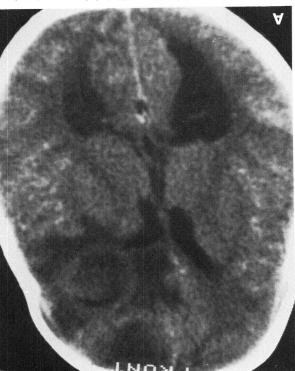

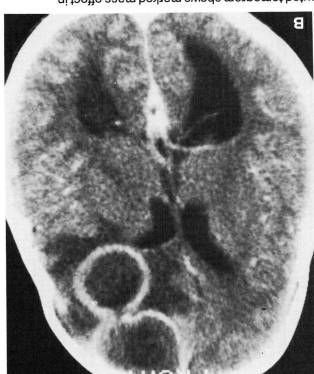

Figure 11-36. **(A)** Axial noncontrast computed tomogram shows marked mass effect in the left frontal lobe. Ringlike areas of isodense tissue are surrounded by low-density edema. **(B)** Axial computed tomographic section at the same level performed after administration of intravenous contrast medium shows enhancement of the periphery of a multiloculated abscess cavity. The patient had a right-to-left cardiac shunt.

important in this regard to emphasize that on both CT and MRI, enhancement of the capsule may persist for some time despite adequate treatment.

Subdural and Epidural Empyema

Although suppurative infections in the subdural or epidural space are uncommon, it is important that they be recognized, because if untreated they are associated with high mortality. Most infections of this nature occur in association with osteomyelitis of the skull, sinusitis, meningitis, or penetrating trauma. In general, on CT scans these lesions appear as areas of hypodensity over the surface of the brain; they may extend into the interhemispheric fissure or along the margins of the tentorium. They are, unless very small, associated with mass effect. Following administration of intravenous contrast medium, variable enhancement is seen about the margins of both subdural and epidural empyemas. Hypodensity is often present within the brain adjacent to this type of infection.[48,82] Subdural empyemas, like

subdural hematomas, are limited by the attachments of the dura; this may be the only way to distinguish an epidural from a subdural suppurative process.

Herpes Simplex

Herpes simplex virus type I causes a severe encephalitis that can occur at any age but is most often seen in adults. If untreated it is often fatal and those persons who survive are frequently left with severe neurologic deficits. Most adults in the general population have antibodies to the herpes simplex type I virus; this organism is also known to exist in a latent form within the trigeminal ganglia of many asymptomatic people. It is not certain whether the encephalitis caused by this agent represents spread from this site or is the result of a new infection.[16]

The CT scan findings of this type of encephalitis are not specific; however, when seen in the appropriate clinical setting they are often characteristic enough to suggest the definitive diagnostic study, that is, brain

biopsy. One important characteristic of herpes simplex type I encephalitis is its tendency to involve the temporal lobes, orbital surfaces of the frontal lobes, and insular cortex, while sparing the nuclei of the basal ganglia. Although not commonly seen, small areas of hemorrhage are also typical. On scans performed without administration of intravenous contrast medium the lesions are seen as areas of reduced attenuation. Early in the infection, enhancement is minimal, if present; later, it often becomes striking. A gyral configuration of the abnormal enhancement is said to be characteristic.[18, 31]

MRI is more sensitive for detection of the changes of herpes simplex type 1 encephalitis than CT, especially in its early stages.[38, 40] Areas of abnormality are seen as reduced-signal intensity on T1-weighted images and as high-signal intensity on T2-weighted scans. Mass effect may be present. The pattern of enhancement is similar to that seen on contrast-enhanced CT scans.

Herpes simplex type 2 encephalitis is most commonly seen in the newborn, frequently in association with a maternal type 2 genital infection and usually as part of a systemic infection. This type of herpes encephalitis does not have the typical geographic distribution that is seen with a type I herpes infection. There are no specific imaging findings, the most typical manifestation being widespread areas of involvement that, on CT scans, appear as reduced density and on MRI as areas of T1 and T2 prolonged relaxation.

Human Immunodeficiency Virus

Clinically manifest neurologic involvement occurs in well over 50% of those individuals infected by the Human Immunodeficiency Virus (HIV); CNS abnormalities are even more commonly present on postmortem examinations of those infected by the HIV. The spectrum of lesions associated with this disease is broad and includes abnormalities directly related to the virus itself (i.e., AIDS encephalitis, neoplasms), and a large variety of secondary viral and nonviral infections. All of these processes are likely to be detected earlier and be seen more clearly with MRI than with CT. A complete discussion of the effects of HIV on the brain is available elsewhere.[62]

AIDS encephalitis is the most common CNS manifestation of infection with HIV; it is believed to result from the direct effects of the virus itself. On both CT and MRI, the most common manifestation of AIDS encephalitis is cortical and central atrophy. White-matter involvement is best detected on T2-weighted MRI images, where it appears early as focal areas of high-signal intensity; later, as the disease progresses, these become more prominent and tend to coalesce. Mass effect is not a feature of AIDS encephalitis.

A large variety of secondary viral and nonviral infectious processes are also commonly seen in individuals with AIDS. None of these produce characteristic or specific findings, and, in many instances, multiple infectious processes exist simultaneously. Toxoplasmosis, cryptococcus, cytomegalovirus, progressive multifocal leukoencephalopathy (papoviruses), and cysticercosis are among the more commonly encountered infectious agents. Toxoplasmosis is the most commonly experienced nonviral secondary infection of the CNS seen in individuals with AIDS, and typically is seen on CT or MRI examinations as either single- or multiple-mass lesions that have a ring enhancement pattern on contrast enhanced scans.

Non-Hodgkin's primary CNS lymphoma also occurs with an increased incidence in individuals with AIDS and may closely mimic many of the infectious complications mentioned above.

CONGENITAL MALFORMATIONS

Congenital malformations are defined as structural defects present at birth. These are characterized by evidence of arrested or abnormal development and occurrence of the defect during the intrauterine period. Using these criteria, as many as 2% of neonates have these lesions; at least one third of them involve the brain or spinal cord. The availability of CT, ultrasound, and MRI has greatly simplified the evaluation of patients with congenital malformations. These techniques have also advanced our understanding about the nature of many of these lesions. While a comprehensive discussion of CNS malformations is beyond the scope of this text, several relatively common specific malformations warrant some comment.

Chiari Malformation

The neuroanatomic complex known as the Chiari malformation consists of three types of brain stem and cerebellar abnormalities of unproved etiology. A complete description of the points that separate these types is beyond the scope of this text; however, important differences are as follows. Type I consists of variable degrees of downward displacement of the inferior cerebellum and cerebellar tonsils without any gross abnormality of the medulla or fourth ventricle; type II also has similar caudal displacement of the cerebellum, but the medulla and fourth ventricle are also abnormal; and, type III has malformations in which the medulla, fourth ventricle and most of the cerebellum are displaced into an occipital and cervical encephalomeningocele.

Type I malformations are usually asymptomatic until adulthood and are not usually associated with a myelomeningocele. They become clinically apparent for a variety of reasons, prominent among which are visual complaints, ataxia, and cervical pain. Segmentation abnormalities of the cervical spine are seen in as many as half of the patients found to have a type I Chiari malformation. The caudal displacement of the cerebellum, which constitutes this lesion, is easily and best recognized on MR images (Fig. 11-37). When MRI is not available, a CT scan performed with water-soluble contrast medium in the subarachnoid space provides an alternate method of diagnosis. Hydromyelia is commonly seen in association with a type I Chiari malformation.

Type II malformations are the most common variety and are nearly always associated with myelomeningocele. MRI, CT, and ultrasonography are all useful in the evaluation of these patients. In principle, MRI is ideal because it allows clear visualization of the multiple facets of this lesion. CT and ultrasonography remain of value, however, in evaluation of patients with this lesion. The CT manifestations of a typical Chiari II malformation include (1) failure to visualize the fourth ventricle, (2) a posterior concavity of the surfaces of the petrous bones, (3) a beaked appearance of the tectum of the midbrain, (4) a heart-shaped appearance of the cerebellum at its upper level, (5) interdigitation of the

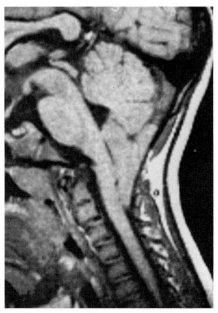

Figure 11–37. Sagittal T1-weighted MR image from a patient with a Chiari I malformation. The cerebellar tonsils are dysplastic and are displaced caudally through the foramen magnum. The fourth ventricle has a normal position.

cerebral hemispheres along the interhemispheric fissure, and (6) hydrocephalus with inferior pointing of the frontal horns of the lateral ventricles (Fig. 11-38). These appearances are seen to even better advantage on MR images. They have been discussed in detail by Naidich and his associates in a now classic series of articles on this subject.[51]

Dandy Walker Cyst

This malformation of unproved etiology has as its principal features aplasia of the cerebellar vermis and cystic dilatation of the fourth ventricle; generally, there is associated hydrocephalus. The CT and MRI scan appearance of a Dandy Walker cyst is characteristic, indicated by small cerebellar hemispheres, dilatation of the fourth ventricle, absence of at least a large portion of the cerebellar vermis, a high position of the tentorium, and a large posterior fossa. Dandy Walker variants are lesions in which the degree of cerebellar hemispheric and vermian dysgenesis is less severe. This lesion should be differentiated from an arachnoid cyst of the posterior fossa because the treatment of the two may be quite different.

Agenesis of the Corpus Callosum

Agenesis of the corpus callosum may occur as an isolated abnormality or may be seen in association with a host of other congenital abnormalities of the brain. Agenesis may be either partial or complete; when partial, the defect most often involves the splenium. The CT scan appearance of callosal agenesis is typical; in the classic example, there is deformity and separation of the lateral ventricles and upward herniation of the third ventricle. Because of its multiplanar capability alone, MRI is superior to CT scanning for demonstration of this malformation. In children with open fontanelles, ultrasound provides another method for recognition of this defect.

Hydrocephalus

Hydrocephalus is defined as an abnormal accumulation of fluid within the cranial cavity. This definition, however, is too inclusive to be of real use, and the term is now generally reserved for those conditions that produce an imbalance between the rate of production and absorption of the cerebrospinal fluid. Implied is the presence of increased intraventricular pressure; usually there is also an associated increased volume of cerebrospinal fluid within the ventricular system. Hydrocephalus normally occurs as the result of obstruction to the flow and thus the absorption of cerebrospinal fluid. Instances resulting from overproduction of

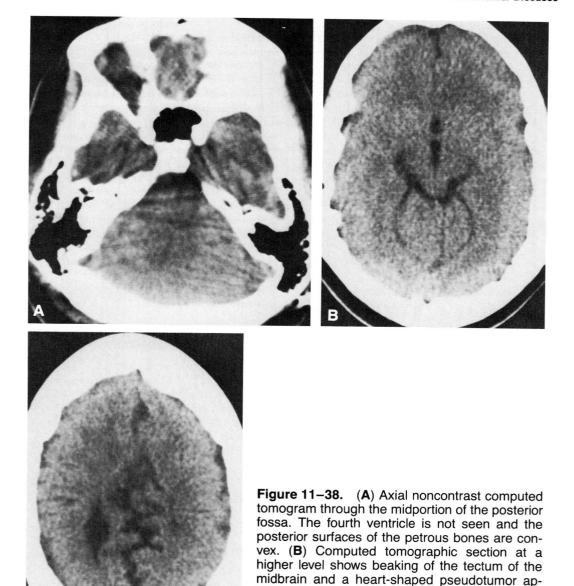

Figure 11–38. **(A)** Axial noncontrast computed tomogram through the midportion of the posterior fossa. The fourth ventricle is not seen and the posterior surfaces of the petrous bones are convex. **(B)** Computed tomographic section at a higher level shows beaking of the tectum of the midbrain and a heart-shaped pseudotumor appearance of the upper portion of the cerebellum. **(C)** Computed tomographic section at a higher level shows interdigitation of the medial surfaces of the cerebral hemispheres.

cerebrospinal fluid are very rare. Hydrocephalus may be either congenital or acquired.

After its production by the choroid plexus, arterial pulsations as well as other forces generated by respiration and gravity result in the pulsatile flow of cerebrospinal fluid. The pathway normally taken is from the lateral ventricles through the interventricular foramina, third ventricle, and aqueduct of Sylvius into the fourth ventricle, and then into the basal cisterns by way of the paired lateral foramen of Luschka and the midline foramen of Magendie. From the basal cisterns, the fluid passes superiorly through the subarachnoid space to reach its site of absorption at the arachnoid villi, which lie over the convexities of the cerebral hemispheres. Hydrocephalus may occur if blockage of this flow occurs at any site along this route. It is known that alternate, though much less efficient, routes of cerebrospinal fluid absorption exist by way of both the ventricular ependyma and the arachnoid membrane.

The term *communicating hydrocephalus* has been used to refer to instances in which there is a blockage of cerebrospinal fluid flow outside the ventricular system; *noncommunicating hydrocephalus* refers to the presence of a blockage within the ventricular system. *Hydrocephalus ex vacuo* indicates the presence of increased cerebrospinal fluid volume as a compensatory measure occurring in response to the loss of brain tissue. All of these terms are incomplete and are potentially confusing. Because essentially all forms of hydrocephalus are due to obstruction of cerebrospinal fluid flow, the use of these terms should be replaced with descriptions that indicate the location at which the blockage occurs. This classification system has been discussed in detail by Harwood-Nash and Fitz, and more recently by Floodmark.[21, 34] The development of hydrocephalus in children is usually associated with an increase in head size. This is unusual in adults.[19]

Acquired Hydrocephalus

As already mentioned, it is possible to develop obstruction of the flow of cerebrospinal fluid anywhere between its site of production and its point of absorption. Many pathologic conditions, including inflammatory, infectious, traumatic and neoplastic disorders, can thus cause hydrocephalus. The presence of increased intraventricular or intracranial pressure can rarely be diagnosed accurately using imaging techniques. In instances of suspected hydrocephalus it is the goal of the imaging evaluation to identify any abnormality of the ventricular or subarachnoid space morphology and, if ventriculomegaly is present, to demonstrate the site and nature of any blockage to the flow of cerebrospinal fluid that may be present. MRI is the best available imaging method with which to achieve this goal.

Most patients with hydrocephalus have enlargement of some part of their ventricular system; that portion above an obstruction being dilated while that below is of normal size. Even in the face of increased intraventricular pressure, however, all portions of the involved ventricular system may not dilate equally. For example, in response to an obstruction that occurs in the basal cisterns, the temporal and occipital horns of the lateral ventricles dilate earlier and to a greater degree than the third and fourth ventricles. When there is significant obstruction of the circulation of cerebrospinal fluid, its passage through the ependymal lining of the ventricles into the adjacent white matter of the cerebral hemispheres occurs as an attempt to correct the imbalance between the rate of production and absorption. On CT scan this is manifested by periventricular hypodensity, which is often more pronounced in the parietal and occipital region than in the frontal area. On MRI, this periventricular increase in white-matter water content is seen best on T2-weighted images, where it appears as a bilateral smooth band of high-signal intensity.

In children with patent anterior fontanelles, ultrasound is an ideal way to assess ventricular size, and, when possible, should be used instead of CT scanning for this purpose. Because of the advantages discussed previously, MRI is supplanting CT as the technique of choice for evaluation of patients with hydrocephalus. This technique shows considerable promise for allowing direct visualization of CSF flow, rather than the mere demonstration of the secondary effects occurring because of impaired CSF circulation. For example, on T2-weighted images, the low-signal intensity of flowing CSF in the cerebral aqueduct stands out in contrast to the higher-signal intensity of the adjacent tectum of the mesencephalon. This is a useful sign of aqueductal patency.[4]

Congenital Hydrocephalus

The potential causes of congenital hydrocephalus include all those conditions listed under the discussion of acquired hydrocephalus. In most instances, however, no identifiable etiology can be defined and the fault seems to lie in some defect of the cerebrospinal fluid absorption mechanism.

The clinical diagnosis of congenital hydrocephalus is usually made with difficulty, so imaging evaluations, CT, ultrasound, and MRI are frequently required to confirm the diagnosis, to establish the severity of ventricular dilation, and to follow the progress of treatment.

Normal Pressure Hydrocephalus

The term "normal pressure hydrocephalus" (NPH) was originally used to describe the syndrome of dementia, gait disturbances, and urinary incontinence occurring in patients with ventricular enlargement and normal cerebrospinal fluid pressure. The diagnosis subsequently has been applied with such indiscretion that there is now great confusion in the literature about the pathogenesis, pathophysiology, and treatment of the condition. While a full discussion of this subject is beyond the scope of this text, a few general comments are warranted.

The finding of large ventricles and normal or small cortical sulci in the presence of normal cerebrospinal fluid pressure has been called NPH by some. This does not reflect the original use of the term, and its use should be discouraged because these observations may be seen in a host of clinical settings, an important one of which is normal variation.

The apparent paradox of progressive ventricular enlargement with normal intraventricular pressure has been explained by this theory: after single or multiple episodes of intermittent increased ventricular pressure, the ventricles dilate, thereby increasing their surface area. Then, according to Pascal's law (force = pressure × area), further dilatation can occur because of this increased surface area, even in the presence of now normal intraventricular pressure. While appealing, this explanation oversimplifies the situation because it does not account for the influence of other factors such as alterations in the elasticity and integrity of the periventricular white matter that are known to occur when there are changes in ventricular volume and pressure.

The success of surgical treatment of NPH (i.e., shunting), varies greatly among reported series. Improvement is most likely when treatment is reserved for those patients who show evidence of progression of mild dementia, ataxia, and urinary incontinence, and who are shown to have lateral ventricular enlargement and small or obliterated cortical sulci.[39] Recent MRI studies suggest that improvement is most likely to occur in those patients with the appropriate clinical findings (i.e., recent and slowly progressive dementia), gait ataxia, and urinary incontinence, as well as evidence of rapid CSF flow in their fourth ventricle and cerebral aqueduct. This flow is seen best as low-signal intensity on heavily T2-weighted images.

VASCULAR DISEASE

Extracranial Occlusive Disease

In 1914 Ramsey Hunt first suggested that stenosis of a carotid artery in the neck could cause a stroke. Since that time a clear relationship between thromboembolic stroke and vascular disease of the carotid and vertebral arteries has been established. Current evidence suggests that at least as many ischemic episodes are caused by embolization of platelet debris from atherosclerotic lesions within these arteries as those that result in impairment of blood flow by hemodynamically significant stenosis. Ischemia of the brain may therefore result either from diminished blood flow occurring as the result of a significant stenosis or because of arterial blockage occurring as a sequel to embolization.

Although the incidence and type of atherosclerotic lesions present in the extracranial arteries of asymptomatic persons is unknown, it is established that advanced lesions of this nature are sometimes present in the cervical arteries of neurologically asymptomatic people. This observation in part explains the controversy and lack of guidelines for diagnostic evaluation and management of patients with asymptomatic atherosclerotic disease. It seems prudent to regard these abnormalities as only part of a more generalized vasculopathy affecting arteries throughout the body, and to direct therapy at the underlying cause of the disorder rather than to marshall all efforts toward correction of morphologic abnormalities found in isolated arterial segments.

The diagnostic evaluation and management of those patients with symptomatic vascular disease is less controversial. Optimal application of established guidelines, however, depends on an accurate assessment of the type of arterial lesion that is present as well as precise characterization of the type of neurologic dysfunction. Once it has occurred, the course of an ischemic stroke is largely refractory to therapy, and the end result is persistent neurologic dysfunction or death in a majority of patients. An effective therapy must therefore be prophylactic, a restriction requiring recognition of the population at risk before they suffer neurologic damage. Risks known to be important in this regard are the presence of all degrees of arterial hypertension, smoking, and a history of intermittent episodes of neurologic dysfunction (i.e., transient ischemic attacks).

Asymptomatic Vascular Disease

Many patients with asymptomatic vascular disease, for a variety of reasons, have a carotid bruit. Although there is an increased incidence of stroke associated with an asymptomatic bruit, the risk is not confined to the arterial territory from which the bruit originates. Because the natural history of asymptomatic vascular disease of this nature has not been completely defined, there is no way in which the value of any prophylactic therapy can be assessed. Some data indicate that those bruits originating from hemodynamically significant lesions are more significant as a risk factor for stroke than are those that occur because of less severe disease.

Duplex ultrasonography offers a method for the accurate noninvasive screening of patients in this category. When properly used, this technique allows recognition of hemodynamically significant lesions (reduction of the arterial lumen by at least 80%) in the cervical portion of the carotid arteries about 95% of the time. If warranted, further evaluation may then be carried out using arteriographic techniques described in the following section.

Symptomatic Vascular Disease

Guidelines for the diagnostic evaluation of patients with specific symptoms of extracranial vascular disease, such as carotid artery territory transient ischemic attacks and evolving or completed strokes, are reasonably well defined. Guidelines for the care of patients with nonspecific symptoms are much more ambiguous and are beyond the scope of this text.

It has recently been established through a carefully performed multicenter randomized trial that carotid endarterectomy is highly beneficial in patients with carotid artery transient ischemic attacks and an ipsilateral stenosis greater than 70%.[54] There is also general agreement that this procedure is also indicated for those individuals who have either recurrent carotid distribution transient ischemic attacks while on appropriate medical therapy, or a stenosis less than 70% associated with a contralateral carotid occlusion. Carotid endarterectomy is not believed to be indicated for patients who have an evolving carotid distribution stroke. One requirement for optimal application of this therapy is precise characterization of the morphologic status of both the intracranial and extracranial arteries. In the past, duplex ultrasonography, as well as other noninvasive techniques, have had little place in the evaluation of these patients because they did not allow assessment of the intracranial vasculature. Recent improvements in transcranial Doppler techniques (TCD) and magnetic resonance angiography (MRA) are, however, making it possible in some situations to modify previous guidelines stating that all symptomatic patients be evaluated with standard catheter arteriography. MRA and TCD will soon assume increasingly important roles in the evaluation of the patient with symptomatic as well as asymptomatic extracranial vascular disease.

Arteriography, when required, may be performed using intravenous digital subtraction, arterial digital subtraction, or standard film–screen techniques. Except for the unusual patient in whom arterial access is either impossible or very hazardous, there is now little place for the use of intravenous digital subtraction arteriography. If necessary, however, most patients can be studied in a definitive manner using intravenous digital techniques (Fig. 11-39).

The use of digital subtraction techniques in conjunction with the intraarterial injection of contrast medium offers significant advantages over standard methods of arteriography. These include reductions in total contrast medium dose required, time to per-

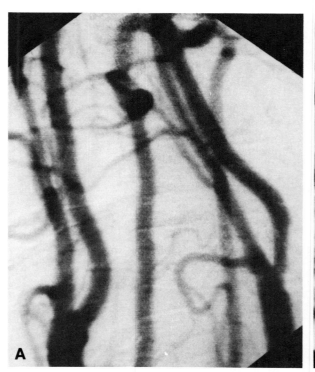
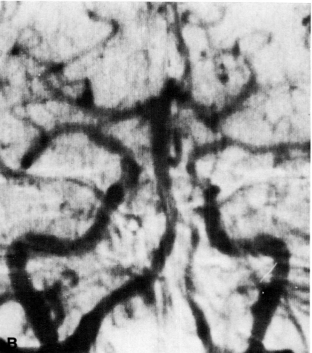

Figure 11–39.   **(A)** Oblique projection of an intravenous digital subtraction arteriogram. The cervical portions of both carotid arteries and the vertebral arteries are well demonstrated. **(B)** PA projection of an intravenous digital subtraction arteriogram showing the intracranial circulation. Arteries to the level of the circle of Willis are clearly demonstrated.

form a study, and film required to record the results of an examination. Although the spatial resolution of digital angiography is lower than that available with standard angiography, this difference has not been of clinical significance. For intraarterial digital subtraction arteriography, the concentration of contrast medium is usually diluted to one third of that employed for standard arteriography.

Atherosclerotic vascular lesions occur most often at regions of hemodynamic stress, particularly at points of major arterial bifurcations. The principal sites of atherosclerotic lesions of the extracranial cervical vasculature are the origins of the brachiocephalic vessels, the carotid bifurcations, and the origins of the vertebral arteries. Stenosis produced by an atherosclerotic plaque tends to narrow the lumen of the involved artery in an eccentric fashion (Fig. 11-40). Small discrete areas of calcification often can be seen adjacent to and within a plaque extending into a narrowed artery. The angiographic diagnosis of arterial occlusion is usually not difficult, the abnormality being characterized by a sudden termination of the arterial lumen. The configuration of an arterial occlusion varies with the artery, sometimes being rounded and at other times being quite angular. Arterial ulceration cannot be detected accurately using any currently available imaging technique other than those that employ radioactive platelets. Arterial ulceration may even go undetected on direct inspection of the involved vessel. Radiographic assessment of arteries involved by atherosclerosis should be limited to description of the vessel as smooth or irregular, and to the degree of narrowing that may be present.

Brain Infarction

Brain infarction may occur as the end result of a large number of pathologic processes, by far the most common of which is atherosclerosis. Approximately 60% of ischemic brain infarcts are etiologically related to atherosclerotic disease of the extracranial segment of the internal carotid artery. A significant percentage of all embolic brain infarctions also result from emboli that originate within the heart. Other causes of brain infarction, besides atherosclerotic vascular disease, include other primary arterial diseases such as fibromuscular hyperplasia, arterial dissections, and arteritis; venous occlusive disease and a host of more unusual diseases such as septic and tumor embolizations may also be associated with infarction of the brain.

Although CT continues to be the most commonly employed imaging technique for evaluation of patients with suspected strokes, MRI has been shown to be a superior method both in permitting earlier detection of ischemic changes and in allowing identification of infarcts not visible on CT scans. These advantages arise from the superior ability of MRI to detect edema and its freedom from artifact caused by the bone and air at the skull base. Most symptomatic infarctions can be recognized with MRI within 12 to 24 hours of their occurrence. MRI is especially useful in demonstrating ischemic changes that involve the brain stem or cerebellum. In most instances, the use of intravenous contrast medium is not required for the diagnosis of infarct, either with CT scanning or MRI. The suggestive evidence that the use of contrast-enhanced CT scans in evaluation of cerebral infarcts is associated with increased damage to neural structures provides added incentive to avoid contrast administration when possible.

The CT scan findings seen following an infarct depend on the size of the abnormality, whether the infarct is associated with hemorrhage, the amount of time that has elapsed between the occurrence of the infarct and the CT scan, and, to a lesser degree, the location of the infarct within the brain. CT scans performed in the initial 24 hours following a nonhemor-

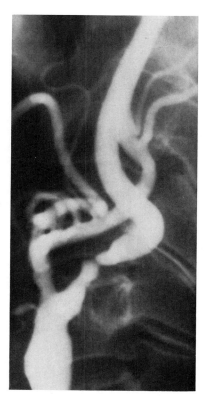

Figure 11–40. Lateral selective common carotid arteriogram. There is an irregular stenosis of the internal carotid artery. From this study, one cannot be sure whether ulceration is present.

rhagic infarct may be normal, especially if the lesion is small or if it is located in the brain stem or cerebellum. In typical examples, scans performed after an interval of more than 24 hours show an area of reduced density that can be related to a single vascular distribution. The character of the infarct evolves from an area of poorly defined inhomogeneous reduced density, which causes mass effect, to one with no mass effect, sharp margins, and homogeneous attenuation values approaching those of cerebrospinal fluid (Fig. 11-41). The subarachnoid space and ventricle adjacent to an old infarct are usually dilated. These changes have a variable time course; however, it is highly unusual for an infarct to have significant mass effect after it has been present for two weeks, and within three weeks its margins should be clearly defined. If intravenous contrast medium is given, a variable pattern of enhancement may be seen from four to five days following occurrence of the infarct for as long as six weeks after its origin. Although the configuration of abnormal enhancement in a brain infarct often assumes a gyral pattern, this is not specific and may be seen in numerous other pathologic conditions. The distribution of abnormal enhancement does not correlate with the amount of brain parenchyma that will ultimately be destroyed.

MRI provides a means for demonstrating ischemic changes in the brain earlier than any other imaging technique, abnormalities having been shown in as little as one hour following experimental arterial occlusion. On T1-weighted images, areas of infarction are seen as an area of decreased signal intensity with a loss of the normal signal differences between gray and white matter. On T2-weighted images, areas of infarction appear as high-signal intensity (Fig. 11-42). In pathologic studies, small areas of hemorrhage into infarcts are very common; these small hemorrhages are often not apparent on high-resolution CT scans, but are frequently seen on MRI studies. Depending upon the stage of evolution of the hemorrhage, their signal intensities are variable, ranging from predominantly low-signal intensities on both T1 and T2-weighted images in acute hemorrhages, to high-signal intensities on T1 and T2-weighted images in subacute hemorrhages, and then again to low signal intensities in longstanding hemorrhages. For details of the evolution of the pattern of MRI signal intensities in parenchymal hemorrhages, see the following section.

Nontraumatic Intracranial Hemorrhage

Most intracranial hemorrhages are the result of trauma and have been discussed in a previous section. Nontraumatic causes of intracranial hemorrhage include hypertension, aneurysms, and vascular malformations.

Careful analysis of the CT scan and MRI findings often allows determination of the likely cause of a nontraumatic hemorrhage.

Hypertensive Hemorrhages

Hypertension is an important etiologic factor in intracranial hemorrhages. If chronic, it results in the presence of structural arterial changes that in themselves predispose to the development of hemorrhages. The presence of elevated blood pressure is also thought to increase the risk of hemorrhage from other nonrelated vascular abnormalities such as aneurysms and arteriovenous malformations.

Hypertensive hemorrhages occur most often in the external capsule. This location is followed in frequency by the thalamus, the internal capsule, the cerebellum and pons, and the lobar white matter of the cerebral hemispheres (Fig. 11-43). Hematomas of this nature frequently rupture into the ventricular system, but rarely are seen in association with subarachnoid hemorrhage. This feature helps in distinguishing these lesions from traumatic hematomas in which the opposite combination is the case. Although the use of contrast-enhanced CT scans is usually not indicated in evaluation of these lesions, it should be noted that as they resolve, hematomas of any nature may be enhanced to simulate closely other mass lesions (i.e., neoplasms and inflammatory abnormalities).

As is the case for hematomas of any etiology, hypertensive hemorrhages appear on CT scans as areas of high density with sharply defined borders. Unless there is still active bleeding or impairment of coagulation, the density of a hematoma is homogeneous. Acutely, on CT scans, edema is not seen in association with a hypertensive hematoma. Over a period of several days following the initial hemorrhage, however, edema develops and low density is commonly seen peripheral to the margin of a hypertensive hematoma. Over a period of several weeks, the density of a hematoma changes from high density to isodense and finally to hypodense, the end stage being an area of encephalomalacia having attenuation values similar to those of CSF.

The MRI appearance of a hematoma is variable depending upon a large number of interrelated factors. These include, among others, the age of the hemorrhage, and, thus, the stage of degradation of both its cellular (erythrocytes) and noncellular (hemoglobin) elements; its location (i.e., parenchymal, subarachnoid, subdural, or epidural); the presence or absence of an associated abnormality (i.e., an arteriovenous malformation or neoplasm); and, the magnetic field strength and pulse sequence used to obtain the image. A complete description of these variables and their

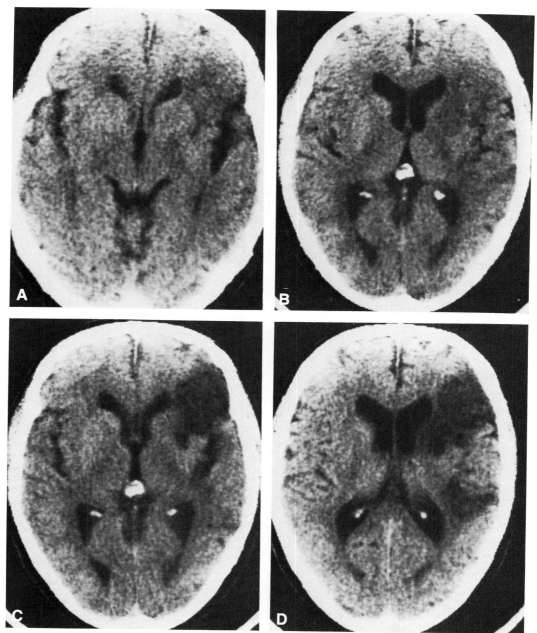

Figure 11–41. (**A** and **B**) Axial noncontrast computed tomograms performed three days following a left middle cerebral infarct. There is an area of low density extending from the lateral aspect of the left frontal lobe into the basal ganglia. (**C** and **D**) Axial noncontrast computed tomograms of the patient shown in *A* and *B*. These scans were done several weeks later. The density within the area of infarction has decreased and the borders of the abnormal tissue are much more clearly defined.

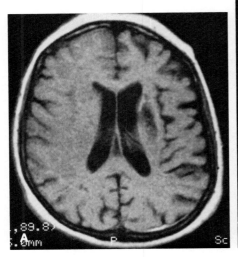 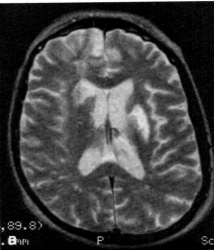

Figure 11–42. (**A**) Axial T1- and (**B**) T2-weighted images from a patient with acute and old infarcts. The acute infarct is in the right basal ganglia. On the T1-weighted image it is seen only as an area of vague mass effect. Contrast this with the old infarct in the left basal ganglia, which, because of the changes of encephalomalacia, is clearly seen as an area of low-signal intensity. The old infarct has no mass effect.

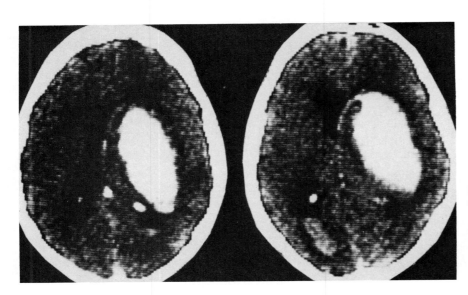

Figure 11–43. Axial noncontrast computed tomogram showing a large hematoma in the left basal ganglia that has ruptured into the lateral ventricle and is causing marked subfascial herniation.

effects on the MR image is beyond the scope of this text. For a further discussion, see Bradley.[5]

In spite of the complexities and variations associated with the MRI appearance of hemorrhages, however, several relatively consistent observations are noteworthy. On MR scans performed within several hours of the onset of a hemorrhage, a hematoma not associated with an underlying lesion appears similar to most other brain lesions (i.e., slightly hypointense on T1-weighted images and hyperintense on T2-weighted images). During the first 24 hours, this appearance changes so that the hematoma is of definite low-signal intensity on both T1 and T2-weighted images. Unlike

on CT scans, surrounding edema (high-signal intensity on T2-weighted sequences) may often be visualized on MR images obtained during this stage of a hematoma's evolution. During the first week after its occurrence, a hematoma becomes of predominant high-signal intensity on both T1 and T2-weighted images. This change in signal intensity from low to high is due to the development of methemoglobin within the lesion and occurs gradually from the periphery of the hematoma to its center, so that there is a steady replacement of low-signal areas by high-signal areas. The rim of a hematoma at this stage of evolution is seen as a sharply defined zone of very low-signal intensity; this is the result of accumulation of hemosiderin, the end product of hemoglobin degradation. After several weeks or even months, a hematoma loses its mass effect and assumes signal intensities similar to those of the adjacent brain and CSF. Small areas of both high- and low-signal intensity may persist, however, almost indefinitely.

Intracranial Aneurysms

An aneurysm is a dilatation of an artery. Most aneurysms within the calvarium are acquired and are classified as saccular (i.e., berry aneurysms). Other types of aneurysms include atherosclerotic, mycotic, and post-traumatic. Berry aneurysms most often become symptomatic during adult life through rupture, which results in subarachnoid and often intraparenchymal hemorrhage. Almost all berry aneurysms occur at points of major arterial branching, the three most common sites being the proximal segment of the middle cerebral artery, the anterior communicating artery, and the junction between the internal carotid artery and the posterior communicating artery. Aneurysms vary in size from those less than 1 mm in diameter to those that exceed 3 cm; those greater than 2.5 cm in diameter are designated giant aneurysms.

The first imaging study done on a patient with a suspected subarachnoid hemorrhage should be an unenhanced CT scan. Although less sensitive than lumbar puncture, a CT scan not degraded by artifact will allow detection of blood within the subarachnoid space of most patients in whom an aneurysm has ruptured. CT scanning also provides a good means for detection of other abnormalities that may be associated with the clinical presentation of a subarachnoid hemorrhage (i.e., arteriovenous malformations, neoplasms, and spontaneous hemorrhages). In instances in which there is significant clinical suspicion of a subarachnoid hemorrhage and the CT scan shows no evidence of subarachnoid blood, a lumbar puncture should be performed. MRI is not an adequate technique for the detection of acute subarachnoid hemorrhage.

While there is no absolute correlation between the location of subarachnoid blood and that of a ruptured aneurysm, the accumulation of blood predominantly on one side of the cranial cavity or primarily above or below the tentorium provides some evidence as to where the lesion is most likely located (Fig. 11-44). It is impossible to distinguish with certainty a parenchymal hematoma that results from an aneurysm rupture from one of another etiology; however, the presence of associated subarachnoid hemorrhage favors the diagnosis of an aneurysm. Intraventricular hemorrhage without associated parenchymal hemorrhage occurring as the

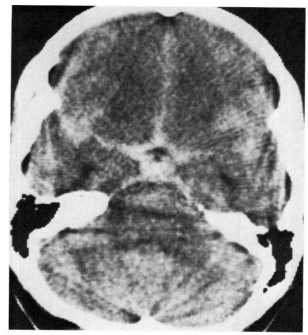

Figure 11–44. Axial noncontrast computed tomogram shows blood opacifying the subarachnoid space and basilar cisterns. The greatest amount of blood is in the right sylvian fissure. This is one indication that the hemorrhage may have occurred from an aneurysm arising from the right middle cerebral artery.

result of an aneurysm rupture most often is the result of an anterior communicating artery aneurysm; less likely is hemorrhage from one of the posterior inferior cerebellar arteries.

In spite of the recent advances in MRA, standard catheter angiography is still required to exclude the presence of an intracranial aneurysm. It is also needed as a measure to allow planning of the treatment of the lesion. Because of the occurrence of multiple aneurysm in as many as 30% of patients, the angiographic evaluation in suspected subarachnoid hemorrhage should include visualization of the entire intracranial circulation. Once an aneurysm is identified, special projections are often needed to define the aneurysm's neck as well as to provide clear depiction of its relationship to adjacent vascular structures (Fig. 11-45). Angiographic signs of aneurysm rupture include mass effect adjacent to the aneurysm, irregularity of the aneurysm surface, and the presence of focal vasospasm. In the presence of multiple aneurysms, the larger aneurysm is likely to be the site of rupture more frequently than the smaller one. On occasion, no abnormality is demonstrated on

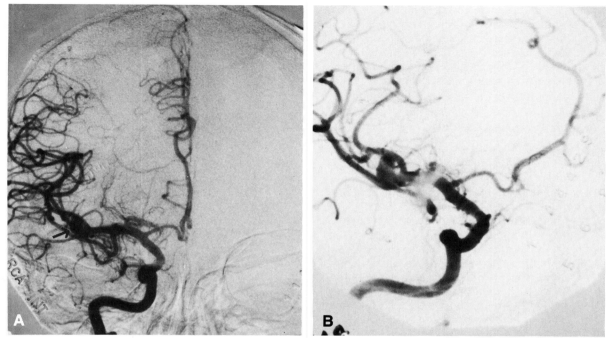

Figure 11–45. (A) AP projection of a right internal carotid angiogram. Although an aneurysm of the right middle cerebral artery is seen (*arrow*), the relationship of its neck to the adjacent branches cannot be appreciated fully. (B) An oblique projection allows visualization of the neck of the aneurysm.

an angiogram performed as a result of the occurrence of subarachnoid hemorrhage. Under these circumstances the study should be repeated after an interval of 7 to 10 days.

Vascular Malformations

Vascular malformations are developmental anomalies that have been classified in a variety of ways. McCormick's widely used classification separates these lesions into four principal types: 1) arteriovenous malformations, 2) telangiectases, 3) cavernous malformations, and 4) venous malformations. Venous angiomas, a type of venous malformation, are by far the most common, a fact not often appreciated because of their tendency to remain asymptomatic. Though far less frequent, arteriovenous malformations are more familiar. They often become symptomatic because of their tendency to hemorrhage and to produce venous hypertension or a steal effect.

Venous Angiomas

Most venous malformations are asymptomatic and are found as a result of an examination, usually a CT or MRI scan done for other reasons. There are instances, however, in which venous angiomas are associated with hemorrhage as well as with more indirect symptoms such as headache or seizures. Venous angiomas are composed of abnormally dilated veins without any associated arterial or capillary abnormalities. The neural parenchyma in and around a venous malformation is histologically normal. There are no guidelines as to how to determine if a particular venous malformation is likely to become symptomatic or is more or less likely to hemorrhage.

Venous angiomas are most frequently found in the white matter of the cerebral hemispheres but also occur regularly in the white matter of the cerebellum. On CT scans performed without the use of intravenous contrast medium, they may not be apparent or may be seen as small, well-defined areas of increased density. Contrast-enhanced scans show them as tubular areas of increased density extending from the deep white matter of the cerebral hemispheres or cerebellum to reach veins of either the subependymal or cortical drainage system (Fig. 11-46). The reliable CT diagnosis of a venous malformation requires that one be able to trace the lesion from its nidus to either the ventricular or subarachnoid surface of the involved portion of the brain.

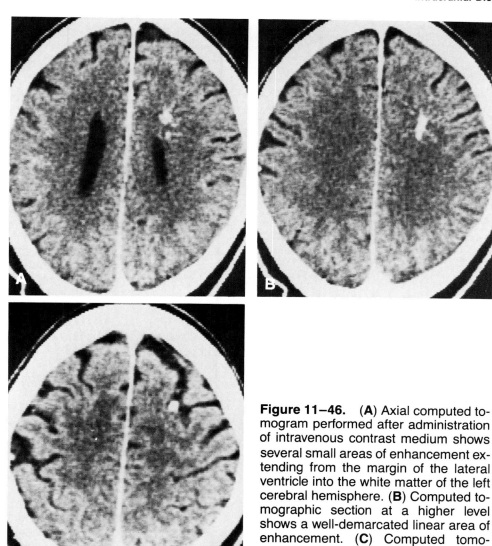

Figure 11–46. (**A**) Axial computed tomogram performed after administration of intravenous contrast medium shows several small areas of enhancement extending from the margin of the lateral ventricle into the white matter of the left cerebral hemisphere. (**B**) Computed tomographic section at a higher level shows a well-demarcated linear area of enhancement. (**C**) Computed tomographic section at a still higher level shows a small tubular enhancement deep within the superior frontal sulcus.

Angiography reveals venous malformations as a cluster of enlarged deep medullary veins draining through one or more veins, emptying into a cortical or subependymal vein (Fig. 11-47). The draining veins of these lesions are enlarged, but neither they nor the nidus of the malformation causes mass effect. Some have compared the angiographic appearance of venous malformations to that of a caput medusae. Venous malformations are best seen in the late venous phase of an angiogram; no abnormality is present in the arterial phase of such a study.

Arteriovenous Malformations

Arteriovenous malformations are anomalous collections of histologically abnormal arteries and veins that may occur in any part of the CNS. They are most common within the distribution of the middle cerebral artery but are by no means unusual in other parts of the brain; most of them occur above the tentorium. These lesions may rupture and produce intracranial hemorrhages; they are also frequently a cause of headache, and at times they may produce neurologic signs and

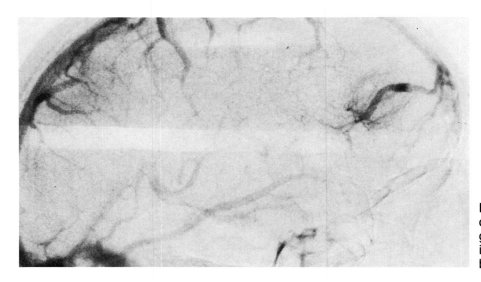

Figure 11–47. Venous phase of an internal carotid arteriogram. The venous angioma in the left frontal lobe resembles a caput medusae.

symptoms as the result of either a vascular steal effect or venous hypertension. Arteriovenous malformations have been classified according to the source of their arterial supply into pial, mixed pial and dural, and dural types. Of these, the pure pial malformations are the most common. There is frequently calcification in and around the vessels of an arteriovenous malformation; the adjacent area of the brain is often atrophic.

CT scans often provide clear evidence of the presence of an arteriovenous malformation. Lesions that have not caused hemorrhage have a variable appearance and may be seen on noncontrast scans as areas either of low density or of mottled high and low density. Small or superficial malformations may not be apparent on noncontrast scans. Following administration of intravenous contrast medium, arteriovenous malformations show striking enhancement, the classic pattern being an irregular central area of increased density from which extend multiple, well-defined serpentine structures of various sizes (Fig. 11-48). These structures represent the dilated feeding arteries and draining veins of the malformation. The enhancement of an arteriovenous malformation is the result of both the increased blood pool within the lesion and impairment of the BBB of the adjacent neural parenchyma. The CT scan appearance of an arteriovenous malformation that has hemorrhaged is often less characteristic, because the resulting hematoma masks the features of the vascular malformation. The presence of vascular calcification and prominent calvarial vascular grooves and foramina, in association with an intracranial hematoma, suggests the diagnosis of an arteriovenous malformation. This diagnosis should also be suspected when intracranial hematomas are found in young normotensive patients who have no other historic feature (e.g., trauma to explain the etiology of their hemorrhage).

MRI is superior to CT both for the diagnosis of arteriovenous malformations and for determining their exact relationship to adjacent neural structures. The feeding arteries, nidus, and draining veins appear in most instances as areas of signal void on both T1- and T2-weighted sequences. The high-signal intensity sometimes caused by slow or turbulent blood flow and the frequent occurrence of calcification in these lesions often result in heterogeneous signal intensities, however, and make it difficult to determine with MRI whether there is either recent or old hemorrhage in the malformation.

Although the diagnosis of an arteriovenous malformation can usually be made on the basis of CT or MRI scan findings alone, angiography is required to make a decision regarding the treatment of the lesion. Proper angiography requires the selective study of all arteries that may supply tissue in the area where the malformation is located. Because of the prominent arteriovenous shunting that occurs in these malformations, rapid sequence filming is essential to allow definition of the exact morphology of the abnormality. The typical angiographic appearance of an arteriovenous malformation is that of several dilated tortuous arteries supplying a tangle of abnormal vessels, from which emerge one or more enlarged draining veins (Fig. 11-49). Arteriovenous malformations do not produce mass effect unless there has been a recent hemorrhage or there is an associated venous varix formation.

Vein of Galen Malformations (Aneurysms)

This is a particular subtype of arteriovenous malformation that derives its name from the fact that the vein of Galen serves as the venous outflow of the lesion. The term "vein of Galen aneurysm" used in the older litera-

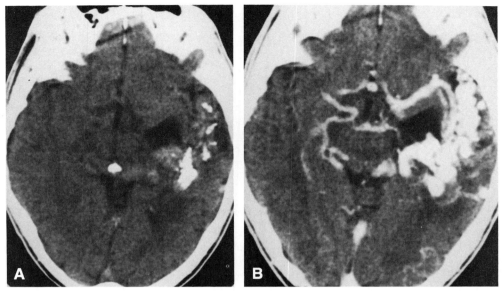

Figure 11–48. (A) Axial noncontrast computed tomogram shows areas of calcification and increased density in the left temporal lobe. There is slight mass effect. The left temporal horn is dilated. (B) Axial computed tomogram at the same level performed after administration of intravenous contrast medium. There is enhancement of the large feeding arteries, nidus, and draining veins of this temporal lobe arteriovenous malformation.

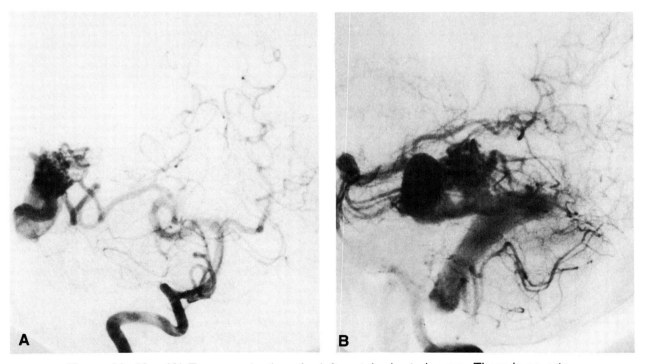

Figure 11–49. (A) Towne projection of a left vertebral arteriogram. There is an arteriovenous malformation in the medial surface of the left temporal lobe. The enlarged feeder, the nidus, and the dilated draining vein are all seen on this film. (B) This lateral projection of a left vertebral arteriogram provides better visualization of the relationship of the draining veins to the nidus of the malformation seen in *A*.

463

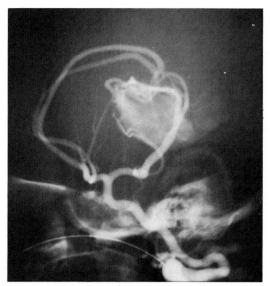

Figure 11–50. Lateral projection of an internal carotid arteriogram. Enlarged anterior cerebral and posterior choroidal arteries are seen entering the nidus of Vein of Galen malformation. There is also opacification of the dilated Vein of Galen.

ture is misleading because the aneurysmal enlargement of the vein of Galen is only a secondary manifestation of the arteriovenous malformation. This lesion usually manifests during childhood. Large lesions with high flow cause high-output cardiac failure in newborns; less severe lesions typically are noted because of the occurrence of hydrocephalus. The arterial component of vein of Galen malformations is usually derived from the choroidal arteries and the anterior cerebral arteries (Fig. 11-50). With current embolization techniques, many of these lesions can be treated effectively.

Dural Arteriovenous Fistula/Malformations

Pure dural fistula/malformations result either from the persistence of normal embryonic dural arteriovenous fistula or from the creation of this fistula during the recanalization of a thrombosed dural sinus. The arterial supply of this type of lesion is derived from dural branches of the internal and external carotid artery and the vertebral artery; the venous drainage is in common with the brain. These abnormalities are associated with a wide variety of clinical presentations; some are incidental findings, others cause only a bruit, and still others are associated with severe symptoms because

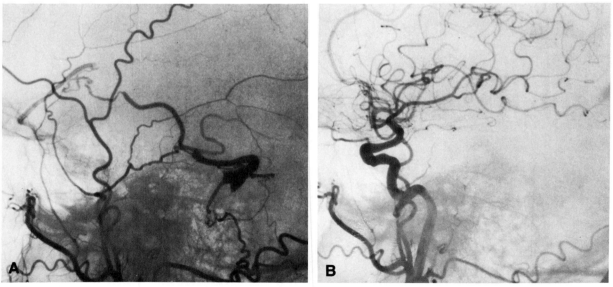

Figure 11–51. (**A**) Lateral projection of left external carotid arteriogram. There is early opacification of the sigmoid sinus and adjacent veins. The arterial supply to this dural arteriovenous fistula comprises the posterior branch of the middle meningeal artery and the transmastoid branch of the occipital artery. (**B**) Lateral projection of a left common carotid arteriogram done following embolization of the dural arteriovenous fistula shown in A. The arteriovenous shunts have been obliterated and the proximal segments of the feeding arteries have been preserved.

of intracranial hemorrhage, venous hypertension, or steal phenomenon. Dural arteriovenous fistula cannot be consistently diagnosed using either CT or MR scanning. Angiography is required both for diagnostic purposes and as a means to allow planning of optimal treatment. Interventional techniques (i.e., embolization), play an important role in the management of many of these lesions (Fig. 11-51).

REFERENCES AND SELECTED READINGS

1. ALBERT A, LEE BC, SAINT-LOUIS L, ET AL: MRI of the optic chiasm and optic pathways. AJNR 7:255, 1986
2. ATLAS, SW: Magnetic Resonance Imaging of the Brain and Spine. New York, Raven Press, 1991
3. BILANIUK LT, ZIMMER RA, LITTMAN P, ET AL: Computed tomography of brainstem gliomas in children. Radiology 134:89, 1980
4. BRADLEY WG, KORTMAN KE, BURGOYNE B: Flowing cerebrospinal fluid in normal and hydrocephalic states: Appearance on MR images. Radiology 159:611, 1986
5. BRADLEY WG: Hemorrhage and vascular abnormalities. In MRI Atlas of the Brain. New York, Raven Press, 1990
6. BRAFFMAN BH, TROJANOWSKI JO, ATLAS SW: The aging brain and neurodegenerative disorders. In Magnetic Resonance of the Brain and Spinal Cord. New York, Raven Press, 1991
7. BRITT RH, ENZMANN DR, YEAGER AS: Neuropathological and computerized tomographic findings in experimental brain abscess. J Neurosurg 55:590, 1981
8. CARROLL BA, LANE B, NORMAN D, ET AL: Diagnosis of progressive multifocal leukoencephalopathy by computed tomography. Radiology 122:137, 1977
9. CLAVERIA LE, SUTTON D, TRESS B: The radiological diagnosis of meningiomas, the impact of EMI scanning. Br J Radiol 50:15, 1977
10. CLIFFORD RJ, REESE DF, SCHEITHAUER BW: Radiographic findings in 32 cases of primary CNS lymphoma. Am J Roentgenol 146:271, 1986
11. CORNELL SH, GRAF CJ, DOLAN KD: Fat–fluid levels in intracranial epidermoid cysts. Am J Roentgenol 128:502, 1977
12. DELL LA, BROWN MS, ORRISON WW, ET AL: Physiologic intracranial calcification with hyperintensity on MR imaging: Case report and experimental model. AJNR 9:1145, 1988
13. DEBRUN G: Treatment of carotid cavernous and vertebral fistulas. In Fein JM, Flamm ES (eds): Cerebrovascular Surgery, Vol 4. New York, Springer–Verlag, 1985
14. DRAYER BP, ROSENBAUM AE, KENNERDELL JS, ET AL: Computed tomographic diagnosis of suprasellar masses by intrathecal enhancement. Radiology 123:339, 1977
15. EDWARDS MK, BONNIN JM: White Matter Disease in Magnetic Resonance Imaging of the Brain and Spine. New York, Raven Press, 1991
16. ENZMANN DR: Imaging of infections and inflammations of the central nervous system: Computed tomography, ultrasound and nuclear magnetic resonance. New York, Raven Press, 1984
17. ENZMANN DR, BRITT RH, PLACONE R: Staging of human brain abscess by computed tomography. Radiology 146:703, 1983
18. ENZMANN DR, RANSOM B, NORMAN D, ET AL: Computed tomography of herpes simplex encephalitis. Radiology 129:419, 1978
19. FISHMAN RA: Cerebrospinal Fluid in Diseases of the Nervous System. Philadelphia, WB Saunders, 1980
20. FITZ CR, WORTZMAN G, HARWOOD-NASH DC, ET AL: Computed tomography in craniopharyngioma. Radiology 127:687, 1978
21. FLOODMARK O: Hydrocephalus. In Putnam CE, Ravin C: Textbook of Diagnostic Imaging. Philadelphia, WB Saunders, 1986
22. GANTI SP, ANTONES JL, LOUIS KM, ET AL: Computed tomography in the diagnosis of colloid cyst of the third ventricle. Radiology 128:385, 1981
23. GANTI SR, HILAL SK, STEIN BM, ET AL: CT of pineal region tumors. AJNR 7:97, 1986
24. GEBARSKI S, GABRIELSEN TO, ET AL: The initial diagnosis of multiple sclerosis: Clinical impact of magnetic resonance imaging. Ann Neurol 17:469, 1985
25. GENTRY LR, MENEZES AH, TURSKI PA: Suprasellar arachnoid cyst; 2. Evaluation of CSF dynamics. AJNR 7:87, 1986
26. GENTRY LR: Primary Neuronal Injuries in Current Concepts in Imaging of Craniofacial Trauma. In Neuroimaging Clinics of North America. Philadelphia, WB Saunders, 1991
27. GEORGE AE, DE LEON MJ: Computed tomography and positron emission tomography in aging and dementia. In Latchaw RE: Computed Tomography of the Head, Neck and Spine. Chicago, Year Book Medical Publishers, 1985
28. GOLDBERG HI: Extraaxial Brain Tumors in Magnetic Resonance Imaging of the Brain and Spine. New York, Raven Press, 1991
29. GEORGE AE, RUSSELL EJ, KRICHEFF II: White matter buckling: CT sign of extra-axial intracranial mass. AJNR 1:425, 1980
30. GRAEB D: Intracranial trauma. In Putnam C, Ravin C: Textbook of Diagnostic Imaging. Philadelphia, WB Saunders, 1986
31. GREENBERG SB, TABER L, SETIMUS E, ET AL: Computerized tomography in brain biopsy proven herpes simplex encephalitis. Arch Neurol 38:58, 1981
32. HAIMES AB, ZIMMERMAN JRD, MORGELLO S, ET AL: MR imaging of brain abscesses. AJNR 10:279, 1989
33. HARA T, KISHIKAWA T, MIYAZAKI S, ET AL: Central nervous system complications in childhood leukemia. Correlation between clinical and computed tomographic findings. Am J Pediatr Hematol Oncol 6:129, 1984

34. HARWOOD-NASH DC, FITZ CR: Neuroradiology in Infants and Children. St. Louis, CV Mosby, 1976

35. HAUGHTON VM, ROSENBAUM AE, WILLIAMS AL, ET AL: Recognizing the empty sella by CT: The infundibulum sign. AJNR 1:527, 1980

36. HEALY ME, HESSELINK JR, PRESS GA, MIDDLETON MS: Increased detection of intracranial metastases with intravenous Gd-DTPA. Radiology 165:619, 1987

37. HAYMEN LA, HINCK VC: Water soluble iodinated contrast media. In Latchaw RE: Computed Tomography of the Head, Neck and Spine. Chicago, Year Book Medical Publishers, 1985

38. HESSELINK JR: Infectious and inflammatory diseases. In Neuroimaging Clinics of North America. Philadelphia, WB Saunders, 1991

39. HUCKMAN MS: Normal pressure hydrocephalus: Evaluation of the diagnostic and prognostic tests. AJNR 2:385, 1981

40. JORDAN J, ENZMANN DR: Encephalitis. In Neuroimaging Clinics of North America. Philadelphia, WB Saunders, 1991

41. KILGORE DP, STROTHER CM, STARSHAK RJ, HAUGHTON VM: Pineal germinoma: MR imaging. Radiology 158:435, 1985

42. KINGSLEY DPE, BROOKS GB, LEUNG AW, JOHNSON MA: Acoustic neuromas: Evaluation by magnetic resonance imaging. AJNR 6:1, 1985

43. KINGSLEY DPE, KENDALL BE: Cranial computed tomography in leukemia. Neuroradiol 16:543, 1978

44. LEE Y, TASSEL P, BRUNER J, MOSER R, SHARE J: Juvenile pilocytic astrocytomas: CT and MR characteristics. AJNR 10:363, 1989

45. LEE Y, TASSEL PV: Intracranial oligodendrogliomas: Imaging findings in 35 untreated cases. AJNR 10:119, 1989

46. LEO JS, PINTO RS, HULVAT GF, ET AL: Computed tomography of arachnoid cyst. Radiology 130:675, 1979

47. LOUIZOU LA, KENDALL BE, MARSHALL J: Subcortical arteriosclerotic encephalopathy: A clinical and radiological investigation. J Neurol Neurosurg Psychiatry 44:294, 1981

48. LUKEN MG, WHELAN MA: Recent diagnostic experience with subdural emphyema. J Neurosurg 52:764, 1980

49. MENDENHALL NP, THAR TL, AGEE OF, ET AL: Primary lymphoma of the central nervous system: Computerized tomography scan characteristics and treatment results for 12 cases. Cancer 52:1993, 1983

50. NAIDICH TP, LIN JP, LEEDS NE, ET AL: Primary tumors and other masses of the cerebellum and fourth ventricle: Differential diagnosis by computed tomography. Neuroradiology 14:153, 1977

51. NAIDICH TP, PUDLOWSKI RM, NAIDICH JB: Computed tomographic signs of Chiari II malformations: I. Skull and dural partitions. II. Midbrain and cerebellum. III. Ventricles and cisterns. Radiology 134:65, 391, 657, 1980

52. NEW PFJ, ARONOV S, HESSELINK JR: National Cancer Institute study: Evaluation of computed tomography in diagnosis of intracranial neoplasms. IV. Meningiomas. Radiology 136:665, 1980

53. NEWTON TH, POTTS DG: Radiology of the skull and brain, 4 vols. St. Louis, CV Mosby, 1978

54. NORTH AMERICAN SYMPTOMATIC CAROTID ENDARTERECTOMY TRIAL COLLABORATORS. Beneficial effect of carotid endarterectomy in symptomatic patients with high-grade carotid stenosis. N Engl J Med 325;445, 1991

55. PAGANI JJ, LIBSHITZ HI, WALLACE S, ET AL: Central nervous system leukemia and lymphoma: Computed tomographic manifestations. Am J Roentgenol 137:1195, 1981

56. PARK TS, HOFFMAN HJ, HENDRICK EB, ET AL: Medulloblastoma: Clinical presentation and management; experience at the Hospital for Sick Children, Toronto, 1950–1980. J Neurosurg 58:543, 1983

57. PINTO RS, KRICHEFF II: Neuroradiology of intracranial neuromas. Semin Roentgenol 19:44, 1984

58. PINTO RS, KRICHEFF II, BERGERON RT, ET AL: Small acoustic neuromas: Detection by high resolution gas CT cisternography. AJNR 139:129, 1982

59. POTTS DG: Brain tumors: Radiologic localization and diagnosis. Radiol Clin North Am 3:511, 1965

60. POTTS DG, ABBOTT GF, VON SNEIDERN JV: National Cancer Institute study: Evaluation of computed tomography in the diagnosis of intracranial neoplasms. III. Metastatic tumors. Radiology 136:657, 1980

61. ROPPOLO HM, LATCHAW RE, MEYER JD, ET AL: Normal pituitary gland: 1. Macroscopic anatomy, CT correlation. AJNR 4:927, 1983

62. ROVIRA MJ, POST MJD, BOWEN BC: Central nervous system infections in HIV-positive persons. In Neuroimaging Clinics of North America. Philadelphia, WB Saunders, 1991

63. RUSSELL DS, RUBINSTEIN LJ: Pathology of Tumors of the Nervous System, 4th ed. Baltimore, Williams & Wilkins, 1977

64. RUSSELL EJ, KIRCHEFF II, BUDZILOVICH GN, ET AL: Atypical computed tomographic features of intracranial meningioma: Radiological-pathologic correlation in a series of 130 consecutive cases. Radiology 135:673, 1980

65. SAVOIARDO M, HARWOOD-NASH D, TADMOR R, ET AL: Gliomas of the intracranial anterior optic pathways in children. Radiology 138:601, 1981

66. SPOTO G, PRESS G, HESSELINK J, SOLOMON M: Intracranial ependymoma and subependymoma: MR manifestations. AJNR 11:83, 1990

67. SEEGER JF, BURKE BP, KNAKE JE, ET AL: Computed tomographic and angiographic evaluation of hemangioblastomas. Radiology 138:65, 1981

68. STROTHER CM, SACKETT JF: Digital subtraction angiography. In Newton TH, Potts DG: Advanced Imaging Techniques, pp 311–322. San Anselmo, CA, Clavadel Press, 1983

69. SWARTZ JD, RUSSELL KB, BASILE BA, ET AL: High resolution computed tomographic appearance of the intrasel-

lar contents in women of childbearing age. Radiology 147:115, 1983

70. TRESS BM: The need for skull radiography in patients presenting for CT. Radiology 146:87, 1983

71. TURSKI PA, NEWTON TH, HORTON B: Anatomic correlation with complex motion tomography in 100 sphenoid specimens. AJNR 2:331, 1981

72. TURSKI PA, NEWTON TH, HORTON B: Sellar contour: Anatomic polytomographic correlation. Am J Roentgenol 137:213, 1981

73. VONOFAKOS D, BARCU H, HACKER H: Oligodendrogliomas: CT patterns and emphasis on features indicating malignancy. J Comput Assist Tomogr 3:783, 1979

74. WEINSTEIN MA, MODIC MT, KEYSER CK: Diseases of the white matter. In Latchaw RE: Computed Tomography of the Head, Neck and Spine. Chicago, Year Book Medical Publishers, 1985

75. YOCK DH: Techniques in imaging of the brain. Part 1: The Skull. In Rosenberg RN: The Clinical Neurosciences, Vol 4. New York, Churchill Livingstone, 1984

76. ZIMMERMAN RA, BILANIUK LT: Age-related incidence of pineal calcification detected by computed tomography. Radiology 142:659, 1982

77. ZIMMERMAN RA, BILANIUK LT: Computed tomography in pediatric head trauma. J Neuroradiol 8:157, 1981

78. ZIMMERMAN RA, BILANIUK, LT: Computed tomography of choroid plexus lesions. J Comput Assist Tomogr 3:93, 1979

79. ZIMMERMAN RA, BILANIUK LT, GENNERALLI T: Computed tomography of shearing injuries of the cerebral white matter. Radiology 127:393, 1978

80. ZIMMERMAN RA, BILANIUK LT, PAHLAJANI H: Spectrum of medulloblastomas demonstrated by computed tomography. Radiology 126:137, 1978

81. ZIMMERMAN RA, FLEMING CA, SAINT-LOUIS LA, ET AL: Magnetic resonance imaging of meningiomas. AJNR 6:149, 1985

82. ZIMMERMAN RD, LEEDS NE, DANZIGER A: Subdural empyema: CT findings. Radiology 150:417, 1984

Paul and Juhl's Essentials of Radiologic Imaging,
Sixth Edition, edited by John H. Juhl and
Andrew B. Crummy. J.B. Lippincott Company,
Philadelphia, © 1993.

CHAPTER **12**

The Spinal Cord and Related Structures

Joseph F. Sackett

The radiographic diagnosis of congenital and acquired lesions, including tumors of the spinal cord and its coverings and herniation of intervertebral disks are considered in this chapter. Also, brief reference to the findings in certain inflammatory lesions and vascular malformations is included. Examination for the detection of these conditions is discussed under several headings: development of the spinal column with plain film demonstration of common anomalies; the demonstration of acquired lesions of the spinal column with myelography, or intrathecal contrast examination of the spinal canal; computed tomographic (CT) scanning both with and without intrathecal contrast medium; and magnetic resonance imaging (MRI).

DEVELOPMENT OF THE SPINAL COLUMN

EMBRYOLOGY

Because of its importance in radiographic interpretation, a summary of the development of the spine as described by Ehrenhaft is given here. The column of cells derived from the entoderm around which the vertebrae develop is called the notochord. During the early weeks of embryonic life, this forms a long rounded column extending from the hypophyseal pouch to the lower end of the primitive spine. It is the central structure around which the vertebrae are formed. Without going into more precise details concerning vertebral development, it is sufficient to recall

that the mesenchyme surrounding the notochord undergoes segmentation with the formation of zones of densely packed cells, called scleromes, separated by less dense zones. The scleromes develop processes that form the anlagen for the vertebral bodies, the neural arches, and the transverse processes or ribs. Eventually the notochord is completely surrounded by the processes arising from the scleromes, and the primitive vertebrae are formed. With further development, the notochord becomes more and more squeezed into the regions that will become the intervertebral disks. The anlage for the vertebral body is divided initially into two lateral halves by an extension of the perichordal sheath. Centers of chondrification begin on either side of the sheath. The cartilage centers fuse but, for a time, there is left a remnant of the sheath in the center of the cartilaginous body known as the mucoid streak. This is continuous with the remnants of notochord that come to lie within the disk regions. These masses of notochordal cells, with the addition of mucoid material, fibrous tissue, and hyalin cartilage cells, form the nucleus pulposus of the fully developed disk. Notochordal cells can be identified in the nucleus until the age of adolescence or even later. During early life and until about the age of 25 to 30 years, the nucleus forms a semifluid, noncompressible substance that is of great importance in absorbing shocks and in distributing the stresses to which the spine is subjected. During the period of its development, the intervertebral disk is supplied by blood vessels derived from the periosteum as well as by some extending into the disk from the vertebral bodies. The latter vessels penetrate the cartilage plate surrounding the nucleus pulposus. Along with other degenerative changes that begin in the disk shortly after birth, these vessels regress and disappear. Where the vessels penetrated the cartilage plates of the disk, defects in chondrification result, and these may persist throughout life. They form weakened areas through which protrusion of disk material into the vertebral body can occur. These herniations are known as Schmorl's nodes (Fig. 12-1). The disks become avascular during the third decade of life, and the nucleus pulposus gradually is replaced by fibrous tissue.

Although the remnants of notochord enclosed within cartilage will disappear as the disk becomes avascular, there are areas where small masses of fetal notochord may persist throughout life. These are found most frequently in the region of the clivus at the base of the skull and in the sacrococcygeal area. It is in these locations that a tumor known as chordoma is prone to develop. Remnants of notochord sometimes persist where the mucoid streak entered the disk. These are visible radiographically as smooth, cup-shaped, or concave defects centrally situated on the disk surface of one or more of the vertebral bodies. Usually the defects are multiple, and they are seen most frequently in

the lower part of the thoracic and upper part of the lumbar spine. Such defects represent weakened areas with thinning or, at times, a complete deficiency of the cartilage plates of the disk. They are in effect a congenital or developmental type of Schmorl's node. In some instances, larger masses of notochordal tissue remain, causing larger defects on the disk surface of the vertebral bodies. Gaps in chondrification of the disk may be formed by vessels arising from the vertebral body. These weak areas predispose to traumatic protrusion of disk material. So long as the herniated material is composed only of cartilage, the defect may be difficult or impossible to visualize in roentgenograms. Usually, with the passage of time, reactive sclerosis forms around the herniated cartilage nodule, and it then becomes visible. Traumatic Schmorl's nodes usually occur near the center of the disk surface of the body but may be situated eccentrically. The defect is concave, and the wall of sclerosis usually is distinct. Thinning of the intervertebral disk space may or may not accompany herniation of disk material. Thinning of the disk in these patients is caused not so much by the actual loss of disk material as it is by the associated degenerative changes that may either precede or follow the herniation. With degeneration, the disk loses turgor and elasticity, and its total volume is reduced.

Ossification of the vertebral body begins from two separate centers at $3^{1}/_{2}$ to 4 months of fetal life. These do not correspond to the two centers of chondrification mentioned earlier but rather are situated dorsally and ventrally. Shortly after their appearance, they fuse to form a single center for each vertebral body. The neural arch ossifies from two centers, one for each lateral half. At birth the vertebra consists of three separate ossification areas, one for the body and two for the arch; these are separated by zones of cartilage. Shortly after birth, the two halves of the laminae unite, beginning first in the lumbar area and ascending to the cervical area. Union of the arches to the bodies begins during the third year of life and is completed by about the seventh year. In this instance, fusion begins in the cervical region and is completed in the lumbar region. At the time of puberty, secondary ossification centers appear for the tips of each of the vertebral processes, and a ringlike epiphyseal plate for the upper and lower edges of the bodies also begins to ossify (Fig. 12-2).

FUSION OF VERTEBRAE

Fusion or partial fusion of two or more vertebral bodies is a frequent occurrence. Usually such fusion can be differentiated from that resulting from disease by the fact that the sum in height of the combined fused bodies is equal to the normal height of two vertebrae

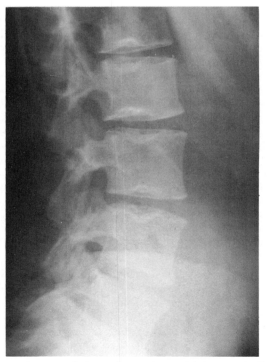

Figure 12–1. Schmorl's nodes, which are shallow and concave in the upper and lower disk surfaces of several lumbar vertebrae.

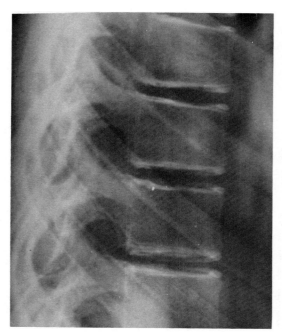

Figure 12–2. Normal "ring" epiphysis of the vertebrae. Lateral view of midthoracic spine of an adolescent.

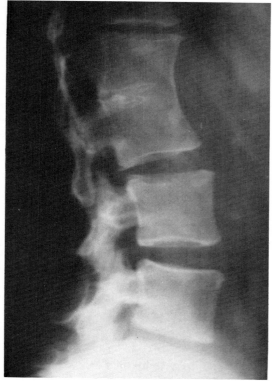

Figure 12–3. Congenital fusion of two lumbar vertebrae ("block vertebrae"). A remnant of the intervertebral disk is present posteriorly.

less the intervertebral disk space. The bony structure is normal except for the fusion. In cases of partial fusion, it is the anterior aspect that fuses while a rudiment of the disk remains in the posterior portion. This condition is called block vertebra (Fig. 12-3). Clinical symptoms ordinarily are not associated with vertebral fusion except as listed under the two following headings.

OCCIPITOCERVICAL FUSION

This consists of a fusion or partial fusion of the atlas and the occiput. Associated with this there usually is deformity of the foramen magnum, which is often decreased in size and irregular in shape, and frequently a platybasia deformity of the skull. In most normal individuals, the upper edge of the odontoid process of the second cervical vertebra lies below a line drawn between the posterior margin of the hard palate and the posterior rim of the foramen magnum (Chamberlain's line) in a lateral radiograph of the skull and cervical spine, or midsagittal MR examination at the skull base.[28] At times, in the normal individual, the odontoid projects slightly above this level, perhaps as much as 5 to 7 mm. When there is fusion of the first cervical vertebra and the occiput, the odontoid also is situated close to the occiput and will extend above this line. In

some cases, there is almost complete assimilation of the first cervical segment into the occiput with complete bony fusion of these structures. Because of the narrowing that results in the upper cervical spinal canal and at the level of the foramen magnum, pressure on the cord and medulla may result, and these patients often develop symptoms simulating multiple sclerosis, lateral sclerosis, syringomyelia, and other neurologic disorders. Other bony anomalies lower in the cervical spine may cause cord compression leading to neurologic disorders. Computed tomographic scan is used in detection of arch anomalies of this type, because bone protruding into the spinal canal is readily observed.

KLIPPEL-FEIL SYNDROME

This syndrome is essentially an extensive fusion of the cervical spinal segments.[33] There is numeric variation in the cervical vertebrae with more or less complete fusion into one bony mass or with multiple irregular ossified segments present. The upper dorsal vertebrae may be affected in the same way, and there often are spina bifida defects as well as other skeletal anomalies. Males and females are affected equally. The classic physical signs include apparent absence or shortening of the neck with a lowering of the hairline on the back of the neck and limitation of motion of the head. Other signs and symptoms that may be present include torticollis, mirror movements, facial asymmetry, dorsal scoliosis, difficulty in breathing or swallowing, and hearing deficiencies. Klippel-Feil syndrome is sometimes associated with congenital elevation of the scapula (Sprengel's deformity.)

NARROWING OR STENOSIS OF THE SPINAL CANAL

Narrowing of the spinal canal may be caused by local overgrowth, or hypertrophy or thickening of the laminae and pedicles. In some instances, the narrowing or stenosis may involve several segments such as in the narrow lumbar spinal canal syndrome in which there is developmental narrowing of the anteroposterior and interpediculate diameters of the lower two or three lumbar vertebrae. In the latter instances, the laminae tend to be oriented vertically with a small interlaminar space. This latter syndrome does not appear to be familial. An anteroposterior diameter of 16 mm or less on the standard lateral lumbar spine film, which reflects an actual diameter of less than 13 mm, is used by Robertson and associates in the diagnosis of this syndrome.[38] Similar narrowing may occur in the cervical canal and less commonly in the thoracic canal.

HEMIVERTEBRA

Failure or improper development of a lateral half of a vertebral body results in a hemivertebra. Embryologically, the fault probably lies in an absence of one of the lateral centers of chondrification. A hemivertebra has a triangular shape when viewed in the anteroposterior roentgenogram; it causes an acute lateral angulation of the spine. A hemivertebra in the thoracic region has only one rib, that on the side of the ossified center. Associated with a hemivertebra there may be numeric variations in the ribs, fusion of two or more ribs, and rudimentary development of some of the others. Except for the scoliotic deformity that it causes, a hemivertebra is of no clinical importance (Fig. 12-4).

VERTEBRAL CLEFTS

Rarely the two lateral centers of chondrification for a vertebral body fail to fuse, and a cleft persists in the midsagittal plane, dividing the body into two lateral halves. More frequently the cleft is only partial, resulting in a rather characteristic shape that is described as

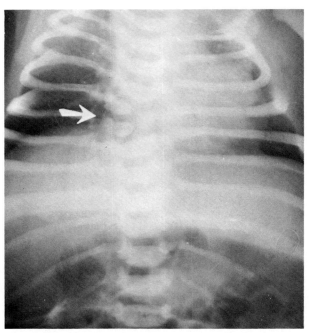

Figure 12–4. Congenital hemivertebrae in the thoracic spine of an infant. Three hemivertebral segments are visualized.

"butterfly vertebra" (Figs. 12-5 and 12-6). Another anomaly consists in a partial or complete cleft in the coronal plane, separating the vertebral body into anterior and posterior portions. Either the anterior or posterior half of a vertebral body may fail to develop, and the result is a ventral or a dorsal hemivertebra. A dorsal hemivertebra is more common and, because of its wedge shape and absence of normal ossification anteriorly, a sharp gibbus deformity is noted in the spine.

Anterior midline cleft of the C1 arch may simulate a vertical odontoid fracture.[36] This is extremely rare and is presumably associated with the presence of two centers for the anterior arch rather than the usual single center. Failure of fusion of the two centers results in the cleft.

The presence of a vertical cleft or ossification defect in the midline of a vertebral arch is common in the lumbosacral region or at other transitional areas in the spine. This condition is known as spina bifida manifesta when there are associated soft-tissue defects or when there is a meningocele, and spina bifida occulta when no visible soft-part malformation exists. Spina bifida occulta is frequent in the cervical spine where it involves the axis (C1) in 3% of all spines. Rarely there may be absence of all of the posterior arch of C1 except for a small ossification in the region of the posterior tubercle. Only slightly less common is spina bifida occulta of the first thoracic vertebra. Rarely an anterior

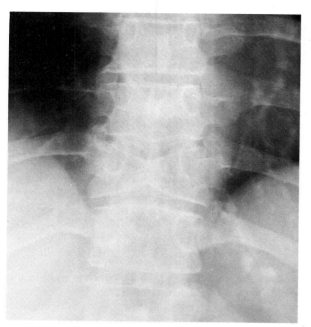

Figure 12–5. Partial sagittal cleft of the tenth thoracic vertebra ("butterfly vertebra").

cleft of the atlas associated with a posterior defect results in a bipartite first cervical vertebra. Spina bifida occulta is also very frequent in the lumbosacral region, affecting either the arch of the fifth lumbar or the first sacral segment. It is doubtful if any symptoms are caused by the defect in most cases. If there is an

associated anomalous development of the articular processes or a partial fusion of adjacent vertebral bodies, such as sacralization of the fifth lumbar or lumbarization of the first sacral segment, it is possible that localized weakness of the spine may result and become manifest after severe exertion. Some orthopedists place more emphasis on this condition than others, and its importance as a cause of low-back disability is not entirely settled.

NEURAL ARCH DEFECTS

Cleft formation between the superior and inferior articular processes of a vertebra is frequent, the incidence being reported as from 6% to 7%. The clefts usually are bilateral, and they predispose to the forward displacement of one vertebra on the other. When clefts exist without displacement, the condition is known as *spondylolysis*. If displacement is present, it is termed *spondylolisthesis* (Figs. 12-7 and 12-8).

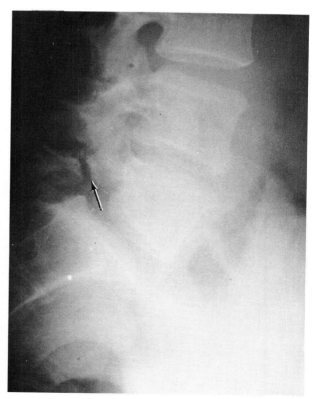

Figure 12–7. Spondylolisthesis. Lateral view of the lumbosacral area showing a forward displacement of the fifth lumbar vertebra on the sacrum. Note the clefts in the arch between the upper and lower articular processes (*arrow*). The anteroposterior diameter of L5 is smaller than that of the other vertebrae.

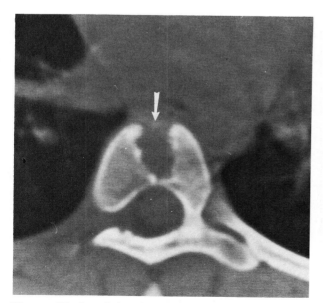

Figure 12–6. Axial CT scan showing midsagittal cleft or a butterfly vertebral body.

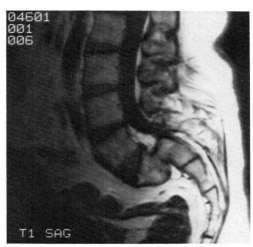

Figure 12–8. Magnetic resonance scan (T1-weighted sagittal) demonstrating fourth-degree spondylolisthesis.

This condition is observed most frequently in the arch of the fifth lumbar; occasionally the fourth lumbar is affected. Rarely, spondylolysis occurs in the cervical spine, usually associated with spina bifida at the same level. Spondylolisthesis may also be present when the defect is bilateral. C6 is the most common cervical site. The amount of displacement varies widely in different cases. Meyerding's classification of the degree of spondylolisthesis is a useful one (Fig. 12-9). In a lateral radiograph, the superior surface of the sacrum is divided into four equal parts. A forward displacement of the fifth lumbar up to one fourth the thickness of the sacrum is called a *first-degree spondylolisthesis*, half the thickness a *second-degree spondylolisthesis*, and so

on. Complete displacement of the fifth lumbar on the sacrum with the body of the fifth actually lying in front of the upper sacrum can happen. This is termed a *fourth-degree spondylolisthesis*. Because the clefts are present between the superior and inferior articular masses, the arch is not attached to the vertebral body by bone; it is described as a "floating arch." When clefts are present, the vertebral body often is decreased in size, particularly in its anteroposterior diameter. The arch may be generally small and poorly developed. Midline spina bifida is sometimes present. Most investigators are now of the opinion that lateral arch defects of this nature are acquired rather than being of developmental origin and have considered birth trauma with a failure of bony union at the sites of the arch fractures as a possible etiologic factor. Also, a chronic stress or fatigue fracture has been implicated in some cases, whereas, in others, acute injury is the likely cause. Those who have described these defects as being of developmental origin consider them to result from the presence of two ossification centers for each side of the arch with subsequent failure of fusion. However, the accumulated evidence indicates an acquired origin in some cases.

UNFUSED CENTER FOR ARTICULAR PROCESS

A small, triangular bony mass may be found at the tip of one or more of the inferior articular processes of the vertebrae. This represents an ununited ossification center, and it can be confused with a fracture. Isolated fracture of this process is very unusual without an associated fracture of the body or neural arch. A similar center occasionally is seen for the superior articular process but is much less frequent.

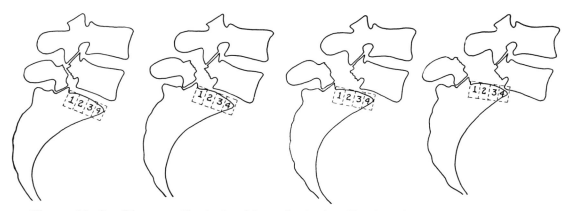

Figure 12–9. Diagrams illustrating Meyerding's classification of spondylolisthesis. The superior surface of the sacrum is divided into four zones. The diagrams (*left* to *right*) illustrate first-, second-, third-, and fourth-degree spondylolisthesis.

TRANSITIONAL VERTEBRA

At the junctions of the various major divisions of the spine, a vertebra may take on part of the characteristics of both divisions. This is most frequent at the dorsolumbar and the lumbosacral areas. The first lumbar, and rarely the second, may have rudimentary ribs articulating with the transverse processes. The fifth lumbar may be partially sacralized, often with one transverse process fused with the sacrum, the other being free and with only a rudimentary disk between them (Fig. 12-10). The first sacral segment may become partially lumbarized in the same manner. When the transition is complete, there will be 6 lumbar vertebrae, or 13 dorsal and 4 lumbar or various combinations. As a rule, an addition of a segment to one division of the spine will be corrected at another level.

The seventh cervical vertebra may have ribs attached to its transverse processes. The ribs may be only short, nubbinlike structures or they may be long enough to articulate with the sternum. Frequently the rib is fused with the first dorsal rib, or it forms a pseudarthrosis with it. Even when the rib is short, a fibrous band may extend from its tip to the first rib or to the sternum, and be a source of pressure on the brachial plexus or the subclavian artery. There may be only one rib, or the condition may be bilateral.

DIASTEMATOMYELIA

This is a rare anomaly of the vertebrae and the spinal cord, usually consisting of a vertical division of the cord or the cauda equina, the two portions being separated by an osseous or fibrocartilaginous septum. This septum is attached anteriorly to one or more of the vertebral bodies. Frequently there is anomalous ossification of the vertebrae; the interpediculate spaces are widened at the site of the defect. Diastematomyelia is found most frequently in the lumbar spine, less commonly in the thoracic region. The lesion is clinically significant, and the patient will show evidence sooner or later of impaired innervation to the lower extremities. Dimpling of the skin, local pigmentation, or excessive hair may be present over the area at birth. Occasionally there is an associated meningocele. Radiographs of the spine show widening of the neural canal over several segments, and often a fusion or partial fusion of vertebral bodies. Other abnormalities commonly associated include kyphosis, scoliosis, spina bifida, hemivertebrae, abnormal fusion of laminae, and narrowing of intervertebral spaces. If the septum dividing the cord is ossified it may be visualized in anteroposterior views as a vertical thin bony plate lying in the midline of the neural canal. Computed tomographic scanning with intrathecal contrast medium defines the septum and divided spinal cord.

SACRAL AGENESIS (CAUDAL REGRESSIVE SYNDROME)

Absence of part or all of the sacrum is an uncommon but not rare anomaly.[24] There is a high incidence of neurogenic bladder in these infants with the complications of vesicoureteral reflux, hydronephrosis, and infection. Occasionally, patients with agenesis of the sacrum or of the lumbar vertebrae or both show a severe neurologic deficit below the level of the vertebral anomaly, which may be complete. The changes associated with sacral agenesis have been termed the *caudal dysplasia syndrome.*[12] In addition to neurogenic bladder, in the more severe cases there may be abduction and flexion deformities of the lower extremities with popliteal webbing so that the legs cannot be straightened. The appearance of the lower extremities has been described as "froglike" or as having a "stuck-on" appearance. Most patients have an equinovarus defor-

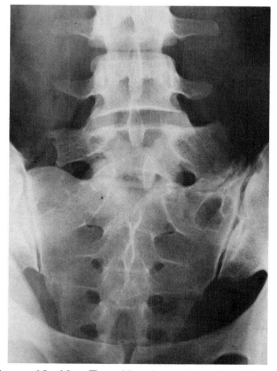

Figure 12–10. Transitional vertebra. The fifth lumbar is partially sacralized. Its left transverse process is broad and articulates with the sacrum. The right transverse process remains free.

mity of the feet and, less frequently, dislocation of the hips. Anomalies in other systems that may be present include renal agenesis, congenital heart disease, imperforate anus, cleft lip or palate, and microcephaly. The upper extremities usually are normal. Increased frequency of this syndrome occurs in infants with diabetic mothers.

MISCELLANEOUS ANOMALIES

Many other variations in development may be found in the spine.[9] The vertebral bodies may be abnormally tall, or one or more may show an increased height with the adjacent ones normal. Occasionally a vertebra may be of unusual height in its posterior aspect, whereas the anterior part is normal. This causes it to appear wedge shaped in the lateral view and to resemble the deformity produced by a fracture. Recognition of the increased height, together with the normal texture and appearance of the bone, will aid in avoiding error. Secondary ossification centers appear at the tips of all the vertebral processes; occasionally one or more of these fail to unite and will persist into adult life as a separate bony fragment. Anterior herniation of the nucleus pulposus may cause a separation of a triangular, smooth, bone fragment, which apparently represents the ring apophysis. It then fails to unite. This results in a triangular bony mass along the anterior border with a corresponding defect in the adjacent vertebral body and is known as limbus vertebra (Fig. 12-11).[14] The vertebral bodies may be unusually wide for their height, the condition being termed *platyspondyly*. This is often associated with other anomalies, particularly of the spinal cord.

Absence or hypoplasia of a pedicle is occasionally observed in the cervical spine. Absence of a lumbar pedicle with compensatory hypertrophy of the opposite pedicle has been reported but is exceedingly rare. The hypertrophy of the opposite pedicle differentiates this anomaly from acquired pedicular lesions. Furthermore, there are other associated congenital anomalies such as persistent synchondrosis between the two halves of the arch, short vertical cleft in the opposite pedicle or an adjacent one, and usually, hypoplasia of ipsilateral arch elements. The intervertebral foramen is widened, and there is posterior displacement of the maldeveloped lateral mass. Absence or hypoplasia of a pedicle must be differentiated from erosions caused by neurofibromatosis, metastatic tumors, vertebral artery aneurysm, and arch fractures.

Moderate to severe local flattening or thinning of a pedicle at the 12th thoracic or 1st lumbar level, either unilaterally or bilaterally, is a common anatomic variant.[1] The inner margin may be straight, convex, or

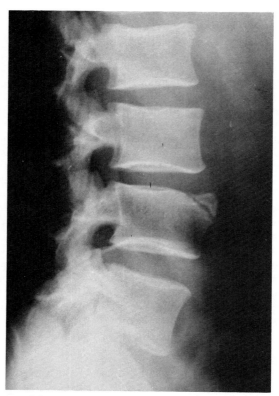

Figure 12–11. Limbus vertebra. There is an unfused ossification center along the upper anterior border of the fourth lumbar vertebra. This should not be mistaken for fracture. It is found most frequently in the lumbar area.

occasionally, concave, whereas the outer margin may be flat or concave. A slight increase in the interpediculate distance at the involved level is common, despite the absence of mass within the spinal canal.

Several anomalies may involve the lamina chiefly in the thoracic and lumbar spine including absence of an inferior articular process, hypoplasia of an inferior articular process, absence of the lamina, and a notch in the inferior lamina, which is usually present bilaterally.

METHODS OF EXAMINATION

PLAIN RADIOGRAPHS

Radiographs of the spinal column can be helpful when a lesion of the cord or intervertebral disks is suspected. These studies may reveal positive evidence of considerable value in many cord tumors, but also they are useful in excluding or in demonstrating infections, tumors, degenerative changes, and injuries involving the vertebrae. In many cases, the examination can be limited to a single anteroposterior and a lateral view. In others, it may be necessary to use multiple projections including oblique views or roentgenograms obtained with the patient flexing or extending the spine. Plain radiographs will also determine if there is a segmentation anomaly or transitional vertebra that will correctly locate the spinal level.

Variations in size of the spinal canal are very important in determining the likelihood of spinal cord compression owing to small defects produced by bony ridges or spurs, small intervertebral disk herniations, or tumors. Developmental narrowing or stenosis may involve several segments. Although single vertebral involvement occurs rarely, it may cause significant local stenosis. Normal measurements are listed in Lusted and Keats.[28]

As is true with other anatomic parts, when observing radiographs of the vertebral column, the student should develop an orderly system of viewing the structures so that small changes from the normal will not be overlooked. It makes little difference how one proceeds as long as all parts are observed carefully.

MYELOGRAPHY

Myelography consists of an introduction of a contrast substance into the spinal subarachnoid space to render it visible on radiographs or CT scanning.[40] It is used to confirm the presence of a lesion that is strongly suspected clinically; to identify the lesion's extent, size, and level; and to find, or exclude, the possibility of multiple lesions. Myelography is used to study patients with suspected degenerative lesions of the spinal cord or atrophic change of the spinal cord. More accurate techniques to assess spinal cord size are axial CT scanning following intrathecal injection of a water-soluble contrast medium or MRI. Postsurgical (laminectomy) complications or persistent pain may also be studied, but the presence of arachnoiditis may preclude accurate interpretation in some of these patients. Historically, gas and an oily contrast medium (Pantopaque) have been used as contrast media to opacify the subarachnoid space. Newer media have been developed over the past decade that are water soluble and nonionic: These have fewer side effects than those previously used. In some unusual instances, Pantopaque may still be used as a contrast medium. If there is blood present within the spinal canal, this is an absolute contraindication to the use of Pantopaque. It has been proved that blood potentiates the irritating effect of this material. The newer media are iopamidol, iohexol, and iotril. They are probably safe to use in the presence of blood in the spinal canal.

The new water-soluble myelographic contrast agents have less acute and chronic neurotoxicity than previously used water-soluble agents. There has been no instance of post myelographic adhesive arachnoiditis following the use of these media in humans. Currently these agents are the positive contrast substances of choice for either film or CT myelography. Their advantages include (1) they are absorbed and need not be removed; (2) the subarachnoid space can be visualized in greater detail than with Pantopaque; and (3) it is safe to use to examine the lumbar nerve roots, spinal cord, and intracranial structures.

Water-Soluble Myelography. Metrizamide (Amipaque) was introduced in the late 1970s for use in North America. It has been used in many examinations, and although it has a few acute side effects, it has no documented long-term ill affects.[17] Metrizamide has been replaced with three new agents with similar physical properties. They are iohexol, iopamidol, and iotrol. Because these agents are miscible with cerebrospinal fluid, care must be taken to ensure that the contrast medium does not become too diluted in the subarachnoid space when special detail on film myelography is required. For CT myelography, however, it is best to have more diluted contrast medium so appropriate resolution of the subarachnoid space is seen on CT scanning.[40] The technique of examination for lumbar myelography involves injection of the water-soluble media and a proper concentration to visualize exiting nerve roots.[22] A 22-gauge spinal needle is used for the lumbar puncture, and the contrast medium is injected under fluoroscopic control to ensure a subarachnoid placement of the contrast medium (Fig. 12-12). For cervical myelography, it is often best to inject the contrast medium by way of lateral C1–C2 spinal puncture with the patient prone.[23] This technique is safe and easy to perform with lateral fluoroscopy. It is advisable to use fluoroscopic control when the contrast medium is injected, once again, to ensure that the medium is entering the cervical subarachnoid space. Thoracic myelography can be performed either by prone lumbar spinal puncture or by supine C1–C2 lateral puncture. In either instance, contrast medium surrounds the thoracic spinal cord with the patient in a supine position. Frontal and lateral radiographs, or axial CT scanning will adequately evaluate the cord and surrounding structures.

COMPUTED TOMOGRAPHIC SCANNING

Computed tomographic scanning has proved to be an excellent technique for evaluating the spinal bony canal as well as certain intraspinal structures.[3, 13] With a good quality axial lumbar CT scan, one can accurately

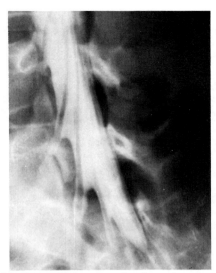

Figure 12–12. Oblique projection of water-soluble lumbar myelogram with good definition of lumbar nerve roots. A normal examination.

diagnose ventral and lateral disk herniation. In the thoracic or cervical region, because of the very narrow subarachnoid spaces, it is difficult to see intraspinal detail without the introduction of low-dose water-soluble contrast medium. Better anatomic relationships are seen if the axial CT sections are performed perpendicular to the central axis of the spinal canal. Another technique for getting anatomic orientation is using computer reformatting of the image resulting in tomographic sections in frontal or sagittal planes.[15] There is some loss of resolution using reformatting with thin sections, but the combination of fine detailed axial images with the more conventional frontal and lateral projections with reformatted images gives excellent orientation and spatial resolution.

MAGNETIC RESONANCE IMAGING

In 1983, MRI was introduced for spinal studies, and experience has confirmed its efficacy. Magnetic resonance imaging is excellent for detecting epidural as well as intramedullary abnormalities.[29, 30, 32] With the recent release of vascular paramagnetic agents (Gadolinium DTPA) MRI is also very sensitive with intradural diseases. The MRI examination must be tailored to the suspected disease process.

DISCOGRAPHY

Discography consists of the direct injection of a water-soluble contrast material, such as Conray 60 or preferably non-ionic contrast agent as is used in myelography,

into the intervertebral disk and the making of suitable roentgenograms. The contrast material is injected through a needle that has been inserted by way of oblique lumbar puncture through the posterior annulus fibrosis into the disk substance. First introduced by Lindblom of Sweden in 1950, this method has received some acceptance in this country. Many believe that discography is of little diagnostic value in patients older than 35 years of age.

ARTERIOGRAPHY OF THE SPINAL CORD

This examination requires bilateral selective catheterization of vertebral and costocervical trunks to outline the vascular supply at the cervical and high thoracic levels of the cord.[5, 6] Selective bilateral intercostal and lumbar arteriography from T8 to L2 will identify the great anterior radicular artery of Adamkiewicz. The upper and midthoracic blood supply is from small radicular feeding arteries. Percutaneous transcatheter embolization has been used successfully in treatment of vascular malformations. This is a valuable alternative when surgical excision is not feasible.

Arteriovenous malformation of the cord is the major indication for spinal arteriography. Of the tumors involving the cord, hemangioblastoma and hypervascular glioma show the most striking findings of tumor vessels and stain, as well as displacement of the anterior spinal artery and rapid arteriovenous shunting.

HERNIATION OF AN INTERVERTEBRAL DISK

When an intervertebral disk ruptures, it may herniate into the vertebral body. When the rupture occurs along the posterior or posterolateral surface of the disk, the mass of herniated disk material projects into the spinal canal or an intervertebral foramen. It may impinge on a nerve root and is a frequent cause of low-back pain with sciatic radiation. The diagnosis of a herniated intervertebral disk often can be made with considerable assurance from the clinical history and physical findings. However, many clinicians believe that the diagnosis should be confirmed by myelography, CT scanning, or MRI. Clinical localization may not always be possible or completely reliable, the diagnosis may be in doubt, and other lesions can give rise to clinical findings resembling those of a herniated disk. The indications for the procedure must be definite, however. The possible risks of myelography include headache, nausea, and even acute brain syndrome.

Most herniated disks occur in the lumbar spine, and most of these affect either the fourth or fifth disk. Only a small percentage of lumbar disk herniations are found above the fourth interspace level. The lesion is uncommon in the thoracic area except for an occasional case encountered in the lower thoracic disk interspaces. Posterior disk herniation in the cervical area is not infrequent, although less common than in the lumbar spine.

Because varied terminology used in discussions concerning herniated disks is somewhat confusing; to avoid misunderstanding, in the present discussion the following usage is implied:

1. *Posterior disk herniation and ruptured intervertebral disk* are terms used synonymously to denote a rupture of the posterior part of the annulus fibrosus with extrusion of a small amount of disk substance that projects into the spinal canal.
2. *Posterior disk protrusion or ridging* is a condition in which the annulus fibrosus is intact, but there is a smooth, ridgelike bulging of the disk posteriorly. This condition is usually associated with, and a part of, degenerative disease affecting the spine. In association with a weakened annulus and a posterior bulging of the disk, there frequently is hypertrophic bony spurring or osteophyte formation along the posterior or posterolateral edges of the adjacent vertebral bodies, resulting in a bony ledge projecting into the canal.

PLAIN RADIOGRAPHS OF THE SPINE

Radiographs of the spine may reveal no abnormality when a herniated intervertebral disk is present. More often there are one or more abnormal findings, which, although suggestive of the presence of disk degeneration, are not specific for this condition. A combination of these signs is more significant than any one alone. These include:

Straightening or reversal of the lumbar lordotic curve. This abnormality is usually the result of muscle spasm. Because there are many causes for spasm of the low-back muscles, it is of limited value as an isolated observation.

Listing of the lumbar spine to one side. This finding also is the result of muscle spasm. The list may be toward the side of the hernia or away from it.

Narrowing of the disk interspace. The amount of disk material that has been extruded is seldom enough to cause a discernible thinning of the intervertebral disk space as seen in roentgenograms. When thinning of the interspace is present in association with a disk hernia, it is an indication of degenerative disease of the disk. This may have preceded the herniation, or it may have followed it. Because localized thinning of an intervertebral disk, usually the fourth or the fifth lumbar, is a very frequent observation in this area without an associated hernia, thinning cannot be relied on as a good diagnostic sign. It is not at all infrequent to find a thinned disk at one lumbar interspace and to demonstrate, by myelography and at subsequent surgery, a herniation at a different level where the height of the disk space was normal.

Posterior offset of the fifth lumbar vertebra on the sacrum. Associated with a reversal of the lumbar lordotic curvature, the posterior surface of the fifth lumbar vertebra may appear to lie slightly behind the corresponding surface of the upper sacrum (reverse spondylolisthesis). This finding too is not specific for a herniated disc but, when combined with some of the other observations as has been noted, it becomes of greater significance.

Calcification of the extruded disk material. This is a very reliable sign but is not observed very often. Calcified disk material in the spinal canal is found in a higher percentage of thoracic than lumbar disk ruptures. Thoracic protrusions are uncommon, and are usually central or slightly eccentric; lateral protrusion occurs rarely.

Posterior Osteophytes on the Vertebral Bodies. Spurs or osteophytes may be found along the posterior or posterolateral edges of the vertebrae contiguous to a disk hernia. The presence of such spurs is positive evidence that at least a posterior bulging or protrusion of the disk is present, but they do not indicate whether there has been an actual rupture of the annulus fibrosus with extrusion of disk material. These osteophytes are a manifestation of degenerative disease.

FILM MYELOGRAPHY

Because a herniated disk is a space-taking mass that encroaches on the subarachnoid space, it will cause a filling defect when radiopaque medium is injected into the space. Characteristically, the defect is seen as a sharply outlined, smooth, unilateral indentation or notch in the opaque shadow along the anterolateral aspect of the spinal canal. The axillary root pouch is either obliterated at the site of the defect, or else it is displaced or distorted. Oblique views often bring out the defect to best advantage because they show it tangentially. Lateral decubitus views are valuable in detecting the more laterally placed lesions. Some typical examples of lumbar disk hernias are shown in Figures 12-13 and 12-14. Herniation at the fourth lumbar interspace usually causes a clear-cut and characteristic defect because the meninges are closely approxi-

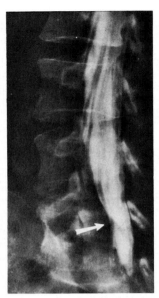

Figure 12–13. Water-soluble lumbar myelogram demonstrating a large extradural defect at the lumbosacral intervertebral disk space (*arrow*). The contrast column has been displaced away from the anterolateral margin of the spinal canal indicating a large lumbosacral disk herniation.

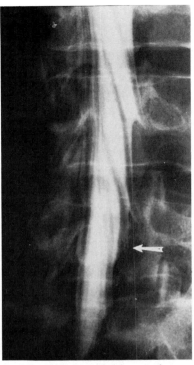

Figure 12–14. Water-soluble myelogram in which the myelographic signs of anterolateral disk herniation are subtle. There is flattening of the exiting S1 root and nonfilling of its axillary root sleeve (*arrow*). These findings indicate a small anterolateral disk herniation.

mated to the anterior and lateral bony walls of the spinal canal, and encroachment on the space by the hernia readily deforms the opaque column. Because the lumbosacral cul-de-sac narrows gradually to a smooth rounded or pointed termination, there may be considerable space in the canal outside the dural sac at the level of the lumbosacral disk (Fig. 12-15). The defect of a hernia often is less obvious at this interspace than when a mass of similar size has herniated at the level of the fourth disk. At times, a lumbosacral defect is quite inconspicuous, being limited to a slight anterolateral indentation on the opaque column with slight elevation of the axillary root pouch. Even a minor defect of this nature at this interspace must be viewed with considerable suspicion, especially when clinical findings indicate nerve root compression on that side and level. When there is clinical suspicion and a wide epidural space in front of the contrast column at the lumbosacral junction, it is necessary to perform CT scanning following the myelogram to look for CT signs of disk herniation (Figs. 12-16 and 12-17).

Occasionally a very large herniation will completely or almost completely obstruct the canal and may mimic a tumor very closely. In fact a herniated disk, being an extradural mass, can cause myelographic changes similar to those of a tumor such as a small neurofibroma. It

is chiefly the characteristic location of the lesion that is significant in diagnosis. At other times, the extruded cartilage will become separated completely from the disk and lie free in the subarachnoid space. It may be displaced from its site of origin. In these cases, the defect may be found behind a vertebral body rather than at a disk interspace and, in rare instances, it will be found along the posterior aspect of the canal rather than the anterior. It may be impossible to exclude the possibility of a neoplasm as a cause for such a defect. Axial CT scanning is helpful for detecting a migrated disk fragment.[41] The location of such an epidural process can be well seen with CT scanning. It is often difficult to separate this lesion from an epidural neoplasm.

In the cervical region, disk hernias are found most frequently at the fifth and sixth interspaces. The defect caused by the herniation may be large and notchlike and resemble that of a lumbar herniation. In other patients, the herniation is small and laterally placed, and produces a unilateral small, rounded, or triangular

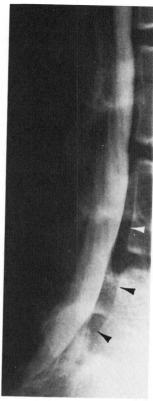

Figure 12–15. A lateral view of a water-soluble myelogram shows the wide epidural space (*arrowheads*) between the contrast column and the posterior margin of the vertebral bodies. This is greatest at the lumbosacral junction.

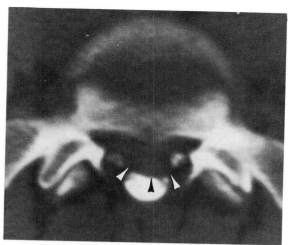

Figure 12–16. A postmyelogram axial CT scan at the lumbosacral junction shows high-density disk material effacing the thecal sac from a large disk herniation (*arrowheads*).

flava is frequently associated. As a result of these changes, pressure on a spinal nerve root may cause signs and symptoms suggestive of a herniated disk. The lesion may be found in any part of the spine but is infrequent in the thoracic area. In the cervical and lumbar areas, multiple disk ridging often is present.

defect that obliterates the root sleeve at the affected level. In some cases, the chief manifestation is a deformity of the axillary root pouch (Fig. 12-18). Because the hernia projects into a spinal foramen, the clinical signs of nerve root impingement may be severe; the small size of a myelographic defect does not necessarily indicate a clinically insignificant lesion. Magnetic resonance imaging is a very accurate technique to evaluate a patient with suspected cervical disk disease.[31, 39]

FURTHER OBSERVATIONS

Transverse Disk Ridging. Posterior bulging of a disk without actual herniation of disk material is known as "posterior disk protrusion" or "ridging." The lesion is a frequent accompaniment of degenerative joint disease of the spine. Also, hypertrophy of the ligamenta

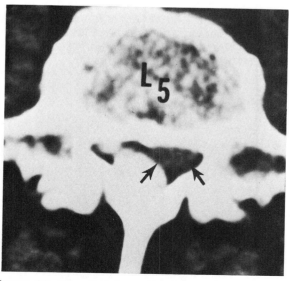

Figure 12–17. Axial computed tomographic scan following myelography through the midbody of L5. A soft-tissue defect within the spinal canal (*arrows*) is a migrated herniated disk fragment.

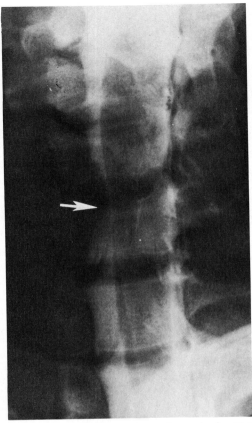

Figure 12–18.   Oblique view of cervical water-soluble myelogram by way of C1–C2 puncture. At the fifth cervical interspace there is amputation of the axillary root sleeve, compression of the opaque column, and even displacement of the spinal cord (*arrow*). Findings indicate disk herniation.

Neurosurgeons frequently speak of ridging as a "hard disk" in contrast to the "soft disk" of a true herniation. The bony marginal osteophytes are particularly prone to encroach on the contiguous spinal foramen.

Radiographic Findings.   Disk-space thinning, and posterior or posterolateral spurs may be noted on plain roentgenograms. However, disk ridging can occur without significant plain-film findings, although this is unusual. Often one can postulate the presence of the lesion from these plain-film findings. On myelography, disk ridging causes a transverse lucent defect in the opaque column. If lateral cross-table views are obtained with the patient prone, a smooth, anterior indentation on the opaque column will be seen at the affected disk level (Fig. 12-19). In posteroanterior views, the ridge may cause a transverse bandlike lucency (Fig. 12-20). Also, bilateral indentations may be seen causing an hourglass type of deformity. If there is associated hypertrophy of the ligamenta flava, these defects are accentuated. Herniated disk may be present at the same level as the ridge but more often it exists alone. It accentuates the filling defect on the side of the herniation, and elevates and compresses the corresponding nerve root more than is seen with ridging alone. At times it is difficult to determine if both conditions are present or not. Computed tomographic scanning following film myelography will usually separate "hard" from "soft" disk disease.

The significance of such ridging is difficult to determine. In the cervical region, it is related to the anteroposterior diameter of the spinal canal. If this diameter is reduced to 13 mm or less, there are often signs of cord compression, and the lesion is significant. In the lumbar region as well, the clinical symptoms determine the significance of the ridging; therefore history

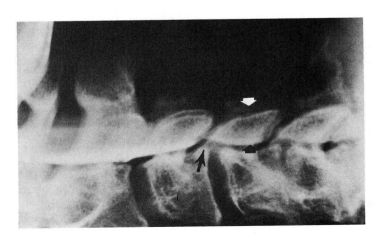

Figure 12–19.   Lateral view of film myelogram in the cervical region. Contrast has been injected by way of C1–C2 puncture. At the third cervical interspace there is osteophyte formation (*black arrow*) with compression of the contrast column at that level. In addition, this patient has a narrow sagittal bony canal that is congenital (*white arrow*).

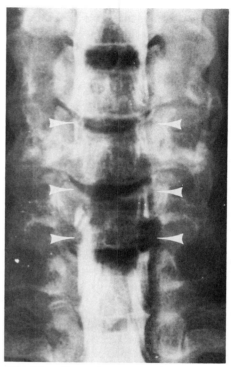

Figure 12–20. Frontal view of cervical water-soluble myelogram. There are narrow canal and ridge defects at the third, fourth, fifth, and sixth cervical interspaces from hypertrophic degenerative change and a congenitally narrow cervical bony canal.

SPINAL COMPUTED TOMOGRAPHIC SCANNING

In the lumbar region, axial CT scanning is very accurate to detect disk herniation. Using half-centimeter thin sections parallel to the intervertebral disk, one can diagnose ventral and lateral disk herniation. Disk material has greater attenuation coefficient than the thecal sac or epidural fat within the spinal canal. In addition to excellent detail involving the intraspinal structures, axial CT scanning gives an excellent view of the bones surrounding the exit foramina (Fig. 12-21). There are other processes that can mimic lumbar disk herniation that can usually be diagnosed with CT scanning and most accurately with CT scanning following injection of intrathecal contrast medium. A conjoined nerve root will have a lower attenuation than the higher density of a herniated disk.[20] A synovial cyst of the facet joint will be in relationship with the facet joint, and there will be degenerative change of the facet joint.[27] Radicular pain in the lumbar region can be caused by either soft disk herniation or compression of the nerve roots in and about the neural foramina because of osteophyte formation from lumbar spondylosis and superior articular facet hypertrophy from degenerative change of the facet joints (Figs. 12-22 and 12-23). Computed tomographic scanning is excellent to detect this abnormality.[3, 18, 19] Lumbar pain and intermittent cauda equina compression can be secondary to lumbar spinal steno-

and physical findings must be correlated with myelographic findings in these cases.

The Postoperative Myelogram. The interpretation of myelograms performed after laminectomy and surgical removal of a herniated disk is difficult and often unsatisfactory. In many patients, there is irregularity and deformity of the opaque column at the level of the previous surgery, which are only the result of adhesions in the subarachnoid space. In some cases, a filling defect resembling a herniated disk is found but, at reoperation, there is no evidence of recurrent hernia. In patients with the severest deformity, there may be a complete obstruction to the flow of contrast medium at the level of the previous hernia and laminectomy. Slight to moderate irregularities in filling that do not show the characteristic notch defect of a herniated disk are most likely the result of adhesions. If a defect that fulfills the criteria for a herniated disk is found, one is justified in interpreting it as evidence for recurrent disk herniation.

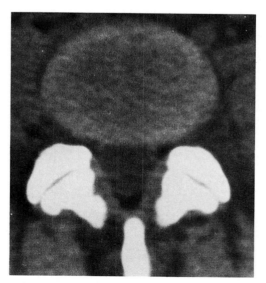

Figure 12–21. A normal CT scan through the fourth lumbar intervertebral disk. Notice the higher density of the intervertebral disk relative to the intrathecal cerebrospinal fluid and epidural fat.

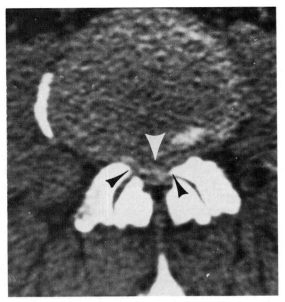

Figure 12–22. Axial CT scan through the fourth lumbar intervertebral disk. The spinal canal is completely compromised by a diffusely bulging intervertebral disk (*white arrow*) and hypertrophic change of the facet joints posterolaterally (*black arrows*). This patient had signs of cauda equina compression.

sis. This is often a combination of a congenitally narrow canal with superimposed hypertrophic degenerative change. Computed tomographic scanning is excellent at detecting such a compromise of the spinal canal.

In the cervical region, axial CT scanning is excellent for determining bony relationships involving the cervical spinal cord or exiting nerve roots (Figs. 12-24 and 12-25). If an epidural defect is detected on film myelography, follow-up CT scanning will be beneficial in separating hypertrophic bony change from soft disk herniation.

MAGNETIC RESONANCE IMAGING

Magnetic resonance imaging has a place in detecting herniated disks.[7, 16, 25] Large disk herniations can be seen in cervical or lumbar regions (Figs. 12-26 and 12-27). Both axial and parasagittal sections can be used to locate or confirm the presence of a disk herniation. It is best to obtain T_1, proton density, and T_2 images to assess for disk herniation fully. The herniated intervertebral disk fragment can migrate away from the disk space. The term used for this is migrated or sequestered disk fragment (Fig. 12-28).[25] The use of paramagnetic contrast agents has assisted in separating postoperative scar from recurrent disk herniation in patients with previous surgery.[2]

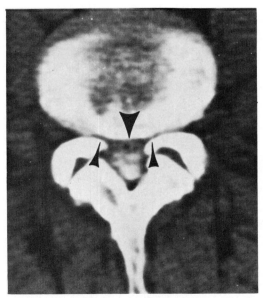

Figure 12–23. Lumbar spondylosis with hypertrophic osteophyte formation from the intervertebral disk (*large arrow*) as well as superior articular facets posterolaterally (*small arrows*). A small amount of contrast medium remains within the subarachnoid space.

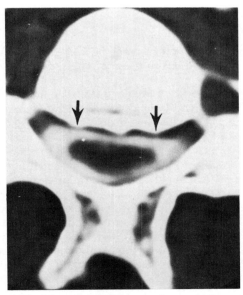

Figure 12–24. Axial CT scan through the cervical spinal column. There is a ventral bony ridge (*arrows*) compromising the sagittal dimension of the canal in deforming the cervical spinal cord.

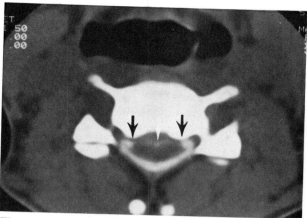

Figure 12–25. Uncinate process hypertrophy has compromised the spinal canal (*black arrows*), and a soft midline disk herniation (*white arrow*) has deformed the cervical subarachnoid space.

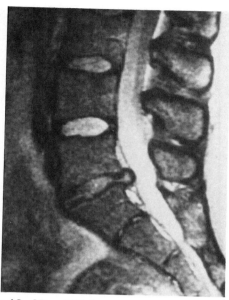

Figure 12–27. MR image (T1-weighted) through the lumbar region showing a large disk herniation.

CHOICE OF AN IMAGING MODALITY FOR LUMBAR DISK DISEASE

The competing modalities used to assess suspected lumbar disk disease include plain CT (without intrathecal contrast medium), CT myelography (CT performed following water-soluble myelography), and MR

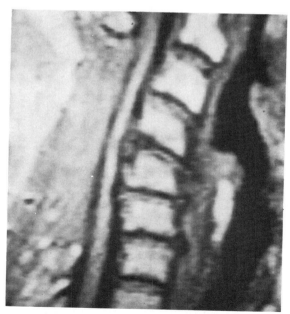

Figure 12–26. MR image (T1-weighted) through the cervical region showing a large cervical disk herniation.

imaging. A recent study by Thornbury and coworkers[44] found that the three were of almost equal diagnostic accuracy (84% to 86%) in the diagnosis of disk-caused nerve root compression. In lower probability type cases, plain CT is equally accurate as MRI in this diagnosis and is thus more cost-effective. In high-probability type cases CT myelography and MRI are essentially equal in accuracy for disk-caused nerve root compression. Because cost is about equal and CT myelography is invasive, the authors recommend MRI be performed as the initial imaging examination.

SPINAL CORD TUMORS

Primary tumors of the spinal cord and its coverings can be classified as intramedullary, extramedullary intradural, or extradural.[8] Such a breakdown is important, not only from the standpoint of operability but because of differences in roentgen findings in the three groups. The histologic types of tumors in the order of frequency are as follows: neurofibroma, meningioma, ependymoma, astrocytoma, glioblastoma, and a miscellaneous group including infrequent lesions such as dermoid and epidermoid cysts, epidural cysts, lipomas, and hemangiomas. In addition to the group of primary tumors, metastatic neoplasms cause compression of the cord very frequently. Metastasis may be from extension of a focus in a vertebral body or its arch; less frequently,

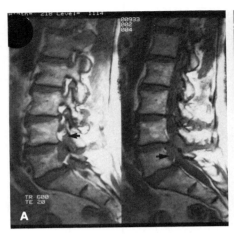
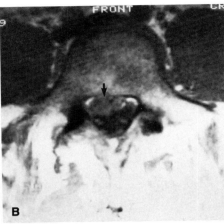

Figure 12–28. **(A)** Sagittal view lumbar spine showing migrated disk fragment (*arrow*). **(B)** Axial magnetic resonance imaging scan of the L5 vertebral body. An extradural migrated disk fragment (*arrow*) compresses the thecal sack.

the metastasis is directly to the cord or the meninges. Any malignant tumor can metastasize in this way.

Myelographic findings usually permit differentiation between the three major types of masses observed within the spinal canal. The *intramedullary* tumor usually causes a fusiform enlargement of the cord (Fig. 12-29), which usually does not cause complete block. The spinal canal may be uniformly widened. *Intradural-extramedullary* masses are usually eccentric and tend to displace the cord and widen the ipsilateral subarachnoid space between the cord and the dura above and below the tumor site. The subarachnoid space is narrowed contralaterally at the level of the mass and to varying degrees above and below it as a result of cord displacement (Fig. 12-30). Below the level of the spinal cord, intradural masses will deviate the nerve roots of the cauda equina (Fig. 12-31). Complete obliteration of the subarachnoid space associated with complete block is not infrequent. *Extradural* masses may surround the dura and produce complete block, or they may be eccentric and cause partial or complete block. The dura, cord, and the surrounding subarachnoid space are displaced by the latter type of lesion in a rather typical manner (Fig. 12-32). Below the cord, the major finding is an indentation of the thecal sac corresponding to the site and size of the extradural mass.

EXTRAMEDULLARY TUMORS

NEUROFIBROMA

Neurofibroma is an extramedullary tumor that can be either intradural or extradural in location, with the majority lying within the dura. Neurofibromas arise from the spinal nerve roots. In the lumbar area, the tumor often is completely within the dural sac. In the thoracic and cervical regions, the lesion tends to be of

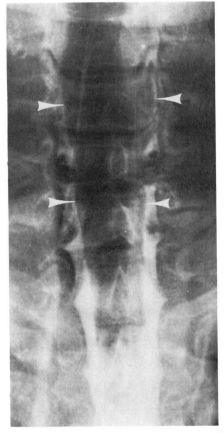

Figure 12–29. Film myelogram by way of lumbar injection. In the cervical region there is diffuse widening of the cervical spinal cord secondary to intramedullary glioma.

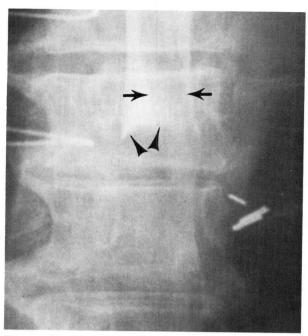

Figure 12–30. Thoracic myelogram. Contrast medium injected by C1–C2 puncture. Spinal cord is displaced to the left (*arrows*), and there is a rounded intradural extramedullary filling defect (*arrowheads*), a thoracic meningioma.

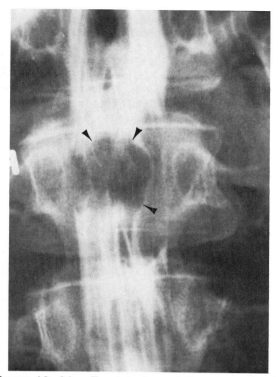

Figure 12–31. Frontal view of the upper lumbar subarachnoid space following lumbar injection of water-soluble contrast medium. There is one large rounded intradural filling defect (*arrows*) as well as nodular enlargement of nerve roots from subarachnoid seeding in metastatic disease.

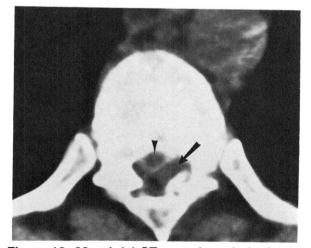

Figure 12–32. Axial CT scan through the lumbar region after low-dose intrathecal injection of water-soluble contrast medium. The spinal cord is displaced anteriorly (*arrowhead*) from a posterolateral epidural process representing extradural lymphoma (*arrow*).

dumbbell type with an intraspinal portion and an extraspinal extension through an intervertebral foramen. In the thoracic area, the extraspinal portion of the tumor often is visible because of the contrast afforded by the air-filled lungs. In the cervical region, a mass is rarely demonstrated. In the lumbar spine, the extraspinal part of the tumor may, if very large, cause an outward bulge of the psoas muscle margin. The intraspinal part of the tumor leads to erosion of the pedicle on one or both sides. Normally the pedicles are seen end-on in anteroposterior roentgenograms as vertical ovoid ringlike shadows. The inner surface usually is convex but may vary from a flattened surface to one slightly concave. Pressure erosion from a neurofibroma causes a thinning of the pedicle with or without a loss of its inner cortical margin. Because of the variations in the contour of normal pedicles, Hinck and colleagues measured the difference between the inner surfaces of the two pedicles of each vertebra, called the interpediculate distance, and published the results in the form of a chart.[21] Erosion from a neurofibroma usually is limited to one or two vertebrae, and comparison of the pedicle shadows above and below the lesion will clearly indicate the presence of abnormality without the need for measurement in most cases. If very large, an intraspinal neurofibroma will cause a smooth, pressure type of erosion of the posterior surface of the vertebral body so that it will have a concave contour as seen in the lateral roentgenogram. A dumb-bell tumor will erode the upper and lower surfaces of the pedicles bounding an intervertebral foramen. Bone changes occur in about 20% of neurofibromas. In patients with neurofibromatosis, posterior scalloping of the vertebral bodies, with concavity resembling pressure erosion as has been described, may be present at several levels in the absence of tumor. There may be associated interpediculate widening, also in the absence of tumor. The changes are presumably caused by dural ectasia. Severe and sharply angulated scoliosis may also be present in these patients.

Neurofibroma as an intraspinal mass is rare in children, but neuroblastoma or ganglioneuroma may produce an hourglass type of lesion with a paraspinal mass in addition to an extradural tumor compressing the cord. There may be bone changes, such as rib or vertebral erosion, producing pediculate thinning and posterior vertebral scalloping. Punctate calcification may be visible in these tumors.

Myelographic signs of an intradural neurofibroma include a sharply outlined, round, or oval-shaped filling defect (Fig. 12-33). Because the tumor often is large enough to block the canal completely, obstruction to the flow of contrast medium is easily demonstrated, and the end of the opaque column has a sharp concave margin as it caps the end of the tumor. Although this type of defect is not specific for a neurofibroma, it is always most suggestive of this tumor and, if erosive changes in the pedicles also are present, the diagnosis is more certain. Sometimes it is important to know the upper limits of a neurofibroma that is above the level of lumbar contrast medium injection. This can be obtained by injecting a small amount of the contrast medium above the lesion, using a lateral puncture at the C1–C2 level and allowing the opaque medium to flow down to the level of the lesion by gravity. Then it will cap the superior surface, and the entire extent of the lesion can be established. The MRI findings are the same as those seen with film myelography, the spinal cord is displaced, and there is a rounded intradural filling defect (Fig. 12-34).

MENINGIOMA

Meningiomas are second only to neurofibromas in frequency and are the most common tumor encountered in the thoracic region. Approximately 80% occur in women averaging 40 to 50 years of age. They are usually intradural-extramedullary in location but occasionally may have an extradural component.

Meningiomas of the spinal canal resemble their counterparts within the cranial cavity in being slowly growing tumors; symptoms usually extend over a period of several years or even longer before the diagnosis is established. Positive findings on plain films of the spine are not common in meningiomas. Although cal-

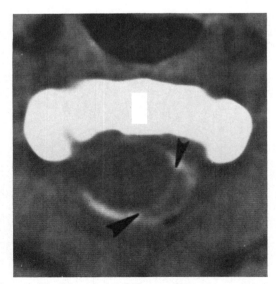

Figure 12–33. Axial CT scan following myelogram with water-soluble contrast medium. A large rounded intradural filling defect is a neurofibroma with the spinal cord shown as the effaced compressed crescentic filling defect outlined laterally. The arrows outline the cleft between the large intradural neurofibroma and the compressed spinal cord.

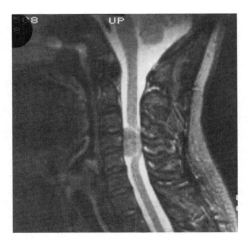

Figure 12–34. Cervical T2-weighted MRI scan demonstrating a large intradural extramedullary lesion compressing the spinal cord, a neurofibroma. (Courtesy of G. H. Brister, MD, Wausau, WI.)

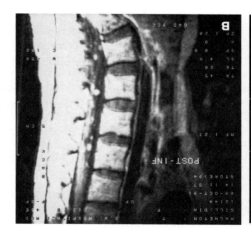

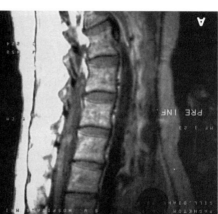

Figure 12–36. **(A)** Preinfusion. **(B)** Postinfusion of gadolinium diethylenetriaminepenta-acetic acid (paramagnetic contrast medium). The multiple intradural extramedullary lesions are seen to enhance. These are multiple neurofibromas in a patient with neurofibromatosis. (Courtesy of Shelah M. O'Connor, MD, Chicago, IL.)

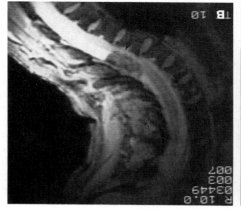

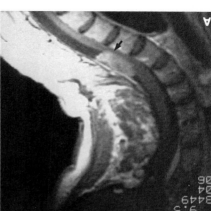

Figure 12–35. MRI scan. **(A)** T1-weighted with gadolinium diethylenetriaminepenta-acetic acid (paramagnetic contrast medium). **(B)** T2-weighted images of the cervical spine demonstrating an intradural extramedullary meningioma (arrow).

cification in the tumor is common in pathologic specimens, it is an infrequent finding in roentgenograms. This is due, in part, to the rather small amount of calcification and, in part, to the difficulty of visualizing small hazy calcific shadows within the thoracic portion of the spinal canal. If it is visible, calcification within the tumor is virtually pathognomonic of meningioma in the adult. Meningiomas do not erode pedicles or vertebral bodies very often, and this sign, of great help in detecting neurofibromas, is not available. The diagnosis is accurate with MRI; the lesions are dural based and can be seen to be intradural in location (Fig. 12-35).

Myelographic signs with meningioma are either partial or complete obstruction to the flow of contrast medium. When the block is partial, the opaque column often narrows slightly just below the lesion and then ends with a fairly sharp cutoff (Fig. 12-30). In other cases the opaque column is effaced more gradually. If the block is incomplete, the contrast medium that passes by the defect does so along one side of the canal only, and the column has the appearance of being

squeezed off rather than sharply cut off as with a neurofibroma. The myelographic signs alone seldom are sufficiently characteristic to make a diagnosis of meningioma, when taken in conjunction with the clinical history and the thoracic location of the lesion, the diagnosis is frequently possible.

The use of intravascular paramagnetic contrast medium enhances the accuracy of MRI. Multiple intradural lesions are seen to best advantage following the use of such contrast media. This technique has replaced the use of water-soluble contrast myelography in the detection of subarachnoid seeding from metastatic neoplasm or the detection of multiple intradural lesions of other origin (Fig. 12-36).

OTHER EXTRAMEDULLARY TUMORS

Intraspinal *dermoid* or *epidermoid* tumors are very rare. Usually they are present in childhood and often are associated with spinal dysraphism. There may be pediculate erosion caused by the tumor. Epidural

INTRAMEDULLARY TUMORS

As a group, the intramedullary tumors are uncommon lesions that resemble one another rather closely in their roentgenographic findings. Ependymomas are the most frequent. In the lumbar region, they arise from the conus medullaris. An ependymoma is more likely than the other lesions in this group to erode the vertebral pedicles and may cause roentgen findings similar to those observed in neurofibroma. On myelography, it may be impossible to distinguish between the lesions because an ependymoma of the conus medullaris is usually a well-circumscribed mass, and the myelographic defect may resemble that of an intradural neurofibroma. Ependymoma of the conus medullaris is intramedullary, but presents as an intradural-extramedullary mass on myelography. When the spinal cord is involved by any of the tumors of this group, the myelogram often is clearly indicative of the intramedullary location of the lesion. Obstruction of the flow of contrast medium may be either partial or complete. When partial, the spinal cord will be seen to widen out at the level of the tumor with thin streaks of opaque medium on either side of the widened cord. When the obstruction is complete, the opaque shadow widens slightly and is effaced gradually without the sharp cutoff characteristic of an intradural-extramedullary mass.

Other intramedullary tumors include astrocytoma, hemangioblastoma, and oligodendroglioma. Intramedullary hematoma may simulate tumor. Sarcoidosis has also been reported as a rare cause of spinal cord widening. Magnetic resonance imaging has a major role in detection of intramedullary mass lesions (Fig. 12-37). T_1, T_2, and contrast-enhanced T_1 imaging will separate cystic change of the spinal cord from intramedullary neoplasm. Hematoma within the cord will have the well-known paramagnetic MRI signal of the degenerating blood products; that is, subacute hematoma will be high signal on both T_1- and T_2-weighted sequences. These MRI features give this technique the best advantage in detecting spinal cord injury following trauma (Fig. 12-38).[4,11]

METASTATIC NEOPLASMS

Extradural metastatic tumors, usually metastatic carcinomas, are frequent lesions compressing the cord by extension from a focus in a vertebra (Fig. 12-39) or as an extension of a paravertebral tumor such as a plasma cell myeloma and the round-cell tumors of childhood.

Hematogenous metastases may result in the attachment of multiple small masses to the cord, the pia

masses may compress the cord and produce myelographic changes that may be similar in several different lesions. These include osteochondroma, particularly in patients with hereditary multiple exostoses, which may be diagnosed on plain-film study. Rarely, other cartilaginous tumors such as enchondroma, chondromyxoid fibroma, and chondroblastoma may project into the spinal canal as an extradural mass. Cervical chordoma may also compress the cord; it is usually associated with clearly defined erosion of the posterior aspect of the adjacent vertebrae and may extend over several segments. Extramedullary hematopoiesis has also been reported as a very rare cause of extradural masses.

Lipoma. Intraspinal lipomas are rare, but they produce fairly characteristic roentgenographic findings. Their most frequent site is the thoracic area, but some involve the low cervical and thoracic areas, and others may involve the low thoracic and lumbar areas. Erosion with thinning of the pedicles results in widening of the interpediculate distance at the level(s) of involvement. At times the lesion may extend over several segments. The pediculate erosion occurs in about one half of these patients, and there may be some erosion of the posterior surface of the adjacent vertebral bodies resulting in widening of the anteroposterior diameter of the spinal canal. The tumors are often adherent to the cord surface, usually in the posterior position.[34] Despite the size of the mass, complete subarachnoid block is not always evident on myelography. In some instances, the tumor may be completely or partially extradural and may then be associated with spina bifida. Many of these tumors are associated with congenital anomalies of the spine; this suggests a developmental origin. Myelography can be used to outline the extent of the lesion. MRI scanning will show the typical fat characteristic of the lipoma; that is, high signal on T_1 images and low signal on T_2 images. When these lipomas are associated with spinal dysraphism, the term lipomeningocele is used. These tumors are both intradural and extradural.

Sarcoma. Sarcomas arising in the epidural area are rare. Plain films may show a paraspinal mass, particularly when the lesion is in the thoracic area. When it invades a vertebral body, irregular destruction may be observed, but this is usually a late manifestation. Myelography demonstrates the extradural lesion, which may partially or completely block the flow of oil. As with other epidural tumors, the final diagnosis depends on biopsy, usually performed at the time of surgical decompression and excision.

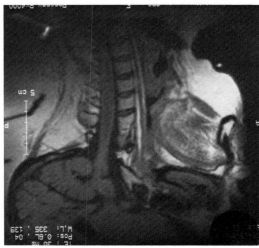

Figure 12-37. Cervical intramedullary expansion of the spinal cord. The MRI scan is not specific for the cause of the intramedullary mass lesion. In this instance this proved to be a glioma of the cervical spinal cord.

arachnoid, or the filum terminale and nerve roots. Carcinomatous and lymphomatous meningeal seeding by way of the cerebrospinal fluid may occur in patients even though they are on systemic chemotherapy. Multiple small-filling defects that represent the tumor masses may be observed at myelography. Involvement

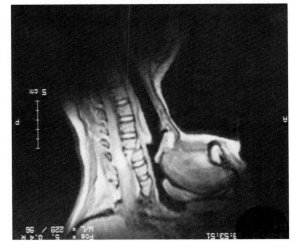

Figure 12-38. Post-traumatic spinal cord injury. C4 has subluxed anteriorly on C5 with epidural hematoma. The bright signal in the spinal cord is a combination of edema and hemorrhage causing paraplegia.

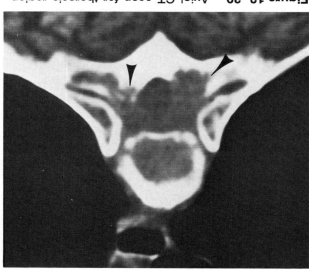

Figure 12-39. Axial CT scan for thoracic region. There is little metastatic change involving pedicles and laminae (*arrowhead*). In addition, there is epidural compromise from metastatic disease to the osseous structures and epidural space.

of the nerve root may present as nodular or a fusiform thickening. More commonly, neurogenic tumors such as medulloblastoma and ependymoma, disseminate by way of the spinal fluid to form multiple nodules similar to those just described. Rarely, sarcoidosis may produce multiple intradural-filling defects similar to those owing to metastases. Radiographs of the spine may reveal the lesion as an area of destruction. Metastatic lesions that cause clinical signs of cord or nerve root compression often have developed in the vertebral arch, and the roentgen findings may be minimal and difficult to visualize. A loss of outline of one pedicle sometimes is the only clue to the presence of the lesion.

Myelography. A metastatic lesion large enough to cause clinical signs and symptoms of cord compression will produce some degree of obstruction to the flow of radiopaque contrast medium and, in many cases, this is complete. If the tumor is extradural, the opaque column narrows slightly where the dura is being compressed by the mass. The end of the column tapers gradually. If the block is only partial, contrast medium may flow upward on one side of the canal when the patient's head is lowered. Occasionally a metastatic nodule is intradural and extramedullary; rarely it is intramedullary in location. Unless there are associated signs in the vertebrae that clearly indicate the nature

of the tumor, it usually is impossible from myelograph-ic evidence to determine whether a given defect is caused by a metastatic or primary tumor.

COMPUTED TOMOGRAPHIC SCANNING IN SPINAL NEOPLASMS

Epidural spinal neoplasms are well evaluated with ax-ial CT scanning. Because CT scanning cannot detect subarachnoid lesions, it is necessary to introduce wa-ter-soluble positive contrast medium to detect sub-arachnoid or intramedullary spinal neoplasms. Nu-clide bone scanning is the most sensitive technique for detecting osseous bony metastatic disease. If it is nec-essary to determine what additional epidural neoplasm may be compromising the spinal cord or nerve root, positive contrast medium in CT scanning is an excel-lent technique. An epidural process will displace the contrast medium away from a bony spinal canal and determination of associated osseous lytic destruction is also well seen with this technique (see Figs. 12-30 and 12-32).

Intraspinal tumors that are extramedullary can be studied with water-soluble low-dose CT scanning (see Fig. 12-31). The spinal cord can be seen displaced away from the lateral margin of the subarachnoid space from a rounded intradural-extramedullary filling defect. Intraspinal expansion can also be diagnosed with low-dose water-soluble CT scanning. An expansion of the spinal cord can be seen with axial CT scanning. Delayed CT scanning is a technique that is sensitive for detecting cystic change within the spinal cord.

MAGNETIC RESONANCE IMAGING

Magnetic resonance imaging has a role in detecting spinal cord neoplasm.[35] Using either a partial satura-tion sequence or a multiple spin-echo sequence, epi-dural involvement of the spinal column with infection or tumor is readily detected. The association of epi-dural compression of the subarachnoid space is well seen with MRI. Vertebral marrow replacement and epidural mass effect is well seen (Fig. 12-40). Other epidural lesions without bone involvement are also best assessed with MRI (Fig. 12-41). Intradural extra-medullary tumors such as neurofibroma and men-ingioma are well evaluated with MRI if paramagnetic contrast medium is used (gadolinium diethylenetri-amine penta-acetic acid).

Intramedullary abnormalities are probably best evaluated using MRI. Expansion of the spinal cord can be seen with T_2-weighted images where the spinal cord is outlined by cerebrospinal fluid with a high signal. In addition to the intramedullary expansion, the structure within the spinal cord can be well evaluated. Cysts of

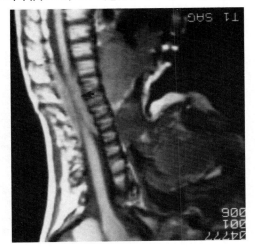

Figure 12-41. Cervical MRI scan in a child demon-strating epidural extension of neuroblastoma com-pressing the cervical subarachnoid space *(arrow)*.

the spinal cord have characteristics similar to cere-brospinal fluid and can be readily detected on MRI.

OTHER CONDITIONS

ADHESIVE ARACHNOIDITIS

Arachnoidal adhesions arise from several causes in-cluding inflammatory processes and chemical irrita-tion. In some patients, the cause remains obscure. The

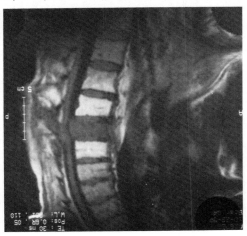

Figure 12-40. Metastatic disease to the spinal col-umn. The bright signal of the normal marrow has been replaced with tumor. There is intraspinal exten-sion of tumor with displacement of the spinal cord and resulting paraparasis.

adhesive process can be localized or widespread. There are no plain-roentgen findings in adhesive arachnoiditis. If, during myelography, the adhesive process is localized, obstruction to the flow of contrast medium may be complete. More often the block is incomplete and the contrast medium passes through the region, outlining a rather tortuous channel with irregular filling defects with poor filling of axillary root sleeves. One must be certain that the contrast medium has been injected properly into the subarachnoid space rather than subdurally or epidurally. The latter injections cause artifacts and defects that may resemble those of arachnoid adhesions. One must also be certain that defects suggesting arachnoid adhesions are not merely associated findings secondary to some other lesion such as a herniated disk or a spinal cord tumor. A peculiar form of arachnoiditis has been described in which the only myelographic manifestation is failure of filling of the root sleeves. These blunted root sleeves are now believed to represent the mildest form of adhesive arachnoiditis.

HEMANGIOMA
ARTERIOVENOUS MALFORMATIONS

Hemangioma is a rather rare lesion involving the spinal cord and meninges. A cavernous hemangioma causes irregular tortuous linear defects in the opaque column of contrast medium. There may be some interference with contrast medium flow but seldom a complete obstruction. The symptoms of arteriovenous malformations appear to be caused by ischemia or recurrent hemorrhage. In hemangioblastoma, spinal cord compression appears to produce the symptoms. As a complication of a cavernous hemangioma, there may be a sudden rupture of one of the vessels with the development of a subdural or epidural hematoma. This causes the rapidly progressive signs of pressure on the spinal cord. Myelography is useful in demonstrating the site of the hematoma.

Angiography is now used to demonstrate hemangiomas and other vascular lesions such as arteriovenous malformations and hemangioblastomas. Selective catheterization of the major feeder vessels is done to define the lesion and its nature clearly.

DiChiro and associates describe three basic patterns of pathologic vessels as follows: type I—a single coiled vessel fed by one artery.[5] Type II—the glomus type in which there is a localized plexus of small coiled vessels confined to a short segment of cord and fed by a single artery; the flow is slow, and draining vessels are seldom seen. Type III—the juvenile type found mainly in children, with multiple large feeding arteries supplying a tumorous malformation, which may fill the spinal canal; the flow is rapid, and draining veins are greatly dilated. These may be outlined myelographically but must also be studied angiographically if surgical removal is contemplated.

Arteriovenous malformations cause myelographic changes similar to those owing to cavernous hemangiomas, and differentiation may be impossible. Even on angiography, it may be difficult to decide which of these lesions is present.

SPINAL EPIDURAL HEMATOMA

Spinal epidural hematoma may occur as a complication of arteriovenous malformations as indicated previously. Bleeding into the epidural space may also occur secondary to trauma, coagulopathy, anticoagulant therapy, or recent surgery, or it may be spontaneous with no apparent cause. Myelography shows varying degrees of block caused by an epidural mass, usually at the level of the spinal cord but occasionally lower at the level of the cauda equina. History of sudden onset of symptoms with rapid progression leading to paresis or paralysis suggests the cause, but hemorrhage into a tumor may also result in similar clinical findings. The paramagnetic properties of degenerating blood allow excellent detection with T_1 MRI.

PERINEURIAL CYSTS

As originally described by Tarlov, perineurial root cysts consist of one or more cystlike spaces surrounding the nerve roots, usually in the sacral area.[43] The cysts may or may not communicate with the subarachnoid space of the spinal canal. If they do not, roentgen diagnosis is not possible. With the larger cysts, a rounded area of smooth erosion along one or more of the sacral foramina may be demonstrated. When the cysts communicate with the spinal subarachnoid space, they fill with contrast medium during myelography, and then are visualized as rounded pockets close to the sacral cul-de-sac and contiguous to the sacral nerve roots (Figs. 12-42 and 12-43). Failure to demonstrate a root cyst during immediate myelographic examination does not exclude the possibility of its presence. Similar cystlike extensions of the arachnoid along the nerve roots have been found, rarely, in the lower cervical and upper thoracic regions. Most, if not all, cysts of this type are asymptomatic and of no clinical significance. Occasionally they may cause nerve root compression resulting in pain.

MENINGEAL CYSTS AND MENINGOCELES

Intra-arachnoid cysts are usually found in the thoracic region and cause no symptoms. They may fill with contrast medium on myelography and produce a pouchlike

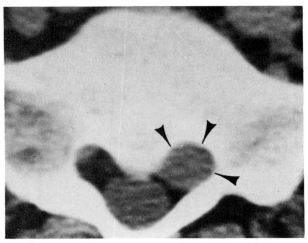

Figure 12–42. Axial CT scan through the sacrum demonstrates an enlarged sacral foramen (*arrowheads*). This could represent perineurial cyst or neurofibroma.

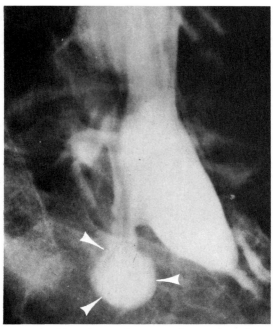

Figure 12–43. A myelogram shows that the osseous change observed in Figure 12–42 was caused by a perineural cyst (*arrows*).

defect that may retain the medium for a time, or may empty with positional change. If not filled, they appear as radiolucent filling defects in the thoracic area. Rarely, they become large enough to compress the spinal cord and require surgical decompression.

An *epidural cyst* is a rare lesion found chiefly in the thoracic region. Here it results in the gradual development of a progressive spastic paraplegia. The patient usually is an adolescent, and the history usually indicates a gradually progressive lesion. Erosion of the pedicles of multiple vertebrae is common. In some cases, there have been findings indicative of a *vertebral epiphysitis of Scheuermann's type* with irregularity of disk surfaces, anterior wedging of the vertebra, and a kyphotic deformity in the spine. This has been thought to be due to disturbance of the blood supply to the vertebrae as a result of the cyst. Myelograms reveal obstruction of extradural type with compression of the opaque column (see Fig. 12-30). Some epidural cysts communicate with the subarachnoid space and fill with contrast medium during myelography. Others do not, and the myelographic signs then are those of an extradural mass.

Small *meningoceles* may present as a cystlike lesion in the lumbosacral area. We have observed patients in whom a small meningocele eroded the sacral laminae. Meningoceles are not to be confused with the perineurial cysts described in the preceding section. The sacral meningocele may fill with contrast medium and its nature thus becomes apparent.

In addition to the more common lumbosacral men-

ingocele usually associated with spinal dysraphism (spina bifida), a meningocele may appear as an intrathoracic posterior mediastinal mass. Most intrathoracic meningoceles occur in association with neurofibromatosis, are on the right side, may enlarge the intervertebral foramen, and, therefore, may resemble neurofibromas. Communication with the subarachnoid space demonstrated on myelography confirms the diagnosis. Rarely, anterior herniation through a sacral defect results in an anterior sacral meningocele. A pelvic mass in conjunction with partial or total sacral agenesis suggests the diagnosis, which is confirmed on myelography. Meningocele must be differentiated from teratoma in some instances.

AVULSION OF CERVICAL ROOTS

Traumatic arachnoid cysts or diverticula in the cervical and upper thoracic areas may result from brachial plexus avulsion or avulsion of cervical roots. When they occur intraspinally, compression of the cord may cause paresis or paralysis. Most of them extend out along the nerve roots to lie lateral to the spinal canal. Myelography outlines the cysts, which fill with contrast media. The injury and subsequent cyst formation are usually unilateral. We have observed similar small cystlike lesions in patients with no known antecedent trauma and no symptoms; these lesions are probably anatomic variants and may be bilateral. Rarely the same type of post-traumatic cyst is found in the lumbosacral area, but protection by the bony pelvis usually prevents root avulsion and meningeal tears in this region.

Pseudomeningoceles or diverticula have also been reported as relatively transient findings following cervical laminectomy and section of dentate ligaments.

HYDROMYELIA

This condition is usually a result of obstruction of the outlets of the fourth ventricle. The central canal serves to aid in decompression of the ventricular system. It dilates diffusely, widening the entire spinal cord in all diameters. This is often associated with the Arnold-Chiari malformation. Myelographic findings consist of uniform dilatation or widening of the entire cord. Magnetic resonance imaging is an excellent technique to assess cystic change of the spinal cord (Fig. 12-44).[26, 42]

SYRINGOMYELIA

Syringomyelia is a condition characterized by cavities considered to be a diverticula of the central canal; it may be caused by rupture of the canal within the cervical cord. Fluid dissects into the tissues producing the cavities that extend within the cord apart from the central canal. The cavity is lined by altered glial elements in contrast to hydromyelia in which the central

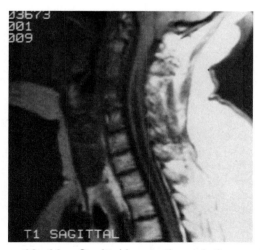

Figure 12–44. Sagittal image through the cervical region showing low cerebellar tonsils and an intramedullary hydromyelia in an adult Chiari malformation.

canal is lined by ependyma. Syringomyelia is commonly observed in the cervical area where the myelographic findings resemble those of intramedullary tumor. Some workers have recommended cyst puncture to make the differentiation between syringomyelia and hydromyelia. Recently, computerized axial tomography has been used in conjunction with a water-soluble contrast agent to outline the cervical cord. Difference in density may provide an outline of the cavitation, but myelography is often necessary for complete evaluation. As with most intramedullary disease processes, MRI is the study of choice. Acquired cystic spinal cord change is well seen with MRI. The acquired cystic change can be secondary to neoplasm or trauma.[37]

THE TETHERED CONUS

This congenital anomaly consists of low position of the conus, which is held in a posterior position. External signs of spinal dysraphism, including hypertrichosis, subcutaneous lipoma, dermoids, and sinus tracts, are present in about one half of these patients. Intradural abnormalities such as lipomas, dermoids, and widening of the dural sac were found in 10 of 24 patients reported by Fitz and Harwood-Nash.[10] Myelography performed with the patient supine shows the dorsally tethered conus in a low position as well as a small lipoma, or cysts of the conus and a thick filum terminale. The widened dural sac, usually found when the conus is at the L4–L5 level, is readily observed at myelography.

EPIDURAL ABSCESS

Epidural abscess may occur with any infection of the vertebrae or intervertebral disks. A common cause of chronic epidural abscess or granuloma is tuberculosis. In addition to chronic lesions, an acute suppurative infection can develop in the epidural space, either by direct extension from an acute osteomyelitis of a vertebra or as a primary focus of infection in the epidural tissues. Because the lesion is a serious one that may compromise the blood supply of the cord, early diagnosis is imperative. The plain radiographs of the spine often are unrevealing. In the thoracic region, one may see a widening of the soft-tissue paraspinal shadow indicative of the paraspinal abscess. If caused by an acute osteomyelitis, it will be several weeks after the onset of symptoms before radiographic signs of the disease become evident in the vertebral body or disk. Nuclide bone scanning is a cost-effective technique to detect bone involvement. However, MRI has proved to be the most sensitive examination to detect spinal osteomyelitis and epidural abscess (Fig. 12-45).

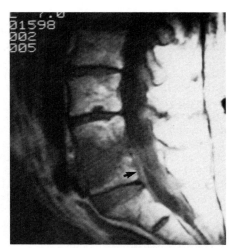

Figure 12–45. MRI scan of the lumbar spine demonstrating disk infection with osteomyelitis of the two adjacent L4 and L5 vertebral bodies. Epidural abcess is present below the involved intervertebral disk space (*arrow*).

REFERENCES AND SELECTED READINGS

1. BENZIAN SR, MAINZER F, GOODING CA: Pediculate thinning: A normal variant at the thoracolumbar junction. Br J Radiol 44:936, 1971

2. BUNDSCHUH CV, MODIC MT, ROSS JS, ET AL: Epidural fibrosis and recurrent disk herniation in the lumbar spine: MR imaging assessment. Am J Roentgenol 150:923, 1988

3. CARRERA GR, HAUGHTON VM, SYVERTSON A, ET AL: Computed tomography of the lumbar facet joints. Radiology 134:145, 1980

4. CHAKERES DW, FLICKINGER F, BRESNAHAN JC, ET AL: MR imaging of acute spinal cord trauma. AJNR 8:5, 1987

5. DICHIRO G, DOPPMAN JL, OMMAYA AK: Radiology of spinal cord arteriovenous malformations. Prog Neurol Surg 4:329, 1971

6. DOPPMAN JL: Arteriography of the spinal cord. Semin Roentgenol 7:231, 1972

7. EDELMAN RR, SHOUKIMAS GM, STARK DD, ET AL: High-resolution surface-coil imaging of lumbar disk disease. Am J Roentgenol 144:1123, 1985

8. EPSTEIN BS: Spinal canal mass lesions. Radiol Clin North Am 4:185, 1966

9. EPSTEIN BS: The spine: A radiologic text and atlas, 4th ed. Philadelphia, Lea & Febiger, 1976

10. FITZ CR, HARWOOD-NASH DC: The tethered conus. Am J Roentgenol 125:515, 1975

11. FLANDERS AE, SCHAEFER DM, DOAN HT, ET AL: Acute cervical spine trauma: Correlation of MR imaging findings with degree of neurologic deficit. Radiology 177:25, 1990

12. GELLIS SS, FEINGOLD M, TUNNESSEN WW JR, ET AL: Caudal dysplasia syndrome (picture of the month). Am J Dis Child 116:407, 1968

13. GENANT HK, CHAFETZ N, HELMS CA: Computed tomography of the lumbar spine. San Francisco, University of California, Printing Department, 1982

14. GHELMAN B, FREIBERGER RH: The limbus vertebra: An anterior disc herniation demonstrated by discography. Am J Roentgenol 127:854, 1976

15. GLENN WV JR, RHODES ML, ALTSCHULER EM, ET AL: Multiple display computerized body tomography applications in the lumbar spine. Spine 4:282, 1979

16. HAN JS, KAUFMAN B, EL YOUSEF SJ, ET AL: NMR imaging of the spine. Am J Roentgenol 141:1137, 1983

17. HAUGHTON VM, HO KC: Effect of blood on arachnoiditis from aqueous myelographic contrast media. Am J Roentgenol 139:569, 1982

18. HAUGHTON VM, SYVERTSEN A, WILLIAMS AL: Soft tissue anatomy within the spinal canal as seen on computed tomography. Radiology 134:649, 1980

19. HAUGHTON VM, WILLIAMS AL: Computed tomography of the spine. St Louis, CV Mosby, 1982

20. HELMS CA, DORWART RH, GRAY MB: CT appearance of conjoined nerve roots and differentiation from a herniated nucleus pulposus. Radiology 144:803, 1982

21. HINCK VC, CLARK WM, HOPKINS CE: Normal interpediculate distances (minimum and maximum) in children and adults. Am J Roentgenol 97:141, 1966

22. HIRSCH C, ROSENCRANTZ M, WICKBOM I: Lumbar myelography with water-soluble media with special reference to the appearances of root pockets. Acta Radiol (Diagn) (Stockh) 8:54, 1969

23. JOHANSEN JG, ORRISON WW, AMUNDSEN P: Lateral C1-2 puncture for cervical myelography. Radiology 146:391, 1983

24. KOONTZ WW JR, PROUT GR JR: Agenesis of the sacrum and neurogenic bladder. JAMA 203:481, 1968

25. KOSTELIC JK, HAUGHTON VM, SETHER LA: Lumbar spinal nerves in the neural foramen: MR appearance. Radiology 178:837, 1991

26. LEE BCP, ZIMMERMAN RD, MANNING JJ, ET AL: MR imaging of syringomyelia and hydromyelia. Am J Roentgenol 144:1149, 1985

27. LIU SS, WILLIAMS KD, DRAYER BP, ET AL: Synovial cysts of the lumbosacral spine: Diagnosis by MR imaging. Radiology 154:163, 1990

28. LUSTED LB, KEATS TE: Atlas of roentgenographic measurement, 3rd ed. Chicago, Year Book Medical Publishers, 1973

29. MARAVILLA KR, LESH P, WEINREB JC, ET AL: Magnetic resonance imaging of the lumbar spine with CT correlation. AJNR 6:237, 1985

30. MODIC MT, MASARYK T, BOUMPHREY F, ET AL: Lumbar herniated disk disease and canal stenosis: Prospective

diagnosis by surface coil MR, CT and myelography. AJNR 7:709, 1986

31. MODIC MT, WEINSTEIN MA, PAVLICEK W, ET AL: Magnetic resonance imaging of the cervical spine: Technical and clinical observations. AJNR 5:15, 1984

32. MODIC MT, WEINSTEIN MA, PAVLICEK W, ET AL: Nuclear magnetic resonance imaging of the spine. Radiology 148: 757, 1983

33. MORRISON SG, PERRY LW, SCOTT LP III: Congenital brevicollis (Klippel-Feil syndrome). Am J Dis Child 115:614, 1968

34. NAIDICH TP, MCLONE DG, MUTLUER S: A new understanding of dorsal dysraphism with lipoma (lipomyeloschisis): Radiologic evaluation and surgical correction. Am J Roentgenol 140:1065, 1983

35. NORMAN D, MILLS CM, BRANT-ZAWADSKI M, ET AL: Magnetic resonance imaging of the spinal cord and canal: Potentials and limitations. Am J Roentgenol 141:1147, 1983

36. PAUL LW, MOIR WW: Non-pathologic variations in relationship of the upper cervical vertebrae. Am J Roentgenol 62:519, 1949

37. QUENCER RM, SHELDON JJ, POST MJD, ET AL: MRI of the chronically injured cervical spinal cord. Am J Roentgenol 147:125, 1986

38. ROBERTSON GH, LLEWELLYN HJ, TAVERAS JM: The narrow lumbar spinal canal syndrome. Radiology 107:89, 1973

39. RUSSELL EJ: Cervical disc disease: State of the art. Radiology 177:313, 1990

40. SACKETT JF, STROTHER CM: New Techniques in myelography. Hagerstown, MD, Harper & Row, 1979

41. SCHELLINGER D, MANZ HJ, VIDIC B, ET AL: Disc fragment migration. Radiology 175:831, 1990

42. SHERMAN JL, BARKOVICH AJ, CITRIN CM: The MR appearance of syringomyelia: New observations. Am J Roentgenol 148:381, 1987

43. TARLOV IM: Cysts (perineurial) of the sacral roots. JAMA 138:740, 1948

44. THORNBURY JR, FRYBACK DG, TURSKI PA, ET AL: Comparison of MR versus CT myelography and plain CT in the diagnosis of disk-caused nerve compression in acute low back pain patients. Radiology 186:731, 1993

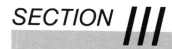

The Abdomen and Gastrointestinal Tract

Paul and Juhl's Essentials of Radiologic Imaging, Sixth Edition, edited by John H. Juhl and Andrew B. Crummy. J.B. Lippincott Company, Philadelphia, © 1993.

CHAPTER *13*

The Abdomen

Michael Davis

THE ABDOMEN

Multiple options are available for radiologic study of the abdomen. Many, such as the barium enema, are directed at one organ. Plain films, however, allow one to view the entire abdomen before proceeding to a more specific investigation.[4]

INDICATIONS

Abdominal distention, abdominal pain, vomiting, diarrhea, and abdominal trauma are the most common reasons for obtaining plain films. The presence of a palpable abdominal mass warrants imaging by computed tomography (CT) or ultrasonography.[8]

NORMAL ABDOMINAL ORGANS

The liver forms a homogeneous shadow in the right-upper quadrant of the abdomen. Its upper border is limited by the right leaf of the diaphragm, which is confluent with the superior surface of the liver. The superior surfaces of the hemidiaphragms are outlined by aerated lung. The right-lateral margin of the liver is usually separated from the density of the abdominal wall by a thin layer of fat. The lower edge of the right lobe of the liver is seen because of the radiolucency of the adjacent omental and pericolic fat. Gas in the hepatic flexure and in the transverse colon also helps identify the lower margin of the liver. The inferior margin of the left lobe of the liver is not visible. The liver's complex shape interferes with determining the presence of hepatomegaly until the liver becomes quite large.

The entire spleen or part of it can usually be seen in the left-upper abdomen. The normal spleen, about 10 to 14 cm long, is about the same size as the kidney. In rare instances the spleen is unusually mobile and may be found medial to the splenic flexure of the colon.

The kidneys lie on either side of the lumbar spine. Visualization depends on perirenal fat; thus their outlines may be lost in patients with markedly diminished body fat. The pancreas cannot be seen on plain films. The outer margins of the psoas muscles can usually be seen because of the fat surrounding them. A loss of body fat or a tapered lateral margin of the muscles may obscure visualization. Less attention is now being paid to the psoas margins in detecting retroperitoneal abnormalities because of the normal variations that exist.[9]

The lateral margins of the peritoneum often are bound externally by thin layers of fat sufficient to cause a radiolucent stripe. The three layers of abdominal musculature can be seen laterally to that stripe. The urinary bladder usually is visible if it contains urine and is surrounded by fat. In women the abdominal fat may allow visualization of the uterus.

Supine films may show a mass created by accumulation of stomach fluid in the fundus. When the patient is in an upright position, the gastric fluid shifts to the antrum and the gas to the fundus.

NORMAL ABDOMINAL GAS

Swallowed air is the source of the gas that is normally seen in the stomach. Some of that gas passes through the small bowel to the colon; it is common to see gas in limited quantities in nondistended small-bowel loops (Fig. 13-1). The colon normally contains gas and feces, which can be easily recognized. Bacterial gas production has been found to be a significant source of colonic gas. The intestinal gas pattern of infants differs from that of adults in that gas is normally present throughout the small bowel. Within a few hours after birth, gas can be seen throughout the intestinal tract.

ABDOMINAL CALCIFICATIONS

Calcified mesenteric lymph nodes are observed most often in the right-lower quadrant or in the lower-central part of the abdomen (Fig. 13-2). Calcification in nodes is believed to be secondary to granulomatous disease. Aortic and arterial calcifications are an almost inevitable consequence of aging and are seen frequently. This calcification often allows estimation of the diameter of the vessel. Aortic and iliac artery aneurysms are the most prevalent and can be confirmed and measured by ultrasonography if necessary (Fig. 13-3). Venous calcification in the pelvis is very common. These round phleboliths often have a radiolucent center that distinguishes them from urinary tract stones. Nodular hepatic and splenic calcifications are seen in individuals who have lived in endemic areas of histoplasmosis (Fig. 13-4A). Simple splenic cysts often calcify and may be large (Fig. 13-4B, C). The episode that led to the calcification usually cannot be determined.

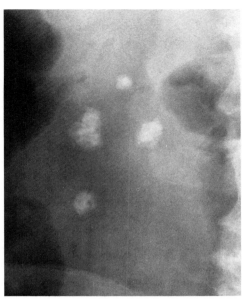

Figure 13–2. Calcified mesenteric lymph nodes. Calcified nodes are mottled areas of density lateral to the right margin of the third and fourth lumbar vertebrae.

Pancreatic calcification, which is actually pancreatic lithiasis (Fig. 13-5A), occurs secondary to pancreatitis. Most patients with pancreatic calcifications have a history of alcoholism. About 10% of gallstones contain enough calcium to be visible on plain film. Often the calcification is ringlike, and it may be faceted (Fig.

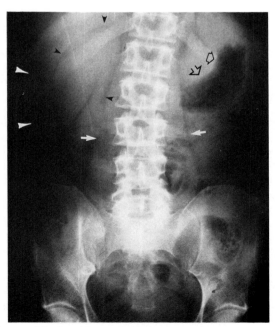

Figure 13–1. Normal abdomen. Some stomach gas (*open arrows*), psoas muscles outlined by fat (*arrows*), liver edge (*white arrowheads*), and kidneys (*black arrowheads*).

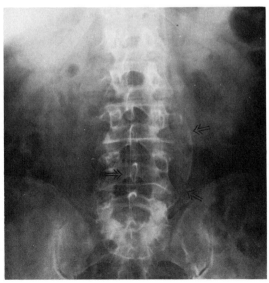

Figure 13–3. Abdominal aortic aneurysm. The diameter of the aneurysm can be measured because of the calcification within the aortic wall (*arrows*).

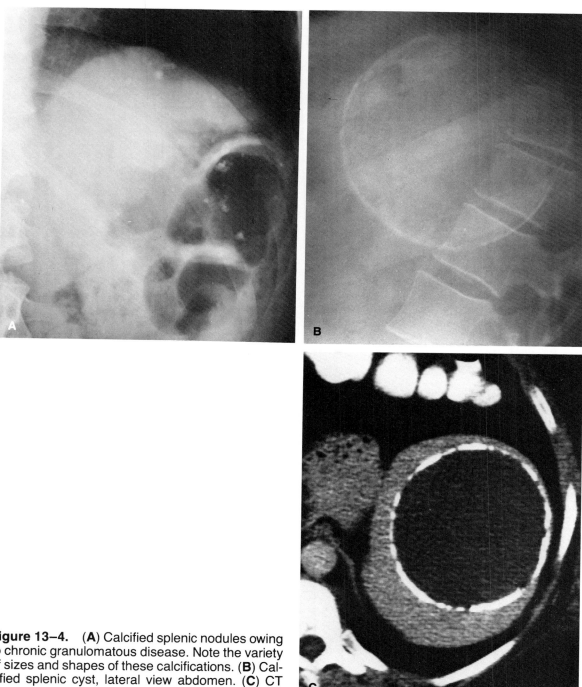

Figure 13–4.　(**A**) Calcified splenic nodules owing to chronic granulomatous disease. Note the variety of sizes and shapes of these calcifications. (**B**) Calcified splenic cyst, lateral view abdomen. (**C**) CT examination of the calcified splenic cyst.

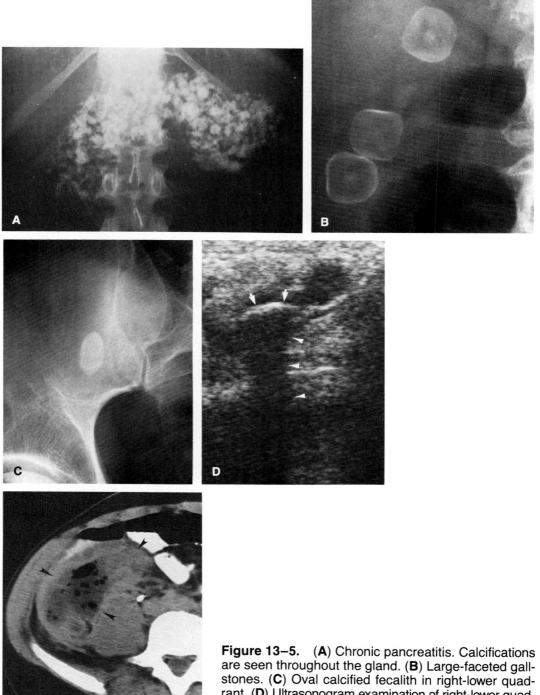

Figure 13–5. **(A)** Chronic pancreatitis. Calcifications are seen throughout the gland. **(B)** Large-faceted gallstones. **(C)** Oval calcified fecalith in right-lower quadrant. **(D)** Ultrasonogram examination of right-lower quadrant shows bright echo of fecalith (*arrow*) and acoustical shadowing (*arrowheads*). **(E)** CT scan shows appendiceal abscess in right-lower quadrant (*arrowheads*).

13-5*B*). Most urinary tract stones are calcified. Intestinal contents that remain at one site for too long may calcify, forming fecaliths or enteroliths. There is a strong association of appendiceal fecaliths with acute appendicitis. Rupture of the appendix may allow the fecalith to move freely in the peritoneal space (Fig. 13-5*C*, through *E*). Enteroliths occur in Meckel's diverticulum and chronic, partially obstructing lesions of the small bowel and colon. Seed pits may sometimes provide the nidus for the enterolith. Adrenal gland calcification may be a consequence of tuberculosis or of hemorrhagic infarction that occurred when the patient was an infant (Fig. 13-6). Many intra-abdominal cysts, which may calcify, can be found in the spleen, liver, adrenal gland (Fig. 13-7*A*), kidney, and mesentery. Echinococcal cysts of the liver calcify, but amebic cysts

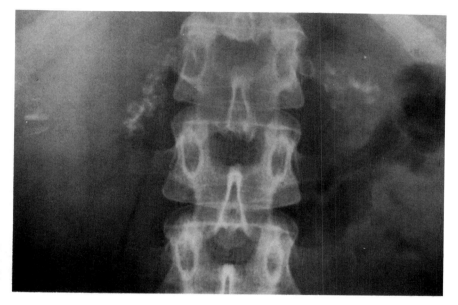

Figure 13–6. Calcification in the adrenal glands is clearly defined on either side of the first lumbar vertebra.

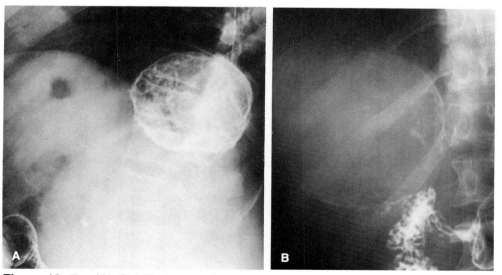

Figure 13–7. (**A**) Calcified cyst of the right adrenal gland. The large cyst with a densely calcified wall is noted to lie directly above the right kidney. (**B**) Large round peripherally calcified hepatic cyst that was considered echinoccal.

do not (Fig. 13-7*B*). Ovarian teratomas may have calcification within them that simulates teeth and bone. These tumors often contain lipid material as well, which can be identified because of its radiolucency (Fig. 13-8*A*, *B*). A tumor that often calcifies is uterine leiomyoma (Fig. 13-9*A*, *B*), whose characteristic mottled "mulberry" calcification occurs as a result of de-

generation. Other malignant tumors in the abdomen may also exhibit calcification. The mucin-producing carcinomas of the stomach and colon are an example. Degenerative calcification may occur in hypernephroma. The psammomatous calcification within ovarian carcinomas can occasionally be seen. Neuroblastomas in children frequently contain calcifications.

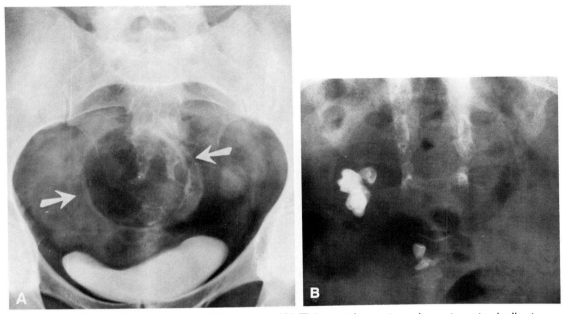

Figure 13–8.   Dermoid cyst of the ovary. (**A**) This cyst has a translucent center indicating its fatty content. The wall is seen as a thin, circular density (*arrows*). The bladder contains contrast material from a previous intravenous urogram. (**B**) This cyst contains a cluster of teeth.

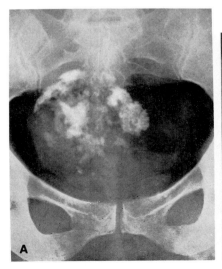
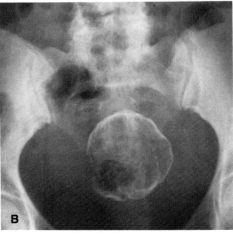

Figure 13–9. (**A**) Calcified uterine leiomyoma. (**B**) More homogeneously calcified uterine leiomyoma.

Meconium peritonitis may occur as the result of intestinal atresia or meconium ileus with bowel perforation. Then calcification may be widely distributed throughout the peritoneal space (Fig. 13-10). Occasionally meconium will be calcified while still within the bowel lumen.

MECHANICAL SMALL-INTESTINE OBSTRUCTION

Abdominal pain, distention, and vomiting occurring in a patient with a history of previous abdominal surgery directs attention to the possibility of obstruction. A film of the chest combined with upright and supine films of the abdomen is a good routine to use in evaluating this situation. The upright chest film decreases the possibility of missing perforation of the gut manifested by subdiaphragmatic air and also allows assessment of the status of the lungs. In a simple obstruction, the intestinal lumen is occluded at a single point without any significant interference with its blood supply. Most often an adhesive band is responsible for the obstruction, though neoplasm, gallstone, or internal hernia may be the cause (Table 13-1).

Within 3 to 5 hours after the onset of an obstruction, gas and fluid accumulate proximally and can be seen on the abdominal film. On the upright film, distended bowel loops with gas-fluid levels are present (Fig. 13-11A through D). In the very early stage or if the obstruction is partial, only a few gas-distended loops may be seen. With the passage of time, the caliber and the number of visible loops increase. The small-bowel loops are distinguished from the colon by their central location in the abdomen and by characteristic small-bowel folds that are close together and extend completely around the circumference of the bowel. This is unlike the colon, where the folds are not circumferential and are widely separated. If the obstruction of the small bowel is complete and enough time has elapsed for colon evacuation, little or no gas may be present in the colon. If the bowel obstruction is incomplete, there may be a normal amount of gas in the colon.

Rarely, the obstructed bowel is entirely filled with fluid. This is likely to occur in proximal jejunal obstruction. In this instance the instillation of a small amount of contrast material through a nasogastric tube will demonstrate the distended, fluid-filled small bowel (Fig. 13-12).

Criteria to distinguish strangulation obstruction were developed many years ago but, unfortunately, have not withstood the test of time. Currently, the ability of ultrasonography and CT to detect the bowel-wall thickening that goes with strangulation has proved more useful than plain films (Fig. 13-13).[5]

MECHANICAL COLON OBSTRUCTION

Colonic obstruction is usually caused by cancer or diverticulitis. Volvulus, hernia, and fecal impaction are other causes. The symptoms of obstipation and abdominal distention direct attention to the colon. In the presence of a competent ileocecal valve, colon obstruction is manifested by gaseous distention of the colon from the cecum to the site of obstruction (Fig. 13-14). A varying amount of fluid is present but usually is not as

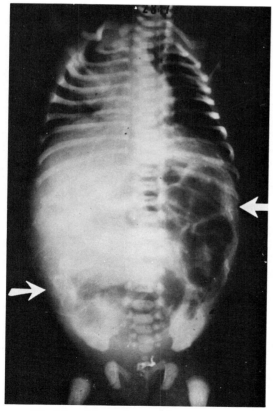

Figure 13–10. Meconium peritonitis in a newborn. There are scattered, small, irregular calcifications along peritoneal surfaces (*arrows*).

Table 13–1. Common Causes of Small-Bowel Obstruction in Adults

Adhesions

Hernia

Malignancy

Inflammatory bowel disease

Miscellaneous (Crohn's disease, volvulus, appendiceal abscess, and gallstone ileus)

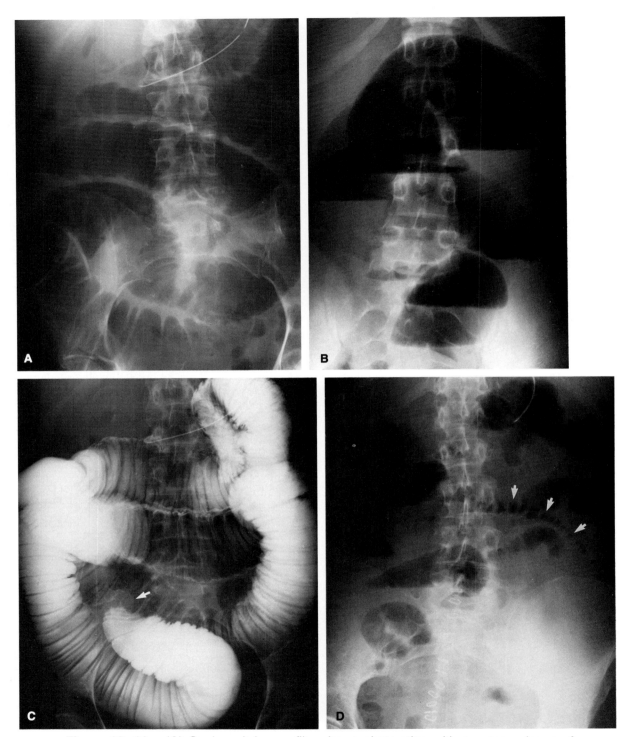

Figure 13–11. (**A**) Supine abdomen film shows obstruction with numerous loops of small bowel dilated. (**B**) Upright abdomen with small-bowel obstruction. Note different level of fluid in each loop that differentiates it from small-bowel ileus. (**C**) Barium study shows site of obstruction caused by adhesion (*arrow*). (**D**) Upright abdomen film in advanced small-bowel obstruction with "string-of-beads" sign (*arrows*).

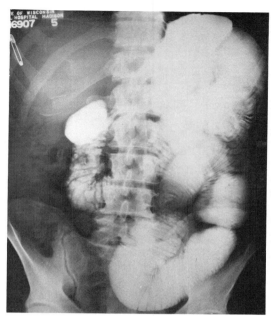

Figure 13–12. Adhesive band. In this film, exposed after the patient had a barium meal, the jejunal loops are noted to be considerably dilated. The mucosal folds have not been obliterated even though there is distention; the appearance resembles that of stacked coins.

prominent as in small-bowel obstruction. If the ileocecal valve is incompetent, the colonic gas may move into the small bowel and partially decompress the colon. The key observation is that there continues to be a disproportionate enlargement of the colon in relation to that of the small bowel.

With sigmoid volvulus, two parallel gas-distended colonic loops are seen rising out of the pelvis (Fig. 13-15A, B). With cecal volvulus, attention is usually directed to the left-upper quadrant, where the gas-distended cecum, which may mimic a gas-filled stomach, is observed (Fig. 13-16).

When plain films suggest colonic obstruction it should be confirmed by endoscopy or barium enema. Prompt decompression will avert cecal perforation.

PARALYTIC (ADYNAMIC) ILEUS

Laparotomy and other types of trauma may lead to impairment of intestinal motility. Hypothyroidism, drugs that inhibit intestinal motility, and hypokalemia also may cause an ileus pattern. Plain films usually show a proportionate distention of small bowel and

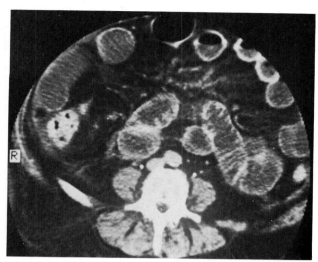

Figure 13–13. Computed tomogram of venous infarction of the small bowel. Intravenous contrast material fills the intramural portion of the markedly thickened small-bowel loops.

colon (Fig. 13-17). Early in the process, the upright films show little fluid in the bowel. Occasionally, the paralytic process only involves the colon. The films then suggest colonic obstruction, but endoscopy or barium enema will eliminate this possibility. As with mechanical obstruction, colonic ileus may result in cecal perforation. Cecal diameters in the range of 12 cm are reason for concern. Either cecostomy or colonoscopy can be used for decompression.

INTESTINAL WALL GAS

In benign pneumatosis intestinalis there is a collection of gas in the bowel wall that usually involves an extensive length of bowel (Fig. 13-18A, B) (Table 13-2). It often appears as multiple gas cysts. Patients usually are not acutely ill. This is in contrast to patients with necrotic bowel and a linear or mottled gas pattern in the wall (Fig. 13-19A, B). They are often desperately

Table 13–2. Some Causes of Portal Venous Gas

Ischemic bowel disease
Diverticulitis
Mechanical small-bowel obstruction
Pneumatosis intestinalis
Pelvic and intra-abdominal abscess
Hemorrhagic pancreatitis

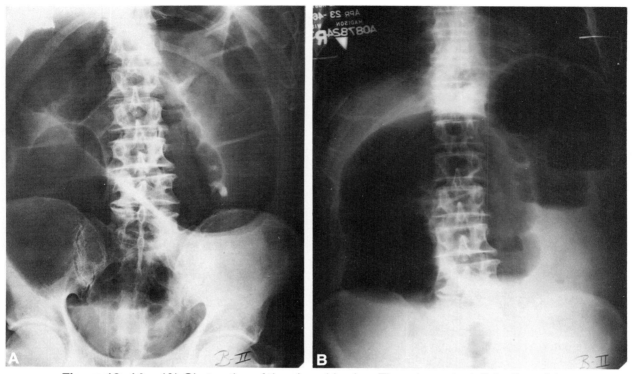

Figure 13–14. (A) Obstruction of the sigmoid colon. There is marked distention of the proximal colon to the region of the splenic flexure. No appreciable amount of gas is present in the small bowel, indicating a competent ileocecal valve. The obstruction in this patient was in the sigmoid. The end of the gas column shown on a single film of this type does not necessarily indicate the site of obstruction. In this patient the cecum is greatly distended; it ruptured shortly after this roentgenographic study was made. (B) Upright film of the patient shown in (A).

ill; sometimes gas is visible in the portal veins within the liver on plain films and on CT scans (Table 13-3) (Fig. 13-20A through C).

THE PERITONEAL SPACE

The peritoneal space has little significance in health because it is actually a potential space. It is extremely important in disease and has been a problem in diagnostic radiology for many years. The peritoneal space was studied directly by performing a pneumoperitoneum, but was used infrequently and is now virtually obsolete. Another way to determine peritoneal-space disease is to look for displacement or other abnormality of the contrast-filled gut. This is not a reliable method.

INDICATIONS

Abdominal distention that might be caused by intraperitoneal blood or another fluid warrants study of the peritoneal space. In the presence of fever or other signs

Table 13–3. Some Common Causes of Pneumatosis Intestinalis

Mesenteric vascular occlusive disease
Pulmonary disease with pneumomediastinum
Iatrogenic trauma (endoscopy, biopsy)
Intestinal obstruction
Collagen vascular disease
Abdominal trauma
Idiopathic

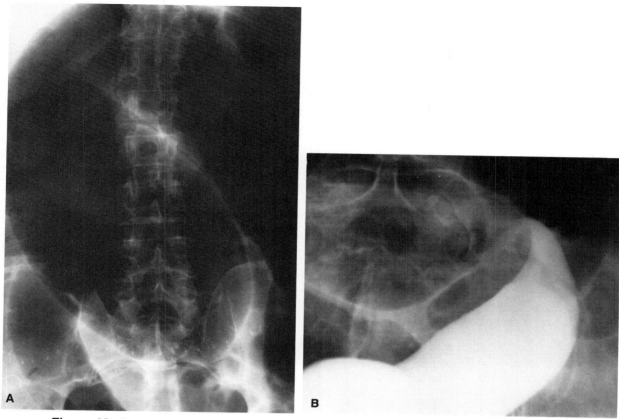

Figure 13–15. **(A)** Sigmoid volvulus. The distended, twisted loop of sigmoid colon fills the entire abdomen giving an inverted U shape to the sigmoid colon. **(B)** Barium given rectally shows the "bird's beak" appearance at the site of the volvulus.

of an intra-abdominal abscess, the peritoneal space must be surveyed. The need to know the extramural extent of a process that also involves the gut wall is also an indication.

ANATOMY

The contour of the peritoneal space is extremely complex.[6] This continuous mesothelial-lined space is best defined by its adjacent structures. Areas have thus been named accordingly (subdiaphragmatic, subhepatic, paracolonic). A pouchlike area (the lesser sac) lies behind the stomach. The peritoneal space extends down into the pelvis; the area in front of the rectum is the cul-de-sac. Another structure that is not gut but is surrounded by peritoneum is the greater omentum.

CONGENITAL ANOMALIES

Congenital defects in the peritoneum are rare. Occasionally there is persistence of the embryonic pleuroperitoneal canal, leading to herniation of abdominal organs into the thorax (Bochdalek's hernia). The most common anomaly is mesenteric cyst, which may be quite large, may be present at any age, displaces the bowel, and creates a visible mass (Fig. 13-21). This mass may not be palpable and is usually asymptomatic. Ultrasonography is an excellent method to identify the cystic nature of these lesions.[2]

In gastroschisis the anterior peritoneum and the other anterior wall structures are absent. In other disorders the peritoneum may be intact, but the lack of

(*text continues on page 515*)

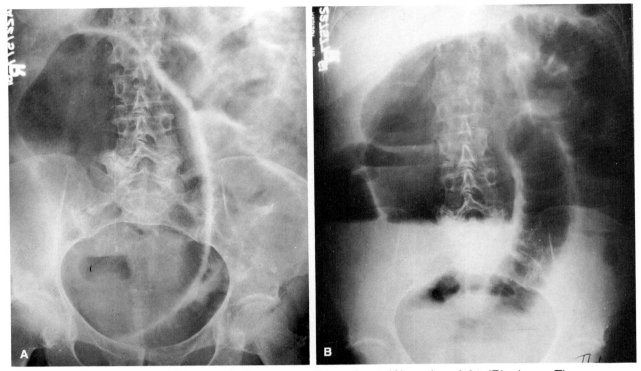

Figure 13–16. Volvulus of the cecum. Recumbent (**A**) and upright (**B**) views. The distended cecum forms an oval-shaped radiolucency with the tip pointed upward and to the right. There is gas distention of the small intestine in the left lateral portion of the abdomen. There is a gas-fluid level in the cecum and smaller levels in loops of small bowel noted in (B). In the central abdomen, air-fluid levels are noted in the cecum and in the small bowel.

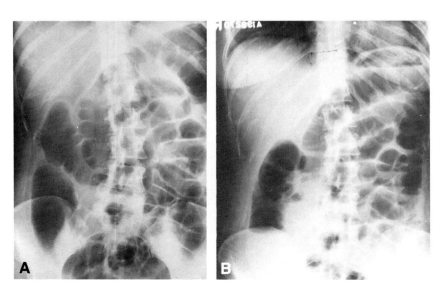

Figure 13–17. (**A**) Adynamic ileus. Recumbent (**A**) and upright (**B**) projections show a considerable amount of gas in the small bowel and colon. Fluid levels are inconspicuous except in the cecum.

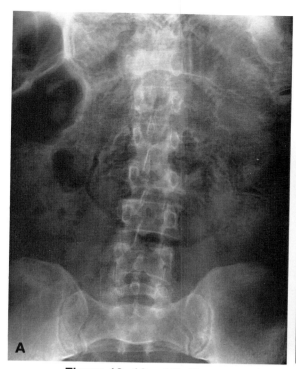

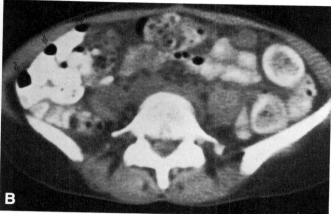

Figure 13–18. (**A**) Pneumatosis cystoides intestinalis. The plain film shows serpiginous collections of gas in the intestinal wall. (**B**) A computed tomograph in a different patient shows the gas cysts (*arrows*) encroaching on the barium-filled bowel.

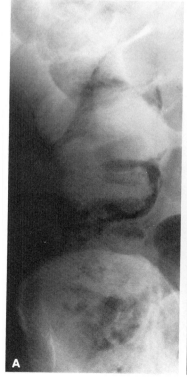

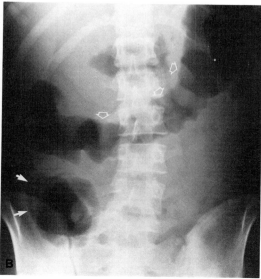

Figure 13–19. (**A**) Right-colon infarction. Intramural linear collections of air that have a mottled appearance. (**B**) Colon infarction. Supine abdomen shows some pneumatosis in right-lower quadrant (*arrows*) and markedly thickened mucosal folds caused by edema and hemorrhage (*arrowheads*).

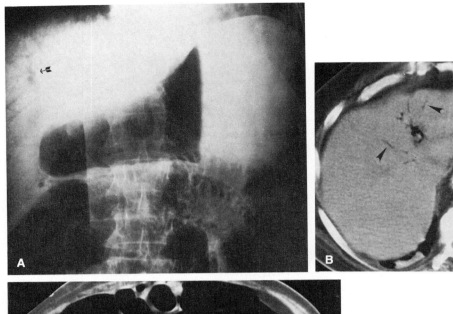

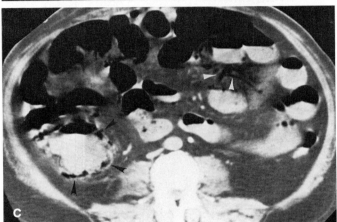

Figure 13–20. **(A)** Portal venous gas. This decubitus film of the abdomen shows the branched gas pattern in the liver (*arrow*). The presence of this quantity of gas in the portal vein is almost always indicative of intestinal infarction. **(B)** CT scan through liver shows portal venous air (*arrowheads*). **(C)** CT scan through lower abdomen shows pneumatosis in intramural location (*black arrowheads*) and in mesenteric veins (*white arrowheads*).

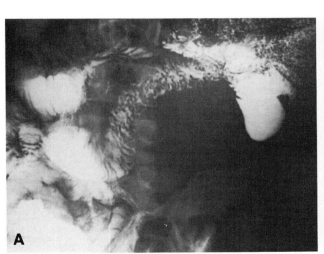

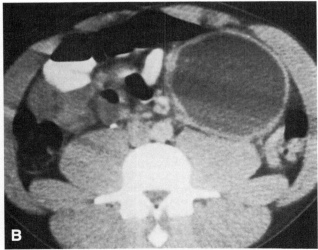

Figure 13–21. Mesenteric cyst. **(A)** Small-bowel loops are displaced by the extrinsic mass in the left side of the abdomen. **(B)** CT clearly identifies the well-encapsulated fluid collection.

supporting structures leads to all types of hernias. Omphalocele and the prune-belly syndrome are examples of this, as well as the more common inguinal hernias. Internal hernias may occur in the paraduodenal areas and as a consequence of defects in the diaphragm. The severest of these results is the entire mobile gut moving to the thorax (Fig. 13-22).

INFLAMMATION

Abscesses in the peritoneal space ordinarily are either postoperative or secondary to gut rupture, particularly appendicitis or diverticulitis. Abscesses are also seen in association with severe inflammatory bowel disease, such as granulomatous enterocolitis. At times plain films of the abdomen are diagnostic. Gas-forming organisms and the inflammatory reaction form a recognizable roentgenographic appearance (Fig. 13-23). When the abscess is filled only with fluid or contains only a little gas, CT and ultrasonography are useful. Both modalities are excellent for identifying and delineating these fluid collections (Fig. 13-24). Real-time ultrasound distinguishes these collections from fluid-filled bowel because the abscess lacks motility. Computed tomography is aided by either a location of the abscess that is incompatible with the bowel or lack of intestinal contrast material in the abscess. The latter may be a problem if there is a large communication

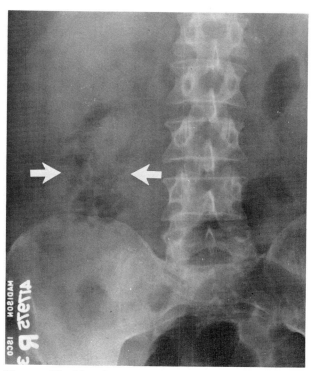

Figure 13–23. Intra-abdominal abscess secondary to perforation of a carcinoma of the colon. The accumulation of mottled gas shadows (*arrows*) is extraluminal as shown by constancy in several other examinations and confirmed by surgical exploration.

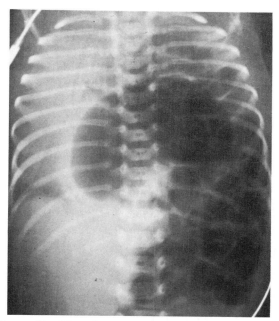

Figure 13–22. Congenital left diaphragmatic hernia. The gas-filled stomach and small bowel are seen in the left hemithorax displacing the heart to the right side.

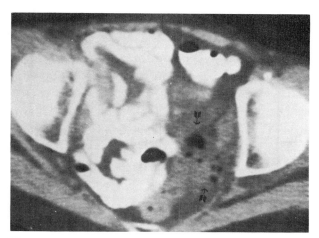

Figure 13–24. Abdominal abscess. Multiple small gas pockets can be seen in the multiloculated left pelvic abscess (*arrows*).

between gut and abscess that allows the ingested contrast material to fill the abscess. Computed tomography is important in planning the percutaneous drainage of these pockets. It is also used as a guide to find a safe, effective drainage route.

Primary peritonitis is prone to occur in patients with severe liver disease. Finding fluid in the peritoneal space with either ultrasonography or CT, both of which are more sensitive than plain films, can be followed by diagnostic aspiration of the fluid.

NEOPLASMS

Mesothelioma represents a primary malignant neoplasm of the peritoneum. Like the pleural form, it is believed to be related to asbestos exposure. The CT appearance is far from characteristic but may provide enough information to justify biopsy. Pseudomyxoma peritonei is perhaps too elaborate a name for what really is a low-grade metastatic malignancy commonly secondary to an appendiceal tumor. Metastases from breast, ovary, colon, and carcinoid tumors may show extensive peritoneal implants and cause ascitic fluid.

PNEUMOPERITONEUM

Although pneumoperitoneum is a natural consequence of surgical exploration of the abdomen, it is distinctly abnormal under other circumstances and usually indicates rupture of either the stomach, duodenum, or colon. Upright plain films or cross-table decubitus films can detect very small quantities of peritoneal gas; additional studies such as CT usually are not necessary (Fig. 13-25A, B) (Table 13-4).

PERITONEAL FLUID

It is no longer necessary to rely on plain films to detect ascites and hemoperitoneum. Positive plain-film findings require the presence of an abundance of peritoneal fluid. Fluid-filled loops of bowel in the pelvis can

Table 13-4. Common Causes of Pneumoperitoneum

Ulcer perforation
Iatrogenic perforation (endoscopy, enemas, etc)
Neoplasm perforation
Pneumatosis intestinalis
Inflammatory bowel disease
Diverticulitis
Foreign-body perforation
Postoperative leakage

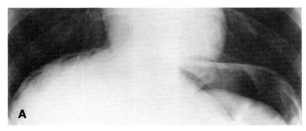
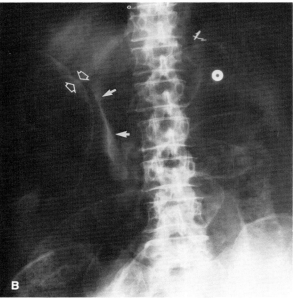

Figure 13–25. (**A**) Upright abdomen film shows free air beneath both hemidiaphragms. (**B**) Supine abdomen film shows falciform ligaments (*arrows*) outlined by free air and "double-wall" sign (*arrowheads*) from the same cause.

be confused with free fluid. Ultrasonography is an extremely sensitive diagnostic modality and can detect very small amounts of free fluid or blood. The free fluid accumulates in the dependent areas of the pelvis and upper abdomen, and changes with the patient's position (Fig. 13-26A through C).

IATROGENIC DISEASE

Unfortunately, any of the implements used in a laparotomy may be left inadvertently in the peritoneal space. Because all sponges and pads are equipped with radiopaque markers, they can be identified by taking a portable abdominal film in the operating room (Fig. 13-27). Occasionally, large items such as scissors, needleholders, and hemostats are left in the abdomen.

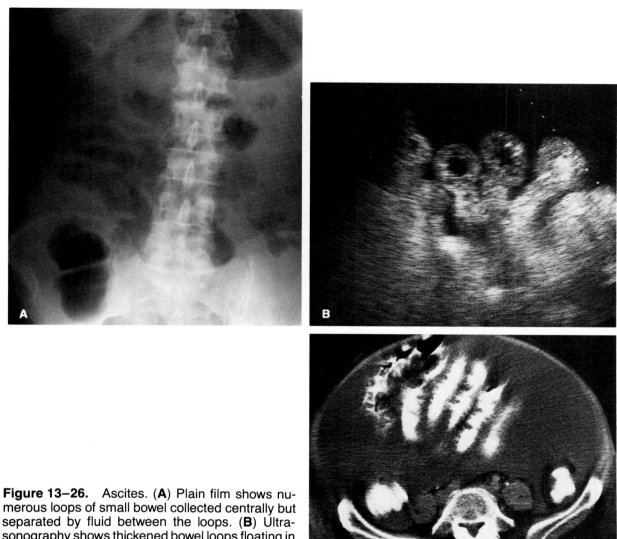

Figure 13–26. Ascites. (**A**) Plain film shows numerous loops of small bowel collected centrally but separated by fluid between the loops. (**B**) Ultrasonography shows thickened bowel loops floating in ascites. (**C**) CT scan shows massive ascites with barium-filled loops of small bowel.

Figure 13–27. Foreign-body–laparotomy pad without radiopaque marker. (**A**) The pad had been left in the abdomen several months before this film was made and appears as a calcified mass. (**B**) A barium study shows the foreign body as an extrinsic mass displacing and kinking the adjacent bowel.

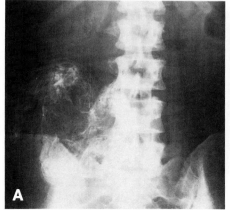

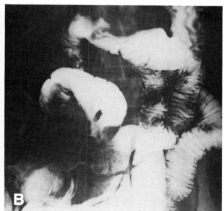

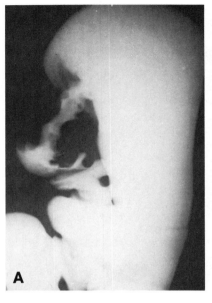 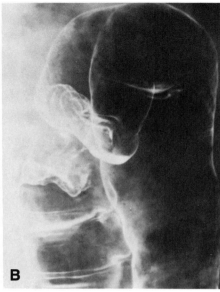

Figure 13–28. Narrowed bowel lumen. **(A)** A solid-column barium enema shows the narrowing caused by an adenocarcinoma of the colon (apple-core configuration). **(B)** In the same patient the air-contrast examination again shows the lesion.

PRINCIPLES OF EXAMINATION BY CONTRAST, ULTRASONOGRAPHY, AND COMPUTED TOMOGRAPHY

CONTRAST

Regardless of the kind or combination of contrast agents, the principles in evaluating the gut are similar.[1, 3]

Gut Caliber. Narrowing of the gut usually implies inflammation or neoplasm, and ordinarily is an intrinsic process (Fig. 13-28). Widening of the gut reflects either obstruction or muscle weakness (Fig. 13-29).

Outpouching. Both diverticula and the various manifestations of mucosal ulceration create outpouchings (Fig. 13-30). Despite the inability to detect the presence or absence of mucosa in these outpouchings by radiologic methods, their morphologic characteristics make them easy to distinguish. Ulcerations vary from small erosions to giant ulcers that may form fistulas. As a rule they are slightly more irregular than diverticula, because mucosa is intact in the latter.

Local Protrusion into the Lumen. Small intraluminal projections are usually neoplastic, and either may be in the wall of the bowel or may arise from the mucosa. Small lesions tend to be benign (Fig. 13-31). Malignant lesions almost always ulcerate as they increase in size (Fig. 13-32); thus, an ulcer within a mass is most often a malignant lesion. Mucosal lesions, such

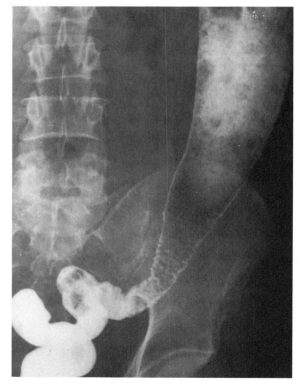

Figure 13–29. Widened bowel lumen above a mild stricture.

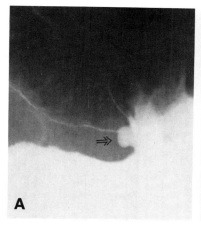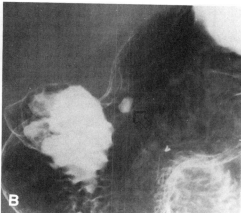

Figure 13–30. Outpouching from the gut lumen. (**A**) A gastric ulcer is seen in profile (*arrow*). (**B**) The same ulcer is seen en face (*arrow*).

as polyps, project into the lumen and may have a broad base or a narrow pedicle. Carcinomas also project into the lumen, are usually broad based, and are irregular or ulcerated and may be circumferential. Intramural lesions tend to be smooth but may have central ulceration, usually are not circumferential, and are less likely to obstruct than are mucosal masses. Differentiation is not always possible, however, because of wide variability in the appearance of the masses. Also it may be difficult to differentiate tumor arising in the bowel wall from inflammatory disease. Tumor edges tend to be more clearly defined and are often overhanging. The limits of inflammatory masses are usually more tapering and difficult to define.

Gas in the Gut Wall. Gas occasionally can occur within the gut wall as a benign, idiopathic process. The

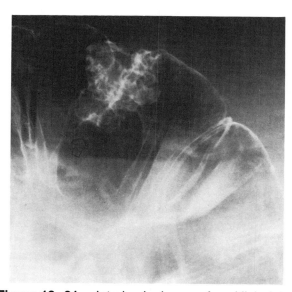

Figure 13–31. Intraluminal mass. A multilobulated polypoid carcinoma (*arrow*) can be seen attached to the colonic wall.

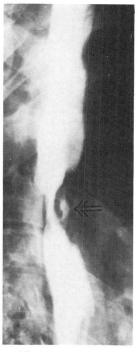

Figure 13–32. Ulcerated mass. This carcinoma of the esophagus creates an intraluminal mass, but the center of it is ulcerated and filled with barium (*arrow*).

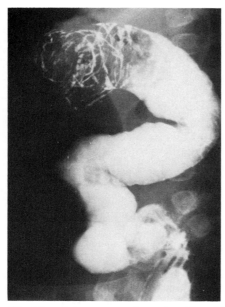

Figure 13–33. Intussusception. In this child with an ileocolic intussusception, the retrograde filling of the colon shows the barium between the prolapsing ileal mass and the colon, creating the "coilspring" appearance.

major concern, however, must always be whether the gas is there because of dead bowel.

Displacement of the Gut. Because most of the gut is not fixed in position, extrinsic disease—whether inflammation or neoplasm—will move the gut away from its normal position.

Miscellaneous. Intussusception (Fig. 13-33), volvulus, colonic urticaria (Fig. 13-34), hernia, webs, and sphincters are all unique to the gut. The ability to recognize them with the aid of contrast material is not difficult because findings are usually characteristic.

ULTRASONOGRAPHY

The use of ultrasonography in bowel disease is of primary value in studying processes that extend beyond the gut wall. The ability to identify fluid collections is particularly valuable. Small amounts of free fluid in the peritoneal space can be detected, and nonpalpable abdominal masses can be found.

COMPUTED TOMOGRAPHY

Computed tomography, like ultrasonography, is a powerful imaging technique for evaluating nonmucosal disease.[7] Because a standard cross-sectional format is used, the images are easier to understand than ultrasonography. The addition of contrast material to the gut lumen provides a marker. Intravenous contrast material is helpful in many ways. It allows identification of vascular structures, and the enhancement of solid organs may demonstrate pathologic changes. The use of CT has been helpful in evaluating the pancreas and the abdominal lymph nodes. Intra-abdominal abscesses not only can be found, but also their exact anatomic position and extent can be defined, an invaluable aid in planning treatment. CT also permits study of the extent of lesions that involve the gut lumen.

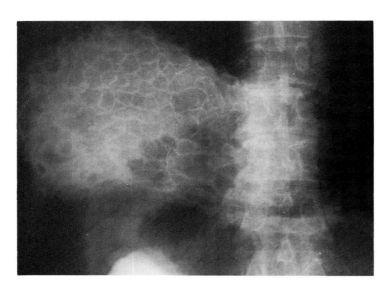

Figure 13–34. Edema of the colonic mucosa. The contrast material coats the colon mucosa and brings out the polygonal pattern that reflects submucosal edema.

REFERENCES AND SELECTED READINGS

1. EISENBERG RL: Gastrointestinal radiology: A pattern approach. Philadelphia, J.B. Lippincott, 1983
2. HANEY PJ, WHITLEY NO: CT of cystic abdominal masses in children. Am J Roentgenol 144:49, 1984
3. MARGULIS AR, BURHENNE JH (EDS): Alimentary tract radiology. St Louis, CV Mosby, 1983
4. MCCORT JJ, MINDELZUN RE, FILPI RG, RENNELL C (EDS): Abdominal radiology. Baltimore, Williams & Wilkins, 1981
5. MEGIBOW AJ, BALTHAZAR EJ, CHOCK C, ET AL: Bowel obstruction: Evaluation with CT. Radiology 180:313, 1991
6. MEYER MA: Dynamic radiology of the abdomen. New York, Springer-Verlag, 1982
7. MOSS AA, GAMSU GG, GENANT HK: Computed tomography of the body. Philadelphia, WB Saunders, 1983
8. SIMEONE JF, NOVELLINE RH, FERRUCCI JT JR, ET AL: Comparison of sonography and plain films in the evaluation of the acute abdomen. Am J Roentgenol 144:49, 1985
9. WILLIAMS SM, HARNED RK, HULTMAN SA, ET AL: Psoas sign: Reevaluation. Radiographics 5:525, 1985

Paul and Juhl's Essentials of Radiologic Imaging,
Sixth Edition, edited by John H. Juhl and
Andrew B. Crummy. J.B. Lippincott Company,
Philadelphia, © 1993.

CHAPTER **14**

The Gallbladder, Biliary Ducts, and Liver

Michael Davis

THE HEPATOBILIARY AREA

There is an extensive menu for investigating the hepatobiliary area. From the simplicity of the plain film to the expense of magnetic resonance imaging to the invasiveness of percutaneous transhepatic cholangiography, all modalities can contribute to the goal of a correct diagnosis. Not all are needed in each patient; thus a careful evaluation of the clinical needs is required before proceeding. It is also apparent that changes are occurring rapidly. The current importance of gallbladder ultrasonography and computerized tomography is well known. Oral cholecystography, however, has made a resurgence because of new methods that treat gallstone diseases (eg, bile acid therapy, lavage chemolysis, and extracorporeal shock-wave therapy). These new methods of treatment require information that is best obtained by oral cholecystography (OCG).[10] Because not all modalities are available in all communities, it is important to tailor the diagnostic algorithm to local skills and equipment.

IMAGING TECHNIQUES

The *abdominal plain film* is of value in finding gas or calcium in the biliary tract. Approximately 10% to 15% of gallstones are calcified and readily identifiable as gallstones on plain films (Fig. 14-1). At times there may be an accumulation of calcium in the gallbladder that simulates contrast material (milk of calcium bile) (Fig. 14-2). Occasionally the gallbladder wall is calcified (porcelain gallbladder), which is important because of the association of this abnormality with gallbladder carcinoma (Fig. 14-3).

Gas may be seen in the center of gallstones in a triangular pattern (Mercedes-Benz sign) (Fig. 14-4). Gas in the biliary ducts implies an abnormal connection between the gut and the gallbladder or common bile duct (Fig. 14-5). This may be caused by penetration of a duodenal ulcer into the biliary tract or gallstone erosion into the stomach, duodenum, or colon. It is more often a consequence of surgical anastomosis of the gut to the biliary tract or to sphincteroplasty of the sphincter of Oddi.

Gas is occasionally seen in the ducts as a manifestation of cholangitis caused by a gas-forming organism. Gas in the gallbladder and its wall (emphysematous cholecystitis) is the manifestation of a similar infection (Fig. 14-6) and usually occurs in diabetics, secondary to occlusion of the cystic artery caused by diabetic angiopathy. Gas in the portal vein, seen peripherally in the liver, implies necrotic bowel, but it may occur with severe cholecystitis-cholangitis (Fig. 14-7).

Oral cholecystography was first accomplished seven decades ago and was revolutionary. The ingestion of a nontoxic iodinated organic compound that is absorbed in the small bowel, excreted by the liver, and concentrated in the bile provides the opportunity to discover noncalcified gallstones preoperatively. In addition to gallstones, other intraluminal abnormalities of the gallbladder can be detected (Fig. 14-8).

Gallbladder ultrasonography (GB-US) has made an

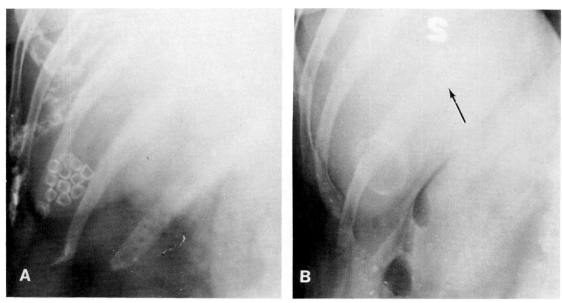

Figure 14–1. Opaque gallstones. (**A**) Several faceted calculi with radiolucent centers are seen. (**B**) A single, large, ring-contoured calculus with a transparent center is evident (*lower arrow*). The smaller calculus (*upper arrow*) is impacted in the cystic duct.

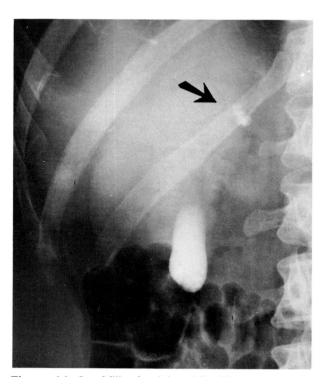

Figure 14–2. Milk of calcium bile. The gallbladder is very dense. A dense calculus was impacted in the cystic duct (*arrow*). The patient had been given no iodinated contrast material.

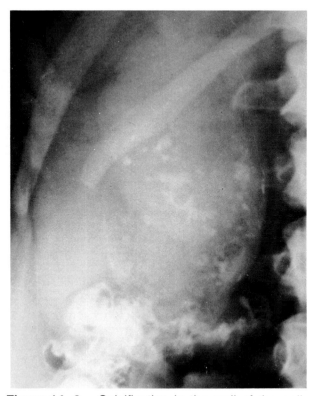

Figure 14–3. Calcification in the wall of the gallbladder. There is an incomplete shell formed by irregular plaques of calcium in the gallbladder wall (porcelain gallbladder). The barium in the colon is a residual of an earlier study of the colon.

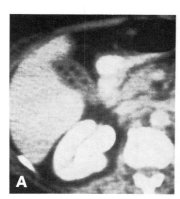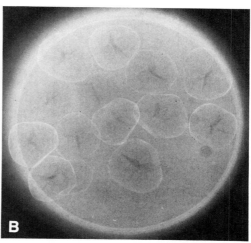

Figure 14–4. (A) Gallstones containing gas. Six gallstones containing gas can be seen in the bile-filled gallbladder on the computed tomogram. (B) This radiograph of gallstones in vitro shows the usual configuration of the gas within the stones (Mercedes-Benz sign).

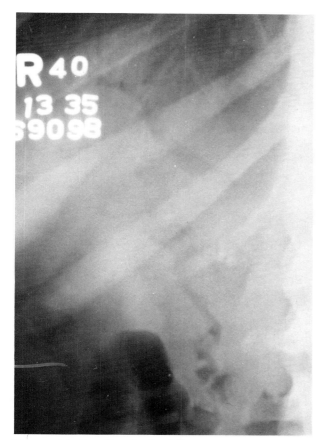

Figure 14–5. Gas in the biliary ducts. The patient had a carcinoma of the head of the pancreas with a fistula between the common duct and duodenum.

enormous impact on biliary tract diagnosis. It has replaced OCG as the primary imaging method because it offers several advantages. There is neither radiation exposure nor a need to ingest contrast material and wait for the opacification process. Jaundice does not interfere with the examination. The ability to determine bile duct size, and to evaluate the parenchyma of the liver and pancreas are enormously beneficial. A skilled ultrasonographer is required for maximum yield. Ultrasonography shows only pathologic anatomy rather than pathophysiology, whereas OCG shows both. Because so many people have asymptomatic gallstones, there is a degree of uncertainty that the stones seen by GB-US are the cause of the patient's complaints. Gallbladder ultrasonography can detect smaller stones than OCG. Ultrasonography is also used to find intraluminal masses other than stones such as adenomas, cholesterol polyps, and carcinoma of the gallbladder.

Cholescintigraphy has been developed as a dynamic study of pathophysiology of the biliary system. Intravenous injection of technetium-labeled imminodiacetic acid compounds allows immediate imaging of the gallbladder, and the radioactivity can be followed into the duodenum. A lack of filling of the gallbladder is indicative of cystic duct obstruction and is a highly reliable sign of acute cholecystitis. Cholescintigraphy has also been advocated as a procedure that can detect bile duct obstruction before duct dilatation occurs and is visible by ultrasonography.[4] It is useful to detect biliary atresia in neonates and bile leaks from any cause.

Endoscopic retrograde cholangiography (ERC) al-

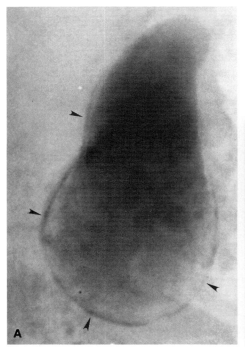

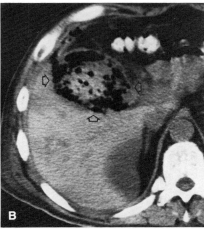

Figure 14–6. Emphysematous cholecystitis. (**A**) Linear collections of air within the wall of the gallbladder (*black arrowhead*) and extensive amount of gas formation within the gallbladder. (**B**) Empyema. Extensive amount of gas formation in and around the gallbladder (*open arrows*).

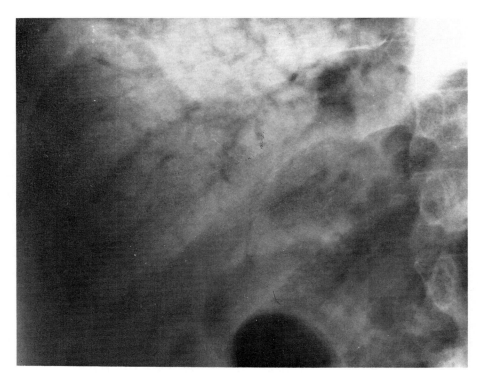

Figure 14–7. Gas within the portal vein secondary to intestinal necrosis. The gas is seen as branching translucent shadows extending into the periphery of the liver.

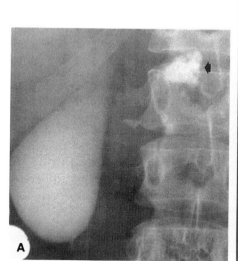
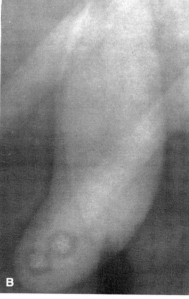
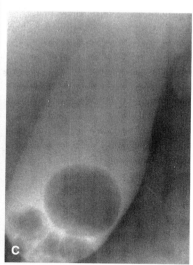

Figure 14–8. (**A**) Normal oral cholecystogram. Gallbladder is well opacified with contrast material. Incidental note of large pancreatic calculus (*arrowhead*). (**B**) Cholelithiasis. Note two gallstones in the dependent portion of the gallbladder with central calcifications surrounded by a lucent halo representing cholesterol formation. (**C**) Cholelithiasis. Numerous small cholesterol stones in the dependent portion of the gallbladder with a large single cholesterol stone above them.

lows direct injection of the common bile duct with contrast material. It is of special value in detecting common duct stones, and both inflammatory and neoplastic ductal abnormalities. Papillotomy, biopsy, stone retrieval from the bile ducts, stricture dilatation, and placement of nasobiliary stents to relieve obstruction are all possible by ERCP.

Percutaneous transhepatic cholangiography is accomplished by injecting contrast material under fluoroscopic vision through a narrow gauge needle placed in the parenchyma of the liver. It is valuable for the same reasons as ERC and has the advantage of allowing the operator to institute biliary drainage if necessary. It is increasingly reserved for patients with biliary obstruction who need permanent or temporary biliary drainage. Needle biopsy of masses, drainage of fluid collections, and placement of external and internal drainage (choledochoduodenal) stents all can be accomplished percutaneously.

Computed tomography (CT) is of less value in evaluating the gallbladder and ductal system than the other methods, but is useful in studying the liver parenchyma for neoplasm. It also is more sensitive than plain films in detecting portal vein gas.[2] CT is sensitive in the detection of calcifications and in determining stone composition.

Angiography is important in the study of hepatic parenchymal lesions.

Magnetic resonance imaging (MRI) of the liver, gallbladder, and ducts is in its infancy. Early evidence suggests that it may be definitive in the diagnosis of hemangiomas. Ionizing radiation is not used in this examination, an important consideration.

INDICATIONS

Right-upper quadrant pain provides the most cogent reason to investigate the gallbladder. Other symptoms such as bloating and dyspepsia brought on by fatty foods are less specific but often lead to imaging studies. Jaundice that is thought to be caused by biliary obstruction is an important indication.[12, 14]

ANATOMY

The normal gallbladder is a thin-walled cystic structure attached to the inferior and medial aspect of the right lobe of the liver. Occasionally, it is intrahepatic in location. The cystic duct joins the gallbladder and common hepatic duct to form the common bile duct. The cystic duct has characteristic spiral (Heister's) valves, which persist even with marked dilatation of the duct. The site of the junction of cystic and common hepatic ducts can vary considerably. The common bile duct courses caudally in close relationship to the head of the pancreas and terminates at Vater's papilla in the duodenum. The pancreatic duct usually merges with the common bile duct proximal to the papilla. Except distally, biliary ducts have an elastic tissue rather than a muscular wall. Distally there is a muscular (Oddi's) sphincter involving the ducts in a short area just proximal to the papilla.

PHYSIOLOGY

The gallbladder functions as a site for the storage and concentration of bile. The contraction of the gallbladder and the relaxation of Oddi's sphincter is mediated by the hormone cholecystokinin, which is released from the duodenal wall as a response to intraluminal fat and amino acids.

CONGENITAL ANOMALIES

The gallbladder may be congenitally absent or may be intrahepatic in location (Fig. 14-9). Computed tomography is the best imaging modality for making these diagnoses. The lack of complete tubulation of the gallbladder can result in adenomyomatous masses within the wall as well as septations of the gallbladder. Adenomyomatosis with its formation of Aschoff-Rokitanksy sinuses and cholesterolosis have been lumped together under the term *hyperplastic cholecystoses*, which are of little clinical significance (Fig. 14-10).

There are many different anomalies of the ducts. Small hepatic ducts going directly through the gallbladder wall may exist. The right hepatic duct may join the cystic duct rather than join with the left hepatic duct. This is one of the more frequent anomalies (Fig. 14-11).

An anomaly of great significance is choledochal cyst (Fig. 14-12). It was formerly thought that the dilatation of the common bile and hepatic ducts was the anomaly, but the discovery that the common bile duct joins the pancreatic duct abnormally at right angles proximal to the papilla at least suggests that the choledochal cyst may be secondary to abnormal dynamics created by this altered anatomy (Fig. 14-13). Patients with choledochal cysts are prone to develop bile duct carcinoma, and recently the anomalous pancreaticobiliary union has been found to be associated with gallbladder carcinoma.[5] Choledochal cysts may be palpated in infants. Gallbladder ultrasonography and CT are excellent diagnostic modalities at any age. Operative cholangiogra-

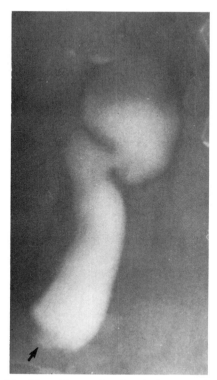

Figure 14–10. Hyperplastic cholecystosis. In this gallbladder, a partial septum divides the gallbladder into two sections (compartmentalized gallbladder). There is also a deformity of the fundus (*arrow*) that has been called adenomyomatosis.

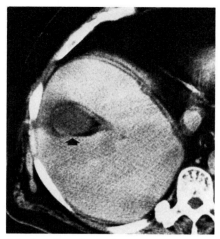

Figure 14–9. Intrahepatic gallbladder. CT scan demonstrates the gallbladder (*arrow*) to be well within the parenchyma of the liver.

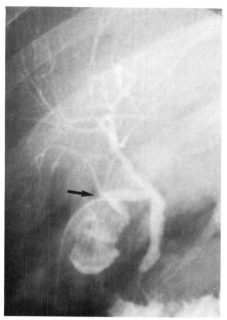

Figure 14–11. A branch of the right hepatic duct anomalously joins the cystic duct (*arrow*).

phy can be used to demonstrate the abnormal common duct–pancreatic duct junction. True cysts or diverticula of the common duct occur but are rare.

Biliary duct atresia is a lesion incompatible with life unless surgical correction can be done. Because ductal patency usually cannot be restored, some patients are now receiving liver transplants.

Caroli's disease is a congenital cystic dilatation of the intrahepatic ducts. Computed tomography, GB-US, transhepatic cholangiography (THC), and ERC are all effective in demonstrating this often asymptomatic anomaly (Fig. 14-14).

Choledochoceles may occur as congenital lesions. A dilated distal common bile duct appears as a mass in the duodenum.[18] There is usually some degree of biliary tract obstruction. Choledochoceles may also develop secondary to papillary stenosis or carcinoma at the papilla (Fig. 14-15).

INFLAMMATION AND GALLSTONES

The most common malady of the gallbladder is cholelithiasis. Gallbladder ultrasonography is very effective in finding stones and is more sensitive than OCG in that it is able to detect smaller-sized stones (Fig. 14-16). If the cystic duct becomes chronically obstructed by a stone, the mucus formed in the gallbladder may distend it to enormous proportions, a condition known as hydrops of the gallbladder. A similar degree of distention may develop secondarily to obstruction of the common bile duct by pancreatic carcinoma.

Computed tomography and US can detect intrahepatic ductal dilatation of any cause (eg, stone, tumor or stricture) (Fig. 14-17). One of the most difficult diagnostic problems is the patient with acalculous cholecystitis. The GB-US may show edema and thickening of the gallbladder wall, but it may be normal and then reliance must be placed on cholescintigraphy.[20] The lack of uptake of radioactive material in the gallbladder is very supportive of the clinical diagnosis (Fig. 14-18).

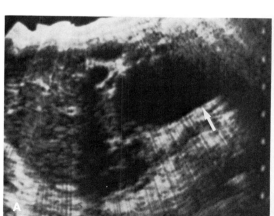

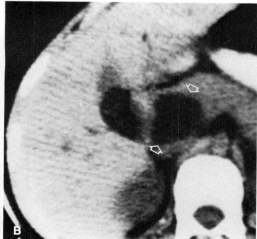

Figure 14–12. **(A)** Choledochal cyst. A longitudinal ultrasound scan shows a large fluid-filled structure (*arrow*) caudal to the liver. **(B)** Choledochal cyst. CT scan through the level of the pancreas shows a large lucent defect in the head of the pancreas (*arrows*).

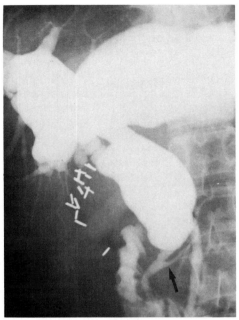

Figure 14–13. Choledochal cyst. The anomalous junction of the pancreatic and common bile ducts proximal to the papilla (*arrow*) is shown by cholangiography.

The use of indium-labeled leukocytes also may be of diagnostic assistance (Fig. 14-19).

After cholecystectomy, recurrent or retained common bile duct stones can be readily demonstrated with either ERCP or THC (Fig. 14-20). The ability of the noninvasive ultrasound examination to find choledo-

cholithiasis has also been improving (Fig. 14-21). Formerly the GB-US examination was mainly of value in seeing ductal dilatation, but now because of improved techniques, the stones are often detected.[7]

Sphincter of Oddi stenosis is a difficult diagnosis because there is no configuration of the distal duct that can be considered too narrow. Reliance is placed on ductal dilatation, abnormal sphincter pressures, biochemical abnormalities, and delayed bile-duct-to-bowel cholescintigraphic dynamics.[8, 21]

Sclerosing cholangitis is a process most often associated with chronic idiopathic ulcerative colitis, though it may occur independently of this disease. Both ERC and THC demonstrate the narrowed and irregular ductal pattern (Fig. 14-22). Differentiating this process from multicentric cholangiocarcinoma can be difficult, particularly because malignant degeneration has been found to develop in patients with sclerosing cholangitis.[9]

Parasites may invade the biliary ducts. Ascaris may be demonstrated with either ERC or THC. Clonorchis of the ducts is common in the Orient.

MOTILITY DISORDERS

Biliary dyskinesia is a term that has been used for a long time, but solid criteria for establishing a diagnosis have not been developed. Patients suffer right-upper-quadrant pain after meals that simulates biliary colic, but no abnormality can be found. Cholecystography after intravenous cholecystokinin injection does not cause a contraction pattern that separates symptomatic patients from asymptomatic ones. Manometry of the sphincter is now being used to investigate these patients.

(*text continues on page 534*)

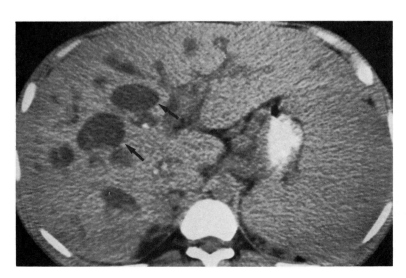

Figure 14–14. Congenital intrahepatic bile-duct dilatation (Caroli's disease). Computed tomogram shows the dilated ducts (*arrows*). Splenomegaly is also present.

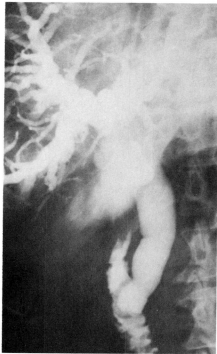

Figure 14–15. Choledochocele. A mass in the duodenum is caused by the distal part of the dilated common bile duct.

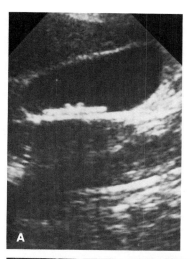

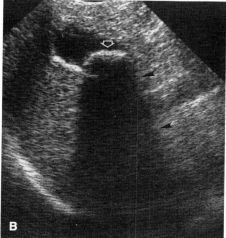

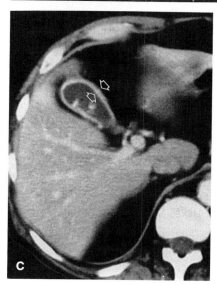

Figure 14–16. (**A**) Gallstones. A longitudinal ultrasound scan shows multiple stones in the gallbladder that cause shadowing of the ultrasound beam below them. (**B**) Cholelithiasis. Ultrasonogram shows large echogenic defect in the gallbladder (*open arrow*) with acoustical shadowing (*black arrowhead*). (**C**) Cholecystitis. CT scan through the level of the gallbladder on contrast-enhanced scan shows enhancement of the gallbladder wall from inflammation (*arrows*). Incidental note of two gallstones within the gallbladder.

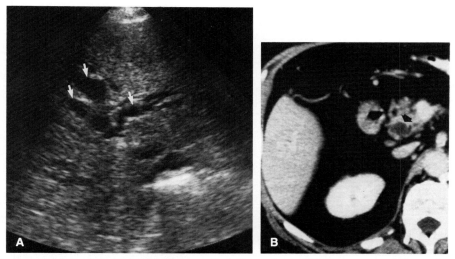

Figure 14–17. (A) Dilated intrahepatic biliary ducts. Ultrasonogram through the right lobe of the liver shows numerous tubular structures representing dilated bile duct (*arrows*) secondary to impacted stone in common bile duct. (B) Dilated common bile duct. Lucent defect in the head of the pancreas (*arrow*) represents dilated common bile duct caused by adenocarcinoma of the ampulla of Vater.

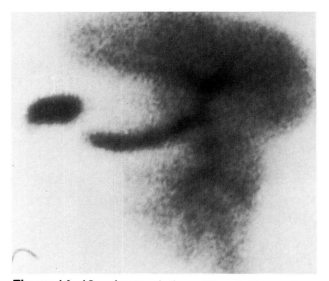

Figure 14–18. Acute cholecystitis. A *N*-para-iso-propylacetanilide-iminodiacetic acid scan shows that the radionuclide is in the liver, bile ducts, and duodenum but does not enter the gallbladder. This is evidence of cystic duct obstruction.

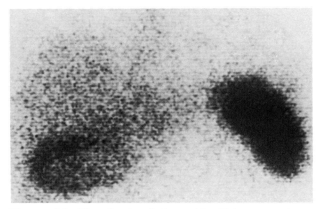

Figure 14–19. Acute cholecystitis. This scan, done with indium-labeled white blood cells, shows that the cells have moved to the site of inflammation in the gallbladder. The splenic activity is normal.

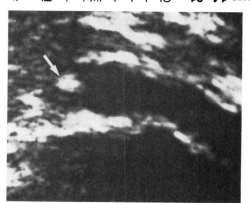

Figure 14–21. Choledocholithiasis. The ultrasonic image shows the bright echo (*arrow*) indicating the stone within the tubular, fluid-filled common bile duct. There is shadowing of the ultrasound beam beneath the stone as in Figure 14–16B.

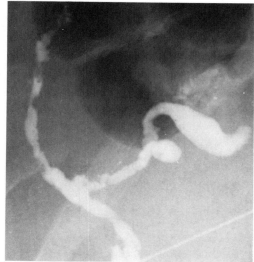

Figure 14–22. Sclerosing cholangitis. A transhepatic cholangiogram demonstrates the marked irregularity of the bile ducts.

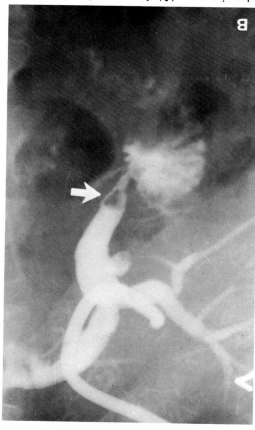

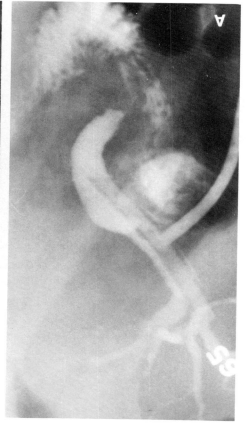

Figure 14–20. Postoperative T-tube cholangiogram. (**A**) An example of a normal study. The contrast material outlines the common duct and some of its hepatic tributaries. Some contrast material is noted in the duodenum. (**B**) In this patient, there is a residual stone in the lower end of the common duct (*arrow*). Obstruction is not complete because there is some contrast material in the duodenum.

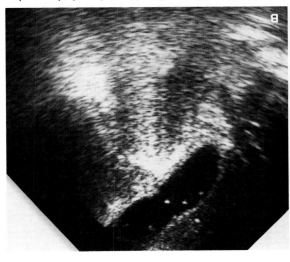

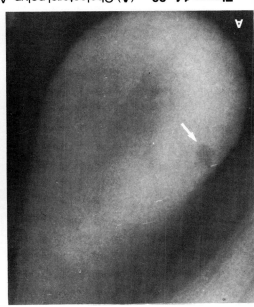

Figure 14-23. (A) Cholesterol polyp. An upright film of the gallbladder taken during oral cholecystography shows a nonmovable filling defect (*arrow*) in the gallbladder. (B) Cholesterolosis. Ultrasonogram shows numerous bright echogenic defects within the gallbladder.

NEOPLASMS

Within the gallbladder, papillomas and adenomas may create nonmovable filling defects, but the most common condition of this type is the nonneoplastic cholesterol polyp.[12] These lesions of the gallbladder wall can be seen with both GB-US and OCG (Fig. 14-23).

Adenocarcinoma of the gallbladder usually occurs in association with gallstones. The diagnosis is generally made late, at a time when surgical cure is not possible. Both GB-US and CT can identify the mass that replaces the normal gallbladder (Fig. 14-24).[17, 19] Metastases to the gallbladder may occur in patients with diffuse melanoma.

In the bile ducts, cholangiocarcinoma causes narrowing of the ducts and eventual obstruction (Fig. 14-25). Usually the lesion has a morphologic appearance similar to a stricture, but at times it causes a discrete filling defect. The tumor may be multicentric and then may be indistinguishable from sclerosing cholangitis. A villous adenoma or a carcinoid may also occur in the ductal system (Fig. 14-26). Computed tomography can delineate liver masses in great detail (Fig. 14-27).

MISCELLANEOUS

The gallbladder may have a significant mesentery and herniate through Winslow's foramen into the lesser omental sac.

Diverticula of the gallbladder (Aschoff-Rokitansky sinuses) are normal microscopic findings in the gallbladder. In association with gallstones and inflammation, these become macroscopic and can be seen with OCG. Cholesterol deposition may be quite extensive within the gallbladder wall (strawberry gallbladder) and can be large enough to cause cholesterol polyps that can be seen by GB-US and OCG. Computed tomography is useful in detecting iron metabolism abnormalities (Fig. 14-28). Collateral vascular channels are best seen with CT scan (Fig 14-29).

IATROGENIC DISEASE

At the time of cholecystectomy the bile duct may be either ligated or damaged. Sometimes the bile duct strictures that form do not cause symptoms for many months. If the duct is completely ligated, jaundice

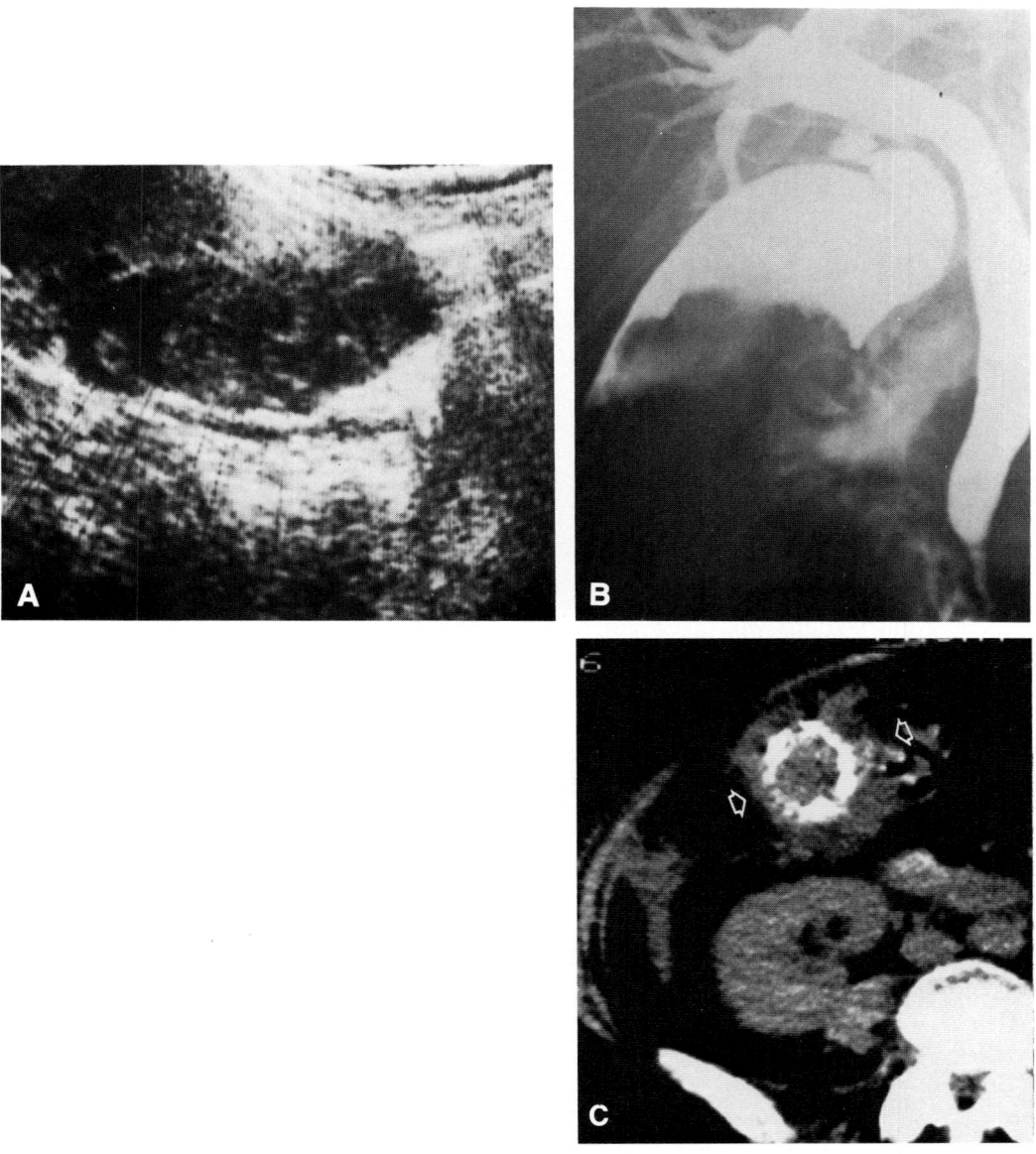

Figure 14–24. (**A**) Carcinoma of the gallbladder. The ultrasound image of the gallbladder shows numerous echogenic foci within the lumen rather than the usual sonolucent appearance. (**B**) Carcinoma of the gallbladder. A transhepatic cholangiogram in a different patient shows a large filling defect in the gallbladder. (**C**) Carcinoma of gallbladder. Computed tomographic scan through the gallbladder shows calcified gallbladder with tumor extending throughout and beyond the gallbladder wall (*arrows*).

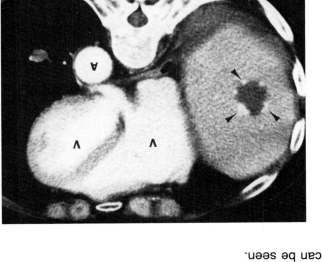

Figure 14–27. (A) Liver hemangioma. CT scan through the right lobe of the liver shows peripheral enhancement consistent with hemangioma (*arrowheads*). A, contrast-enhanced aorta. The ventricles of the heart also show enhancement (V). (B) Metastatic carcinoid to liver. CT scan shows numerous lesions of varying sizes scattered throughout both lobes of the liver. (C) Metastatic carcinoma of the gallbladder to the liver. CT scan shows large irregular low-density mass lesion in the right lobe of the liver.

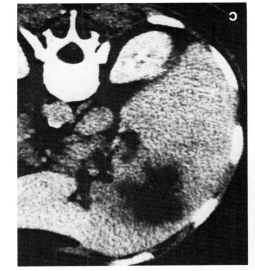

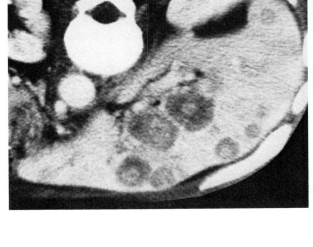

Figure 14–25. Cholangiocarcinoma. In the transhepatic cholangiogram, the narrowing of the right and left hepatic ducts as well as the common hepatic duct can be seen.

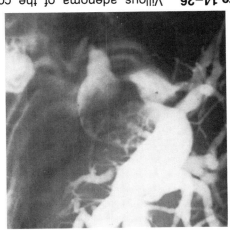

Figure 14–26. Villous adenoma of the common bile duct.

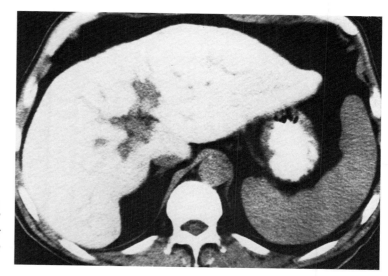

Figure 14–28. Hemochromatosis—liver. CT scan through the liver shows "white" liver representing iron deposition. The liver should have CT density comparable to the spleen.

develops immediately. Both THC and ERC are excellent methods to locate the stricture site.

Endoscopic sphincterotomy may lead to a defective bile pathway with extravasation into the periduodenal tissues. Fluoroscopic evaluation of the bile duct postsphincterotomy can be helpful in recognizing this problem.[4]

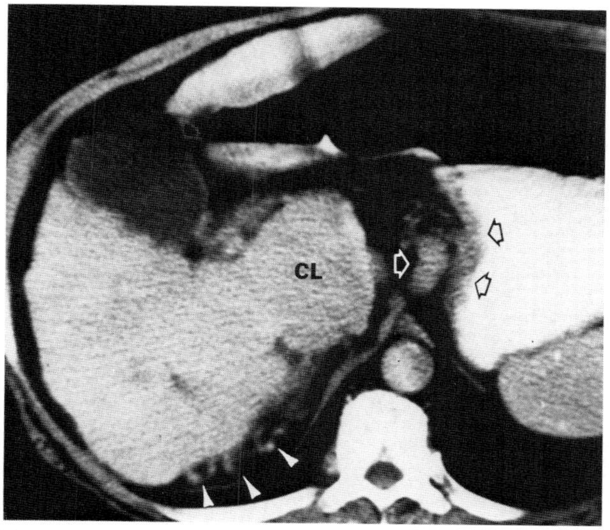

Recently the infusion of chemotherapeutic agents via a catheter in the hepatic artery has resulted in several complications. Chemical cholecystitis, gallbladder infarction, sclerosing cholangitis, and bile duct necrosis have been reported.[2, 7, 11, 15]

Figure 14–29. Cirrhosis with esophageal varices and collaterals. CT scan through the liver shows enlarged caudate lobe (*CL*), large gastric and esophageal varices (*arrows*), and other collateral channels that have developed on the under surface of the liver (*arrowheads*).

REFERENCES AND SELECTED READINGS

1. CARRASCO CH, FREENY PC, CHUANG VP, ET AL: Chemical cholecystitis associated with hepatic artery infusion chemotherapy. Am J Roentgenol 141:703, 1983

2. DENNIS MA, PRETORIUS D, MANCO-JOHNSON ML, ET AL: CT detection of portal venous gas associated with suppurative cholangitis and cholecystitis. Am J Roentgenol 145:1017, 1985

3. GREENBERG HM, GOLDBERG HI, SHAPIRO HA, ET AL: The importance of radiographic monitoring of endoscopic sphincterotomy. Radiology 141:295, 1981

4. KAPLUN L, WEISSMAN HS, ROSENBLATT RR, ET AL: The early diagnosis of common bile duct obstruction using cholescintigraphy. JAMA 254:2431, 1985

5. KIMURA K, OHTO M, SAISHO H, ET AL: Association of gallbladder carcinoma and anomalous pancreaticobiliary ductal union. Gastroenterology 89:1258, 1985

6. KURODA C, IWASAKI M, TANAKA T, ET AL: Gallbladder infarction following hepatic transcatheter arterial embolization. Radiology 149:85, 1983

7. LAING F, JEFFREY RB, WING VW: Improved visualization of choledocholithiasis by sonography. Am J Roentgenol 143:949, 1984

8. LEE RGL, GREGG JA, KOROSHETZ AM, ET AL: Sphincter

of Oddi stenosis, diagnosis using hepatobiliary scintigraphy and endoscopic manometry. Radiology 156:793, 1985

9. MacCarty RL, LaRusso NF, May GR, et al: Cholangiocarcinoma complicating primary sclerosing cholangitis: Cholangiographic appearances. Radiology 156:43, 1985

10. Maglinte DDT, Torres WE, Laufer I: Oral cholecystography in contemporary gallstone imaging: A review. Radiology 178:49, 1991

11. Makuuchi M, Sukigara M, Mori T, et al: Bile duct necrosis: Complication of transcatheter hepatic arterial embolization. Radiology 156:331, 1985

12. Matzen P, Malchow-Møller A, Brun B, et al: Ultrasonography, computed tomography, and cholescintigraphy in suspected obstructive jaundice—a prospective comparative study. Gastroenterology 84:1492, 1983

13. McGregor JC, Cordiner JW: Papilloma of the gallbladder. Br J Surg 61:356, 1974

14. O'Connor KW, Snodgrass PJ, Swonder JE: A blinded prospective study comparing four current noninvasive approaches in the differential diagnosis of medical versus surgical jaundice. Gastroenterology 84:1498, 1983

15. Pien EH, Zeman RK, Benjamin SB, et al: Iatrogenic sclerosing cholangitis following hepatic arterial chemotherapy infusion. Radiology 156:329, 1985

16. Shapero TF, Rosen IE, Wilson SR, et al: Discrepancy between ultrasound and oral cholecystography in the assessment of gallstone dissolution. Hepatology 2:587, 1982

17. Smathers RL, Lee JKT, Heiken JP: Differentiation of complicated cholecystitis from gallbladder carcinoma by computed tomography. Am J Roentgenol 143:255, 1984

18. Venu RP, Geenen JE, Hogan WJ, et al: Role of endoscopic retrograde cholangiopancreatography in the diagnosis and treatment of choledochocele. Gastroenterology 87:1144, 1984

19. Weiner SN, Koenigsberg M, Morehouse H, et al: Sonography and computed tomography in the diagnosis of carcinoma of the gallbladder. Am J Roentgenol 142:735, 1984

20. Weissman HS, Badia J, Sugarman LA, et al: Spectrum of 99m-Tc-IDA cholescintigraphic patterns in acute cholecystitis. Radiology 138:167, 1981

21. Zeman RK, Burrell MI, Dobbins J, et al: Postcholecystectomy syndrome: Evaluation using biliary scintigraphy and endoscopic retrograde cholangiopancreatography. Radiology 156:787, 1985

Paul and Juhl's Essentials of Radiologic Imaging, Sixth Edition, edited by John H. Juhl and Andrew B. Crummy. J.B. Lippincott Company, Philadelphia, © 1993.

CHAPTER **15**

The Pancreas and Abdominal Interventional Procedures

Michael Davis

THE PANCREAS

Although the pancreas continues to present a challenge surgically, diagnostic capabilities have improved greatly because of cross-sectional imaging procedures and endoscopic retrograde cholangiopancreatography (ERCP). These modalities combined with the ability to biopsy pancreatic masses percutaneously have removed the need for using the barium-filled gut to imply pancreatic disease.

IMAGING TECHNIQUES

Plain film of the abdomen is of value in finding pancreatic lithiasis (Fig. 15-1) and gas within pancreatic abscesses. The pancreas cannot be visualized normally on plain abdominal radiographs. Pancreatic ultrasonography is particularly satisfactory for examination of the head and body of the gland; however, intestinal gas often obscures the tail. Computed tomography (CT) provides the best images of the entire gland and its relationship to other structures (Fig. 15-2). Endoscopic retrograde pancreatography is invaluable for the detail this procedure provides in visualizing the pancreatic duct (Fig. 15-3). Its disadvantage is that a skillful endoscopist is required to cannulate the duct, and there is a risk of pancreatitis if the duct is overfilled. At the moment magnetic resonance imaging (MRI) is still in development regarding pancreatic imaging.

ANATOMY

The pancreas is the product of the fusion of the dorsal pancreas with its duct (Santorini) and the ventral pancreas with its duct (Wirsung). Wirsung's duct and the common bile duct usually join and form a common channel at the major papilla (Vater). The distal dorsal pancreatic duct, which in embryonic life enters the duodenum at the minor papilla, is usually atretic at birth.

PHYSIOLOGY

The pancreatic parenchyma consists of the exocrine and endocrine portions. The exocrine portion secretes digestive enzymes and the bicarbonate ion through the pancreatic duct into the duodenum. The endocrine islet cells are important as the source for insulin, though they also secrete other hormones (glucagon, somatostatin, pancreatic polypeptide, vasoactive intestinal peptide, and others).

CONGENITAL ANOMALIES

Annular pancreas occurs when the dorsal and ventral pancreatic segments fail to rotate and fuse. The result is a ring of pancreatic tissue surrounding the duodenum, which may be asymptomatic, but can narrow

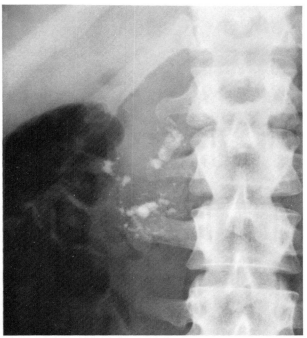

Figure 15–1. Chronic pancreatitis. There is a scattering of calculi in the region of the enlarged head of the pancreas.

the lumen and cause partial or complete duodenal obstruction (Fig. 15-4).

Pancreas divisum occurs when the ducts of Santorini and Wirsung do not join, which leaves a small ventral pancreatic segment and a duct that joins the common bile duct at the major papilla. The larger dorsal pancreatic segment drains through the minor papilla as in embryonic life. It is important to recognize this anomaly at ERCP so as not to overfill the acini with contrast material (Fig. 15-5). There is much controversy about the importance of this anomaly in pancreatitis, particularly those in whom alcohol is not the underlying cause.[10]

PANCREATITIS

Hereditary pancreatitis is seen in children and young adults. The pancreatic ducts are normal, and pancreatic calcification occurs. The etiology of this condition is not known.

Acute pancreatitis may result from a variety of causes. Alcohol abuse is that most frequently cited, but

other causes, such as choledocholithiasis (gallstone pancreatitis), must be excluded because they may be correctable. Both pancreatic ultrasonography and CT show an enlarged edematous gland during the acute phase (Fig. 15-6).[15, 16] In the subacute phase pseudocysts, phlegmons, and abscesses may form (Fig. 15-7).[7] Pancreatic ascites may occur. The cross-sectional imaging methods are very effective in delineating these abnormalities. They are also of value in following the resolution of these complications.

Chronic pancreatitis is manifested by calcifications and a ductal system that shows multiple irregularities of the lumen and beading with saccular dilation of the branches (Fig. 15-8).

NEOPLASM

Benign nonfunctioning neoplasms of the pancreatic parenchyma are quite rare. They may attain considerable size before detection because they do not interfere with any physiologic mechanisms. Examples of these are cystadenoma and papillary epithelial neoplasm (Fig. 15-9).[1, 12, 18] Benign tumors of the islets are more common and can be divided into those with and those without endocrine function.[20] There are insulinomas, glucagonomas, gastrinomas, and so forth. These can be benign as well as malignant with spread to lymph nodes and liver. Computed tomography is an excellent method to find these tumors, and angiography has also been effective (Fig. 15-10).[3, 5, 11]

The most common pancreatic tumor is the adenocarcinoma. Sometimes all modalities may have to be used to establish the diagnosis. The tumor may be detected by pancreatic ultrasonography or CT when it is quite small if there is encroachment on the bile duct and jaundice develops. Tumors in the body and tail develop without symptoms when small and then cause pain as they involve the parapancreatic nerves. Endoscopic retrograde pancreatography shows ductal obstruction as the usual finding in pancreatic carcinoma (Fig. 15-11). The duct proximal to the cancer becomes dilated and can be seen by both ultrasonography and CT (Fig. 15-12).[2, 14]

TRAUMATIC LESIONS

Fracture, contusion, and pseudocyst may occur as the consequence of either blunt or penetrating trauma to the abdomen. Diagnosis and follow-up are best done with CT.[13] Fracture can be confirmed with ERCP (Fig. 15-13).

(text continues on page 545)

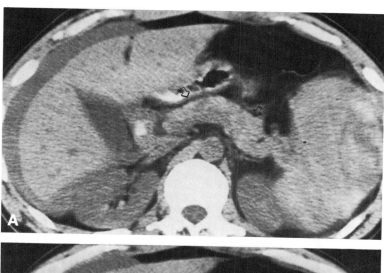

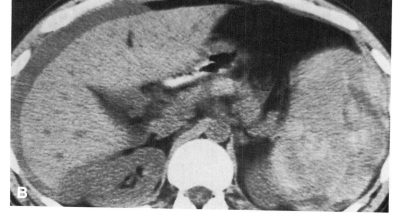

Figure 15–2. Normal computed tomogram of the pancreas in a patient with intrasplenic and peritoneal hemorrhage following trauma. **(A)** Head and body of the pancreas can be seen (*arrows*). Barium is seen anteriorly in the stomach and to the right in the duodenum. **(B)** Tail of the pancreas, which is a section at a slightly more cephalic level (*arrow*).

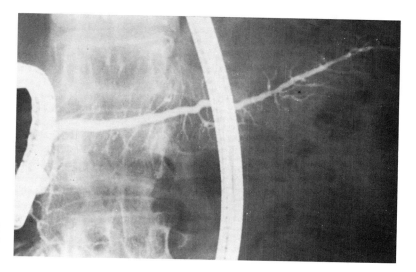

Figure 15–3. A normal pancreatic duct visualized by endoscopically guided injection.

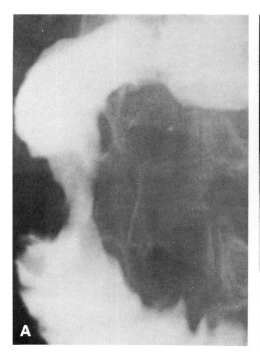

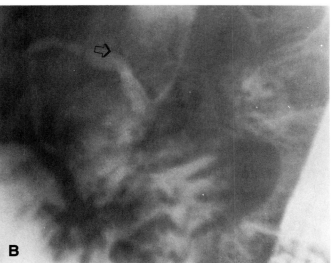

Figure 15–4. (**A**) Annular pancreas causing indentation in the lateral wall of the descending duodenum. (**B**) Annular pancreas. The ventral pancreatic duct and the common bile duct which contains a large stone (*arrow*) are observed.

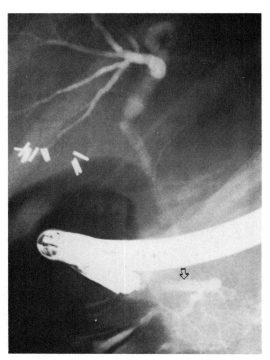

Figure 15–5. Pancreas divisum. Only the ventral pancreatic duct (*arrow*) and the common bile duct are filled through the major papilla. The dorsal pancreatic duct empties separately at the minor papilla and thus is not visualized by this injection.

Figure 15–7. (**A**) Pseudocyst in the tail of the pancreas (*arrow*). (**B**) Pancreatic pseudocyst. Large pancreatic pseudocyst in midabdomen and left abdomen. Note thick mature wall of pancreatic cyst (*arrows*). (**C**) Pancreatic phlegmon. Large amorphous low dense mass in region of head and body of pancreas consistent with large inflammatory mass (phlegmon) (*arrows*). The phlegmon is nonenhancing, which indicates lack of vascularity. (**D**) Pancreatic abscess. Huge amorphous mass with debris and extensive gas collections represent abscess (*open arrows*). The abscess has extended to the spleen(s).

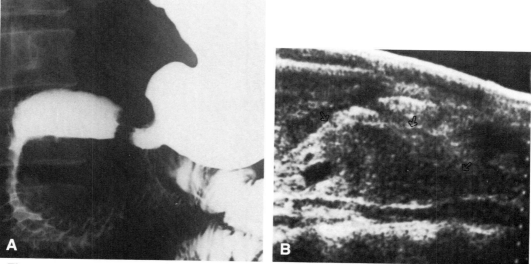

Figure 15–6. **(A)** Acute pancreatitis. The inflammation in the head and body of the pancreas has extended to the second and third parts of the duodenum. The duodenal folds are enlarged because of the submucosal edema, and the lumen is narrowed because of the enlarged pancreas. **(B)** Acute pancreatitis. A longitudinal ultrasonogram shows a sonolucent mass (*arrows*) anterior to the vena cava. This represents the enlarged edematous pancreas.

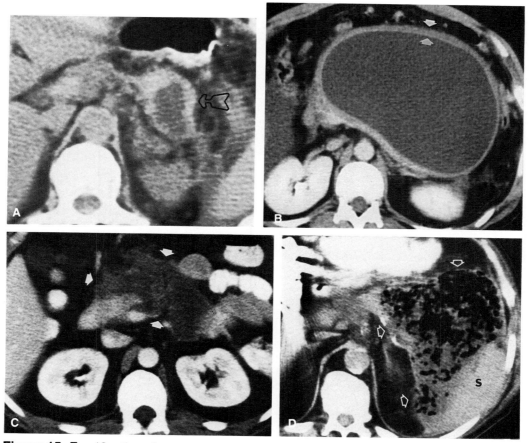

Figure 15–7. (*Continued*)

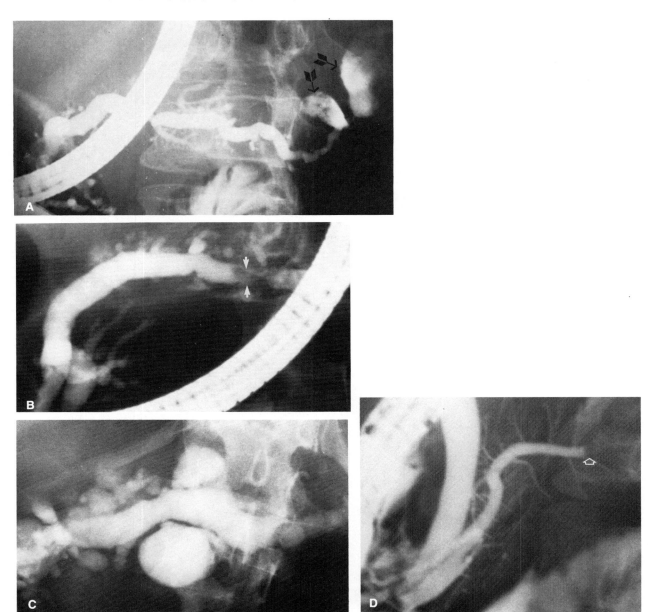

Figure 15–8. (**A**) Chronic pancreatitis. The main pancreatic duct is dilated and tortuous in its course. The side branches are dilated (compare with Fig. 15–3). Two small pancreatic pseudocysts are filled with contrast material (*arrow*). (**B**) Chronic pancreatitis with impacted stone. The main pancreatic duct is dilated, and its branches show dilatation, irregularity, and cystic changes. An oblong stone is lodged in the mid-duct (*arrows*). (**C**) Severe chronic pancreatitis. The main pancreatic duct and its branches show marked dilatation, distortion, and extensive cystic changes. (**D**) Obstructing pancreatic duct stone. The pancreatic head and proximal portion of the body is normal; however, there is an abrupt obstruction from lodged stone (*open arrow*).

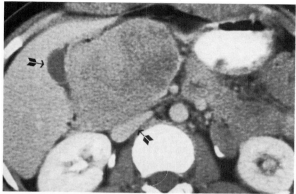

Figure 15–9. Large papillary epithelial neoplasm of the pancreas occurring in a young woman. Note the compression of the gallbladder and inferior vena cava (*arrows*).

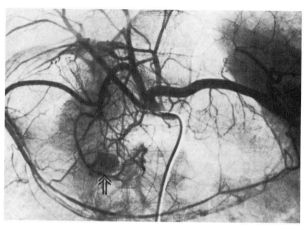

Figure 15–10. Insulinoma of the pancreas demonstrated by celiac artery angiography (*arrow*).

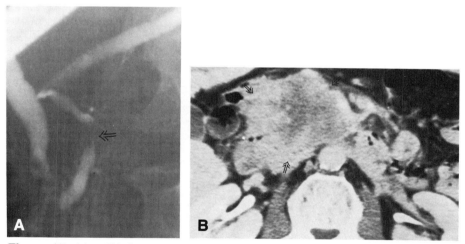

Figure 15–11. (**A**) A small pancreatic carcinoma causing a localized narrowing and partial obstruction of the pancreatic duct (*arrow*). (**B**) A large pancreatic carcinoma involving the body of the gland (*arrows*).

ABDOMINAL INTERVENTIONAL PROCEDURES

INTRODUCTION

A few years ago angiography was the main invasive radiologic procedure for evaluation of pancreatic and other masses. There is now an ever-increasing list of procedures that can be used not only for diagnosis but

also for treatment. They may be accompanied by morbidity or mortality, but they are clinically acceptable alternatives to surgical methods.

BIOPSY

Percutaneous biopsy of almost any abdominal mass can be performed and is of value in pancreatic lesions to avoid laparotomy. Enlarged adrenals are also access-

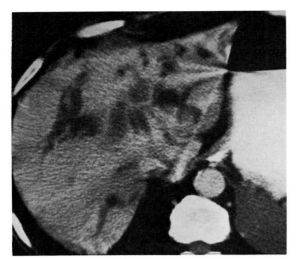

Figure 15–12. Biliary tract obstruction manifested by intrahepatic bile duct obstruction in a contrast-enhanced computed tomogram of the liver.

ible (Fig. 15-14). Quite often these are aspiration biopsies, and correct interpretation of the material obtained requires a skilled cytopathologist.[17]

ABDOMINAL FLUID COLLECTIONS

It is usually possible to drain fluid collections within the abdomen, using ultrasonography or CT guidance.

Abscesses and pancreatic pseudocysts are lesions that have been treated successfully (Fig. 15-15).[9]

OSTOMY

Feeding gastrostomies can be established using a percutaneous approach (Fig. 15-16). A similar technique can be used for cecal decompression in patients with colonic ileus who are in danger of cecal perforation. Cholecystostomy can be done as an emergency procedure in acute cholecystitis or as an elective measure to gain access to the biliary tract for stone dissolution or removal.[6]

BILIARY DRAINAGE

Following transhepatic cholangiography, a biliary catheter can be put in place to drain the bile externally.[4] If the obstruction can be passed with a guide wire, it is often possible to put a stent across the lesion and drain the bile internally (Fig. 15-17). This may be done as a preoperative measure, allowing time to improve the patient's general condition, or permanently as a palliative measure, aiding the patient who has nonresectable disease.

STONE REMOVAL

Percutaneous common duct stone removal using the T-Tube tract began many years ago. Similar techniques are now used in the urinary tract.

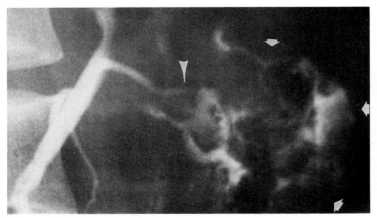

Figure 15–13. Transection pancreatic duct. Proximal pancreatic duct normal. There is an abrupt change in caliber of the main pancreatic duct (*arrowhead*) with extravasation into the peripancreatic tissues (*arrows*). This transection of the pancreatic duct was secondary to a kick to the abdomen.

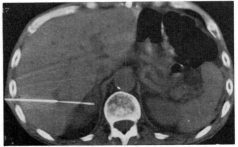

Figure 15–14. CT–guided biopsy of a right adrenal gland mass. A similar technique can be used for percutaneous biopsy of any nonvascular abdominal mass.

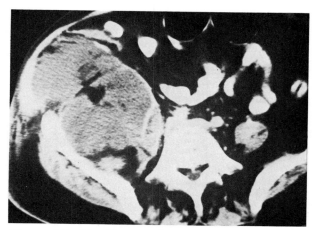

Figure 15–15. Psoas abscess that was drained percutaneously. Fluid collections related to the liver, pancreas, appendix, colon, and so on can be treated in a similar way.

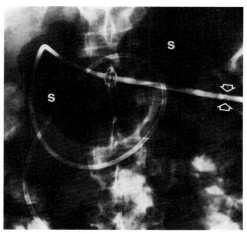

Figure 15–16. Feeding gastrostomy tube. A percutaneous feeding tube (*open arrows*) enters the gas filled stomach(*s*) and then loops in the duodenum and extends into the ileum.

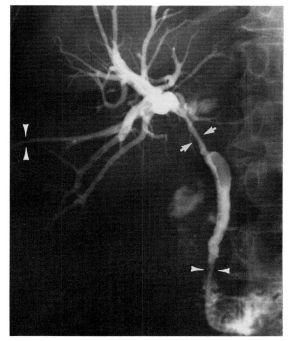

Figure 15–17. Percutaneous biliary drainage catheter placement. Percutaneous catheter extends medially to enter the biliary tree and traverses a tumor site (*arrows*). Continuing through biliary system terminating in the duodenum distally. Catheter (*arrowheads*).

DILATATION

Any narrowing in the gut or biliary tract can be dilated. Dilatation of the biliary tract is particularly helpful in treating patients who have sclerosing cholangitis or biloenteric anastomoses.[8,19] It is also used in the presence of esophageal strictures as well as an overly narrow gastric opening after gastric plication.

REFERENCES AND SELECTED READINGS

1. BALTHAZAR EJ, SUBRAMANYAM BR, LEFLEUR RS, ET AL: Solid and epithelial neoplasm of the pancreas. Radiology 150:39, 1984

2. BERLAND LL, LAWSON TL, FOLEY WD, ET AL: Computed tomography of the normal and abnormal pancreatic duct: Correlation with pancreatic ductography. Radiology 141:715, 1981

3. BREATNACH ES, CHAMPAULT G, PHARABOZ C, ET AL: CT evaluation of glucagonomas. J Comput Assist Tomogr 9:25, 1985

4. DOOLEY JS, DICK R, GEORGE P, ET AL: Percutaneous transhepatic prosthesis for bile duct obstruction. Gastroenterology 86:905, 1984

5. EELKEMA EA, STEPHENS DH, WARD EM, ET AL: CT features of nonfunctioning islet cell carcinoma. Am J Roentgenol 143:943, 1984

6. EGGERMONT AM, LAMERIS JS, JEEKEL J: Ultrasound-

guided percutaneous transhepatic cholecystostomy for acute acalculous cholecystitis. Arch Surg 120:1354, 1985

7. FEDERLE MP, JEFFREY RB JR, CRASS RA, ET AL: Computed tomography of pancreatic abscesses. Am J Roentgenol 136:879, 1981

8. GALLACHER DJ, KADIR S, KAUFMAN SL, ET AL: Nonoperative management of benign postoperative biliary strictures. Radiology 156:625, 1985

9. GERZOF SG, JOHNSON WC, ROBBINS AH, ET AL: Percutaneous drainage of infected pancreatic pseudocysts. Arch Surg 119:888, 1984

10. GOLD RP, BERMAN H, FAKHRY J, ET AL: Pancreas divisum with pancreatitis and pseudocyst. Am J Roentgenol 143:1343, 1984

11. GUNTHER RW, KLOSE KJ, RUCKERT K, ET AL: Islet cell tumors: Detection of small lesions with computed tomography and ultrasound. Radiology 148:485, 1983

12. ITAI Y, MOSS AA, OHTOMO K: Computed tomography of cystadenoma and cystadenocarcinoma of the pancreas. Radiology 145:419, 1982

13. JEFFREY RB JR, FEDERLE MP, CRASS RA: Computed tomography of pancreatic trauma. Radiology 147:491, 1983

14. LAWSON TL, BERLAND LL, FOLEY WD, ET AL: Ultrasonic visualization of the pancreatic duct. Radiology 144:865, 1982

15. LAWSON TL: Acute pancreatitis and its complications. Radiol Clin North Am 21:495, 1983

16. MENDEZ G JR, ISIKOFF MB, HILL MC: CT of acute pancreatitis. Am J Roentgenol 135:463, 1980

17. MILLER DA, CARRASCO CH, KATZ RL, ET AL: Fine needle aspiration biopsy: The role of immediate cytologic assessment. Am J Roentgenol 147:155, 1986

18. PERSSON M, BISGAARD C, NIELSEN BB, ET AL: Solid and epithelial neoplasm of the pancreas presenting as a traumatic cyst. Acta Chir Scand 152:223, 1986

19. RUSSELL E, HUTSON DG, GUERRA JJ, ET AL: Dilatation of biliary strictures through a stomatized jejunal limb. Acta Radiol [Diagn] 26:283, 1985

20. ROSSI P, BAERT A, PASSARIELLO R, ET AL: CT of functioning tumors of the pancreas. Am J Roentgenol 144:57, 1985

*Paul and Juhl's Essentials of Radiologic Imaging,
Sixth Edition,* edited by John H. Juhl and
Andrew B. Crummy. J.B. Lippincott Company,
Philadelphia, © 1993.

CHAPTER 16

The Pharynx and Esophagus

Michael Davis

THE PHARYNX

INDICATIONS

Reasons for pharyngeal examination by radiologic methods include coughing; choking; dysphagia; varying degrees of aspiration; nasopharyngeal reflux; a sensation of food "sticking"; a "lump" or tightness in the pharynx; a change in swallowing following head trauma, stroke, or brain tumor; or the inability to handle secretions.

ANATOMY AND PHYSIOLOGY

Structures observed on the pharyngeal swallow examination include lips, tongue, soft palate, epiglottis, valleculae, pyriform sinuses, and cricopharyngeus muscle. The myriad muscles supporting these structures and their nerve innervation is complex, and a detailed knowledge is required for thorough understanding of swallowing abnormalities.[13] A normal swallow begins with closed lips and trapping of the barium on the superior aspect of the tongue followed by a muscular wave within the tongue that propels the barium to the oropharynx. The soft palate elevates and closes the nasopharynx, the barium bolus fills the valleculae, and a contraction of the oropharynx occurs with depression of the epiglottis and closure of the glottis with a propulsion of the barium to the hypopharynx followed by contraction of the cricopharyngeus muscle (which is not normally seen except at the end of the swallow), and passage of the barium into the cervical and thoracic portions of the esophagus. All of the steps of the swallowing sequence must occur in an organized, coordinated fashion for a normal swallow to occur. Distortion of the normal anatomy or neuromuscular dysfunction will result in swallowing abnormalities.

Examination of the esophagus after a pharyngeal study is often required, especially if the etiology of the swallowing abnormality is not clear. Esophageal tumors, strictures, involvement by extrinsic structures, motility disorders, and gastroesophageal reflux disease may all refer symptoms to the pharyngeal area.

METHODS OF EXAMINATION

The pharynx may be evaluated by routine barium-swallow studies. This is best done by the use of video fluoroscopic swallowing procedures where the motion dynamics of the swallowing mechanism are recorded on video tape at 30 frames per second. Tape recorders capable of variable speeds and freeze frame are invaluable. Fluoroscopic rapid spot-film cameras (100-mm cut film or 105-mm roll film) that film at a rate of at least 6 frames per second are also used. Newer digital computerized fluoroscopic equipment can now acquire images at a rate of up to 30 frames per second. The use of high-density barium (200% W/V) will give excellent mucosal coating and outline the anatomic structures of the mouth and pharynx, which should be examined in frontal and lateral projections. In patients with large upper torsos that would obscure the hypopharynx, a slightly oblique view may be necessary.

Patients are usually examined in the upright position, but if a patient is unable to stand, he or she may be examined sitting in specialized chairs that can be placed between the fluoroscopic imaging intensifier and the x-ray table; by fluoroscopic C-arm units with the patient in a wheelchair or on a stretcher; or on an x-ray table with an imaging tube mounted for cross-table lateral imaging with patients in the supine position. Some investigators recommend that patients be examined in supine position.[18] Other investigators recommend oblique projections to augment the standard views.[35]

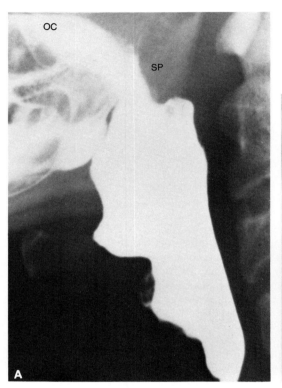

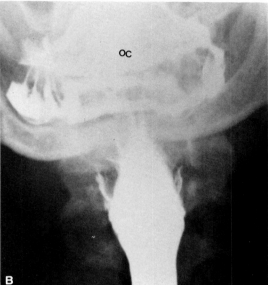

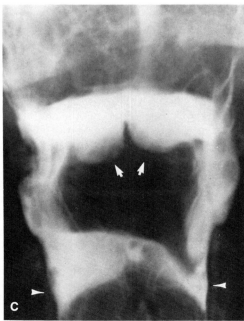

Figure 16–1. (**A**) Normal lateral pharynx, oral cavity (*OC*), soft palate (*SP*). (**B**) Normal frontal pharynx, oral cavity (*OC*). (**C**) Frontal view of pharynx shows pooling of barium in the valleculae (*arrowheads*) and piriform sinuses (*arrows*), consistent pharyngeal paresis (*C*).

RADIOLOGIC PHARYNGEAL ABNORMALITIES

MOTOR AND NEUROSENSORY DISORDERS

Pooling of barium in the valleculae and pyriform sinuses is a common finding, especially with age, and may be considered a form of paresis, where the neuromuscular function is inadequate to express barium from these structures (Fig. 16-1A through C). Nasopharyngeal reflux of varying degrees and laryngeal aspiration are easily identified. Dysfunction of the cricopharyngeus muscle (upper esophageal sphincter) is also a common abnormality that may occur in older patients or may reflect a protective mechanism in patients with gastroesophageal reflux disease (Fig. 16-2A). Cricopharyngeal (zenker's) diverticula occur just proximal to the cricopharyngeus muscle. The hypertonic cricopharyngeus muscle increases the pressure in the hypopharynx, and with time, a mucosal herniation through a triangular zone of sparse musculature can occur. These diverticula can grow to be sizable, and may contain food and saliva and put the patient at risk for aspiration (Fig. 16-2B).[12]

CONGENITAL PHARYNGEAL WEBS

Congenital pharyngeal webs are usually singular, but may be multiple, and may involve a portion or all of the circumference of the pharynx at its level of origin (Fig. 16-3).

EXTERNAL IMPINGEMENT

Cervical spine osteophytes are one of the most common causes of external pharyngeal impingement, although other masses such as lymph nodes, tumors,

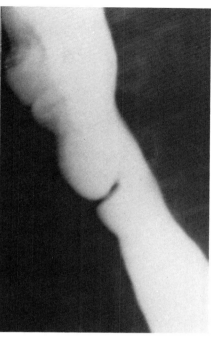

Figure 16–3. Lateral view of midpharynx and hypopharynx shows a thin mucosal web that extends from the anterior wall of the pharynx.

and enlarged thyroids may also deform the pharynx (Fig. 16-4).

TRAUMA

Swallowed sharp foreign bodies, penetrating trauma, caustic agents, and iatrogenic injuries are common causes of pharyngeal trauma (Fig. 16-5).

Figure 16–2. **(A)** Lateral view of hypopharynx shows curvilinear filling defect representing prominent cricopharyngeus muscle visualized throughout the swallow. **(B)** Moderately large cricopharyngeal (Zenker's) diverticulum containing barium exerts narrowing effect on the cervical esophagus.

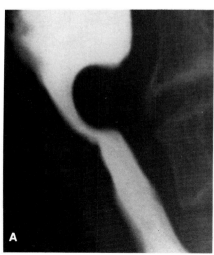
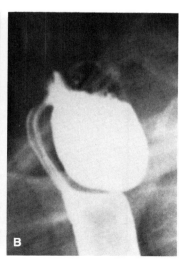

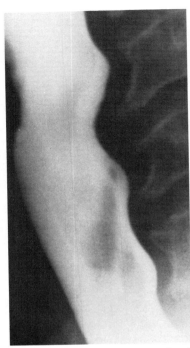

Figure 16–4. Cervical osteophyte impingement. Lateral view of lower pharynx shows large osteophytes impinging on the posterior wall of the pharynx.

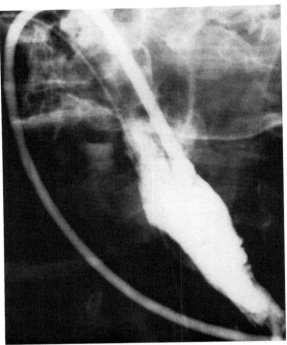

Figure 16–5. Slightly obliqued frontal view shows nasal intubation of feeding tube that perforated the left piriform sinus. The barium is extending along the cervical fascial plane that surrounds the piriform sinus.

INFLAMMATION

The Plummer-Vinson syndrome or Paterson-Kelly syndrome is manifested by iron deficiency anemia, glossitis, pharyngeal webs, and dysphagia.[7] Four to sixteen percent of patients with this disease have been reported to have hypopharyngeal or esophageal carcinoma. These tumors are almost always associated with webs located inferior to the cricoid cartilage (Fig. 16-6).

BENIGN TUMORS

Benign tumors are uncommon and are usually composed of existing mesenchymal tissue. As they grow in size, dysphagia becomes the presenting symptom (Fig. 16-7).

MALIGNANT TUMORS

The most common malignant tumor of the pharynx is squamous-cell carcinoma. Persons with long-term history of alcohol and tobacco use are at increased risk for developing this malignancy. Carcinomas may develop at the base of the tongue, epiglottis, pyriform sinuses,

valleculae, and the palatine tonsils. Enlargement of the tonsils may simulate carcinoma. Double-contrast technique appears to be the best conventional method for diagnosing malignancy where asymmetric or irregular surface mass lesions are detected. Ulcerations and asymmetry caused by the mass leads to the detection of these tumors. If the carcinoma is large enough, single-contrast technique can identify the lesion (Fig. 16-8A). Computed tomography is helpful, not only in identifying the tumor but also in detecting invasion of adjacent structures (Fig. 16-8B). When examining patients with known tumors of the pharynx and larynx, it is important to examine the esophagus for the presence of a synchronous esophageal carcinoma, which may exist in up to 5% of patients with head and neck cancer.

ESOPHAGUS

INDICATIONS

The most common symptoms that lead to examination of the esophagus are heartburn from gastroesophageal reflux disease, followed by difficult (dysphagia) or pain-

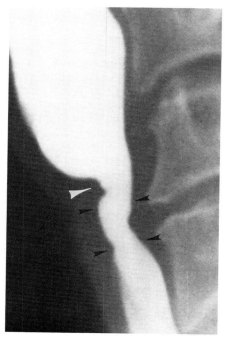

Figure 16–6. Large web indenting anterior wall (*white arrowhead*) with associated stricture (*black arrowheads*). Note distended upper pharynx secondary to the stricture.

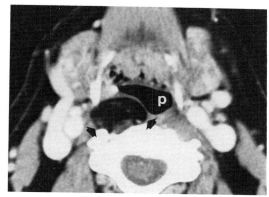

Figure 16–7. Lipoma. CT scan through pharynx shows hypodense, smoothly marginated, fatty lesion representing a lipoma (*arrows*), which deforms the pharyngeal airway (*p*).

ful (odynophagia) swallowing. Motility disorders, when severe enough, may give the patient a feeling of chest discomfort or pain. Strictures of the esophagus (usually from gastroesophageal reflux disease) may cause the sensation of food "sticking."

ANATOMY AND PHYSIOLOGY

The cervical esophagus begins below the cricopharyngeus muscle (upper esophageal sphincter) and becomes the thoracic esophagus at the thoracic inlet, which then continues to the level of the lower esophageal sphincter, which may be 1 or 2 cm below the diaphragm. In the thorax, the distended esophagus is indented on the left side by the aortic arch and the left mainstem bronchus (Fig. 16-9). With age, a dilated thoracic aortic arch may significantly narrow the lumen of the esophagus causing dysphagia. As the thoracic aorta elongates and extends into the left chest, it may displace the esophagus, especially if aneurysms have formed. Cardiac chamber enlargement, in particular of the left atrium and the left ventricle, will show an extrinsic compression involving the lower anterior esophageal wall (Fig. 16-10). The lower esophageal ring (mucosal ring or B-ring) can be seen as a dia-

phragmlike structure in the distended distal esophagus when a sliding hiatal hernia is present.[25] It corresponds to the squamocolumnar mucosal junction.

As a response to swallowing, the primary wave of esophageal motility that carries forth the bolus of barium signals the lower esophageal sphincter to open and then close immediately after the swallowed material passes into the stomach. The transport of food and fluid from the mouth to the stomach is aided by gravity in the upright position, but can be accomplished by peristalsis alone in the recumbent position. Radiologic studies are used to study both anatomic alterations and motility disorders.

METHODS OF EXAMINATION

Plain films of the chest are of limited utility, but are indicated in certain situations, such as when an opaque foreign body, perhaps a bone or a coin has become lodged in the esophagus. Cervical or mediastinal emphysema is visible on plain films and usually indicates disruption of either the esophagus or a site in the respiratory tract. This finding may lead to a contrast examination.

At fluoroscopy, the esophagus may be imaged by the single-contrast, double-contrast or mucosal-relief techniques, using large spot films, fluoroscopic spot-film camera, and video-recording techniques. Usually with overhead filming techniques, only single-contrast examination is done. The single-contrast technique uses a medium density barium (50 to 60 W/V), whereas double-contrast examination employs a heavy or dense barium (200 + % W/V) in conjunction with an effervescent powder that is given with water just before barium ingestion. In mucosal relief technique the esophagus is

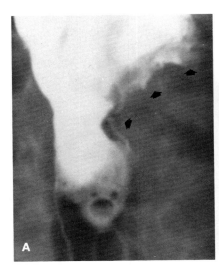

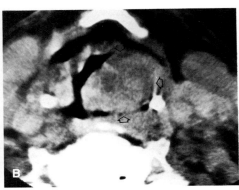

Figure 16–8. (A) Pharyngeal carcinoma. Frontal view of single-contrast swallow examination shows large irregularly shaped mass that involves the left aspect of the hypopharynx (*arrows*). (B) Computed tomogram of same patient shows large homogeneous mass that protrudes into the airway (*arrows*), but shows no significant infiltration into adjacent soft tissues.

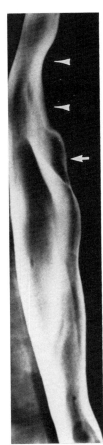

Figure 16–9. Normal double-contrast esophagram shows indentation by aorta (*arrowheads*) and left mainstem bronchus (*arrow*).

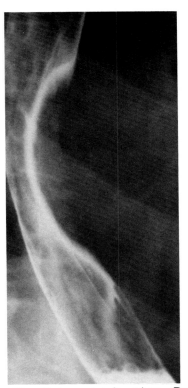

Figure 16–10. Enlarged left atrium. Double-contrast esophagram shows extrinsic compression of the anterior wall of the lower esophagus.

filmed after barium has passed, and the mucosal folds are collapsed yet remain visible.

Other special barium examinations of the esophagus require the use of food substances such as marshmallows, pieces of bagel, cracker or cookie impregnated with barium, barium paste, and barium tablets. Esophageal strictures and esophageal motility disorders are better evaluated with these techniques than with liquid barium alone. Alternatives to barium sulfate are the water-soluble solutions of iodinated organic compounds that may be used when perforation of the esophagus is suspected. These alternative solutions prevent permanent deposition of barium in the soft tissues where it remains as foreign material. The disadvantage of ionic water-soluble contrast is that it is irritating to the tracheobronchial mucosa, and is undesirable if either aspiration or tracheoesophageal fistula is suspected. Barium sulfate is nonreactive in the tracheobronchial tree. Computed tomography has value in studying the extent of processes beginning in the esophagus and extending into the mediastinum.

ALTERNATIVE NONRADIOLOGIC METHODS

Esophageal endoscopy is an accurate method used to view the mucosal surface of the esophagus. It has the advantage of allowing immediate biopsy of pathologic areas, but it is not a good method to study motility. Currently, it has the disadvantage of being more costly than radiologic methods and has the potential of causing iatrogenic trauma. Measuring intraluminal esophageal pressures (manometry) and recording pH can be accomplished with tubes placed in the esophagus. There is no substitute for the information obtained this way. The ingestion of radioisotope-labeled food is another method of studying esophageal transport, gastroesophageal reflux, and gastric emptying.

CONGENITAL ANOMALIES

The least severe manifestation of the failure of tubulation is the esophageal web, whereas the severest form is esophageal stenosis. Esophageal atresia occurs in multiple forms, but the most common is when the esophagus communicates with the trachea below the atretic segment. Other forms have a fistula above the atresia, or both above and below the atresia. There may be atresia without a tracheoesophageal fistula. An indication that something may be wrong with the esophagus occurs with the first feedings. Chest films may show the effects of pulmonary aspiration. These abnormalities, however, can be diagnosed in utero with ultrasonography, which can detect polyhydramnios and absence of stomach fluid. After birth, if an infant with esophageal atresia has a fistula in the normal lower

esophagus, an abundance of air will be seen in the gut. If there is no fistula, the gut will be airless. A lateral film of the chest taken after placing an opaque tube in the esophagus may show the tube coiled in the proximal esophagus and yield enough information for a diagnosis (Fig. 16-11). If necessary, a small amount of barium sulfate suspension may be injected through the tube with the patient in the upright position. The atresia will then be quite evident. After the radiographs have been obtained, the contrast material should be removed to prevent aspiration. Surgical repair of these defects is very successful. As these patients are studied postoperatively, they may not transmit a peristaltic wave

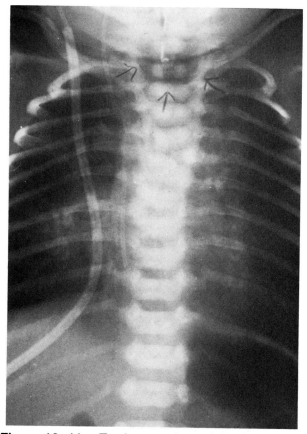

Figure 16–11. Tracheoesophageal fistula. The tip of the nasogastric tube is seen in the air-distended upper esophagus (*arrows*). The tube could not be passed into the stomach, establishing the diagnosis of upper-esophageal atresia. The presence of air in the stomach established the presence of a fistula between the airway and the distal esophagus below the atretic segment. The right pulmonary infiltrate is secondary to the flow of orally ingested fluid into the right lower lobe.

normally through the anastomotic area.[16] Ordinarily, this is not a clinical problem. There may be associated anomalies of the vertebrae and ribs. Less commonly, there are cardiovascular or other gastrointestinal abnormalities.

FOREGUT SEPARATION FAILURE

Occasionally, the separation of the cervical esophagus from the airway may not occur and contrast material demonstrates a single cavity. When this cleft is present there is massive aspiration with either feeding or contrast ingestion.

H-TYPE FISTULA WITHOUT ATRESIA

The H-type of tracheoesophageal fistula can be extremely difficult to demonstrate with a conventional feeding esophagram. The injection of contrast through an esophageal tube with the patient prone is the recommended approach (Fig. 16-12). In this way, each segment can be examined under fluoroscopic observation, and good distention of each segment with contrast

material can be achieved. Tracheomalacia is usually present.

Duplications of the esophagus usually do not communicate with the esophageal lumen. Their presentation is that of a mediastinal or paraesophageal mass. Their cystic nature may be identified with computed tomography (CT).[19]

INFLAMMATION

Regardless of etiology, the radiologic manifestations of inflammatory disease are quite similar. With a mild degree of inflammation of the esophagus, there are no radiologic abnormalities. As the process becomes severer, there is or may be a combination of any of the following: nodularity, thickened folds, erosions, ulceration, spasm, and edema.

GASTROESOPHAGEAL REFLUX DISEASE

Both acid and pepsin and alkaline bile gastroesophageal reflux may occur and lead to esophagitis. Acid reflux is the most common and is related to inappropriate relaxation or incompetence of the lower esophageal sphincter.[5, 10, 11] This scenario usually occurs in the presence of a hiatal hernia. The severity of esophagitis depends on the frequency of reflux and the length of time the refluxed fluid in the esophagus remains before being cleared by primary and secondary peristaltic waves. The pH of the reflux fluid, whether acid or alkaline, also is a factor in the development of esophagitis. In addition to showing the radiopathologic changes caused by the inflammation, the radiologic examination can occasionally reveal the esophageal reflux.[9, 26]

Observation of gastroesophageal reflux at the time of fluoroscopy is of limited value unless substantial reflux has occurred, and there is delayed clearing.

Radiographic changes of reflux esophagitis are varied depending on the severity of the disease. Early changes of erythema are not visible radiographically as they are endoscopically. Radiologic changes of esophagitis include erosions, nodularity, thickened folds, luminal narrowing, diffuse ulceration with strictures, or any combination of these (Fig. 16-13).

Columnar lined esophagus (Barrett's esophagus) is a manifestation of chronic gastroesophageal reflux disease, where normal squamous epithelium has been denuded by inflammation and replaced by columnar epithelial lining. Barrett's esophagus is almost always an acquired condition that leads to metaplasia of the columnar mucosa.[31, 32] Barrett's esophagus occurs in 10% to 20% of patients with significant gastroesophageal reflux disease.[29] Barrett's esophagus may present radiographically with a large, deep ulcer. Barrett's

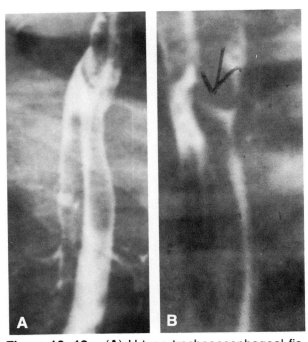

Figure 16–12. **(A)** H-type tracheoesophageal fistula. Catheter injection of contrast material into the thoracic esophagus fills the trachea as well as the esophagus. **(B)** H-type fistula. A film taken in the lateral projection shows the narrow fistulous tract (*arrow*) extending in a slightly cephalad direction from esophagus to trachea.

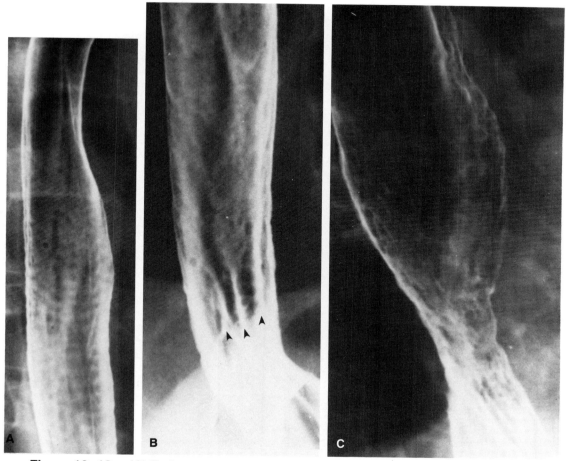

Figure 16–13. (**A**) Early esophagitis. Double-contrast esophagram shows diffuse nodularity of mucosal surface. (**B**) Moderate changes of esophagitis. Lower esophagus shows thickened folds (*arrowheads*) and nodularity in distal esophagus. (**C**) Severe esophagitis. Diffuse mucosal ulcerations with stricture formation.

ulcers may heal with stricture formation distally or in the upper esophagus. A high esophageal stricture or ulcer in the presence of gastroesophageal reflux disease is strongly suggestive of Barrett's esophagus (Fig. 16-14*A, B*). An increased incidence of adenocarcinoma results from Barrett's esophagus. The approximate incidence of Barrett's esophagus with adenocarcinoma is about 15% (Fig. 16-14*C*).[20]

EXTRINSIC AGENTS

Either acid or alkaline can cause severe inflammatory changes. In infants and children, an accidental ingestion is usually the problem, whereas in adults it is usually part of a suicide attempt.[24] Caustic ingestion may cause long, permanent strictures with an increased incidence of carcinoma after three and four

decades (Fig. 16-15*A*). Radiation therapy is often responsible for severe symptomatic esophagitis, and stricture may occur many years later (Fig. 16-15*B*). A variety of oral medications may cause mucosal irritation and ulceration when they adhere to the mucosa, usually because not enough oral fluids are taken with the medication. Antibiotic medications, such as tetracycline and doxycycline, are well known to cause this problem; other medications include potassium chloride, quinidine, vitamin C tablets, and oral ferrous sulfate.[8]

INFECTIOUS ESOPHAGITIS

Immunosuppression and general debilitation are generally the background for herpes simplex,[21, 30] cytomegaloviruses,[33] and Candida infection.[22, 23] Candida

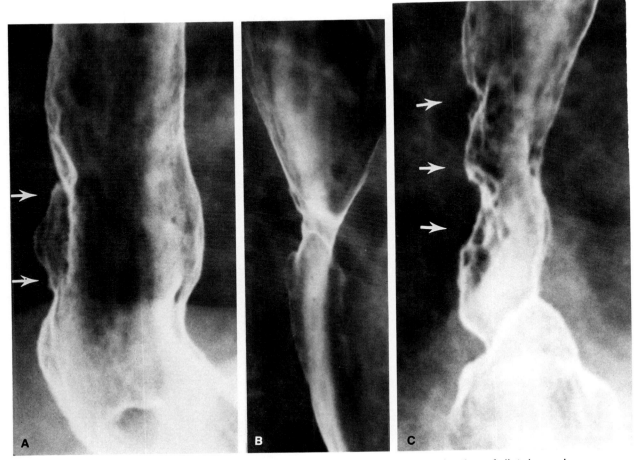

Figure 16–14. **(A)** Barrett's esophagus. Double-contrast examination of distal esophagus demonstrates presence of large deep ulceration involving posterolateral wall of distal esophagus (*arrows*). **(B)** Smooth midesophageal stricture from healed Barrett's ulcer. **(C)** Adenocarcinoma in Barrett's esophagus. Double-contrast examination of distal esophagus shows luminal narrowing, mucosal irregularity, and indentation along one wall of the esophagus where adenocarcinoma has formed (*arrows*).

infection is by far the most common. It is best seen on double-contrast esophagrams, which demonstrate plaquelike lesions often oriented in vertical fashion. When the disease is diffuse, the mucosa becomes markedly irregular or ragged in appearance. If Candida and viral esophagitis occur together, the Candida lesion may obscure the ulceration of the viral disease, which otherwise is quite obvious (Fig. 16-16).

Numerous ulcerations with a lucent rim of edema are seen both in profile and en face. The ulcers are represented en face by collections of barium with surrounding lucent halos of edema. Any esophageal infection may heal and return to normal, but it may also produce permanent esophageal stricture. Tuberculous

esophagitis is rare and usually seen only in advanced cases of pulmonary and mediastinal tuberculosis, which are seen increasingly as acquired immunodeficiency syndrome (AIDS) complications. Tuberculous infections have a tendency to form fistulas.

MISCELLANEOUS

Two conditions that have similar manifestations are pemphigus and epidermolysis bullosa.[36] Smooth filling defects indicative of an intramural process are seen in addition to ulcerations and scarring often followed by stricture. Crohn's disease rarely involves the esophagus but when present may show aphthous ulcers, a

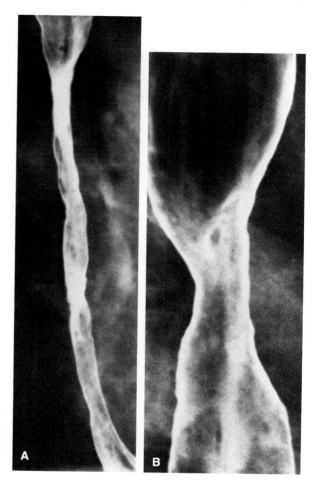

Figure 16–15. (A) Caustic ingestion stricture. At least two thirds of the esophagus demonstrates marked narrowing from ingestion of caustic agent years before. (B) Radiation stricture. Double-contrast esophagram shows smooth stricture midesophagus.

corrugated mucosal pattern, and even pseudopolyps. Behçet's syndrome is another disease that may show an irregular ulcerated mucosal pattern. Eosinophilic gastroenteritis may have esophageal involvement with fine ulcerations and a nodular mucosa. Glycogenic acanthosis is a common benign condition.[6, 15] Multiple white plaques are seen at endoscopy, and they create a nodular appearance on double-contrast esophagrams. It is a degenerative phenomenon seen in the aging process where glycogen is stored in surface cells.

MOTILITY DISORDERS

Presbyesophagus. The most common motility change observed in the esophagus is that related to aging. This disorder is usually asymptomatic because the failure of muscular transport can be compensated by gravity. Therefore, it may not be noted that esophageal function is diminished until some other disease process makes it necessary to take food and fluids in the recumbent position. The components of presbyesophagus observed radiographically are (1) failure of a primary peristaltic wave to pass completely along the esophagus to the stomach; (2) nonperistaltic (simultaneous, tertiary) contractions in response to swallowing (Fig. 16-17); (3) aperistalsis, that is, no muscular response to swallowing; and (4) either an absence of any contraction of the lower esophageal sphincter or a failure of relaxation of the sphincter with swallowing. All these components, except absence of contraction of the sphincter, can be observed at fluoroscopy.

Achalasia. Achalasia is an interesting but uncommon abnormality of the lower esophageal sphincter. The process is slow and insidious in its development. The patient frequently has a dilated esophagus before becoming symptomatic. Sometimes the diagnosis is first made on the basis of seeing a dilated esophagus on a plain chest film that has been made for an entirely different purpose. On the upright chest film an air-

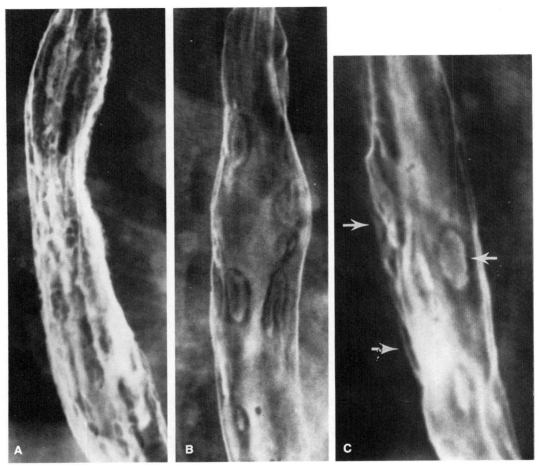

Figure 16–16. (**A**) Advanced Candida infection. Double-contrast esophagram demonstrates markedly irregular mucosal surface pattern in which plaquelike formation tends to run in vertical fashion. (**B**) Herpes esophagitis. Several oval discrete ulcerations with normal intervening mucosa. (**C**) Cytomegalovirus esophagitis with ulcers seen en face and in profile (*arrows*).

fluid level can be seen in the thoracic esophagus. When barium is given there is a normal peristaltic wave down to the thoracic inlet but not beyond. The barium suspension outlines the fluid-filled, dilated esophagus and passes by gravity to the level of the lower sphincter. This area will often have a bird's-beak appearance (Fig. 16-18). Observing the beak while the patient swallows shows a momentary relaxation of the sphincter, allowing a small amount of barium to enter the stomach. Occasionally, weak tertiary contractions can be observed in the body of the esophagus.

The pathophysiology of achalasia involves two features. The first is a hypertonic lower esophageal sphincter that relaxes incompletely with swallowing. The second is a lack of peristalsis in the body of the esophagus. Because the changes in the body are irre-

versible, treatment is directed at releasing the obstruction at the lower esophageal sphincter. An esophagomyotomy can be accomplished by either balloon dilatation or surgery. The simple dilatation that is effective for inflammatory strictures may not relieve the patient who has achalasia. After esophagomyotomy the radiographic picture improves only slightly despite genuine symptomatic relief. Occasionally, treatment will cause an esophageal perforation or enough destruction of the sphincter to allow free gastro-esophageal reflux. Because the esophagus cannot generate secondary peristalsis and there is acid-pepsin reflux from the stomach, esophagitis may be very severe. There is a suspicion that carcinoma of the esophagus is more common in patients with achalasia, but there is insufficient data to support this.

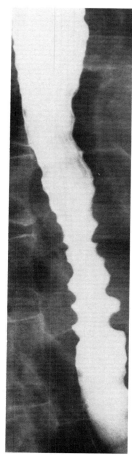

Figure 16–17. Presbyesophagus. Single-contrast esophagram demonstrates numerous tertiary contractions in the middle and lower portion of the esophagus without significant advancement of the barium bolus.

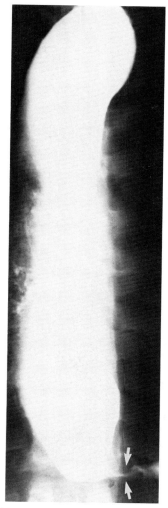

Figure 16–18. Achalasia. Single-contrast esophagram shows dilated barium-filled esophagus with small abrupt "birdlike" beak distally (*arrows*).

Chagas' Disease. A picture like that of achalasia can result from infection by *Trypanosoma cruzi*. This disease is endemic in parts of South America.

Diffuse Esophageal Spasm, the "Nutcracker" Esophagus, and the Hypertonic Lower Esophageal Sphincter. A variety of conditions fall into the category of esophageal dysmotility. Classification is difficult and changes regularly. Accurate diagnosis requires intraluminal esophageal manometry. At the present time there are no reliable radiologic criteria to sort out these conditions, because their diagnosis depends on knowledge of the intraluminal pressure. They are important conditions because they may cause chest pain that may mimic myocardial ischemia (Figs. 16-19*A, B*).

Scleroderma. As part of the progressive systemic sclerosis, the vascular supply to the esophagus may be impaired and muscle function lost. This usually involves a lower two thirds of the thoracic esophagus, the striated muscle portion, including the sphincter. When barium is given there is normal peristalsis down to, but not beyond, the aortic arch level. Because the lower esophageal sphincter is involved, there is easy flow into the stomach in the upright position. When the patient is in the recumbent position, esophageal transport is markedly delayed; when the patient has a full stomach, free gastroesophageal reflux may be observed. Peptic esophagitis and stricture can be a severe problem in scleroderma. Most often the esophageal changes are only part of an obvious clinical picture of

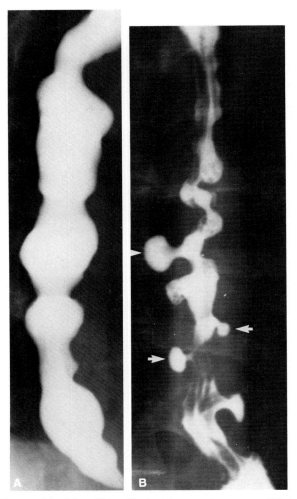

Figure 16–19. (A) Probable corkscrew "Nutcracker" esophagus. Numerous deep and wide contractions throughout the esophagus in patient with simultaneous chest pain. (B) Diffuse esophageal spasm. Marked spasm throughout distal two thirds of esophagus caused formation of pseudodiverticula (*arrows*) that disappear with relaxation.

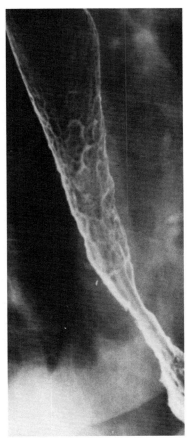

Figure 16–20. Scleroderma. Double-contrast examination shows distal esophageal stricture with unusual surface pattern that may reflect the underlying atrophy and fibrosis of the smooth muscle.

progressive systemic sclerosis. It is rare that the esophageal symptoms occur first (Fig. 16-20).

Esophageal Diverticula. Esophageal diverticula are common and are the result of esophageal motor disorders.[14] Diverticula may occur throughout the esophagus, but frequently occur in the middle and lower third. With distal esophageal strictures, an epiphrenic diverticulum may develop (Fig. 16-21A). Diverticula usually are formed by increased intraluminal pressure with eventual pulsion (Fig. 16-21B).

Miscellaneous. Rheumatoid arthritis, systemic lupus erythematosus, and alcoholism may have associated esophageal dysmotility. The easiest manifestation to recognize is aperistalsis. Unusual peristaltic patterns have also been described in diabetes.

VARICES

Most esophageal varices are produced by either liver disease with portal hypertension or thrombosis of the splenic-portal trunk. The varies occur in the distal esophagus. If they are large enough and bulge into the lumen, they are readily detected on radiographic examination (Fig. 16-22A). Because bleeding esophageal varices may not be detectable radiographically, endoscopy is considered a more sensitive and specific diagnostic test. Current enthusiasm for the treatment of

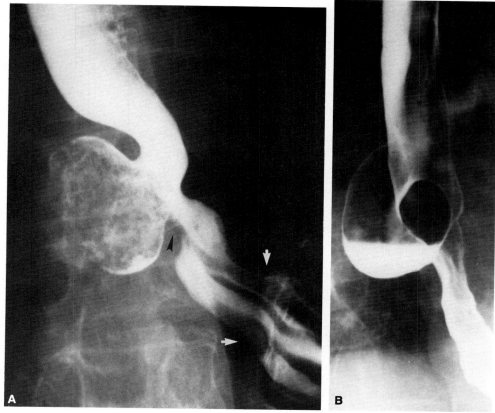

Figure 16–21. (**A**) Epiphrenic diverticulum. Single-contrast examination shows epiphrenic diverticulum with inspissated food material. The diverticulum is just above a distal esophageal stricture (*arrowhead*). Hiatal hernia is also present (*arrows*). (**B**) Double-contrast esophagram of distal half of esophagus shows wide-mouth diverticulum containing barium-fluid level.

varices by endoscopic sclerosis is conducive to combined diagnostic and therapeutic methods. After sclerotherapy the thrombosed veins may ulcerate and create a distinctive radiographic appearance (Fig. 16-22B).[1] Thrombosis in the superior vena cava may lead to the dilatation of collateral veins in the upper esophagus, which have been aptly named "down-hill varices." Computed tomography and barium esophagram have a similar ability to detect esophageal varices. Computed tomography has the advantages of imaging paraesophageal varices and other manifestations of portal hypertension.[4]

FOREIGN BODIES

Children can, and do, ingest a variety of foreign objects. Because of an object's size or configuration, it may become lodged in the esophagus. If a foreign object is radiopaque, plain films are adequate for localization. Barium given orally is necessary for a nonradiopaque object. Detection is difficult in the cervical esophagus, where the bolus may pass so rapidly that a small object, such as a bone impaled in the mucosa, may be missed. Cotton balls soaked with barium have been used effectively to detect small foreign bodies. Endoscopy can be used as well for search and removal of foreign bodies. Removal of many objects in children can be accomplished by inflating a balloon catheter distal to the foreign body and then withdrawing it through the mouth. This is best done under fluoroscopic control.

In adults the most common foreign object to become lodged in the esophagus is an oversized piece of meat, sometimes occurring when an individual is inebriated or engrossed in conversation. Dentures or lack of teeth can promote the swallowing of large boluses. Efferves-

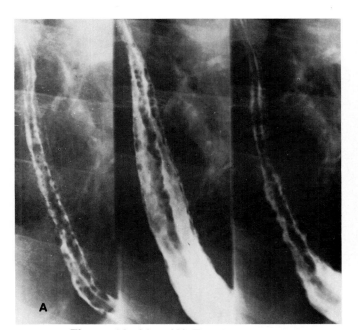
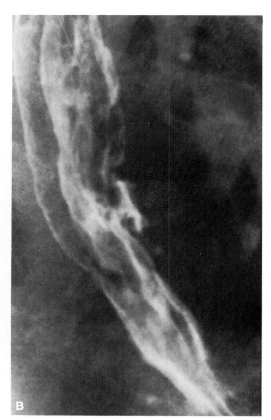

Figure 16–22. **(A)** Esophageal varices. These large varices are easily distinguished from normal esophageal folds because of their tortuous contours. **(B)** Esophageal varices after sclerotherapy. The thrombosed veins are well visualized, and there is also ulceration of a thrombosed varix (*arrow*).

cent powders in conjunction with intravenous glucagon have been tried with some success in treating such impacted foreign bodies. The balloon catheter method used in children is seldom applicable in adults because the foreign body often totally occludes the lumen (Fig. 16-23). Endoscopic removal may be necessary.

NEOPLASMS

Benign. The most common benign esophageal tumors are leiomyomas, most of which are asymptomatic and found incidental to the search for another process. Leiomyomas in the esophagus do not ulcerate and bleed as do those in the stomach. They have the characteristic appearance of an intramural mass with their margins at relatively obtuse angles in relation to the vertical lumen of the esophagus (Fig. 16-24). Other benign intramural masses such as esophageal duplication cyst or lipoma may produce a similar appearance. Epithelial polyps of the esophagus are quite rare. In-

fluenced by esophageal peristalsis, they may develop a long pedicle. The stalk is occasionally long enough to allow the patient to regurgitate the mass into the oral cavity.

Malignant

Primary. Squamous-cell carcinoma is the most common histologic type found in the esophagus. Adenocarcinoma is also found, and it is thought to develop in the setting of dysplastic mucosa associated with Barrett's esophagus. Malignant esophageal tumors rarely bleed significantly, so they must attain a size sufficient to interfere with food transport before they are symptomatic. They begin as plaques, become polypoid or begin circumferentially, spreading and eventually causing long irregular strictures. They may ulcerate, develop a serpiginous vertical infiltrative pattern that resembles varices (varicoid carcinoma), and occasionally begin by superficial spreading of multiple nod-

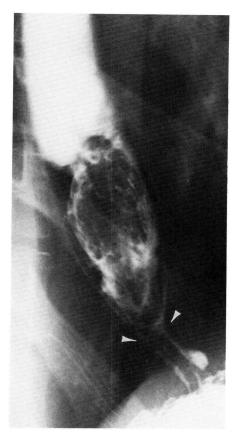

Figure 16–23. Reflux esophagitis stricture. Food bolus is impacted just proximal to a distal esophageal stricture (*arrowheads*). Note that the impacted food is obstructing the passage of barium.

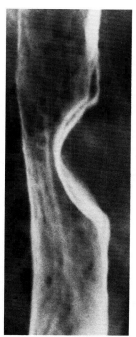

Figure 16–24. Esophageal leiomyoma. Double-contrast examination shows typical appearance of intramural leiomyoma. Note the obtuse mucosal angle characteristic of an intramural lesion.

ules throughout the mucosa of an involved segment (Fig. 16-25*A-E*). Their circumferential growth eventually narrows the lumen enough to block passage of a bolus and cause symptoms of dysphagia.

Radiographic detection of the early flat lesion can be difficult if not impossible. Later growth makes the lesion much easier to see. Sometimes during the course of the disease or following treatment, a fistula to the trachea or bronchus may develop. It is important to limit the volume of contrast material given in this situation. Staging of esophageal cancer using CT is useful.[28] Computed tomography may clearly identify adenopathy that is not amenable to resection (Fig. 16-26*A, B*). Computed tomography should be done for preoperative staging of esophageal carcinoma because it has greater than 90% accuracy in detecting mediastinal invasion.[17] Magnetic resonance imaging has the same accuracy as CT in demonstrating nonresectability of esophageal carcinoma.[34] Liver metastases may also

be shown. Computed tomography is less accurate in determining the local limits of the tumor when patients have a marked weight loss, and the fat planes that aid CT often are not present. Rarely, a primary lymphoma of the esophagus occurs (Fig. 16-27). An interesting but unusual tumor is the spindle-cell tumor,[2] which is also known as carcinosarcoma or pseudosarcoma. Evidence suggests that this tumor is of connective tissue origin. This neoplasm often presents a bulky intraluminal mass (Fig. 16-28).

Metastatic Disease. Lung cancer can invade the esophagus directly, but even in the face of the present epidemic it rarely occurs as a clinical problem. Breast and renal tumors also may metastasize to the esophagus.[3] Melanoma spreads so widely throughout the body that it can involve any part of the gastrointestinal tract (Fig. 16-29). The same is true of Kaposi's sarcoma, which is now seen in patients with AIDS.

TRAUMA

The esophagus may rupture in association with major trauma, but more often rupture occurs secondarily to

(*text continues on page 568*)

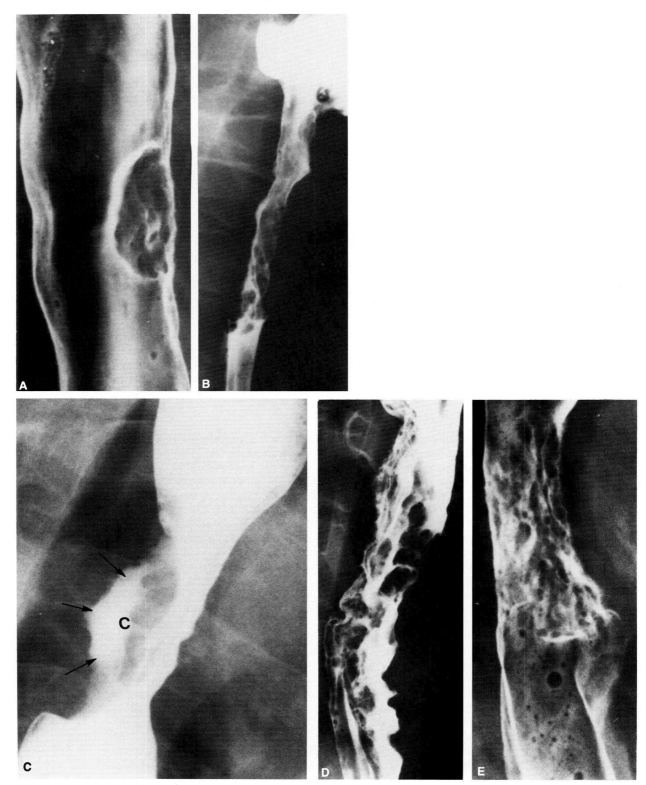

Figure 16–25. *(Continued)*

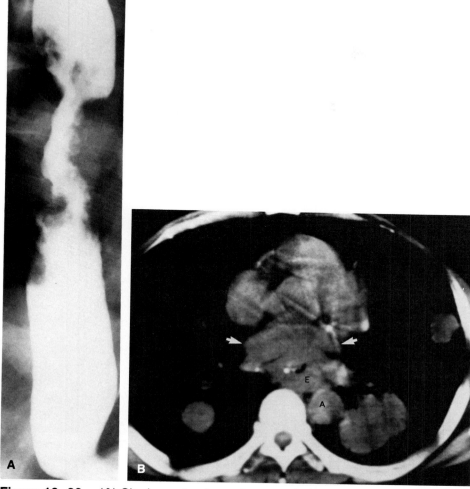

Figure 16–26. (**A**) Single-contrast esophagram demonstrates advanced circumferential infiltrating squamous cell carcinoma of esophagus. (**B**) CT scan through central portion of lesion shows markedly thickened esophageal wall (*E*), adjacent adenopathy (*arrows*), and several lung metastases that are obvious. *A*, aorta.

◄**Figure 16–25.** (**A**) Plaque carcinoma with small central ulceration. (**B**) Long segment of circumferential carcinoma of the proximal esophagus. (**C**) Large ulcerated carcinoma, proximal esophagus. Ulcer (*U*). (**D**) Varicoid carcinoma (note serpiginous folds of the tumor that simulate esophageal varices). (**E**) Numerous superficial carcinomatous nodules involving the mucosa at the level of the aorta arch. The smaller, darker round defects at the lower portion of the image represent residual bubbles.

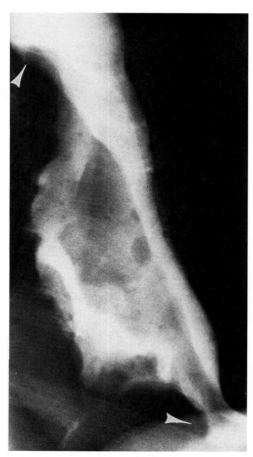

Figure 16–27.   Lymphoma. Single-contrast esophagram shows widening of the lumen of the distal esophagus with irregular margins and leading edges of the tumor proximally and distally (*arrowheads*).

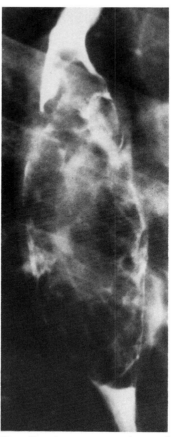

Figure 16–28.   Carcinosarcoma. Large bulky mass expands lumen of midesophagus.

severe vomiting (Boerhaave's syndrome). The rupture tends to occur on the left side of the lower esophagus and may extend into the left pleural space. Eventually, swallowed air dissects into the mediastinum. Plain films show a combination of a lower mediastinal density with or without a pleural effusion or mediastinal emphysema. Fluoroscopic examination with a small amount of water-soluble contrast material will confirm the diagnosis, showing extravasation in the area of the rupture (Fig. 16-30).

Instrumentation.   Any type of instrument introduced

into the esophagus may perforate that structure. Dilatation of the esophagus for the treatment of stricture or achalasia is the usual cause of perforation.

Surgery.   Mild dysphagia may develop after truncal vagotomy, but it usually is self-limited. Mild esophageal narrowing is observed. The anastomosis of stomach to esophagus is technically difficult and suture line leaks will occasionally occur. Water-soluble contrast material is preferred to study suspected perforation.[27]

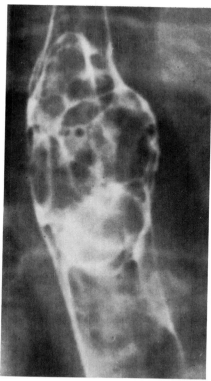

Figure 16–29. Metastatic melanoma of the esophagus creating a multinodular polypoid mass.

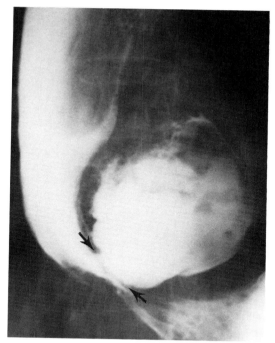

Figure 16–30. Boerhaave's syndrome—esophageal rupture. Single-contrast examination with water-soluble material fills a rounded area just adjacent to the distal esophagus. Site of rupture clearly seen (*arrows*).

REFERENCES AND SELECTED READINGS

1. AGHA FP: The esophagus after endoscopic injection sclerotherapy: Acute and chronic changes. Radiology 153:37, 1984

2. AGHA FP, KEREN DP: Spindle-cell squamous carcinoma of the esophagus: A tumor with biphasic morphology. Am J Roentgenol 145:451, 1985

3. ANDERSON MF, HARRELL GS: Secondary esophageal tumors. Am J Roentgenol 135:1243, 1980

4. BALTHAZAR EJ, NAIDICH OP, MEGIBOW AJ, ET AL: CT evaluation of esophageal varices. Am J Roentgenol 148:131, 1987

5. BEHAR J: Reflux esophagitis: Pathogenesis, diagnosis and management. Arch Intern Med 136:560, 1976

6. BERLINER L, REDMOND P, HOROWITZ L, ET AL: Glycogen plaques (glycogenic acanthosis) of the esophagus. Radiology 141:607, 1981

7. CHISHOLM M: The association between webs, iron and post-cricoid carcinoma. Postgrad Med J 50:215, 1974

8. CRETEUR V, LAUFER I, KRESSEL HY, ET AL: Drug-induced esophagitis detected by double-contrast radiography. Radiology 147:365, 1983

9. CRETEUR V, THOENI RF, FEDERLE MP, ET AL: The role of single and double contrast radiography in the diagnosis of reflux esophagitis. Radiology 147:71, 1983

10. DENT J, DODDS WJ, FRIEDMAN RH, ET AL: Mechanism of gastroesophageal reflux in recumbent asymptomatic human subjects. Clin Invest 65:256, 1980

11. DODDS WJ, HOGAN WJ, MILLER WN: Reflux esophagitis. Digest Dis 21:49, 1976

12. DODDS WJ, LOGEMANN JA, STEWART ET: Radiologic assessment of abnormal oral and pharyngeal phases of swallowing. Am J Roentgenol 154:965, 1990

13. DODDS WJ, STEWART ET, LOGEMANN JA: Physiology and radiology of the normal oral and pharyngeal phases of swallowing. Am J Roentgenol 154:953, 1990

14. ENTERLINE H, THOMPSON J (EDS): Diverticula and diverticulosis, in Pathology of the esophagus. New York, Springer-Verlag, 1984, pp. 43–54

15. GLICK SN, TEPLICK SK, GOLDSTEIN J, ET AL: Glycogenic acanthosis of the esophagus. Am J Roentgenol 139:683, 1982

16. GUNDRY SR, ORRINGER MR: Esophageal motor dysfunction in an adult with a congenital tracheoesophageal fistula. Arch Surg 120:1082, 1984

17. HALVERSON RA JR, THOMPSON WM: Computed tomographic staging of gastrointestinal tract malignancies: I. Esophagus and stomach. Invest Radiol 22:2, 1987

18. JONES B, DONNER MW: Examination of the patient with dysphagia. Radiology 167:319, 1988

19. KUHLMAN JE, FISHMAN EK, WANG K, ET AL: Esophageal duplication cyst: CT and transesophageal needle aspiration. Am J Roentgenol 145:531, 1985

20. LEVINE MS, CAROLINE DF, THOMPSON JJ, ET AL: Adenocarcinoma of the esophagus: Relationship to Barrett's mucosa. Radiology 150:305, 1984

21. LEVINE MS, LAUFER I, KRESSEL HY, ET AL: Herpes esophagitis. Am J Roentgenol 136, 1981

22. LEVINE MS, MACONES AJ, LAUFER I: Candida esophagitis: Accuracy of radiographic detection. Radiology 154:581, 1985

23. LEVINE MS, WOLDENBERG R, HERLINGER H, ET AL: Opportunistic esophagitis in AIDS: Radiographic diagnosis. Radiology 165:815, 1987

24. MUHETALER CA, GERLOCK AJ, DE SOTO J, ET AL: Acid corrosive esophagitis: Radiographic findings. Am J Roentgenol 134:1137, 1980

25. OTT, DJ, GELFAND DW, WU WC: Esophagogastric region and its rings. Am J Roentgenol 142:281, 1984

26. OTT DJ, GELFAND SW, WU WC: Reflux esophagitis: Radiographic and endoscopic correlation. Radiology 130:583, 1979

27. OWEN JW, BALFE DM, DOEHLER RE, ET AL: Radiologic

evaluation of complications after esophagogastrectomy. Am J Roentgenol 140:1163, 1983

28. PICUS D, BALFE DM, KOEHLER RE, ET AL: Computed tomography in the staging of esophageal carcinoma. Radiology 146:433, 1983

29. SARR MG, HAMILTON SR, MAWRONE GC, ET AL: Barrett's esophagus: Its prevalence and association in adenocarcinoma in patients with symptoms of reflux. Am J Surg 149:187, 1985

30. SHORTSLEEVE MJ, GAUVIN GP, GARDNER RC, ET AL: Herpetic esophagitis. Radiology 141:611, 1981

31. SJÖGREN RW, JOHNSON LF: Barrett's esophagus: A review. Am J Med 74:313, 1983

32. SPECHLER SJ, GOYAL RK: Barrett's esophagus. N Engl J Med 315:362, 1986

33. ST. ONCE G, BEZAHLER GH: Giant esophageal ulcer associated with cytomegalovirus. Gastroenterology 82:127, 1982

34. TAKASHIMA S, TAKEUCHI N, SHIOZAKI H, ET AL: Carcinoma of the esophagus: CT vs. MR imaging in determining resectability. Am J Roentgenol 156:297, 1991

35. TAYLOR AJ, DODDS WJ, STEWART ET: Pharynx: Value of oblique projections for radiographic examination. Radiology 178:59, 1991

36. TISHLER JM, HAN SW, HELMAN CA: Esophageal involvement in epidermolysis bullosa dystrophica. Am J Roentgenol 141:1283, 1983

*Paul and Juhl's Essentials of Radiologic Imaging,
Sixth Edition*, edited by John H. Juhl and
Andrew B. Crummy. J.B. Lippincott Company,
Philadelphia, © 1993.

CHAPTER **17**

The Stomach and Duodenum

Michael Davis

THE STOMACH AND DUODENUM

INDICATIONS

Symptoms of epigastric pain raise the possibility of
peptic ulcer disease and lead to an examination of the
stomach and duodenum. Hematemesis or melena is
also a strong indication. The nausea-vomiting complex
on a subacute or chronic basis raises the possibility of
an obstructive lesion. A palpable mass in the upper
abdomen may involve the stomach. Weight loss and
anorexia are less specific symptoms but can occur with
gastric cancer. All intra-abdominal structures can now
be seen directly using computed tomography (CT) or
ultrasound. Nevertheless, barium and other contrast
materials remain invaluable in detecting alimentary
tract diseases.

ANATOMY

The stomach and duodenum are divided into segments
that do not have sharply defined margins. The cardia,
fundus, body, antrum, and pyloric canal are commonly
used terms to identify the position of gastric lesions
(Fig. 17-1*A* through *D*). In the duodenum it is the
bulb, second, third, and fourth portions (Fig. 17-2).
The stomach itself varies considerably in size and position. The asthenic habitus is associated with a vertically
oriented body and antrum, with the stomach often
dipping into the pelvis. Stouter patients have stomachs
with a transverse orientation. The duodenum has few
anatomic variations mainly because most of it is retro-

peritoneal and fixed in position. Occasionally, there is
some redundancy in the postbulbar area. The mucosal
folds in the duodenum are relatively constant in size,
(Fig. 17-3*A*, *B*), but there is a large range in the size of
normal gastric folds. Gastric folds are particularly
prominent along the greater curvature and in the
fundus (see Fig. 17-1*D*).

PHYSIOLOGY

The primary digestive process begins in the stomach
where the secretion of acid and pepsin create an environment for both protein breakdown and peptic ulcer
disease. Stomach content is carried to the duodenal
bulb where the pH drops to more neutral levels. The
stomach and duodenum also have endocrine-type activity with gastrin released from cells in the antrum and
cholecystokinin released from the duodenal cells. Gastric motility is a complex process, but it can be divided
into a churning phase and an emptying function. The
stomach empties fluids much more rapidly than solids.

METHODS OF EXAMINATION

The fluoroscopic-radiographic examination of the upper gut with barium sulfate suspension has been standard for years. The single-contrast examination uses
180 to 300 ml of medium-density barium (50% to 60%
W/V) (see Fig. 17-1*A*, *D*). Effervescent powders are
given in conjunction with heavy or dense barium
(200% W/V +) to create the double-contrast examina-

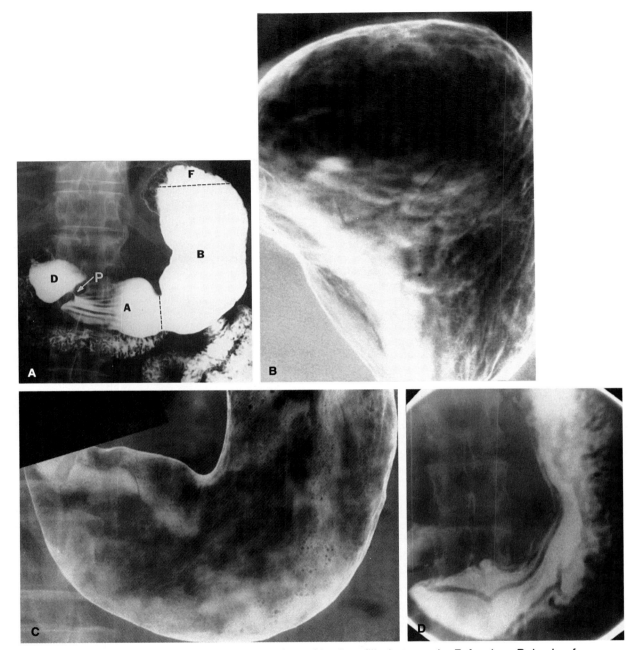

Figure 17–1. (**A**) Posteroanterior view of barium filled stomach. *F*, fundus; *B*, body of stomach; *A*, antrum; *P*, pylorus; *D*, duodenal bulb. (**B**) Double-contrast examination of body and fundus of stomach. (**C**) Air-contrast examination of lower body and antrum of stomach. (**D**) Stomach partially filled with barium outlining the rugal folds. Note the abundance of rugal folds along the greater curvature.

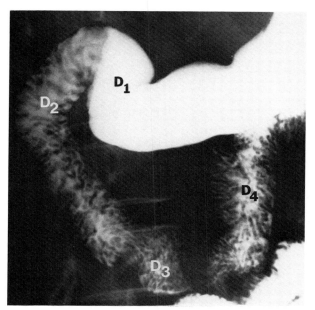

Figure 17–2. Normal duodenum. Duodenal segments indicated by numbers.

tion (see Fig. 17-1*B*, *C*). The double-contrast method provides improved visualization of the mucosal surface. This is particularly important in finding shallow erosions and small polypoid lesions. Some investigators employ the biphasic examination, which encompasses aspects of both the single- and double-contrast techniques.[18, 25] Water-soluble contrast material is used if perforation of the stomach or duodenum is suspected. The use of glucagon in small doses to inhibit motility temporarily can be helpful.[10, 19] Computed tomography and ultrasonography may demonstrate a large gastric mass quite well, but they are not considered the prime modes of detecting gastroduodenal lesions. Computed tomography is particularly of value in the preoperative staging of malignant lesions.[21, 30]

ALTERNATE NONRADIOLOGIC METHODS

Fiberoptic endoscopy is a magnificent method for visualizing the mucosa of the stomach and duodenum. Repeated studies show increased sensitivity compared with the radiologic method. In some parts of the world it has replaced the radiologic method as the primary

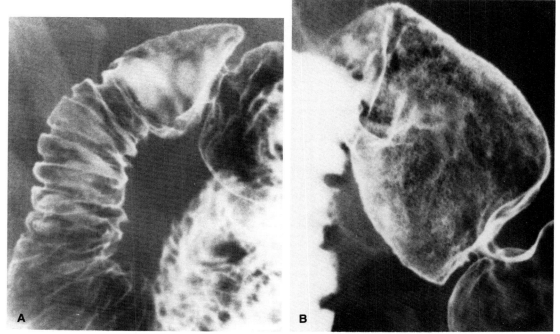

Figure 17–3. (**A**) Double-contrast examination of duodenal bulb and descending duodenal segments. Folds are normal in thickness. (**B**) Double-contrast examination of duodenal bulb. This magnified view shows the velvety mucosal surface representing the duodenal villi.

examination. In others the disparity in costs for the two studies has kept the radiologic method primary.

CONGENITAL ANOMALIES

Failures of Tubulation. Duodenal atresia is discovered quickly after birth. Upright plain films showing air-fluid levels in the stomach and duodenum and no gas in the rest of the intestine are characteristic of obstruction but similar findings may also be seen with the duodenal bands associated with malrotation and with volvulus of the small bowel. It is not usually necessary to do contrast studies under these circumstances. A web as a manifestation of incomplete tubulation can manifest itself in the stomach as an antral diaphragm. This may not be symptomatic. In the duodenum a nearly complete web can produce a complicated roentgenographic appearance. The web may balloon caudally like a wind sock. This appearance has been given the name *intraluminal diverticulum*. The web is primary, and the diverticulum develops later.

Dextroposition. The stomach may be on the right, associated with total situs inversus. Rarely, there will be only dextroposition of the stomach or situs inversus of only the abdominal viscera.

Duplication and Diverticula. Diverticula of the cardia of the stomach that arise posteriorly are the only common gastric diverticula (Fig. 17-4). Perhaps these are a throwback to the multiple stomachs of the ruminants. Gastric and duodenal duplication cysts are rare (Fig. 17-5). Duodenal diverticula are extremely common, particularly the inner aspect of the descending portion, and are rarely of any pathologic significance (Fig. 17-6).

Congenital Rests. Aberrant pancreatic tissue can occur in the gastric antrum and proximal duodenum. Although it has the configuration of an intramural mass, it may have a small central depression at the site of a miniature excretory duct (Fig. 17-7).

Microgastria. A very small midline stomach may be found, but this is rare. It is usually associated with other congenital anomalies. There is often gastroesophageal reflux and esophageal dilatation.

Congenital Hypertrophic Pyloric Stenosis. Persistent vomiting in an infant at the age of 3 to 5 weeks suggests the possibility of pyloric stenosis. At times the hypertrophied pyloric muscle can be palpated; it can also be visualized ultrasonographically. The standard method of diagnosis is with oral barium sulfate. The

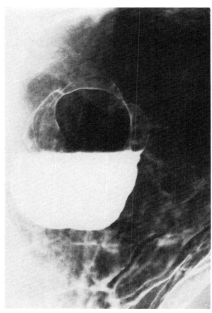

Figure 17–4. Double-contrast examination of the proximal stomach where a large wide-mouth diverticulum is present. Barium is pooling in the dependent portion of the diverticulum.

diagnosis rests on seeing an elongated pyloric canal (Fig. 17-8) often with thick muscle bulging into the base of the duodenal bulb. A delay in gastric emptying is not adequate for diagnosis because it can occur normally. Rarely, pyloric stenosis is found in the adult;

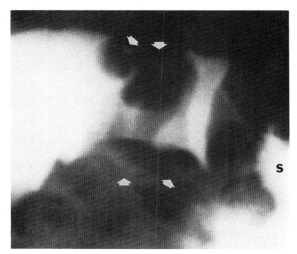

Figure 17–5. Single-contrast examination of the duodenal bulb demonstrates a duplication cyst (*arrows*). S, distal stomach.

The Stomach and Duodenum 575

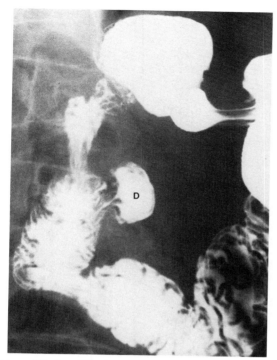

Figure 17–6. Single-contrast examination of duodenal sweep. The outpouching involving the medial wall of the descending duodenum represents a diverticulum (*D*).

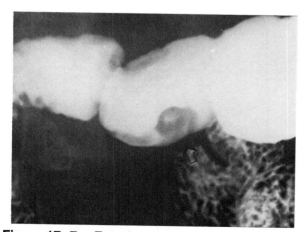

Figure 17–7. Ectopic pancreatic tissue in the gastric wall. The dimple in the mass is the ductal region and is quite characteristic.

it must be differentiated from circumferential antral carcinoma.

Annular Pancreas. Fusion of the ventral and dorsal pancreas so that it completely surrounds the duodenum is rare, but if it does occur it may cause partial or complete duodenal obstruction (Fig. 17-9).

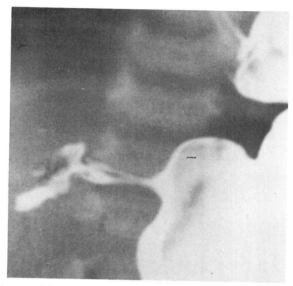

Figure 17–8. Hypertrophic pyloric stenosis in an infant. The elongated pyloric canal is well demonstrated.

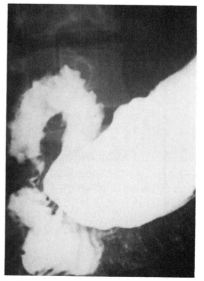

Figure 17–9. Annular pancreas causing lateral compression of the descending duodenum.

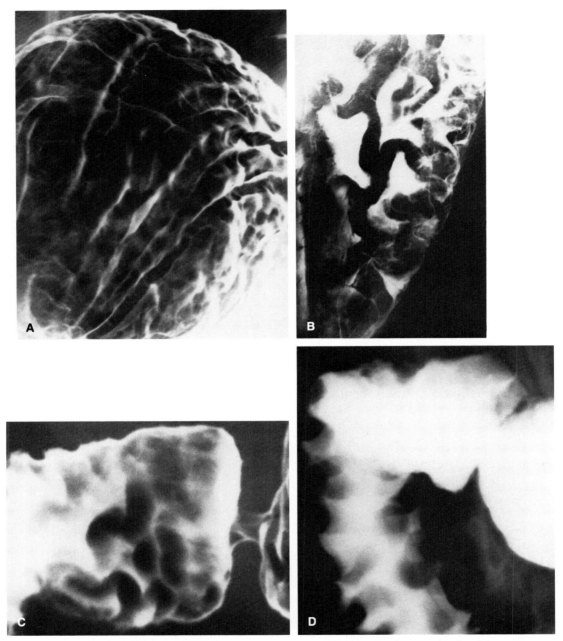

Figure 17–10. (**A**) Double-contrast examination of fundus and upper body of the stomach shows thickened gastric rugal folds consistent with gastritis. (**B**) Another example of gastritis. (**C**) Double-contrast examination of duodenal bulb shows thickened folds representing peptic duodenitis. (**D**) Single-contrast examination shows thickened folds in the duodenal bulb and descending duodenal segments consistent with duodenitis.

PEPTIC ULCER DISEASE

Fold Enlargement and Mucosal Distortion. The earliest changes of peptic disease in the stomach and duodenum may be hypertrophy or enlargement of folds (Fig. 17-10A through *D*). In some instances the mucosal surface pattern can become irregular (Fig. 17-11). Neither fold enlargement or mucosal changes are specific for peptic disease.

Erosions. Gastric and duodenal erosions are the most minimal manifestations of peptic ulcer disease that can be detected. Sometimes there is a small mound of associated edema, whereas at other times only the erosion is present. The double-contrast technique is particularly effective in demonstrating these small lesions (Fig. 17-12). Such erosions can be responsible for both epigastric pain and bleeding. Because they are quite small, they will heal quickly with treatment.

Ulcers. It is difficult to define the difference between an ulcer and an erosion, and indeed the spectrum is continuous. Ulcers are erosions that have penetrated more deeply into the mucosa, and ordinarily their diameter is greater than that of other erosions. The increase in size allows more ready radiologic detection. Ulcers, like erosions, may be seen anywhere in the stomach or proximal duodenum, but they are most

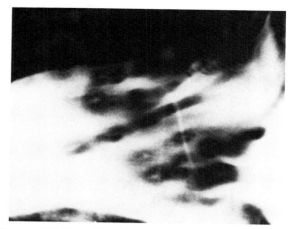

Figure 17–12. Double-contrast examination of antrum shows numerous elliptic-shaped lucencies with central collections of barium representing gastric erosions.

common in the antrum, pyloric canal, and duodenal bulb (Figs. 17-13 and 17-14).[3] The lesser curvature of the body of the stomach is also a prevalent site, but ulcers may occur on the greater curvature as well. Very large benign ulcers found on the greater curvature are often caused by ingestion of drugs such as nonsteroidal anti-inflammatory compounds. The major sign is the ulcer crater, which usually projects beyond the gastric wall. There is often a smooth rim of edema at the edge of the crater (Hampton line). Mucosal folds are often observed extending to the rim or edge of the crater. Greater curvature ulcers are more varied in appearance and may resemble malignant lesions. In such cases, careful follow-up or biopsy is indicated. The radiologic method is not only valuable for detecting these ulcers but also for evaluating the effects of treatment.

Perforated Ulcers. A gastric or duodenal ulcer, often with few premonitory symptoms, may perforate into the peritoneal space. The symptoms then become quite dramatic. Plain films are indicated in this situation. Upright films will show free air under the diaphragm. If the upright position cannot be achieved, an anteroposterior film of the abdomen with the patient's left side down will demonstrate air between the liver and the right lateral peritoneum.

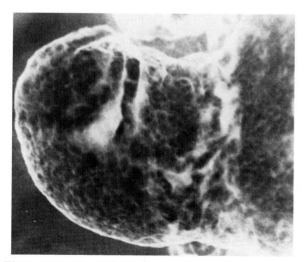

Figure 17–11. Double-contrast examination of gastric antrum demonstrates some thickened folds and a markedly irregular, coarse mucosal surface pattern consistent with inflammation.

Scarring. While erosions leave no demonstrable scar, medium and large ulcers may heal with a con-

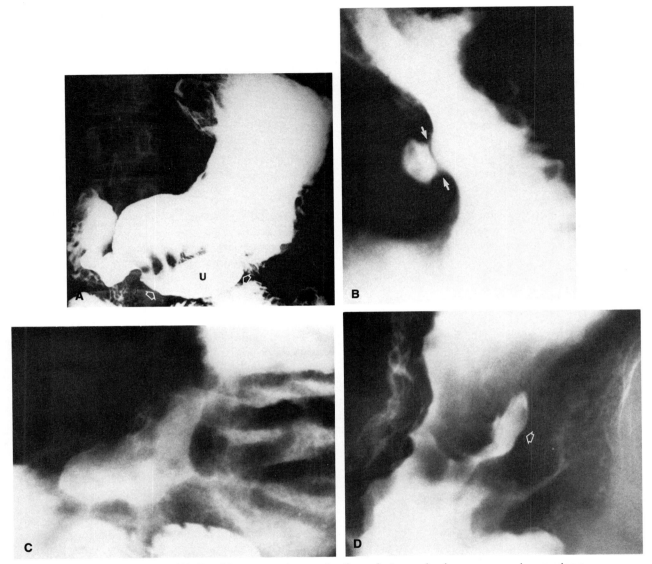

Figure 17–13. **(A)** Double-contrast examination of stomach shows a very large ulcer protruding from the lumen of the greater curvature (*arrows*) *U*, ulcer crater. **(B)** Single-contrast examination shows a gastric ulcer protruding from the lesser curvature of the body of the stomach. The thin lucent line indicated by the white arrows represents Hampton's line, indicative of a benign ulcer. **(C)** A single-contrast examination shows a large flat ulceration along the lesser curvature of the stomach. Note the large uniform gastric folds radiating to the ulcer crater with abrupt termination. This is consistent with benign ulcer. **(D)** Shows an elliptic-shaped ulcer crater (*open arrow*). The ulcer is considered indeterminate because there are no radiographic criteria to identify it as benign or malignant.

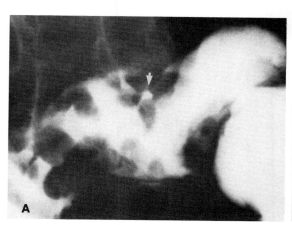

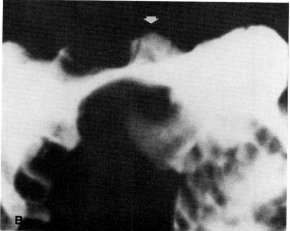

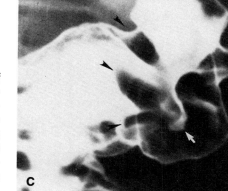

Figure 17–14. (**A**) Single-contrast examination of duodenal bulb shows a tiny ulceration (*arrow*) surrounded by edematous folds. (**B**) Active peptic ulcer. Single-contrast examination shows ulcer collection protruding from superior aspect of the apex of the duodenal bulb (*arrow*). (**C**) Benign peptic ulcer demonstrated in this double-contrast examination. Note the radiating folds (*black arrowheads*) toward the ulcer crater (*white arrow*).

siderable deformity. In the stomach, gastric folds radiating toward a central point are indicative of a healed ulcer (Fig. 17-15A, B). In the duodenum the craters tend to occur in the midbulb just beyond the pyloric canal, and they leave a characteristic "cloverleaf" or "butterfly" deformity (Fig. 17-16). Scarring in the pyloric canal area can produce a double channel between the stomach and the duodenum (Fig. 17-17). Scarring of the pylorus and duodenum may become severe enough to cause partial or complete gastric outlet obstruction.

Hypergastrinism. A particularly severe form of peptic ulcer disease can be associated with gastrinomas or other sources of gastrin. The ulcers may be multiple and may involve the small bowel as well. The excessive gastric secretion may be evident in both the stomach and the small bowel. The inflammatory insult

to the duodenum may cause edematous folds and eventual atony (megaduodenum) (Fig. 17-18). These radiographic findings are indications for obtaining serum gastrin levels.

INFLAMMATORY DISEASES

Extrinsic Agents. Several agents, when combined with the acid-pepsin milieu of the stomach, can cause erosion and ulceration. Alcohol and anti-inflammatory drugs are the most common offenders. Whether steroids are causative agents has not been resolved. Either alkali or acid taken in strong concentration can cause severe gastric damage leading to a gastric stricture or multiple areas of constriction (Fig. 17-19). The ingestion of ferrous sulfate tablets may cause severe

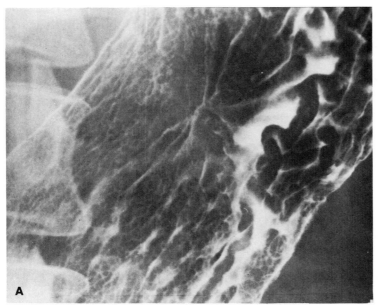

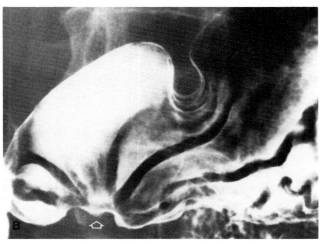

Figure 17–15. **(A)** Gastric ulcer scar. Radiating folds toward the site of the previous ulcer are observed. The normal polygonal "area gastrica" pattern of the stomach mucosa is especially well demonstrated along the lesser curvature. **(B)** Double-contrast examination shows folds converging toward the greater curvature in the distal antrum from an ulcer scar (*open arrow*).

gastric damage in infants and small children. Although many medications seem to cause gastric symptoms, it is unusual to find radiologic changes.

Specific Infections. Tuberculosis and syphilis of the stomach are now uncommon entities; they cause thickening and rigidity of the gastric wall (linitis plastica). Strongyloidiasis is still seen, particularly in South America. Debilitated and immunosuppressed patients may have the usual range of opportunistic organisms, such as the herpes virus, which may cause gastritis.[12] Anisakiasis of the stomach, with the roundworms causing threadlike filling defects, has been described by Nakata and colleagues in Japan.[22]

Crohn's Disease. There is a tendency to have pyloroantral and duodenal involvement in Crohn's disease (Fig. 17-20 *A, B*). This can occur without any manifest disease in the jejunum. The radiographic features are as similar and varied as in other parts of the bowel. Ulceration, nodularity, and luminal narrowing mimic both peptic ulcer disease and neoplasm such as lymphoma. Upper gastrointestinal involvement as the initial presentation of Crohn's disease is uncommon, so the key to the diagnosis is to find the characteristic changes in the more distal gut.

Gluten Enteropathy. The radiologic findings of sprue begin in the duodenum and extend into the jejunum

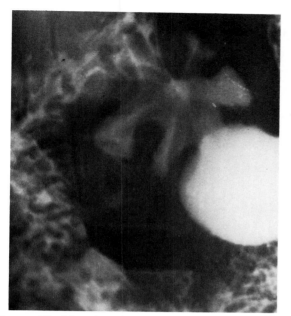

Figure 17–16. A posterior wall duodenal ulcer associated with the classical ("cloverleaf," "butterfly") deformity of chronic duodenal ulcer disease.

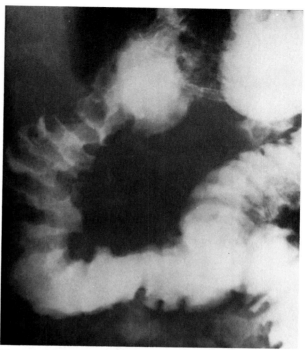

Figure 17–18. Hypergastrinism (Zollinger-Ellison syndrome). The severe duodenitis with markedly edematous mucosal folds is secondary to the gastric hypersecretion.

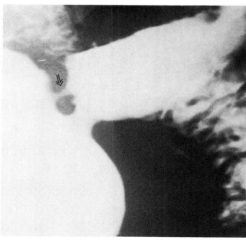

Figure 17–17. "Double pylorus." This actually represents the normal pylorus plus a fistula (*arrow*) between antrum and bulb as a residual of a healed antral ulcer.

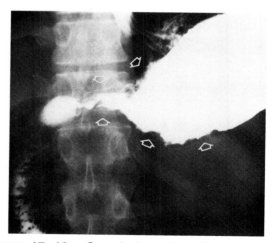

Figure 17–19. Caustic ingestion. Single-contrast examination shows irregularity of the mucosa and narrowing of the gastric antrum caused by the ingestion of caustic material. Lesser changes are seen involving the duodenum with nodularity and thickened folds.

(Fig. 17-21). Dilatation is the most reliable finding and may be so severe in the duodenum that it warrants the description *megaduodenum*. At times the mucosal folds are enlarged. It should be emphasized that when sprue is diagnosed promptly by small-bowel biopsy there may be no abnormal radiographic findings.

Rarely, there are radiographic and biopsy findings of sprue in patients without symptoms.

Miscellaneous Disorders. Ménétrier's disease is a syndrome of protein-losing enteropathy associated with huge gastric rugal folds. These large folds involve

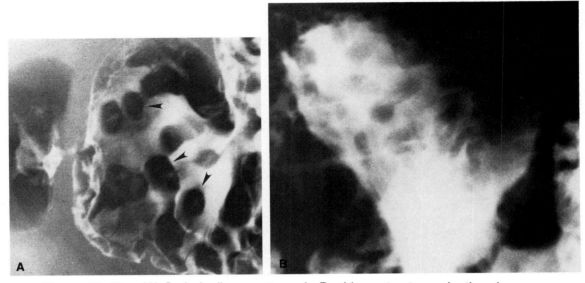

Figure 17–20. (A) Crohn's disease stomach. Double-contrast examination shows numerous rounded lucencies with central barium collection representing Crohn's aphthous ulcerations. (B) Crohn's disease of duodenal bulb. Numerous aphthous ulcerations present.

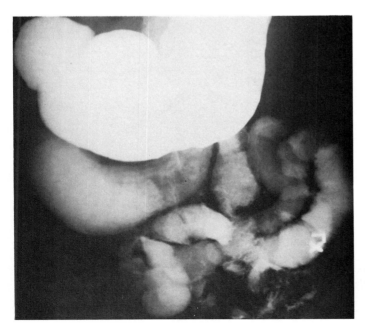

Figure 17–21. Collagenous sprue. Megaduodenum, dilated small bowel, and loss of small bowel mucosal folds are the findings in this severe form of nontropical sprue.

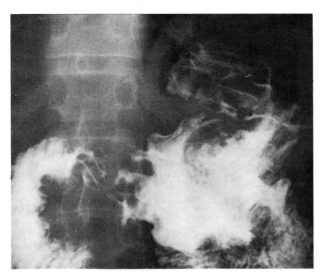

Figure 17–22. Ménétrier's disease. Huge gastric folds are present. In this patient, it is unusual that the antral folds are also large.

the fundus and body of the stomach rather than the antrum (Fig. 17-22). *Eosinophilic gastroenteritis* is a diffuse process that may manifest itself with large distal gastric and small-bowel folds. At times, a cobblestone appearance predominates. Gastric manifestations of *scleroderma* are uncommon. There may be diffuse hypotonia causing prolonged emptying time and a smooth gastric outline caused by effacement of mucosal folds. Thick tenacious secretions found in cystic fibrosis may cause megaduodendum (Fig. 17-23). Pancreatitis may cause inflammatory changes in the stomach and duodenum (Fig. 17-24).

MOTILITY DISORDERS

The stomach rarely loses its motility function. Gastroparesis can be seen in the diabetic, and it can be a clinical problem. Patients after truncal vagotomy have a disorder that may combine lack of motility and diminished gastric acid secretion. As a consequence, food bezoars may form in the stomach, and they often are composed of food with high cellulose content such as lettuce and oranges (Fig. 17-25). There are no identifiable conditions of gastric hypermotility.

VASCULAR DISORDERS

Gastric Varices. Gastric varices may coexist with esophageal varices or may be isolated, especially in cases of splenic vein thrombosis. In splenic vein thrombosis the splenic drainage is through the short gastric veins and thence through normal channels to the portal vein. Such gastric varices can be mistaken for either a mucosal or intramural gastric tumor (Fig. 17-26).

Duodenal Varices. Duodenal varices are rare, but they can be large enough to deform the duodenum and mimic peptic ulcer disease.[13] It is important to recog-

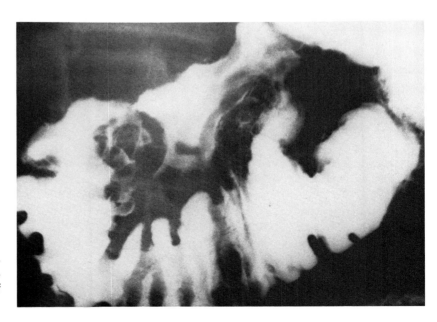

Figure 17–23. Cystic fibrosis duodenum. Single-contrast examination shows marked enlargement of duodenum with thickened folds.

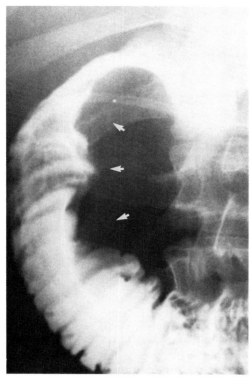

Figure 17–24. Pancreatitis. The medial wall of the duodenum is narrowed by pancreatic enlargement. There is also duodenal fold thickening.

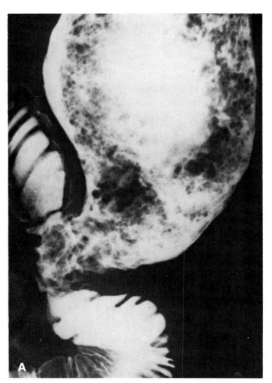

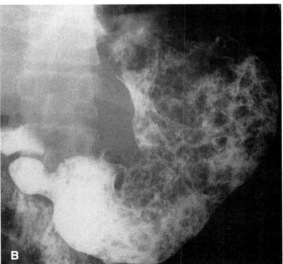

Figure 17–25. (**A**) Gastric phytobezoar following vagotomy, partial gastrectomy, and gastrojejeunostomy. (**B**) Intact stomach enlarged by bezoar in a patient with diabetes mellitus.

nize this possibility when studying a cirrhotic patient with gastrointestinal bleeding.

Angiodysplasia. The limits of the barium examination does not permit detection of angiodysplasia. Success has been reported with angiography.[27] Endoscopically, these have been described as the "watermelon lesion."[14]

EXTRINSIC DEFORMITY

The stomach or duodenum may be displaced or deformed by any adjacent organ or process (ie, abscess, cyst) that becomes large enough (Fig. 17-27).

FOREIGN BODIES

Foreign bodies are less common in the stomach than in the esophagus. Often they will pass spontaneously through the rest of the gut. Mentally deranged patients can swallow a great variety of objects. Occasionally, a trichobezoar will form from ingested hair. Persimmons have long been known to form gastric phytobezoars. They appear as large irregular intragastric masses (see Fig. 17-25A, B).

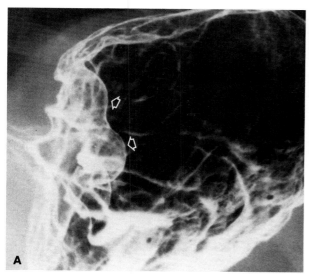

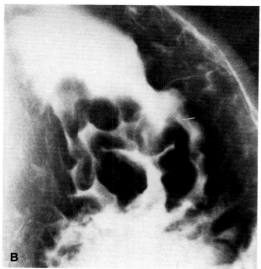

Figure 17–26. (**A**) Gastric varices. Double-contrast examination shows the gastric varices in profile (*arrows*). (**B**) Gastric varices seen en face.

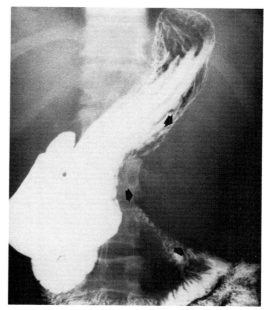

Figure 17–27. Extrinsic deformity of stomach. Single-contrast examination shows stomach being displaced toward the midline from the left by a greatly enlarged spleen (*arrows*).

NEOPLASMS

PRIMARY BENIGN

Benign Adenomatous and Inflammatory Polyps and Villous Adenomas. These mucosal lesions, which can occur in the stomach and duodenum (see Fig. 17-26),[22] may be single or multiple (Fig. 17-28).

Benign Intramural Tumors. Benign intramural tumors constitute another major group. Lipomas, neurofibromas, and leiomyomas are found in the gastroduodenal wall. Most often they are small and asymptomatic. An exception is the leiomyoma, which can attain a large size, and in the process the mucosa may ulcerate and bleed (Fig. 17-29). Some leiomyomas are calcified, which allows their histologic diagnosis based on radiographic analysis.

Polyposis Syndromes. Gastric lesions have been observed in the polyposis syndromes (familial colonic polyposis, Gardner's syndrome, Peutz-Jeghers syndrome, Cronkhite-Canada syndrome) (Fig. 17-30).[7] Enlarged, nodular rugal folds have been seen in Cronkhite-Canada syndrome.[15] In the other conditions polypoid masses are found. A case of gastric carcinoma in Gardner's syndrome has been reported.[5]

PRIMARY MALIGNANT

Adenocarcinoma of the stomach starts as a small plaquelike lesion.[8, 11] This may or may not ulcerate. Great strides in the understanding and detection of small lesions have been made in Japan, where the disease is prevalent. Exquisite air-contrast studies are

(*text continues on page 589*)

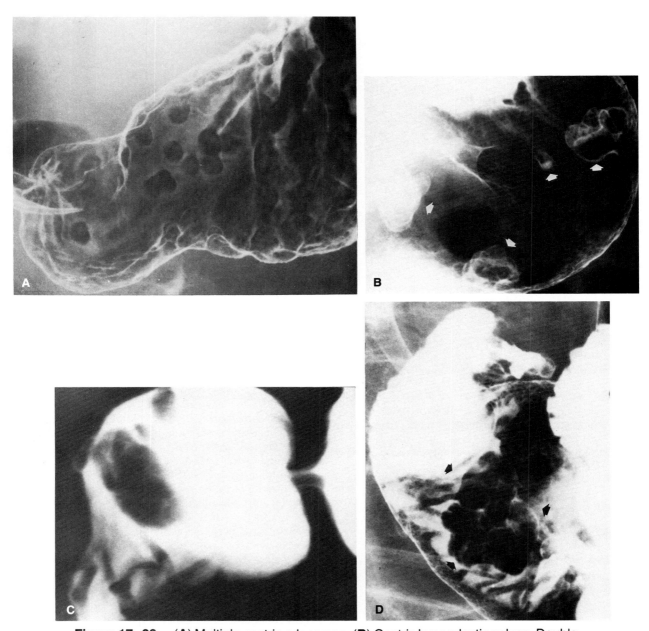

Figure 17–28.   (A) Multiple gastric adenomas. **(B)** Gastric hyperplastic polyps. Double-contrast examination shows numerous polypoid defects protruding into the lumen (*arrows*). **(C)** Hyperplastic polyp duodenum. Single-contrast examination shows large filling defect at the apex of the bulb. **(D)** Duodenal adenoma. Barium examination demonstrates large polypoid defect in the descending segment of the duodenum (*arrows*).

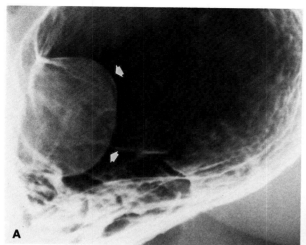

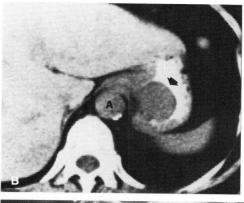

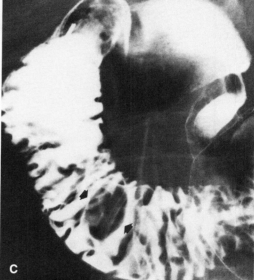

Figure 17–29. (**A**) Gastric leiomyoma. Profile view of large smooth mass (*arrows*). (**B**) Gastric leiomyoma. CT examination through level of stomach shows smooth intraluminal filling defect (*arrow*). *A*, aorta. (**C**) Duodenal lymphangioma. Elliptic lucent mass in descending duodenum (*arrows*).

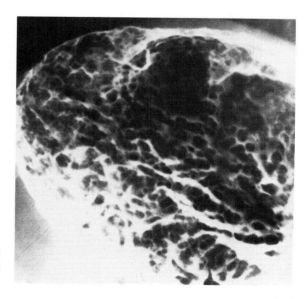

Figure 17–30. Gastric polyposis in a patient with familial polyposis. Double-contrast examination shows numerous small rounded polyps carpeting the gastric mucosa.

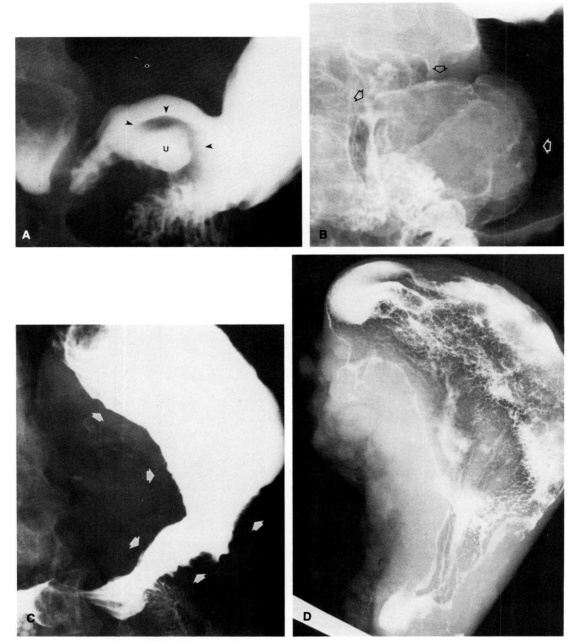

Figure 17–31. (**A**) Gastric adenocarcinoma. Large mass in antrum of stomach (*arrowheads*) with central ulceration. *U*, ulcer. (**B**) Gastric adenocarcinoma. Large polypoid mass (*arrows*) in antrum of stomach. (**C**) Gastric adenocarcinoma. Distal half of stomach narrowed and irregular (*arrows*). (**D**) Gastric adenocarcinoma. Resected specimen of lesion in Figure 17–31*C*. Note the extensive infiltration beyond the wall of the stomach that is not visible on barium examination. (**E**) Gastric adenocarcinoma. CT examination shows two large polypoid lesions projecting into the stomach lumen (*arrows*). Metastases to the liver shown as rounded low-dense areas (*arrowheads*). (**F**) Gastric adenocarcinoma. Single-contrast examination of dilated esophagus shows marked narrowing distally (*arrows*) representing submucosal infiltration of distal esophagus from fundal adenocarcinoma. (**G**) Gastric adenocarcinoma. Double-contrast examination of antrum shows flattening and retraction of the lesser curvature (*open arrow*) and margins of the spreading tumor (*white arrows*).

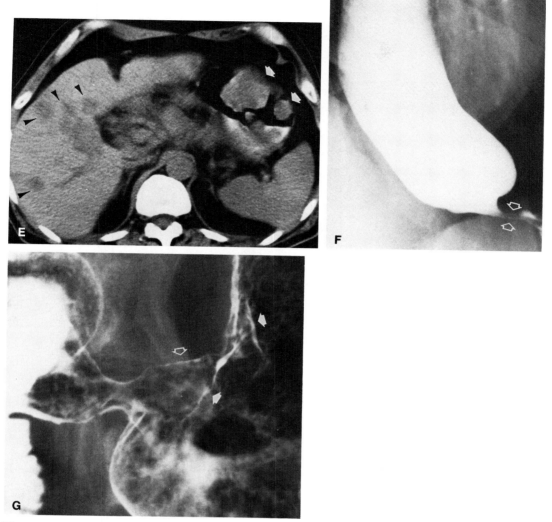

Figure 17–31.   (*Continued*)

required to image the lesions. As the cancer grows it may become polypoid and be easy to detect. Infiltrative lesions that just stiffen the gastric wall without causing either a mass or ulceration are the most difficult to detect.

These infiltrative or scirrhous carcinomas are being detected in the proximal part of the stomach in greater numbers rather than in the classic form involving the distal stomach. Endoscopy has significant limitations in confirming the diagnosis with positive pathologic findings in only 70% of cases.[17]

The end result of this may be a diffusely involved nondistensible ("leather bottle," linitis plastica) stomach (Fig. 17-31A through G). Occasionally, the neo-

plasm is primarily ulcerative and can be identical in appearance to a benign ulcer. In the past many roentgen criteria were used to distinguish benign from malignant ulceration. Almost all were based on identifying a mass and preferably an irregular mass associated with the ulcer. On a practical level this has largely disappeared. If endoscopy and biopsy are not done, trial therapy is given. Ulcers that do not heal are then subject to biopsy. Adenocarcinomas of the duodenum are rare and usually are not found until they have grown enough to cause partial obstruction (Fig. 17-32A through C). Mucinous adenocarcinomas of the stomach may have calcification in either the primary tumor or the metastases.

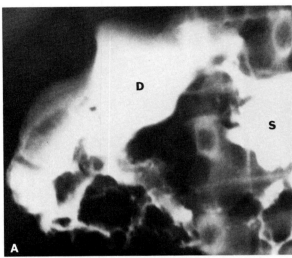

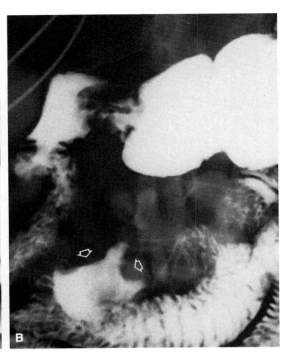

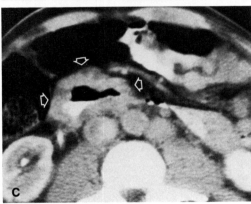

Figure 17–32. **(A)** Duodenal adenocarcinoma. Markedly irregular infiltrated lesions in second, third, and fourth portions of duodenum. *S,* stomach; *D,* duodenal bulb. **(B)** Duodenal adenocarcinoma. Irregular barium collection at junction of second and third portions of duodenum (*open arrows*). **(C)** Duodenal adenocarcinoma. CT examination of the lesion depicted in Figure 17–32*B.* Note marked wall thickening (*arrows*).

Leiomyosarcoma. Leiomyosarcomas start in the intramural portion of the stomach and become bulky tumors, often with huge ulcerations of their gastric surfaces.[23] They do not mimic the infiltrative type of adenocarcinoma.

Lymphoma. The usual lymphoma of the stomach mimics the adenocarcinoma completely. Rarely, there is a lymphoma that is manifested by only large gastric folds and some rigidity of the stomach (Fig. 17-33A through *F*).

Carcinoid. The carcinoid tumors of the stomach may mimic all the benign and malignant lesions.[2] There

is no roentgen appearance that allows a correct prebiopsy diagnosis.

METASTATIC TUMORS

Melanoma, lymphoma, Kaposi's sarcoma, and breast carcinoma are the metastatic processes that involve the stomach more often than others. None is really common; they are submucosal lesions and may ulcerate. Melanoma, lymphoma, and Kaposi's sarcoma all may present with multiple gastric nodules that may be ulcerated. Breast carcinoma can infiltrate the entire stomach and mimic the leather-bottle appearance of a primary cancer (Fig. 17-34A through *D*).

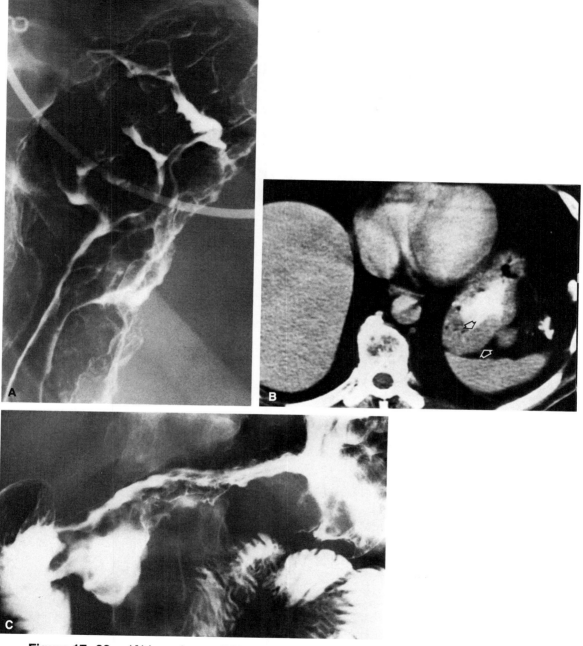

Figure 17–33.   (**A**) Lymphoma. Diffusively enlarged and irregular folds throughout body and fundus of the stomach. (**B**) Lymphoma. CT scan through proximal stomach shows marked wall thickening by lymphoma (*arrows*). (**C**) Diffusively narrowed distal body and antrum of stomach caused by extensive submucosal infiltration of lymphoma. (**D**) CT scan shows diffusely thickened wall surrounding opacified lumen as depicted in Figure 17–33C. (**E**) Single-contrast examination of duodenum shows marked widening of the duodenal sweep. (**F**) CT examination in the area of duodenal sweep shows massive lymphadenopathy caused by lymphoma (*arrows*). This is the patient depicted in Figure 17–33E. D, duodenum.

(*continued*)

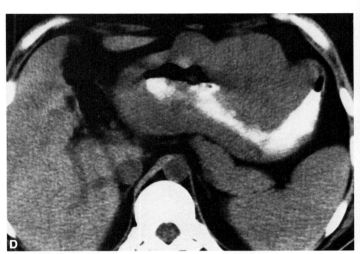

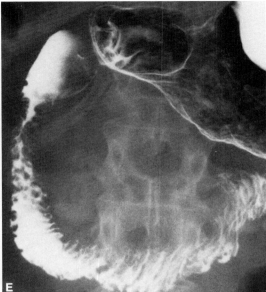

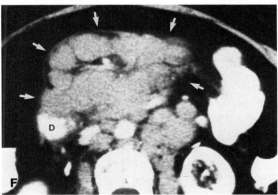

Figure 17–33. *(Continued)*

COMPUTED TOMOGRAPHY AND ULTRASONOGRAPHY

Although these modalities may actually detect a gastric or duodenal lesion, they are more useful for tumor staging. Computed tomography can be used to detect lymphadenopathy, but it does not accurately image the true extent of pathology in patients with gastric carcinoma and should not be used routinely for staging purposes.[29] Both modalities are effective in finding liver metastases.

TRAUMA

The stomach has a very thick wall, and because it is on a mesentery it can move. Thus it is rarely damaged by blunt trauma, and is more likely to be injured by a knife

or a bullet (Fig. 17-35). Although the stomach may not be damaged by blunt trauma, a tear of the diaphragm may occur that allows the stomach to move into the thorax (Fig. 17-36). Contrast material will confirm that the hiatus is intact, and the gastroesophageal junction is in a normal location. The stomach above the diaphragmatic rent is then easily appreciated. The duodenum, conversely, is fixed retroperitoneally and lies just in front of the spine. As a consequence of its anatomy, both hematoma and rupture may occur with blunt trauma (Fig. 17-37). Computed tomography is valuable in getting a global idea of the damage. Water-soluble contrast material is an excellent choice in trying to detect duodenal rupture. Patients with hematomas of the duodenum may have partial obstruction caused by the intramural mass. The resolution of the hematoma can be followed with barium studies, ultrasound, or CT.

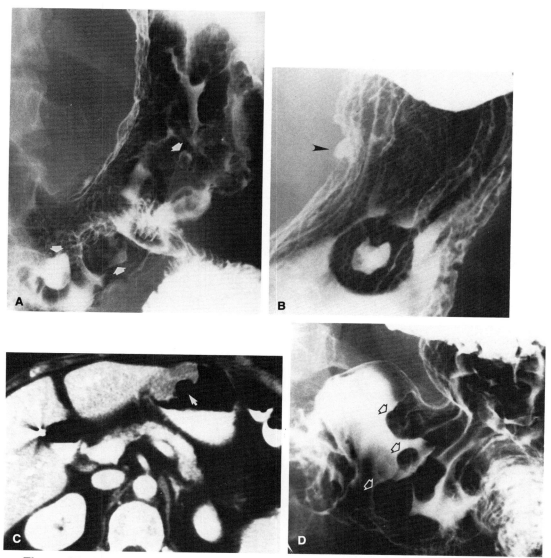

Figure 17–34. (**A**) Double-contrast examination of stomach shows markedly irregular folds and numerous ulcerations (*arrows*) caused by metastatic breast carcinoma. (**B**) Two metastatic lesions in stomach from carcinoma of lung. Larger metastasis is seen en face, and smaller metastasis is seen in profile (*arrowhead*). (**C**) CT examination through stomach shows mass lesion along the anterior wall of stomach with central ulceration (*arrow*) representing metastatic melanoma. (**D**) Numerous large polypoid gastric-filling defects (*open arrows*) represent stomach involvement with Kaposi's sarcoma.

HIATAL HERNIA

Undoubtedly more attention is paid to the diagnosis of small hiatal hernias than they deserve. A strong argument can be made that they are normal or are variations accompanying aging. The simplest radiographic crite-

rion for the diagnosis is to see if the tube (esophagus) meets the bag (stomach) above or below the diaphragm. Because the diaphragm is a moving structure, even this is arbitrary. An additional criterion is whether gastric folds can be seen in the thorax. Because the lower esophageal (Schatzki) ring represents the squa-

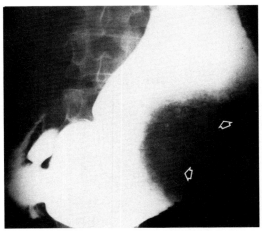

Figure 17–35. Gastric hematoma. Single-contrast examination shows large filling defect long greater curvature (*open arrows*) representing intramural hematoma in blunt trauma.

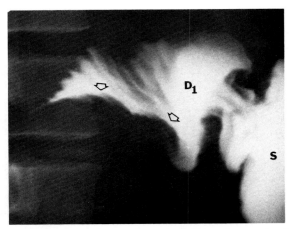

Figure 17–37. Second portion of duodenum is obstructed by large rounded masses (*open arrows*) representing duodenal hematoma in blunt trauma. *S,* stomach; *D₁,* duodenal bulb.

mocolumnar mucosal junction, the visualization of the ring above the diaphragm represents a third criterion (Fig. 17-38A through E).

Hernias have also been defined as sliding, paraesophageal, and mixed. In the sliding type the gastroesophageal junction is the main element displaced

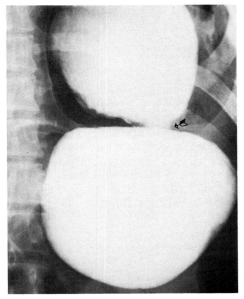

Figure 17–36. Rupture of the diaphragm. A small traumatic tear of the diaphragm (*arrow*) allowed the stomach to herniate into the thorax.

cephalad. The paraesophageal hernia has the stomach displaced cephalad alongside a normally positioned esophagus. The mixed version is a combination of the other two. These descriptions have no clinical utility, and they cannot be used with precision.

There are hiatal hernias with clinical significance. These are the hernias that usually occur in later life. The entire stomach is found above the diaphragm. Sometimes the transverse colon may also herniate through the hiatus. In this situation volvulus of the stomach may occur, not only obstructing the flow of food and secretions, but also interfering with the blood supply to the stomach and resulting in gastric infarction. Plain films in this situation may show multiple air-fluid levels above the diaphragm (Fig. 17-39). Barium will nicely demonstrate the obstruction.

IATROGENIC CONDITIONS

INSTRUMENTATION

Intubation of the stomach rarely results in rupture; if it does, the thick, healthy gastric wall is self-sealing. Pneumoperitoneum has occurred after endoscopy and anesthesia with no patient morbidity.

SURGICAL

There is a fairly lengthy list of postsurgical complications, most of which can be identified by radiologic study. Because vagotomy and pyloroplasty have been in vogue, the complications have been less than when

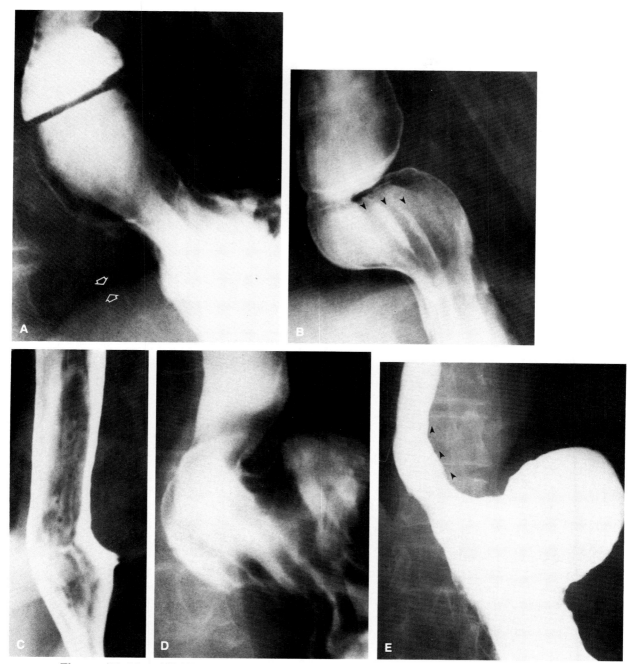

Figure 17–38. (A) Hiatal hernia with mucosal ring (Schatzki's ring). Diaphragm delineated by open arrows. (B) Hiatal hernia shows gastric folds protruding beyond the diaphragm (*arrowheads*). (C) Normal double-contrast examination of esophagus but a sliding hiatal hernia (D) develops in same patient seconds later. (E) Demonstration of gastroesophageal reflux.

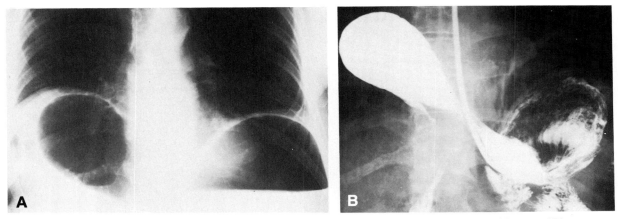

Figure 17–39. (A) Plain film shows herniation of bowel into the right hemithorax. (B) Barium study shows that the antrum of the stomach has herniated through the esophageal hiatus.

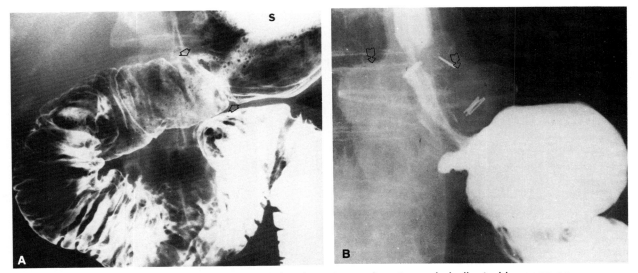

Figure 17–40. (A) Billroth-I gastroduodenostomy. Anastomosis indicated by open arrows. S, stomach. (B) Angelchik prosthesis (*arrows*) can be identified as a soft-tissue density containing a circular radiopaque marker. This doughnut-shaped device is used to reduce gastroesophageal reflux and is ordinarily seen below the diaphragm. In this patient the prosthesis herniated through the hiatus into the thorax.

gastric resection and gastroduodenostomy (Fig. 17-40A) or gastrojejunostomy were done. Immediately after vagotomy, gastric emptying may be slow or absent for several weeks. This delayed emptying almost always ceases spontaneously. Recurrent ulceration is the most common reason to study a patient after the immediate postoperative period. A gastric resection is necessary

for gastric cancer. In this situation a search for recurrence in the remaining stomach is important.

Gastric operations for the treatment of obesity recently have been done. Gastric diversion involves stapling the proximal stomach closed and performing a gastrojejunostomy. The prime difficulty is making the gastric reservoir too big or too small.[16, 20, 26] In a gastroplasty the proximal stomach is stapled closed and then enough staples are removed to allow a narrow passage to the distal stomach. In this procedure a problem arises if the narrowing in the stomach is either too small or too large.[1, 28] The inflated gastric (Garren) balloon is being tried as an artifical bezoar to cause weight reduction.[9]

A Teflon doughnut (Angelchik) prosthesis wrapped around the cardia of the stomach has been used as a treatment for gastroesophageal reflux–hiatus hernia. Erosion of the gut by the prosthesis and its migration both cephalad and caudad have been described (Fig. 17-40B).[4, 6]

REFERENCES AND SELECTED READINGS

1. AGHA FP, ECKHAUSER FE, STRODEL WE, ET AL: Mason's vertical banded gastroplasty for morbid obesity: Surgical procedure and radiographic evaluation. Radiology 150:825, 1984

2. BALTHAZAR EJ, MEGIBOW A, BRYK D, ET AL: Gastric carcinoid tumors: Radiographic features in eight cases. Am J Roentgenol 139:1123, 1982

3. BROWN P, SALMON PR, BURWOOD RJ, ET AL: The endoscopic, radiological, and surgical findings in chronic duodenal ulceration. Scand J Gastroenterol 13:557, 1978

4. BURHENNE LJW, FRATKIN LB, FLAK B, ET AL: Radiology of the Angelchik prosthesis for gastroesophageal reflux. Am J Roentgenol 142:507, 1984

5. COFFEY RJ JR, KNIGHT CD JR, VAN HURDEN JA, ET AL: Gastric carcinoma complicating Gardner's syndrome in a North American woman. Radiology 153:321, 1984

6. CURTIS DJ, BENJAMIN SB, KERR R, ET AL: Angelchik antireflux device: Radiographic appearance of complications. Radiology 151:311, 1984

7. DENZLER TB, HARNED RK, PERGRAM CJ: Gastric polyps in familial polyposis coli. Radiology 130:63, 1979

8. DEKKER W, OP DEN ORTH JO: Early gastric cancer. Radiologia Clinica 46:115, 1977

9. EDELL SL, WILLIS JS, GARREN LR, ET AL: Radiographic evaluation of the Garren gastric bubble. Am J Roentgenol 145:49, 1985

10. FECZKO PJ, SIMMS SM, IORIO J, ET AL: Gastroduodenal response to low-dose glucagon. Am J Roentgenol 140:935, 1983

11. GOLD RP, GREEN PHR, O'TOOLE KM, ET AL: Early gastric cancer: Radiographic experience. Radiology 152:283, 1984

12. HOWILER W, GOLDBERG HI: Gastroesophageal involvement in herpes simplex. Gastroenterology 70:775, 1976

13. ITZCHAK Y, GLICKMAN MG: Duodenal varices in extrahepatic portal obstruction. Radiology 124:619, 1977

14. JABBARI M, CHERRY R, LOUGH JO, ET AL: Gastric antral vascular ectasia: The watermelon stomach. Gastroenterology 87:1165, 1984

15. KILCHESKI T, KRESSEL HY, LAUFER I, ET AL: The radiographic appearance of the stomach in Cronkhite-Canada syndrome. Radiology 141:57, 1981

16. KOEHLER RE, HALVERSON JD: Radiographic abnormalities after gastric bypass. Am J Roentgenol 138:267, 1982

17. LEVINE MS, KONG V, RUBESIN SE, ET AL: Scirrhous carcinoma of the stomach: Radiologic and endoscopic diagnosis. Radiology 175:151, 1990

18. LEVINE MS, RUBESIN SE, HERLINGER H, ET AL: Double-contrast upper gastrointestinal examination: Technique and interpretation. Radiology 168:593, 1988

19. MILLER RE, CHERNISH SM, GREENMAN GF, ET AL: Gastrointestinal response to minute doses of glucagon. Radiology 143:317, 1982

20. MOFFAT RE, PELTIER GL, JEWELL WR: The radiological spectrum of gastric bypass complications. Radiology 132:33, 1979

21. MOSS AA, SCHNYDER P, MARKS W, ET AL: Gastric adenocarcinoma: A comparison of the accuracy and economics of staging by computed tomography and surgery. Gastroenterology 80:45, 1981

22. NAKATA H, TAKEDA K, NAKAYAMA T: Radiological diagnosis of acute gastric anisakiasis. Radiology 135:49, 1980

23. NAUERT TG, ZORNOZA J, ORDONEZ N: Gastric leiomyosarcomas. Am J Roentgenol 139:291, 1982

24. OP DEN ORTH JO, DEKKER W: Gastric adenomas. Radiology 141:289, 1981

25. OP DEN ORTH JO: Use of barium in evaluation of disorders of the upper gastrointestinal tract: Current status. Radiology 173:601, 1989

26. POULOS A, PEAT KW, LORMAN JG, ET AL: Gastric operation for the morbidly obese. Am J Roentgenol 136:867, 1981

27. ROBERTS LK, GOLD RE, ROUTT WE: Gastric angiodysplasia. Radiology 139:355, 1981

28. SMITH C, GARDINER R, KUBICKA RA, ET AL: Gastric restrictive surgery for morbid obesity: Early radiologic evaluation. Radiology 153:321, 1984

29. SUSSMAN SK, HALVORSEN RA JR, ILLESCAS FF, ET AL: Gastric adenocarcinomas: CT versus surgical staging. Radiology 167:335, 1988

30. THOMPSON WM, HALVORSEN RA, FOSTER WL JR, ET AL: Computed tomography for staging esophageal and gastroesophageal cancer: Reevaluation. Am J Roentgenol 141:951, 1983

Paul and Juhl's Essentials of Radiologic Imaging, Sixth Edition, edited by John H. Juhl and Andrew B. Crummy. J.B. Lippincott Company, Philadelphia, © 1993.

CHAPTER **18**

The Small Intestine

Michael Davis

THE SMALL BOWEL

INDICATIONS

The presence of an abdominal mass or the suspicion of partial small-bowel obstruction leads to examination of the small bowel. Unexplained diarrhea, malabsorption, and unexplained intestinal bleeding are also indications. Abdominal pain or tenderness may justify a small-bowel examination. Usually a search is made first for diseases of the upper gastrointestinal tract and colon before studying the small bowel. This is done because the frequency of a symptomatic abnormality of the small intestine is much less than that of the upper gastrointestinal tract and colon.

ANATOMY

The jejunum and ileum are termed the *mesenteric small intestine.* The small bowel is not fixed within the peritoneal space, and thus considerable shift of any individual segment can occur. The fold pattern in the jejunum is caused by the valvulae conniventes. These are normally 1 to 2 mm in width and regularly spaced. In the ileum the fold pattern becomes less regularly spaced though fold thickness remains at the same width.

PHYSIOLOGY

As the chyme goes through the small intestine the processes of digestion and absorption occur. Reabsorption of bile salts and water are important functions of the ileum. Motility of the small bowel has two active phases. One is a churning phase in which distal transport of chyme is random. A second phase is related to the migrating motor complex. This pacemaker of the bowel starts its activity in the stomach and gradually sweeps through the entire small intestine. It is extremely effective in delivering all the material in the small bowel to the colon. There is also a quiescent phase in which no motor activity occurs.

METHODS OF EXAMINATION

Barium Studies. The conventional method of studying the small bowel with barium sulfate is to extend the examination of the stomach and duodenum. Ordinarily, the patient drinks a total of 480 to 600 ml of a medium-density barium (50 to 60 W/V). Overhead and fluoroscopic spot films of the small bowel are done at 20- to 30-minute intervals until the colon fills. During fluoroscopy, the small bowel is manipulated to observe the mobility of the loops, and to detect any abnormal focal process such as an adhesion, mass, or hernia. This cycle is repeated until barium is seen in the colon when fluoroscopic spot films of the terminal ileum are done (Fig. 18-1).

Thickening, straightening, dilatation, nodularity, or a combination of these fold patterns are found in several focal and diffuse small-bowel conditions. A precise diagnosis usually depends on correlation with clinical and laboratory findings. Biopsy may be necessary for final confirmation. At times, however, the correlation of the clinical findings and small-bowel studies results in a reliable diagnosis.

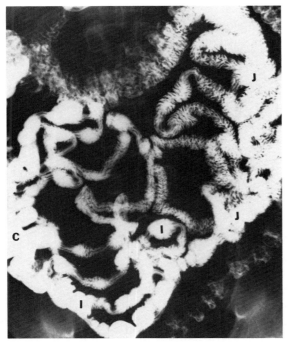

Figure 18–1. Normal small-bowel series. *J*, jejunum; *I*, ileum; *C*, colon. Note the increased number of mucosal folds in the jejunum in the left-upper quadrant and midabdomen. Mucosal folds are decreased in the ileum in the midabdomen and right-lower quadrant.

Enteroclysis. Placing a nasointestinal tube with the tip at or preferably just beyond the duodenal-jejunal junction and infusing barium at a rate about 100 ml/minute far exceeds the rate of gastric emptying. With this method, there is no overlap of the stomach on the small bowel, and there is complete control of the flow of barium during the examination. Infusing the barium into the small intestine can quickly overcome restrictions such as masses or adhesions that normal peristalsis only overcomes slowly. In addition, methylcellulose may be infused after the barium to provide a "see-through" or double-contrast effect for better visualization of the mucosal folds. During the filling of the bowel, each segment can be observed with the fluoroscope. This small-bowel enema (enteroclysis) has the disadvantages of increased patient discomfort associated with nasal intubation and usually more radiation exposure. There is disagreement regarding the efficacy of the conventional peroral small-bowel examination versus enteroclysis (Fig. 18-2*A* through *C*).[24] The dedicated or detailed small-bowel examination and enteroclysis show comparable sensitivities for common disor-

ders. Enteroclysis better visualizes focal lesions and partial bowel-obstructive processes such as adhesions.[25]

Peroral Small-Bowel Examination with Pneumocolon. Examination of the ileocolic area may be enhanced by introducing air into the rectum as barium arrives at the ileocecal area.

Reflux Small-Bowel Examination. During barium enema examination, reflux into the small intestine through an incompetent ileocecal valve can opacify the small intestine. The entire small bowel may be filled this way, usually with some discomfort to the patient (Fig. 18-3).

Water-Soluble Studies. The use of water-soluble contrast agents to examine the small bowel is indicated if perforation is suspected. In all other instances its use compromises the examination.[5] The dilution of the material that occurs in the fluid-filled bowel, and the osmotic effect of the hypertonic solution interferes with the identification of pathologic anatomy. Water-soluble material is suitable as a radiopaque marker to determine passage of intestinal contents to the colon. It is also used effectively as a method to opacify the intestine for computed tomographic (CT) scanning, though it has no detectable advantage over dilute barium sulfate.

In the presence of a palpable abdominal mass examination either ultrasonography or CT is generally more informative, and is done without earlier barium study.

Nuclear medicine studies are of value in locating Meckel's diverticula that contain acid-secreting cells. The localization of small-bowel bleeding is another contribution made by nuclear studies.

ALTERNATIVE NONRADIOLOGIC METHODS

The development of fiberoptic tubes that can examine the entire small intestine is in its infancy. The present instruments can reach the duodenojejunal junction and enter the terminal ileum in a retrograde manner at colonoscopy. Laparoscopy can be used to explore the peritoneal space, but its use has been sharply limited since CT, and percutaneous biopsy is most often a preferable substitute.

CONGENITAL ANOMALIES

Tubulation Defects. As in the duodenum, atresia and stenosis of the small bowel can occur. They may be multiple and diffuse as well as being localized. Symptoms usually occur immediately following birth, and

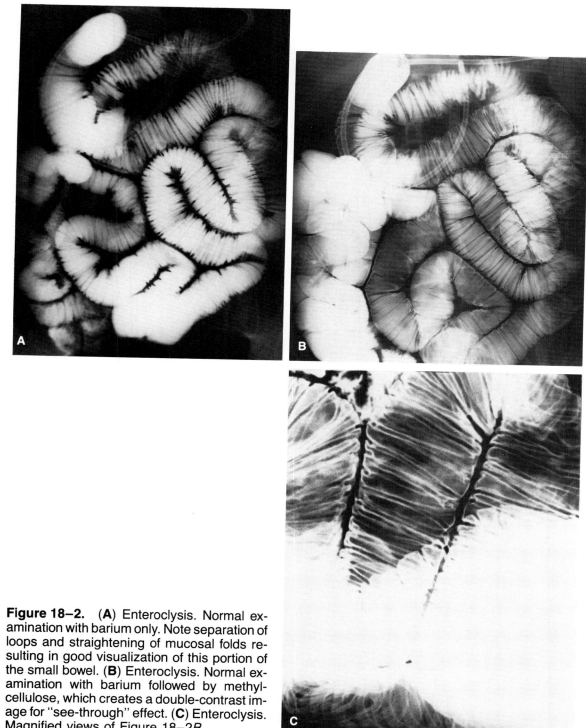

Figure 18–2. (**A**) Enteroclysis. Normal examination with barium only. Note separation of loops and straightening of mucosal folds resulting in good visualization of this portion of the small bowel. (**B**) Enteroclysis. Normal examination with barium followed by methylcellulose, which creates a double-contrast image for "see-through" effect. (**C**) Enteroclysis. Magnified views of Figure 18–2*B*.

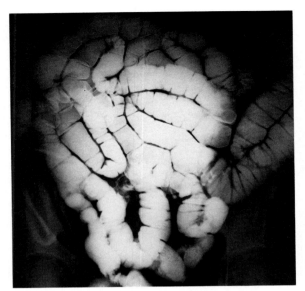

Figure 18–3. Normal reflux small-bowel examination during barium enema.

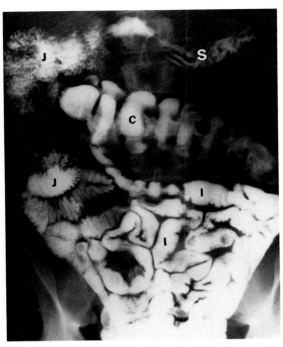

Figure 18–4. Nonrotation. *S*, stomach; *J*, jejunum; *I*, ileum; *C*, colon. See Figure 18–1. The jejunum is normally in the left-upper quadrant, (LUQ); the ileum in the midabdomen and the right-lower quadrant, and the right colon in the right-lower quadrant.

plain films of the abdomen show dilated, fluid-filled small bowel. Barium studies are often unnecessary.

Rotation Anomalies. The herniation of sac-encased intestine through a defect in the anterior abdominal wall at the level of the base of the umbilical cord (*omphalocele*) is one manifestation of lack of proper fetal development. Because this is such a visible process, radiographic studies are unnecessary. This anomaly may be identified in utero by ultrasonography.

Nonrotation can result in the entire small bowel being on the right side of the abdomen and the entire colon on the left. Frequently the third and fourth portions of the duodenum are not fixed retroperitoneally and also are on the right side. There may be no associated symptoms (Fig. 18-4).

A condition that is symptomatic is *midgut volvulus*. This occurs as a complication of a mesentery that is unduly long, allowing excess mobility of the intestine. This condition may be complicated by infarction of the bowel. Peritoneal bands or veils that compromise the duodenal lumen also may be part of this anomaly. Barium studies can be done in these patients if the plain films do not provide enough justification for an exploratory laparotomy (Fig. 18-5).

Duplication Cysts and Diverticula. *Duplication cysts* can occur any place along the bowel. Because they are fluid-filled, ultrasonography is particularly effective in diagnosis. *Multiple diverticula* of the small bowel may occur and not be symptomatic until bacterial

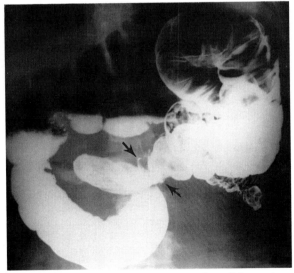

Figure 18–5. Midgut volvulus. Small-bowel series shows twisted loops of bowel with obstruction (*arrows*).

overgrowth in these pockets creates enough bile salt deconjugation or vitamin B_{12} consumption to cause the classical symptoms of diarrhea, steatorrhea, and megaloblastic anemia. The diverticula are readily visualized with barium. It is important to understand that occasional jejunal and ileal diverticula are seen without causing symptoms (Fig. 18-6).

Meckel's diverticulum deserves special attention because of its frequency and propensity to cause symptoms. This diverticulum represents the persistence of the omphalomesenteric duct. It is present in up to 4% of the population and most often is totally asymptomatic. It may cause problems as a site of volvulus or intussusception with resultant small-bowel obstruction. Inflammation and a perforation similar to that seen in the vermiform appendix may occur. The diverticulum may contain acid-secreting cells that may cause ulceration of the sensitive ileal mucosa and subsequent hemorrhage. Enteroclysis is the only barium method that has had consistent success in finding these ileal diverticula (Fig. 18-7).[21] Technetium studies are helpful in patients who are bleeding and have ectopic gastric mucosa in the diverticulum. Rarely, the diverticula are very large, and sometimes they contain calcified enteroliths.

INFLAMMATORY CONDITIONS, INFESTATIONS AND INFECTIOUS DISEASES

Extrinsic Agents. Because the esophagus, stomach, and duodenum are buffers for damaging extrinsic agents, the small bowel is largely spared. At one time enteric coated potassium chloride tablets resulted in several cases of localized ulceration and stricture of the small bowel. Reformulation of the medication has virtually eliminated this problem.

Floxuridiene, a pyrimidine used for treatment of carcinoma of the colon and rectum that has metastasized, can be infused into the hepatic arterial system or systemically by intravenous infusion. This drug causes severe diarrhea. Radiographic findings include thickening of the mucosal folds with effacement or segmental narrowing, usually in the terminal ileum. Radiographic findings are reversible when the drug is discontinued.[17]

Nonsteroidal anti-inflammatory drugs may cause strictures in the small intestine. The findings resemble Crohn's disease.[19]

Flucytosine is an antifungal drug used for the treatment of cryptoccocal meningitis and other fungal diseases. Ulcerative enterocolitis may develop in patients receiving this drug. Radiographic findings include ulcerations, strictures, and thickening of the bowel wall.[27]

Radiation enteropathy of the small bowel is less frequent now because CT can better estimate the tumor mass volume. This results in more accurate radiotherapy doses and less radiation to nontumor tissue.[14] Radiation effects occur late, with stricture and intestinal obstruction being the clinical manifestations. Early radiographic findings include edema and wall thickening, followed by narrowing, fixation, and sometimes kinking (Fig. 18-8).

Specific Organisms. Intestinal parasites are extremely common worldwide. The mature ascaris

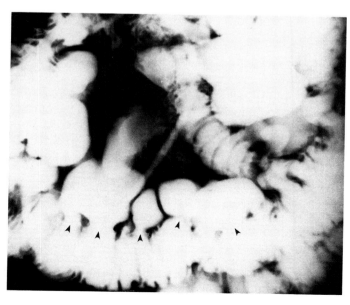

Figure 18–6. Diverticulosis of small bowel (*arrowheads* identify several of the many diverticula present).

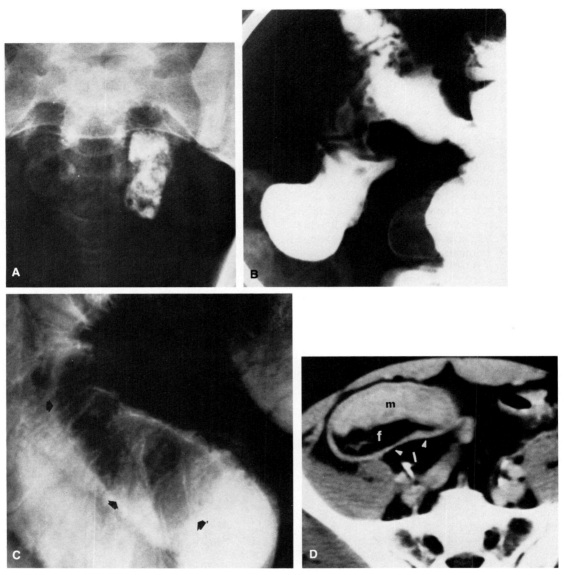

Figure 18–7. (A) Calcified enterolith within Meckel's diverticulum. (B) Barium-filled blind pouch represents Meckel's diverticulum. (C)Intraluminal small-bowel mass represents intussusception of Meckel's diverticulum (*arrows*). (D) CT scan of Meckel's intussusception. *F,* mesenteric fat; *M,* inverted Meckel's diverticulum (intussusceptum); *I,* intussuscipiens (*arrowheads*).

(round) worm can be easily identified within the small bowel as a round or elongated filling defect in the bowel lumen (Fig. 18-9). The same is true with a tapeworm infestation (Fig. 18-10). *Campylobacter* and *Giardia lamblia* can cause an acute illness with recognizable small-bowel edema,[2] usually in the upper jejunum (Fig. 18-11). In its chronic phase giardiasis may not have any radiographic abnormalities. *Strongyloides stercoralis* can cause severe small-bowel symptoms and radiographic findings. These findings are most prominent in the jejunum with edema, nodularity, and stricture being the radiographic findings (Fig. 18-12). The findings mimic Crohn's disease and are chronic in nature.

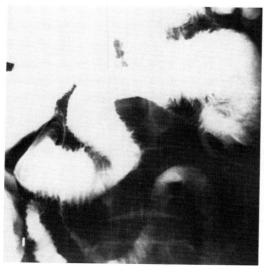

Figure 18–8. Radiation enteritis. Several loops of small bowel show luminal narrowing, wall thickening, and mucosal irregularity.

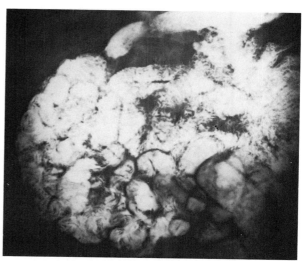

Figure 18–10. *Taenia saginata.* The beef tapeworm creates thin longitudinal filling defects that are most easily seen in the ileum.

Tuberculosis of the small bowel is most common in the ileocecal area. Either the bovine or the human form may be responsible. The radiographic findings are not specific; the final stages usually are those of stricture, which quite often involves the cecum (Fig. 18-13).

Yersinia enterocolitica can cause an acute disease with changes in the terminal ileum that simulate Crohn's disease, but it is a self-limited process, and the bowel usually returns to normal in about 6 weeks.[6]

Patients who are immunodeficient may develop *cryptosporidiosis* of the gastrointestinal tract.[1,4] This same group may have *Mycobacterium avium-intracellulare* infection. The radiographic findings are those of small-bowel edema, causing thickened mucosal folds.

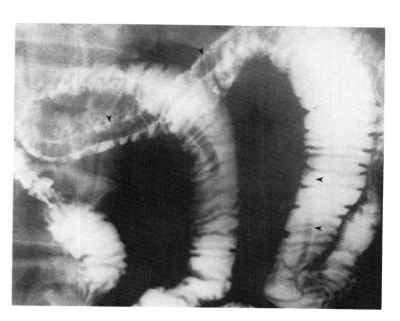

Figure 18–9. Ascariasis. Two worms present (*arrowheads*).

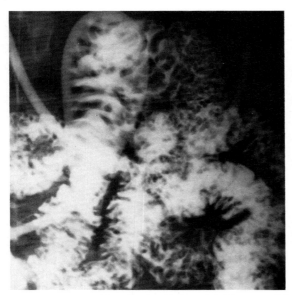

Figure 18–11. Giardiasis. Jejunal folds are thick and irregular.

Whipple's Disease. The success of antibiotic therapy in this disease suggests a bacterial etiology, but this has yet to be proved. The radiographic findings are mucosal fold thickening and irregular fold distortion without dilatation. Small-bowel biopsy shows the characteristic periodic acid-Schiff (PAS) positive material in the macrophages.

Crohn's Disease. Crohn's disease continues to be a very important abnormality in the United States. No etiologic agent has been discovered. The involvement of the small intestine usually begins in the ileum, and eventually it can involve all parts of the small bowel. It may be spotty in its distribution with normal segments of bowel (skip areas) interspersed between pathologic segments. The radiographic manifestations of Crohn's disease begin with aphthous ulcerations, mucosal fold thickening, and mucosal fold distortion (Fig. 18-14A).[10] This can then progress to deep linear ulceration, a nodular cobblestone mucosal pattern, and eventual stenosis (Fig. 18-14B). Longer segments of involvement can occur (Fig. 18-14C). Fistulas and sinus tracts occur (Fig. 18-14D, E). Abdominal abscesses can be very large (Fig. 18-14F). Barium examinations can give a good estimate of the extent and severity of disease, though it is important to know that the correlation of roentgenographic findings and symptoms is often poor in this disease. Computed tomography can add much to the understanding of the extent of disease.[12] It is of particular value in identifying abscesses and fistulas.

Recently there have been more observations of malignancy developing in areas of Crohn's disease—similar to the situation in long-standing chronic ulcerative colitis.[18]

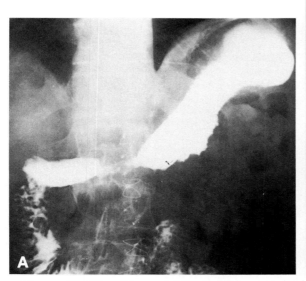
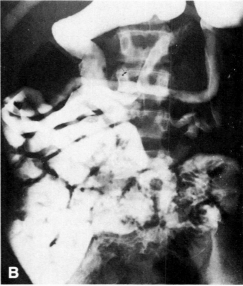

Figure 18–12. Strongyloidiasis. This parasite invades the wall of the gastrointestinal tract and can cause permanent fibrosis in both the stomach (**A**) and small bowel (**B**).

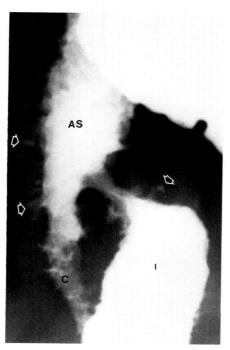

Figure 18–13. Ileocecal tuberculosis. Coning of cecum with mucosal ulcerations and stricture of ileum. *C*, cecum; *AS*, ascending colon; *I*, terminal ileum. Ulcerations (*arrows*).

MOTILITY DISORDERS

Scleroderma. The intestinal manifestations of progressive systemic sclerosis may be severe. The bowel becomes dilated, and the small bowel and colon may have outpouchings of mucosa (sacculations) that are characteristic for scleroderma (Fig. 18-15A, B). The lack of transport in the small bowel may lead to bacterial overgrowth with the same symptoms as seen in the blind loop syndrome and multiple intestinal diverticula.

Intestinal Pseudo-Obstruction. This condition is of unknown etiology. The plain films strongly suggest mechanical small-bowel obstruction, but neither radiologic studies nor laparotomy demonstrate an anatomic lesion. Although the small-bowel manifestations are predominant, it has been pointed out that motility in the other parts of the gastrointestinal tract may also be abnormal.

Myxedema. Another condition that may simulate mechanical small-bowel obstruction is chronic hypothyroidism. Fortunately, this condition is reversible with replacement therapy.

Paralytic Ileus. This most common motility disorder occurs after surgery or injury. The small bowel and colon dilate with gas, and transport is inhibited. The diagnosis of this condition is easily made in the proper clinical setting with plain supine and upright films. Usually there is equal distention of both small bowel and colon (Fig. 18-16). Unlike mechanical small-bowel obstruction, air-fluid levels in the bowel only occur if the process persists from 5 to 7 days. Paralytic ileus is usually a self-limited process, and radiographic improvement is preceded by the passage of flatus. Postoperative potassium deficiency is the most common electrolyte imbalance in patients with adynamic ileus.

Transit Time. Although barium might seem to be a good marker to measure small-bowel motility from stomach to colon, it is actually of little value. Occasionally barium may reach the cecum inside of 5 minutes without any clinical signs to suggest hypermotility. On the opposite end of the spectrum, transit times in the 5- to 6-hour range can be seen as normal phenomena.

VASCULAR DISEASES

Intestinal Ischemia. One of the most serious problems involving the small bowel is infarction. Plain-film findings have been notoriously unreliable in making this diagnosis until gas is present in the intestinal wall. Computed tomography is of more help because the dilated, thick-walled, fluid-filled loop is enough to suggest the correct diagnosis.[8, 11] Similar observations may be made with ultrasonography.[8] Ischemia without infarction may occur, and in this instance barium studies may show a narrowed irregular lumen secondary to the submucosal edema and hemorrhage. Patients with postprandial pain and weight loss caused by ischemia often have normal barium studies. Angiography should be performed when this diagnosis is suspected. Generally, at least two of the three mesenteric vessels need to be compromised. The exception to this is when the superior mesenteric artery is obstructed distal to the pancreaticoduodenal and middle colic arteries.

Intestinal Wall Hemorrhage and Edema. Conditions that result in submucosal hemorrhage or edema all have the same radiographic manifestations. The fold pattern becomes prominent and eventually may be effaced (Fig. 18-17). The process can be localized or diffuse. Examples of conditions with edema are hypoproteinemia from any cause, hereditary angioneurotic edema, and graft-versus-host disease. Sources of submucosal hemorrhage are anticoagulant overdose, mesenteric venous infarction, and hemorrhagic disorders

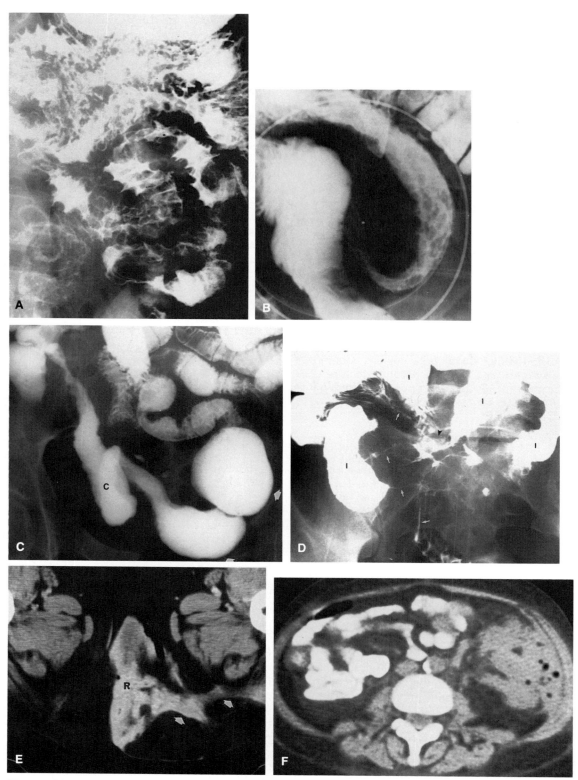

Figure 18–14.

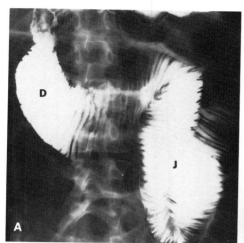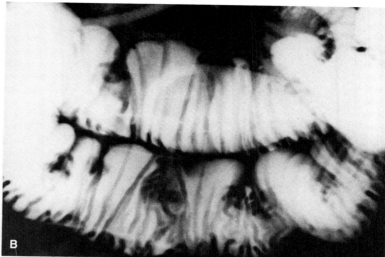

Figure 18–15. **(A)** Scleroderma. Jejunum (*J*) shows dilatation with thin, straight folds. **(B)** Scleroderma. Magnified view of small bowel shows several sacculations. Mucosal folds extend throughout sacculation.

such as hemophilia, and both thrombocytic and non-thrombocytic purpura.[14]

FOREIGN BODIES

Bezoars. Bezoars occasionally leave the stomach and become obstructing objects in the small bowel (Fig. 18-18). This is particularly prone to occur in a patient with a gastrojejunostomy where the anastomosis provides less restraint than the normal pyloric canal.

Drugs. The use of ingested drug-filled condoms to illegally transport drugs across national borders results in a recognizable radiographic appearance. The condom may break, and the smuggler then becomes toxic. Abdominal films can be helpful in identifying the condoms because most contain some gas.

Enteroliths. Enteroliths can occur not only in Meckel's diverticulum, but also anywhere there is a partial small-bowel obstruction. Enteroliths are calcified and thus detectable on plain films. Seeds may be the nidus for enteroliths (See Fig. 18-7A).

Gallstone. Large gallstones may enter the duodenum through a cholecystoduodenal fistula. For unknown reasons the stone can fail to move beyond the midileum or become impacted at the ileocecal valve and thus cause intestinal obstruction. Air in the gallbladder and bile ducts combined with small-bowel obstruction (gallstone ileus) are characteristic diagnostic findings (Fig. 18-19A, B).

Miscellaneous Foreign Bodies. Animal bones and toothpicks are examples of sharp objects that may enter the small bowel and cause perforation. The combina-

◄ **Figure 18–14.** Crohn's disease. **(A)** Early changes of nodularity, fold thickening, and mucosal irregularity in jejunum. **(B)** The "cobblestone" pattern is a reflection of deep longitudinal ulcerations leaving islands of edematous, nonulcerated mucosa. **(C)** Long segment of involvement. Note absence of mucosal folds and areas of dilatation (*arrows*). *C*, cecum. **(D)** Like spokes of a wheel, multiple fistulous tracts (*arrows*) are seen leading to an extraluminal barium collection (*arrowhead*). *I*, ileal loops. **(E)** CT scan shows fistula to left gluteal area from rectum (*arrows*). *R*, rectum. **(F)** Computed tomogram demonstrates an abscessed area on the left side of the abdomen. The multiple small circular air collections that do not fill with contrast material are easily distinguished from the normal bowel appearance in the right abdomen.

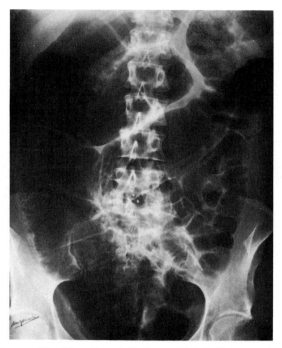

Figure 18–16. Paralytic ileus. This is the usual appearance with proportionate gaseous distention of large and small bowel.

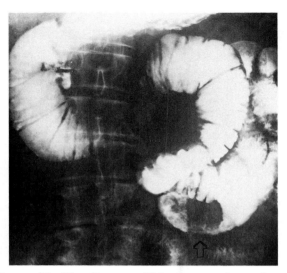

Figure 18–18. Bezoar. This bezoar (*arrow*) occurred in a patient after vagotomy and antrectomy and caused a partial small-bowel obstruction.

tion of plain films and CT can assist in identifying the area of perforation and associated abscesses.

METABOLIC, ALLERGIC, AND MISCELLANEOUS IDIOPATHIC DISEASES

Nontropical Sprue. It is now understood that this disease is caused by gluten hypersensitivity. Malabsorption of fat and hypoproteinemia occur. The hypoproteinemia is responsible for the edematous mucosal folds seen in this condition. The bowel may be dilated and fluid filled. Intestinal loops contract poorly. Segmentation and flocculation of barium are not observed with the newer suspending agents. The diagnosis is established by a small-bowel biopsy that shows villous atrophy. At the present time the diagnosis is often established before there are any radiographic findings. Patients with a long history of sprue have an increased risk for developing lymphoma. Except in the case of collagenous sprue in which submucosal collagen is present, treatment is usually effective in reversing both the mucosal and radiographic changes (Fig. 18-20A, B).

Dysgammaglobulinemia. Prominent lymphoid follicles may be seen normally in the terminal ileum, but this is an abnormal finding in the jejunum. The radiographic finding has been seen to correlate with immunoglobulin A deficiency (nodular lymphoid hyperplasia).

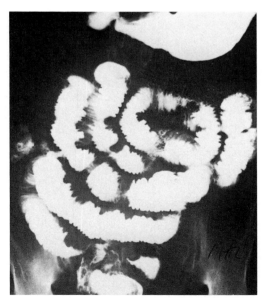

Figure 18–17. Intramural fluid. The accumulation of any substance diffusely in the bowel wall coarsens the mucosal folds and separates the loops. In this instance, there was diffuse hemorrhage into the bowel wall related to anticoagulant overdose.

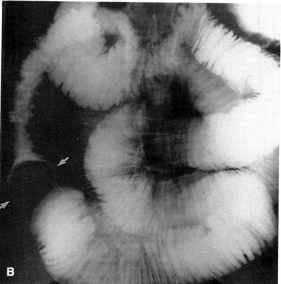 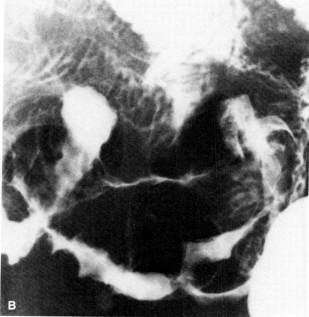

Figure 18–19.   (**A**) Gallstone obstruction. An intraluminal filling defect in the jejunum is suspected to be a gallstone because the contrast material shows a fistula to the gallbladder (*arrow*). (**B**) Gallstone ileus or obstruction. Large gallstone impacted in distal ileum where the obstruction usually occurs (*arrows*).

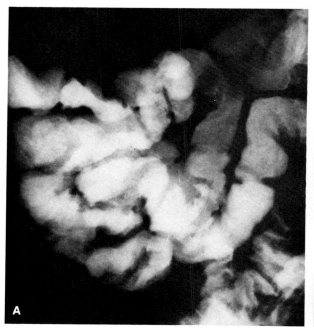 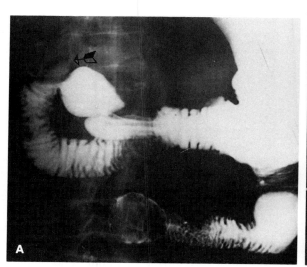

Figure 18–20.   (**A**) Sprue. Note decreased number of mucosal folds and mucosal effacement. (**B**) Development of lymphoma in same patient years later. Note dramatic change in appearance of small-bowel pattern.

Large mucosal folds can be seen in Waldenström's macroglobulinemia. Systemic mastocytosis may cause nodulation resembling lymphoid hyperplasia.

Eosinophilic Gastroenteritis. These patients may or may not have peripheral eosinophilia. The radiographic manifestation is fold enlargement from the antrum of the stomach, through the duodenum and into the small bowel.

Abetalipoproteinemia. This extremely rare condition is manifested by a lack of beta lipoproteins and clinical manifestations that include steatorrhea. Mucosal fold enlargement may be seen.

Amyloidosis. Recognizable amyloidosis of the small bowel is rare. Thickened folds have been observed in this condition. They may be symmetric and uniform in appearance, or irregular with nodular defects.

Cystic Fibrosis. The submucosal glands become distended with the very viscous secretions associated with cystic fibrosis. The distended glands create a nodular deformity of the mucosal pattern from duodenum through the colon. Because respiratory symptoms predominate, a diagnosis is usually made by the time the intestine has been studied.

Cavitating Lymph Node Syndrome. A group of patients with chronic diarrhea, splenic atrophy, and flat intestinal mucosa has been described.[22] The characteristic feature of this syndrome is large, cavitated, fluid-filled intra-abdominal lymph nodes. The CT appearance is diagnostic.

Behçet's Syndrome. Ileal ulceration has been observed in this disease. More often there is colonic ulceration simulating chronic ulcerative colitis.[23]

Lymphangiectasia. Lymphangiectasia can be the source of malnourishment because there is leakage of lymph back into the intestine. Pedal lymphangiography can demonstrate flow from the thoracic duct to the intestinal lumen. Barium studies show large edematous small-bowel folds caused by the hypoproteinemia[7] and possibly the enlarged lymphatics (Fig. 18-21).

Whipple's Disease. The success of antibiotic therapy in this disease suggests a bacterial etiology, but this has yet to be proved. The radiographic findings are mucosal fold thickening and irregular fold distortion without dilatation. Small-bowel biopsy shows the characteristic PAS positive material in the macrophages (Fig. 18-22).

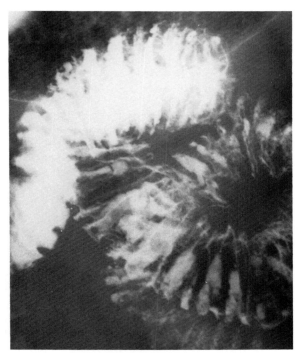

Figure 18–21. Lymphangiectasia. Thickened, nodular folds proximal jejunum.

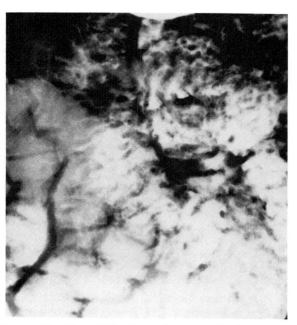

Figure 18–22. Whipple's disease. Nodular, distorted folds in jejunum.

NEOPLASMS

BENIGN

Solitary. Adenomatous polyps in the small bowel are rare, whereas intramural tumors that originate in connective tissue are common. Fortunately, connective tissue tumors are small, do not continue to grow, and are usually only a curiosity seen at autopsy. Leiomyomas occasionally may become large enough to be palpable. When smaller they can cause an intussusception with bowel obstruction (Fig. 18-23). Carcinoid tumors may occur as solitary intramural tumors in the distal small bowel. They are usually small and are rarely detected on routine examination of the small bowel. They may become malignant, and when they produce a desmoplastic response after extension into the mesentery, there may be local distortion, separation, angulation, and fixation of the bowel (Fig. 18-24).

Multiple. Lipomatosis of the small bowel has been reported. In Peutz-Jeghers syndrome multiple small-bowel polyps can be found (Fig. 18-25). They may also be found in the colon. Intussusception may occur. The presence of the characteristic circumoral melanin pigmentation confirms the diagnosis. It is believed that the polyps are hamartomatous in nature.

Gastrointestinal polyposis, alopecia, skin pigmentation, and atrophy of the fingernails and toenails are the hallmarks of the Cronkhite-Canada syndrome. The

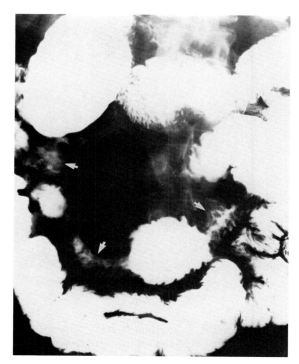

Figure 18–24. Carcinoid. Segmental narrowing of small bowel (*arrows*) and mesenteric involvement noted by separation of bowel loops.

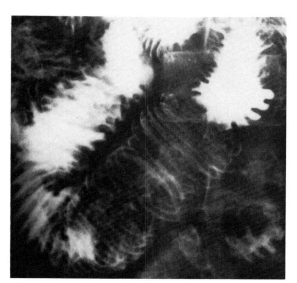

Figure 18–23. Intussusception caused by leiomyoma. The tumor is not visible, but the "coiled-spring" appearance is characteristic of intussusception.

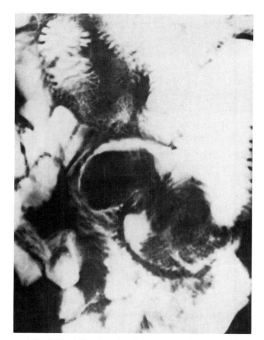

Figure 18–25. Peutz-Jeghers syndrome. The large hamartomatous polyps are seen in the distal jejunum. Intussusception and partial small-bowel obstruction occurred in this patient.

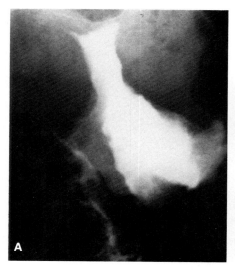

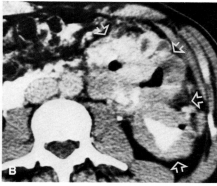

Figure 18–26.   Leiomyosarcoma. **(A)** Barium-filled irregular cavity. **(B)** CT scan of tumor (*arrows*).

polyps are thought to be inflammatory in origin, and this is supported by a recent report of total regression of the polyps.

MALIGNANT

Primary. Adenocarcinomas of the small bowel are rare, with bulky leiomyosarcomas occurring more often. When large, they may become necrotic, and when filled with barium, these necrotic cavities appear amorphous and irregular. Computed tomography shows the thickness of the tumor best. Adenocarcinoma, leiomyosarcoma, and lymphoma may be indistinguishable (Fig. 18-26A, B). The most frequent lesion is non-Hodgkin's lymphoma, which may present in myriad ways.[15] There may be an intussuscepting mass, and there may be an annular constricting lesion. Most confusing of all, lymphoma may resemble a dilated segment of small bowel (Fig. 18-27). Crohn's disease may be difficult to distinguish from lymphoma. In addition to barium studies, CT is of great benefit in determining the extraluminal extent of the tumor (Fig. 18-28).

Metastatic. Metastatic lesions from breast, lung, kidney, melanoma, and from Kaposi's sarcoma may occur (Figs. 18-29 and 18-30). In addition there is the local spread from primary tumors of the uterus, ovaries, bladder, and colon.[26] Metastatic carcinoid tumors characteristically spread to the peritoneum and small bowel. Barium studies of the small bowel are often very helpful in detecting these lesions.

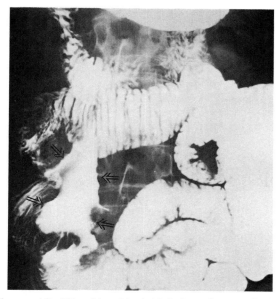

Figure 18–27.   Non-Hodgkin's lymphoma. A mass with a large ulceration (*arrows*) within it can be seen in the right-lower quadrant. The dilated proximal small gut is a reflection of an incomplete small-bowel obstruction.

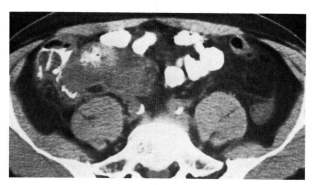

Figure 18–28. Non-Hodgkin's lymphoma. A large soft-tissue mass incorporating loops of small bowel is seen on the right side of the abdomen, anterior to the psoas muscle.

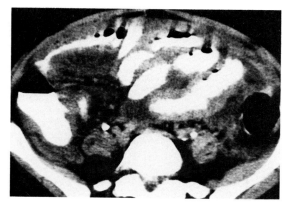

Figure 18–30. Kaposi's sarcoma. CT scan of barium-filled small bowel shows nonspecific mural thickening.

HERNIAS

The small bowel has more of a tendency to enter right inguinal hernias than left. It is unusual to see small bowel above the diaphragm except in the case of a congenital absence of the diaphragm. A type of hernia that is very difficult to diagnose is the paraduodenal hernia. In this condition the small bowel goes through a defect in the posterior peritoneum and is entrapped in a retroperitoneal location. It is difficult on barium studies to appreciate this encapsulation (Fig. 18-31). Computed tomography holds the greatest hope as an accurate diagnostic tool. The small bowel may slip in and out of the hernia, and partial or complete small-bowel obstruction can occur. Herniation through a mesenteric defect may occur, but it is usually detected

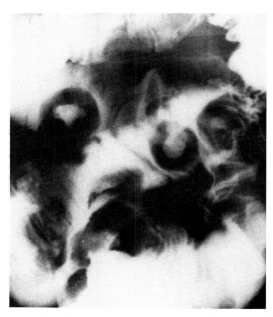

Figure 18–29. Melanoma. Metastatic "target" or "bull's-eye" lesions where the central barium collections represent necrosis or ulceration.

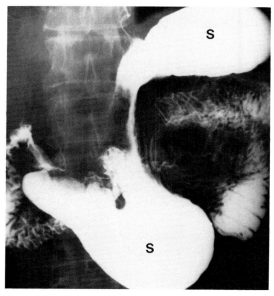

Figure 18–31. Left paraduodenal hernia. Proximal small bowel contained in the left-upper quadrant deforms greater curvature of stomach (*S*).

only when obstruction is produced. Even then, the cause of obstruction may not be evident on small-bowel studies.

TRAUMA

Radiographic methods are not of much use in the types of trauma that damage the small bowel. These are usually knife and gunshot wounds, and the nature of the injury demands surgical exploration.

IATROGENIC CONDITIONS

Adhesions. Laparotomy almost inevitably leads to intraperitoneal adhesions. These fixed adhesions and the mobile small bowel may lead to intestinal obstruction, a process that slowly becomes symptomatic as food and fluid can no longer reach the colon. By the time patients with complete obstruction appear for medical care, the radiographic findings on the supine and upright films are diagnostic. The small bowel is distended, and air-fluid levels are seen proximal to the obstruction. There usually is little or no gas in the colon because it has been evacuated in the presymptomatic phase. If the obstruction is partial, the findings are less striking (Fig. 18-32). The small-bowel distention is less, although fluid levels are present. There may be the normal amount of gas and feces in the colon. The site and cause of partial obstruction can sometimes be determined on barium study. Closed-loop obstructions

may be complicated by intestinal ischemia or infarction. Because of this they present earlier and with severer systemic symptoms. In this situation plain films may be normal, but the obstruction can easily be demonstrated with contrast material.

Ileostomies. The current trend for patients with a permanent ileostomy is to create a reservoir that can be emptied periodically. This "continent" ileostomy is subject to mechanical problems that create a partial small-bowel obstruction. Barium instilled through the ileostomy is an excellent method of studying the problem.

Benign Pneumatosis Intestinalis. For unknown reasons gas will sometimes be observed in the wall of the small bowel (Fig. 18-33). It has been seen in patients with blind loops associated with jejunoileal bypass in patients with morbid obesity. It also has been reported with catheter feeding into the jejunum.

Graft-versus-Host Disease. Although the gastrointestinal reaction following bone-marrow transplantation may involve the entire gut, the findings in the small intestine are striking. Narrowed, tubular, separated small-bowel loops are seen. It is thought that this reflects marked small-bowel edema (Fig. 18-34).

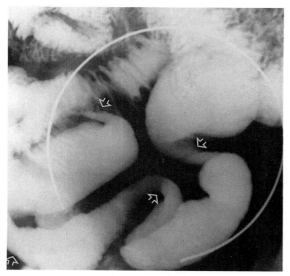

Figure 18–32. Adhesions. Several areas of narrowing caused by adhesions (*arrows*) resulting in incomplete obstruction between adhesions.

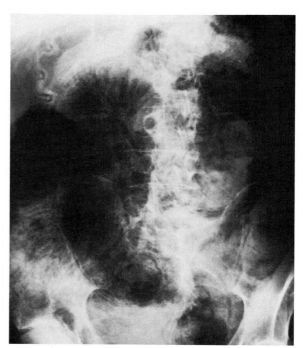

Figure 18–33. Pneumatosis cystoides intestinalis. Gas is observed in the wall of the entire small bowel and colon.

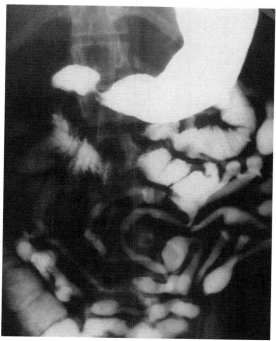

Figure 18–34. Graft-versus-host disease. Narrowed, tubular appearance of long segments of small bowel.

REFERENCES AND SELECTED READINGS

1. BERK RN, WALL SB, MCARDLE CB, ET AL: Cryptosporidiosis of the stomach and small intestine in patients with AIDS. Am J Roentgenol 143:549, 1984

2. BLASER MJ, RELLER LB: Campylobacter enteritis. N Engl J Med 305:1444, 1981

3. CLUCK WL, AKWARI OE, KELVIN FM, ET AL: A reversible enteropathy complicating continuous hepatic artery infusion chemotherapy with 5-fluoro-2-deoxyuridine. Cancer 56:2424, 1985

4. CURRENT WL, REESE NC, ERNST JV, ET AL: Human cryptosporidiosis in immunocompetent and immunodeficient persons. N Engl J Med 308:1252, 1983

5. DUNN JT, HALLS JM, BERNE TV: Roentgenographic contrast studies in acute small-bowel obstruction. Arch Surg 119:1305, 1984

6. EKBERG O, SJÖSTRÖM B, BRAHME F: Radiological findings in *Yersinia ileitis.* Radiology 123:15, 1977

7. FARTHING MJG, MCLEAN AM, BARTRAM CI, ET AL: Radiologic features of the jejunum in hypoalbuminemia. Am J Roentgenol 136:883, 1981

8. FEDERLE MP, CHUN G, JEFFREY RB, ET AL: Computed tomographic findings in bowel infarction. Am J Roentgenol 142:91, 1984

9. FLEISCHER AC, MUHLETALER CA, JAMES AE JR, ET AL: Sonographic assessment of the bowel wall. Am J Roentgenol 136:887, 1981

10. GLICK SN, TEPLICK SK: Crohn disease of the small intestine: Diffuse mucosal granularity. Radiology 154:313, 1985

11. GLUCK WL, AKWARI OE, KELVIN FM, ET AL: Computed tomographic findings in bowel infarction. Radiology 159:570, 1986

12. GOLDBERG HI, GORE RM, MARGULIS AR, ET AL: Computed tomography in the evaluation of Crohn disease. Am J Roentgenol 140:277, 1983

13. GRENDELL JH, OCKNER RK: Mesenteric venous thrombosis. Gastroenterology 82:358, 1982

14. HERLINGER H, MAGLINTE D: Clinical radiology of the small intestine. Philadelphia, WB Saunders, 1989, pp. 466–467

15. IKE BW, ROSENBUSCH G: Gastrointestinal malignant lymphoma: Roentgenographic features and pathologic and morphologic correlations. Diagn Imaging 50:66, 1981

16. KELVIN FM, GEDGAUDAS RK, THOMPSON WM, ET AL: The peroral pneumocolon: Its role in evaluating the terminal ileum. Am J Roentgenol 139:115, 1982

17. KELVIN FM, GRAMM HF, GLUCK WL, ET AL: Radiologic manifestations of short-bowel toxicity due to floxuridine therapy. Am J Roentgenol 146:39, 1986

18. KERBER GW, FRANK PH: Carcinoma of the small intestine and colon as a manifestation of Crohn disease: Radiologic manifestations. Radiology 150:639, 1984

19. LANGMAN MJ, MORGAN L, WORRALL A: Use of anti-inflammatory drugs by patients admitted with small or large bowel perforations and hemorrhage. Br Med J 290:347, 1985

20. MAGLINTE DDT, HALL R, MILLER RE, ET AL: Detection of surgical lesions of the small bowel by enteroclysis. Am J Surg 147:225, 1984

21. MAGLINTE DDT, ELMORE MF, ISENBERG M, ET AL: Meckel diverticulum: Radiologic detection by enteroclysis. Am J Roentgenol 134:925, 1980

22. MATUCHANSKY C, COLIN R, HEMET J, ET AL: Cavitation of mesenteric lymph nodes, splenic atrophy, and a flat small intestinal mucosa. Gastroenterology 87:606, 1984

23. MCLEAN AM, SIMMS DM, HOMER MJ: Ileal ring ulcers in Behçet syndrome. Am J Roentgenol 140:947, 1982

24. OTT DJ, CHEN YM, GELFAND DW, ET AL: Detailed peroral small bowel vs enteroclysis. Radiology 155:29, 1985

25. OTT DJ: Efficacy of small-bowel examination. In Chen MYM, Zagoria RJ, Ott DJ, Gelfand DW (eds): Radiology of the small bowel. New York, Igakar-Shoin, 1992, p. 457

26. ROSE HS, BALTHAZAR EJ, MEGIBOW AJ, ET AL: Alimentary tract involvement in Kaposi sarcoma: Radiographic findings in 25 homosexual men. Am J Roentgenol 139:661, 1982

27. WHITE CA, TRAUBE J: Ulcerating enteritis associated with flucytosine therapy. Gastroenterology 83:1127, 1982

*Paul and Juhl's Essentials of Radiologic Imaging,
Sixth Edition,* edited by John H. Juhl and
Andrew B. Crummy. J.B. Lippincott Company,
Philadelphia, © 1993.

CHAPTER **19**

The Colon and Appendix

Michael Davis

THE COLON AND APPENDIX

INDICATIONS

The major reasons for studying the large bowel relate to colon cancer and inflammatory bowel disease. Both bright red rectal bleeding and chemical evidence of hemoglobin products in the stool are strong indications. Subacute or chronic diarrhea suggests the possibility of inflammatory bowel disease. Other symptoms and signs that may indicate the presence of colonic disease include a change in caliber of the stool, constipation, and weight loss, but most often no organic bowel disease is found in these patients. Severe anemia is sometimes seen with right-colon neoplasms. Abdominal distention raises the possibility of colonic obstruction. The presence of a left-lower-quadrant mass with tenderness suggests diverticulitis or tubo-ovarian abscess, and the same findings in the right-lower quadrant can occur with an appendiceal or tubo-ovarian abscess. The colon is often studied in patients with genitourinary malignancies to exclude invasion of the gut.

ANATOMY

The mobile portions of the colon are the sigmoid and transverse portions because they have a longer mesentery and thus can shift more in position. The cecum also may be mobile if it has a long mesentery—a situation that may lead to cecal volvulus. The rest of the colon has a short mesentery and is fixed in position. The rectum is an extraperitoneal structure and has a fixed position. There is considerable variation in the position of the appendix. Although it usually is in the right-lower quadrant, it can move with the cecum, may be retroceal, and occasionally will be long with the tip extending into the subhepatic region.

PHYSIOLOGY

Water absorption occurs in the right colon, but the main function of the colon is one of the storage and transport of feces. The contraction waves in the colon are not ordinarily a subject of radiologic study. The anal sphincter is under voluntary control.

METHODS OF EXAMINATION

Plain films of the abdomen have great value in detecting colonic obstruction, colonic ileus, and the toxic megacolon syndrome in inflammatory bowel disease. The dilated colon can be readily appreciated in all these conditions.

Single- and double-contrast examinations with barium sulfate are the usual methods used to study the colon. In these combined fluoroscopic-radiographic procedures the contrast agents are introduced through the rectum under fluoroscopic observation. A controversy exists concerning single- versus double-contrast studies, but the prevailing opinion is that smaller lesions of the colon, such as aphthous ulcers and small polyps, can be detected better with the double-contrast method.

Of vital importance in barium enema studies is a clean colon. All combinations of cathartics and enemas have been tried. The regimens that work best include a purgative or laxative with copious amounts of oral liquids (the latter acting as a flush).[15] Water-soluble–contrast enemas are indicated if colonic perforation is suspected and are occasionally used to soften a fecal impaction. Ultrasonography can be of great help in identifying abscesses and bowel-wall thickening that may accompany inflammatory disease. Occasionally, nonpalpable abdominal masses are also found by ultrasonography. Because of the presence of colonic gas, ultrasonography is not often a useful method for detecting the ordinary intraluminal lesions. Computed tomography (CT) is valuable in determining the presence and extent of extracolonic disease. Abscess, fistula, diverticulitis, and lymphadenopathy can be detected by CT.

Alternative Nonradiologic Methods. Colonoscopy is a competitive alternative to barium studies of the colon. There is a distinct advantage in being able to view the mucosa directly and to biopsy suspicious lesions at the time of this examination. The current disadvantages of colonoscopy are the inability to see the entire colon in some patients and the costs, which are considerably more than a radiologic study. Sigmoidoscopy continues to be a supportive and complementary adjunct to radiologic studies. The detection of anal canal lesions in particular is much better accomplished by direct observation.

CONGENITAL ANOMALIES

TUBULATION DEFECTS

While any part of the colon may be atretic, the most common clinical problem is anorectal atresia. By allowing intestinal gas to reach the sigmoid colon, the proximal site of the obstruction can be determined. Fistulas to the vagina and bladder can occur in the imperforate anus syndrome. Knowing the length of the atresia helps in planning reparative surgery.

COLONIC DUPLICATION

Duplication of the colon is rare. The duplication may or may not communicate with the functioning colon. Barium studies may show a double lumen (Fig. 19-1). Ultrasonography can determine the cystic nature of a noncommunicating duplication anomaly.

FAILURES OF ROTATION

Nonrotation places the entire colon on the left side of the abdomen. Incomplete rotation and fixation of the colon may leave the cecum unusually mobile and prone to volvulus (Fig. 19-2A,B).

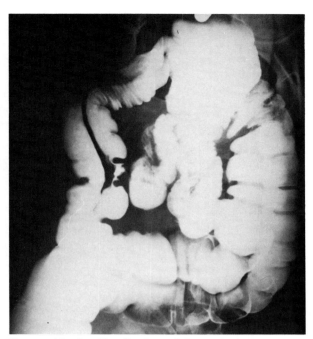

Figure 19–1. Duplication of the colon.

AGANGLIONIC MEGACOLON

Aganglionosis of the colon causes the colon to be functionally partially obstructed at the site where the aganglionosis begins. This site can be anywhere from the cecum to the rectum. Progressive dilatation of the colon occurs; barium enema and biopsy lead to the correct diagnosis. The colon may appear normal as it is filled with barium, but there is a failure to evacuate the barium through the aganglionic area (Fig. 19-3). The most difficult type to detect is aganglionosis involving only the anal canal area. These patients will commonly have the meconium plug syndrome at birth. The rectal meconium will be obstructive until passed spontaneously or aided by an enema. Later the infant's constipation becomes apparent, and the colonic dilatation down to the anus is detected. Biopsy then confirms the aganglionosis. Functional megacolon may simulate aganglionosis of the anal canal on barium enema except that dilatation is usually greatest in the rectum in the functional type.

INFLAMMATORY DISEASES

EXTRINSIC AGENTS

It is rare for individuals to introduce damaging agents into the rectum, but colonic damage has been reported in children who were repeatedly given detergent en-

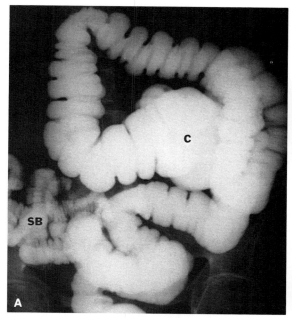

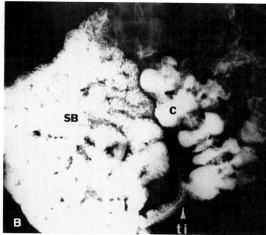

Figure 19–2. **(A)** Incomplete rotation of colon. Note high position of cecum (*C*). Small bowel (*SB*) seen in right-lower quadrant. **(B)** Nonrotation of colon. *C*, colon; *TI*, terminal ilium; *SB*, small bowel. Note entire small bowel in right abdomen and all of colon in left abdomen.

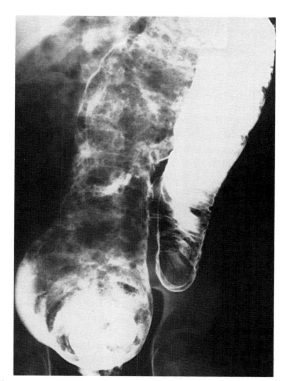

Figure 19–3. Aganglionic megacolon. Note hugely distended rectum filled with feces. Note abrupt tapering in distal rectum.

emas. Adults can have the cathartic colon syndrome,[45] in which the haustrations of the colon are obliterated, leaving a very smooth internal contour (Fig. 19-4). It usually involves the right colon more than the left, and is caused by long-standing laxative abuse. Radiation damage to the rectum and sigmoid following treatment of genitourinary malignancies is now rare. The strictures that occur are caused by damage to the small blood vessels. The radiographic findings are stricture or lack of normal distensibility.

SPECIFIC ORGANISMS

The organisms that cause acute and self-limiting colitis are rarely studied radiologically. The same holds true for most types of subacute colitis. Amebiasis and tuberculosis are more chronic diarrheal diseases that are often studied radiologically. Tuberculosis classically involves the ileocecal area with ulceration and stricture formation (Fig. 19-5). Amebiasis tends to be a cecal inflammatory process with the cecum sometimes completely obliterated after healing occurs (Fig. 19-6).[27] Amebic granulomas can occur anywhere in the colon and mimic neoplasm. Both tuberculosis and amebiasis may manifest themselves as a diffuse ulcerating colitis. Schistosomiasis can produce a chronic ulcerative colitis and go on to pseudopolyp formation manifested by multiple small filling defects projecting into the colonic lumen. Yersinia can mimic idiopathic inflammatory

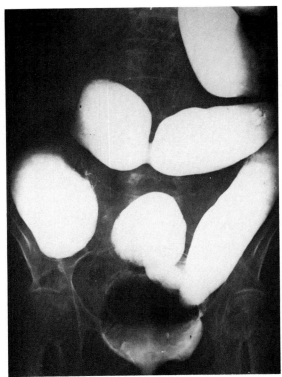

Figure 19–4. Cathartic colon. The dilated colon without a haustral pattern is a consequence of long-standing laxative abuse.

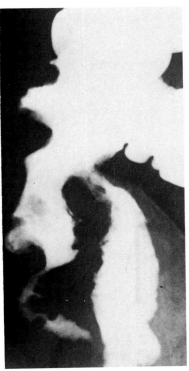

Figure 19–5. Tuberculosis. Classically, there is ileocecal involvement with both ulceration and luminal narrowing in intestinal tuberculosis.

bowel disease because it causes a subacute colitis.[28, 39] *Clostridium septicum* and *Clostridium perfringens* have been observed to cause severe ulcerative colitis with gas formation in the colonic wall; these patients often have malignant neoplasms.[36, 37] Herpes simplex can cause deep aphthous and collar-button ulcers of the anus and rectum.[40] Herpes zoster rarely can cause small ulcerations in short segments of the colon. The colonic involvement is accompanied by the typical skin lesions. Recently, *Campylobacter* was recognized as an organism frequently causing a subacute colitis in man.[3] The radiographic findings are those of ulceration and edema not unlike those in ulcerative colitis. The lack of immune competence may lead to colitis caused by unusual organisms such as the cytomegalovirus or *Candida*.[14, 41] Venereal-related colitis, usually proctitis, can be caused by gonococcus and many other organisms, such as *Mycoplasma* and *Entamoeba* in addition to herpes simplex.[17, 42] *Lymphogranuloma venereum* infection can result in edema and ulceration followed by extensive strictures in the anorectal area. Pseudomembranous colitis has now been found to be a result of a toxin liberated by *Clostridium difficile*. Be-

cause this organism frequently overgrows the colon after antibiotic therapy, this condition was previously called antibiotic colitis. The radiographic pattern is slightly different from the usual ulcerative process, because mucosal edema predominates (Fig. 19-7). The colonic surface may appear irregular and shaggy, caused by the pseudomembrane and superficial ulceration. The disease usually involves the entire colon, but cases of rectal sparing are now being reported.[35] When the disease is severe, barium enema is contraindicated.

APPENDICITIS

Obstruction of the appendix leads to a sequence of inflammation, perforation, and abscess formation. Although appendicitis is a very common condition, the use of imaging techniques for diagnosis is rare. Early in the disease process, plain films may be normal or may show slight gaseous distention of the ileum. With perforation and abscess the terminal ileum may be involved enough to resemble a partial or complete small-bowel obstruction. A stone in the appendix suggests

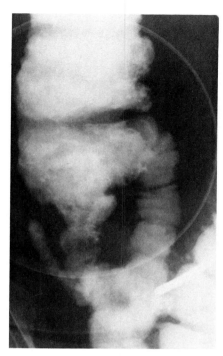

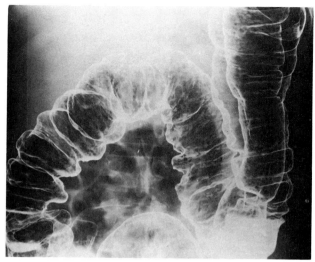

Figure 19–7. Pseudomembranous colitis. The marked mucosal irregularity is caused by the edematous colonic mucosa.

Figure 19–6. Amebiasis. The cecum is cone shaped in this instance and may become very small after healing.

the diagnosis. Barium studies in simple appendicitis have been somewhat controversial. It is agreed that the lack of appendiceal lumen filling can occur normally and does not justify a positive diagnosis. The filling of the entire appendix does exclude appendicitis. Some believe that there is spasm of the terminal ileum and cecum in appendicitis and that it can be detected at fluoroscopy. Because this is such a subjective observation, it is difficult to assess.[9] With abscess formation, ultrasonography, CT, and barium studies are all helpful in identifying the morphologic changes (Fig. 19-8).

IDIOPATHIC COLITIDES

Ulcerative colitis (Fig. 19-9*A,B*) and granulomatous colitis (Fig. 19-10*A*, through *D*) can most often be distinguished by radiographic changes (Table 19-1). In a small percentage of cases a clear distinction is not possible even with microscopic study of the colon. Toxic megacolon, pseudopolyposis, and an increased risk of colon carcinoma occur in both conditions but are more common in idiopathic ulcerative colitis.[29] Barium studies aid the primary diagnosis and, with ultrasonography and CT, are helpful if complications de-

velop. CT can directly image the bowel wall, lymph nodes, and adjacent mesentery for complications such as abscess, fistula, sinus tract, perirectal changes; and hepatobiliary, genitourinary, and musculoskeletal complications.[18] Identifying early carcinoma in ulcerative colitis requires colonoscopy and biopsy.

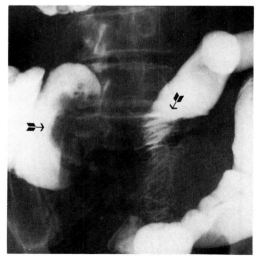

Figure 19–8. Appendiceal abscess. The extraluminal abscess deforms both the cecum and adjacent ileum (*arrows*).

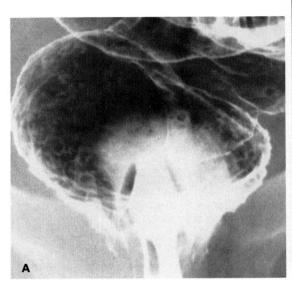
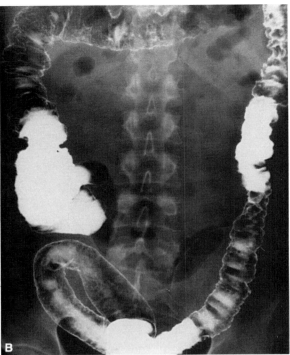

Figure 19–9.   **(A)** Acute early ulcerative colitis. Note numerous ulcerations throughout the mucosa. **(B)** Ulcerative colitis involves entire colon.

Diversion colitis is an ulcerative change that can be seen in that portion of the bowel from which the fecal stream has been diverted.[26,38] *Behçet's syndrome* is a rare condition with buccal and genital ulcerations as well as skin and ocular manifestations. The colon and small bowel may have changes of inflammation mimicking the more common colitides.[16,43] Behçet's syndrome tends to mimic Crohn's disease more than ulcerative colitis, although the ulcers of Behçet's syndrome are often larger than those of Crohn's disease. Hemorrhage and perforation are frequent complications. *Neutropenic colitis* is a complication of acute leukemia, aplastic anemia, or cyclic neutropenia. Cecal wall thickening and intramural gas have been observed on CT examination.[12] *Colitis cystica profunda* is most often seen in young adults and is characterized by the presence of mucous cysts in the muscularis mucosa. The importance is that the segmental proliferative changes that are usually present in the rectum or sigmoid should not be mistaken for adenocarcinoma.[25] On barium enema a narrowed irregular lumen is seen (Fig. 19-11). The cysts may produce intraluminal filling defects. *Solitary rectal ulcer syndrome* is a localized abnormality in the rectum that has both a polypoid and an ulcerative phase[8,10] and may produce stricture. Treatment is palliative, and it is important not to confuse this process with neoplasm. *Solitary colonic ulcers* occur in areas other than the rectum; because of associated spasm and fibrosis, the lumen is narrow so it can simulate an annular carcinoma.[13,31] Colonoscopy is valuable in distinguishing these lesions and avoiding laparotomy. Spontaneous healing may occur, but bleeding and perforation requiring resection have been reported.

Table 19–1. Radiographic Characteristics of Ulcerative and Granulomatous Colitis

ULCERATIVE COLITIS	GRANULOMATOUS COLITIS
Involves rectum	Frequently spares rectum
Continuous disease	May have normal skipped areas
Minimal "backwash" ileal changes	Frequent ileal disease
Colonic shortening may occur	Bowel shortening is unusual
Circumferential bowel involvement	Eccentric bowel involvement
Sinus tracts and fistulas are rare	Fistulas and sinus tracts may occur
Shallow ulcers	Deep ulcers
May have free peritoneal perforation	Free perforation is rare

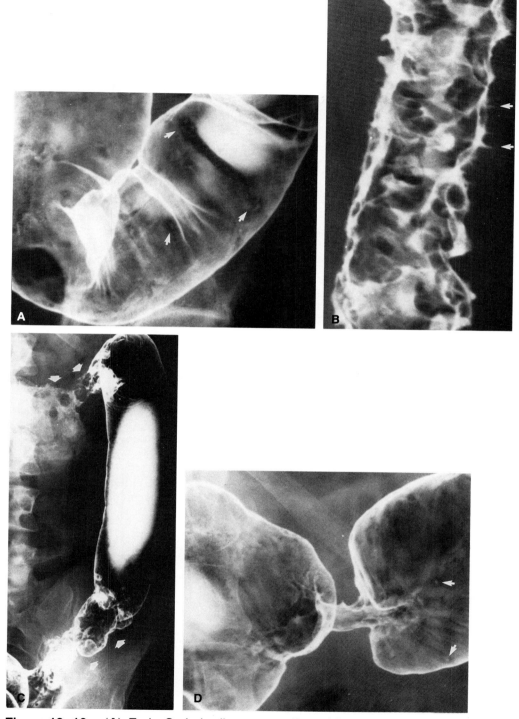

Figure 19–10. (**A**) Early Crohn's disease manifested by numerous small aphthous ulcerations (*arrows*). (**B**) Advanced Crohn's disease. Deep penetrating ulcers of the lateral wall ("Rose-thorn" ulcerations) (*arrows*). (**C**) Crohn's disease shows two advanced areas of involvement (*arrows*) with long segment of relatively normal intervening colon. (**D**) Crohn's disease with short stricture that simulates adenocarcinoma. Reactivation of disease indicated by aphthous ulcerations (*arrows*).

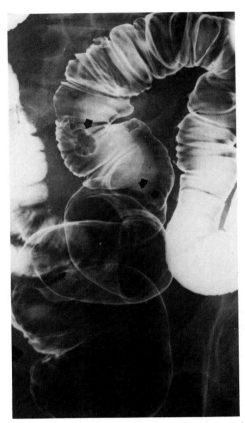

Figure 19–11. Colitis cystica profunda and adenomatous polyps. The irregularity on the right side of the rectum (*large arrow*) represents colitis cystica profunda. Multiple polyps are present proximal to this area (*arrows*).

MOTILITY DISORDERS

The contribution of radiologic methods to the diagnosis of spastic colon, constipation, incontinence, and diabetic diarrhea has been exclusion of other diseases. In scleroderma, wide-mouthed diverticula (sacculations) are seen as a characteristic finding but are unrelated to colonic motility (Fig. 19-12).

VASCULAR DISEASE

NECROTIZING ENTEROCOLITIS

Increasing survival rates of premature infants has led to more cases of necrotizing enterocolitis. It is proposed that this condition is caused by poor perfusion of the bowel wall. Pathologic changes range from mucosal ulcerations to transmural necrosis. Radiologic findings start with intestinal distention followed by gas in the bowel wall and then evidence of bowel perforation (Fig. 19-13). Contrast studies usually are not necessary because laparotomy is done only if perforation occurs. This can usually be detected by finding free air in the peritoneal space.

ISCHEMIC COLITIS

Poor perfusion of the colon in adults can cause intramural edema and hemorrhage. The process usually results in some mucosal necrosis as well. Bright red rectal bleeding is the common presenting symptom. Barium studies are characteristic. The intramural hemorrhage distorts the inner colonic contour and creates a thumbprint pattern (Fig. 19-14A,B). Ischemic colitis usually is completely reversible, but occa-

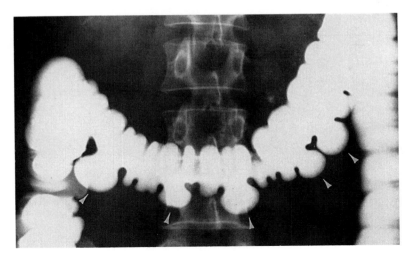

Figure 19–12. Scleroderma. Numerous large sacculations (*arrowheads*) seen only in scleroderma.

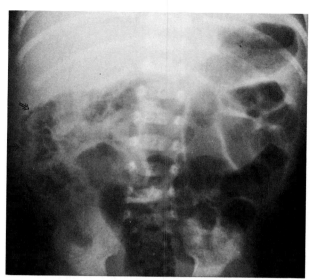

Figure 19–13. Necrotizing enterocolitis. The linear gas collection (*arrows*) in the wall of the ascending colon is a manifestation of a loss of mucosal integrity.

sionally the damage is severe enough to result in a smooth stricture. Transcatheter embolization, vasopressin therapy, and ethanol infarction of other abdominal organs have all been associated with colonic ischemia.[7, 24, 34]

FOREIGN BODIES

In what can be characterized as deviant behavior, miscellaneous foreign bodies are introduced into the rectum. Many of these objects are radiopaque (vibrators, bottles) and can be recognized on plain films. The rectum is also a site used by drug smugglers, and radiographs at the customs stations are often diagnostic; the condoms usually used are visible on plain films.

DIVERTICULOSIS AND DIVERTICULITIS

The low-residue diet associated with the refined grain products customarily consumed today is blamed for the high incidence of colonic diverticulosis. Despite almost universal diverticulosis in the older population, the incidence of diverticulitis is not very high. Infec-

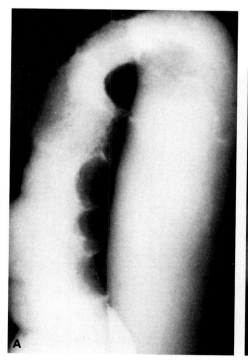
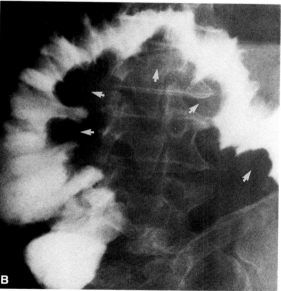

Figure 19–14. (**A**) Ischemic colitis. Thumbprinting of distal transverse colon represents early stage of ischemic colitis. (**B**) Ischemic colitis. Large thumbprinting is seen in ascending and transverse colon segments (*arrows*).

tion is a common complication, however, which leads to diverticulitis. The diagnosis of diverticulitis can usually be made on clinical grounds, but if necessary the imaging methods can demonstrate both intraluminal and extraluminal changes. With barium, evidence of an extrinsic mass narrowing the lumen is the most common observation (Fig. 19-15). Occasionally, a sinus tract from the colon to the pericolonic mass will be seen. Rarely, a fistula to the bladder or uterus can be demonstrated. Direct communication of the ruptured diverticulum with the mesenteric veins has been observed. Both ultrasonography and CT confirm the existence and extent of the inflammatory reaction around the colon.[21] The diagnosis and treatment of diverticulitis have been improved remarkably by CT examination. CT should be the initial examination when the clinical features are atypical for sigmoid diverticulitis.[6, 30] The usual site for diverticulitis is the sigmoid colon, but any part of the colon may be involved. One of the problems in diagnosis is distinguishing an annular carcinoma from diverticulitis; when that cannot be done radiographically it is important to obtain a biopsy. All series of colonic carcinoma contain cases that were originally diagnosed as diverticulitis. The giant sigmoid diverticulum is an unusual variant,[23] which likely represents an old diverticular abscess that has spontaneously drained into the colon but remains open. Giant sigmoid diverticula will be filled with gas on the plain film and may fill with barium at the time of the enema (Fig. 19-16). Often they are asymptomatic.

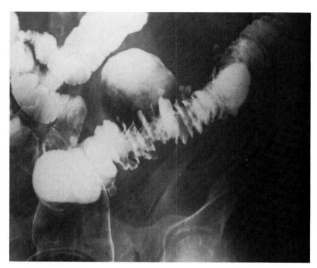

Figure 19–16.   Giant sigmoid diverticulum.

NEOPLASMS

Benign Polyps. Both adenomatous and hyperplastic polyps occur frequently in the colon. Inflammatory polyps are rarely larger than 5 mm, whereas adenomatous polyps can attain a size of several centimeters. Because evidence suggests that adenomatous polyps can become adenocarcinomas, it is important to

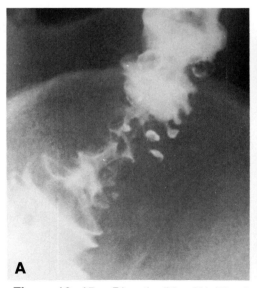
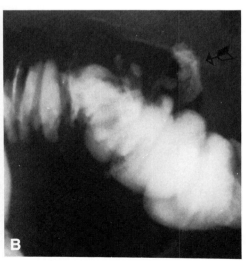

Figure 19–15.   Diverticulitis. (**A**) The intramural inflammatory process causes a localized narrowing of the lumen of the sigmoid colon. (**B**) The diverticular abscess (*arrow*) is filled at the time of the barium enema.

find and remove these lesions. Air-contrast study of the colon is the most sensitive radiographic examination in finding polyps (Fig. 19-17 A through D).

Polyposis Syndromes. Familial colonic polyposis (Fig. 19-18 A through C) and the variant associated with soft-tissue tumors (Gardner's syndrome) are of most serious consequence.[5] Malignancy of the colon develops in individuals usually before age 30. There is also a less well-defined group that has multiple polyps but the number of polyps is much less than in familial polyposis. Colon cancer is not inevitable in this group and develops later in life. The rare combination of intracerebral tumors (usually glioblastomas) and colon polyps is called Turcot syndrome. Colon polyps are found in both the *Peutz-Jeghers* (hamartomas) and the *Cronkhite-Canada* (Juvenile polyp histology) syndromes (see Chap. 18).

Juvenile Polyps. Hamartomatous polyps that may cause bleeding or intussusception can occur in children (Fig. 19-19). These lesions have no malignant poten-

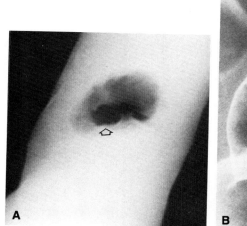

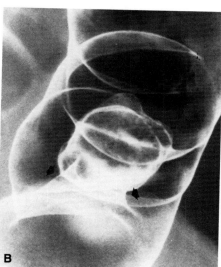

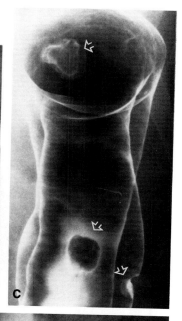

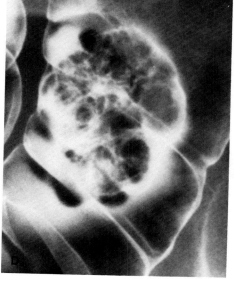

Figure 19–17. **(A)** Adenomatous polyp. Single-contrast enema shows moderate-size filling defect with central dark area representing polyp's stalk (*open arrow*). **(B)** Adenomatous polyp. Moderate-size adenomatous polyp seen en face with stalk clearly delineated (*black arrows*). **(C)** Multiple adenomatous polyps (*arrows*). **(D)** Villous adenoma. A variety of adenomatous polyps represented by large polypoid mass with ill-defined irregular surface pattern.

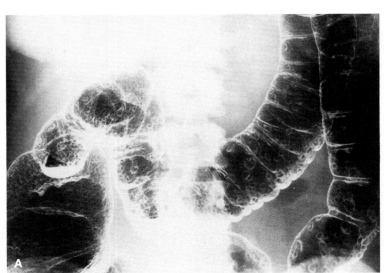

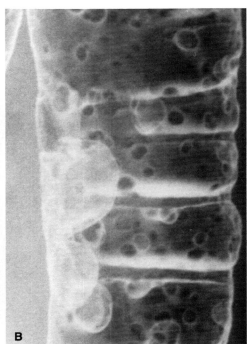

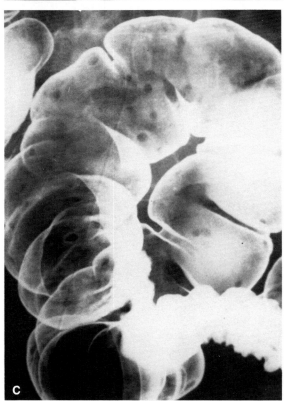

Figure 19–18. (**A**) Familial polyposis. Entire mucosa carpeted with varying size polyps. (**B**) Familial polyposis. Magnified view shows variation in size of familial polyps. (**C**) Gardner's syndrome. Numerous small polyps scattered throughout the mucosa. Note the decreased number of polyps compared with familial polyposis.

tial, so removal is not necessary unless bleeding becomes a problem.

Lymphoid Hyperplasia. Double-contrast studies of the colon can demonstrate slightly enlarged lymphoid follicles on the colonic mucosal surface (Fig. 19-20). They are seen most frequently on the right side of the colon,[22] and their clinical significance is unknown. Although there is some speculation that they are reactive changes related to inflammation of the colon, they can be seen in patients without symptoms.

Intramural Tumors. In the colon lipomas are the most common type of mesenchymal tumor (Fig. 19-21). Lipomas may be quite large, and the extraluminal aspect may predominate. In addition to characteris-

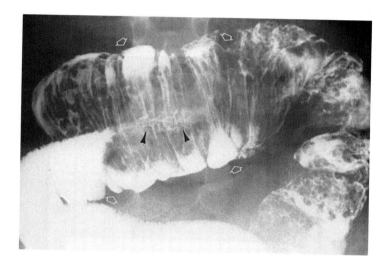

Figure 19–19. Ileocolic intussusception caused by a benign polyp. Intussusceptum (*black arrowheads*) and intussuscipiens (*open arrows*).

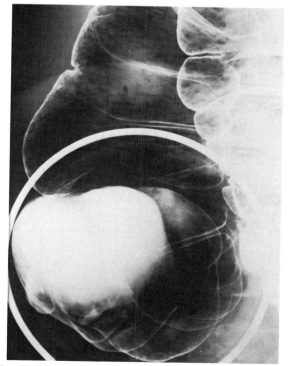

Figure 19–20. Benign nodular lymphoid hyperplasia in the ascending and transverse colon.

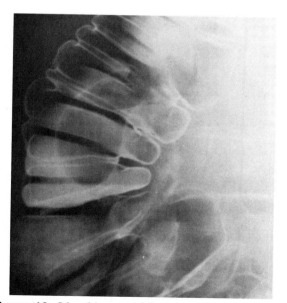

Figure 19–21. Lipoma of the ascending colon. This large smooth mass without ulceration suggests an intramural lesion. CT has been successful in identifying the fatty nature of these colonic masses.

tic barium studies outlining a submucosal mass, CT can prove that the tumor is composed of fat.[20, 32] Multiple fatty tumors may occur.

Adenocarcinoma. There are about 150,000 new cases of carcinoma of the colon and rectum reported each year. There is an adenoma-to-cancer sequence that takes several years to develop. The polyp spreads at its base, ulcerates, and may surround the bowel and eventually obstruct it. The radiographic diagnosis can be made at any of these stages (Fig. 19-22A through D). Computed tomography is of value in detecting spread

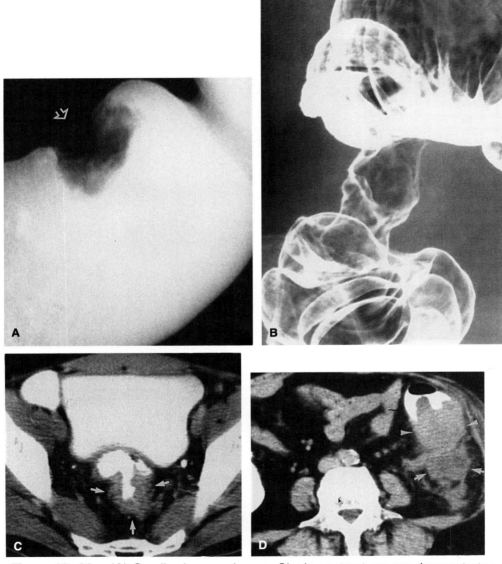

Figure 19–22. (**A**) Small adenocarcinoma. Single-contrast enema demonstrates an irregular polypoid mass that shows wall invasion (*arrow*). (**B**) Adenocarcinoma. Double-contrast enema demonstrates "apple-core" lesion consistent with advanced infiltrating carcinoma. (**C**) Adenocarcinoma. CT examination of rectum shows infiltrating mass (*arrows*) representing adenocarcinoma. (**D**) Adenocarcinoma with recurrence. CT examination shows large mass lesion in left colon (*arrowheads*) with marked extension away from recurrence into pericolic tissues (*arrows*).

to the lymph nodes and liver as well as showing the local extent of the primary lesion.[11] The sensitivity, specificity, and accuracy for staging primary carcinoma varies 48% to 100%. The mean accuracy in detecting recurrent tumor is 90%.[44] Because synchronous carcinomas exist in about 4% of cases, a thorough search of the colon for other filling defects is essential. Rarely, scirrhous carcinoma can involve the colon. This tumor spreads longitudinally as well as around the lumen, producing an elongated area of narrowing. Often the mucosal surface is normal in a portion of the lesion.

Non-Hodgkin's Lymphoma. Lymphoma of the colon can be a primary process. Frequently, the radiographic appearance is no different from that of adenocarcinoma. It can be multinodular and involve the entire colon (lymphomatous polyposis) (Fig. 19-23A, B).[46] Also, it may be solitary and resembles a polypoid carcinoma.

Extrinsic Neoplasm. Any of the malignant tumors of the genitourinary tract, including the kidneys, may invade the colon. Direct extension of gastric and pancreatic tumors down the mesentery of the transverse colon creates an identifiable contour change, often a fixed irregularity. Endometriosis is another condition that can involve the wall of the pelvic colon. Rarely there will be rectal bleeding in synchrony with menstruation so that the diagnosis can be made or suspected. Usually, some narrowing of the colon at the site of the lesion is observed. The mucosa is intact, so the narrowing is smooth and often tapered. At times it may resemble annular carcinoma, however. A local endometrioma resembles any other submucosal mass (Fig. 19-24). The lesions are usually in the lower sigmoid colon or rectum.

Appendiceal Tumors. A chronically obstructed non-inflamed appendix may dilate and fill with mucus. This

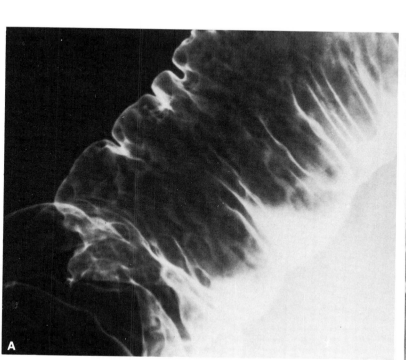
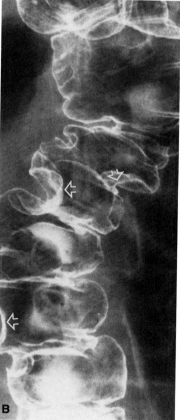

Figure 19–23. (**A**) Non-Hodgkin's lymphoma. The nodular pattern is similar to benign nodular hyperplasia, but the nodules are larger. Slight umbilication of these nodules is manifested by the barium collections at the center of the filling defects. (**B**) Lymphomatous polyposis. Scattered large polypoid masses of the right colon (*arrows*).

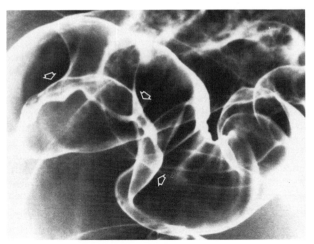

Figure 19–24. Endometriosis. Double-contrast enema shows large mass infiltrating the wall and protruding into the lumen (*open arrows*).

appendiceal mucocele is often caused by a low-grade adenocarcinoma. Occasionally, the contents of the mucocele may calcify (myxoglobulosis). Carcinoid tumors of the appendix are most often discovered by the pathologist sectioning an appendix removed for inflammation. The appendix is an unusual site for a malignant carcinoid tumor.

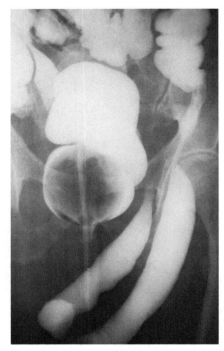

Figure 19–25. Inguinal hernia. The sigmoid colon frequently will be found in left inguinal hernias.

HERNIAS

Because the sigmoid and transverse portions of the colon are on a long mesentery, they are the segments that are involved in hernias. The transverse colon may normally move to a position between the right hemidiaphragm and liver, and if there is a defect in the diaphragm it can herniate into the chest. Morgagni's hernia is more common and results from an anterior defect in the diaphragm. The transverse colon may also enter the thorax by way of the esophageal hiatus. Anterior abdominal wall incisional hernias may contain colon. The sigmoid colon seemingly has a penchant for left inguinal hernias (Fig. 19-25), which must be reduced before barium enema, because distention of the colon in the hernial sac may prevent retrograde passage of barium to the remaining colon. The spigelian hernia associated with the defect in the fascia of the rectus muscle laterally may contain sigmoid colon. The colon herniates through the transverse and internal oblique muscles, but is contained by the external oblique, so may not be palpable.

PNEUMATOSIS COLI

A striking radiographic appearance is created with multiple, small air cysts in the colon (Fig. 19-26). The etiology is unknown, and it is benign and self-limited. Treatment with 100% oxygen may help resolve the cysts but is probably unnecessary.

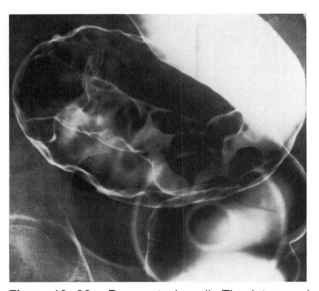

Figure 19–26. Pneumatosis coli. The intramural collections of gas indent the lumen but are easily identifiable as gas (*arrows*) rather than soft-tissue masses.

TRAUMA

Because the colon is more fixed in position than the small bowel, it is also more prone to rupture secondary to blunt trauma. The rectum may also be damaged by impalement. These circumstances mandate the use of water-soluble contrast material when studying the colon.

IATROGENIC CONDITIONS

Catheter Therapy. Both catheter embolization and infusion of vasopressin to halt colonic bleeding have been associated with ischemia and infarction. Similarly, the colon has been damaged when ethanol infarction of a renal cell or other carcinoma resulted in reflux of the agent into the aorta.

Surgical Anastomoses. Colocolic surgical anastomoses are not initially water tight, and gross disruption can occur, particularly in rectal anastomoses after anterior colonic resection. Strictures at anastomotic sites are unusual, but a diaphragmlike obstruction has been reported following a stapled anastomosis in the rectosigmoid region.

Ileoanal Reservoirs. The principles of the continent ileostomy have now been applied to the anal area in an attempt to avoid an anterior ostomy. The anatomy and function of these reservoirs can be easily studied with either barium or water-soluble contrast material (Fig. 19-27).

Rectal Perforation Associated With Barium Enema. Rectal perforation still occurs occasionally with barium enemas despite the use of soft catheter material.[19, 33] Balloon retention catheters can also be responsible for a perforation. Extreme care must be exercised not to inflate the balloon beyond the size of the rectal ampulla. If perforation occurs above the peritoneal reflection, surgical repair is usually necessary to decrease morbidity and mortality. Therefore, early diagnosis of extravasation of barium or air into the peritoneal cavity is very important.

Toxic Megacolon. A hugely distended colon was first observed as a very serious complication of idiopathic ulcerative colitis (Fig. 19-28). It has also been seen in granulomatous colitis. A patient whose psoriasis was being treated with methotrexate developed an acute megacolon that took almost 3 weeks to resolve.[1] It

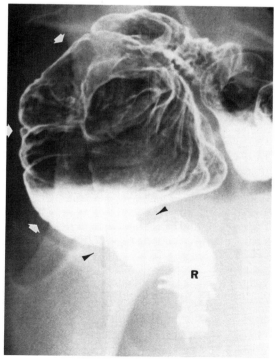

Figure 19–27. Ileoanal-ileorectal reservoir. Double-contrast enema shows ileal reservoir (*white arrows*) and the ileoanal reservoir–rectal anastomoses (*black arrowheads*). *R*, rectum.

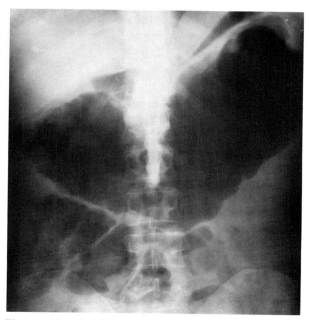

Figure 19–28. Toxic megacolon. Plain film of abdomen shows markedly widened transverse colon with nodular margins in patient with acute ulcerative colitis.

seems likely that other chemotherapeutic agents could cause a similar syndrome. Introduction of any contrast material into the colon in these conditions is contraindicated because of the danger of perforation. Patients with colonic ileus (Ogilvie's syndrome) will have similar radiographic features, but their clinical course is more benign.[2] In colonic ileus, contrast studies are not contraindicated and are of value in excluding mechanical colonic obstruction.

REFERENCES AND SELECTED READINGS

1. ATHERTON LD, LEIB ES, KAYE MD: Toxic megacolon associated with methotrexate therapy. Gastroenterology 86:1583, 1984

2. BACHULIS BL, SMITH PE: Pseudo-obstruction of the colon. Am J Surg 136:66, 1978

3. BRODEY PA, FERTIG S, ARON JM: Campylobacter enterocolitis: Radiographic features. Am J Roentgenol 139:1199, 1982

4. BURRELL MI, HYSON EA, SMITH GJW: Spontaneous clostridial infection and malignancy. Am J Roentgenol 134:1153, 1980

5. BUSSEY HJR, VEALE AMO, MORSON BC: Genetics of gastrointestinal polyposis. Gastroenterology 74:1325, 1978

6. CHO KC, MOREHOUSE HT, ALTERMAN DD, ET AL: Sigmoid diverticulitis: Diagnostic role of CT—comparison with barium enema studies. Radiology 176:111, 1990

7. COX GG, LEE KR, PRICE HI, ET AL: Colonic infarction following ethanol embolization of renal-cell carcinoma. Radiology 145:343, 1982

8. FECZKO PJ, O'CONNELL DJ, RIDDELL RH, ET AL: Solitary rectal ulcer syndrome: Radiologic manifestations. Am J Roentgenol 135:499, 1980

9. FEDYSHIN P, KELVIN FM, RICE RP: Nonspecificity of barium enema findings in acute appendicitis. Am J Roentgenol 143:99, 1984

10. FORD MJ, ANDERSON JR, GILMOUR HM, ET AL: Clinical spectrum of the "solitary ulcer" of the rectum. Gastroenterology 84:1533, 1982

11. FREENY PC, MARKS WM, RYAN JL, ET AL: Colorectal carcinoma evaluation with CT: Preoperative staging and detection of postoperative recurrence. Radiology 158:347, 1986

12. FRICK MP, MAILE CW, CRASS JR, ET AL: Computed tomography of neutropenic colitis. Am J Roentgenol 143:763, 1984

13. GARDINER GA, BIRD CR: Nonspecific ulcers of the colon resembling annular carcinoma. Radiology 137:331, 1980

14. GEDGAUDAS-McCLEES RK: Aphthoid ulcerations in ileocolic candidiasis. Am J Roentgenol 141:973, 1983

15. GELFAND DW, CHEN MYM, OTT DJ: Preparing the colon for the barium enema examination. Radiology 178:609, 1991

16. GOLDSTEIN SJ, MACKENZIE CROOKS DJ: Colitis in Behçet's syndrome. Radiology 128:321, 1978

17. GOODELL SE, QUINN TC, MKRTICHIAN E, ET AL: Herpes simplex virus proctitis in homosexual men. N Engl J Med 308:868, 1983

18. GORE RM: CT of inflammatory bowel disease. Radiol Clin North Am 27:717, 1989

19. HAN SY, TISHLER JM: Perforation of the colon above the peritoneal reflection during the barium-enema examination. Radiology 144:253, 1982

20. HEIKEN JP, FORDE KA, GOLD RP: Computed tomography as a definitive method for diagnosing gastrointestinal lipomas. Radiology 142:409, 1982

21. HULNICK DH, MEGIBOW AJ, BALTHAZAR EJ, ET AL: Computed tomography in the evaluation of diverticulitis. Radiology 152:491, 1984

22. KENNEY PJ, KOEHLER RE, SHACKELFORD GD: The clinical significance of large lymphoid follicles of the colon. Radiology 142:41, 1982

23. KRICUN R, STASIK JJ, REITHER RD, ET AL: Giant colonic diverticulum. Am J Roentgenol 135:507, 1980

24. LAMBERT M, DE PEYER R, MULLER AF: Reversible ischemic colitis after intravenous vasopressin therapy. JAMA 247:666, 1982

25. LEDESMA-MEDINA J, REID BS, GIRDANY BR: Colitis cystica profunda. Am J Roentgenol 131:529, 1978

26. LUSK LB, REICHEN J, LEVINE JS: Aphthous ulceration in diversion colitis. Gastroenterology 87:1171, 1984

27. MARTINEZ CR, GILMAN RH, RABBANI GH, ET AL: Amebic colitis: Correlation of proctoscopy before treatment and barium enema after treatment. Am J Roentgenol 138:1089, 1982

28. MILLER VE, HAN SY, WITTEN DM: Reticular mosaic (urticarial) pattern of the colonic mucosa in yersinia colitis. Radiology 146:307, 1983

29. MUNYER TP, MONTGOMERY CK, THOENI RF, ET AL: Postinflammatory polyposis (PIP) of the colon: The radiologic-pathologic spectrum. Radiology 145:607, 1982

30. NEFF CC, VAN SONNENBERG E: CT of diverticulitis diagnosis and treatment. Radiol Clin North Am 27:743, 1989

31. ONA FV, ALLENDE HD, VIVENZIO R, ET AL: Diagnosis and management of nonspecific colon ulcer. Arch Surg 117:888, 1982

32. ORMSON MJ, STEPHENS DH, CARLSON HC: CT recognition of intestinal lipomatosis. Am J Roentgenol 144:313, 1985

33. PETERSON N, ROHRMANN CA JR, LENNARD ES: Diagnosis and treatment of retroperitoneal perforation complicating the double-contrast barium-enema examination. Radiology 144:249, 1982

34. ROSENKRANTZ H, BOOKSTEIN JJ, ROSEN RJ, ET AL: Post embolic colonic infarction. Radiology 142:47, 1982

35. RUBESIN SE, LEVINE MS, GLICK SN,, ET AL: Pseudomembranous colitis with rectosigmoid sparing on barium studies. Radiology 170:811, 1989

36. RUDIKOFF JC: Clostridium-produced gas gangrene of the colon. Radiology 124:26, 1977

37. SCHAAF RE, JACOBS N, KELVIN FM, ET AL: Clostridium septicum infection associated with colonic carcinoma and hematologic abnormality. Radiology 137:625, 1980

38. SCOTT RL, PINSTEIN ML: Diversion colitis demonstrated by double-contrast barium enema. Am J Roentgenol 143:767, 1984

39. SEAMAN WB, CLEMENTS JL JR: Urticaria of the colon: A nonspecific pattern of submucosal edema. Am J Roentgenol 138:545, 1982

40. SHAH SJ, SCHOLZ FJ: Anorectal herpes: Radiographic findings. Radiology 147:81, 1983

41. SHAO-RU C, TISNADO J, LIU C, ET AL: Bleeding cytomegalovirus of the colon: Barium enema and angiography. Am J Roentgenol 136:1213, 1981

42. SIDER L, MINTZER RA, MENDELSON EB, ET AL: Radiographic findings of infectious proctitis in homosexual men. Am J Roentgenol 139:667, 1982

43. STANLEY RJ, TEDESCO FJ, MELSON GL, ET AL: The colitis of Behçet's disease: A clinical-radiographic correlation. Radiology 114:603, 1975

44. THOENI RF: CT evaluation of carcinomas of the colon and rectum. Radiol Clin North Am 27:731, 1989

45. URSO FP, URSO MJ, LEE CH: The cathartic colon: Pathological findings and radiological/pathological correlation. Radiology 116:557, 1975

46. WILLIAMS SM, BERK RN, HARNED RK: Radiologic features of multinodular lymphoma of the colon. Am J Roentgenol 143:87, 1984

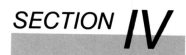

The Urinary and Female Genital Tracts

Paul and Juhl's Essentials of Radiologic Imaging, Sixth Edition, edited by John H. Juhl and Andrew B. Crummy. J.B. Lippincott Company, Philadelphia, © 1993.

CHAPTER **20**

The Urinary Tract

Fred T. Lee, Jr
John R. Thornbury

Introduction of new methods and enhancement of traditional radiologic methods have greatly influenced the use of imaging to diagnose and treat patients who have urinary tract disease. In the past, plain films of the abdomen and excretory urography were the starting point in the diagnostic imaging process. Today, computed tomography (CT), ultrasonography, or magnetic resonance imaging (MRI) may be requested initially. Choosing the appropriate method has become more complex because of the variety that confronts the physician.

If physicians think critically about the selection of patients before requesting an imaging examination, they can improve their use of such examinations.[47] First, the physician must hypothesize a differential diagnosis. Then, based on personal experience and knowledge of the literature and before deciding whether to request the examination, the physician should answer two questions.

1. Is this examination going to affect my diagnostic certainty about the differential diagnosis I am considering, and, if so, how much?
2. Will the information I expect to receive from this examination change my diagnostic thinking enough to affect my choice of treatment?

Particularly important is the action of linking the use of the diagnostic test to the choice of treatment.

The following paragraphs present the most frequently used (or most useful) examinations for the specific diagnostic problem situations that are discussed subsequently.

METHODS OF EXAMINATION

THE PLAIN-FILM ROENTGENOGRAM

Roentgenographic examination of the urinary tract should begin with a plain film of the abdomen, exposed with the patient in a supine position, that includes the kidneys and the ureteral and bladder areas. This "scout" film, which must be obtained before contrast medium is given for the excretory urogram, reveals the renal shadows and permits assessment of the size, shape, and position of the kidneys. The presence of calcium in cysts, tumors, or stones can be detected along with vascular or lymph node calcification in the area. Psoas muscle shadows are usually well outlined, and asymmetry or other abnormalities can be noted. The ureters cannot be defined, but radiopaque calculi may be detected along the course of the ureter. The shadow cast by the urinary bladder can often be identified. Vesical calculi can be outlined. Vascular calcifications, including phleboliths and arterial plaques, are frequently seen in the pelvis and must be differentiated from urinary calculi. Doing so may require other examinations, such as intravenous pyelography or even CT.

EXCRETORY UROGRAPHY

Preparation of the Patient

Excretory urography (intravenous pyelography), the most frequently used imaging examination for general assessment of the urinary tract, requires intravenous injection of radiopaque contrast material. Serial films are then obtained over 15 to 25 minutes as contrast is excreted by the kidneys for visualization of the renal collecting systems, ureters, and bladder. Patient preparation before an elective examination often involves bowel cleansing, with use of cathartics such as castor oil, senna preparations (X-Prep), or bisacodyl (Dulcolax). Catharsis is particularly helpful in bed-ridden patients to remove gas and fecal matter from the colon, both of which obscure the renal areas. In ambulatory patients, gas and feces are not as much of a problem.

Many variations of the approach just described are in use. Satisfactory urography often can be obtained with no preparation, particularly in ambulatory out-patients. There are situations in which adequate hydration is clearly important. In patients who have multiple myeloma, renal failure, or insulin-dependent diabetes mellitus, or in those who are critically ill (including neonates), the preparation is altered to fit each patient's needs, and dehydration is avoided.

Contrast Material

The contrast media are organic iodides that depend on their iodine content for radiopacity.[139] Currently there are two types of contrast material in use: ionic and nonionic. The former has been standard for more than 40 years and has been either diatrizoate or iothalamate medium. The low-osmolality, nonionic mediums were introduced in Europe for general use in the late 1970s. In 1986, after initial European experience and subsequent U.S. testing documented much lower toxicity, with decreased reaction rates (including deaths), the Food and Drug Administration approved two new nonionic mediums, iopamidol and iohexol, for intravascular and myelographic use.

Clinical experience[46, 75] indicates that the non-ionic mediums have overall reaction rates of about one third to one fourth that of the ionic mediums (3.13% vs 12.66%). Severe reactions for ionic agents were encountered in 0.22% of patients, and in 0.04% of patients given nonionic agents. The death rate generally considered representative by most experts for traditional ionic contrast agents intravenously injected is about 1 in 40,000.[5] Estimates for the non-ionic mediums are that the death rate may be as low as 1 in 168,000.[75]

For ionic contrast agents, a meglumine diatrizoate medium is often used in a dose of 0.5 ml per pound of body weight. Our method delivers 0.34 mg of iodine per kilogram of body weight, which is usually a satisfactory dose for patients with reasonably good renal function. These contrast agents are excreted almost entirely by glomerular filtration with very little, if any, tubular resorption of contrast. In children, dose ranges

have been recommended that are based on body surface area.[34] The upper limit of dose is 4ml/kg body weight for infants weighing less than 2.5 kg. Dose may be decreased in thin patients or increased in obese patients. A nomogram for dose determination has been provided by Diament and Kangerloo.[34]

In premature and newborn infants, relatively larger doses of contrast are required (up to 4 ml/kg body weight), which will enhance opacification of vascular and soft-tissue structures. It can therefore be used in the differential diagnosis of abdominal masses, both intrarenal and extrarenal. Currently, however, ultrasonography or CT (computed tomography) may be used initially to evaluate abdominal masses in premature and newborn infants.

Contraindications to intravenous urography include (1) hypersensitivity to the contrast agent, (2) the presence of combined renal and hepatic disease, (3) oliguria, (4) a serum creatinine level over 2.5 to 3.0 mg/100 ml, (5) diabetes mellitus (insulin dependent with renal insufficiency), and (6) multiple myeloma (unless the patient can be kept well hydrated during and after the study). All these contraindications are relative, and the value of potential information to be obtained must be weighed against the risk in each patient.

The urographic contrast media may produce reactions of varying severity.[5, 71, 106] Minor reactions are the most common, having an incidence of about 5% to 10% of injections using ionic contrast material. Incidence of minor reactions to nonionic agents is less by approximately a factor of 6.[75, 99] The most common signs and symptoms are urticaria, itching, nausea, and vomiting. These are usually self-limited, but on occasion may require antihistamine treatment for more comfortable recovery. Minor reactions are more common in patients having a history of allergy. It is not clear whether a history of minor reaction to a contrast medium causes that patient to be at significantly greater risk for a life-threatening major reaction from a subsequent injection.

Severe major reactions are rare with a reported incidence ranging from about 3 to 5 times the death rate. Reported death rates for ionic agents range from about 1 in 30,000 to 1 in 75,000. The Katayama study of nonionic agents reported an even lower severe reaction rate, 0.045%.[75] Major reactions most often feature sudden onset of cardiovascular collapse, which can rapidly progress to cardiac arrest if not promptly and successfully treated. Less frequently, respiratory system collapse or central nervous system disaster is the predominant feature initially and also can progress rapidly to death.

Unfortunately, the precise mechanism of these major reactions remains obscure. These reactions are clearly not classic antigen-antibody–type allergic reactions. Thus, there are no pretesting methods (including use of an intravenous test dose) that will identify patients who are likely to have a major reaction.[45] Some types of patients, however, seem to have an increased risk of severe reaction and death. Such patients include those with (1) prior severe reaction to contrast media, (2) asthmatics, (3) severe cardiac or renal disease, (4) hyperviscosity conditions (such as macroglobulinemia or multiple myeloma), (5) advanced dehydration, and (6) anxiety states.[86]

The radiologist should have a plan for response to a serious reaction. The equipment, the medication, and the personnel trained to manage severe reactions must be immediately available whenever and wherever contrast mediums are injected. If a major reaction appears to be developing, treatment should begin at once and an emergency call for skilled help should be made. Maintenance of an adequate airway is essential, and oxygen should be given in all major reactions. Table 20-1 indicates the various types of reaction and the method of treatment and lists the representative drugs and their doses.

The prophylactic use of drugs to decrease reaction risk is controversial. Some authors advise the prophylactic use of antihistamines in patients with a history of allergy, although there is no solid evidence to indicate that it has a definite value. In patients with asthma or severe allergy, prednisone in 30- to 50-mg doses for 3 days before the examination may be useful. A blinded, randomized study demonstrated the protective effect of 32 mg of methylprednisolone given 12 and 2 hours before contrast administration, and lack of protection from a single dose given 2 hours before injection.[89] It is important to realize, however, that prophylactic steroid treatment does not guarantee nonreaction.[23, 89]

Radiopaque contrast mediums also have a potential toxic effect on the kidney. The risk is very low in normal, healthy young adults but begins to increase slightly in elderly patients with otherwise normal (for age) renal function. By age 65, about one fourth of normally functioning nephrons have been destroyed by the aging process. Insulin-dependent diabetes mellitus, chronic renal parenchymal diseases (such as glomerulonephritis), shock from trauma or sepsis, renal ischemia, or other clinical problems with renal components (such as heart failure) considerably increase the risk of contrast-induced renal failure.[99] Such risk factors must be balanced against expected diagnostic value when one decides whether to request excretory urography.

Advanced Renal Failure. Until the advent of high-quality ultrasound imaging of the kidneys in the

Table 20–1. Acute Management of Anaphylaxis

REACTION: TREATMENT COURSE

Urticaria:
1. No treatment needed in most cases.
2. Diphenhydramine: 50 mg IV, IM, or PO, if severe.

Facial/laryngeal edema:
1. Evaluate airway. Intubate, if needed.
2. Epinephrine: 0.1–0.3 ml 1:1000 SQ; every 15 min × 3, prn (total of 1 mg).
   If patient does not respond, proceed to:
3. Cimetidine: 300 mg IV in D5W over 15 min.
4. Diphenhydramine: 50 mg IM or IV.

Bronchospasm:
1. O_2 2 l via nasal cannula or mask.
2. Epinephrine: 0.1–0.3 ml 1:1000 SQ; every 15 min × 3, prn (total of 1 mg).
   If patient does not respond, proceed to:
3. Aminophylline: 250 mg IV in D5W over 10–20 min, then 0.4–1.0 mg/kg/hr, prn; or terbutaline: 0.25–0.5 mg IM or SQ; and/or beta-agonist inhalers (i.e., metaproterenol or albuterol).
4. Cimetidine: 300 mg IV in D5W over 15 min.
5. Diphenhydramine: 50 mg IV or IM.

Severe hypotension:
1. Large volumes of isotonic fluid (i.e., 0.9% [normal] saline).
2. O_2 2 l via nasal cannula or mask.
   If patient does not respond, proceed to:
3. Epinephrine: 1–3 ml 1:10,000 IV or 1–3 ml added to 7–9 ml saline and given intratracheally, every 5–10 min × 3, prn.
   If patient does not respond, proceed to:
4. Cimetidine: 300 mg IV in D5W over 15 min.
5. Diphenhydramine: 50 mg IM or IV.
6. Dopamine: 2–20 µg/kg/min IV.
7. Atropine: 0.5–2.0 mg IV.

Note—Doses given are routinely used doses for an adult of average weight. Please see text for further discussion of suggested dose ranges. Steroids probably do not affect the acute course of an anaphylactic reaction, but can be given acutely and continued for 1–2 days (to prevent a recurrence of symptoms once the acute episode has been successfully treated). H1 and H2 antihistamines can be continued for 1–2 days after an acute reaction if symptoms do not completely subside or recur. With permission of authors and the American Roentgen Ray Society. From Cohen RH, et al. AJR 151:264, 1988.

mid-1970s, high-dose excretory urography was used to evaluate patients with moderate renal insufficiency. Tomography of the kidneys done at the time of urography produced roentgenograms that revealed even faintly opacified urine excreted by chronically diseased kidneys. The combined studies usually allowed one to determine the existence of obstruction and renal parenchymal atrophy, while eliminating the need for more risky, expensive retrograde pyelography that required cystoscopy. Reports of renal failure worsened by the nephrotoxicity of high-contrast doses,[139] along with the improving diagnostic quality of ultrasonography, quickly persuaded physicians and radiologists to abandon high-dose urography in favor of ultrasonography.

Ultrasonography has also replaced excretory urography in imaging of patients with renal failure to exclude hydronephrosis.[74] When renal failure is caused by obstruction, usually both kidneys are blocked, because a unilateral obstruction would leave a functioning contralateral kidney. Ultrasonography is very sensitive and specific in detection of chronic hydronephrosis, but serial examinations may have to be performed to exclude acute hydronephrosis. The renal size and cortical thickness can also be evaluated by ultrasonography. These parameters are important to the clinician because normal-sized kidneys may have a reversible cause, whereas small kidneys usually imply more chronic disease. The echogenicity of both kidneys is diffusely increased in medical renal disease, regardless of the specific etiology, although the sensitivity of this finding has been questioned.[121]

Nuclear medicine renal scintigraphy is also valuable in the work-up of renal failure. Renal blood flow, acute tubular necrosis, glomerular filtration rate, renal function, and obstructive or reflux nephropathy can all be evaluated with the appropriate radionuclide. When the cause and level of obstruction are still unclear, retrograde pyelography may be necessary, requiring cystoscopy for ureteral catheter placement.

Technique of Examination

Following intravenous injection of the contrast substance, it is desirable to obstruct the ureters slightly with an abdominal compression band. Doing so retains some opacified urine in the kidneys and produces better visualization of the pelvis and calyces. Compression is not advised in patients with urinary obstruction (eg, suspected acutely impacted ureteral calculus). In patients with known aortic aneurysms, the use of compression is unwise.

The first roentgenogram is obtained about 1 minute after injection and a second is obtained at 5 minutes. Decision about compression is made on review of the 5-minute roentgenogram. The compression band is then applied, and small frontal and oblique views of the kidneys are obtained at approximately 10 minutes. The compression band is released and a postrelease view of the abdomen is taken at about 15 minutes. We use tomography on most patients, usually between 1 and 5 minutes after injection of a bolus of contrast medium. A minimum of three tomographic cuts is obtained at 1-cm intervals. Additional tomograms are obtained as needed and each film is monitored as the examination progresses.

Alterations in the procedure are made when indicated. Additional exposures of the bladder area may be necessary in some instances. We obtain a postvoiding film of the bladder in patients older than 40 years of age, and in those with incontinence. Oblique films are of value in patients with suspected ureteral calculi and in those in whom questionable calyceal abnormalities are observed on anteroposterior films. When it is important to visualize the ureters, a film with the patient in right or left prone oblique position is useful, because the ureters fill better in the prone than in the supine position.

If excretion of contrast material is delayed, it may be necessary to obtain roentgenograms for periods up to several hours after injection. In patients with acute ureteral obstruction (eg, a ureteral calculus being passed), there is often a delay in excretion on the involved side. Delayed roentgenograms may show opacification of the renal pelvis and ureter down to the level of obstruction when the immediate roentgenograms will reveal only increased density of the renal parenchyma. In patients with decreased renal function, preliminary tomograms are necessary as a baseline with which to compare the faint opacification of renal parenchyma (nephrogram), or calyces and pelves. Calyceal appearance time is normally within 3 minutes after the contrast medium is injected. Several variations of this technique are used, such as hypertensive urography (see Renovascular Hypertension).

RETROGRADE PYELOGRAPHY

Retrograde pyelography, another method used in the examination of the upper urinary tract, is generally used when the excretory urogram has been unsatisfactory or inconclusive. Cystoscopy and catheterization of the ureters are necessary for this examination. Roentgenograms are obtained following direct instillation of contrast material into the pelves via the catheters. Mediums available for intravenous use are diluted to 20% or 30% and are then satisfactory for retrograde pyelography. Roentgenograms are obtained after 3 to 5 ml of a contrast medium are slowly introduced through the ureteral catheter into the renal pelvis. The catheters are withdrawn and another roentgenogram is obtained. Oblique views and delayed frontal views may also be necessary in some patients. The contrast medium may be injected by syringe or may be introduced by gravity with a vessel containing the medium no higher than 45 cm above renal level.

Care should be taken to avoid overdistending the collecting system because the high pressure may produce backflow into the renal tubules, interstitium, lymphatics, or veins. The chief advantage of retrograde pyelography is that a dense contrast substance can be injected directly under controlled pressure so that visualization is good. The extent of impairment of renal function that may be present does not influence the degree of visualization. Excretory urography is a simpler, less risky procedure because cystoscopy is not necessary.

RENAL ANGIOGRAPHY

There are several methods for the radiographic study of the renal arteries. The use of a vascular catheter, introduced percutaneously into the femoral artery by the Seldinger technique, permits wide variability in techniques. A midstream aortic injection is made first, using 40 to 60 ml of an organic iodide. This examination indicates the location and number of renal arteries and may define abnormal lumbar vessels in patients with metastatic tumor (Fig. 20-1A).

Selective renal arteriograms are then obtained by manipulation of the catheter tip under fluoroscopic control into the desired renal artery followed by injection of small amounts (10 to 15 ml of the opaque medium) into the artery. The advantage is dense opacification of the renal artery and its branches, which is needed in a detailed study of the vessels. The disadvantages are that a small accessory vessel may be missed, and multiple injections are required when multiple vessels are present. Simultaneous study of both renal arteries can be obtained by midstream aortic injection with the catheter tip above the orifices of the renal arteries. This method fills accessory arteries that may be present and provides simultaneous visualization, allowing comparison of the renal vessels on the normal and abnormal sides.

Rapid film changers are used, programmed to radiograph arterial, nephrographic, and venous phases of the examination. Magnification techniques may be used to study vascular detail in one or both kidneys. Epinephrine may be used to improve accuracy in the diagnosis of renal masses.[19] As a rule, normal vessels constrict while tumor vessels do not, making tumor identification easier. Inflammatory neovascularity tends to constrict slightly. Digital subtraction angiography has begun to replace traditional cut-film angiography and has the advantage of lower-contrast dose.

TRANSLUMBAR AORTOGRAPHY

This examination has been largely supplanted by the Seldinger technique of percutaneous transfemoral catheterization, which permits aortography and selective renal arteriography at the same time. The translumbar approach is used only in patients with advanced arteriosclerotic disease when transfemoral catheterization is hazardous or impossible. Following local anesthesia, a long needle is inserted directly into the abdominal aorta from a point just below the 12th rib on the left posteriorly. After making certain that the needle or catheter is in the aorta, contrast medium is

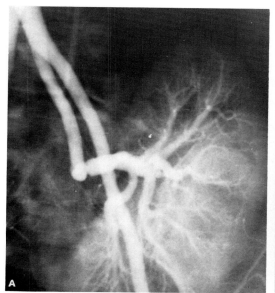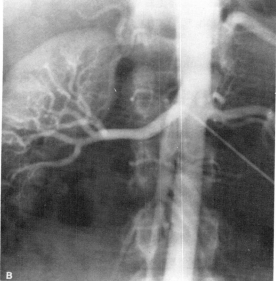

Figure 20–1. **(A)** Angiogram in the study of renal transplant. The percutaneous catheter technique was used to demonstrate the renal artery, which is anastomosed to the internal iliac artery. **(B)** Translumbar aortogram of a normal person. The needle tip is near the orifice of the right renal artery, which is well filled and clearly defined. There is some filling of the left renal, the splenic, the hepatic, and the superior mesenteric arteries as well as the aorta.

injected and roentgenograms are obtained using automatic changers (Fig. 20-1*B*).

RENAL VENOGRAPHY

Retrograde renal venography is performed by introducing a catheter into the femoral vein with the Seldinger technique, advancing the catheter through the vena cava into the main renal vein to the region of the point of division of segmental veins. The retrograde injection of contrast medium is not very effective because of the strong pressure of venous flow. Because of this, the patient is asked to perform the Valsalva maneuver during the injection to aid in retrograde flow of contrast. Amounts of about 20 ml of iodinated contrast are given over 2 to 3 seconds. Filming sequence varies with individuals, but digital subtraction techniques are now commonly employed. The examination is performed after a renal arteriogram has been secured so that the patency of the renal vein can be determined. Although they occur infrequently, renal vein valves may cause technical difficulty. Renal venography is used to assess inflammatory disease; to differentiate congenital absence of a kidney from a small, contracted, nonfunctioning kidney; to confirm the presence of renal vein thrombosis; and to detect avascular tumors. In other words, it may be used to make a definitive diagnosis when arteriography has failed to do so. Digital subtraction angiography is replacing the cut-film type of renal venography.

PERCUTANEOUS ANTEGRADE PYELOGRAPHY (PERCUTANEOUS NEPHROSTOMY)

A needle is placed percutaneously into the renal pelvis from a posterolateral approach, and either fluoroscopic or ultrasonic guidance is used. After a sample of urine is obtained for analysis, a contrast medium can be injected to evaluate the pelvocalyceal system and ureter. Subsequently, conventional percutaneous nephrostomy, brush biopsy, stent placement, stone dissolution or extraction, physiologic pressure-flow study, or dilatation of a stenosis can be performed using the access gained to the collecting system from the initial needle placement.

Percutaneous nephrostomy is most often used for emergency drainage of the obstructed upper urinary tract. For temporary, acute drainage, a standard percutaneous catheter with external drainage is effective. For chronic drainage, a Foley catheter or ureteral stent can be used. Percutaneous nephrostomy can also be used to introduce solutions such as sodium bicarbonate to dissolve uric acid stones. Using the percutaneous route, calculi can be treated by basket removal[8] or by the use of an ultrasonic lithotriptor. Percutaneous nephrostomy can provide palliation in patients with terminal neoplastic disease and has been used in renal transplants for diagnosis and therapy.

VOIDING CYSTOGRAPHY OR CYSTOURETHROGRAPHY

This examination is used in the study of patients suspected of having lower urinary tract obstruction or vesicoureteral reflux, and in children with persistent or recurrent urinary tract infection in whom vesicoureteral reflux is suspected. The examination consists of filling the bladder with radiopaque material to the point of urge to void, so that the voiding process subsequently can be imaged.

The patient is examined before, during, and after urination. Voiding cystography should be performed on unanesthetized patients who have not had recent instrumentation. Bladder filling is monitored as contrast is instilled. Image intensification fluoroscopy is necessary to obtain an adequate examination. In addition, spot film (70- or 90-mm or conventional spot films) are used to record the findings. The examination can be recorded on video tape if desired, because no additional radiation is used. Films are exposed with the patient in a lateral or an extreme posterior oblique position for best visualization of the bladder neck and urethra. If there is vesicoureteral reflux, films are obtained to show the amount and level of ascent of reflux, and also the size of the ureters and renal collecting systems.

CYSTOGRAPHY

Retrograde cystography is another method of studying the bladder. Following voiding, a urethral catheter is inserted and the bladder is filled with opaque contrast material. Rarely, a small amount of contrast medium is absorbed from the bladder. Among the indications for cystography are the study of trauma victims with suspected bladder rupture, and patients with bladder tumors, diverticula, or calculi. Ultrasonography of the bladder in many situations now has largely supplanted cystography.

COMPUTED TOMOGRAPHY

Initially, a scout film of the abdomen and pelvis is obtained by incrementally moving the patient through the CT scanner. The approximate locations of the kidneys (from T12 to L3), the ureters, and the bladder can be estimated from the scout view. The kidneys are usually scanned with contiguous 1-cm sections during partial expiration with the patient supine. Scans without intravenous contrast allow detection of renal or ureteral calculi. Enhanced scans utilizing a bolus injection of 50 to 100 ml of a 60% contrast agent are useful to evaluate attenuation changes from a mass, inflammation, or ischemia; surrounding vascular anatomy; excretion into the pelvocalyceal system and ureter; and trauma to the kidney with extravasation. Such scans also enable one to differentiate parapelvic cysts from hydronephrosis. Thinner sections (1.5 to 5 mm) can be used to evaluate small lesions. Dynamic scanning can also be useful, especially in evaluating the renal vessels or the vascularity of a mass.

The bladder can be evaluated using the low attenuation of urine as an in situ contrast agent. To obtain better distention of the bladder, a Foley catheter can be inserted and sterile saline or water introduced. Alternatively, air or CO_2 can be introduced via the Foley catheter with the patient placed in a position so that the air is adjacent to the region of abnormality. Intravenous contrast should still be given at some point to identify the ureters.

ULTRASONOGRAPHY

The kidneys can usually be adequately imaged with real-time, high-resolution sector scanners. The right kidney can be scanned in a supine or decubitus position (left side down) with longitudinal, transverse, and coronal images. The left kidney can be imaged in the supine or decubitus position (right side down) with similar views. Occasionally, a prone position may prove useful. The best images are obtained with the patient's respiration suspended; frequently, the end of partial or full inspiration brings the kidney into better view. A 5-MHz transducer is preferable to optimize resolution. If this does not provide adequate acoustic penetration, a 3.5-MHz transducer can be used. Duplex and color Doppler technology is becoming increasingly available and can be used to assess renal vasculature. This is particularly important in the evaluation of the renal transplant patient. This will be discussed in greater detail in a subsequent section.

In cases of hydronephrosis, it may be difficult to follow dilated ureters to the point of obstruction. Varying the patient's position may provide a better view along with imaging in coronal, longitudinal, or oblique planes. The distal ureters often can be visualized through a full bladder. The distended bladder is optimally viewed from a suprapubic approach with the patient supine. Transrectal transducers can also be used, especially to view the bladder neck, distal ureters, and prostate. When the suprapubic approach is used, the gain should be adjusted so that there are no echoes within the bladder.

RENAL SCINTIGRAPHY

The most common radionuclides used to image the kidney are technetium (Tc-99m) DTPA and iodine (I-131-hippuran). These are used to evaluate overall renal function. Renal perfusion and glomerular filtration can be assessed by Tc-99m-DTPA, and renal plasma flow and tubular function by I-131-hippuran. A new tubular agent, Tc-99m-Mertiatide has recently become available and can be used much like I-131-hippuran. The collecting systems can be evaluated by all of these radionuclides, although DTPA and Mertiatide are the preferred agents because of better imaging properties. Tc-99m-Glucoheptonate is an agent that can evaluate both glomerular and tubular function. Radionuclides such as Tc-99m-DMSA, which permit evaluation of renal cortical morphology are rarely used.

Intravenous injections consist of 10 to 15 mCi of Tc-99m-DTPA, and images are obtained by a gamma camera at 3-second intervals for approximately one half minute. These dynamic images allow evaluation of renal perfusion. Subsequent serial static images over the next 30 minutes with delayed views as needed allow assessment of renal function and the collecting systems.

For the hippuran renogram, 150 μCi of I-131-ortho-iodohippurate is injected intravenously with simultaneous gamma camera and computer acquisition over the next 30 minutes. Using a region of interest over renal parenchyma, one can generate a time activity curve (renogram) for each kidney. The renogram has three phases: (1) vascular phase, (2) cortical transit phase, and (3) excretory phase. Similar data can be obtained after injection of Mertiatide. The usual dose is 5 to 10 mCi injected intravenously.

A diuretic (Lasix) renogram is frequently performed, especially in children, to distinguish functional from mechanical obstruction. Intravenous administration of 1 mg/kg body weight of Lasix (children) and 20 mg (adults) is given when retention of activity is demonstrated within the renal pelvis. The renogram is most frequently performed with DTPA although Lasix can also be used with hippuran or Mertiatide.

A nonobstructed pelvocalyceal system (such as an extrarenal pelvis) will respond with a brisk diuresis and a decrease in radionuclide activity in the region of the pelvis. If a true mechanical obstruction is present, there will be no diuresis or change in radionuclide activity.

Renal transplants can be evaluated with a Tc-99m-DTPA perfusion study and an I-131-hippuran or Tc-99m-Mertiatide renogram with static images. Usually, a baseline study is obtained within the first day following the transplantation. Serial studies are then obtained as needed to evaluate transplant status.

ROENTGENOGRAPHIC ANATOMY

THE KIDNEY

The normal kidney is a bean-shaped structure that lies on either side of the lower thoracic and upper lumbar spine, usually between the upper border of the eleventh thoracic and the lower border of the third lumbar vertebrae. In the upright position, the kidney descends 2 or 3 cm. The right kidney lies approximately 2 cm lower than the left. Both move moderately with respiration and with change in position. The long axis is directed downward and outward, parallel to the lateral border of the psoas muscle on either side. In the lateral plane, the axis is directed downward and anteriorly, so that the lower pole is 2 to 3 cm anterior to the upper pole. When the patient is supine, the renal pelvis and proximal ureters lie well posterior to the anterior edge of the vertebral bodies (shown well on CT). At L3 the average ureter is three fourths of a vertebral width from the posterior vertebral margin. It then curves anteriorly to the level of the anterior vertebral border at L4; at L5 it is anterior to the vertebral body about one-fourth of the anteroposterior diameter of this vertebral body.

Normal renal size varies. Normal range of renal length in adults is 11 to 15 cm. The right kidney is usually shorter than the left, with an upper limit of a 1.5-cm variation in length. There is a relationship between vertebral body height and renal length. As a rule the kidney length is 3.7 ± 0.37 times the height of the second lumbar vertebra measured on the same film using the posterior margins of the vertebral body. According to Batson and Keats,[11] 97% of normal kidneys are within the range between the height of L1 through L3 and the height of L1 through L4. In children between 1½ and 14 years of age, the renal length is about equal to the length of the first four lumbar bodies including the three intervening disks + 1 cm. In infants the renal size is relatively greater. In children the normal difference in renal length on the two sides may be up to 1 cm.

There is some variation in renal shape, particularly on the left side. Fetal lobulations may persist on one or both sides, producing rather clearly defined indentations or notches along the lateral aspect of the kidney. The left kidney may be generally triangular in shape with a local bulge or convexity along the left midborder sometimes termed a *dromedary hump*. This may be related to the position of the spleen, may be a form of fetal lobulation, or may be both. The kidney is visualized in roentgenograms mainly because of the presence of perirenal fat. The increased radiolucency of fat makes the outline of the kidney stand out from the surrounding soft tissues. If there has been much wasting caused by chronic illness or malnutrition, the renal outlines may be very indistinct or completely invisible due to loss of perirenal fat. The kidneys are contained within the renal capsule and surrounded by perirenal fat, which is enclosed within Gerota's (perirenal) fascia. Perirenal hemorrhage, pus, or urine tend to be contained within this fascia and can be detected with CT or ultrasonography.

There are three anatomic spaces around each kidney: perirenal, anterior pararenal, and posterior pararenal (Fig. 20-2). The perirenal space is bounded by the anterior and posterior portions of the perirenal (Gerota's) fascia. The leaves of fascia fuse superiorly,

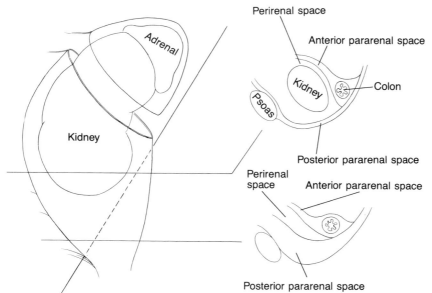

Figure 20–2. Anatomic spaces around the kidney. With permission of author and W.B. Saunders, Co., Philadelphia; Radiol Clin N Amer 17:323–324, 1979.

laterally, and medially, enclosing the kidney, adrenal gland, renal vasculature, and emerging portion of the proximal ureter. This fascial envelope is functionally open caudally to just above the pelvic brim. At that point it communicates with the caudal extent of the anterior and posterior pararenal spaces. The ureter emerges from the perirenal space about midlumbar spine level to course caudad in the anterior pararenal space and ultimately reach the bladder.

The anterior pararenal space is bound posteriorly by the anterior portion of the perirenal fascia, anteriorly by the posterior parietal peritoneum, and laterally by the lateral conal fascia. It contains the pancreas; the second, third, and fourth portions of the duodenum; the ascending and descending colon; and the vascular supply to the spleen, liver, pancreas, and duodenum. The posterior pararenal space is bound posteriorly by the transversalis fascia and anteriorly by the posterior portion of Gerota's fascia. It contains only fat and scattered vessels and nerves. All three spaces potentially communicate caudally near the bony pelvic brim. Thus, blood or an infected fluid collection in the perirenal space can track caudally and then involve either or both ipsilateral pararenal spaces (see Fig. 20-2).

THE URETERS

The ureters normally course downward from the most dependent portion of the pelves to the midsacral region, then turn posterolaterally and course in an arc downward and then inward and anteriorly to enter the trigone of the bladder on either side of the midline. Slight redundance is common, and alteration in size is frequently noted. Therefore, it is necessary to exercise care in making the diagnosis of ureteral stricture, displacement, or dilatation. There are three areas where normal narrowing of the ureter can be observed when it is filled with radiopaque material: the ureteropelvic junction, the ureterovesical junction, and the bifurcation of the iliac vessels. These are sites where calculi often lodge in the course of passage. A common normal variant is symmetric deviation medially of the ureters as they enter the bony pelvis. The narrower the bony pelvis, the more medial the position of the ureters.

THE BLADDER

The normal urinary bladder is transversely oval or round; the inferior aspect normally projects 5 to 10 mm above the symphysis pubis. Its floor parallels the superior aspect of the pubic rami, and its dome is rounded in the male and flat or slightly concave in the female due to the presence of the uterus above it. The size and shape of the normal bladder vary considerably. The internal aspect of the wall of the normal bladder is smooth as outlined by opaque material used in urography or cystography. The bladder is in a higher position in children than in adults and is slightly higher in males than in females. The bladder is relatively larger in children than in adults. A common normal variant is the anterior prolongation type, which results in a pear-shaped appearance.

THE NORMAL UROGRAM

The renal pelvis varies considerably in size and shape but is usually roughly triangular with the base parallel to the long axis of the kidney (Figs. 20-3 and 20-4). It may be conical with the apex contiguous to the upper ureter. The range of normal is wide; some pelves are long narrow tubes while others are large and globular. There is also a considerable variation in position of the pelvis in relation to the kidney. It may be almost completely within the renal outline (intrarenal) or almost completely extrarenal. The former is usually small, whereas the latter is large. The average normal pelvis is partially intrarenal and partially extrarenal. Bifurcation or duplication of the pelvis is very common and is considered an anatomic variant rather than a congenital anomaly.

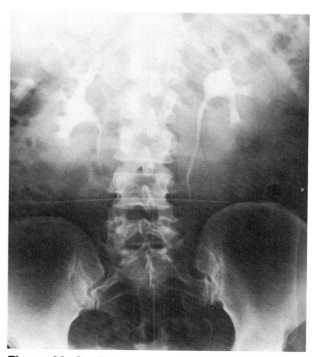

Figure 20–3. Intravenous urogram of a normal person showing good filling of the pelves, calyces, and ureters down to about the level of the compression device, the superior portion of which overlies the lower fourth lumbar vertebra.

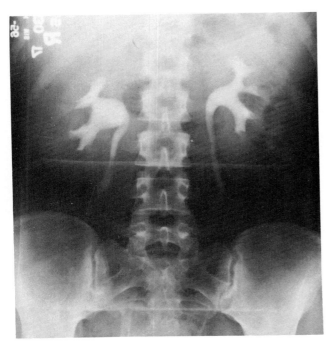

Figure 20–4. Intravenous urogram of a normal person. The use of compression has resulted in a little blunting of the calyceal fornices. Note that there is some asymmetry on the two sides.

The calyceal system consists of major calyces that begin at the pelvis and extend into the kidney to the junction with the minor calyces. Each major calyx may be divided into a base adjacent to the pelvis, and an infundibulum that is more or less tubular and extends from the base to the apex, or distal portion, from which one or more minor calyces project. The minor calyx consists of a body or a calyx proper, beginning at the junction with the major calyx, and the fornix that surrounds the conical renal papilla and into which the latter appears to project. The anatomic shape of the minor calyx is fairly constant, but since this structure is projected in various planes in the urogram there is considerable apparent variation. When viewed en face, it resembles a circular life preserver with a dense periphery and a relatively radiolucent center. In profile the appearance of a minor calyx is somewhat triangular with the apex of the triangle pointing toward the major calyx; the base is pointing away from it and is sharply concave or cupped. By contrast, there is marked variation in the shape of the major calyces, which can be long and narrow, or short and broad. There are usually two major calyces and 6 to 14 minor calyces, but the number can vary widely. The calyceal system is not always bilaterally symmetric, which makes interpretation difficult in some instances.

There is coordinated peristalsis that begins in the calyceal system of the kidneys. The collecting systems alternately fill and contract, activity that accounts for the variable appearance of the collecting system during intravenous urography. The discharge of urine from the pelvis into the ureter is accompanied by ureteral peristalsis. This occurs as broad waves at variable intervals (from 4 to 12 per minute). Ureteral peristalsis causes the ureter to have a variable caliber in different portions at the same time and a variation in contour in serial roentgenograms. The waves are visible as smooth areas of constriction or complete absence of filling that may separate one or more areas of slight dilatation. The effects of calyceal and ureteral peristalsis must be taken into account in the interpretation of excretory urograms.

Renal Backflow

The term *backflow* was initially applied to the escape of contrast material from the renal pelvis and calyces during retrograde pyelography as a result of an increase in intrapelvic pressure. The pressure is increased in excretory urography owing to osmotic diuresis and use of compression devices. Acute ureteral obstruction also results in increased intrapelvic pressure. Because similar phenomena occur in these instances, the term backflow has been carried over to describe changes observed in excretory urography. Backflow occurs in the normal kidney, and its recognition and differentiation from changes owing to disease of the kidney are therefore important.

There are two major types, pyelotubular and pyelointerstitial (pyelosinus). Pyelolymphatic and pyelovenous backflow are merely stages of the pyelointerstitial form. Pyelotubular backflow is the most frequent type; when it occurs during excretory urography it represents stasis in the tubules in the papilla rather than actual backflow. Roentgenographic findings consist of a brushlike tuft of opacity radiating into the papilla from the minor calyx (Fig. 20-5). Pyelointerstitial (pyelosinus) backflow begins with minute rupture (painless) of the fornix of a calyx, permitting the escape of contrast material or urine into the renal sinus, which is the loose adipose and connective tissue surrounding the pelvis and calyces and supporting a venous plexus. When the amount of extravasation increases it extends medially into the peripelvic area, into the perirenal fat within Gerota's fascia, and downward along the ureter. The extravasated material may enter the lymphatics to produce pyelolymphatic backflow. A much less common occurrence is pyelovenous backflow in which, presumably, the material enters the arcuate and other veins. Some investigators believe that the arcuate shadows observed in this condition are produced by

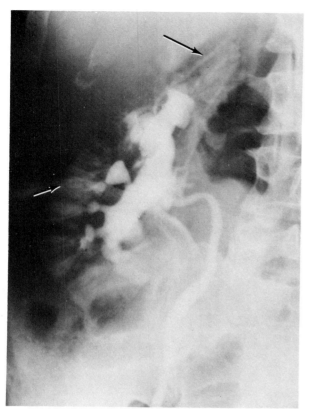

Figure 20–5. Backflow. This retrograde pyelogram shows a marked amount of pyelolymphatic backflow (*upper arrow*). Pyelotubular backflow is outlined (*lower arrow*). There is also some extravasation in the vicinity of the ureteropelvic junction representing interstitial backflow.

perivascular extension of pyelosinus extravasation, not by filling of the veins. All forms of backflow may be observed at one time (Fig. 20-5).

The roentgenographic findings in the early extravasation of the pyelointerstitial backflow consist of a hornlike projection of opaque medium extending from the fornix away from the papilla into the renal substance. As more material is extravasated it extends medially to the hilum and along the upper ureter, producing poorly defined densities in these areas. Pyelolymphatic backflow is manifested by opacification of lymphatic channels that extend from the hilum of the kidney medially toward the para-aortic nodes. These channels tend to be redundant, somewhat tortuous, and branched.

Extravasation of medium into the renal parenchyma also results when the catheter penetrates a calyx in retrograde pyelography. The roentgenographic ap-

pearance is variable, depending on the amount and distribution of the extravasated material.

Arterial and Venous Impressions

Arterial impressions or indentations on the renal pelvis and infundibula were found in 18% of 150 patients studied by Nebesar and colleagues.[111] They occur three times more often on the right than on the left. The most common site is the superior infundibulum on the right. The impressions consist of smooth transverse or oblique indentations on the infundibulum or pelvis. Most of the involved vessels are ventral to the collecting system. They usually cause no symptoms and are significant only in that they must be differentiated from pathologic processes (Figs. 20-6 and 20-7). Rarely, partial infundibular obstruction is produced, leading to dilatation of calyces and pain and occasionally to infection. Oblique as well as frontal projections are needed to make the diagnosis. Confirmation by angiography may be necessary when other causes are suspected. Occasionally a slightly tortuous renal artery, renal artery aneurysm, or bulbous renal vein simulating a renal sinus mass (pseudotumor) is observed, particularly on a tomogram. The appearance is that of a round or oval mass in the renal sinus that is usually recognized as vascular, but angiography may be needed for differentiation in some instances.

Venous impressions of the superior infundibulum are not as common as those produced by arteries. Urographic findings are quite characteristic[101] and include a wide, smooth filling defect of the proximal part of the superior infundibulum that is usually best shown on the prone film. Venography can be used to confirm the diagnosis but is seldom necessary. Real-time ultrasound is a simple noninvasive method for further assessing vascular impressions.

THE NORMAL CYSTOGRAM

The normal cystogram outlines the contrast-opacified urine in the smooth-walled, rounded, or oval bladder. The urinary bladder is usually filled to some extent during excretory urography, and this examination is often sufficient to outline gross lesions. When additional study of the bladder is needed, cystography is used (Fig. 20-8). Films are exposed in frontal, lateral, and oblique projections; if necessary, upright and postvoiding roentgenograms may be obtained.

COMPUTED TOMOGRAPHY, ULTRASONOGRAPHY, MAGNETIC RESONANCE IMAGING, AND RADIONUCLIDE ANATOMY OF THE KIDNEY

On CT the kidneys appear as elliptical or round soft-tissue structures of soft-tissue density with the central renal sinus predominantly composed of fat density.

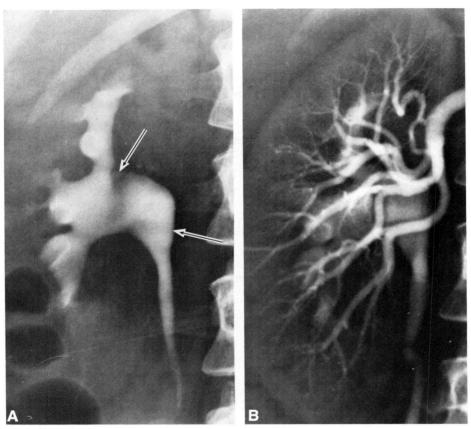

Figure 20–6. **(A)** Urogram showing arterial indentations producing a vertical lucency on the lateral aspect of the pelvis (*upper arrow*) and horizontal pelvic indentation (*lower arrow*). **(B)** Selective renal arteriogram, on the same patient shown in **A**, demonstrating the relationship of arteries to the indentations noted in **A**.

Because of the surrounding perirenal fat, the margin of each kidney is visible and should be smooth (Fig. 20-9). The cortex and medullary portions cannot be distinguished on unenhanced scans, but can be demarcated with a rapid intravenous bolus. The collecting system is best seen on enhanced scans because of the high attenuation values of the contrast. The renal vessels are best seen with dynamic scans; the renal veins are usually larger than the arteries. The anterior pararenal, posterior pararenal, and perirenal compartments can usually be distinguished (see Fig. 20-2). Normally, Gerota's fascia is imperceptible or is seen as a thin fascial band. With certain pathologic processes (eg, pancreatitis) Gerota's fascia becomes thickened and is more easily seen. Coronal and sagittal reformations allow estimation of renal size and volume.

The most prominent feature of the normal kidney on ultrasonography is the central renal sinus. This is quite

echogenic, mainly because of the fat surrounding the pelvo-calyceal system (Fig. 20-10). The amount of fat is variable depending on the individual, and there is an increase in fat and the echogenicity of the renal sinus with age.[127] There may be mild dilatation of the pelvis as a normal variant, but dilated calyces do not usually accompany this. Normal calyces are not usually seen. Vascular branching may mimic hydronephrosis. A vessel should not directly abut the renal pyramid as a dilated calyx in hydronephrosis would. Color Doppler examination can more definitively identify vessels in questionable cases. The peripheral cortex contains low-level echoes, whereas the pyramids are hypo- or anechoic. The bright, small, circular echoes in the region of the corticomedullary junction represent the arcuate arteries. The perinephric fat and capsule are seen as an echogenic region surrounding the kidney. The normal ureter is usually not visible. The renal

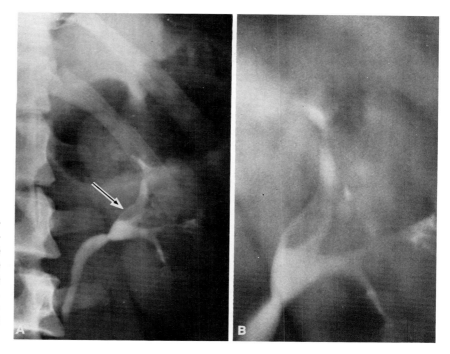

Figure 20–7. (**A**) Unusual vascular indentation causing a persistent elongated defect in the upper pole infundibulum on the left (*arrow*). (**B**) Close-up of the defect, which was persistent. Subsequent selective arteriogram showed a renal arterial branch causing the defect.

veins are readily visualized, but the arteries are more difficult to see.

MRI anatomy of the kidney is similar to that described for CT in the axial plane, but MRI has the advantage of multiplanar display (Fig. 20-11). On T1-weighted images, the cortex has medium to high signal intensity, and the medulla has low signal intensity.

Because of this, the corticomedullary junction is usually well seen. T2-weighted images have less signal contrast between the cortex and medulla.[95] Vessels in the renal hilum are easily identified, and associated flow void assures vascular patency.

The normal perfusion image with Tc-99m-DTPA shows counting rates that are nearly equal over both kidneys. Static images at 0, 5, and 10 minutes and later as needed reveal activity in the renal parenchyma and excretion into the collecting systems (Fig. 20-12). The

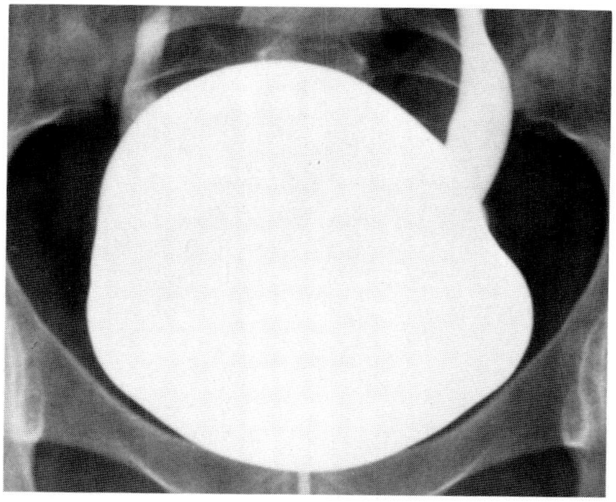

Figure 20–8. Cystogram showing bilateral vesicoureteral reflux. The bladder outline appears normal.

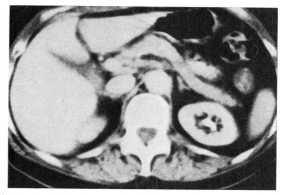

Figure 20–9. Normal left renal anatomy. Enhanced CT shows smooth contour of left kidney.

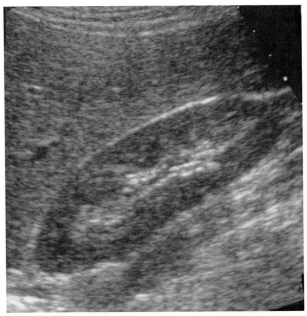

Figure 20–10. Normal renal anatomy. Longitudinal ultrasound of right kidney in which the echogenic central renal sinus is visible. The renal parenchyma is isoechoic or hypoechoic to adjacent normal liver. (Courtesy of Deborah Krueger, RDMS.)

normal ureters are only occasionally visualized. Activity can be demonstrated in the bladder as early as the 5-minute image, although more often it is seen on the 10-minute image. The normal hippuran renogram demonstrates an initial rise in counts due to activity in the extrarenal and renal vessels during the vascular phase. The counts continue to increase gradually dur-

ing the cortical transit phase because of the accumulation of I-131-hippuran or Tc-99m-Mertiatide by the renal tubular cells. The peak occurs when the rate of uptake equals the rate of excretion into the collecting system. The counts then gradually decrease during the excretory phase because of the excretion of hippuran into the collecting system (Fig. 20-13).

ANOMALIES

Anomalies of the kidney and ureter result from errors in development.[78] The kidneys arise from a mass of renal mesenchyme at the upper end of the ureteral buds, which in turn rise from the lower end of the mesonephric (wolffian) ducts. The mesonephron is the excretory organ lower in the phylogenetic scale, and in the human it functions for a short time in early embryologic development before becoming part of the male genital system. The ureteral buds grow dorsally, lying close together as the renal mesenchyme differentiates. Each bud bifurcates into an upper and lower sprout to form the major calyces. The ureter is anterior to the kidney as the latter ascends from the upper sacral area to its position in the lower-thoracic–upper-lumbar region. As it ascends the kidney rotates to bring it lateral to the ureter in the midlumbar region. The renal blood supply is attained after the kidney reaches its normal adult position. The lower end of the ureter loses its relation to the wolffian duct and opens into the bladder in a higher and more lateral position. The wolffian duct migrates distally and its orifices are eventually situated in the distal portion of the floor of the prostatic urethra to become the ejaculatory ducts in the male. The orifices of the wolffian duct become vestigial structures in the female.

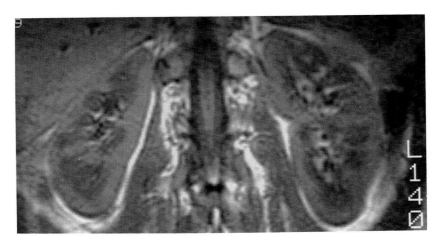

Figure 20–11. Normal renal anatomy. Coronal T1-weighted MRI. Multiplanar capability allows wide range of imaging planes.

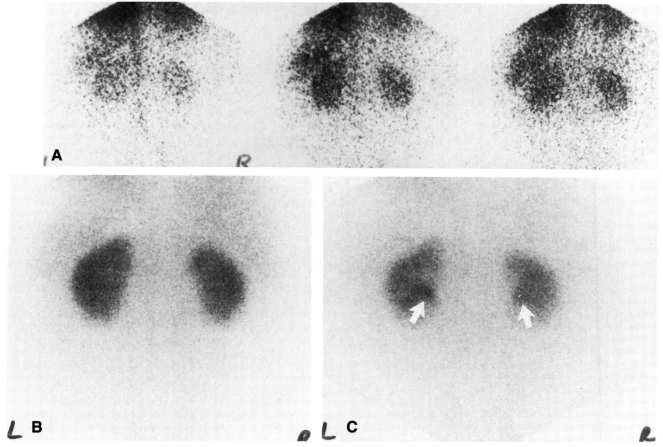

Figure 20–12. **(A)** Normal perfusion scan of aorta and kidneys, also showing spleen and lung bases, at 3 seconds per frame. **(B)** Diethylenetriaminepenta-acetic acid (DTPA)—immediate static image. **(C)** DTPA—static image at 10 minutes. Note excretion into collecting systems (*arrows*).

ANOMALIES IN NUMBER

Renal Agenesis (Single Kidney)

The occurrence of a single kidney is a rare anomaly. Care must be taken when making a radiographic diagnosis of unilateral renal agenesis because a contralateral nonfunctioning kidney may not be readily visible. The single kidney tends to be larger in patients with agenesis of one kidney than in patients with secondary compensatory renal hypertrophy. Radiographic signs are an absence of a renal shadow on one side with an unusually large kidney on the other side. The trigone is usually deformed with the ureteral orifice missing on the involved side, so that cystoscopy may confirm the diagnosis. At times, however, a portion of the lower ureter may be present in renal agenesis; therefore, the trigone may have no deformity. Angiog-

raphy confirms the absence of the renal artery, but renal venography is said to be more reliable than arteriography in making the diagnosis of renal agenesis. Other anomalies such as congenital heart disease and a neuromuscular deficit accompanied by a small pelvic outlet, sacral agenesis, and bladder hypoplasia (caudal regression) may be associated with renal agenesis. With the advent of CT and ultrasonography, the diagnosis of renal agenesis has become much easier, and angiography is no longer routinely used.

Supernumerary Kidney

Supernumerary kidney is a rare anomaly. The usual finding is that the anomalous kidney is small and rudimentary, and the other kidney on the same side is often smaller than the normal kidney on the opposite side.

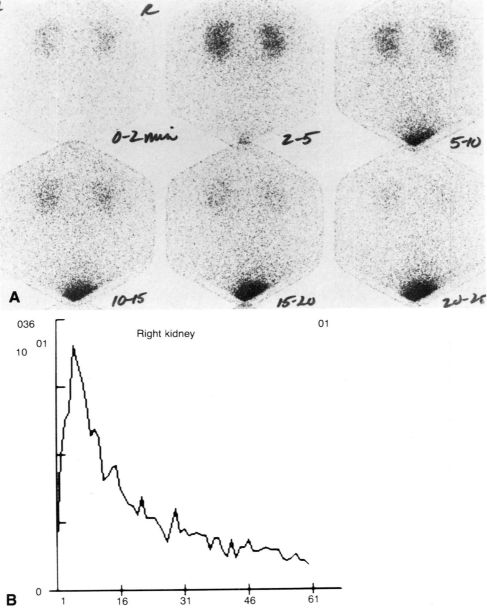

Figure 20–13. (A) Gamma camera scans of hippuran renogram. (B) Normal time-activity curve for hippuran (x axis in minutes).

Demonstration of the presence of a separate pelvis, ureter, and blood supply is necessary to make the diagnosis. Excretory urography can be used to outline the collecting system of the supernumerary kidney if it is functioning. Aortography will show the blood supply if that is necessary to confirm the diagnosis. Computed tomography and ultrasonography are less invasive and may be helpful.

ANOMALIES IN SIZE AND FORM

Hypoplasia

Anomalies of renal size and form are more common than anomalies in number. Hypoplasia on one side is usually associated with hyperplasia on the other. The hypoplastic or infantile kidney functions normally so that it can be seen on excretory urograms. It must be differentiated from the acquired atrophic kidney, which is small and contracted because of vascular or inflammatory disease. In congenital hypoplasia the calyceal system and pelvis are small, and there is a normal relationship between the amount of parenchyma and the size of the collecting system (Fig. 20-14). In the secondarily contracted kidney, the pelvis and calyces tend to be normal in size so that the decrease in renal size is due to a parenchymal deficit. Furthermore, the function of the latter tends to be impaired. Despite these differences, it is often very difficult to distinguish between the two conditions without the use of renal arteriography. The size of the orifice of the renal artery is important; in hypoplasia it is small; in an atrophic kidney it is normal, but may taper to a very small size near the orifice.

Hyperplasia

The other anomaly in size, hyperplasia, is associated with agenesis or hypoplasia on the opposite side. Enlargement of the kidney is usually caused by conditions other than agenesis or hypoplasia, however, and is then more properly termed *compensatory hypertrophy.* Several disorders may cause renal enlargement; these include obstructive hydronephrosis, polycystic disease, other cystic or dysplastic disorders, neoplasm, renal vein thrombosis, acute infection, Waldenström's macroglobulenemia, hemophilia, acute arterial infarction, and duplication of the renal pelvis.[85] Often the enlargement is bilateral, however, and there are clinical, laboratory findings and urographic findings that help to make the differentiation. Conditions that characteristically cause bilateral renal enlargement include (1) acute glomerulonephritis, (2) lymphoma, (3) leukemia in children, (4) systemic lupus erythematosus, (5) polycystic disease, (6) bilateral renal vein thrombosis, (7) amyloidosis, (8) sarcoidosis, (9) sickle cell disease, (10) lipoid nephrosis, (11) lobular glomerulonephritis, (12) glycogen storage disease, (13) hereditary tyrosinemia, and (14) total lipodystrophy.

FUSION ANOMALIES

Fusion anomalies represent an alteration in form of the kidneys and can often be recognized or at least suspected on plain roentgenograms of the abdomen. Computed tomography provides more complete information about these anomalies than does excretory urography. Ultrasonography likewise provides better assessment of the renal parenchyma.

Horseshoe Kidney

The horseshoe kidney is the most common type of fusion anomaly. In this condition the lower poles of the kidney are joined by a band of soft tissue, the isthmus, which varies from a thick parenchymatous mass as wide as the kidneys themselves to a thin stringlike band of fibrous tissue. The upper poles are rarely in-

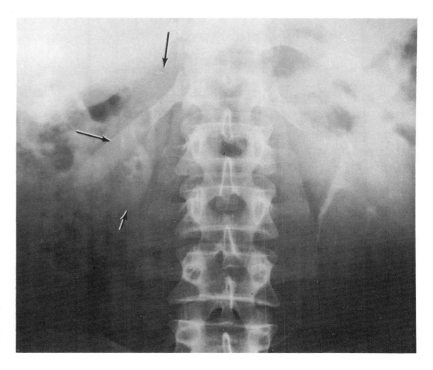

Figure 20–14. Hypoplasia of the right kidney. Note the marked difference in size of the two kidneys. Function is present on the right kidney despite its small size; its limits are outlined (*arrows*).

volved. The long axis of the kidney is reversed in this anomaly so that the lower pole is nearer the midline than the upper. There is also an associated rotation anomaly on one or both sides that varies in degree, usually more on the left. The calyces are directed backward or posteromedially rather than laterally. As a result they are seen on end or obliquely, which alters their appearance considerably (Fig. 20-15A). The ureters tend to be somewhat stretched over the isthmus and partial obstruction on one or both sides is not unusual. This leads to dilatation of the pelvis and calyces and may also lead to chronic inflammatory disease and the formation of calculi. The roentgenographic diagnostic features on plain film are (1) alteration in the axis of the kidneys, (2) mass observed connecting the lower poles, (3) renal enlargement if present, and (4) calculi if present. Urographic findings confirm these findings; in addition there are (1) malrotation, with the pelves anterior or anterolateral in position, (2) nephrographic demonstration of the parenchymal isthmus connecting the lower poles (if present), (3) often varying degrees of dilatation of the collecting system on one or both sides, (4) possible nonfunction of one kidney because of massive obstructive hydronephrosis, (5) possible partial obstruction of both kidneys, usually at or near the ureteropelvic junction, and (6) upper ureteral displacement, which varies with the amount of malrotation. These findings are often particularly strik-

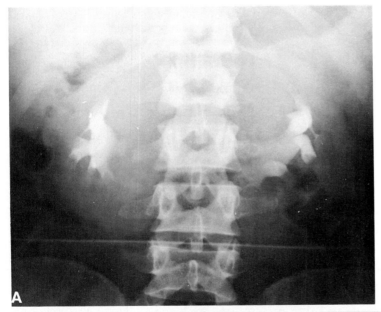

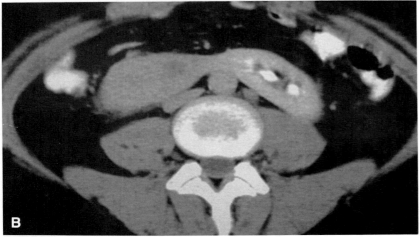

Figure 20–15. Horseshoe kidney. **(A)** Note the reversal of the long axis of the kidneys. There is rotation anomaly. The fusion inferiorly is faintly visualized on this reproduction. **(B)** Enhanced CT in a separate patient shows isthmus crossing the midline.

ing on CT (Fig. 20-15B) or MRI. Horseshoe kidneys are frequently supplied by multiple arteries, and the isthmus is often supplied by anomalous branches of the common iliac artery on one or both sides.

Crossed Ectopy

Crossed ectopy with fusion, the unilateral fused kidney, is an anomaly of form that is much less common than the horseshoe kidney. It consists of fusion of the kidneys on the same side; the lower one is ectopic and its ureter crosses the midline to enter the bladder normally on the opposite side. Both kidneys are often lower in position than normal, and various rotation anomalies as well as a wide variation in shape and type of fusion are noted. This anomaly is also frequently associated with partial obstruction, which results in inflammation and often in calculus formation. The "pancake" kidney is a variation in which there is fusion of both upper and lower poles; with failure of rotation, the calyces are directed posteriorly. The renal mass lies in or near the midline and is low in position, often overlying the sacrum. The ureters enter the bladder normally. Several descriptive terms have been applied to other rare forms of fusion. All these forms tend to

result in obstruction, which is turn causes hydronephrosis, infection, and calculus formation. These ectopic kidneys usually have an aberrant blood supply, often with multiple arteries.

Extrarenal calyces occur rarely if the portion of the ureteric bud fails to invaginate the ectopic nephrogenic mass. The extrarenal calyx is large, probably because there is no supporting parenchyma, and mimics the blunt calyx due to obstruction or infection. Computed tomography and ultrasonography usually are more informative than urography.

ANOMALIES IN POSITION

Anomalies of renal position are common. Malrotation has been described in the foregoing as being almost constantly present in fusion anomalies, but it also occurs as a single anomaly (Fig. 20-16). It results from incomplete or excessive rotation, and urographic study will indicate the degree of anomaly. Rotation anomalies are usually of little clinical significance unless associated with obstruction, but it is important to recognize these as innocuous anatomic variations that do not produce symptoms. Retroperitoneal tumor masses may displace the kidneys and produce an alteration in

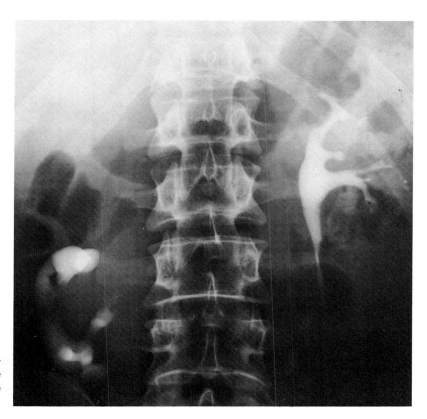

Figure 20–16. Ectopic and malrotated right kidney. The calyces are dilated as compared with those in the normal left kidney.

rotation that must be differentiated from congenital rotation anomalies. Crossed ectopy may occur without fusion, and the findings are similar to those described in the preceding section except for the lack of fusion. The ectopic kidney is lower than the normal one in position and is usually described as a sacral or pelvic kidney, depending on its position. Failure to visualize the kidney in its normal position should lead one to suspect ectopy and to look for it, because agenesis of a kidney is rare. In many instances the kidney can be visualized only when contrast material outlines it, so that excretory urography, radionuclide scanning, or retrograde pyelography may be necessary to indicate its position. A simpler way to assess such an ectopic kidney is by CT or ultrasonography. If it is nonfunctioning, aortography may be used to identify the aberrant artery (arteries) to a pelvic kidney, which may or may not appear as a pelvic mass on plain film. The pelvic mass representing an ectopic kidney may be discovered on study of the small bowel or colon as an extrinsic mass displacing bowel. Characteristically, the ureter of an ectopic kidney is only long enough to reach from the renal pelvis to the bladder, and this aids in distinguishing displacement of a normal kidney downward from one that developed in an abnormally low position. Superior ectopia of the kidney (or "intrathoracic" kidney) is probably more common than reports in the literature would indicate. The possibility of intrathoracic kidney should be considered in the differential diagnosis of masses of appropriate size projecting into the posterior thorax from below the diaphragm. An intrathoracic kidney is usually unilateral. It may be associated with herniation through the foramen of Bochdalek or a congenital eventration of the diaphragm posteriorly. Excretory urography or ultrasonography will readily identify the position of the kidney in these cases.

Nephroptosis is the term applied to abnormal downward displacement of the kidney. Roentgenograms obtained with the patient in the upright position normally show downward displacement of the kidney equal to the height of up to two lumbar vertebra. When the kidney is displaced more than this, ptosis is said to be present. The condition is more common on the right side than on the left; it is frequent in females but rare in males. It is of doubtful clinical significance because obstruction ordinarily is not produced and surgical intervention is rarely, if ever, indicated. roentgenographic demonstration of this condition can be accomplished by obtaining an additional exposure during urography with the patient in an upright position. In the low position the kidney often rotates on its horizontal axis; the lower pole then lies more anterior than normal. Oblique views are necessary to measure true

renal length when this occurs. Rarely, there is enough mobility so that the kidney (usually the right) will move across the midline when a patient is in the appropriate lateral decubitus position. Also, one kidney may be displaced across the midline by an extrarenal mass, an acquired abnormality.

OTHER RENAL ANOMALIES

Aberrant Papilla

Aberrant papilla occurs occasionally. The papilla projects directly into the lumen of the infundibulum as a smooth, conical mass that appears round or oval when viewed en face. It bears no resemblance to a minor calyx in which a normal papilla projects. Other anomalies include *multiple papillae* entering a single calyx, which may simulate a blood clot or nonopaque stone.[15]

Megacalyces

The term *megacalyces* describes an anomaly consisting of enlargement of calyces in one or both kidneys associated with underdeveloped renal pyramids. There is no evidence of obstruction, and function is normal. Because of calyceal size, there may be stasis with a tendency for stone formation, which may result in infection that can alter the urographic findings.[144]

Benign Cortical Nodule

Cortical nodules are a normal variation resulting from the presence of more cortical tissue than usual in a portion of the kidney. Based on location, there are three types of cortical nodules: (1) subcapsular, (2) hilar lip, and (3) septa of Bertin. The patterns of urographic appearance of cortical nodules have been described by Thornbury[149] based on the elegant anatomic correlation work done by Hodson. When the cyst/tumor/cortical nodule differential diagnoses question is raised on excretory urography, ultrasonography is the most direct way to resolve the question when simple cyst is the most likely diagnosis. When tumor or cortical nodule seems more likely, dynamic contrast CT examination of the kidney usually provides the most definitive information to distinguish tumor from normal variant.

A focal prominence of one or more columns of Bertin can mimic a mass lesion due to tumor or inflammation. However, it has a fairly easily recognized roentgenographic appearance in most cases.[149] It is caused by a variant of normal renal development where there is more cortical tissue in an area than usual. Depending on its location this cortical nodule can distort the adjacent calyces and the adjacent surface of the kidney.

Solitary Renal Calyx

A solitary renal calyx is an extremely rare anomaly in which one or both kidneys have a single calyx that drains the entire kidney into a somewhat bulbous tube that represents the pelvis. Several other mammalian kidneys have a solitary calyx. This anomaly does not necessarily indicate renal disease, but other congenital anomalies may be associated with it.

ANOMALIES OF THE RENAL PELVIS AND URETER

Ureteropelvic Junction Anomalies

Ureteropelvic dysfunction or obstruction, the most common congenital anomaly of the urinary tract, is usually bilateral but not always symmetrical. The left side is often more severely involved than the right. The amount of hydronephrosis depends on the severity of obstruction. In the neonate, when obstruction is marked it may be the cause of massive unilateral or bilateral renal enlargement. There is some controversy as to the cause of this anomaly. The majority appear to be the result of an intrinsic wall abnormality. Occasionally the cause may be an extrinsic abnormality such as an aberrant vessel or band of fibrous tissue, either of which may angulate the ureter and tend to hold it in place while the pelvis dilates. Rarely, an intrinsic mucosal fold or web may be present.[2] If infection occurs, secondary fibrosis may aggravate the condition.

Urographic findings vary with the severity of the condition. Caliectasis and pyelectasis are observed along with a somewhat rectangular extrarenal type of pelvis that is rather characteristic. Often the ureteropelvic junction is not dependent as in the normal individual, so the insertion of the ureter is high and posterior. Diuretic-influenced radionuclide study often will help determine whether the ureteropelvic narrowing is functionally significant.[153]

Duplication of the Pelvis and Ureter

Incomplete double ureter is formed when the renal bud divides too early or the division extends into the ureter.[59] The division varies from an exaggeration of the length of major upper- and lower-pole calyces to duplication of the ureter for most of its length. Complete duplication of the ureter may also occur. Each ureter has its own vesical orifice; the upper ureter usually drains the upper third of the kidney, whereas the ureter that drains the lower pelvis drains the lower two thirds of the kidney (Fig. 20-17). The ureter that drains the upper pole is ventral to the lower one but crosses over and empties into the bladder in a lower and more

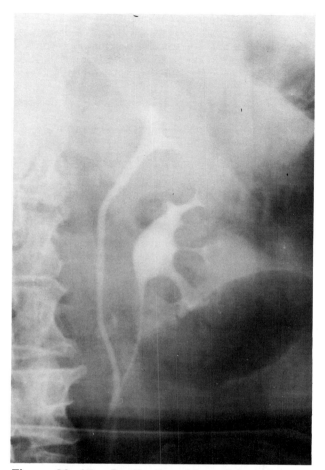

Figure 20–17. Duplication of the pelvis and ureter. The upper pelvis drains the upper pole of the kidney, whereas the lower pelvis drains the central portion of the kidney as well as the lower pole.

medial position (Weigert-Meyer rule); when one of the ureters empties in an extravesical location it is the one that drains the upper pelvis. Urographic recognition of duplication is simple when both pelves and ureters are opacified. Duplication should be suspected if only one of them fills, because there will then be a segment of kidney without apparent drainage. These anomalies of the pelvis and ureter may be unilateral or bilateral, with a tendency to be asymmetrical. Multiple budding will occasionally result in multiple short upper pelves and ureters that are extrarenal in type. In this anomaly, each of several major calyces will have its own pelvis and upper ureter, which usually joins with the others to form a common lower ureter. It is not infrequent for half of a double ureter to be obstructed.

Several abnormalities are related to duplication of the kidney and ureters, the most common being vesicoureteral reflux, ureterocele, and ectopic ureteral orifice. All may be associated with infection, and obstruction may complicate ureterocele and ectopic ureteral orifice. The upper pole ureter is prone to obstruction, whereas the lower pole is subject to vesicoureteral reflux.

When obstruction and infection result in nonfunctioning of the upper pole, the roentgenographic findings are varied. If there is a nonobstructive inflammatory lesion resulting in nonfunction, the findings are those of a calyceal system that drains only the central and lower pole of the kidney so the calyces are fewer than normal in number and the most superior calyx does not extend into the upper pole of the kidney. To make this determination, one must obtain clear visualization of the outline of the upper pole. If there is a hydronephrotic mass, the upper pole will be enlarged, and the lower calyces that are filled may be displaced by the large upper pole mass ("drooping lily sign"). There may also be some rotation of the kidney, the amount depending on the size of the mass. If the mass is very large, the entire kidney and upper ureter may be displaced laterally. Calculi may occur in the obstructed or infected upper pole.

Anomalies in Position of Ureteral Orifice

There are several possible anomalies in position of the ureteral orifice. This variation is usually better studied by cystoscopy than by radiographic means. In the male, the ureter may open into the seminal vesicles, the vas deferens, the ejaculatory duct, or the posterior urethra. In the female, the abnormal ureter may open into the urethra, beneath the urethral orifice near the hymen, or into the lateral vulvar wall, the uterus, the vagina, or, rarely, into the rectum. Although ectopic ureteral insertion is present in all patients with ureteral duplication, it also occurs in patients with a single ureter. The sites, symptoms, and radiographic findings are similar except that there is no duplication.

Ureteral Jet Phenomenon

The ureteral jet phenomenon is caused by a jet of opaque medium propelled by ureteral peristalsis, which may occasionally extend across the base of the bladder to the opposite side. The jet maintains the caliber of the ureter and simulates an anomalous ureter that opens on the opposite side of the trigone (Fig. 20-18). When present, it excludes the possibility of significant vesicoureteral reflux.[82] When there is a

question about the cause of an apparent anomaly, another film will reveal a normal lower ureter in these patients.

Retrocaval Ureter

Postcaval or retrocaval ureter is limited to the right side except in situs inversus. It is caused by failure of the right subcardinal vein to atrophy and persists as the adult vena cava. Normally, the right supracardinal vein persists as the vena cava. The abnormal relationship may cause partial obstruction, leading to hydronephrosis, infection, and calculus formation. The ureter passes to the left behind the inferior vena cava, then turns toward the right and courses downward in its normal position. In some cases there is redundancy of the ureter proximally, so that an S-type, or fish-hook, or inverted J-type of deformity is produced. The site of narrowing or obstruction, if present, is proximal to the vena cava and at the lateral edge of the psoas, and it is caused by the pressure of the retroperitoneal fascia over the muscle. In other cases of retrocaval ureter with no redundancy, obstruction is less common and when present coincides with the lateral margin of the inferior vena cava.

The diagnosis can usually be made on urography. In addition to the abnormal course of the right ureter in the frontal projection, its posterior position in the lat-

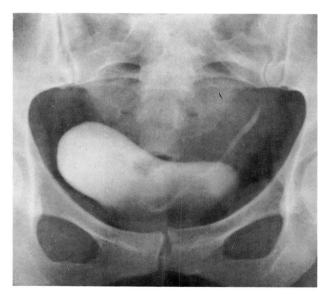

Figure 20–18. Ureteral jet phenomenon. Note the apparent extension of the ureter across the midline. Cystoscopy revealed a normal position of the ureteral orifice on the left.

eral view can be observed. The diagnosis can be confirmed by inferior vena cavography with an opaque catheter in the ureter but is more easily demonstrated by CT. The medial swing is usually maximum at L4–L5 and occasionally as high as L3. There may be partial obstruction at the level of the lateral wall of the vena cava. Medial deviation of the ureter (medial to the vertebral pedicles) may also be related to psoas muscle prominence associated with a narrow pelvic inlet. Retroperitoneal fibrosis and abdominal aortic aneurysm may also cause medial deviation. The deviations in the retroperitoneal fibrosis are bilateral, and there is no S- or J-shaped redundancy. Retroperitoneal masses (such as lymphoma) with ureteral displacement must also be differentiated, and CT is particularly helpful in doing so.

Ureterocele

There are two types of ureterocele, simple and ectopic.[148] The simple ureterocele consists of an intravesical dilatation of the ureter immediately proximal to its orifice in the bladder. It usually results from a combination of ureteral orifice stenosis and a deficiency in the connective tissue attachment of the ureter to the bladder. It varies in size from a scarcely perceptible dilatation to one that is moderately large and resembles a cobra head (or spring onion) in shape. There may be partial obstruction resulting in ureterectasis. In general the simple ureterocele is smaller than the ectopic ureterocele. It occurs with equal frequency in males and females and is usually discovered incidentally. A calculus in the intramural portion of the ureter may produce dilatation simulating ureterocele, but the calculus produces pain and is usually visible on plain film. A tumor of the bladder, either primary or secondary, may also cause dilatation simulating simple ureterocele, a so-called pseudoureterocele.

The ectopic type of ureterocele is usually discovered in childhood and is much more common in females (6 or 7 to 1) than in males. It is more likely to be associated with severe hydronephrosis, ureterectasis, or infection than the simple type. Both types tend to occur in the presence of duplication of the ureter; the ectopic type is almost always associated with this anomaly. The ectopic ureterocele consists of the submucosal passage of the distal portion of the involved ureter within the vesical wall to terminate in the urethra rather than in the bladder, as in the simple type. The submucosal portion of the ureter dilates and bulges anteromedially into the bladder to form the ureterocele. It may prolapse through the urethra to form a vulvar "cyst" and usually extends posteriorly to the vesical neck and proximal urethra. It invariably involves the ureter from the upper pole of the kidney (Fig. 20-19).

The roentgenographic appearance of the simple type depends on whether the opaque medium fills the ureterocele. If it is filled, the lesion is outlined by a radiolucent wall that stands out in contrast to the filled bladder as well as to the filled, dilated, distal ureter. When the ureterocele is not filled with opaque material it appears as a radiolucent mass within the opacified bladder in the region of the ureteral orifice. The shape may be somewhat fusiform with a narrow lower end resembling a cobra's head, but the larger ones tend to be more rounded in shape. When a calculus is present in the ureterocele, it is noted to lie on one side of the midline and remains there despite changes in the patient's position.

Ectopic ureteroceles are larger than the simple ones and often extend to the anterior bladder wall when viewed in the lateral projection. The contact with the floor of the bladder is broad and extends to the internal urethral orifice. Obstruction of the other ureter is frequent, and the extravesical portion may distort the bladder. Several conditions may simulate ectopic ureterocele. These include hydrometrocolpos and "cyst" of the seminal vesicle produced when an ectopic ureter inserts into the seminal vesicle. The condition is less frequent in males than in females, but in males the incidence of infection is higher, the malformation is more complex, and the frequency of a single collecting system is greater than in females. Eversion is also more common in males, and the tendency to prolapse into the posterior urethra causing bladder outlet obstruction is greater.

Excretory urography is the roentgenographic method of choice in diagnosis of ureterocele. An eccentric mass encroaching on the bladder floor in a patient with duplication of the ureter is virtually pathognomonic.

There is an acquired condition, called a *pseudoureterocele*, that simulates a simple ureterocele.[151] It is usually encountered on excretory urography. The contrast-delineated distal ureter simulates a simple ureterocele. On closer inspection, however, usually this dilatation is slightly asymmetric. There may even be a very small eccentric beaked appearance of the tip of the contrast column in the ureter. It is important to distinguish a pseudoureterocele from a true ureterocele because the pseudoureterocele may be the first indication of a neoplasm. Usually this is a transitional cell carcinoma of the bladder or invasion of the trigone area by carcinoma of the cervix. Benign conditions can also cause a similar appearance and include fibrosis of the ureteral orifice secondary to prior transient impaction of a ureteral calculus or injury from previous transurethral resection of bladder pathology. Cystoscopy

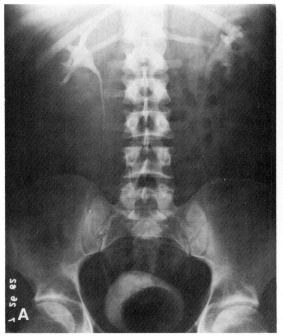

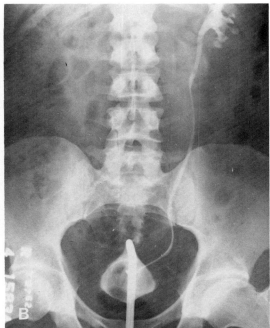

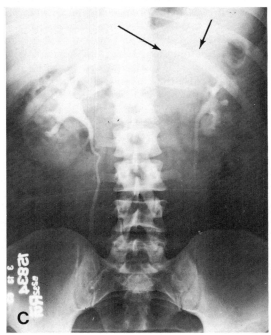

Figure 20–19. Ectopic ureterocele. (**A**) Note the large, rounded mass encroaching on the bladder, chiefly on the left side. The collecting system on the left drains the lower left kidney. (**B**) Retrograde pyelogram in which a ureteral orifice in the normal position was catheterized, shows drainage of the lower kidney. The ectopic ureter draining into the ureterocele could not be catheterized. It drained the upper pole in the left kidney and was obstructed so that no function was present at the time of the urogram. (**C**) Upper pole of the kidney on the left (*arrows*).

and reexamination of the patient following discovery of the pseudoureterocele will usually reveal its cause.

Ureteral Diverticula

A single ureteral diverticulum is probably a congenital anomaly and may represent a dilated rudimentary branched ureter.[28] When the diverticulum is filled with contrast medium, the diagnosis is easily made because the appearance is similar to that of a diverticulum elsewhere. Some of these diverticula have the appearance of a blind-end duplication without much dilatation and almost certainly are rudimentary or partially duplicated ureters. They are best demonstrated by retrograde pyelography, but may be apparent on an excretory urogram. Many diverticula are acquired; most authorities believe that multiple diverticula are almost always acquired and are indicative of previous infection. They appear as ureteral outpouchings of various sizes and numbers, best seen on a retrograde pyelogram, but with good ureteral filling they may also be clearly defined on an excretory urogram.

Other Ureteral Anomalies

Transverse Ureteral Folds. In infants, a corkscrew appearance may be demonstrated in the upper ureters on an excretory urogram. This appearance is caused by thin, transverse folds that represent inward projections of the full thickness of the ureteral wall. They appear as horizontal folds measuring about 1 mm in thickness on the urogram, probably represent persistence of fetal tortuosity of the ureter, are of no clinical significance, and represent a minor anatomic variant that occasionally persists into adolescence.

Vertical Ureteropelvic Striations. The vertical striations occasionally observed in the pelvis and upper ureter usually are associated with reflux and are probably secondary to infection and mucosal edema. In rare instances, however, they appear to be a minor anatomic variant. They may be observed on excretory urograms or retrograde pyelograms.

Ureteral Valves. A ureteral valve is a very unusual anomaly that is manifested by the following: (1) anatomically demonstrable transverse folds of ureteral mucosa containing bundles of smooth muscle fibers; (2) obstruction above the valve and a normal ureter below it; and (3) no other evidence of mechanical or functional obstruction. A ureteral valve is usually unilateral and may be annular with a pinpoint opening or may be cusplike in appearance. It may occur anywhere in the ureter, although it is slightly more common in the lower ureter than elsewhere. The cause of this anomaly is uncertain.[2]

Patent Urachus and Urachal Cyst

The urachus represents the intra-abdominal remnant of the allantoic duct or caudal extension of it, which is continuous with the vesical portion of the urogenital sinus in embryologic development. Normally it constitutes the middle umbilical ligament. The allantois extends from the primitive urinary bladder through the umbilicus to the placenta. Four types of anomalies are possible: (1) complete patency, (2) patency at umbilical end or blind external type, (3) patency at vesical end or blind internal type, and (4) patency between bladder and umbilicus, which gives rise to the urachal cyst. Urachal prominence or urachal remnant is observed fairly often in patients with high intravesical pressure dating from birth or before birth. Examples are patients with myelomeningocele or posterior urethral valves. The blind external type and complete patency are usually recognized on inspection when the umbilical cord sloughs off but may be suspected earlier. Roentgen visualization can be obtained by using contrast materials that can be injected into the umbilical end of the urachus. Cystography is needed to demonstrate the effect of a urachal cyst or patent urachus. The findings are those of a smooth-walled tubular structure lying in the anterior midline that extends into the plane of a line between umbilicus and the bladder. The bladder may be distorted and elevated. The cyst may extend from the bladder to the umbilicus or end blindly when it begins at either end. When a cyst of the urachus is present without internal or external communication, roentgenographic findings may depend on its size. If large, it may be noted as a midline, soft-tissue mass lying between the bladder and the umbilicus in the anterior abdominal wall. Gas-filled small intestine may be displaced and study of the small bowel by means of barium meal will show comparable displacement. Rarely, calculi may form in a patent urachus or urachal cyst. Computed tomography and ultrasonography now provide more complete assessment of the extent of this urachal anomaly.[84]

HYDRONEPHROSIS (OBSTRUCTIVE UROPATHY)

Regardless of its cause, chronic obstruction of the urinary tract leads to hydronephrosis, which indicates dilatation of the pelvis and calyces with potential progressive destruction of renal parenchyma. The terms *pyelectasis, caliectasis, ureterectasis,* and *hydroureter* are more accurate in designating the location of the dilatation. The obstruction that produces hydronephrosis may be unilateral or bilateral, depending on the site of the lesion producing it. Unilateral obstruction is caused by a lesion at or above the ureterovesical junction, whereas bilateral obstruction may be caused by a lesion distal to that point. Enlargement of the urinary collecting system including pelves, calyces, ureters, and bladder may result from causes other than obstruction, however.

NONOBSTRUCTIVE HYDRONEPHROSIS (URINARY STASIS)

Several nonobstructive conditions may cause dilatation of the renal pelvis, calyces, and ureters. Diabetes insipidus may be associated with relatively moderate hydronephrosis. Nephrogenic diabetes insipidus tends to cause severer dilatation, often with tortuosity of the ureters in addition to the dilatation. In this condition there is a tubular abnormality with insufficient absorption of water, leading to a large volume of hypotonic urine.[102] Urinary tract infection tends to cause segmental or generalized dilatation of the ureter with poor or reversed peristalsis leading to pyelectasis and caliectasis. This may be augmented by vesicoureteral reflux, which is commonly found in association with urinary infections. The changes may decrease or disappear when the infection is successfully treated. Dilatation with stasis in the absence of urinary tract abnormality may also be caused by intraabdominal inflammatory disease such as appendicitis or peritonitis, a finding similar to that of adynamic ileus involving the gut in patients with peritonitis. Excessive fluid intake (overhydration) may cause some dilatation. A variety of neurologic disorders is also associated with dilatation without obstruction. An adynamic, short segment of upper ureter may also cause some dilatation of the pelves and calyces; this appears on a urogram as a short, narrow ureteral segment with dilatation above it.

CONGENITAL HYDRONEPHROSIS

Congenital hydronephrosis is the most common cause of an abdominal mass in neonates. It is caused by a variety of lesions. In anomalies of position it is usually due to the abnormal relationship of the upper ureter to the kidney. Congenital strictures, bands, aberrant vessels, ureteroceles, and valves may also produce hydronephrosis. In addition, there are instances of congenital hydronephrosis in which the cause is obscure; many of these are "neurogenic" in that they are associated with lesions of the spinal cord and with congenital

megacolon. The dilatation is usually bilaterally symmetrical in patients with congenital megacolon. Congenital abnormalities then may result in either obstructive or nonobstructive uropathy. In neonates, ascites at birth may indicate obstructive uropathy, often secondary to posterior urethral valves, but a variety of lesions may cause the obstruction.[54] Obstruction of the bladder outlet, ureteral atresia, presacral neuroblastoma, complex caudal anomalies including urethral and anorectal atresia, ureterocele, vesical neck valve, and myelomeningocele have also been reported as rare causes of neonatal ascites secondary to obstructive uropathy. If congenital hydronephrosis is severe, oligohydramnios may develop. This can lead to pulmonary hypoplasia. Pneumomediastinum can result with attempts to ventilate these patients.

Rarely, ureteropelvic junction obstruction may produce intermittent hydronephrosis related to overhydration in patients who may have an extrarenal-type pelvis. In patients with symptoms of intermittent hydronephrosis, urography at the time of acute dilation following overhydration, may clinch the diagnosis. As indicated earlier, duplication with ectopic ureteral insertion into the urethra often results in hydronephrosis of the upper collecting system. This is a congenital anomaly, but acquired disease such as infection may be the major cause when obstruction is observed in the adult. Rarely, there is lower-pole hydronephrosis in a duplicated kidney.

ACQUIRED HYDRONEPHROSIS (OBSTRUCTIVE UROPATHY)

Acquired hydronephrosis is caused by a variety of lesions, among which are tumors, calculi, strictures, radiation therapy, operative procedures, and prostatic enlargement. Ureteropelvic junction obstruction is the most common type of bilateral obstruction above the bladder. It may be asymmetric. Congenital narrowing appears to be the most common cause of the obstruction. Pregnancy in the third trimester is often associated with hydronephrosis that tends to be more severe on the right than on the left. Ureters are dilated to the pelvic brim. The most likely cause is mechanical pressure from the enlarging uterus. Hydrocolpos and hydrometrocolpos also tend to cause ureteral obstruction. Abdominal aortic aneurysm may compress the ureter, or retroperitoneal bleeding (associated with aneurysm) may cause fibrosis leading to ureteral stricture and hydronephrosis. Granulomatous (Crohn's) disease of the small intestine or colon occasionally causes distal ureteral obstruction. There are all degrees of dilatation, and progression of the changes can be noted on serial examinations if the obstruction is not relieved.

Urographic Findings

The earliest urographic change in hydronephrosis is a flattening of the normal concavity of the calyx and blunting of the sharp peripheral angle produced by the papilla as it juts into the calyx. This early change is reversible and is readily produced by a small increase in pressure. The pelvis enlarges gradually with increasing or prolonged obstruction, but pelvic and calyceal dilatation are not necessarily parallel. The next calyceal change is that of "clubbing," in which the concavity produced by the papilla is reversed (Figs. 20-20 and 20-21). Calyces then gradually enlarge with progressive destruction of parenchyma and enlargement of the collecting system of the kidney until the kidney becomes a nonfunctioning hydronephrotic sac in which the normal anatomy is obliterated (Fig. 20-22).

Occasionally, acute obstruction leads to rupture of the collecting system, usually at a calyceal fornix. Extravasation of urine into the retroperitoneum occurs and can track along the psoas muscles. These patients do well clinically if the obstruction is promptly removed. Long-standing obstruction and urine leakage can lead to sizable urine collections (urinomas) that

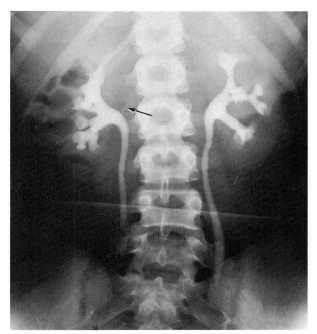

Figure 20–20. Minimal bilateral hydronephrosis. The pelves are not enlarged, but there is a little blunting of the calyces. Note the minimal pyelolymphatic backflow on the right (*arrow*).

may need percutaneous or surgical drainage, particularly if complicated by superimposed infection.

Renal function may be greatly diminished in severe hydronephrosis, and there is accumulation of opaque material in the parenchyma adjacent to the grossly dilated calyces. This forms crescentic areas of faint opacification termed the *crescent sign of hydronephrosis* (Fig. 20-23). Later there may be faint opacification of the calcyes themselves. Infection may be a complicating factor, tending to accelerate parenchymal destruction. When present, infection produces more irregularity in the dilated calyces than is seen in uncomplicated hydronephrosis. Also there may be bleeding with clots in the dilated collecting system that may resemble intrapelvic tumor. In the evaluation of patients with dilatation of the pelvis and calyces, particularly in children, it is important that the bladder be emptied before the urogram is obtained. A distended bladder may result in a false hydronephrosis.[13] When the bladder is empty, the hydronephrosis disappears. This finding is also seen during ultrasound examinations of the kidneys, and thus the bladder should be empty before the diagnosis of hydronephrosis is made. Vesicoureteral reflux may accentuate the dilatation of the upper urinary tract in these patients but does not appear to be the major cause.

When severe obstruction persists, there is usually increasing hydronephrosis with so-called hydronephrotic atrophy resulting in loss of renal parenchyma of varying degrees. In some instances, function will return following relatively long periods of obstruction, providing a reasonable amount of renal parenchyma remains. A combination of obstruction and ischemia occasionally may result in decreased renal size after the obstruction is relieved. Computed tomography often gives more specific information than urography as to the cause of obstruction, particularly when the cause is extraureteral (such as metastatic tumor). Ultrasonography is valuable and reliable in demonstrating hydronephrosis and can be especially helpful when contrast is not excreted by the kidney (Fig. 20-24). Ultrasound is also useful in assessing the amount of renal parenchymal atrophy or scarring in long-standing cases of hydronephrosis.

RENAL AND URETERAL CALCULI

It is thought that upper urinary tract calculi originate as Randall's plaques deep in the lining of the collecting ducts in the renal papillae.[150] These may detach and pass into the renal collecting system. Calculi may lodge in the pelvis, often in the region of the papillae

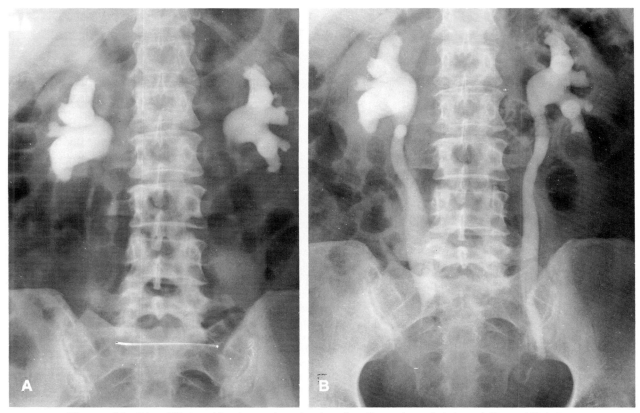

Figure 20–21.   Bilateral hydronephrosis showing the value of delayed films. **(A)** Intravenous urogram, obtained 15 minutes after injection of a contrast medium, shows dilatation of pelves and calyces with no definite ureteral opacification. **(B)** This film, exposed 90 minutes after injection of the medium, shows dilatation of ureters extending down to stricturelike narrowing, which is a little higher on the right than on the left.

and calyces. The calculi may remain within the pelvis and gradually increase in size to form a cast of the pelvis and calyces, representing a staghorn calculus (Fig. 20-25). Multiple calculi may form within the calyceal system and may be similar or may vary considerably in size. Urinary stasis and infection are important factors in promoting the formation of calculi, but the exact cause is not certain in many instances. Calculi tend to be asymptomatic until they cause obstruction. Then typical renal or ureteral colic symptoms are produced. About 90% of upper tract calculi contain enough calcium to be visualized on roentgenograms. Calcium phosphate, calcium oxalate, and magnesium ammonium phosphate (struvite) stones are the most common. Stones usually are composed of a mixture of chemical compounds because pure stones are relatively rare. Diamonium calcium phosphate and magnesium phosphate stones are uncommon. Cystine,

urate, and xanthine stones are rare and often of low density.

Matrix calculi are a combination of about two thirds mucoprotein and one third mucopolysaccharide; they are radiolucent and usually form in the presence of Proteus infection. This amorphous mucoprotein is present in stone formers, but, since it is not present in normal urine, it probably plays a role in the formation of renal calculi. Hyperparathyroidism and other conditions with hypercalcemia, including some that cause dissolution of bone, may also be associated with calculi. These include osteolytic metastases, leukemia, multiple myeloma, and sarcoidosis. Gout and other conditions associated with high serum uric acid and hyperuricosuria increase the incidence of uric acid stones. Hyperoxaluria, whatever the cause, also tends to promote formation of renal calculi. There is some evidence to indicate that calculi may also result from renal artery

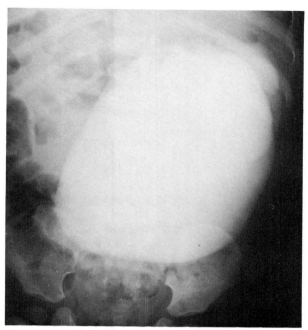

Figure 20–22. Massive hydronephrosis in a child. The greatly dilated pelvis is opacified. It nearly fills the entire left abdominal cavity. Physical findings were those of a large, somewhat fluctuant abdominal mass on the left.

stenosis; the vascular insufficiency may cause parenchymal injury leading to calculus formation.

Roentgenographic Findings

The roentgenographic findings are those of an opacity of varying size and shape overlying the urinary tract. Often the plain-film diagnosis is easily made, particularly when the calculus forms a cast of the pelvis or calyces or both. Subsequent excretory urography is often used for localization and to determine the condition of the calyceal system. Oblique views may be necessary in addition to frontal projections to localize a calculus definitely. Urography is necessary to find radiolucent low-density calculi. These calculi appear as negative shadows displacing the opaque medium. In patients with renal or ureteral colic there is usually delayed excretion by the involved kidney. With the acute obstruction produced by the passage of a ureteral stone, the intrapelvic pressure increases to the point at which there is decreased glomerular filtration of contrast material. Increasing density of the kidney (nephrogram) is due to slowed flow of urine through the collecting ducts in the parenchyma, and ongoing obligatory tubular water resorption in the nephrons results in increasing concentration of opacified urine.[143] Eventually there is usually some opacification of the calyces, pelvis, and ureter. It is, therefore, important to obtain

Figure 20–23. Hydronephrosis, the crescent sign. (**A**) Selective left renal arteriogram shows grossly stretched, narrow vessels with very few branches. Note the vessels stretched over the large renal pelvis medially. (**B**) Later film shows the crescent sign caused by opacification in the thin rim of remaining renal tissue. Surgical removal confirmed the diagnosis of severe hydronephrosis. (Courtesy of Thomas L. Carter, MD, and Richard Logan, MD.)

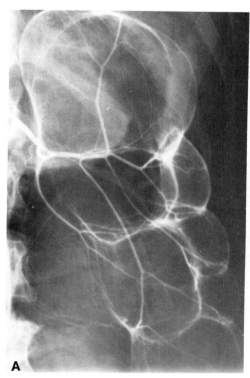

A

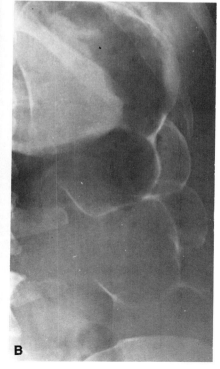

B

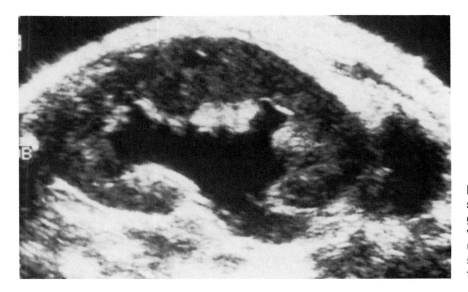

Figure 20–24. Hydronephrosis in a renal transplant. Sonogram shows the dilated pelvocaliceal system and proximal ureter. The small anechoic space adjacent to the kidney is the bladder.

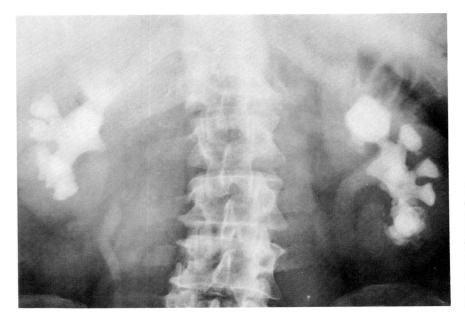

Figure 20–25. Staghorn calculi. Note the calcification forming a cast of the pelvis and calyces on each side. Renal function was so poor that very little additional density was observed on these urograms. The ureters are faintly opacified, however.

films until opacification is adequate to make the diagnosis. If the urogram shows a prolonged density on the involved side, it is likely that serial films exposed at 30-minute or progressively longer intervals will show enough opacification to localize the site of the obstructing ureteral calculus and confirm its presence within the ureter (Fig. 20-26). Prone and upright films can also be obtained to aid in localizing the sight of obstruction. Rarely, it may be necessary to do cystoscopy and place an opaque catheter. The calculus can be localized in relation to the ureteral catheter by means of frontal and oblique roentgenograms.

The most common lodging site for ureteral calculi is at or above the ureterovesical junction in the pelvic portion of the ureter. Occasionally a calculus will have passed before the examination is completed and no obstruction is then visible. When the calculus has lodged at the ureterovesical junction for any length of time, it is not uncommon to note a localized radiolucent indentation on the bladder owing to edema of the

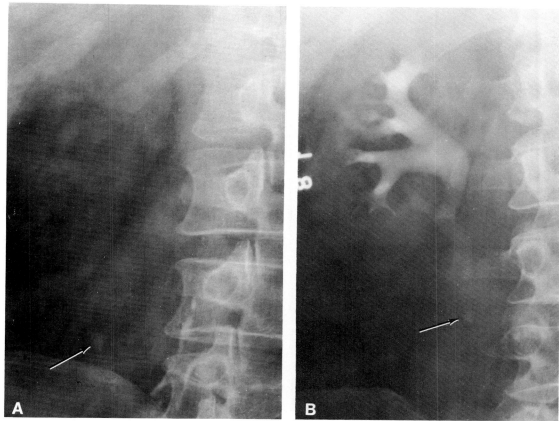

Figure 20–26. Right ureteral calculus. (**A**) Note the density (*arrow*) just above the right iliac crest in this right posterior oblique projection. (**B**) Urogram shows slight dilatation of the ureter extending down to the site of the calculus. This roentgenogram was obtained at 90 minutes following the intravenous injection of contrast material. Earlier films showed no excretion on the right side, demonstrating that delayed films were essential to confirm the diagnosis of ureteral calculus in this patient.

trigone above the ureteral orifice, even though the calculus may have been passed. Ureteral calculi are usually small in size (1 to 3 mm in diameter). In general, these small stones pass quickly down the ureter to lodge at or near the ureterovesical junction. The great majority of stones pass in 72 to 96 hours.[150] The stones tend to be parallel to the course of the ureter when they are oval or elongated. Most lie above a line drawn through the ischial spines. It should be recognized, however, that angulation of the roentgen-ray tube or alteration of position of the pelvis may project these calculi lower in position. Larger calculi are not as likely to leave the renal pelvis and to become lodged in the ureter.

Ureteral calculi tend to be round or oval in shape. If the calculus remains within the ureter for a long time,

it may become elongated and increased in size from deposition of urinary sediment. Large stones found within the ureter usually mean that these have been present for a considerable period of time (Fig. 20-27). In patients with acute colic caused by an obstructing ureteral calculus, urography may demonstrate the classic findings of hydronephrosis as described earlier. In addition, pyelointerstitial backflow may be seen. Occasionally, forniceal rupture can lead to urine extravasation and urinoma formation as previously discussed.

Differential Diagnosis

Suspected renal or ureteral calculus must be differentiated from other calcifications that may occur in the renal areas and along the course of the ureters. Gall-

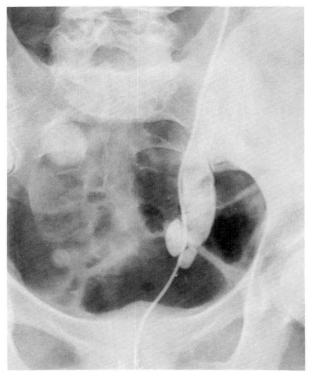

Figure 20–27.   Multiple large ureteral calculi on the left. The ureteral catheter indicates the relationship of the calculi to the ureter. The bladder is outlined by air.

stones are usually multiple, tend to be faceted, and often exhibit typical concentric rings of calcium. Oblique roentgenograms will show their anterior position. Common duct and cystic duct stones may be opaque, but they also lie anteriorly to the kidney and ureter. Calcification of costal cartilages is common and usually readily identified. Oblique projections will show the relationship of such shadows to the anterior lower thoracic wall if there is any doubt about their nature. Calcified mesenteric nodes and calcifications in the appendices epiploica usually move enough from one position to another to be differentiated from urinary calculi. The same is true of opaque material in the gastrointestinal tract. Pancreatic calculi usually conform to the shape and location of the pancreas and can be identified readily. Calcification in cysts and tumors of the kidney and elsewhere in the abdomen must also be differentiated. The contour of the cyst wall can usually be identified and when a calcified tumor is present, it is usually large enough to be visualized as a soft-tissue mass. Occasionally the lateral tip of a transverse process of one of the lumbar vertebrae may be easily visible in comparison to the remainder of the

process and resemble a ureteral calculus; close inspection will suffice to make the differentiation.

Vascular calcification, either in pelvic arteries or in veins (phleboliths) are generally the most difficult problems. Arterial calcification is usually along the course of a large artery and tends to be elongated and to outline the arterial walls, forming a ringlike density when seen in cross section and parallel lines when seen in longitudinal section. Phleboliths often have a fairly typical appearance with a radiolucent central area and tend to be more rounded in contour than calculi; some may have a central calcific nidus surrounded by a zone of lesser density, which in turn is surrounded by a denser periphery. Roentgenograms obtained in anteroposterior and oblique projections are often sufficient to exclude the possibility of urinary calculus as the cause for the density or densities present. If not conclusive, excretory urography with oblique and special views including delayed roentgenograms or fluoroscopy usually will provide the diagnosis. If there still is doubt, cystoscopy with introduction of a radiopaque catheter into the ureter usually solves the problem. The ureteral stone stays in relation to the contrast medium in the ureter in all projections.

In any patient having symptoms suggestive of ureteral colic, importance should be attached to any calculus density, no matter how small, occurring along the course of the ureter, particularly if it is found in the region of the distal part of the ureter. Conversely, in a patient with no symptoms suggestive of ureteral colic, small rounded calcifications in the lateral aspect of the pelvis can usually be disregarded because they most likely represent phleboliths. Occasionally, impacted ureteral calculi do not cause dilatation of the ureter or collecting system.[162]

RENAL MILK OF CALCIUM

The term *milk of calcium* refers to a suspension of fine sediment containing calcium that is observed most often in a calyceal diverticulum or hydrocalyx with little or no drainage or in a so-called pyelogenic or calyceal cyst.[110] Films exposed with the patient erect show a horizontal level indicating that the calcium is in suspension. The appearance is similar to that observed in the milk-of-calcium gallbladder. Similar suspension of liquid or semisolid calcium has been observed in association with renal cysts. Rarely, it has been seen associated with hydronephrosis. On upright films, several levels of calcium are noted in calyces.

Findings in plain films that suggest the diagnosis include (1) a somewhat peripheral location as compared to the central location of stones in the collecting system, (2) an unusually large area, (3) circular, or nearly circular, configuration, (4) faint calcification, particularly in relation to size, (5) diminishing density toward the periphery, and (6) indistinct margins. When these findings suggest the possibility, an upright or decubitus film can be obtained to confirm the diagnosis.

NEPHROCALCINOSIS

Nephrocalcinosis refers to multiple calcium deposits within the renal parenchyma. Two forms of nephrocalcinosis have been described: cortical and medullary types. The cortical type, which is the more uncommon of these conditions, is associated with hypotension (often from obstetric complications), chronic renal transplant rejection, chronic glomerulonephritis, Alport's syndrome (chronic hereditary nephritis), and oxalosis. This group is represented by patients with renal disease in which calcium is precipitated in damaged tissue. Normal blood calcium levels are usually present. Calcinosis is rare in chronic glomerulonephritis; when present the findings of tiny granular calcifications scattered throughout the cortex of small kidneys are very suggestive of the diagnosis.

Medullary nephrocalcinosis is found in association with several diseases characterized by abnormally high concentrations of calcium or phosphorus resulting in precipitation of calcium phosphate in healthy renal tissue. Primary hyperparathyroidism is the best example of this group, and nephrocalcinosis occurs in approximately 25% of patients with the disease. Renal lithiasis, however, is more common than nephrocalcinosis. When the latter occurs, tiny calcifications confined to the medulla are usually present with occasional larger calcifications occurring in the renal pyramids. Hypercalciuria of undetermined cause, hyperchloremic acidosis, hypervitaminosis D, milk-alkali syndrome, sarcoidosis, renal tubular acidosis, hyperoxaluria, carcinoma metastatic to bone, regional enteritis with secondary enteric hyperoxaluria, and idiopathic hypercalcemia are other conditions producing this type of nephrocalcinosis. Medullary sponge kidney can also cause medullary nephrocalcinosis and will be discussed in detail in a later section.

Roentgenographic findings depend on the extent of calcification, which varies from faintly visible granular densities to stippled calcification in the renal papilla and cortex (Fig. 20-28). The findings are relatively rare, and it has been shown that there are many instances of histopathologically proved renal calcification in which the calcium cannot be visualized radiographically in the living subject. Films of good quality in the low-kilovoltage range (70 to 76 kVp) exposed before a contrast medium is given are necessary to demonstrate small amounts of calcium. Coned views to include only the renal area as well as oblique views are often necessary to localize the calcium within the kidney. Tomography and CT are also very helpful in demonstrating and localizing calcifications in the kidney. At times, calcification is seen on tomograms or CT when it is not visible on the plain film. This is particularly true of low-density stones, which are best confirmed on CT.

Renal Tubular Acidosis

Nephrocalcinosis and nephrolithiasis are the radiographic findings in patients with renal tubular acidosis.[27] The nephrocalcinosis is manifest by dense calcium deposits in the medullary portion of the kidney. Those patients who lose calcium also have osteomalacia. The calcifications occur chiefly in patients with distal tubular acidosis and not in those with only slight hypercalciuria. Radiographically, the dense

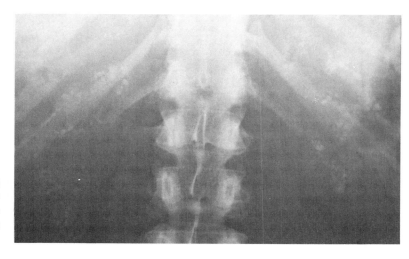

Figure 20–28. Nephrocalcinosis. Note the bilateral stippled renal calcific densities in a patient with renal tubular acidosis. There is overlying calcification of the costal cartilages.

medullary calcifications are somewhat similar to those observed in medullary sponge kidney, but the individual calcifications are larger in renal tubular acidosis and have less tendency to be oval or elongated than in medullary sponge kidney. Also, the calcification is somewhat more widespread in some patients.

LOW-DENSITY OR NONOPAQUE CALCULI

Although 85% to 90% of upper urinary calculi are opaque and readily seen on the roentgenogram, the remainder are not. These calculi are most often predominantly cystine, uric acid, or xanthine. Stones reach the ureter, cause colicky pain, and become impacted, causing varying degrees of obstruction. Excretory urography will show the effects of the obstruction, but the deformity of the end of the ureteral contrast column often simply indicates an intraluminal radiolucent defect. This could be due to calculus, tumor, or blood clot. In the past, retrograde pyelography usually was necessary to make diagnostic distinctions. However, presently CT is the most reliable and anatomically depicting way to distinguish tumor from calculus from clot. Computed tomography tends to enhance even minimal low-density calcifications, and CT numbers will measure in the 75 to 140 Hounsfield units range. Tumor or other soft-tissuelike materials will measure less than 60 Hounsfield units. There is very little overlap so that tumor can usually be excluded with great confidence when the CT number exceeds about 70 Hounsfield units.[136]

INFECTIONS AND RELATED CONDITIONS

ACUTE PYELONEPHRITIS

Acute nontuberculous pyelonephritis, which is among the most frequently encountered acute renal infections, is the least serious of a spectrum of related acute nontuberculous infectious problems. This spectrum extends from acute pyelonephritis to acute bacterial nephritis to acute renal abscess, and to acutely infected pre-existing spaces such as renal cysts or hydronephrotic kidneys. The pathogenesis is similar in all these entities. Bacteria reach the kidney via hematogenous route or by the ascending route from the bladder via the ureter. The course of the acute renal infection is then determined by the aggressiveness of the infectious agent, the immune response of the patient, and predisposing conditions (such as urinary obstruction).

The ordinary case of uncomplicated acute pyelonephritis is readily diagnosed from the clinical presentation of acute onset of flank pain and tenderness accompanied by sudden onset of substantial fever. These findings coupled with bacteriuria and pyuria on urinalysis will usually confirm the diagnosis. No imaging is necessary to make treatment decisions unless the infection does not respond promptly to the usual antibiotic therapy. In that event, dynamic computed tomography is used to determine if the disease has progressed beyond simple acute pyelonephritis. Specifically, predisposing and complicating conditions such as obstruction, occult calculus, or renal abscess needs to be excluded.

Acute pyelonephritis shows positive urographic findings in about 25% of uncomplicated cases in which urography is done.[147] Findings include renal enlargement, diminished intensity of the nephrogram, decreased calyceal contrast density, delayed calyceal appearance time, distortion and attenuation of the calyces and infundibula, and pyelocaliectasis. Renal enlargement is the most common finding, usually on the symptomatic side. Occasionally, the contralateral kidney is also enlarged.

Computed tomography better demonstrates positive findings. Unenhanced scans may be normal or may show regions of slightly decreased attenuation within the parenchyma. Contrast enhanced scans demonstrate radially oriented or wedge-shaped low attenuation regions that extend from the collecting system to the renal surface.[66] Computed tomography is more sensitive than urography in detecting acute infectious parenchymal changes and is the imaging nodality of choice.[147] Ultrasonography also has been found diagnostic, and has the advantage of not requiring contrast administration or exposure to ionizing radiation.[159] Ultrasound findings include renal enlargement and decreased echogenicity of the renal parenchyma, which may be diffuse or regional.

Occasionally, the acute pyelonephritic process may only involve a portion (or lobe) of the kidney. This is termed *acute focal pyelonephritis*. On urography the only suggestive findings are a focal parenchymal contrast blush and focal renal enlargement. Computed tomography and ultrasonography demonstrate the findings previously described for pyelonephritis in a more focal distribution.

Emphysematous pyelonephritis is a rare special form of acute pyelonephritis affecting diabetics or patients with urinary tract obstruction. The finding of gas in and around the kidney in an acutely ill patient suggests the diagnosis. The affected kidney usually does not function well. Gas-forming organisms recovered include *Escherichia coli* and *Proteus vulgaris*. Emphysematous pyelonephritis should be regarded as a complication of a severe necrotizing infection, usually indicating extensive destruction of renal parenchyma, with a poor prognosis (Fig. 20-29).

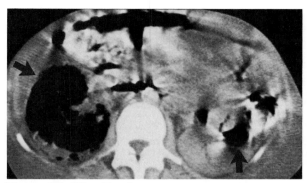

Figure 20–29. Emphysematous pyelonephritis. Unenhanced CT showing bilateral collections of air in the kidneys (*arrows*). The right kidney is almost totally replaced with air.

RENAL ABSCESS

Acute suppurative abscess of the renal parenchyma is rare, is usually hematogenous in origin, and begins in the cortex. Unless recognized and treated early, there is often extensive destruction of renal parenchyma. The most frequent causative organism is staphylococcus. When one or more small cortical abscesses develop in the parenchyma, no roentgenographic manifestations are present. If these small abscesses coalesce to form a large abscess, a plain-film roentgenogram often shows local enlargement of the kidney. The perirenal fat is blurred in the area of involvement so that the renal outline tends to be indistinct. The involved kidney may be fixed during inspiration and expiration. The psoas muscle is often indistinct. There may be scoliosis with the concavity toward the involved side; this suggests the complication of perirenal abscess. Excretory urography is of value if there is enough function to outline the calyceal system. The findings are those of compression and displacement or obliteration of the calyces owing to the tumorlike mass produced by the abscess. The cortical abscess may break through into the collecting system, to appear as a cavity communicating with a calyx and simulating tuberculosis. A peripheral abscess may also break through the renal capsule and produce a perirenal abscess. When multiple acute renal abscesses coalesce this is termed a *renal carbuncle*. Clinical signs of infection may not be present in some patients, particularly when the course is prolonged and the infection is chronic. Therefore, the differentiation from tumor may be difficult.

The imaging diagnosis can best be established by use of CT.[63] Renal ultrasonography may be an alternative if contrast use is contraindicated or the patient's condition does not warrant CT.[159] On CT the findings of acute renal abscess are (1) round or ovoid regions of low attenuation, (2) an irregular wall that may exhibit varying degrees of enhancement, (3) a central fluid component that shows little or no enhancement, (4) extension into the perirenal space or pelvis, and (5) gas within the fluid collection. Only the finding of gas is specific for an abscess. On ultrasonography the findings highly indicative of acute abscess are (1) irregular margin, (2) fluid component (anechoic or low-level internal echoes), and (3) bright echoes representing gas. The distinction between acute focal pyelonephritis and renal abscess is important because an abscess must be drained either percutaneously or surgically. When findings are equivocal, selective renal arteriography may be used if a necrotic neoplasm is a reasonable possibility in the patient's clinical context. The arteriographic clue of most reliability is demonstration of tumor vessels. However, inflammatory vessels on the periphery of the abscess can mimic tumor vessels. In that event, percutaneous needle aspiration biopsy of the mass using CT or ultrasound guidance will usually answer the tumor versus abscess question.[120]

Chronic Renal Abscess

Chronic renal abscess is simply a later stage in the development of an acute renal abscess that does not respond to control by treatment or by the patient's immune response. The abscess requires about 10 to 21 days to mature to a chronic state. The focal area of central inflammatory mass necrosis progresses to a more coalescent liquefaction state. The inflammatory parenchymal margin progresses to a definitive thickened "wall" composed predominantly of fibrotic tissue. The imaging approach is basically the same as in the acute abscess, but imaging results often are less certain in distinguishing necrotic tumor from benign chronic abscess. Needle aspiration biopsy and, on occasion, open surgery are required to make a definitive diagnosis.

Perirenal Abscess

Hematogenous infection in the renal parenchyma may also result in perirenal inflammatory disease and abscess formation. Rarely, the infection may actually arise in the perirenal area in addition to extending there as a complication of cortical abscess. Plain-film roentgenograms of perirenal abscess may show an absence of the perirenal fat shadow, causing an indistinctness of the renal margin. When the abscess is confined within the perirenal (Gerota) fascia, the posterior and inferior portion of the perirenal space fills with pus; this may be outlined as a mass that is confined chiefly to the infrarenal area, since the perirenal space is largest in this area.

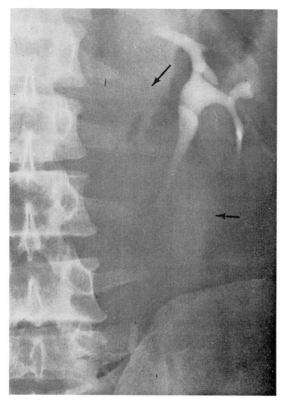

Figure 20–30. Psoas abscess. Note the large psoas mass (*arrows*), which displaces the left kidney and upper ureter. It also compresses the ureter. This is a chronic abscess that is so well localized that the psoas shadow is clearly defined.

Thus, the lower pole of the kidney is obscured. Excretory urography may show upward, anterior, and either medial or lateral renal displacement depending on the site of the abscess. There may be some compression of the collecting system if the abscess is large. Fixation of the kidney by the infection is demonstrated on roentgenograms obtained in inspiration and expiration, which show a failure of the normal movement of the kidney with respiration. The psoas muscle shadow is enlarged and its margin is indistinct adjacent to the area of infection. Lumbar scoliosis with convexity away from the side of the lesion results from muscle splinting and is usually present. The diaphragm is often slightly elevated with areas of linear subsegmental atelectasis in the basal lung manifested by small horizontal densities in the basal lung parenchyma. Computed tomography or ultrasound can show the size and extent of the abscess. Psoas abscess may displace the kidney and ureter, but does not ordinarily spread to involve the kidney (Figs. 20-30 and 20-31).

ACUTE BACTERIAL NEPHRITIS

Davidson and Talner have described the correlation of clinical setting and imaging findings in this rare complication of acute renal infection.[32] This condition is characterized by rapid aggressive hematogenous spread of infection in the kidney overwhelming the patient's immune response. The result is a generalized life-threatening infection featuring renal enlargement owing to severe diffuse inflammatory edema, which severely decreases the parenchymal renal blood supply. The early onset of septicemia in this process ac-

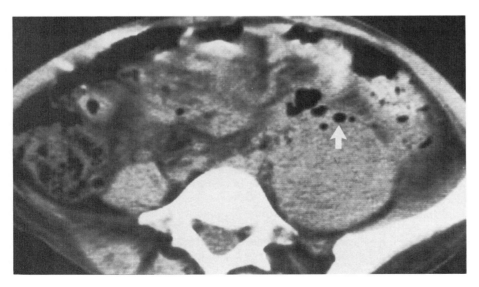

Figure 20–31. Psoas abscess. Unenhanced CT of a patient with Crohn's disease and a left psoas abscess. Note the bubbles of air anteriorly (*arrow*).

counts for the high mortality (30% to 40%) in this rare infection.

The clinical setting is almost pathognomonic. The usual acute pyelonephritis clinical signs and symptoms are exaggerated and the patient often presents in septicemic shock. This occurs almost exclusively in patients with inhibited immune response due to severe insulin-dependent diabetes, chemotherapy for cancer, or drug abuse. It is critical that the diagnosis be established immediately and that appropriate antibiotic and support treatment be initiated.

The imaging examinations used may begin with excretory urography, but usually go on to CT or Doppler ultrasonography to make the distinction between acute bacterial nephritis versus acute renal vein thrombosis, the usual differential diagnosis. The renal veins will be normal in acute bacterial nephritis. Urographic findings are (1) generalized renal enlargement, (2) faint, diminished nephrogram, and (3) delayed and severely diminished calyceal opacification. Computed tomography demonstrates patchy or diffuse regions of low attenuation on enhanced scans. If advanced, there may be progression to frank abscess that can rupture into the subcapsular and perirenal spaces. Ultrasonography is not as sensitive as CT in the detection of acute bacterial nephritis. The involved kidney is enlarged with decreased echogenicity of the renal parenchyma. If there is abscess formation, this can appear as an anechoic focal mass.[31]

ACUTE INFECTION OF PRE-EXISTING RENAL SPACES

In this acute infection of a simple renal cyst or the dilated collecting system of a chronically obstructed kidney, the clinical presentation mimics acute pyelonephritis. The cyst most closely mimics acute renal abscess on imaging examinations. The term *pyonephrosis* is used to describe an infected hydronephrotic renal collecting system. When severe acute infection clinically is associated with such obstruction, percutaneous needle aspiration to make the diagnosis and then to provide a route for percutaneous pyelostomy drainage is the usual approach. Often this is performed in an urgent life-threatening clinical setting.[120]

CHRONIC PYELONEPHRITIS (ATROPHIC PYELONEPHRITIS)

The following criteria for the diagnosis of chronic atrophic pyelonephritis were suggested by Hodson[65, 66]: (1) The disease is centered in the medulla with scarring eventually affecting the whole thickness of renal substance. (2) There is an irregular surface depression over the involved area. (3) The involved papilla is retracted from scarring with secondary dilatation of its calyx. (4) The dilated calyx has a smooth margin but variable shape. (5) Renal tissue adjacent to the involved area is normal or hypertrophied with a sharp definition between normal and abnormal. (6) Distribution is unifocal or multifocal, involving one or both kidneys. (7) There is a decrease in size of the involved kidney.

Chronic bacterial infection of the kidneys usually starts as a focal process in the medulla, causing a localized area of fibrosis or scarring. As it progresses, the infection causes further scarring, resulting in loss of renal parenchyma, irregularity of the renal surface, and distortion of the calyx in the involved area as seen on excretory urography. The calyces involved become clubbed. Renal tissue between involved areas is normal or hypertrophied. Parenchymal loss may progress to the point where there are only a few millimeters of scar tissue between the capsule and the calyx. Unless there is obstruction or significant reflux, the distribution of the lesions is uneven (Fig. 20-32).

The disease usually begins in childhood, but it may not be recognized until early adult life. The earliest roentgenographic sign is a decrease in the amount of renal parenchyma, often in one pole of the kidney. Later, the adjacent calyx or calyces exhibit clubbing. As the disease progresses, the findings become more generalized and are often bilateral but usually not symmetric.

Ureteral reflux and bladder infection as well as focal ischemia probably play a part in the development of changes in the kidney. Scarring and atrophy are most severe in areas in which there is intrarenal reflux in addition to the ureteral reflux into the collecting system.

Hydronephrotic atrophy or obstructive atrophy of the kidney also causes progressive blunting of the calyces and narrowing of the renal parenchyma. However, this tends to be very symmetric in contrast to the irregular distribution of calyceal clubbing and the scars of chronic pyelonephritis. A similar appearance may be observed in patients with vesicoureteral reflux. Infection may be present in both conditions and can cause the focal parenchymal scarring that is found in pyelonephritis. When the disease begins in adult life, there is less scarring of the parenchyma, but the calyceal blunting is similar.

Excretory urography findings feature small, irregular renal shape, clubbed calyces approaching the scarred margin, and interposed focal parenchymal hypertrophy. Computed tomography reflects the same appearance. Ultrasonography demonstrates small shrunken kidneys with increased echogenicity of the kidneys relative to the liver and spleen. The borders of

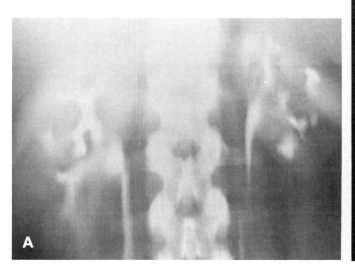

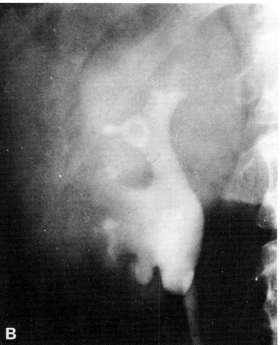

Figure 20–32. **(A)** Pyelonephritis. Chronic pyelonephritis in the left kidney. Note the blunted calyces and the parenchymal loss adjacent to the calyces (greater in the upper pole). **(B)** In another patient with chronic pyelonephritis, the upper-pole calyces appear reasonably normal. Central- and lower-pole calyces are clubbed, and, on the initial film, marked decrease in lower-pole parenchyma could be observed.

the kidneys are difficult to visualize because the irregular, scarred margins scatter the echoes so they do not return to the transducer.[134]

Xanthogranulomatous Pyelonephritis

This form of severe chronic inflammation of the kidney is found predominantly in adult females. The clinical findings consist of a history of easy fatigability and low-grade fever that may antedate urinary symptoms of dysuria, frequency, and a dull, aching flank pain sometimes associated with a palpable flank mass. Recurring attacks may occur. Calculi are common, and there may be parenchymal calcification. The disease is usually unilateral, but the opposite kidney is often involved by pyelonephritis. The pathologic process consists of granulomatous involvement of the renal parenchyma, associated with foam cells, cholesterol slits, extensive fibrotic changes, and atrophic glomeruli. The process may be localized or may involve the entire kidney; at times it may extend to produce a periureteric mass in the upper ureteral region. It may also extend to involve perirenal fat leading to the production of a fixed renal

mass. Chronic obstruction at the ureteral, ureteropelvic, or major calyx level is almost always present. *Proteus vulgaris* is commonly found in the urine but may not be the etiologic agent. Urographic findings consist of calyceal dilatation and blunting with irregularity of papillae, decreased cortical thickness, and ureteral deformity and stricture that may resemble changes due to extensive tuberculosis. The kidney and psoas outlines may be indistinct. Retrograde pyelography reveals dilatation and gross distortion of the pelvis and calyces indicating obstruction. In some patients a local mass resembling carcinoma is present; in others there is a poorly demarcated, diffuse mass, often associated with greatly diminished or no renal function. Calculi are often present as a cause of obstruction. Angiography reveals displacement and stretching of intrarenal arteries with absence of small peripheral branches. Capsular and ureteric branches may be prominent. The nephrogram phase resembles that of hydronephrosis. In many instances the granulomatous mass cannot be differentiated from renal cell carcinoma by angiographic methods. Computed tomography better delineates the total parenchymal process, but often percutaneous aspiration biopsy is required to confirm the diagnosis.[52]

Pyelitis of Pregnancy

The term *pyelitis* is applied to renal infection that may accompany pregnancy. Most pregnancies are associated with some degree of dilatation of the collecting system and ureter. One study found that 90% of the right kidneys and 67% of the left kidneys showed at least mild hydronephrosis.[118] The hydronephrosis is probably caused by mechanical obstruction of the ureters by increased uterine size, although hormonal changes may also play a role. The predominance of hydronephrosis in the right kidney has been attributed to the sharper angulation of the right ureter as it crosses the right iliac artery and ovarian vein at the level of the pelvic brim.[38] The hydronephrosis usually clears 3 to 6 weeks following delivery.

When infection occurs, however, urinary symptoms result from the combination of obstruction and infection. Infection is more common during the last two trimesters. Before use of ultrasonography, urography showed dilated collecting systems and ureters down to the brim of the pelvis (Fig. 20-33). Infection, when present, is usually of recent origin, so that there are no anatomic changes directly related to it unless the patient has had repeated infections in the past or has chronic pyelonephritis.

Ultrasonography provides a safe, easy, and noninvasive means of evaluating hydronephrosis associated with pregnancy. Computed tomography plays less of a role because of the radiation involved, but can be valuable in the postpartum state if hydronephrosis or infection persists.

RENAL PAPILLARY NECROSIS

Renal papillary necrosis, or necrotizing renal papillitis, is characterized by infarction of renal papillae, resulting in necrosis and sloughing of the involved papillary tissue. The necrotic material may be passed in fragments or as a single mass, or it may remain in the calyx. When it remains, it may calcify peripherally to form a rather typical triangular concretion. The etiology of the necrosis is not clear, but it is most likely that medullary ischemia can result from several causes. The condition is usually bilateral and may involve few or many papillae. It is more frequent in females than in males. The abuse of analgesics such as phenacetin over prolonged periods of time is associated with a chronic form of the disease and probably causes it in a large majority of cases. A chronic form also may be associated with sickle cell (homozygous-Ss) disease; with heterozygous-SC hemoglobinopathy, minimal papillary necrosis de-

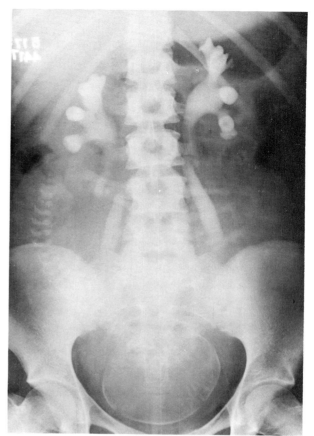

Figure 20–33. Hydronephrosis in pregnancy. The patient had upper urinary tract infection. Combined with pregnancy, this condition is sometimes termed *pyelitis of pregnancy*. A urogram obtained 2 months after delivery showed normal urinary tract. Hydronephrosis is present in the latter period of pregnancy in most gravid patients, but infection is relatively uncommon.

velops without signs or symptoms. An acute fulminating form associated with infection occurs in patients with diabetes mellitus and in patients with obstructive uropathy, particularly when infected. In the acute fulminating form the diminished renal function may make excretory urography useless, but in most instances the diagnosis can be made with this examination. Therefore, retrograde pyelography is seldom necessary. Renal size is normal in the analgesic-abuse group of patients, but in those with the fulminant infectious form, the kidneys may be enlarged and kidney function decreased. Eventually there is enough destruction or atrophy to decrease renal size so that the kidneys become small and smooth. Early papillary swelling may be very difficult to assess by excretory urography. The earliest urographic manifestations suggesting the diagnosis are those of necrosis with formation of tracts extending from the fornix into the parenchyma paralleling the long axis of the papilla.

There are three forms of papillary sloughing.[124] One is the central or partial type in which there is a tract extending inward from the tip of the papilla. The shape of this cavity varies considerably from one calyx to another. In the second form, the necrosis occurs at the base of the papilla, resulting in sloughing of the papilla. The papilla may remain in the kidney or be excreted, and can occasionally become lodged in the ureter causing obstruction. The third form of papillary sloughing is necrosis in situ in which the papilla remains attached, decreases in size, and eventually may calcify; it usually cannot be recognized until calcification occurs. A triangular radiolucent shadow ringed with a dense opaque shadow, the "ring shadow," may be observed when the separated necrotic papilla remains in the calyx. Eventually, a typical concretion may develop; it consists of a dense, calcified shell surrounding a radiolucent center. Late in the disease, scarring may result in some distortion. The diagnosis can be histopathologically confirmed if some of the sloughed material is passed and recovered from the urine.

BILATERAL ACUTE RENAL CORTICAL NECROSIS

This disease is characterized by bilateral, symmetrical, ischemic necrosis of the renal cortex, sparing the subcapsular cortex. It is a cause of acute renal failure and has terminated fatally in most instances. It may be associated with a number of antecedent conditions such as severe burns, multiple fractures, internal hemorrhage, severe infections, transfusions of incompatible blood, peritonitis, and others. It occurs frequently in pregnancy, often associated with abruptio placentae. With the advent of modern treatment, including hemodialysis, several patients have recovered partially from the disease and certain roentgenographic findings have been observed that suggest the diagnosis.

Initially, the kidneys are usually enlarged, which is followed by a decrease in size of varying degrees. Faint cortical calcification is seen on urography in the form of a thin shell-like rim around the periphery of the kidney appearing in 50 to 60 days after onset. This is so faint that tomograms or CT may be necessary for adequate visualization in patients suspected of having the disease. Tram-line or double-line calcification has also been reported. The calcification may extend into the interlobular septa, appearing as diffuse and punctate densities in the remaining cortical tissue.[116] The renal contour may be irregular and the calcification

interrupted, depending on distribution of the disease. The renal pelvis and calyceal system appear normal, but function is usually so decreased following recovery from the acute phase of the disease that retrograde pyelography is necessary to outline the collecting system.

PYELOURETERITIS CYSTICA, PYELITIS CYSTICA, AND URETERITIS CYSTICA

Pyeloureteritis cystica and ureteritis cystica are manifested by small suburethelial cysts that elevate the epithelium of the ureteral wall and sometimes the wall of the renal pelvis. These cysts appear as small radiolucent defects along the course of the ureter when it has been opacified by contrast substance. The appearance of multiple, small, mucosal filling defects is pathognomonic. The defects are usually more numerous in the upper ureter than elsewhere. They may become large enough to produce partial ureteral obstruction and range from microscopic size to 2 cm in diameter. Signs of active infection at the time of urography are often present in these patients, or there may be a history of previous urinary tract infection. Stones in the urinary tract are also common. The pathogenesis is unknown, however. The lesions may be unilateral (70%) or bilateral. The condition is relatively rare in the ureters and renal pelvis and is extremely rare in the infundibula and calyces.[39]

TUBERCULOSIS

Pathology

The kidney is involved by tuberculosis in a manner comparable to involvement of other organs. The infection is hematogenous. The organisms are filtered out by the glomerular capillary bed, where they may produce small tubercles, some of which will heal. However, necrosis may occur and organisms may migrate from the cortex to the region of the renal papilla. There, new tubercles are formed in Henle's loop, leading to destruction of medullary tissue and ulceration. These early lesions are often multiple but do not involve all the papillae. As the disease progresses, involvement of adjacent infundibula often leads to obstruction. Similar stricture formation leading to obstruction is found when there is ureteral involvement. If the disease does not heal spontaneously, the destruction continues, producing irregular cavities adjacent to the calyces. Eventually this leads to virtual destruction of the entire kidney. If ureteral obstruction is not a factor, the kidney may gradually decrease in size or remain normal in size and gradually fill with caseous material along with some calcium to form the so-called putty kidney. If ureteral obstruction occurs before the kidney is destroyed and functionless, the result is a large hydronephrotic kidney in which there are irregular cavities adjacent to the calyces. The anatomic changes are visible on urograms and form the basis for the roentgenographic diagnosis of renal tuberculosis. This diagnosis should always be confirmed, as in pulmonary tuberculosis, by demonstration of the organisms in the urine from the involved kidney. Even though the disease is hematogenous, the initial source, usually lung or bone, may not be detected. Clinical evidence of renal involvement is unilateral in about 75% of patients even though the organisms have presumably been disseminated to both kidneys. Computed tomographic and ultrasound findings are similar to those found at urography.

Roentgenographic Findings

The roentgenographic findings on plain-film examination are those of alteration in size of the kidney and calcification within it due to advanced disease. These are nonspecific findings but may be suggestive, particularly if cloudy flocculent calcification outlines most of the renal shadow, indicative of extensive destruction of parenchyma, so-called autonephrectomy. The calcification may be dense and irregular and may lie within the renal outline, often in the cortical area. In the early stages of cortical involvement, no urographic findings are present, and it is possible to have considerable parenchymal involvement without urographic change. The earliest finding is that of a slight irregularity of the involved calyx caused by ulcerative papillary lesions (Fig. 20-34). Further destruction is manifested by loss of the normal papilla and irregular ragged cavity formation (Fig. 20-35). Often this is associated with a narrowing of the infundibulum to the affected calyx. The infundibulum may later become completely obstructed, so that the diseased area is not visible on retrograde pyelography. A careful evaluation of calyceal distribution in relation to the renal outline is necessary in all patients with suspected renal tuberculosis. Parenchymal destruction may result in cortical scarring with irregular narrowing of the parenchyma and irregularity of the renal outline. When the renal pelvis is involved, the mucosa is irregular because of ulceration. Later local constriction caused by fibrosis is also common, and dilatation results when there is obstruction at or below the ureteropelvic junction. Ureteral involvement may result in stricture formation, often multiple; mucosal infection can also produce small local nodules that appear as filling defects along the ureteral wall. The appearance is quite variable, ranging from that of a beaded to a corkscrew pattern to that of single or multiple strictures in some instances. In advanced in-

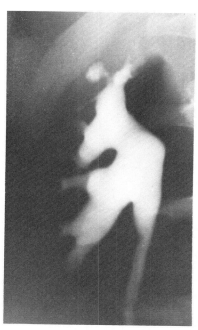

Figure 20–34. Renal tuberculosis. The calyces of the upper pole are involved and are irregular as a result of adjacent parenchymal destruction.

volvement of the ureter it is common to find the ureter unusually straight, extending in a direct line downward from the renal pelvis to the pelvic brim ("pipe stem" ureter) without the usual slight curves seen in the normal ureter. The bladder, seminal vesicles, and vas deferens may also be involved in patients with renal tuberculosis. The bladder wall may be thickened and its capacity diminished. Tuberculous granulation tissue projecting into the bladder may resemble carcinoma in some instances. Irregular mottled calcification in these structures suggests the diagnosis.

Urography is used in renal tuberculosis as a method of making an anatomic diagnosis, to be confirmed by bacteriologic study. It is also of value in following the renal lesion during treatment, in detecting complications, such as ureteral obstruction or infundibular obstruction, and in outlining the opposite kidney.

Differential Diagnosis

Differential diagnosis of calcium deposits must include consideration of renal calculi and nephrocalcinosis as well as cyst and tumor calcification. Calculi are usually more discrete and rounded than the calcification seen in tuberculosis. Tumor calcification often extends beyond the border of the kidney and tends to appear less hazy and flocculent than that in tuberculosis. Calcifica-

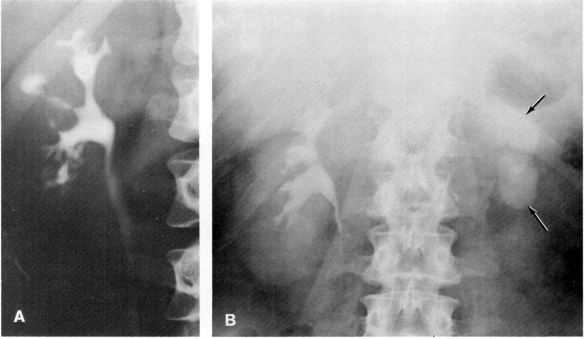

Figure 20–35.   Renal tuberculosis. **(A)** There is extensive involvement with cavity formation superiorly and centrally. There is also irregular narrowing of one of the upper central infundibula. **(B)** The right kidney is relatively normal, but the small, dense, irregular kidney on the left did not change during urography. This left kidney represents the so-called putty kidney.

tion in cysts occurs in the wall and tends to outline it in an arcuate form of varying size. This calcification also tends to extend beyond the shadow of the normal kidney. Urographic changes in chronic pyelonephritis consist of calyceal abnormality that may resemble early tuberculous involvement, but the change is usually more general than in tuberculosis. The same is true in renal papillary necrosis, which is usually bilateral and tends to be more extensive than renal tuberculosis. In some patients, granulomatous changes predominate to the extent that a renal mass is formed, which must be differentiated from other renal masses. Usually other signs are present that aid in the diagnosis of these cases. Brucellosis may produce findings in the kidney identical to those due to tuberculosis, but it is very rare.

RENAL CANDIDIASIS

Because renal candidiasis usually occurs in patients who have a chronic illness or whose immune system has been altered, the following factors are important in its development: acquired immunodeficiency syndrome (AIDS), antibiotic therapy, prolonged use of indwelling intravenous catheters, treatment with steroids or chemotherapy, therapy with immunosuppressive agents, blood dyscrasias, diabetes mellitus, intravenous drug abuse, and chronic disease such as malignant neoplasm.[24] In systemic candidiasis, involvement of the kidney is common. Renal candidiasis may assume three forms that may be different stages of the same disease: (1) acute pyelonephritis in which the fungi proliferate in the renal tubules to form cortical and medullary abscesses with interstitial edema and renal failure, (2) a more chronic process with hydronephrosis and chronic pyelonephritis, and (3) disseminated candidiasis that involves several organs including the kidneys. Excretory urography may demonstrate the multiple fungus balls in the renal pelvis and upper ureter in patients with pyelonephritis, but renal function may be so poor that retrograde studies, CT, or ultrasound may be needed to reveal their presence. The appearance is one of shaggy, irregular filling defects in the renal pelvis, often extending into the infundibula and upper ureter. Acute papillary necrosis resulting from candidiasis is similar to that caused by other acute fulminating infections, except that in candidiasis more debris may be present in the calyces and pelvis representing the sloughed necrotic papilla plus the fungus balls (mycelial masses). Computed tomographic findings are similar, although without corroborating clinical data the findings may be confused with other causes of luminal filling defects, such as transitional cell carcinoma.

TRAUMA

RENAL TRAUMA

The kidney lies in a well-protected area and is not frequently injured. In patients with chronic renal disease, however, relatively minor trauma may cause considerable damage. Direct force over the renal area is the usual cause of injury. Trauma to the kidney is usually manifested by hematuria, which may be gross or microscopic. Hematuria after an injury indicates some type of damage to the kidney or injury to the lower urinary tract. Excretory urography with tomography has been the traditional imaging modality to evaluate *minor* renal trauma. It is a safe procedure and may lead to a definitive diagnosis of the extent of renal injury relatively soon after the trauma. The excretory nephrogram (1- to 2-minute film) is a good indicator of renal function. Radionuclide scintigraphy could also be used to evaluate renal function but is usually not performed in the setting of acute trauma. Excretory urography also allows evaluation of the contralateral kidney if surgical removal of the injured kidney is contemplated. However, there are instances in which extravasation is not shown on the excretory urogram because function is greatly reduced.

CT has proved its value in evaluation of *major* renal trauma. Computed tomography reveals contusions, incomplete and complete lacerations, intra- and extrarenal hematomas, and fractured or shattered kidneys. It is superior to excretory urography in differentiating major from minor renal injuries.[42] Other studies have corroborated that CT is more specific than other noninvasive radiographic studies in demonstrating the nature of blunt renal trauma.[133] The choice of surgical or medical therapy will depend on the severity of injury to the kidney, and CT therefore has a significant impact. It offers the added value of detection of extrarenal injuries in trauma affecting other visceral organs such as the liver or spleen. The CT scan should be performed with intravenous contrast and dynamic technique to optimize detection of lacerations, extravasated urine,

and hematomas. Dynamic CT is superior to conventional CT in assessing parenchymal renal injuries. Dynamic CT correctly diagnosed parenchymal injuries in 129 of 130 cases versus 116 of 130 cases for conventional CT in a study presented by Lang and colleagues.[88]

Injury to the renal pedicle should be suspected if there is delayed or nonvisualization of the kidney on CT or excretory urography after a bolus injection of iodinated contrast material. CT has the advantage over excretory urography of being able to prove definitively the existence or absence of a nonfunctioning kidney in the event of nonvisualization after contrast injection (Fig. 20-36). Patients with renal aplasia, hypoplasia, or other congenital abnormalities may have false-positive studies at excretory urography and receive unnecessary angiography.

Renal angiography is indicated in the posttraumatic period if there is suspicion of injury to the renal pedicle. Subintimal flaps, renal artery thrombosis, arteriovenous fistula, or laceration of the artery may occur. Arteriography is still considered the best modality for demonstrating injuries to the renal artery, although MRI may have a role in the future. Angiography also has the potential of being therapeutic. Transcatheter embolization or balloon occlusion can be used to treat extensive hemorrhage or arteriovenous fistulas.[88] If renal artery damage is demonstrated, immediate surgical correction of the vascular lesion may prevent permanent renal damage in some instances.

The severity of parenchymal injury may vary from rupture of a calyx with extravasation of blood or urine into the parenchyma to more extensive fracture of the parenchyma with subcapsular and parenchymal extravasation. With more extensive injury, the capsule can rupture with perirenal hemorrhage and extravasation of urine. These nonpenetrating injuries can be classified into the following categories: (1) contusion, (2) cortical laceration (often with intrarenal hematoma), (3) calyceal laceration, and (4) fracture with laceration of the renal capsule. A fractured kidney may have associated lacerations of the calyces, infundibula, or pelvis. Nonparenchymal injury, such as rupture of the renal pelvis or rupture of an anomalous extrarenal calyx, may occur. Immediate surgical extirpation of the kidney may be required in some instances when there is extensive fracture with retroperitoneal and intraperitoneal hemorrhage. The opposite kidney should always be studied by means of excretory urography or CT before nephrectomy. Conservative management of the traumatized kidney, whenever possible, is being utilized more often now than in the past.

The radiographic findings depend on the extent of injury. A simple contusion is usually manifest by renal swelling, decreased density of the nephrogram in the

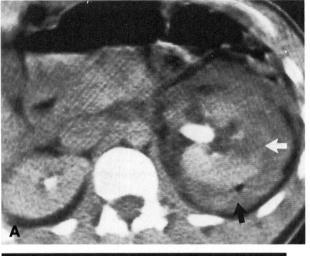

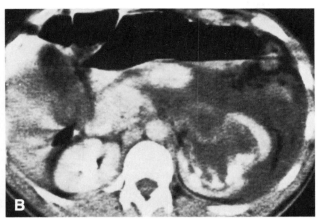

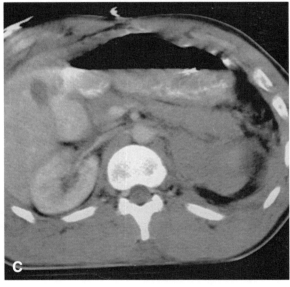

Figure 20–36. Renal trauma. (**A**) Enhanced CT of a laceration in the midportion of the left kidney (*white arrow*) with predominantly perirenal hematoma (*black arrow*). (**B**) Enhanced CT of a different patient with perirenal, pararenal, and central sinus hematomas. (**C**) Enhanced CT of a patient with a renal fracture and pedicle injury. Note lack of contrast enhancement of renal parenchyma on left.

affected portion, and decreased or delayed excretion of contrast into the collecting system. If perirenal hemorrhage is present, the renal shadow, and sometimes the psoas shadow, is obliterated or enlarged on the plain film. At times the hemorrhage remains localized in the perirenal area and produces a localized or generalized enlargement of the kidney. Computed tomography nicely demonstrates perirenal and pararenal hematoma (Fig. 20-36). Kunin has described bridging fibrous septa within the perinephric space, which can act to limit and stop the perirenal hemorrhage by tamponade.[83] Rarely, calcification of a hematoma in or around the kidney may be seen as a late finding in renal trauma. Subcapsular hematoma produces a lenticular

indentation on the renal parenchyma (Fig. 20-37). Accessory signs on plain films are scoliosis (convexity to the opposite side indicating muscle spasm); dilated small-bowel loops in the vicinity of the injury caused by local adynamic ileus; and fracture of an adjacent rib, vertebral body, transverse, or spinous process. Urography demonstrates the amount of extravasation and may show calyceal compression and distortion caused by parenchymal and subcapsular accumulations of blood, urine, or both (Fig. 20-38). Computed tomography provides a better view of the extent of extravasation in many instances (Fig. 20-39). The amount of extravasation is not necessarily proportional to the parenchymal or vascular damage, however. Because post-

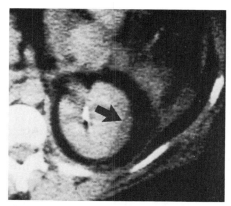

Figure 20–37. Renal trauma. Enhanced CT showing subcapsular hematoma. Note the indentation on the renal parenchyma (*arrow*) from the pressure of the hematoma confined by the renal capsule.

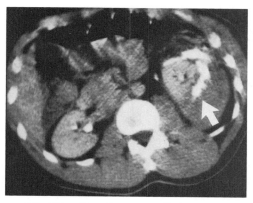

Figure 20–39. Renal trauma. Enhanced CT shows extravasation of contrast (*arrow*) in addition to the hematoma around the left kidney.

traumatic distortion and stricture are important, urographic studies should also be carried out during or following convalescence to outline any residual deformity.

RENAL CYSTIC DISEASE

The classification of renal cystic disease is difficult, and there is much confusion in the literature because of disagreement among pathologists. For our purposes the classification of Elkin,[40] as modified later by Elkin and Bernstein,[41] is most useful (Table 20-2).

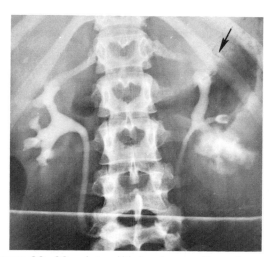

Figure 20–38. Interstitial extravasation of opaque medium in the lower pole of the left kidney caused by trauma. Site of a fracture of the eleventh rib, on the left (*arrow*).

Table 20–2. Classification of Renal Cysts

   I. Renal Dysplasia
      A. Multicystic kidney
      B. Focal and segmental cystic dysplasia
      C. Multiple cysts associated with lower urinary tract obstruction
  II. Polycystic Disease
      A. Infantile polycystic disease
         1. Polycystic disease of the newborn
         2. Polycystic disease of childhood
             a. Congenital hepatic fibrosis
             b. Medullary tubular ectasia
      B. Adult polycystic disease
 III. Cortical Cysts
      A. Trisomy syndromes
      B. Tuberous sclerosis complex
      C. Simply cysts
         1. Solitary
         2. Multiple
      D. Multilocular cysts
 IV. Medullary Cysts
      A. Medullary sponge kidney
      B. Medullary cystic disease
      C. Medullary necrosis
      D. Pyelogenic cyst
  V. Miscellaneous Intrarenal Cysts
      A. Inflammatory
         1. Tuberculosis
         2. Calculous disease
         3. Echinococcus disease
      B. Neoplastic-cystic degeneration of carcinoma
      C. Traumatic intrarenal hematoma
 VI. Extraparenchymal Renal Cysts
      A. Parapelvic cyst
      B. Perinephric cyst

RENAL DYSPLASIA

Multicystic Dysplastic Kidney

Congenital multicystic dysplastic kidney is a rare disorder usually considered to be a severe form of renal dysplasia.[55] The bilateral form results in renal nonfunction, while the unilateral form, which is more common, carries a good prognosis if uncomplicated by other anomalies. There is absence of normal renal parenchyma, the pelvis is small or absent, and the ureter is hypoplastic, stenotic, or atretic. The few nephrons that are present are hypoplastic with arrested development. Blood supply is variable. The kidney consists of a mass of cysts of varying size and is usually very large. The opposite, uninvolved kidney is often hypertrophied, and there is an association with contralateral ureteropelvic junction obstruction. The disease usually presents as a unilateral flank mass in a healthy-appearing infant. The mass may be visible on plain film.

The pattern on excretory urography of a large mass in the renal fossa with opacification of strands of vascularized dysplastic tissue and cyst walls surrounding radiolucent cysts, plus absent nephrogram and no identifiable collecting system or ureter, is virtually diagnostic. This is especially so if cystoscopy and retrograde pyelography have demonstrated absence of one half of the trigone or atretic ureter on the involved side. Shell-like calcification may outline some of the cysts. Occasionally there will be delayed opacification of some irregular cystic spaces. There may be a small amount of functioning renal tissue scattered in the dysplastic kidney to account for this.

Ultrasonography demonstrates unilateral multiple cysts of varying shape and size in the renal fossa. These cysts do not communicate (as opposed to the communicating appearance of hydronephrosis), and the atretic renal pelvis cannot be visualized. Occasionally, ultrasound-guided percutaneous cyst puncture is needed to distinguish renal dysplasia from hydronephrosis. Dysplasia is a benign lesion and need not be removed once the diagnosis is made.

Segmental multicystic renal dysplasia may also occur. In the cases reported by Daughtridge,[30] there was peripheral and central calcification resembling that sometimes observed in renal cell carcinoma. Arteriography often reveals a sharply demarcated, avascular mass with no neovascularity. Differentiation from avascular tumor is difficult in this segmental form of the disease.

POLYCYSTIC DISEASE

There are two general categories of polycystic disease: polycystic renal disease of the young and adult polycystic kidney disease. Both are inherited diseases characterized by multiple cystic abnormalities within both kidneys. Beyond those similarities the two categories differ greatly in many aspects. The micro-dissection research of Osathanondh and Potter[115] in the mid-1960s established the pathogenesis and the embryologic defects that characterize the two basic categories of polycystic disease.

Polycystic Renal Disease of the Young

The pathologic-radiologic hallmark of this disease is grossly elongated, dilated collecting ducts throughout the renal parenchyma. The dilated ducts extend from the papillary tips to the surface of the cortex, and urine flow from nephrons into these ducts is slower than normal. When seen in profile, clusters of these ducts in each renal lobule look like straws seen from the side. When seen on end, the ducts appear like a cluster of straws seen on end. The kidneys are usually symmetrically and uniformly enlarged with correspondingly enlarged, but otherwise normal, collecting systems. The renal vasculature, nephrons, and ureters are normal. The surface of the kidneys is studded with a myriad of 1- to 2-mm vesiclelike protrusions representing the peripheral end of clusters of dilated collecting ducts seen on end.

The embryologic defect is due to abnormal development of the interstitial portion of the ureteral bud occurring in the first trimester of gestation. Genetically this is an autosomal recessive disease. The only cystic involvement of other organs occurs in the liver. It features generalized proliferation of the intrahepatic biliary ducts. Grossly, this appears as generalized ectasia of the ducts and it occurs to a greater or lesser degree in all cases.

The clinical course is determined by the severity of the changes in the kidneys and the liver and the balance of degree of involvement of the kidneys versus the liver. There are four clinical subgroups based on the time the disease becomes clinically manifest.[16] The earliest is the *perinatal group*, in which about 90% of renal collecting ducts are involved. The disease presents at birth with grossly palpably enlarged kidneys. Patients usually die before the age of 6 weeks from rapidly progressive renal failure. The hepatic abnormality does not have time to become clinically manifest. The latest appearance is the *juvenile group*, in whom 10% or fewer renal collecting ducts are involved. The renal disease is usually not clinically manifest, but the liver disease is predominant and usually lethal. Clinical manifestations reflect severe progressive periportal hepatic fibrosis with portal hypertension, gastric and esophageal varices, and hematemesis. Age of clinical onset is usually between 4 and 8 years.

In between the perinatal and juvenile groups are two

intermediate groups: *neonatal*, in whom about 60% of renal ducts are involved, and *infantile*, in whom about 25% are involved. The radiologist, on the basis of urographic findings, can sort the patients into two main groups that Elkin has called (1) polycystic disease of the newborn and (2) polycystic disease of childhood.[40] The former roughly encompasses the pathologic-based perinatal and neonatal groups; the latter, the infantile and juvenile groups.

Use of excretory urography has been replaced by ultrasonography to a large extent. Findings on urography in the newborn category include bilateral massive renal enlargement (with smooth margins), prolonged nephrogram density (up to 72 hours), contrast accumulation in dilated collecting ducts producing a streaky parenchymal pattern, and normal collecting systems and ureters (when seen). In the childhood category, the hepatic component predominates. Urography usually shows mildly enlarged kidneys, a mildly prolonged nephrogram phase, a streaky parenchymal contrast pattern that is predominantly medullary in location, and gross hepatic enlargement.

On ultrasound examination, the kidneys are enlarged and show a diffusely heterogeneous increased echogenicity. The cysts are too small to be seen on ultrasonography as fluid-filled regions, but are large enough to cause echoes, mainly in the medulla. The periphery of the kidneys may be hypoechoic. Cysts may be seen in the liver. The hepatic parenchyma appears more echogenic because of fibrosis.

Adult Polycystic Kidney Disease

This disease is transmitted as an autosomal dominant trait with strong penetrance. Spherical, fluid-filled cysts, usually from 1 to 3 cm in size, are scattered throughout the renal parenchyma. Occasionally the cysts have curvilinear walls or intrarenal punctate calcifications. The superficial cysts produce a knobby appearance of the kidney surface. Between the cysts are scattered islands of normal parenchyma containing normal nephrons and collecting ducts. Kidneys are greatly enlarged with correspondingly larger-than-normal collecting systems that are irregularly compressed by many adjacent cysts. In about one third of patients, large spherical cysts are scattered throughout the liver. These do not communicate with the biliary tree. Spherical cysts occasionally also involve the pancreas, spleen, lungs, and ovaries. There is a modest increased incidence of berry aneurysm of the arteries at the base of the brain.[161] The embryologic abnormality is a sporadic failure of both the ampullary and interstitial portions of the ureteral bud. This results in failure to form normal nephrons and collecting ducts in areas scattered throughout the renal parenchyma.

Clinical manifestations most often appear in adults in the 30- to 50-year age group. Rarely, it occurs in young infants. The most frequent presenting problems include hypertension, microscopic hematuria, and presence of palpable abdominal masses owing to renal enlargement. The disease may be diagnosed on excretory urography, ultrasound, or CT examinations. Urographic findings include enlarged, knobby-surfaced kidneys; round radiolucent nephrogram defects; irregularly distorted collecting systems; and, in some cases, lucent hepatic defects representing cysts as an unexpected nephrogram film finding.

Ultrasonography readily demonstrates the enlarged kidneys containing a multitude of fluid-filled, anechoic cysts. The hepatic cysts, likewise, are easily seen. Computed tomography shows to good advantage all the pathologic cystic findings described earlier in the kidneys and the liver (Fig. 20-40).[57] For follow-up of a known disease, ultrasonography is less expensive, noninvasive, and easy to perform.

CORTICAL CYSTS

Tuberous Sclerosis

Renal cysts are usually small and of tubular origin. Rarely, cortical cysts large enough to produce distortion have been reported. Angiomyolipoma of the kidney is found frequently in association with tuberous sclerosis. (This tumor or hamartoma is described in a subsequent section on benign tumors.)

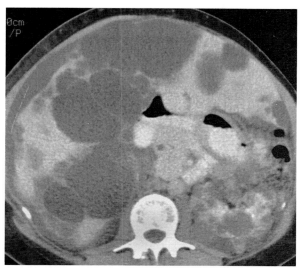

Figure 20-40. Adult polycystic disease. Enhanced CT shows hepatic and bilateral renal cysts.

Simple Cysts

The simple renal cyst is often a "silent" lesion of little or no clinical importance, but it is the most common unifocal renal mass. Simple cysts rarely bleed but may become large enough to be noted as masses that can be palpated through the abdominal wall. They may cause renal damage because of their size, particularly if situated in a region where obstruction of the excretory system can occur. Lesions may be unilateral or bilateral. A cyst may be solitary, but often there are two or more in a kidney. They may be so numerous that differentiation from adult polycystic disease may be difficult. The roentgenographic findings depend on the location. The chief importance of the simple cyst is that it may simulate a tumor in its appearance. Plain-film roentgenograms may outline a smooth, local enlargement of the kidney. Occasionally (less than 1%), there is a thin shell of calcium outlining the cyst wall or a portion of it (Fig. 20-41). It is somewhat more common to see curvilinear calcifications in tumors of the kidney than in cysts. The cysts may reach massive size and actually dwarf the kidney. Urographic findings consist of crescentic defects and stretching of the infundibula and calyces when the lesion arises close to the calyces. When the cyst arises farther away there is less calyceal change, and when the cyst is in a subcapsular position there is little or no pressure deformity on the pelvis or calyces.

The following urographic signs are present in the great majority of cysts. (1) The lesion is peripheral so that it bulges out of the kidney. (2) The wall is very thin and smooth if visible. (3) The mass is quite radiolucent compared with the adjacent parenchyma and sharply demarcated from the renal parenchyma. Often this appears as a beaklike (or "claw") deformity (Fig. 20-42). If all these signs are present, the lesion most likely is a cyst. Following urography suggesting the diagnosis of a cyst, CT or ultrasonography is usually the next imaging examination, provided the patient would be treated if the lesion turned out to be a tumor rather than a cyst. For further discussion on the differentiation of cysts from tumors see the section on renal cell carcinoma.

Multilocular Cysts

This rare condition consists of unilateral solitary cysts that contain numerous loculi that neither intercommunicate nor connect with the renal pelvis.[9] This abnormality is usually found in childhood. The remainder of the kidney is normal. Some consider it a form of renal dysplasia; others believe it to be a benign neoplasm, a multilocular cystic nephroma. Rarely, diffuse calcification is present, resembling that in renal cell carcinoma. Abdominal mass is the usual major presenting complaint. Roentgenographic findings resemble those of simple cyst on the urogram. Arteriography shows the mass to be avascular; vessels around it may be stretched, but no neovascularity or "tumor stain" is demonstrated. Ultrasonography and CT show a multichambered cystic type lesion. Cyst puncture is occa-

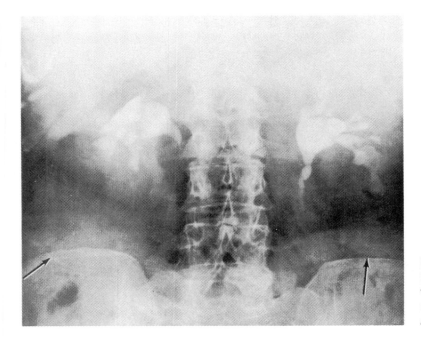

Figure 20–41. Bilateral renal cysts. Note the relatively large size of the cysts with a faint rim of calcification on the right. Inferior aspects of the cysts (*arrows*).

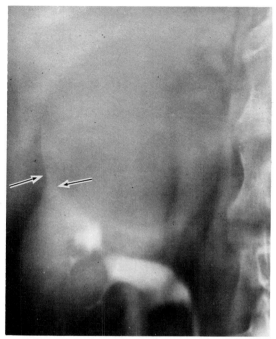

Figure 20–42. The claw sign of a renal cyst (*arrows*). Nephrotomogram clearly outlines the smooth wall of the radiolucent cyst adjacent to the density of the opacified parenchyma.

sionally needed to eliminate the possibility of malignancy.

MEDULLARY CYSTS

Medullary Sponge Kidney

Medullary sponge kidney is a form of cystic disease involving the medulla of the kidney. It is more frequent in males (about 2:1) than females; it has been reported in siblings but does not appear to be hereditary. The changes are confined to the renal medulla and consist of dilatation involving the collecting tubules in the renal pyramids. Calculi can develop in the dilated ducts. The condition may be limited to a single pyramid, but is usually more extensive and is usually bilateral, but not necessarily symmetrical. Renal enlargement may be present when the lesions are general. The defect appears to be a developmental one involving the formation of the collecting ducts. There may be morbidity caused by infection or colic when calculi are passed. Microscopically, the elongated or irregular cysts present a varied appearance. The epithelium varies from transitional to squamous or columnar, normal tubules are reduced or absent, and some degree of inflammatory change is usually present. The dilated ducts may contain calculi or masses of calcified debris.

The urographic findings usually are quite characteristic.[117] The plain film demonstrates the calculi when present. Their medullary position and appearance are often diagnostic but can mimic stones in renal tubular acidosis. The calculi are usually multiple, small, and spindle-shaped, and they occur in clusters or in a fan-like arrangement in the renal pyramids. In the excretory urogram the dilated tubules are seen to be opacified unless infection has impaired renal function. Minimal dilatation produces a fine striated appearance; with increasing dilatation the appearance becomes more cystlike, with rounded or elongated cavities enlarging and often distorting the papilla and minor calyx (Fig. 20-43). Adjacent calyces may show a considerable difference in the degree of involvement.

Medullary Cystic Disease

Nephronophthisis (familial juvenile nephronophthisis, medullary cystic disease of the kidney) is a rare disorder of unknown origin usually found in children and young adults. Anemia, polydipsia, polyuria, salt wasting, and progressive uremia develop insidiously. Growth retardation, bone deformities, and hypocalcemic tetany occur in young patients. Urine has a low, fixed specific gravity with absence of protein or formed elements. Histopathologic findings consist of alternating areas of cystic dilatation and atrophy in the proximal and distal tubules with marked thickening of the basement membrane. Interstitial fibrosis with round-cell infiltration is prominent. Glomeruli show minor focal thickening early, progressing to sclerosis and periglomerular fibrosis.

Urographic study has been of limited value because of poor function. With high-dose urography, minor calyceal blunting, uniform contraction of the kidneys, and cystlike areas of medullary lucency may be observed. Renal angiography shows marked cortical thinning and multiple cysts that spare the thin outer cortex, which is undulating because of the numerous cysts that also displace vessels. The cortex is best seen in the nephrogram phase of angiography.[100] Ultrasonography shows bilateral small echogenic kidneys.[127] A few cysts may be visible as fluid-filled structures. Computed tomography may show small, smooth kidneys with cysts in the medulla or at the corticomedullary junction.

Calyceal Diverticulum
(Pyelogenic or Calycine Cysts)

The term *calyceal diverticulum* refers to the small cystlike spaces that often communicate with a calyx, but that occasionally are observed on urography to opacify despite no apparent connection with the adjacent calyx. This lesion may be a true congenital cyst.

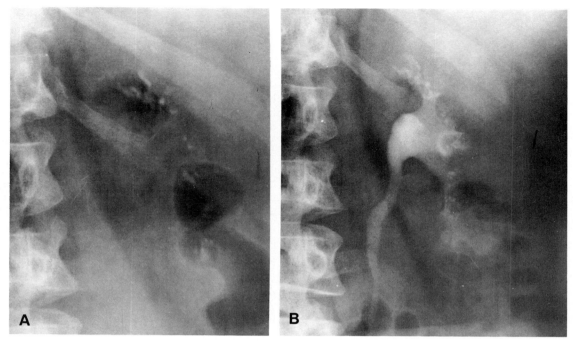

Figure 20–43.   Sponge kidney. **(A)** Preliminary film shows mottled calcifications in the left kidney. **(B)** Urogram of the patient shown in **A** demonstrates the relationship of the calcifications to several of the calyces. These calcifications are in dilated tubules in the renal papillae.

Cystlike structures of similar appearance may result from inflammatory destruction of parenchyma adjacent to a calyx or be associated with sickle cell disease. The diagnosis is made on excretory urography when a small, rounded space fills with opaque medium (Fig. 20-44).[161] The cysts are filled by their own tubules and are visible despite lack of apparent communication with the calyceal system. In contrast to the cysts in the renal pyramids as found in sponge kidney, calycine cysts often arise from the fornix of the calyx and occur laterally rather than centrally in relation to the papilla. These cysts are of little clinical significance unless infected or the site of calculus formation. Rarely, milk of calcium is observed, with a fluid level evident on an upright film (Fig. 20-45).

EXTRAPARENCHYMAL RENAL CYSTS

Parapelvic Cysts

Parapelvic cysts are relatively rare. Unlike simple renal cysts, they do not lie within the renal parenchyma. They are located in, and probably originate in, the hilus of the kidney in close proximity to the pelvis and major calyces. Their origin is obscure. Some authors believe them to be of lymphatic origin; others believe they are congenital cysts that arise from embryonic rests or from remnants of the wolffian body or from mesonephric remnants.

Urographic findings are those of a mass in the renal hilus that causes compression and displacement of the pelvis and distortion and displacement of the major calyces and infundibula. Mild local caliectasis may result from partial obstruction resulting from compression. They do not contain calcium. They resemble renal sinus lipomatosis when the latter results in a focal mass in the renal hilum.

Because there is no renal parenchymal interface with this type of cyst, the nephrographic phase of arteriography or nephrotomography is somewhat different from that seen in the simple cyst. The parapelvic cyst appears as a spherical mass (of lesser density than the opacified renal parenchyma adjacent to it) surrounded by a halo of fat that is more radiolucent than the cyst (Fig. 20-46). Ultrasonography or CT is used to establish a certain diagnosis of parapelvic cyst.

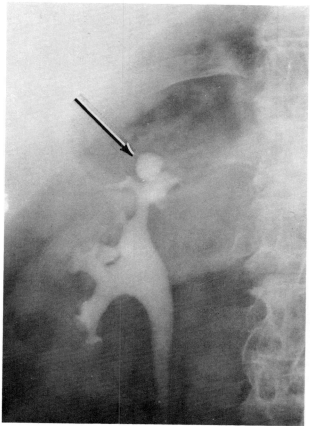

Figure 20–44. Calycine cyst (*arrow*). The cyst communicates with one of the calyces of the upper pole.

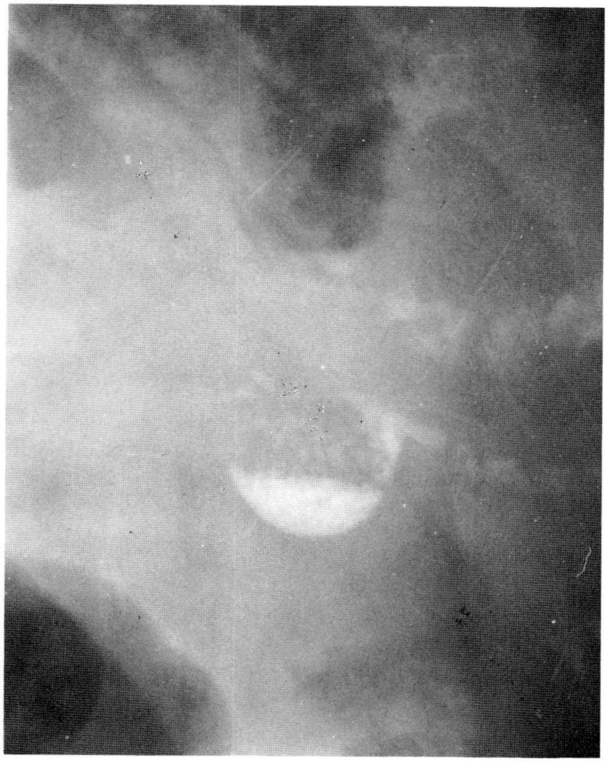

Figure 20–45. Milk of calcium in a renal cyst. This film, exposed with the patient in the upright position, shows calcium, which is somewhat granular in appearance, in a cyst located in the central portion of the left kidney. There is also evidence of calcium in the cyst's wall.

Pararenal Pseudocyst—Urinoma

Pararenal pseudocyst is used to describe a complication of injury of the renal pelvis or proximal ureter. A rent in the renal collecting system or kidney can result in persistent extravasation of urine or blood into the perirenal space. This may produce compression of the pelvis or upper ureter, and resultant hydronephrosis that may lead to eventual loss of renal function. Urographic findings consist of a mass effect that is medial and inferior to the kidney. The mass often displaces the kidney upward and rotates it laterally. Usually, a definite line of separation between the mass effect and the kidney is observed. Excretory urography may opacify the mass (if contrast extravasates into it) and will reveal the displacement of the ureter, kidney, or both. Retrograde study may be necessary to visualize the upper tract distally to the obstructing urinoma.

Ultrasonography or CT will better delineate the extent of the pseudocyst and its relation to the space around the kidney (Fig. 20-47).[60]

ECHINOCOCCAL (HYDATID) CYSTS

The kidney may be involved in patients with echinococcal infestation with formation of cysts similar to those noted in the liver and other parenchymal organs. The cysts may have a calcified wall visible on plain-film study (50% to 80%). The calcification may be similar to that found in tumors or cysts or may resemble renal calculi. Cysts are pear-shaped or round and may be closed, although most eventually open into a calyx and can be outlined by opaque medium with excretory urography or retrograde pyelography. The large cyst often contains daughter cysts that are smaller and resemble a grapelike cluster of masses extending into the

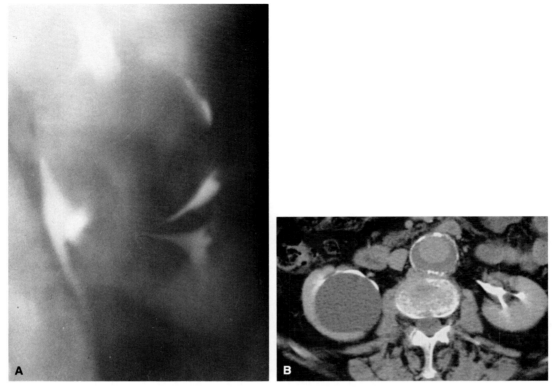

Figure 20–46.   Halo sign of a parapelvic cyst. **(A)** Nephrotomogram shows ill-defined radiolucency caused by compressed renal sinus fat surrounding the smoothly rounded cyst in the renal hilus. **(B)** Enhanced CT of parapelvic cyst. Note that cyst displaces contrast-filled collecting system. This differentiates cyst from hydronephrosis or extrarenal pelvis in which contrast would enter the fluid-filled cavity.

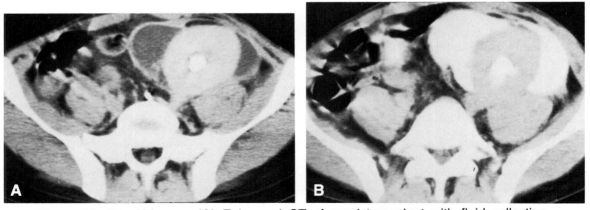

Figure 20–47.   Urinoma. **(A)** Enhanced CT of renal transplant with fluid collection surrounding the kidney. **(B)** Delayed scan now reveals contrast within the urinoma.

larger cyst or adjacent to it. The cysts deform the renal outline and calyceal system in a manner similar to the deformity produced by a simple cyst. They tend to obliterate the minor calyces and deform the major calyces to a somewhat greater extent. They may reach very large proportions and may result in considerable compression of renal parenchyma and distortion of calyces. The discharge of daughter cells into the renal pelvis can produce symptoms of colic. This discharge can be both retroperitoneal and intraperitoneal. When the cyst communicates with the collecting system, it may be seen to fill on excretory urography or CT, so that the grapelike clusters of daughter cysts within it are visible—a highly suggestive sign. Ultrasonography likewise can provide similar strong evidence to make this diagnosis.

RENAL VASCULAR ABNORMALITIES

Renal Artery Aneurysm

Aneurysm of the renal artery is not common but is well known to radiologists because the aneurysm wall can contain calcium. About 25% to 30% of these aneurysms contain enough calcium to be roentgenographically visible. The diagnosis can usually be made on plain-film studies in the calcified group. The rounded, ring-contoured, calcified aneurysm maintains a constant relationship to the renal pelvis in various projections. About two thirds are located at the bifurcation of the renal artery and one third in the segmental branches. About half of those involving segmental arteries are intraparenchymal. They may be congenital, atherosclerotic, or post-traumatic (often false aneurysms). Systemic hypertension is present in about 15% of patients with aneurysm of the renal artery. Renal arteriography or dynamic CT can be used for confirmation and is the only means of diagnosis when the aneurysm is not calcified. Bilateral renal aneurysms are relatively common (about 20%), so arteriography is indicated on the opposite side when an aneurysm, either calcified or noncalcified, is found on one side. Calcified aneurysms generally do not rupture, but the incidence of rupture of uncalcified aneurysms is about 25%. In selected patients surgical repair should be considered for those with noncalcified renal artery aneurysms.[141] Occasionally, such aneurysms are found incidentally on CT or ultrasound examinations. If indicated by the clinical setting (eg, hypertension, size of the aneurysm, etc), arteriography should then be considered.

POLYARTERITIS NODOSA

Multiple, small, intraparenchymal renal aneurysms are commonly observed in polyarteritis nodosa. Similar microaneurysms are present in other viscera involved by this disease. In the kidney, the multiple small aneurysms involving the interlobar and arcuate arteries are associated with scarring, which results from thromboses and infarctions. The aneurysms may rupture to produce renal hemorrhage (Fig. 20-48). Clinically, the infarcts produce pain and hematuria. Renal arteriography outlines the aneurysms, and its use is essential for making the diagnosis. The small aneurysms found in this disease sometimes regress spontaneously.

RENAL ARTERIOVENOUS FISTULA

A renal arteriovenous fistula may be congenital or acquired. The etiologic background is undetermined in some, which may be termed *idiopathic*. The congenital malformations may be very large and may result in high-output cardiac failure, whereas others are very small and are of little clinical significance. Most arteriovenous fistulas in the kidney are acquired, usually following percutaneous biopsy. Others follow blunt or penetrating renal trauma or surgical procedures in the renal area, and some are secondary to renal neoplasms. Renal arterial disease occasionally may result in an arteriovenous fistula. Many form following trauma, including those caused by percutaneous renal biopsy, and heal spontaneously. When the fistulas persist, hematuria and hypertension may occur as complications. Urograms and plain films are usually not very helpful in determining the diagnosis, but plain films may reveal calcification; in the case of a large arteriovenous fistula, the collecting system may be displaced by the mass produced by the fistula. Color Doppler ultrasound can often make the diagnosis noninvasively by directly imaging the fistula. Duplex Doppler interrogation of the renal vein will demonstrate pulsatile, arterial-type flow if the fistula is of adequate size. Arteriography reveals the fistula along with early venous filling and often demonstrates venous dilatation and tortuosity secondary to the arteriovenous shunt. Renal function may be diminished on the side of involvement, depending on the severity of the shunt.

RENAL ARTERY OCCLUSION

Renal arterial occlusion is most frequently caused by embolism in patients with cardiac disease. Thrombosis also occurs, most often secondary to atherosclerosis, but sometimes caused by trauma. Regardless of cause, when a renal artery is occluded function is lost. Partial function may occasionally return in a year or more. The roentgenographic findings in acute renal arterial occlusion consist of urographic evidence of a nonfunctioning kidney of normal size in which retrograde pyelography

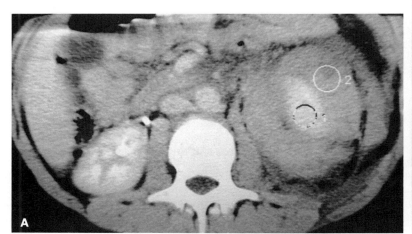
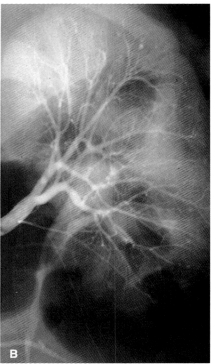

Figure 20–48. Polyarteritis nodosa. **(A)** Enhanced CT scan demonstrates sponta-neous perirenal hemorrhage as measured by cursors. **(B)** Angiogram in same patient. Note multiple microaneurysms.

shows no abnormality. A peripheral rim of opacified cortex may be observed during the nephrographic phase. Presumably, this cortex is supplied by the col-lateral circulation of the renal capsule. Acute segmen-tal infarction may be responsible for either complete nonvisualization on excretory urography or a local fail-ure of calyceal filling. The cause for the complete loss of function in these patients is not certain. It may be that a shower of small emboli accompanies the segmental embolic block.[109] Following total renal infarction with-out infection, the kidney decreases in size and usually remains nonfunctioning. Retrograde study reveals de-crease in size of the calyceal system consistent with renal size. The late findings in segmental infarction are those of local decrease in size, which may distort the kidney locally and cause an irregular contour. Renal arteriography is used to confirm the diagnosis in all types of arterial occlusion. Both left and right sides should be studied because involvement is frequently bilateral. Doppler ultrasound can suggest the diag-nosis of renal arterial occlusion. The role of MRI angi-ography is under investigation. Computed tomog-raphic findings parallel those of urography. However, effects of hemodynamics are better shown.

RENAL VEIN ANOMALIES

Valves are occasionally found in renal veins, as indi-cated previously. Anomalies of the left renal vein, spe-cifically circumaortic or retroaortic left-renal veins, are occasionally seen at CT. Radiographically, it is recog-nized as a bifurcation or retroaortic position of the renal vein as it courses from the kidney to the vena cava. It is important to recognize these vascular anom-alies as incidental findings, and not mistake them for adenopathy or other pathology. Surgeons need to know of the existence of these variants before retroperitoneal surgery.

RENAL VEIN THROMBOSIS

Thrombosis of the renal vein occurs more frequently in children than in adults. In adults, direct invasion, or extrinsic pressure by tumor, and thrombosis of the inferior vena cava are among the more frequent causes. Acute enteritis is considered the chief cause in chil-dren, but any condition that produces dehydration, acidosis, and hemoconcentration may be an inciting factor. In infants who have had intrauterine renal vein thrombosis, a faint lacelike calcification corresponding to intrarenal vascular structures may be observed in the newborn on plain film. Because diagnosis is difficult from a clinical standpoint, radiographic methods are of prime importance. Roentgenographic findings depend on the rapidity of the occlusion and its relation to the development of venous collaterals.

In the acute, complete thrombosis with infarction and perirenal hemorrhage, the kidney is enlarged, and excretory urography shows no excretion of contrast. The renal arteriogram shows delayed flow through narrow, stretched, interlobar arteries. Opacification of the parenchyma is poor, and the nephrogram phase is prolonged. Venous drainage cannot be identified. When the acute occlusion is partial, the kidney also becomes enlarged. Function as demonstrated by excretory urography is gradually regained in about 2 weeks as venous collaterals develop. In gradual occlusion, collateral circulation has time to develop, and the roentgenographic examination may show no abnormality whatsoever. When renal arteriography is carried out, the venous phase may show extensive venous collaterals. Dynamic CT also delineates the process well, when it is in an advanced stage. The role of ultrasound in detection of renal vein thrombosis is unclear. Ultrasound signs include thrombus in the inferior vena cava, loss of corticomedullary junction, and hyperechoic streaks in the interlobar spaces surrounding the medullary pyramids.[87]

When renal vein thrombosis is suspected, excretory urography should be performed. If the diagnosis is supported by absence or decrease of function and increase in renal size, renal arteriography should be the next step in the radiographic study of the patient. Evaluation of the renal arterial supply, intrarenal pathologic state, venous collaterals, or absence of renal vein filling and possibly demonstration of the actual obstructive site can all be accomplished with proper timing of the examination (Fig. 20-49). Inferior venacavography and selective renal venography can alternatively be performed, but catheter insertion adds to the risk of thromboembolism.

RENOVASCULAR HYPERTENSION

Gifford has defined *renovascular disease* as the presence of a stenotic lesion in the renal artery or its branches. Diagnosis depends on demonstrating the stenotic lesion on arteriography. The patient may or

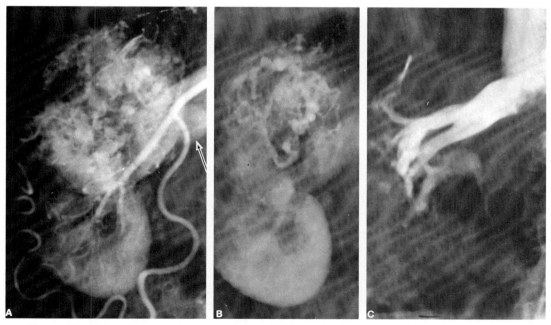

Figure 20–49. Renal vein thrombosis. (**A**) Renal arteriogram at 2 seconds shows a large, vascular mass in the upper pole of the right kidney. Note the renal vein below the artery (*arrow*). (**B**) Five-second film shows a continued opacification of the tumor and clear definition of the renal vein. (**C**) Renal venogram. The tumor thrombus is clearly defined in the inferior aspect of the renal vein at its junction with the vena cava, which is now outlined above the renal vein. Although there is partial obstruction of the renal vein, no collaterals are visible.

may not be hypertensive. By contrast, *renovascular hypertension* connotes the presence of a stenotic renal artery lesion plus relief of the hypertension by revascularization or removal of the affected kidney. In his experience, simultaneous occurrence of essential hypertension and coincidental renovascular disease is far more frequent than true renovascular hypertension.[49]

Gifford has estimated the prevalence of renal artery stenosis caused hypertension in adults at less than 1% of unselected hypertensive patients. The lowest estimate in the literature is from the Mayo Clinic experience, 0.18%. A reasonable average figure from informal survey of vascular surgeons would be about 3%.[152]

Use of modified excretory urography to screen hypertensive patients was begun in the early 1960s to detect patients having unilateral renal artery stenosis. Those with positive examinations would have renal arteriography to determine the presence of a stenotic renal artery lesion. Presence of a stenotic lesion would then elicit a question about whether it was hemodynamically significant. In other words, was it curable using angioplasty or surgery?

The data from the Cooperative Study of Renovascular Hypertension (as reassessed in 1982) indicates that the hypertensive urogram has a false-negative rate of nearly 22% and a false-positive rate of about 13% in detection of unilateral renal artery stenosis. More important, it has poor predictive accuracy regarding which patients would respond to angioplasty or surgery: less than 50% (ie, less than a coin flip).[152]

Strategies have thus been proposed to permit more effective detection. Hillman has concluded that abandoning the hypertensive urogram (HTU), and using renal digital subtraction arteriography, but limiting this to patients having moderate to severe hypertension (diastolic pressure of 105 mm Hg or greater), would be cost effective.[62] Thornbury and colleagues also have recommended that HTU be abandoned and that clinical criteria used by vascular surgeons be used to determine which hypertensive patients should have renal arteriography as a primary imaging examination.[152]

Patients selected for arteriography (digital or conventional) using the operative clinical criteria approach are those not excluded from surgery for other reasons, those whose hypertension is not well controlled on antihypertensive medication, those whose severe hypertension responds well to an angiotensin II–converting enzyme inhibitor or a beta-blocking agent, and those who then fall into one of two subgroups of patients (having all of the following):

Group I

1. Diastolic pressure above 115 mm Hg when first discovered

2. Age less than 45 years, particularly in white women
3. A sudden onset of increased pressure.

Group II

1. Diastolic pressure above 115 mm Hg
2. Age 45 years or older
3. Stigmata of generalized atherosclerotic disease
4. An accelerating or malignant form of hypertension.

Use of this approach, combined with correlation of renal vein renin sampling and arteriographic clues indicative of a hemodynamically significant stenotic lesion, results in very high cure rates by renal revascularization techniques. This approach also results in the lowest number of patients having arteriography from which a subgroup actually goes on to surgery or angioplasty.

This operative criteria approach does not guarantee that every patient who has renal artery stenosis will be detected. It will, however, result in identification of a subpopulation of patients that is as small as practically possible, which, in addition, includes almost all patients with renovascular hypertension (ie, curable by renal revascularization).

For those physicians who feel more comfortable using less restrictive patient selection criteria for renal arteriography, Hillman's approach also appears cost effective but results in more patients having arteriography. The approach is based primarily on limiting arteriography to patients having moderate to severe hypertension (diastolic blood pressure of 105 mm Hg or greater). They favor use of intravenous digital subtraction angiography to show renal artery stenosis. Patients are then selected for transluminal angioplasty or surgery based on the presence of a "significant" stenotic lesion as correlated with renal vein renin studies.

Several new noninvasive methods have become available to study the renal arteries. MR angiography has recently been shown to assess renal artery stenosis accurately when the lesion is proximal (see Fig. 20-50). Current methods to create angiographic effects by MR angiography include two-dimensional time of flight, three-dimensional time of flight, and phase-contrast techniques. It is expected that further technologic improvements will make this an accurate way to study the renal arteries noninvasively. Disadvantages of these techniques include distal or segmental stenoses, and the imaging of multiple renal arteries. In addition, the technology and expertise to perform these techniques is not yet widespread.[33, 76]

Early literature was optimistic for the usefulness of Doppler ultrasound to screen for renal artery stenosis. Criteria for stenosis include increased renal artery velocities (> 100 cm/seconds) and increased renal artery

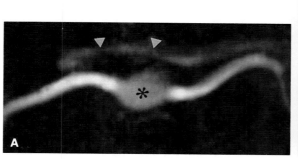

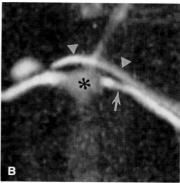

Figure 20–50.   MRI angiography of the renal arteries. **(A)** Normal axial MR using phase-contrast technique. Aorta (*) and left renal vein (*arrowheads*). **(B)** Renal artery stenosis. Note stenosis in proximal left renal artery (*arrow*). Aorta (*) and left renal vein (*arrowheads*) leading to inferior vena cava. (Courtesy of Thomas M. Grist, MD, Madison, WI.)

to aorta velocity ratios (> 3.5). More recent reports are less optimistic in the ability of ultrasound to image the renal arteries consistently and thus question its usefulness as a screening modality.[14]

Radionuclide scanning may also play a role in the evaluation of renal artery stenosis. Scans with Tc-99m-diethylenetriamine penta-acetic acid (DTPA) combined with captopril have yielded sensitivities of 91% with specificities of 93%. Scintigraphy without captopril had much poorer results.[22]

The renal arteries may be studied by three angiographic methods.

1. *Percutaneous arterial vascular catheterization (Seldinger technique).* Catheter tip is selectively placed in the aorta and then each renal artery, using fluoroscopic guidance. Aortic flush injection of contrast material and then bilateral selective renal artery injection is recorded by rapid serial films (conventional arteriography) or by video-displayed digital subtraction imaging and filming methods. This study is the most widely used and accurate of the three methods. Angioplasty can be performed at that time if a significant lesion is found.

2. *Intravenous digital subtraction arteriography (DSA).* A vascular catheter is percutaneously placed in the venous system with its tip either in the inferior vena cava (inguinal approach) or superior vena cava (antecubital fossa approach). Contrast injection is made and subsequent opacified blood flow through the abdominal aorta and renal arteries is recorded by video displayed digital subtraction imaging and filming. If the catheter tip is in the inferior vena cava it can be manipulated under fluoroscopic guidance to obtain renal vein and inferior vena caval renin samples (before injection). This method provides acceptable information about main renal artery lesions (but not about segmental vasculature) in about 90% of examinations. It is not practical to use in young children because they cannot remain as motionless as adults during injection/filming time.

3. *Translumbar aortography.* This requires percutaneous direct needle puncture of the abdominal aorta using a lumbar approach. Contrast injection is made through the needle or an indwelling vascular catheter, and image recording follows on rapid serial films or DSA imaging. This route is used only when it is not possible to use the percutaneous arm or inguinal route.

Atherosclerotic plaque-type lesions are the most common cause of renal artery stenosis. Usually these are short and vary from a smooth circumferential narrowing to an irregular eccentric focal defect in the opacified renal artery (Fig. 20-51). Most often these involve the renal artery orifice or the proximal third of the main renal artery and can progress to complete occlusion.

Also common, but usually in younger female patients, are varying types of fibromuscular dysplasia lesions. The right renal artery is involved more often than the left, and the stenoses are located in the distal two thirds of the renal artery and extend into the segmental branches. Arteriographic appearance varies from a prominent string-of-beads appearance to tubular symmetric or eccentric arterial lumen deformity. These lesions can progress in severity of luminal narrowing (Fig. 20-52).

Other rare renal artery lesions that can cause reno-

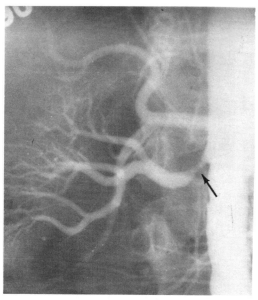

Figure 20–51. Translumbar aortogram with good visualization of the renal artery. Site of a stenotic lesion secondary to arteriosclerosis in a 63-year-old man with hypertension (*arrow*). Note the poststenotic dilatation of the renal artery.

vascular hypertension include those associated with arterial dissections, neurofibromatosis, musculotendinous bands, embolus, thrombosis, encasement by tumors, polyarteritis nodosa, scleroderma, aneurysms, arteriovenous malformations, and effects of renal trauma.

Once a stenotic lesion is found, arteriographic clues must be used to determine whether the lesion is hemodynamically significant. The degree of reduction of the cross-sectional luminal area is a critical element. However, the assessment of this area factor is not precise. In general, cross-sectional area must be reduced about 80% to be significant. This corresponds (if the narrowing is symmetrically circumferential) to about 45% reduction in diameter. Another rule of thumb is that reduction of diameters by about 50% that result in a diameter of less than 1.5 mm usually is associated with a pressure gradient greater than 25 mm Hg.

Pharmacoangiography has been used to bring out another type of clue that, in some investigators' hands, has proved highly predictive of surgical curability.[17] This involves demonstration of change in direction of flow contrast opacified blood in arterial collaterals after the intra-arterial administration of a vasoconstrictor or dilator. These findings are correlated with clinical findings and renal vein renin studies in the decision process regarding surgical treatment.

It is important to note that renovascular disease and hypertension in pediatric patients (up to 17 years of age) vary from that in adults; thus they are assessed differently.[140] Hypertension in pediatric patients is secondary to identifiable specific causes in up to 80% of cases, 24% of which have been reported to have resulted from renal artery stenosis.[80] Renal arteriography is therefore used in a much higher proportion of pediatric hypertensive patients than in adults. Contrary to the situation in adults, hypertensive urography is the appropriate *first* imaging examination in pediatric patients. While results are abnormal in only 27% to 58% of proven renovascular hypertension patients, nonvascular renal causes of hypertension occur often enough in children to justify screening excretory urography.

TUMORS OF THE KIDNEY

BENIGN TUMORS

Most benign renal tumors are small and usually asymptomatic; they are rare, and most are discovered at autopsy. Histologic types include adenoma, fibroma, lipoma, leiomyoma, hemangioma, and hamartoma; the renin-secreting juxtaglomerular cell tumor is very rare and is usually small, but may be seen on arteriography as an avascular mass surrounded by a denser rim of compressed parenchyma. There may be a few dilated, tortuous arteries present and, of crucial importance in the diagnosis, elevation of venous renin from the affected kidney. When the benign renal tumors are small, they may not be detected on excretory urography, although they may be seen on CT or ultrasonography. If they attain sufficient size, a plain-film roentgenogram will reveal enlargement of the renal shadow at the site of the tumor. Urography may then show enough distortion of the pelvocalyceal system to make the diagnosis of renal tumor. The chief importance of these benign renal tumors lies in differentiation between them and malignant tumors, which usually cannot be made with certainty on excretory urography. A leiomyoma arising in the renal capsule may rarely contain calcium resembling that observed in other leiomyomas. Most benign renal tumors are avascular on angiography except for hemangiomas. Malignant tumors may be avascular, and benign tumors may exhibit abnormal vascularity. In current practice CT and ultrasonography should be the imaging modalities used to evaluate renal masses. Angiography can then be used if needed to assess a tumor's vascularity and the renal arteries. Retroperitoneal masses arising near the kidney may be difficult on excretory urography to differentiate from renal tumors, since they may distort the kidney and displace the upper ureter (Fig. 20-53).

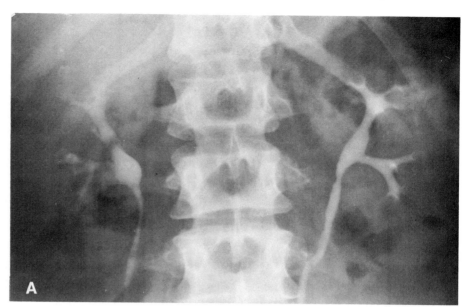

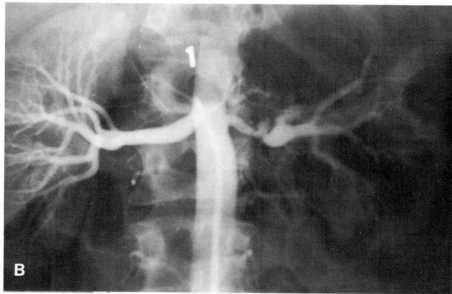

Figure 20–52. Fibromuscular dysplasia in an 18-year-old woman with hypertension. (**A**) This urogram shows very slight hyperconcentration on the left. There are a few minor indentations on the upper-left ureter, suggesting the possibility of collateral vessels. (**B**) This arteriogram shows a normal right renal artery. On the left there are multiple constrictions with poststenotic dilatation. There is great delay in perfusion of the left kidney as compared with the right. Note the collateral arteries in and below the renal hilus.

Computed tomography, ultrasonography, or MRI will allow more accurate differentiation of intra- from extra-renal masses.

Renal Angiomyolipoma

Renal angiomyolipoma (hamartoma) often can be differentiated from other benign tumors and from malignant renal tumors. It is a mixed mesodermal tumor composed of adipose tissue, smooth muscle, and blood vessels in varying proportions. Angiomyolipomas may be associated with tuberous sclerosis, in which case they are usually multiple and bilateral. This hamartoma may also occur as a solitary unilateral tumor, usually found in older women. Clinical manifestations include signs of infection, pain, hematuria, or an asymptomatic abdominal mass. This tumor is prone to bleed, and patients may present in hypovolemic shock.

Urographic findings are those of a mass that enlarges the kidney and distorts and displaces the pelvis and calyces. If much fat is present, the radiolucent areas within the mass suggest the diagnosis. If multiple and

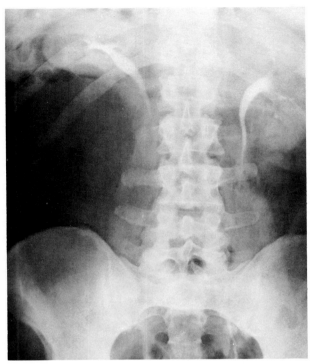

Figure 20–53. Huge radiolucent tumor distorting the right kidney and ureter. This is a large retroperitoneal lipoma.

bilateral, they may simulate polycystic disease. Typically, the angiomyolipoma appears as a focal hyperechoic mass on ultrasonography because of the fatty elements. However, Hartman and colleagues found in a retrospective review that a mixed or hypoechoic pattern could also be found. Renal-cell carcinoma can also

have a hyperechoic pattern, so that this ultrasonic finding can be suggestive but not pathognomonic of angiomyolipoma.[58] The demonstration of fat within a renal tumor on CT is diagnostic of angiomyolipoma (Fig. 20-54). The ease of detection of fat on CT is proportional to the amount of fat in the angiomyolipoma, since partial volume artifacts and bleeding into the tumor can alter density measurements.[18]

The most striking angiographic finding is the presence of many, peculiar, small, regular outpouchings of the interlobar and interlobular arteries resembling berry aneurysms. In some patients, the interlobular arteries terminate in these aneurysms resembling a cluster of grapes, in contrast to the irregular size and contour of the tumor vessels seen in renal cell carcinoma. This appearance is present in the arterial phase and is obscured by the nephrographic phase. Later, there is irregular puddling, indistinguishable from that owing to malignant tumor. The venous phase is normal, not early as in renal cell carcinoma. Differentiation from renal cell carcinoma by angiographic means alone may be difficult.

Lipomatosis of the Renal Sinus

This condition is also called fibrolipomatosis, fatty replacement, fatty transformation, lipomatous paranephritis, and lipoma diffusum renis. Because it may resemble tumor on urographic study, it is considered here. Lipomatosis consists of an excessive amount of fat in the renal sinus that distorts the calyces, infundibula, and renal pelvis to varying degrees. It is usually found as a replacement process in renal atrophy, whatever the cause, but may occur in simple obesity. It is found in older age groups, usually in those older than 50. The urographic appearance may simulate renal tumor,

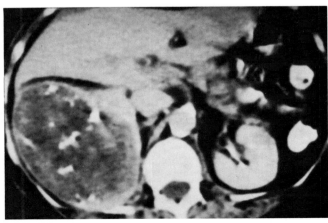 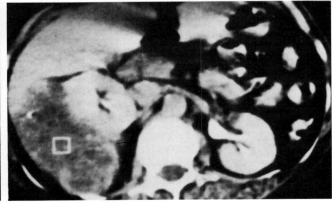

Figure 20–54.   Angiomyolipoma. Enhanced CT at two different levels. Note the very low attenuation areas compatible with fat in the tumor.

parapelvic cyst, or polycystic disease. It is therefore important that differentiation be made since lipomatosis is not a surgical problem.

The condition can usually be suspected on excretory urography, but nephrotomography best outlines the changes and facilitates the diagnosis. The pelvis is flattened or irregularly indented on its lateral aspect; the infundibula are elongated, narrow, and often appear stretched. The calyces may be relatively normal but may be dilated and blunted if pyelonephritis is superimposed.

At times, the deposition of fat is localized so that cyst or tumor may be simulated. The diffuse type can also resemble polycystic disease. The infusion method of urography in conjunction with tomography demonstrates in sharp relief the relationship of the radiolucent fat to the opacified pelvocalyceal system (Fig. 20-55). Computed tomography also nicely demonstrates the parapelvic fat in renal sinus lipomatosis. The fat can be recognized by its low attenuation values with the site and extent of fatty replacement also delineated.[142] On ultrasonography, renal sinus lipomatosis appears hyperechoic, similar to but more so than normal fat in the sinus.

This process may be unilateral or bilateral. When it is bilateral, it is not necessarily symmetric. Involvement on the left is often somewhat greater than on the right. The involved kidney may be enlarged with some thinning of the remaining renal tissue.

Renal Pseudotumor

The kidney is capable of hypertrophy and hyperplasia. A focal mass or pseudotumor may be difficult to differentiate from a tumor. There may be compression of the pelvocalyceal system, splaying of the calyces, and local enlargement with protrusion from the renal surface. Because the calyces do not regenerate, the masses do not contain these structures. In addition to the demonstration of a mass, excretory urography may reveal the signs of renal disease, which results in the regeneration of renal parenchyma including nonobstructive caliectasis and irregular thinning of the cortex. Enlarged Bertin's column is an example of invagination of the renal cortex into the medulla, simulating a tumor. It is often found at the junction of the middle and upper third of the kidney.

Angiography reveals spreading of the arteries, but

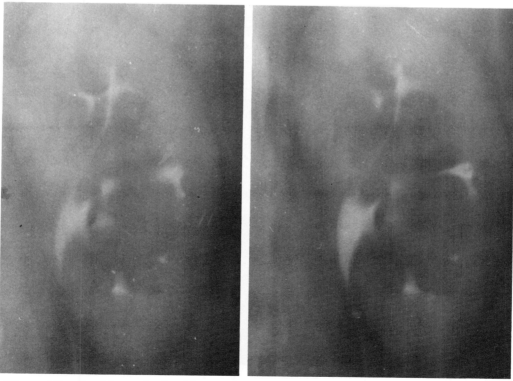

Figure 20–55.   Lipomatosis of the renal sinus. These tomograms show radiolucent fat in the renal sinus with elongation and narrowing of infundibula.

no tumor vessels or arteriovenous shunts are present, so there is no early venous filling. The capillary blush equals or exceeds that of the remaining renal parenchyma, and there is no evidence of a wall or capsule. Ultrasonography, CT, radionuclide studies, or MRI can be used to differentiate pseudotumors from true tumors. Angiography is sometimes used for this indication. Some tumors on ultrasonography can have very similar echogenicity to normal renal parenchyma and could be missed.

A number of other conditions may resemble renal hilar or parenchymal masses. These include fetal lobulations, aneurysm of the renal artery, dilated vein(s), renal abscess, hematoma, xanthogranulomatous pyelonephritis, renal tuberculosis, and, most important and most often, renal cyst.

MALIGNANT TUMORS

Malignant tumors of the kidney can be divided into the following types: (1) renal cell carcinoma (adenocarcinoma or hypernephroma), (2) embryonal tumors (Wilms' tumor), (3) tumors of the renal pelvis (transitional cell carcinoma), (4) mesenchymal tumors (sarcoma), (5) lymphoma, including leukemia, and (6) metastases. The adenocarcinoma or renal cell carcinoma is the most common malignant tumor, and it can arise in any portion of the kidney. The tumor may attain great size before it causes symptoms.

Renal Cell Carcinoma (Hypernephroma) (Adenocarcinoma)

Renal cell carcinoma occurs more frequently in males and is most common in the 40- to 60-year-old age range. Clinically, the patient may present with weight loss, flank pain, palpable mass, or hematuria. Metastases to the lungs, liver, and lymph nodes and tumor extension into the renal vein and inferior vena cava

need to be evaluated. Plain-film findings consist of local or general enlargement of the kidney, which varies with the size of the tumor. The renal border may be preserved (although lobulated or distorted) or it may be irregular and disrupted. The lesions are usually limited by the renal capsule until they are far advanced. It is not uncommon to note calcification within the tumor, which may be irregularly scattered or curvilinear. It may also be rimlike or curvilinear, outlining the periphery of the tumor. Renal displacement or tilting of the axis may result when there is a large medial mass in the upper or lower pole, or the entire kidney may be displaced if the tumor is large. Displacement of neighboring organs occurs when the tumor attains sufficient size. This may be apparent on a plain film, but is best appreciated with CT or MRI.[114, 137]

Urographic changes are due to the distortion produced by the tumor mass. Calyces are elongated, distorted, narrowed, or obliterated. The renal pelvis may be altered similarly. Renal cell carcinoma usually produces more disruption of the calyces or pelvis than a cyst of similar size. This disruption is important because cysts can elongate and compress the pelvocalyceal system, but tend to cause less distortion. Large tumors may cause considerable displacement of the upper ureter and may also partially obstruct the pelvis or upper ureter (Fig. 20-56). There is usually enough function to visualize the calyces and pelvis on excretory urography, in contrast to the loss of function often noted in hydronephrosis (which may produce renal enlargement). At times, infiltration of the kidney by tumor may be so extensive that no function remains. Also, function may be decreased by invasion and thrombosis of a renal vein.

The malignant renal tumor must be differentiated from a renal cyst. In the past, urographic criteria were used to do this. Renal cysts had a "claw sign" in the nephrographic phase and a crowding together of the

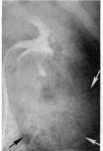
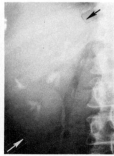
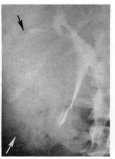
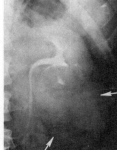
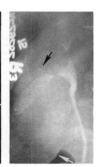

Figure 20–56. These excretory urograms indicate various findings produced by renal carcinoma. Note the considerable distortion of the calyces sometimes associated with the tumor mass. Tumor site in each case (*arrows*).

calyces. Calyces were rarely amputated, and the cyst was attached to the periphery of the kidney. Renal tumors, conversely, demonstrated invasion of the renal pelvis, separation of the calyces, calyceal amputation, and a mass contiguous with the body of the kidney.[128] These criteria, however, were not accurate in distinguishing cyst from tumor. Currently, ultrasonography and CT are used to distinguish cyst from tumor. Pollack and colleagues demonstrated an accuracy rate of 98% for diagnosing a simple cyst when certain criteria were fulfilled on ultrasonography. These criteria include (1) enhancement of sound transmission beyond the cyst, (2) absence of internal echoes, (3) sharp delineation of the far wall, and (4) a spherical or slightly ovoid shape (Fig. 20-57).[123] Computed tomographic criteria for a simple cyst include (1) homogeneous attenuation value near water density, (2) no enhancement with intravenous contrast, (3) no measurable thickness of the cyst wall, and (4) a smooth interface with renal parenchyma (Fig. 20-58).[98] Hyperdense renal cysts can also be diagnosed by CT (Fig. 20-59). These hyperdense cysts meet all the CT criteria for simple cysts, except they have higher density measurements. The high attenuation values are usually due to hemorrhage within a cyst, although they can also be secondary to infection.

Renal cell carcinoma on CT appears as a solid lesion within the kidney that deforms the renal contour. The interface between the tumor and normal renal parenchyma is difficult to define on precontrast scans, but is usually clear after intravenous contrast. Postcontrast

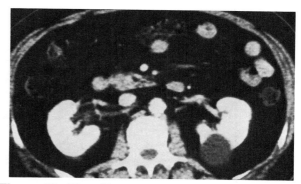

Figure 20–58. Simple renal cyst. Dynamic enhanced CT of a cyst in the posterior aspect of the left kidney. Note the smooth interface with the renal parenchyma and the lack of enhancement within the cyst.

scans usually show the tumor to enhance less than the normal renal parenchyma (Fig. 20-60).[37] Low-attenuation regions within the tumor that do not change after contrast are compatible with necrosis or hemorrhage. Computed tomography can also be used in the staging of renal cell carcinoma. In one study involving 62 cases, CT was more sensitive in detecting lymphadenopathy and perinephric extension compared with angiography, and as good as angiography in detecting renal vein and inferior vena caval involvement.[157] More recently, MRI has been used in the evaluation of renal-cell carcinoma. Most investigators agree that although most renal-cell carcinomas can be detected by MRI, some may be isointense to normal kidney on T1- and T2-weighted sequences. Newer literature suggests that fat-suppression and breath-hold techniques may be as sensitive as CT for detection of renal masses.

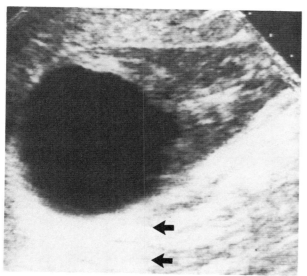

Figure 20–57. Simple renal cyst. Longitudinal ultrasound of a large cyst in the upper pole of the right kidney. Note the absence of internal echoes and the through transmission (*arrows*) beyond the cyst.

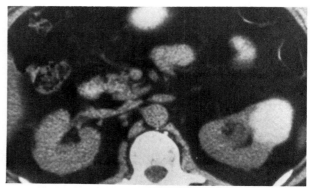

Figure 20–59. Hyperdense renal cyst. Unenhanced CT shows the homogeneous, high-attenuation cyst in the lateral portion of the left kidney.

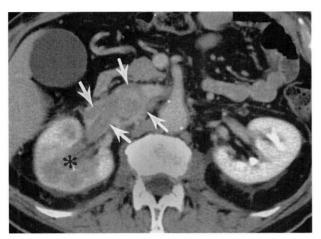

Figure 20–60. Renal cell carcinoma. Enhanced CT shows lack of enhancement of tumor (*) relative to normal parenchyma. Tumor thrombus involves right renal vein and extends into inferior vena cava (*arrows*). (Courtesy of Phillip Murphy, MD, Rochester, NY.)

Magnetic resonance imaging may be more advantageous in evaluating vascular patency (Fig. 20-61), detecting perihilar lymphadenopathy, and assessing direct tumor invasion of adjacent organs.[43, 68]

Both ultrasonography and CT can be used to guide percutaneous biopsies of renal masses for cytopathology or histology. On ultrasonography, renal cell carcinoma can be isoechoic, hypoechoic, or hyperechoic compared with the normal renal parenchyma.[26] Ultrasonography can also be used to evaluate renal vein and inferior vena caval involvement.

Angiography is currently used less often for the diagnosis of renal cell carcinoma. Angiography of renal cell carcinoma may show (1) increased vascularity with irregular pooling, arteriovenous communications with early venous filling (Fig. 20-62), (2) relative avascularity of the entire tumor or a portion of it, (3) abnormal circulation by way of capsular or extrarenal vessels, (4) venous collaterals and abnormal peripheral venous channels around the mass, and (5) lack of constrictor response to epinephrine in tumor vessels. When epinephrine is injected into the renal artery a few seconds

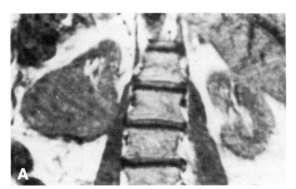

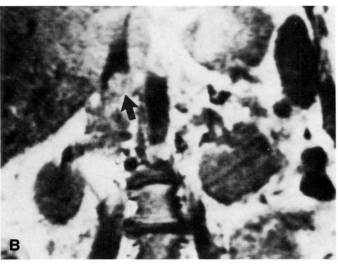

Figure 20–61. Renal cell carcinoma. (**A**) Coronal T1-weighted MRI of a large right renal cell carcinoma. (**B**) Coronal MRI in a different patient shows tumor thrombus (*arrow*) within the inferior vena cava.

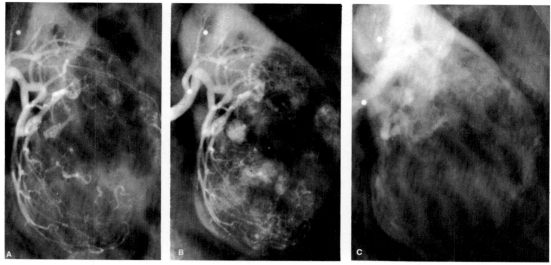

Figure 20–62. Hypernephroma as seen on the selective renal arteriogram. **(A)** At 1.5 seconds there are abnormal vessels within the lower pole mass while arteries surrounding it are stretched. **(B)** At 3 seconds, more puddling and arteriovenous shunting is visible with many abnormal "tumor" vessels. **(C)** At 16 seconds the renal vein is opacified. Note also the abnormal veins lateral to the mass, outside the kidney.

preceding injection of a contrast agent, the normal arteries contract and the tumor vessels that do not respond are more clearly outlined. This differential constriction, unfortunately, may also be observed in renal abscess or carbuncle. Transcatheter embolization of renal cell carcinoma has been performed.[53] It is done preoperatively to aid in surgical removal because the embolization causes tumor vessels to collapse, resulting in a decrease in operating time and blood loss. In patients with inoperable tumors, it is undertaken to relieve symptoms and reduce tumor size. Materials that have been used for embolization include autologous clot, Gelfoam, Ivalon (a polyvinyl alcohol), microspheres, muscle tissue, steel coils, and faromagnetic silicone. Balloon catheter occlusion has also been used.

A renal mass may be first seen on urography, ultrasound, or CT. Excretory urogram should be done with tomography. If a typical cyst is suggested, then ultrasonography should be performed to confirm this finding. If there is an atypical cyst or solid mass, then CT should be performed to evaluate the mass. Percutaneous fine-needle aspiration biopsies can be performed utilizing CT or ultrasonography for guidance on indeterminate lesions and solid masses. Angiography should be reserved for equivocal findings on CT or ultrasonography; angiography or MRI can also be used to assess the renal vascular anatomy. Aspiration with contrast injection of atypical cysts may be required in some cases, but cyst punctures are not performed as often as they once were prior to the use of CT and ultrasonography.

Wilms' Tumor

Wilms' tumor, or nephroblastoma, is the most common abdominal neoplasm of infancy and childhood. Wilms' tumor arises from embryonic renal tissue and tends to become very large. Most Wilms' tumors arise in the first 5 years of life, but are rarely present at birth in contrast to neuroblastoma or the fibromyomatous hamartoma of the kidney. Nephroblastomatosis, or persistence of subcapsular deposits of primitive nephroblastic tissue, is considered to represent a precursor of Wilms' tumor. Wilms' tumor is usually unilateral (although it is bilateral in up to 5% of cases) and presents as an abdominal mass. Hematuria is not common and pain is present in about one fourth of cases. Scout roentgenograms show the outline of the mass with displacement of neighboring structures and elevation of the diaphragm on the side of the lesion. Wilms' tumor may occasionally contain calcifications, in contrast to neuroblastoma (about 50% contain calcifications), which also causes a large tumor mass in infants and children. Urographic findings are those of a large intrarenal tumor that distorts the calyces and pelvis and often displaces and partially obstructs the ureter. The distortion of the calyces tends to be less than with renal-cell carcinoma of similar size but is greater than in neuroblastoma, which often arises adjacent to the kidney and displaces it. Renal function may be impaired, but there is usually enough function to outline some of the calyces on urography and to differentiate this tumor from hydronephrosis causing massive renal enlargement. Ultrasonography usually shows a homogeneous, echogenic, renal mass; there may be small hypoechoic regions that represent cysts within the tumor.[4] Computed tomography is useful in confirming the intrarenal location of Wilms' tumors (Fig. 20-63) and can also demonstrate necrosis or hemorrhage, the absence of vessel encasement (vessel encasement would suggest neuroblastoma), and distortion of the renal calyces. Retrocrural lymphadenopathy, if seen on CT, would suggest neuroblastoma. In one study of 15 patients with Wilms' tumor, no retrocrural lymphadenopathy was seen.[96] Angiography has been done in a few reported cases. Tumor stain is not common and no arteriovenous shunts are present to produce puddling or pooling. The tumor vessels are long and tortuous, resembling a creeping vine. These vessels tend to be discrete, to be of large caliber, and to have an irregular diameter. Invasion, obstruction, or displacement of the inferior vena cava can be detected by cavography, although ultrasonography, MRI, or CT (Fig. 20-64) is more commonly used now. Wilms' tumor tends to metastasize to the lungs and para-aortic lymph nodes and can also extend locally by direct invasion. Calcification in metastases has been reported but is extremely rare.

Tumors of the Renal Pelvis

Tumors of the renal pelvis are of epithelial origin and present a different urographic picture than does renal cell carcinoma. There are two major types of malignant lesions: transitional cell carcinoma and the squamous

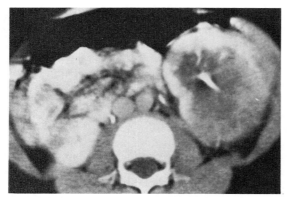

Figure 20–63. Wilms' tumor. Enhanced CT shows the large tumor (with little enhancement) arising in the left kidney.

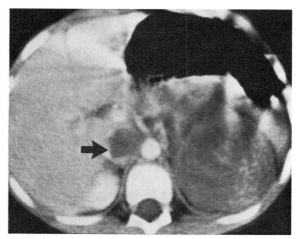

Figure 20–64. Wilms' tumor. Enhanced CT (same patient as in Fig. 20-60) shows involvement of the inferior vena cava (*arrow*) by the low attenuation tumor thrombus. The Wilms' tumor is again seen in the left kidney.

cell epithelioma. Transitional cell tumors, which comprise nearly 90% of malignant tumors of the renal pelvis, tend to be somewhat less invasive than the squamous-cell type. The latter is frequently associated with chronic infection, leukoplakia, or calculi. These tumors produce symptoms of hematuria, pain (obstructive type), and sometimes a palpable mass caused by obstructive hydronephrosis or a large tumor with perirenal extension. On the plain film, there may be no sign of tumor. Because hematuria is an early sign, the patients are usually examined when the lesion is small and therefore difficult to detect in the calyx or pelvis. The tumor causes a filling defect that may be smooth or irregular and may be small or large. These defects are outlined on urograms as radiolucent areas projecting into the opacified calyx or pelvis (Fig. 20-65). Malignant tumors are usually more irregular than benign papillomas of the pelvis, but urographic differentiation of the various cell types of renal pelvis tumors is not possible. The urographic evidence of an infiltrating type of tumor may be minimal, but it can also become very large and produce major alterations in the renal pelvis (Fig. 20-66). Blood clots and radiolucent calculi can produce similar defects. For this reason, it is common practice to follow excretory urography by retrograde pyelography when a filling defect is noted. If a blood clot or calculus caused the defect, the second examination will show disappearance or alteration in the size or position of the defect. Calcification may occur within this type of tumor but is rare. Ureteral and bladder implants occur frequently and produce

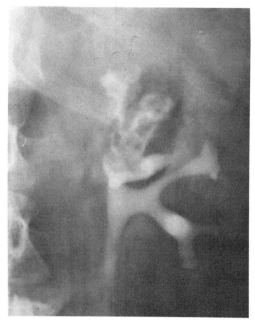

Figure 20–65. Carcinoma of the renal pelvis. Note the irregular filling defects of the upper pole calyces and infundibula. The lesion was a transitional cell carcinoma.

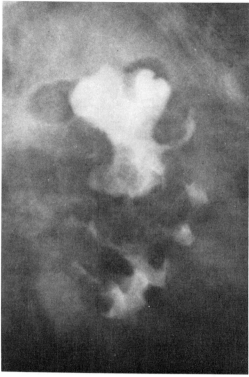

Figure 20–66. Infiltrating carcinoma (transitional cell) of the renal pelvis. Note gross distortion of infundibula and calyces. The pelvis does not opacify because it is full of tumor.

small defects similar to those caused by the primary tumor in the kidney. Occasionally, a tumor may invade and infiltrate the adjacent parenchyma to simulate renal cell carcinoma.

Computed tomography can be used to differentiate a tumor from a radiolucent calculus in the renal pelvis.[136] Baron and colleagues recommend that CT be performed after excretory urography in patients with known or suspected transitional cell carcinomas for diagnosis, preoperative staging, and evaluation of whether limited resection is possible.[10] On CT, transitional cell carcinoma appears as a soft-tissue density within the renal pelvis (Fig. 20-67).[122]

Transitional cell carcinoma is relatively hypovascular on angiography. There is no pooling, arteriovenous shunting, or neovascularity. The residual parenchymal vessels are occluded or encased by tumor and narrowed. These angiographic findings, however, may also be found in metastases to the kidney.

Squamous Metaplasia of the Renal Pelvis. Leukoplakia or squamous metaplasia of the renal pelvis is probably caused by infection or chronic irritation from another source. It is included here because it may resemble carcinoma of the pelvis and often precedes squamous cell carcinoma of the renal pelvis. Infection

is found in 80% of patients, and 40% have had renal calculi. The patient may describe passing tissue or gritty material, and the diagnosis is established by finding keratinized squamous epithelium in the urine. The condition is usually unilateral. Clinically, hematuria may be present with intermittent chills or fever also occurring.

Radiographic findings are varied. Irregular areas in the renal pelvis partially surrounded by contrast material, large laminated masses presenting an onion-skin appearance, irregular plaques or bands producing linear striations, and roughening or wrinkling of the renal pelvis may be found. Any of these findings should suggest the diagnosis, but lucent calculi, hematoma, and carcinoma of the renal pelvis must be considered in the differential diagnosis.

Sarcoma. Sarcomas of the kidney may originate from fibrous elements in either the renal parenchyma or renal capsule or from smooth muscle rests in the parenchyma or blood vessels. Retroperitoneal sarcoma aris-

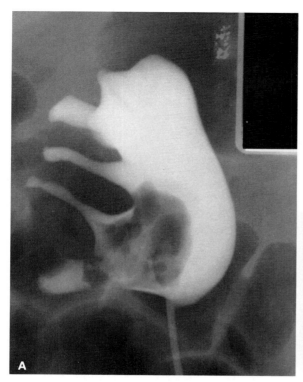

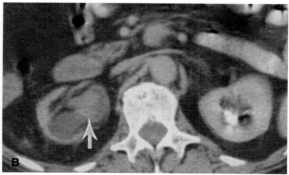

Figure 20–67. Carcinoma of renal pelvis. **(A)** Retrograde pyelogram demonstrates filling defect in the right renal pelvis. **(B)** Enhanced CT scan of same case showing tumor in renal pelvis (*arrow*). Soft-tissue mass definitively excludes low-density renal calculus as cause of filling defect. (Courtesy of Patrick J. Fultz, MD, Rochester, NY.)

ing in or near the kidney often becomes so extensive that it is not possible to determine the site of origin even at autopsy. Renal sarcomas are rare tumors. Fibrosarcoma, liposarcoma, leiomyosarcoma, rhabdomyosarcoma, and even osteosarcoma of the kidney have been reported. Roentgenographic findings are those of a mass in the renal area that is often difficult to outline clearly and may obliterate the psoas shadow in its more cephalad aspect. Urograms tend to show somewhat less distortion of the pelvocalyceal system than is noted in a renal cell carcinoma of similar size. Neifeld and colleagues think that CT is valuable in suggesting more extensive involvement than may be appreciated with other diagnostic modalities or by clinical examination.[113] Computed tomography can also be used to follow patients to look for recurrence of the sarcoma. Liposarcoma is the most common retroperitoneal sarcoma.

Lymphoma and Leukemia

Involvement of the kidneys in patients with chronic leukemia may occur late in the disease. In children with acute leukemia, renal involvement is more common than in the chronic form. The leukemic infiltrate tends to be largely cortical in location. Renal enlargement, usually bilateral, is demonstrated on plain films. Urographic signs in addition to bilateral enlargement consist of enlargement of the renal pelvis (without dilatation or evidence of obstruction), stretching and elongation of the calyces and pelvis, and irregularity of the renal outline. Computed tomography is useful in demonstrating the renal enlargement, associated lymphadenopathy and splenomegaly, and complications such as hemorrhage.[61, 73] Breatnach and colleagues have reported a case of intrarenal chloroma causing obstructive uropathy.[20]

The kidneys can also be involved with lymphoma; most represent secondary involvement. Non-Hodgkin's lymphoma involves the kidneys more frequently than Hodgkin's lymphoma. The distribution of disease is somewhat more varied than in the leukemias. Renal enlargement (caused by infiltration of the kidneys) is a common form of involvement. Other findings include distortion or elongation of the pelvocalyceal system, solitary or multiple tumor nodules, and perirenal masses that may engulf or displace the kidney (Fig. 20-68). The solitary tumor nodules cannot be differen-

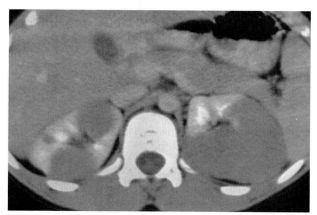

Figure 20–68. Renal lymphoma. Enhanced CT shows large soft-tissue masses involving both kidneys. (Courtesy of Bevan Bastian, MD, Green River, WY.)

tiated from primary renal tumors by urography, CT, or ultrasonography. Multiplicity of tumor nodules should suggest the possibility of lymphoma. Some lymphomas with multiple renal masses may resemble polycystic disease on urography or angiography, but CT or ultrasonography can be used to demonstrate the solid nature of these masses. Retroperitoneal adenopathy along with the CT findings of renal nodules, renal enlargement, or renal infiltration can suggest the diagnosis of renal lymphoma. Computed tomography can also be used to evaluate the course of lymphoma and its response to therapy.[72] On angiography lymphoma can resemble renal cell carcinoma, appear hypovascular, or contain vessels with a straight palisadelike appearance. The nephrotic syndrome has been reported in association with lymphatic leukemia and Hodgkin's lymphoma with renal involvement. Another complication is hypertension caused by obstruction of a renal artery by the tumor.

Metastases to the Kidney

Metastatic tumors to the kidney are twice as common as primary renal tumors. However, most of these are small and are discovered at autopsy. If lymphoma is excluded, lung cancer is the most common metastasis. Breast, stomach, colon, cervix, pancreas, and contralateral renal tumors in addition to melanoma can metastasize to the kidney. These metastases usually are blood borne, but can occur from lymphatic spread or direct extension. In a series of nine patients studied by Mitnick and colleagues, the tumors were usually multiple and bilateral.[104]

Metastases to the kidney may be detected with excretory urography, but the increasing widespread use of CT and ultrasonography in all oncology patients may allow for increased detection rates. The metastases are best seen on dynamic enhanced CT scans as low attenuation regions relative to the normal parenchyma. The appearance on ultrasonography in the series by Mitnick and colleagues varied from hypoechoic to a mixed pattern of hypoechoic and more echogenic regions. The amount of vascularity and the histology of the primary tumor may determine the appearance on ultrasonography.

MISCELLANEOUS RENAL CONDITIONS

Amyloidosis

Renal amyloidosis may be primary or secondary to chronic inflammatory disease. Plain-film findings include bilateral, symmetric renal enlargement with normal collecting systems. Late in the disease the kidneys may become small and have diminished function. Angiographic findings recorded in a few reports include slightly decreased renal artery size, pruning, tortuosity and irregularity of the distal interlobar arteries, a relatively homogeneous nephrogram, nonvisualization of the interlobar arteries, prominent extrarenal arteries, and uneven involvement of the kidneys. Renal vein thrombosis is common. When the disease is restricted to the renal pelvis, linear submucosal calcification outlining the pelvis may be noted. Computed tomographic findings reflect the angiographic features of the venous thrombosis component.

Scleroderma

Renal scleroderma may show changes similar to those found in the kidneys of patients with advanced malignant hypertension. In patients with scleroderma the nephrogram phase of the roentgenographic examination is quite characteristic. Spotty lucencies are seen scattered throughout the kidney with a delay in arterial flow manifested by persistent filling of arteries during the nephrogram phase.[160]

Chronic Glomerulonephritis

Renal cortical calcification somewhat similar to that in patients who survive acute renal cortical necrosis is rarely observed in patients with chronic glomerulonephritis. The kidneys of patients with chronic glomerulonephritis are usually symmetrically small with relatively normal collecting systems.

Multiple Myeloma

In multiple myeloma, renal involvement is the result of precipitation of abnormal proteins in the tubules. Findings are those of bilateral, smooth renal enlargement with normal collecting systems. Parenchymal thickness is increased. Later in the disease, renal failure with oliguria may result in small kidneys. In this disease, it is essential that the patient be well hydrated during excretory urography to decrease the risk of precipitation of abnormal urinary protein in the tubules, causing renal failure.

Agnogenic Myeloid Metaplasia

When extramedullary hematopoiesis occurs in the renal hilus, it may simulate a parapelvic cyst or neoplasm.[154]

Hemophilia

Nonobstructive renal enlargement has been noted in patients with hemophilia, primarily in children.

Sickle-Cell Hemoglobinopathy

Sickle-cell hemoglobinopathy may be a cause of renal papillary necrosis. It may occur in SS, SC, and SA disease. Papillary necrosis in these patients is similar to that in analgesic-abuse patients. Bilateral renal enlargement has also been reported in patients with sickle-cell hemoglobinopathies and in thalassemia, but is not found in many of these patients.

Sarcoidosis

The hypercalcemia frequently observed in patients with sarcoidosis may result in nephrocalcinosis and nephrolithiasis. In addition, the granulomas of sarcoidosis may involve the kidney. The granulomatous disease is usually not severe enough to cause any recognizable alteration, but the nephrocalcinosis as well as renal calculi can be observed in this disease. Usually there is no deformity of the collecting system. There may be some irregularity of the renal outline secondary to scarring related to tubular atrophy in patients with long-standing hyperuricemia.

Radiation Nephritis

Acute radiation nephritis develops after a period of 6 to 12 months following radiation treatment for malignancy. The urogram and CT may show only slight diminution in excretion. In chronic radiation nephritis, there is glomerular damage, tubular atrophy, and interstitial fibrosis as well as damage to smaller arteries and arterioles. Atrophy involves the area irradiated, whether it be a portion of, or the entire kidney, which is then decreased in size. The other finding is diminution in renal excretion, which may be observed when comparison is made with the opposite normal kidney. Hypertension often develops in patients with severe renal damage. In some, the condition progresses to malignant hypertension, which is relieved if the involved kidney is removed. The cause of hypertension in these patients is not entirely clear.

Nephrosclerosis

Nephrosclerosis refers to the alteration in renal parenchyma that results from decreased arterial blood flow due to diffuse arteriosclerosis; therefore, the condition is associated with renal ischemia. Some patients have this small-vessel disease due to predisposing disease such as diabetes mellitus. Nephrosclerosis can lead to local infarction. The imaging findings depend on the type of involvement. The infarcts produce a renal scar that appears as an irregularity indenting the renal cortical margin. The collecting system is usually normal. When the disease is uniform and widespread, the kidney decreases in size and there is also evidence of decrease in function.

Radiology in Renal Transplant Patients

Arteriographic studies are obtained on potential donors for renal transplantation to identify the number of renal arteries, to demonstrate unsuspected disease involving the renal arteries, and to outline the anatomic variations. In the post-transplant period, both radionuclide scintigraphy and ultrasonography are valuable imaging modalities.

Radionuclide scintigraphy can be used to evaluate parenchymal failure in the renal transplant due to rejection or acute tubular necrosis. Tc-99m-DTPA and I-131-orthoiodohippurate are the most commonly used radiopharmaceuticals to evaluate the renal transplant, although Tc-99m-Mertiatide is becoming more frequently used.[145] Evaluation of renal perfusion, parenchymal accumulation, and transit time on serial scans can help to distinguish acute tubular necrosis from transplant rejection. Rejection usually is manifested by progressive deterioration of renal perfusion and function while acute tubular necrosis will show improvement or a plateau in perfusion and function after an initial drop at about 24 to 48 hours post-transplantation.[77] Radionuclide scintigraphy can also help to evaluate mechanical injuries to the blood vessels or problems with urinary drainage in the transplant.

Ultrasonography may demonstrate several findings compatible with post-transplant rejection. Medullary edema, increase in transplant size, increase in cortical echoes, decreased parenchymal echoes, indistinct corticomedullary boundary, and decreased renal sinus echoes have been reported as anatomic features of rejection (Fig. 20-69). Serial scans are again important to document changes from a baseline study. Ultrasonography can also evaluate hydronephrosis and perinephric fluid collections around the transplant such as urinoma, hematoma, or lymphocele.

Doppler ultrasound, both duplex and color, is widely used to evaluate renal transplants. Because of its ability to distinguish flowing blood from other structures, Doppler technology greatly assists in locating and characterizing transplant vascularity. Complications such as arteriovenous fistulas, renal artery stenosis, renal infarction, renal vein thrombosis, and pseudoaneurysms, may be diagnosed by ultrasound, often reducing the necessity for angiography.[138, 146]

Sampling of arcuate and segmental arteries with pulsed Doppler in normal renal allografts yields characteristic low-impedance antegrade flow. This low-impedance flow is characterized by antegrade flow during diastole. Early literature demonstrated that acute rejection could be diagnosed by demonstrating increased vascular impedance leading to decreased or reversed

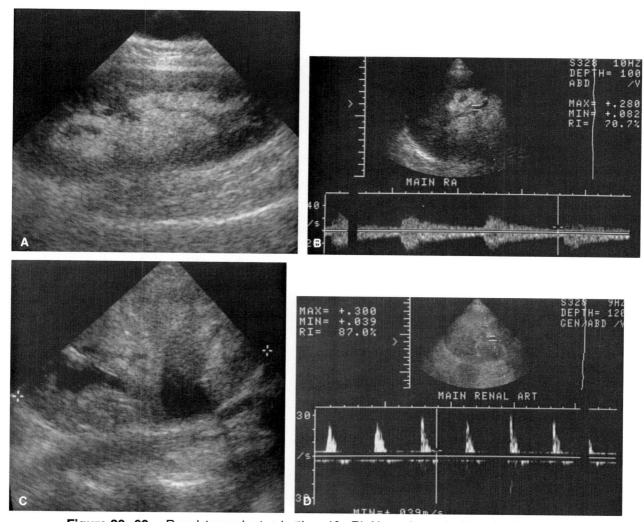

Figure 20–69. Renal transplant rejection. (**A, B**) Normal renal allograft. Ultrasound demonstrates normal renal sinus and cortex. Duplex Doppler study has normal computed resistive index (*RI*) of 70.7%. (**C, D**) Acute rejection. Allograft is now swollen with loss of differentiation between sinuses and parenchyma. Collecting system is more prominent. Computed RI is now 87.0% with noticeable lack of diastolic flow.

flow during diastole.[112, 130] This was quantified by resistive or pulsatility indices.

$$RI = \frac{\text{Peak systolic velocity} - \text{End diastolic velocity}}{\text{Peak systolic velocity}}$$

$$PI = \frac{\text{Peak systolic velocity} - \text{End diastolic velocity}}{\text{Mean velocity}}$$

Pulsatility indices greater than 1.5 or a resistive index greater than 0.9 were thought to be specific signs of acute rejection. A resistive index of 0.8 to 0.89 was thought likely to correspond to rejection.[130] Later work demonstrated that other complications such as acute tubular necrosis, pyelonephritis, external compression, chronic rejection, and renal vein obstruction can also elevate pulsatility or resistive indices. Needle biopsy, often performed under ultrasound guidance, is thus needed to evaluate transplant dysfunction definitively after surgical complications have been excluded.[35, 125, 126]

Excretory urography should play a limited role because of the possibility of renal damage and the availability of ultrasonography and radionuclide scintigraphy. Angiography also plays a more limited role currently because it is an invasive procedure and involves the use of a contrast agent. If an angiographic procedure needs to be performed, a digital subtraction arteriogram may be preferable to evaluate renal artery stenosis or an abnormal vascular pattern.

The role of MRI in renal transplantation is still being evaluated. One study was able to distinguish hematomas from lymphoceles. Patients with acute rejection showed a decrease in cortico-medullary differentiation and a decrease in overall signal intensity compared with a baseline state. The cortico-medullary junction could not be differentiated in chronic rejection.[48] MRI spectroscopy may prove useful in making the specific diagnosis of rejection noninvasively, but remains under investigation.[56]

TUMORS OF THE URETER

Tumors of the ureter are rare, but benign papilloma, hemangioma, benign fibrous polyps, fibrolipoma, leiomyoma, and epithelial carcinoma may arise there. The benign tumors originate from the nonepithelial components of the ureteral wall. Benign fibrous polyps appear to be the most common of the benign tumors.[135] They usually have a core of fibrous tissue that is covered by a layer of transitional epithelium. The polyp is often a long, branched, smooth, intraluminal structure that becomes quite large. The polyp reported by Howard measured 10 by 3 cm.[67] There can be multiple polyps present. Polyps can cause obstruction, but the obstruction may not be as severe as the size of the polyp might indicate. The nonpolypoid tumors are not as common. Endometriosis of the ureter may simulate tumor because the lesion can invade the ureter and penetrate the mucosa. Endometriosis more often is an extrinsic lesion that involves the adventitia. If the ureter is involved, this usually occurs below the pelvic brim. Obstruction may be severe enough to cause symptoms.

Most malignant tumors of the ureter are epithelial. Renal pelvis epithelioma may implant in the ureter. Transitional cell carcinoma is the most common epithelial tumor and is usually papillary in form. The papillary tumors tend to be multiple. When multiple tumors are found, this is usually attributed to a multicentric origin. Roentgenographic findings do not differentiate the various types of epithelial tumors. Obstruction of the ureter is common, leading to hydronephrosis. An intraluminal tumor mass may be seen in addition to the ureteral obstruction on excretory urography. An infiltrating carcinoma occasionally may result in local narrowing of the lumen, simulating a benign ureteral stricture (Fig. 20-70). In some cases there is no ureterectasis above the tumor even if it is large. The ureter is apparently able to dilate locally to accommodate the tumor as it grows so that obstruction does not occur. The entire length of the ureter must be seen in these instances. The only roentgenographic sign is an intraluminal mass appearing as a negative filling defect, which requires outlining by contrast material within the ureter to be visualized. A localized dilatation immediately below the tumor has been described (Fig. 20-71). If retrograde pyelography is attempted, the catheter tip may coil in the region of localized dilatation, the intraluminal mass impeding its upward progress. The coiling of the catheter is then a sign of ureteral tumor, since the local dilatation does not occur below a ureteral calculus unless it is large, calcified, and easily detected. It is difficult to demonstrate both the upper and lower borders of a negative filling defect on one exam. Excretory urography may be required to demonstrate the upper border and retrograde pyelography to demonstrate the lower border in these cases. Tomography of the ureter at the time of urography is helpful in some instances. Computed tomography can be used to detect periureteral extension in patients with transitional cell carcinoma and can demonstrate metastases to enlarged lymph nodes. It cannot, however, distinguish tumors with muscle wall invasion from those limited to the mucosa. The tumors approach soft-tissue density with some of the tumors noted to increase in attenuation values on the enhanced scans.[10]

Metastases to the ureter from tumors outside the urinary tract may cause local involvement with little or

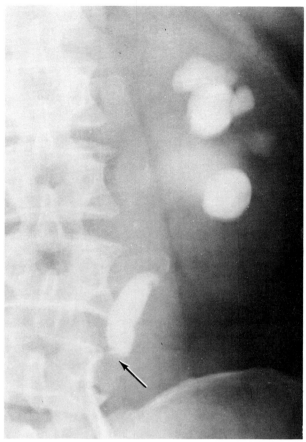

Figure 20–70. Carcinoma of the left ureter (*arrow*) has produced partial obstruction with hydroureter and hydronephrosis above it.

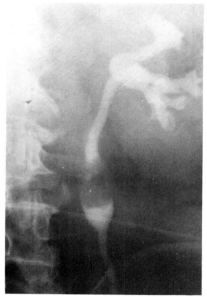

Figure 20–71. Ureteral carcinoma. The tumor produces a filling defect that is somewhat irregular superiorly and demonstrates dilatation below the tumor.

placed in patients with uterine prolapse or procidentia. Primary or secondary tumors or massive lymph nodes may also displace one or both ureters and sometimes will produce obstruction. Fecal impactions in the sigmoid colon may displace the ureter in a manner simulating a pelvic mass. In patients with Crohn's disease, a ureter may be caught in an inflammatory mass and

no extrinsic mass. Alternatively, the ureter may be caught in a retroperitoneal mass, displaced, and narrowed. Metastases to the ureter on CT are demonstrated as soft-tissue thickening or mass in the ureteral wall (Fig. 20-72). There may be associated ureterectasis and hydronephrosis proximal to the lesion. Although selective arteriography can be used to identify ureteral tumors to help differentiate them from strictures, it is rarely used.

OTHER URETERAL ABNORMALITIES

Ureteral Displacement

The ureter may herniate into the inguinal canal, the femoral canal, or the sciatic notch. The relationship of the ureter to these various structures usually determines the diagnosis, and there is often a portion of the bowel extending into the hernia. Ureters are also dis-

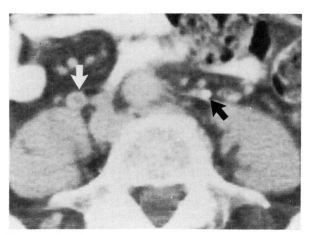

Figure 20–72. Ureteral metastasis. Enhanced CT shows the thickened right ureteral wall (*white arrow*) in this patient with breast cancer. Note contrast in the normal left ureter (*black arrow*).

displaced or obstructed by the accompanying fibrosis. In patients with aortic aneurysm, there may be traction displacement medially of one of the ureters toward the aneurysm. Presumably this is an indication of retroperitoneal bleeding with resultant fibrosis causing the displacement. Pelvic lipomatosis may also result in alteration in the course of the ureters, and in some instances may produce ureteral obstruction. More often there is alteration in the appearance of the bladder, which is elevated and elongated vertically, the so-called pear-shaped bladder.

Schistosomiasis

Schistosomiasis may cause calcification in the ureteral wall as well as medial deviation, a straight lumbar course, or a bowed appearance in the pelvis with medial and upward displacement at the level of the trigone. There may be some stasis and dilatation of the upper urinary tract, owing mainly to fibrosis rather than to mechanical obstruction.

Polyarteritis

Polyarteritis may cause dilatation and nodular irregularity of the ureteral wall simulating a string of pearls.

Amyloidosis

Amyloidosis may involve the ureter, causing a stricturelike defect that may partially obstruct it, producing colicky pain and hematuria as well as ureterectasis above the stricture.[92]

Primary Megaloureter (or Adynamic Distal Ureteral Segment)

This appears to be a specific entity in which there is local dilatation of one or both ureters just above the bladder, often without evidence of anatomic obstruction or reflux.[119] It fails to transmit an effective peristaltic wave. Its cause is not clear. Usually there is no upper ureteral, pelvic, or calyceal dilatation unless infection is present. Maximal dilatation is immediately proximal to the aperistaltic segment, which averages 1.5 cm in length and is relatively narrow. It may not fill on excretory urography. Videotaped fluoroscopy may be used to demonstrate the disturbed peristalsis. The peristaltic activity is normal or vigorous in the proximal dilated ureter, but peristalsis is absent in the distal ureteral segment.

Retroperitoneal Fibrosis

Originally called periureteral fibrosis, this disease is more aptly termed *retroperitoneal fibrosis* because it may involve lymphatic and vascular structures in addition to the ureters. The cause of the disease is unknown, and it is characterized by a fibrosing inflammatory process in the retroperitoneum that may extend from the kidneys caudally to the pelvic brim and spread laterally to involve the ureters. In addition to the idiopathic cases (about 70%), several cases have been reported in patients on long-term methysergide (Sansert) therapy for migraine headaches. If the drug is withdrawn, the process may regress. However, if methysergide therapy is resumed, the process seems to recur. Other drugs such as phenacetin and methyldopa have also been implicated. Patients with retroperitoneal neoplasms (primary or metastatic) may also have a fibrotic reaction similar to that of the idiopathic form.

Fibrosis of the orbit, duodenum, rectosigmoid, common bile duct, and pancreatic duct have been reported in association with retroperitoneal fibrosis. Involvement of the splenic vein, vena cava, celiac axis, superior mesenteric artery, or iliac arteries may also be found. Males are affected twice as often as females and the condition is usually bilateral. Retroperitoneal fibrosis affects patients 8 to 80 years old with the peak incidence in the fifth and sixth decades.[79] The patients can have back, flank, or abdominal pain. A palpable abdominal or rectal mass is noted in 30% of cases.

The radiographic findings may suggest the diagnosis. The normal fat lines may disappear so that the outlines of the psoas muscle are not visible on plain film. Excretory urography may show delayed excretion with varying degrees of hydronephrosis or absence of excretion caused by obstruction. If the ureters are opacified, they gradually taper to the area of maximum stenosis. The involved segment is often 4 to 5 cm in length, usually, but not always, with medial deviation of the tapered ureters at the level of the lower lumbar vertebrae. Some slight redundancy may be observed in the ureter above the stenotic segment. Retrograde pyelography can also reveal the site and length of obstruction and there is often a paradoxical ease of retrograde passage of ureteral catheters. Lymphangiography and inferior vena cavography were also used in the past to demonstrate lymphatic or vascular obstruction but are rarely used at present.

Computed tomography can provide direct information about the fibrosis and also allow evaluation of vascular and urologic structures. The fibrosis is easy to recognize when it appears as a large bulky mass. The appearance is nonspecific and lymphoma, hematoma, sarcoma, and lymph node metastases can cause a similar appearance. The location may be helpful as lymphomas are found higher in the retroperitoneum while the fibrosis is usually located caudal to the renal hilum. The attenuation values on unenhanced scans are in the range of muscle. After intravenous contrast, the density of the fibrosis may markedly increase, simulating a vascular neoplasm.[72] Ultrasonography also will demonstrate a solid retroperitoneal mass, which usually will envelop but not displace the adjacent vascular structures and ureters. MRI is becoming increasingly useful in the diagnosis and follow-up of patients with retroperitoneal fibrosis. In particular, MRI may help assess vascular patency and may be able to help distinguish the malignant from nonmalignant varieties based on signal characteristics. T2-weighted images in the malignant form will show increased signal intensity when compared with T1-weighted images. Benign retroperitoneal fibrosis has low signal intensity on both T1- and T2-weighted images. Unfortunately, some reports have shown overlapping signal characteristics of the different forms, although it is distinctly unusual for malignant retroperitoneal fibrosis to have low signal intensity on T2-weighted images.[3, 6, 108] Early recognition and surgical ureterolysis are important to preserve renal function in idiopathic disease. The vascular obstruction may be more important clinically than the ureteral obstruction in some instances.

THE URINARY BLADDER

CONGENITAL ANOMALIES

Exstrophy

Exstrophy of the bladder is of imaging interest because of the wide separation of the pubic bones anteriorly at the symphysis that accompanies this anomaly. The symphysis is separated approximately the width of the sacrum; this leads to a rather square appearance of the pelvis (Fig. 20-73). Exstrophy consists of an absence of the anterior wall of the bladder and of the lower anterior abdominal wall. The diagnosis is made on observation, so that roentgenographic examination is not necessary but is useful to study the kidneys and ureters, since ureteral obstruction is often associated. A characteristic dilatation of the distal ureters ("Hurley-Stick" ureter) is sometimes noted. Wide separation of the pubic bones is also found in some patients with epispadias.

Duplication of the Urinary Bladder

Duplication of the urinary bladder is extremely rare and is usually associated with urethral duplication (Fig. 20-74). Incomplete duplication may also occur, in which a septum partially divides the bladder and a multilocular or multiseptated bladder has been described. There may occasionally be a partial horizontal septum, sometimes resulting in an hourglass appearance. The ureters empty into the lower compartment. Cystography is often necessary to outline these anoma-

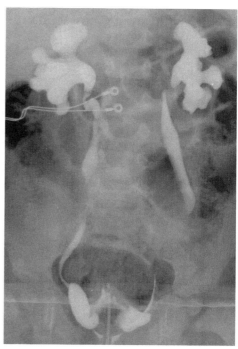

Figure 20–73. Bladder extrophy. Note the wide symphysis pubis and characteristic "Hurley stick" dilatation of the distal ureters.

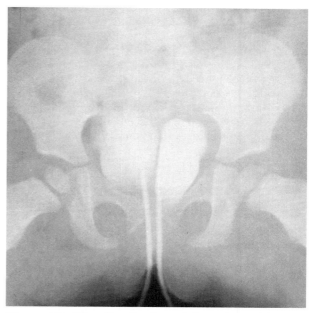

Figure 20–74. Duplication of the urinary bladder. Cystogram outlines the duplication with each bladder drained by its own urethra.

lies, but excretory urography with special films of the bladder may obviate the need for cystography.

Agenesis of the Bladder

Agenesis of the bladder is very rare and is usually incompatible with life, largely because of associated anomalies. Congenital enlargement of the bladder with hydronephrosis and ureterectasis is found in association with congenital absence or hypoplasia of the abdominal muscles, the prune-belly syndrome. This is a rare condition that occurs almost exclusively in males. No obstruction can be demonstrated to account for the dilatation. Associated abnormalities include nondescent of the testes, malrotation of the intestine, and, more rarely, persistent urachus, dislocated hips, clubfoot, harelip, spina bifida, hydrocephalus, and cardiac malformations. The abdomen is distended and the skin wrinkled (prune belly).

Bladder Ears

Lateral protrusions of the bladder caused by extraperitoneal herniations through the internal inguinal ring into the inguinal canal have been observed. They are usually noted in infants and are associated with a high incidence of clinical inguinal hernia. This is not a true bladder anomaly, but is rather a bladder deformity secondary to a large internal inguinal ring. The term *bladder ears* has been used in preference to hernia because the deformity does not usually persist beyond infancy. Roentgenographic findings at cystography or urography consist of anterolateral protrusion of the bladder into the inguinal canal, which is usually bilateral. The protrusion is most often observed in the partially filled bladder and tends to disappear when the bladder is completely filled. Oblique or lateral views show the anterior extent of the protrusion. It is important to be aware of this condition so that surgical misadventures are avoided during inguinal herniorrhaphy.

The Pear-Shaped Bladder

Some patients have this appearance as a normal variant due to anterior prolongation of the bladder. However, the tear-drop or pear-shaped alteration in the shape of the bladder was first described in patients with pelvic hematoma. Other abnormalities that also may result in an elongated bladder with a narrow base include pelvic lipomatosis, hematoma, large iliopsoas muscles, enlarged pelvic nodes, lymphoceles, lymphoma and other pelvic tumors, and inferior vena cava occlusion. When the inferior vena cava is occluded, large venous collaterals may compress the bladder, altering its shape to this configuration.

VESICAL CALCULI

Obstruction and infection are the chief causes of vesical calculi. About half of these calculi are radiopaque and can be easily seen on plain-film roentgenograms (Fig. 20-75). Others contain small amounts of calcium and are poorly visualized on plain film. The condition occurs largely in males.

Cystography with air or with diluted contrast medium can be used to outline radiolucent stones. Computed tomography and ultrasonography also readily delineate vesical calculi. Stones may be single or multiple and tend to lie in the midline except when contained in a bladder diverticulum. In this case the position of the calculus depends on the site of the diverticulum. Bladder calculi must be differentiated from calcification in lymph nodes, fecaliths, calcification in uterine fibroids, and prostatic and seminal vesicle calculi. Radiopaque bladder calculi are often laminated and very dense; when multiple, they may be faceted. Lymph node calcification usually is higher in position and the nodes are mottled and not as uniformly dense as calculi. Uterine leiomyomas that contain calcium are often higher in position than bladder calculi and have a mottled appearance. Fecaliths of the sigmoid are rare, but may simulate bladder calculi closely in texture and position. Oblique views and barium enema will permit differentiation. Prostatic calculi are usually multiple and produce a mottled density in contrast to the uniform or laminated appear-

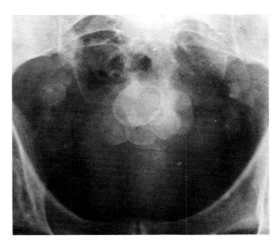

Figure 20–75. Vesical calculi. This roentgenogram of the pelvis obtained without the use of contrast material, outlines five partially calcified bladder stones. Note their midline position.

ance of vesical calculi; they are also lower in position. The same is true of calculi in the seminal vesicles.

Cystography and cystoscopy may be necessary to differentiate bladder calculi from other causes of calcification. A foreign body within the bladder may act as a nidus for deposition of calcium and other salts to form a calculus. Foreign bodies may be introduced by way of the urethra during treatment or by the patient. They also may be introduced through penetrating wounds or left in or near the bladder during surgery. The shape of the calculus then is dependent on the foreign body, which can often be visualized on plain roentgenograms. Foreign bodies in the bladder almost invariably become encrusted with calcium.

Calculi in the prostate usually occur in the form of small granular deposits and are visualized overlying or directly above the level of the symphysis pubis in standard anteroposterior roentgenograms of the lower abdomen. They offer little difficulty in differential diagnosis as a rule because of their position, characteristic small size, and multiplicity (Fig. 20-76).

INFLAMMATION OF THE BLADDER (CYSTITIS)

Acute inflammation of the urinary bladder usually does not produce changes that can be recognized and diagnosed on cystography. Chronic cystitis results in decreased bladder size. The wall may be smooth but sometimes is serrated; when serration is present along with major contraction at the dome, the so-called Christmas-tree bladder of chronic cystitis is formed. A

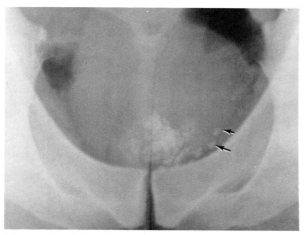

Figure 20–76. Prostatic calculi. The mottled densities above the symphysis pubis are characteristic of prostatic calculi. Their distribution indicates probable prostatic enlargement. The calcifications on the left, which tend to parallel the pubic ramus, are phleboliths (*arrows*).

bladder of this shape, also called pine-tree bladder, is also found in association with neurogenic bladder dysfunction although it may occur with any chronic bladder obstruction. Cystoscopy is more useful than cystography in the examination of bladder infections.

Of interest roentgenologically is *cystitis emphysematosa* (emphysematous cystitis), an inflammatory disease of the bladder in which there is gas in the vesical wall and/or lumen. This condition is caused by gas-forming bacteria, and nearly 50% of the reported cases have occurred in patients with diabetes mellitus. The gas may be present for only a short time, which probably accounts for its low reported incidence. Roentgenographic findings are characteristic. A ring of radiolucency outlines the bladder wall or part of it. There is often gas within the bladder lumen as well. The zone of gas expands and contracts with the bladder and is a transient finding unless the infection fails to respond to therapy. The bladder infection is often benign and transient and may produce very few symptoms.

Schistosomiasis

Schistosomiasis (bilharziasis) is caused by a group of blood flukes, *Schistosoma mansoni*, *S. japonicum*, and *S. haematobium*. The lower urinary tract is involved mainly by *S. haematobium*. Large numbers of ova are deposited in the submucosa of the bladder wall, which becomes thickened, ulcerated, and sometimes papillomatous. In chronic disease, the distal ureters may be involved, leading to stricture, hydronephrosis, and renal damage. Calcification in the bladder wall, which occurs in chronic cases, has a characteristic appearance. When the bladder is empty, thin parallel lines of density are observed. The appearance resembles that of the postvoiding bladder on excretory urography, in which a thin coating of opaque medium outlines the bladder wall. When the bladder is full of contrast medium, a very thin radiolucent line, representing the thickened mucosa, separates the opacified bladder lumen and the thin rim of submucosal calcification (Fig. 20-77). The ova in the bladder wall may calcify. Lower ureteral nodular involvement may produce the roentgenographic findings of ureteritis cystica. Bladder capacity eventually is reduced. The distal ureters may be calcified in a manner similar to that noted in the bladder. Calculi in the bladder, ureters, and kidneys are common.

Candidiasis

Candidiasis may involve the urinary bladder in circumstances similar to those in which the kidney is affected. There may be gas within a fungus ball, giving a laminated appearance. Otherwise, the fungus balls appear

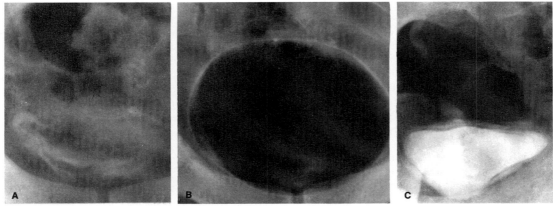

Figure 20–77. Schistosomiasis of the bladder. **(A)** Plain films showing parallel lines of calcific density of the wall of the empty bladder. **(B)** Air cystogram showing a thin rim of calcium in the bladder wall. **(C)** Renografin cystogram showing the thin rim of calcium separated from the lumen by a lucent line representing the thickened bladder wall.

as filling defects that must be differentiated from blood clot, radiolucent calculi, and tumors.

Cyclophosphamide Cystitis

Cytoxan, used in the treatment of leukemia and lymphoma, may produce a hemorrhagic cystitis with hematuria of varying degrees of severity. Blood clots within the bladder may then appear as filling defects. On cystography, minimal mucosal irregularity is noted in addition to the clots. Later, contraction and thumbprinting secondary to edema and submucosal hemorrhage are evident. Ultimately, the bladder may be markedly contracted and, very rarely, calcification may occur in its wall.

Radiation Cystitis

Large doses administered in radiation therapy may produce enough necrosis of the bladder wall to result in calcification that is similar radiographically to that observed in schistosomiasis.

Cystitis Cystica

Cystitis cystica is a form of chronic disease of the bladder in which a number of small cystlike mucosal lesions are noted, mainly in the region of the trigone. In almost all instances, this condition is associated with infection, obstruction, tumor, calculi, or stasis. Its presence in children usually indicates that an associated chronic infection will be difficult to control. Radiographically, multiple filling defects are observed chiefly in the region of the trigone. The irregularity and deformity, if severe, may resemble changes observed in bladder tumors. Although the lesions may be visible on cystography, cystoscopy is the best method of examination in patients with this condition.

Cystitis Glandularis

Cystitis glandularis represents metaplasia of the bladder epithelium induced by a variety of irritants. Most lesions occur in the region of the vesical neck and trigone. They appear as irregular, rounded elevations separated by deep ridges and are usually sharply demarcated from the normal mucosa. When they exist in the dome of the bladder, villouslike proliferations may occur, often several centimeters in size. The lesions appear to be premalignant. Because their radiographic appearance is similar to that in cystitis cystica, cystoscopy and, often, biopsy are required for definitive diagnosis. The condition may also simulate bladder tumor.[29]

Malakoplakia

This rare chronic inflammatory disease is usually confined to the bladder, renal pelvis, and ureters. Malakoplakia may occasionally involve the renal parenchyma on one or both sides, and it causes marked enlargement of the involved kidney(s). When renal infection with gram-negative organisms is an associated finding, xanthogranulomatous pyelonephritis and infected polycystic disease should be considered in the differential diagnosis. Malakoplakia is probably caused by an unusual histiocytic response to infection (usually *E. coli*) and may result in renal failure when bilateral.

The soft plaques formed in the bladder may not produce any recognizable roentgenographic changes on cystography.

OBSTRUCTION OF THE BLADDER

Bladder obstruction may be caused by congenital or acquired lesions. Benign prostatic hyperplasia is the most frequent cause. Prostatic enlargement is difficult to assess by urography. However, when elevation of the bladder floor is accompanied by a J-shaped or hockey-stick appearance of the distal ureters, prostatic enlargement can be inferred. Prostatic carcinoma, acquired urethral stenosis, urethral valves, and neurogenic dysfunction (cord bladder) are other causes. The first change in the bladder wall resulting from obstruction is hypertrophy of the muscles, which can often be observed as a soft-tissue shadow, several millimeters thick, paralleling the opaque shadow of the inner bladder wall in excretory urography or cystography. The normal bladder wall does not ordinarily produce a visible soft-tissue shadow. As the muscle bundles enlarge they cause irregular interlacing bands known as trabeculae. The intervening outpouchings are called cellules (Fig. 20-78). Trabeculation becomes more prominent as obstruction continues, and the cellules may enlarge until diverticula are formed. There also may be reflux of urine into one or both ureters with development of hydronephrosis. It is more likely that reflux is caused by infection, however.

As obstruction develops, the bladder may become decompensated, increasing in size and containing increasing amounts of residual urine, until it presents as a large, lower abdominal mass on physical examination and on roentgenographic study. The plain roentgenogram will demonstrate a large soft-tissue mass extending out of the pelvis, often displacing the bowel upward and posteriorly. Cystography will outline the large bladder with trabeculations standing out in a somewhat reticular manner, with cellule or small-diverticulum formation.

Cystourethrography is used to examine patients with suspected bladder or urethral obstruction as well as patients (usually children) with chronic or recurrent urinary infection. There are differing opinions regarding the mechanisms of roentgenographic findings in the bladder-neck obstruction that is not obviously due to a mechanical-type obstruction such as prostatic enlargement. Such "functional" obstructing problems have been better understood since the recent advent of urodynamic methods for investigating the bladder and urethra. Better understanding of bladder physiology and recognition of the infrequent voiding syndromes have cleared up previous ambiguities.

Diverticulum of the Bladder

A diverticulum of the bladder wall is a localized herniation of mucosa, usually having a narrow neck. These protruding defects, which may be single or multiple, vary in size from a small cellule to a large sac having a capacity greater than the bladder itself. Chronic obstruction is a frequent cause, but some diverticula are of congenital origin. Infection is also a factor in many cases. If the diverticula are small and empty completely, they are usually of no clinical significance. Large diverticula that do not empty completely, however, are often the site of infection that is fostered by stagnation. Calculus formation is also common in this type of large diverticulum. Roentgenographic findings are confined to those diverticula that are noted at cystography or excretory urography unless the diverticulum is large enough to produce an actual mass shadow on a plain roentgenogram. Then the nature of the mass must be determined by means of cystography, cystoscopy, or ultrasonography. When the bladder is examined by means of cystography, the diverticulum is outlined by the opaque substance, and its size, shape, and position, as well as the width of its neck, can be determined (Fig. 20-79). It is often important to assess the presence and the amount of urinary retention in a large diverticulum, and a roentgenogram

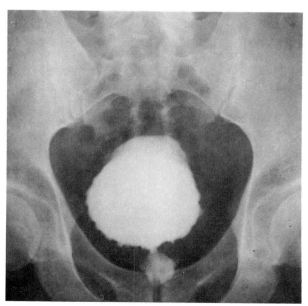

Figure 20–78. Trabeculation of the bladder. Note the irregularity of the inferior and lateral bladder wall shown in this cystogram. The patient has had a transurethral prostatectomy with opacification of the rounded prostatic bed following the operation.

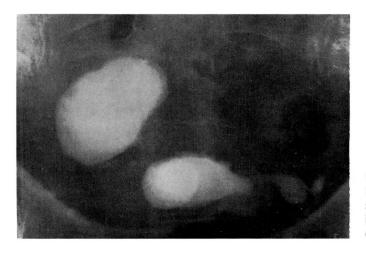

Figure 20–79.   Multiple bladder diverticula. The large opacified diverticulum on the right has a smooth wall in contrast to the trabeculation of the bladder wall. There is also a small diverticulum on the left.

obtained following voiding is usually sufficient for this purpose. If the bladder still contains enough opaque material to obscure the diverticulum partially, a second roentgenogram may be obtained following catheterization of the bladder. A tumor may occasionally occur in a diverticulum. This lesion is often difficult to visualize, but presents as a filling defect on the otherwise smooth wall of the diverticulum. Computed tomography provides more complete assessment of such a tumor.

Neurogenic Bladder Dysfunction

Disease or injury involving the spinal cord or peripheral nerves supplying the bladder results in changes in bladder function that may produce either incontinence or retention of urine. The urographic appearance of the type of neurogenic dysfunction is not related to the type of neurologic lesion producing it. Patients with small, spastic, trabeculated bladders often have upper motor neuron lesions, but simple outlet obstruction may cause the same appearance (pine-tree bladder). In theory, patients with lower motor neuron lesions have large, atonic bladders, but some have small, trabeculated bladders. The large, atonic bladder with little or no trabeculation often is found in association with tabes dorsalis, diabetes, or syringomyelia, but it may also be due to infrequent voiding in patients with no neurologic disease. The following findings may be observed in patients with neurogenic dysfunction: a trabeculated bladder with a circular or pyramidal (pine-tree) pattern; an hourglass bladder; a small, hypertonic trabeculated bladder; a large dilated hypotonic bladder without trabeculation; and variations in the contour of the vesical neck and prostatic urethra in which there may be saccular dilatation, funnel-shaped dilatation or contraction, and spasm of the bladder neck. The diag-

nosis of exact abnormality is based on urodynamic studies. Cystographic study will delineate vesical size, presence or absence of trabeculation, reflux into the ureters, retention or lack of it, vesical-neck dilatation, and the presence of other associated gross anatomic changes.

VESICOURETERAL REFLUX

Vesicoureteral reflux in children is usually due to abnormal anatomy of the vesicoureteral junction. Normally, the ureters enter the bladder at a shallow angle and proceed in the bladder submucosa before emptying into the bladder. This arrangement creates a valve mechanism that allows antegrade flow of urine without reflux. If abnormal anatomy is present, usually a shortened submucosal course of the ureter, vesicoureteral reflux is common. Reflux will often spontaneously resolve as a child ages because of the lengthening of the submucosal portion of the ureter. In general, the worse the reflux at the time of diagnosis, the less likely it will resolve spontaneously and therefore may require surgical intervention.[64, 93]

Infection is the most common adult cause of vesicoureteral reflux, which is also found occasionally in patients with lower-urinary-tract obstruction. The obstructive lesions include posterior urethral valves, urethral stricture, and median bar enlargement of the prostate. Neurologic disorders that result in neurogenic bladder dysfunction, congenital anomalies such as ectopic ureter, and other anomalies of the distal ureter and trigone may also produce reflux.

The study used for detection of reflux is the voiding cystourethrogram. If reflux is present it is manifested by retrograde filling of one or both ureters. The ureters may dilate considerably and there may be marked hydronephrosis associated with reflux. Children with unexplained recurrent urinary tract infection should have a urologic study including cystourethrography. Because evidence of reflux is sometimes fleeting, fluoroscopic spot-film examination or videotaping is important. Radionuclide cystography now provides a more physiologic and lower radiation dose method to assess reflux.

Renal parenchymal scarring, either local with a blunted calyx or extensive, may be seen by ultrasound or at excretory urography. About 60% of adult patients with reflux have extensive scarring. Mucosal striations in the pelvis and upper ureter are also observed in patients with reflux, probably the result of edema and infection.[70]

THE MEGACYSTIS SYNDROME

The definition of this syndrome is somewhat controversial. However, the term *megacystis* refers to a large, thin-walled, smooth bladder. This is usually accompanied by severe vesicoureteral reflux with ureterectasis and recurrent or persistent urinary tract infection. It is usually discovered in childhood and is more frequent in females than in males. The trigone may appear large because the ureteric orifices are situated more laterally than normal. The intramural portions of the ureters are shortened and widened. The nature of the underlying disorder leading to the megacystis syndrome is unclear, but it may represent the most severe end of the vesicoureteral reflux spectrum. The enlarged bladder may be due to the child resetting his or her voiding urge so as to void less frequently. The enlarged bladder can accommodate the large volume of refluxed urine that drains back down into the bladder after micturition, plus the additional urine that the kidneys excrete.[39] There may also be a congenital disproportionate increase in size of the vesical base leading to reflux and infection. Cystography demonstrates the large bladder with vesicoureteral reflux on one or both sides.

VESICAL TUMORS

Benign Lesions

Benign bladder tumors are rare and not as important as malignant epithelial tumors. They include neurofibroma, leiomyoma, fibroma, fibromyoma, myxoma, hemangioma, lymphangioma, paraganglioma (pheochromocytoma), and nephrogenic adenoma. Other heterotopic types include dermoid cyst, rhabdomyoma, and chondroma. There are also other conditions that may produce bladder changes, demonstrable by cystography, which resemble tumor. Endometriosis can involve the bladder wall or present as an extravesicular mass. Hematuria may be present, although cyclic pain, dys-

uria, and frequency are more often present. Granulomatous disease can also involve the colon or small bowel adjacent to the bladder. Occasionally, localized cystitis glandularis and cystitis cystica may simulate bladder tumor. The radiographic findings are those of a mass extending into or indenting the bladder wall. There are no characteristics to distinguish the histologic type. Multiple and extensive masses can be seen in neurofibromatosis; most patients will also have cutaneous involvement. Leukoplakia is associated with chronic urinary infection and is felt to be precancerous. The diagnosis is best made by cystoscopy, because the lesions are not usually demonstrable by cystography.

Malignant Tumors

Some malignant tumors of the bladder arise in the region of the trigone and tend to obstruct the ureteral or urethral orifices. The "benign" papilloma is the most common tumor and is often multiple. This epithelial tumor is malignant or has malignant potential, thus the term "benign" is a misnomer. Many consider it to be a grade-I papillary transitional cell carcinoma. Radiographic detection of the papilloma depends on its size; the small tumors are very difficult to visualize with cystography.

Carcinoma of the bladder is usually of the transitional cell type; squamous-cell carcinoma and adenocarcinoma are fairly rare. Cystography demonstrates an irregular filling defect, usually at the base, often resulting in ureteral obstruction (Fig. 20-80). Calcification may occur in the primary tumor and in metastases from it. The size and shape of these tumors vary widely. Double-contrast cystography can be used to study the bladder mucosa in patients with intravesicular tumors, but is time-consuming and is not warranted if the patient undergoes cystoscopy. Computed tomography will demonstrate bladder cancer as a soft-tissue density involving the bladder wall. The appearance of the tumor will vary depending on its size and whether it is sessile or polypoid (Fig. 20-81). Computed tomography cannot reliably differentiate involvement of the mucosa, lamina propria, and superficial or deep muscle; it is advantageous, however, in detecting extravesicular tumor spread. Computed tomography is also useful in evaluating extension of tumor to the pelvic sidewalls, lymphadenopathy, and hydronephrosis/ureterectasis caused by bladder cancer.

Magnetic resonance imaging of the bladder is most useful for staging known neoplasms (Fig. 20-82). MRI is probably superior to CT in staging early disease, and both techniques are accurate to assess pelvic nodal involvement. Both CT and MRI have limitations in staging local bladder tumors, however, and there are problems of understaging tumors with both

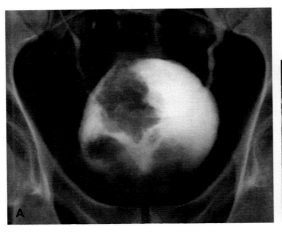

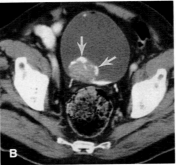

Figure 20–80.   Transitional cell carcinoma. **(A)** Irregular filling defect represents tumor. Impression at bladder base is due to enlarged prostate. **(B)** Enhanced CT scan of same patient. Note rim of calcification involving tumor (*arrows*). (Courtesy of James P. Bronson, MD, Laconia, NH.)

techniques. One study demonstrated understaging of bladder tumors in 32.5% by MRI, though several other studies have demonstrated better results.[21, 69] It is possible that newer pulse sequences and phased-array coils will increase the accuracy of MRI staging in the near future.

Rhabdomyosarcoma occasionally arises in the bladder and usually presents in the first 3 or 4 years of life or in late adulthood. The tumor originates from remnants of the urogenital sinus and wolffian ducts; it may originate in the submucosal or superficial layers, usually at the base. The tumor tends to involve the trigone and can become large enough to displace the ureters laterally. This sarcoma can also bulge upward into the

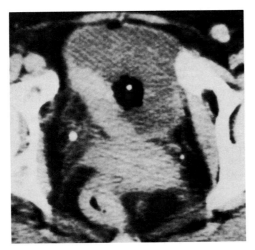

Figure 20–81.   Transitional cell carcinoma. Unenhanced CT shows a sessile tumor along the right posterolateral bladder wall. A Foley catheter balloon filled with air is in the center of the bladder.

bladder to form a lobulated filling defect in it. The tumor nodules may also force their way downward into the urethra, forming a cone of dilatation in the posterior urethra. Some appear as rectal masses; others may protrude through the vulva. Urinary retention caused by bladder obstruction is the most common symptom. Excretory urography often demonstrates ureteral displacement as well as deformity and displacement of the bladder. Biopsy is necessary to make the diagnosis. Rhabdomyosarcomas comprise about 10% of malignant tumors of childhood, and there is a slight male predominance. Most rhabdomyosarcomas arise in the bladder, but they may also arise in the prostate, vagina, spermatic cord, and broad ligament. The tumor is sometimes termed *sarcoma botryoides* because of its polypoid appearance (Fig. 20-83).

Metastases to the Bladder

Three general types of metastases to the bladder may be observed: (1) bladder implant secondary to epithelial tumors of the kidney or ureter, (2) direct extension from primary tumors in the area such as prostatic, uterine, ovarian, and colonic neoplasms, and (3) hematogenous metastases from various sources such as breast, lung, stomach, or from melanoma arising at a distant site. Melanoma is the most common tumor that metastasizes to the bladder.

TRAUMA OF THE BLADDER

Rupture of the bladder may result from a direct blow to a distended bladder as a single injury or may be associated with more extensive injury such as pelvic fracture, penetrating wounds, or gun-shot wounds. Instrumentation may also cause rupture of the bladder or urethra. Bladder rupture may be intra- or extra-perito-

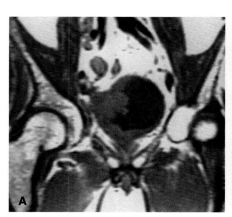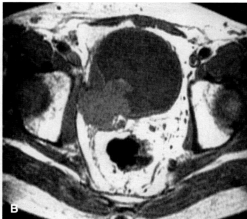

Figure 20–82. (A, B) Transitional cell carcinoma. Coronal and axial T1-weighted MRI demonstrates invasion of the tumor through the perivesical fat to the pelvic sidewall. (Courtesy of Patrick J. Fultz, MD, Rochester, NY.)

neal. Intraperitoneal rupture is more common in children because the bladder is mainly abdominal in location before maturity. Otherwise it is difficult to determine the incidence of intra- versus extraperitoneal rupture because the state of bladder distention is an uncontrollable variable affecting the type of injury and because all pelvic fractures are grouped together when the incidence of bladder injury is determined in many series.[132]

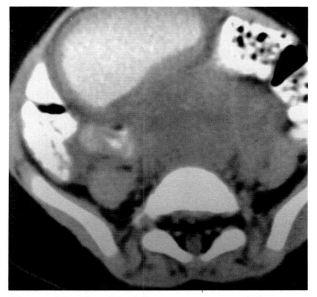

Figure 20–83. Rhabdomyosarcoma of the prostate. Large tumor mass displaces bladder anteriorly.

Retrograde cystography is the preferred imaging modality to evaluate for bladder rupture. Excretory urography is suboptimal because of dilution of the contrast and because small tears may not be demonstrated with the low resting intravesical pressure. Intraperitoneal rupture results in extravasation of contrast into the peritoneal cavity with outlining of the smooth outer walls of the pelvis and the lower abdominal and pelvic viscera. The actual site of rupture may not be visible on the roentgenogram because of overlapping shadows. Extraperitoneal bladder rupture is usually caused by blunt trauma associated with a fractured pelvis and produces a more varied pattern, depending on the site of rupture. The extravasated contrast outlines the tissue planes of the pelvic floor and extends varying distances into the perivesical soft tissues in an irregular, streaky manner. Computed tomography offers the advantage of summary assessment of all pelvic structures and spaces versus cystography (Fig. 20-84). Certain patients, such as those involved in motor vehicle accidents, will also require evaluation of the upper abdomen, and CT of the abdomen and pelvis can be quickly performed in one setting. At times, the differentiation between intraperitoneal and extraperitoneal rupture may be difficult. Rarely, spontaneous rupture of the bladder may occur, usually in patients with severe cystitis, extravesical infection, or malignant disease, or it may be due to overdistention secondary to mechanical obstruction or neurogenic dysfunction. Pelvic and lower abdominal trauma may also result in perivesical hematoma without rupture. Cystography or CT will then show displacement of the bladder, which varies with the size and location of the hematoma.

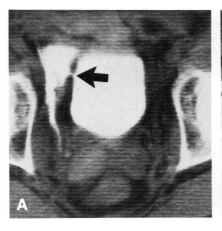 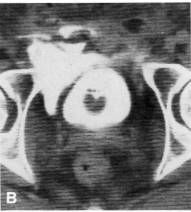

Figure 20–84. Extraperitoneal bladder rupture. (**A**) CT shows the site of bladder rupture (*arrow*) in the right bladder wall. (**B**) A more caudal slice shows the marked extravasation of contrast into the surrounding soft tissues.

FOREIGN BODIES

Foreign bodies in the bladder can be seen on plain-film roentgenograms when radiopaque. Oblique and lateral views may be necessary, however, to verify the position of the foreign body in relation to the bladder. Cystography will outline radiolucent foreign bodies and demonstrate associated changes in the bladder wall. Various oblique and lateral projections are usually necessary to ascertain the location. Ultrasonography is very useful in this situation. Cystoscopy is used for both diagnosis and treatment. A foreign body in the bladder is usually introduced by the patient and has a higher incidence in adults who have mental illness and in children. Occasionally, foreign bodies are introduced at the time of surgery or instrumentation, and they may also result from penetrating wounds. A foreign body may serve as a nidus for the deposition of calcium salts and the formation of a bladder calculus, as indicated previously.

HERNIA OF THE BLADDER

Bladder herniation is said to occur in 10% of all inguinal hernias in men over age 50, but large hernias with descent into the scrotum are unusual.[51] Herniation must be differentiated from diverticulum; this is usually accomplished on the basis of the hernia's location and the direction of its protrusion as well as its relatively wide mouth as compared with the diverticulum. Films with the patient in the erect and prone oblique positions are necessary to demonstrate these findings in most patients.

RETROGRADE URETHROGRAPHY

The retrograde urethrogram is the simplest radiographic method for examination of the urethra. It consists of retrograde injection of a radiopaque contrast into the urethra, after which films are exposed in various projections as the occasion demands. It is occasionally used in the female to demonstrate diverticula that may be missed at cystoscopy. In the male, diverticula, strictures, abscess cavities, fistulas, and prostatic abnormalities and enlargement may be delineated. Videotaping may be used in selected cases when fleeting deformities are expected.

Voiding Urethrography

The male urethra can be demonstrated following excretory urography by having the patient void against the partial obstruction produced by a Zipser penile clamp. Excretory urography is performed, and on completion the patient is asked to drink as much water as necessary to increase the urge to void. The scout film is obtained with the patient in a supine, 45°, posterior-oblique position. A Zipser penile clamp is placed at the base of the glans penis. The patient is then shown how to hold the clamp and asked to void. Voiding against a peripheral resistance slightly distends the urethra and aids in the evaluation of abnormalities involving it. Films are obtained with the patient in both oblique positions if possible. The advantages of this method of examination are the simplicity and ease with which it is carried out and the avoidance of instrumentation or catheterization. Voiding must be sufficient to permit an adequate flow of the urinary stream. Before urography is started, the patient should be asked to void so that the excreted contrast medium is not diluted unduly by residual urine in the bladder.

Seminal Vesiculography

Seminal vesiculography is a specialized urologic-radiologic method of examining the seminal vesicles. The technique and the normal seminal vesiculogram are described by Banner and Hassler.[7]

POSTERIOR URETHRAL VALVES

Posterior urethral valves produce varying degrees of obstruction leading to infection, vesicoureteral reflux, and hydronephrosis, with destruction of the kidneys unless corrected. Valves are found almost exclusively in males, most often in children. Enuresis is a common symptom. Other symptoms and signs are bladder distention, dribbling, a poor stream, and failure to thrive. In the newborn male, signs of flank mass caused by urinary ascites coupled with respiratory distress should suggest the diagnosis.[105] The valves are located in the vicinity of the verumontanum. Voiding cystourethrography is the roentgenograpic method used to demonstrate this lesion.

Roentgenographic findings of the most common type of valve consist of a thin membrane arising near the verumontanum and coursing anteriorly, laterally, and inferiorly. This partially obstructs the urethra during voiding. The posterior urethra must be filled in order to distend the valve; otherwise, it will not be visible. A true lateral projection is also necessary in order to identify the position of the valve. The valve stretches in sail-like fashion to obstruct the urethra. The valve itself may not be visible, but the dilatation of the prostatic urethra and a constricting ring at the vesical neck are characteristic. Rarely, anterior urethral valves may be present; obstruction with proximal dilatation similar to that in posterior valves may be present. The lucent defect of the anterior valve may be visualized on cystourethrography.

MISCELLANEOUS ANOMALIES OF THE URETHRA

Urethral Diverticula. In males some urethral diverticula are congenital, but most follow trauma or infection. The diverticula are visible on urethrography. In females most, if not all, are acquired; they usually result from retention in periurethral glands. Infection and calculi may complicate urethral diverticula. Voiding urethrography usually outlines these abnormalities in females, in whom retrograde urethrography is a difficult technique.

Other Urethral Diseases

Calculi. Calculi are almost always associated with diverticula and infection in females. In males calculi occur proximal to obstruction, often in the prostatic or bulbous urethra. If the area is included on the plain film, the diagnosis can usually be made radiographically.

Trauma. Trauma may result in complete or incomplete urethral rupture or in urethral laceration. Anterior urethral injuries (bulbous and cavernous urethra) are associated with direct blows or straddle injuries. Posterior urethral injuries (membranous and prostatic urethra) usually are due to pelvic fractures or trauma. Urethrography demonstrates the abnormality by showing extravasation of opaque medium. As a rule, when there is complete urethral rupture, no medium injected into the urethra reaches the bladder because of retraction of the ruptured ends of the urethra.

The anterior urethra can be examined despite placement of an indwelling Foley catheter. A small plastic feeding tube is gently inserted through the external meatus and its tip placed about halfway up the anterior urethra, beside the Foley catheter. With the glans compressed adequately, contrast injected gently via this accessory catheter can delineate urethral injuries.

Condyloma Acuminata. (Venereal Warts). Condyloma acuminata occasionally spread into the urethra. Radiographic findings consist of varying numbers of flat verrucous filling defects. Retrograde urethrography occasionally can be used in examining patients with this condition.

Urethral Strictures. Urethral strictures may be caused by infection or trauma and rarely represent a congenital anomaly in males. The site, severity, length, and associated sinus or fistulous tracts can be outlined on urethrography.

Urethral Tumors. Urethral tumors are more common in females than in males. Urethrography is difficult technically and not very successful in demonstrating tumors in females, but is useful in outlining the irregularity and intraluminal masses found in the male with urethral carcinoma. Rarely, polyps may occur in the prostatic urethra of boys and are demonstrated as small, rounded, or oval filling defects on urethrography.

VAS DEFERENS CALCIFICATION

Calcification of the vas deferens is occasionally present in diabetic men, but also occurs in nondiabetic, elderly, and hypercalcemic men. It probably represents a degenerative phenomenon in these patients. Roentgenographic findings are the presence of densely calcified, often bilaterally symmetrical, tubular shadows about 3 mm in diameter in the low midpelvis (Fig. 20-85), which have a distinctive appearance.

THE ADRENAL GLANDS

The right adrenal gland is cephalad and slightly medial to the upper pole of the right kidney. The right adrenal is also just posterior to the inferior vena cava, which serves as a good landmark on CT. The left adrenal

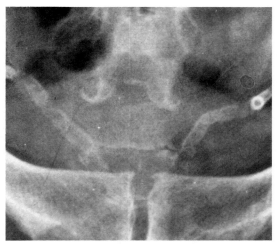

Figure 20–85. Calcification in the vas deferens of a 45-year-old man with a history of diabetes of more than 20 years' duration.

gland is also cephalad to the upper pole of the left kidney, but is located more medially relative to the aorta than the right adrenal (Fig. 20-86). The right adrenal has an inverted V shape, with its two limbs roughly paralleling the diaphragmatic crus. The left adrenal is usually wider and shorter and can have a variety of shapes, but may be shaped similarly to a seagull. The adrenals are small, the combined average weight being 11 to 12 g.

The most common cause of calcification in the adrenal is believed to be hemorrhage, often associated with

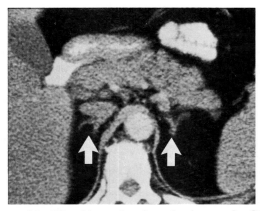

Figure 20–86. Normal adrenals (*arrows*). CT of right adrenal posterior to the inferior vena cava and left adrenal just lateral to the left diaphragmatic crus. The shape of the left adrenal can vary; this left adrenal has the "sea-gull" configuration.

hypoxia or birth trauma, severe maternal infection, hypoprothrombinemia, or increased vascular fragility. Calcification is often found in infants of diabetic mothers. There is a high incidence of abnormal obstetric history, including prematurity, use of forceps, and breech deliveries in children with adrenal calcification. Neonatal adrenal hemorrhage, which may be massive, unilateral, or bilateral, will be seen as a radiolucent suprarenal mass in the total body phase of excretory urography in neonates. Adrenal hemorrhage can have a variable appearance on ultrasonography, depending on when the hematoma is scanned. Acutely, the hematoma can appear echogenic, but as it liquefies it usually assumes a more anechoic or hypoechoic appearance.[103] Calcification occurs rapidly around the periphery a few weeks after the hemorrhage, then contracts slowly to the original size and shape of the gland. If the hemorrhage is unilateral, the right adrenal is more frequently involved. Stippled adrenal calcifications can be found in adults without any signs or symptoms of adrenal insufficiency. The cause in these cases remains obscure. Computed tomography or ultrasonography can document calcifications within the adrenal. Tuberculosis of the adrenal gland is now a rare cause of adrenal insufficiency. About one third of tuberculosis patients develop calcification within the adrenal. The calcification may appear as amorphous granular density within the gland or may entirely outline it.

Adrenal cysts may also contain calcium. Peripheral calcification is present in about 15% of cases. Peripheral calcification is suggestive of a cyst, whereas calcification within an adrenal mass is more suggestive of tumor. Adrenal cysts are rare, and they occur equally on the right and left sides. Their incidence is 50% higher in females than in males. Lymphangiectatic and pseudocysts are the most frequent types, although parasitic, epithelial, and those secondary to hemorrhage or necrosis are also found. These cysts are usually asymptomatic. Cyst puncture is advocated by some physicians in the diagnostic evaluation of adrenal masses, and the procedure can be done under CT or ultrasound guidance. Cysts that do not contain calcium may simulate a tumor on plain film, but are not visible on plain film unless they become large (Fig. 20-87). CT, ultrasonography, and MRI are all useful in the imaging of adrenal cysts.[36]

ADRENAL CORTICAL TUMORS

Adrenal tumors are divided according to their origin into cortical and medullary types. The cortical lesions are glandular in type and are mesodermal in origin. Benign adenoma and carcinoma are the two types that are found, and they can be either functioning or nonfunctioning. When these tumors result in a distur-

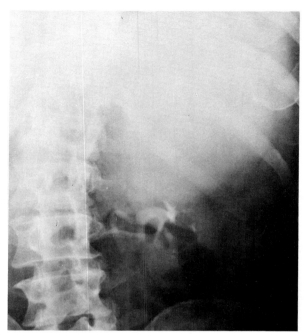

Figure 20–87. Cyst of the left adrenal gland. Note the large mass above and partly overlying the upper pole of the left kidney. The kidney is displaced downward, but is not deformed or distorted significantly.

bance of function, they can affect both cortical and medullary function. Hyperplasia of the adrenal cortex can also disturb cortical and medullary function. The symptoms are varied and may be caused by an excess of androgens, estrogens, adrenocorticotropic hormone, or other hormones. Sex changes and Cushing's syndrome may be present. In some patients no hormonal

disturbance is noted, but this is rare. About 75% of patients with Cushing's syndrome have hyperplastic adrenals and 25% have an adenoma or carcinoma. The hyperplastic gland is enlarged bilaterally and retains its normal shape, whereas tumors tend to be round or oval and produce an alteration in the contour of the adrenal gland (Fig. 20-88). Excretory urography was used in the past to localize suspected adrenal tumors. Computed tomographic scanning and ultrasonography are now the primary diagnostic methods. In one study of suspected adrenal disease, CT had a sensitivity of 84%, specificity of 98%, and accuracy of 90%.[1] Ultrasonography may be somewhat limited in the evaluation of patients with Cushing's syndrome because of the increased adipose tissue. More invasive procedures such as arteriography, venography, or venous sampling may be necessary if CT or ultrasonography cannot demonstrate the adrenal mass. Retroperitoneal pneumography is no longer used. The angiographic signs are similar to those of tumor elsewhere and consist of dilated and displaced vessels, tortuous vascular patterns, and arteriovenous shunts.

Primary aldosteronism or Conn's syndrome consists of hypertension, hypokalemia, hyperkaliuria, and low plasma renin. The renin production is suppressed by the excess aldosterone. Seventy to eighty percent of patients with Conn's syndrome have a unilateral adenoma, which is often less than 2 cm in diameter.[158] Nodular bilateral cortical hyperplasia accounts for most of the remaining patients. Because of the risks of angiographic procedures, CT is preferable for the initial imaging modality. Computed tomography can demonstrate the small adenoma causing the hyperaldosteronism. Venography and radionuclide techniques can also be used to detect these small adenomas. Scintiscanning with (^{131}I) 19-iodo-cholesterol has been used to demonstrate increased radioactivity in the abnormal

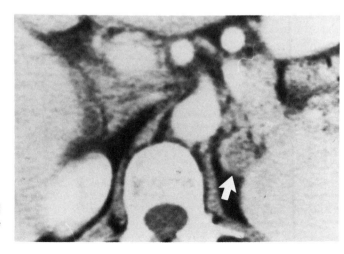

Figure 20–88. Cushing's syndrome. Enhanced CT of a left adrenal adenoma (*arrow*) medial to the spleen.

adrenal gland and to differentiate hyperplasia from cortical adenoma and adenocarcinoma.

Nonfunctioning cortical adenomas and carcinomas also appear as solid masses on CT. Adenomas are usually small (measuring less than 3 cm in diameter) and are unilateral. Because of high lipid content, adenomas often have density measurements that approach water (Fig. 20-89). Carcinomas are usually larger than adenomas and can be bilateral. Most nonfunctioning tumors large enough to produce symptoms are malignant.[36] Myelolipoma is a rare benign tumor of the adrenal gland. It is composed of fat, erythroid, and myeloid elements. If fat is found in an adrenal mass, the diagnosis of myelolipoma can be made with confidence (Fig. 20-90).

MRI can detect adrenal abnormalities with approximately the same sensitivity as CT. Currently, the most widespread use of MRI in adrenal imaging is to separate patients with adrenal metastases from those with nonhyperfunctioning adenomas. Because metastases to the adrenals and nonhyperfunctioning adenomas are both common, this can represent a significant clinical

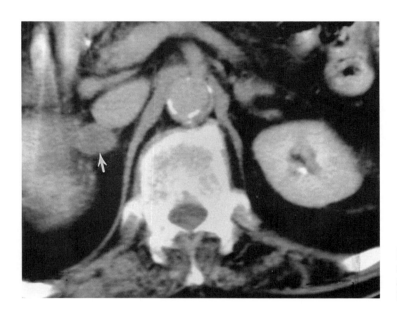

Figure 20–89. Nonhyperfunctioning adrenal adenoma. Incidentally found low-density adrenal adenoma (*arrow*). (Courtesy of Luke E. Sewall, MD, Madison, WI.)

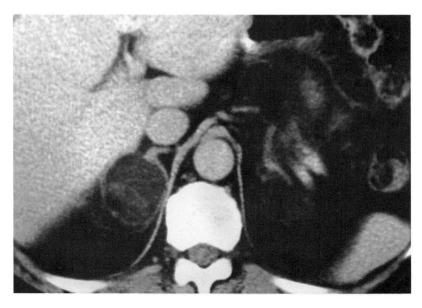

Figure 20–90. Adrenal myelolipoma. Large right adrenal tumor is composed primarily of fat. (Courtesy of Donald R. Yandow, MD, Madison, WI.)

problem. Recent work has shown that in contrast to adenomas, metastases appear brighter on T2-weighted images, enhance more quickly with contrast administration, and stay enhanced for longer periods. Unfortunately, approximately 30% of patients fall into an intermediate category and require biopsy for more definitive evaluation.[36, 50, 81]

ADRENAL MEDULLARY TUMORS

Adrenal medullary tumors are ectodermal in origin. They include ganglioneuroma, ganglioneuroblastoma, neuroblastoma, and pheochromocytoma. Pheochromocytoma clinically is characterized by hypertension (secretion of epinephrine and norepinephrine), which is paroxysmal in nature, with flushing, sweating, tachycardia, and anxiety. The diagnosis is usually made by measuring elevated levels of urine catecholamines. About 10% of pheochromocytomas are bilateral, 10% are extra-adrenal, and 10% are malignant. Pheochromocytomas are usually solitary and more commonly located in the right adrenal. Computed tomography is very accurate in locating pheochromocytomas. In one review study, CT demonstrated the tumor in 52 patients who initially presented and in 8 patients with evidence of recurrence.[156] These tumors are usually greater than 2 cm in size and may be solid or cystic. When the adrenal glands do not have evidence of tumor by CT, then the remainder of the abdomen and pelvis should be scanned. The retroperitoneum in the periaortic region and the organ of Zuckerkandl (located near the aortic bifurcation) are the most common location of pheochromocytomas outside of the adrenal. The neck and chest are other possible sites. Pheochromocytomas are associated with the multiple endocrine adenomatoses (both type I and type II).

MRI is also an effective way to localize suspected pheochromocytomas. CT should be used as the first method of imaging, but MRI can be valuable when the tumor is in an extra-adrenal location, or the patient has had previous retroperitoneal surgery.[36, 44]

Pheochromocytoma is usually a very vascular tumor with arteriovenous lakes and early venous filling. Because of the danger of a precipitous rise in blood pressure in patients with suspected pheochromocytoma, blood pressure and electrocardiogram are continuously monitored. Intravenous injection of iodinated contrast materials can precipitate a hypertensive crisis and should thus be avoided if possible. Phentolamine should be available for immediate intravenous injection if blood pressure rises suddenly. An injection of 5 mg phentolamine is usually sufficient to control the blood pressure, but repeated injections may be necessary in some patients. Angiography usually demonstrates a hypervascular mass with an intense capillary stain (Fig. 20-91). Less frequently, a hypovascular mass can be seen. Adrenal venography can also be used if arteriography is not successful. Ganglioneuroma, which is benign, usually causes no symptoms; the tumor is probably the differentiated form of neuroblastoma. Large ganglioneuromas may be visible on scout radiographs. If not, CT, MRI, venography, or angiography can be used for diagnosis.

NEUROBLASTOMA

Neuroblastoma, the most common malignancy in infants and children, is a tumor of adrenal medullary origin. About 30% of neuroblastomas are diagnosed in children under age 1, another 15% to 20% in children less than age 2, 25% in children between ages 2 and 5, and about 90% in those under age 8. The tumor may arise in cells of the sympathetic nervous system as well as in the adrenal medulla; this type of tumor may thus be found below as well as above the kidney. Neuroblastoma is highly malignant and can attain great size before discovery. Two thirds of children with neuroblastoma will have distant metastases (usually osseous) when they present. Calcification in the mass is common (about 40% to 50% on plain films and 85% on CT) (Fig. 20-92), whereas in Wilms' tumor, from which it must be differentiated, calcium is rare. The calcification has a fine granular or stippled appearance. Urography serves to indicate that the mass is extrarenal with the kidney typically being displaced laterally. The tumor may fill most of the abdomen. Computed tomography is more sensitive for detecting calcification, is superior to urography in defining extent of disease, can evaluate possible involvement of the inferior vena cava, and can be used to evaluate recurrent disease. Ultrasonography is an alternative imaging modality that can provide similar information in the evaluation of neuroblastoma (Fig. 20-93).

Metastases to the liver and lungs as well as bone are common. The osseous metastases are often very extensive and characteristic, being of mixed lytic-blastic character. Often there is extensive involvement of the calvarium with separation of the sutures. Because the tumor may revert to benign ganglioneuroma, spontaneously or during treatment, localization and treatment of the primary tumor are important.

OTHER ADRENAL TUMORS

Other adrenal tumors are rare. They arise in the adrenal stroma and include neuromas, fibromas, lipomas, neurofibromas, hemangiomas, myomas, sarcomas, lymphangiomas, myelolipomas, osteomas, and melanomas. Tumors metastatic from other areas are common in the adrenal glands and should be considered in

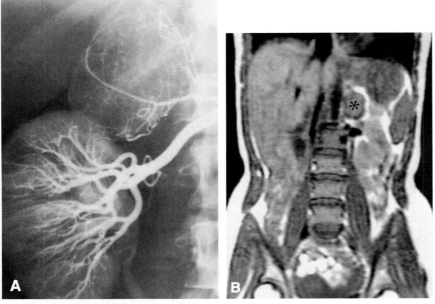

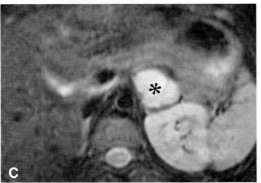

Figure 20–91. Pheochromocytoma. (**A**) Angiogram demonstrates hypervascularity typical of pheochromocytomas. (**B**) T1-weighted coronal MRI. Pheochromocytoma (*) in a separate patient in left adrenal gland. (**C**) T2-weighted axial image shows high signal typical of pheochromocytoma (*).

the differential diagnosis of every adrenal mass. Metastatic lung carcinoma is the most common; breast, colon, and thyroid cancer along with melanoma can also metastasize to the adrenals. Metastases are often bilateral.[36] Computed tomography is the preferred imaging modality for evaluation of adrenal metastases. The CT density is variable and can be solid or have low attenuation values (Fig. 20-94). In patients with adrenal masses in whom proof of metastatic disease will alter therapy, CT- or ultrasound-guided aspiration biopsy can be performed. Melanoma metastatic to the adrenals has been reported to cause curvilinear calcifications simulating those noted in benign adrenal cyst.[155]

MISCELLANEOUS ADRENAL CONDITIONS

Adrenal abscess is very rare but is a possible cause of adrenal enlargement in neonates. It must be differentiated from other adrenal masses such as hematoma and neuroblastoma. Total body opacification was used in the past, but CT or ultrasonography is now preferable in evaluating abscess. It may be difficult to distinguish abscess from hematoma from infected hematoma.

Adrenal milk of calcium is a rare occurrence in which a suspension of calcification, resembling the milk of calcium observed in the gall bladder, accumulates in an adrenal cyst.[107]

THE PROSTATE

Recent innovations in ultrasound and MRI technology have led to increased interest in imaging of the prostate gland. Clinical interest has remained high because of the large numbers of deaths from carcinoma of the prostate, estimated at 30,000 men in 1990. Several factors make diagnosis, screening, and treatment of this disease difficult.

Carcinoma of the prostate mostly affects older men.

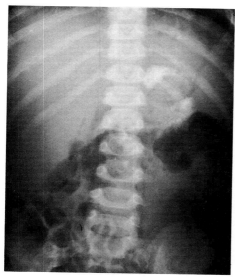

Figure 20–92. Neuroblastoma arising in the left adrenal gland. Note the mottled, somewhat granular calcification in the left upper abdomen, which is typical of the calcification observed in neuroblastoma.

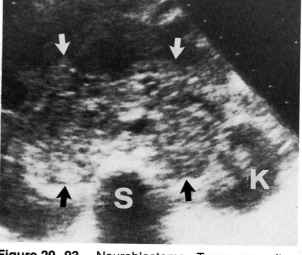

Figure 20–93. Neuroblastoma. Transverse ultrasound demonstrating the lateral displacement of the left kidney (*K*) by the solid retroperitoneal mantle of tumor (*arrows*). *S*, spine.

One autopsy series showed a prevalence of 30% in patients who die of unrelated causes. The question then arises, which patients have clinically significant tumors that will cause morbidity and mortality, and in which patients is the disease largely incidental? This question has not been completely resolved, although several authors believe that tumor volume predicts tumor behavior. Tumors 3 cc or larger are more likely to have extracapsular spread and aggressive histologic types. Thus, even though tumors may be multicentric in one patient, the largest tumor, or index cancer, will most likely have the most aggressive histologic changes, and will most closely predict tumor behavior.

A second confounding factor is the complexity of internal anatomy and the changes the aging prostate normally undergoes. The prostate can be divided into an inner gland (transition zone) and an outer gland (central and peripheral zone). The transition zone, which lies in a periurethral location, is the site of benign prostatic hyperplasia, which can occlude the urethra when severe. The peripheral and central zones lie posterior and lateral to the transition zone. The peripheral zone is the primary tumor site in up to 70% of patients, whereas the transition zone is the primary site in approximately 15%. Tumor is more likely to escape the gland into the seminal vesicles, through the capsule, or into the neurovascular bundles when located in the peripheral zone; therefore, this area needs to be closely scrutinized when imaging the prostate (Fig. 20-95).

Transrectal ultrasound of the prostate (Fig. 20-96) was introduced in the 1970s in Japan by Watanabe and others. Until 1985, it was largely believed that cancer arose centrally in the gland, and was hyperechoic or of mixed echnogenicity. During the late 1980s, whole-mount pathologic studies were performed, and it became clear that cancer was primarily hypoechoic (Fig. 20-97). In addition, most tumors originated in the peripheral zone, a finding similar to the pathologic literature. As tumors enlarged, the histology was more likely to become infiltrative, with tumor "fingers" extending into surrounding tissue. Because of this, echogenicity varied with increasing tumor size.

Transrectal ultrasounded–guided biopsy became widely available during the late 1980s. The combination formed a useful tool in the diagnosis and staging of prostate cancer. Biopsy could now be performed simply and easily in an outpatient setting, and strategically guided biopsies could occasionally prove extraprostatic spread. The positive predictive value for cancer when biopsy is performed of a hypoechoic nodule varies, with one report yielding 41%. This number is probably lower in an unselected population. Recently it has been shown that knowledge of the prostate-specific antigen (PSA) level may help select patients for biopsy.

The role of MRI in prostate cancer is unclear. Imaging of the internal architecture of the gland with body coil technology has been largely unsuccessful, and predicting local spread has had mixed results. Conventional MRI techniques are thus largely limited to

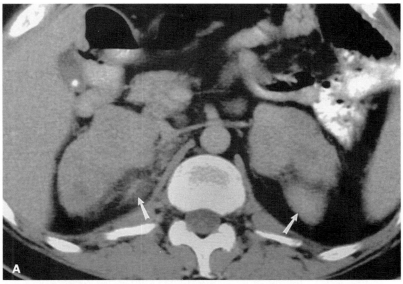

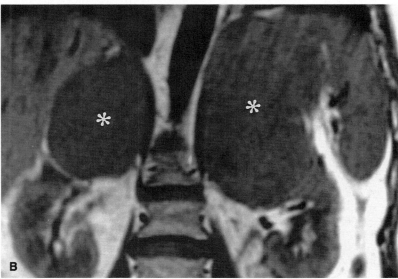

Figure 20–94. (**A**) Enhanced CT of bilateral adrenal metastases in a patient with bronchogenic cancer. Upper pole of kidneys (*arrows*) are separated from adrenal glands by a fat plane. (**B**) Coronal T1-weighted MRI of a patient with non-Hodgkin's lymphoma shows bilateral large adrenal masses (*).

detecting gross extraprostatic spread and detecting enlarged pelvic lymph nodes. Two recent technologic advances may prove fruitful in the diagnosing and staging of local disease: endorectal surface coils and phased array coils (Fig. 20-98 and 20-99). Early work has been encouraging, but more study is needed. CT is largely limited to detecting nodal enlargement in the pelvis and metastatic disease elsewhere. Computed tomography does not play a significant role in evaluating intraprostatic or early extraprostatic disease (Fig. 20-95).[12, 90, 91, 114, 129]

The issue of screening for prostate cancer remains controversial. The role of PSA, ultrasound, and MRI continues to evolve for this indication. Studies are currently under way to try and evaluate the best strategy for screening, or to decide if large-scale efforts are warranted.

THE SCROTUM

Scrotal contents include the testis, epididymis, and spermatic cord. The testicle is covered by a fibrous sheath called the tunica albuginea, and this in turn is surrounded by the tunica vaginalis. The epididymal head is superior to the testis, and the body and tail are

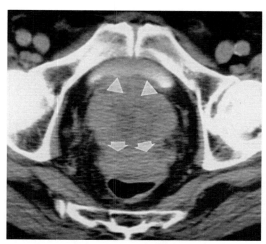

Figure 20–95. Prostate cancer. Enhanced CT scan demonstrates large prostate cancer with bladder (*arrowheads*) and rectal (*arrows*) invasion.

located posteriorly and inferiorly. The blood supply to the testicle derives from the spermatic cord, which contains the testicular artery.

The testicle is imaged using both ultrasound and nuclear medicine techniques.[12, 94, 97, 131] Ultrasound should be performed using a high-resolution, linear-array transducer. Doppler technology is also useful, particularly to assess for torsion or hyperemia associated with injury or infection. Nuclear medicine imaging requires the injection of an adult dosage of approximately 15 to 20 mCi of [99]mTc-pertechnetate intravenously. Flow and static images are performed with the penis taped up to the pelvis.

TESTICULAR TORSION

Testicular torsion usually presents with acute testicular pain in the newborn or adolescent male. The process is caused by a twisting of the spermatic cord, compromising venous and then arterial flow. Diagnosis needs to be made promptly, usually within 6 hours, to assure testicular viability. Nuclear medicine imaging with [99]mTc-pertechnetate has been the traditional imaging method to diagnose testicular torsion. Acutely, decreased flow is seen in the expected position of the testis. If the condition remains untreated for more than 24 hours, a rim of increased activity with a photopenic central area may develop, the so-called halo sign. This sign of delayed torsion can also be seen with testicular abscess, hematoma, or tumor. Recently, Doppler ultrasound has become more widely used to diagnose torsion. Acquisition of an arterial signal from the central portion of the testicle effectively excludes torsion. Before making this diagnosis, it is important to confirm that normal flow is seen in the contralateral testis. This will confirm that the Doppler instrument has sufficient sensitivity to document slow flow for small vessels and that imaging parameters are set correctly. Ultrasound has the advantage over nuclear medicine of being able to image the remainder of the scrotum. Often, if testicular torsion is excluded, ultrasound is able to suggest the proper diagnosis.

EPIDIDYMITIS

Infection of the epididymis is often associated with infection of other portions of the genitourinary tract. The main importance of this condition is differentiating it from testicular torsion, which is a surgical emergency.

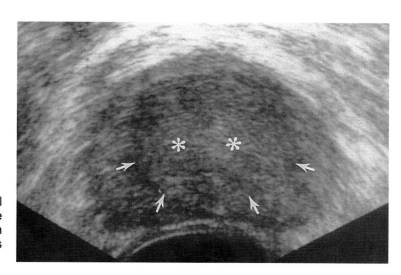

Figure 20–96. Normal axial transrectal ultrasound of the prostate. Transition zone (*) is prominent in this patient with benign prostatic hypertrophy. Peripheral zone is external to surgical capsule (*arrows*).

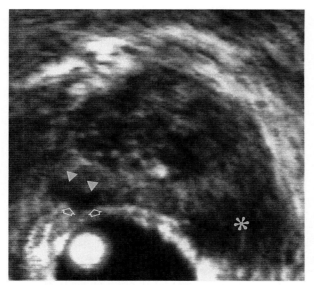

Figure 20–97. Prostate cancer. Axial transrectal ultrasound shows large hypoechoic tumor mass (*) extending into periprostatic tissues. A second small lesion (*arrowheads*) is present on contralateral side of the gland. Note peripheral location and deformity of prostatic capsule (*open arrows*).

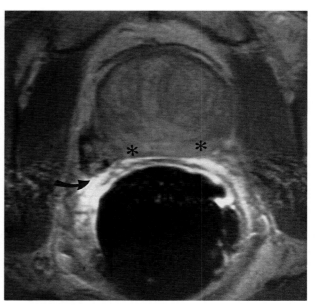

Figure 20–99. Carcinoma of the prostate. Stage C. Endorectal surface coil, MRI. T2-weighted image. TR, 3,000 ms; TE, 90 ms. The tumor involves the entire peripheral zone (*), which normally should be high-signal intensity. On the right side, at the 7-o'clock position, the tumor has extended beyond the capsule to involve the neurovascular bundle (*curved arrow*). (Courtesy of Howard M. Pollock, MD, Philadelphia, PA.)

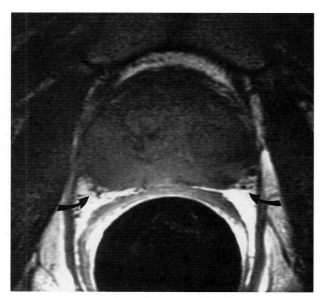

Figure 20–98. Sixty-eight-year-old man. Normal prostate gland, Endorectal surface coil MRI. T1-weighted image. TR, 600 ms; TE, 15 ms. The neurovascular bundles can be seen on each side (*curved arrows*). (Courtesy of Howard M. Pollock, MD, Philadelphia, PA.)

Nuclear medicine imaging in epididymitis reveals increased blood flow to the affected side. No photopenic areas are encountered. Ultrasound shows an enlarged heterogeneous-appearing epididymis with increased flow by Doppler. If orchitis is also present, the testicle is usually swollen, hypoechoic, and hyperemic.

TESTICULAR TUMORS

The main job of the radiologist in evaluating a painless scrotal mass is to decide whether it arises from within the testicle or elsewhere. Testicular abnormalities need to be viewed with a great deal of suspicion, and should be considered tumors until proved otherwise. Testicular tumors are the most common neoplasm in men aged 25 to 35. Malignant testicular tumors may be seminomas, choriocarcinomas, embryonal carcinomas, or teratomas/teratocarcinomas (Fig. 20-100). Other tumors that can affect the testicles include lymphoma, leukemia, and metastases. In general, tumors are hypoechoic to normal testicle, and seminoma is relatively homogeneous in appearance. Predicting the tumor cell

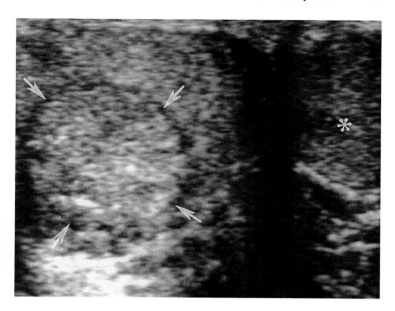

Figure 20–100. Nonseminomatous testicular tumor. Transverse ultrasound demonstrates heterogeneous, centrally placed testicular mass (*arrows*). Comparison with uninvolved testis (*) shows size difference in testicles. (Courtesy of Kathleen Scanlan, MD, Madison, WI.)

type by ultrasound findings has not proved accurate, however. If a testicular tumor is found, the retroperitoneum should be examined, usually with CT, for nodal spread. Involved lymph nodes are initially found at the sites of lymphatic drainage. Tumors from the right testis spread to nodes in the preaortic, precaval, and aortocaval areas. Tumors on the left drain to left para-aortic nodes. Trauma to the scrotum, in particular testicular hematomas, can mimic testicular tumors. It is important to follow cases of suspected hematoma, which should undergo evolution and regress. Tumors will stay stable or enlarge over time.

HYDROCELE

Hydroceles represent fluid collections between layers of the tunica vaginalis. They are often idiopathic, but can be seen with almost any scrotal or testicular pathology including trauma, infection, or tumors.

VARICOCELE

Varicoceles are an abnormal collection of dilated veins of the spermatic cord. They are caused by an abnormal venous valvular mechanism or obstruction to blood return from the testis. The junction of the right spermatic vein and the inferior vena cava form a valvelike mechanism owing to the acute angle of incidence. The left spermatic vein joins the left renal vein at a more obtuse angle, and thus is subject to increased retrograde venous pressure. Therefore, 90% of the idiopathic variety of varicoceles arise on the left. Var-

icoceles may also be found in association with venous obstruction secondary to tumor mass or other retroperitoneal process. If a patient presents with bilateral or unilateral right hydroceles, a search of the retroperitoneum for a causative factor is strongly recommended.

Varicoceles present as dilated vascular structures near the upper pole of the testis. The Valsalva maneuver or scanning the patient upright will cause an increase in size. Varicoceles may be a cause of male infertility because of increased scrotal temperature, and they are amenable to surgical repair, or they can be thrombosed by percutaneous transcatheter placement of coils in the spermatic vein. In this approach, the spermatic vein is accessed by passing a catheter through the left renal vein.

SPERMATOCELE

These are dilatations of efferent ductules, usually found in the head of the epididymis. They are generally asymptomatic and should be differentiated from varicoceles.

REFERENCES AND SELECTED READINGS

1. ABRAMS HL, SIEGELMAN SS, ADAMS DF, ET AL: Computed tomography versus ultrasound of the adrenal gland: A prospective study. Radiology 143:121, 1982
2. ALBERTSON KW, TALNER LW: Valves of the ureter. Radiology 103:91, 1972

3. AMIS ES JR: Retroperitoneal fibrosis. Am J Roentgenol 157:321, 1991

4. AMIS ES JR, HARTMAN DS: Renal ultrasonography 1984: A practical overview. Radiol Clin North Am 22:315, 1984

5. ANSELL G, TWEEDIE MCH, WEST CR: The current status of reactions to intravenous contrast media. Invest Radiol 15:S32, 1980

6. ARRIVE L, HRICAK H, TAVARES NJ, ET AL: Malignant vs. non-malignant retroperitoneal fibrosis: Differentiation with MR imaging. Radiology 172:139, 1989

7. BANNER MP, HASSLER R: The normal seminal vesiculo-gram. Radiology 128:339, 1978

8. BANNER MP, POLLACK HM: Fluoroscopically guided percutaneous extraction of upper urinary tract calculi. Radiol Clin North Am 22:415, 1984

9. BANNER MP, POLLACK HM, CHATTEN J, ET AL: Multi-locular renal cysts: Radiologic-pathologic correction. Am J Roentgenol 136:239, 1981

10. BARON RL, MCCLENNAN BL, LEE JKT, ET AL: Computed tomography of transitional-cell carcinoma of the renal pelvis and ureter. Radiology 144:125, 1982

11. BATSON PG, KEATS TE: The roentgenographic determination of normal adult kidney size as related to vertebral heights. Am J Roentgenol 116:737, 1972

12. BENSON CB, DOUBILET PM, RICHIE JP: Sonography of the male genital tract. Am J Roentgenol 153:705, 1989

13. BERDON WE, BAKER DH: The significance of a distended bladder in the interpretation of intravenous pyelograms obtained on patients with "hydronephrosis." Am J Roentgenol 120:402, 1974

14. BERLAND LL, KOSLIN DB, ROUTH WD: Renal artery stenosis: Prospective evaluation of diagnosis with color duplex ultrasound compared with angiography. Radiology 174:421, 1990

15. BINDER R, KOROBKIN M, CLARK RE, ET AL: Aberrant papillae and other filling defects of the renal pelvis. Am J Roentgenol 114:746, 1972

16. BLYTH H, OCKENDON BG: Polycystic disease of kidneys and liver presenting in childhood. J Med Genet 8:257, 1971

17. BOOKSTEIN JJ, WALTER JF, STANLEY JC, ET AL: Pharmacoangiographic manipulation of renal collateral blood flow. Circulation 54:328, 1976

18. BOSNIAK MA: Angiomyolipoma (Hamartoma) of the kidney: A preoperative diagnosis is possible in virtually every case. Urol Radiol 3:135, 1981

19. BOZNIAK MA, AMBOS MA, MADAYAG MA, ET AL: Epinephrine-enhanced renal angiography in renal mass lesions: Is it worth performing? Am J Roentgenol 129:647, 1977

20. BREATNACH E, STANLEY RJ, CARPENTER JT JR: Intrarenal chloroma causing obstructive nephropathy: CT characteristics. J Comput Assist Tomogr 9:822, 1985

21. BUY JB, MOSS AA, GUINET C, ET AL: MR staging of bladder carcinoma: Correlation with pathologic findings. Radiology 169:695, 1988

22. CHEN CC, HOFFER PB, VAHJEN G, ET AL: Patients at high risk for renal artery stenosis: A simple method of renal scintigraphic analysis with Tc-99m-DTPA and captopril. Radiology 176:365, 1990

23. CHO KJ, THORNBURY JR: Severe reactions to contrast material by three consecutive routes: Intravenous, subcutaneous, and intra-arterial. Am J Roentgenol 131:509, 1978

24. CLARK RE, MINAGI H, PALUBINSKAS AJ: Renal candidiasis. Radiology 101:567, 1971

25. COHEN RH, DUNNICK NR, BASHORE TM: Treatment of reactions to radiographic contrast material. Am J Roentgenol 151:263, 1988

26. COLEMAN BG, ARGER PH, MULBERN CB JR, ET AL: Gray-scale sonographic spectrum of hypernephromas. Radiology 137:757, 1980

27. COUREY WR, PFISTER RC: The radiographic findings in renal tubular acidosis. Radiology 105:497, 1972

28. CULP OS: Ureteral diverticulum: Classification of the literature and report of an authentic case. J Urol 58:309, 1947

29. DANN RH, ARGER PH, ENTERLINE HT: Benign proliferation processes presenting as mass lesions in the urinary bladder. Am J Roentgenol 116:822, 1972

30. DAUGHTRIDGE TG: Segmental, multicystic renal dysplasia. J Can Assoc Radiol 26:149, 1975

31. DAVIDSON AJ: Radiology of the kidney, 2nd ed. Philadelphia, WB Saunders, 1985

32. DAVIDSON AJ, TALNER LB: Urographic and angiographic abnormalities of adult-onset bacterial nephritis. Radiology 106:249, 1973

33. DEBATIN JF, SPRITZER CE, GRIST TM: Imaging of the renal arteries: Value of MR angiography. Am J Roentgenol 157:981, 1991

34. DIAMENT MJ, KANGARLOO H: Dosage schedule for pediatric urography based on body surface area. Am J Roentgenol 140:815, 1983

35. DON S, KOPECKY KK, FILO RS, ET AL: Duplex Doppler ultrasound of renal allografts: Causes of elevated resistive index. Radiology 171:709, 1989

36. DUNNICK NR: Adrenal imaging: Current status. Am J Roentgenol 154:927, 1990

37. DUNNICK NR, KOROBKIN M: Computed tomography of the kidney. Radiol Clin North Am 22:297, 1984

38. DURE-SMITH P: Pregnancy dilatation of the urinary tract. Radiology 96:545, 1970

39. ELKIN M: Radiology of the urinary system, 1st ed. Boston, Little, Brown & Co, 1980

40. ELKIN M: Renal cystic disease—an overview. Semin Roentgenol 10:99, 1975

41. ELKIN M, BERNSTEIN J: Cystic diseases of the kidney—radiological and pathological considerations. Clin Radiol 20:65, 1969

42. FEDERLE MP, KAISER JA, MCANINCH JW, ET AL: The role of computed tomography in renal trauma. Radiology 141:455, 1981

43. FEIN AB, LEE JKT, BALFE DM, ET AL: Diagnosis and staging of renal cell carcinoma: A comparison of MR imaging and CT. Am J Roentgenol 148:749, 1987

44. FINK IJ, REINIG JW, DWYER AJ, ET AL: MR imaging of pheochromocytomas. J Comput Assist Tomogr 9:454, 1985

45. FISCHER HW, DOUST VL: An evaluation of pretesting in the problem of serious and fatal reactions to excretory urography. Radiology 103:497, 1972

46. FISCHER HW, SPATARO FR, ROSENBERG PM: Medical and economic considerations in using a new contrast medium. Arch Intern Med 146:1717, 1986

47. FRYBACK DG, THORNBURY JR: Informal use of decision theory to improve radiological patient management. Radiology 129:385, 1978

48. GEISINGER MA, RISIUS B, JORDAN ML, ET AL: Magnetic resonance imaging of renal transplants. Am J Roentgenol 143:1229, 1984

49. GIFFORD RW JR: Epidemiology and clinical manifestations of renovascular hypertension. In Stanley JC, Ernst CB, Fry WJ (eds): Renovascular hypertension. Philadelphia, WB Saunders, 1984, pp 77–99

50. GLAZER GM: MR imaging of the liver, kidneys and adrenal glands. Radiology 166:303, 1989

51. GOLDIN RR, ROSEN RA: Effect of inguinal hernias upon the bladder and ureters. Radiology 115:55, 1975

52. GOLDMAN SM, HARTMAN DS, FISHMAN EK, ET AL: CT of xanthogranulomatous pyelonephritis: Radiologic-pathologic correlation. Am J Roentgenol 142:963, 1984

53. GOLDSTEIN HM, MEDELLIN H, BEYDOUN MT, ET AL: Transcatheter embolization of renal cell carcinoma. Am J Roentgenol 123:557, 1975

54. GRISCOM NT, COLODNY AH, ROSENBERG KH, ET AL: Diagnostic aspects of neonatal ascites: Report of 27 cases. Am J Roentgenol 128:961, 1977

55. GRISCOM NT, VAWTER GF, FELLERS FX: Pelvoinfundibular atresia: The usual form of multicystic kidney: 44 unilateral and two bilateral cases. Semin Roentgenol 10:125, 1975

56. GRIST TM, CHARLES HC, SOSTMAN HD: Renal transplant rejection: Diagnosis with ^{31}P MR spectroscopy. Am J Roentgenol 156:105, 1991

57. HARTMAN DS, FRIEDMAN AC, DACHMAN A, ET AL: CT of renal cystic disease. In Siegelman SS, Gatewood OMB, Goldman SM (eds): Computed tomography of the kidneys and adrenals, vol 3. New York, Churchill Livingstone, 1984

58. HARTMAN DS, GOLDMAN SM, FRIEDMAN AC, ET AL: Angiomyolipoma: Ultrasonic-pathologic correlation. Radiology 139:451, 1981

59. HARTMAN GW, HODSON CJ: The duplex kidney and related abnormalities. Clin Radiol 20:387, 1969

60. HEALY ME, TENG SS, MOSS AA: Uriniferous pseudocyst: Computed tomographic findings. Radiology 153:757, 1984

61. HEIBERG E, WOLVERSON MK, SUNDARAM M, ET AL: CT findings in leukemia. Am J Roentgenol 143:1317, 1984

62. HILLMAN BJ: Digital imaging of the kidney. Radiol Clin North Am 22:341, 1984

63. HODDICK W, JEFFREY RB, GOLDBERG HI, ET AL: CT and sonography of severe renal and perirenal infections. Am J Roentgenol 140:517, 1983

64. HODSON CJ: Reflux Nephropathy: A personal historical review. Am J Roentgenol 137:451, 1981

65. HODSON J: The radiological contribution toward the diagnosis of chronic pyelonephritis. Radiology 88:857, 1967

66. HOFFMAN EP, MINDELZUN RE, ANDERSON RU: Computed tomography in acute pyelonephritis associated with diabetes. Radiology 135:691, 1980

67. HOWARD TL: Giant polyp of ureter. J Urol 79:397, 1958

68. HRICAK H, DEMAS BE, WILLIAMS RD, ET AL: Magnetic resonance imaging in the diagnosis and staging of renal and perirenal neoplasms. Radiology 154:709, 1985

69. HUSBAND JES, OLLIFF JFC, WILLIAMS MP, ET AL: Bladder cancer: Staging with CT and MR imaging. Radiology 173:435, 1989

70. HYDE I, WASTIE ML: Striations (longitudinal mucosal folds) in the upper urinary tract. Br J Radiol 44:445, 1971

71. JACOBSSON BF, JORULF H, KALANTAR MS: Nonionic versus ionic contrast media in intravenous urography: Clinical trial in 1,000 consecutive patients. Radiology 167:601, 1988

72. JAFRI SZH, BREE RL, AMENDOLA MA, ET AL: CT of renal and perirenal non-Hodgkin lymphoma. Am J Roentgenol 138:1101, 1982

73. JEFFREY RB: Computed tomography of lymphovascular structures and retroperitoneal soft tissues. In Moss AA, Gamsu G, Genant H (eds): Computed tomography of the body, 1st ed. Philadelphia, WB Saunders, 1983

74. KAMHOLTZ RG, CRONAN JJ, DORFMAN GS: Obstruction and the minimally dilated renal collecting system: US evaluation. Radiology 170:51, 1989

75. KATAYAMA H, YAMAGUCHI K, KOZUKA T, TAKASHIMA T, SEEZ P, MATSUURA K: Adverse reactions to ionic and nonionic contrast media: A report from the Japanese committee on the safety of contrast media. Radiology 175:621, 1990

76. KIM DS, EDELMAN RR, KENT KC: Abdominal aorta and renal artery stenosis: Evaluation with MR angiography. Radiology 174:727, 1990

77. KIRCHNER PT, ROSENTHALL L: Renal transplant evaluation. Semin Nucl Med 12:370, 1982

78. KISSANE JM: Congenital malformations. In Hepinstall RH (ed): Pathology of the kidney, vol 1, 2nd ed. Boston, Little, Brown & Co, 1974, pp 69–119

79. KOEP L, ZUIDEMA GD: The clinical significance of retroperitoneal fibrosis: Surgery 81:250, 1977

80. KOROBKIN M, PERLOFF DK, PALUBINSKAS AJ: Renal arteriography in the evaluation of unexplained hypertension in children and adolescents. J Pediatr 88:388, 1976

81. KRESTIN GP, STEINBRICH W, FRIEDMANN G: Adrenal masses: Evaluation with fat gradient-echo MR imaging

and Gd-DTPA enhanced dynamic studies. Radiology 171:675, 1989

82. KUHNS LR, HERNANDEZ R, KOFF S, ET AL: Absence of vesico-ureteral reflux in children with ureteral jets. Radiology 124:185, 1977

83. KUNIN M: Bridging septa of the perinephric space: Anatomic, pathologic, and diagnostic considerations. Radiology 158:361, 1986

84. KWOK-LIU JP, ZIKMAN JM, COCKSHOTT WP: Carcinoma of the urachus: Role of computed tomography. Radiology 137:731, 1980

85. LALLI AF: Renal enlargement. Radiology 84:688, 1965

86. LALLI AF: Urographic contrast media reactions and anxiety. Radiology 112:267, 1974

87. LALMAND B, AVNI EF, NASR A: Perinatal renal vein thrombosis. J Ultrasound Med 9:437, 1990

88. LANG EK, SULLIVAN J, FRENTZ G: Renal trauma: Radiological studies: Comparison of urography, computed tomography, angiography, and radionuclide studies. Radiology 154:1, 1984

89. LASSER EC: Pretreatment with corticosteroids to prevent reactions to IV contrast material: Overview and implications. Am J Roentgenol 150:257, 1988

90. LEE F, LITTRUP PJ, LOFT-CHRISTENSEN L: Predicted prostate specific antigen results using transrectal ultrasound gland volume: Differentiation of benign prostatic hyperplasia and prostate cancer. Cancer 1992

91. LEE F, TORP-PEDERSEN ST, SIDERS DB, ET AL: Transrectal ultrasound in the diagnosis and staging of prostatic carcinoma: State of the art. Radiology 170:609, 1989

92. LEE KT, DEETHS TM: Localized amyloidosis of the ureter. Radiology 120:60, 1976

93. LEONIDEAS JC, MCCAULEY RG, KLAUBER GC: Sonography as a substitute for excretory urography in children with urinary tract infection. Am J Roentgenol 144:815, 1985

94. LERNER RM, MEVORACH RA, HULBERT WC, ET AL: Color Doppler US in the evaluation of scrotal disease. Radiology 176:355, 1990

95. LIPUMA JP: Magnetic resonance imaging of the kidney. Radiol Clin North Am 22:925, 1984

96. LOWE RE, COHN MD: Computed tomographic evaluation of Wilms tumor and neuroblastoma. Radiographics 4:915, 1984

97. LUTZKER LG, ZUCKIER LS: Testicular scanning and other applications of radionuclide imaging of the genital tract. Semin Nucl Med 20:159, 1990

98. MCCLENNAN BL, STANLEY RJ, MELSON GL, ET AL: CT of the renal cyst: Is cyst aspiration necessary? Am J Roentgenol 133:671, 1979

99. MCCLENNAN BL, STOLBERG HO: Intravascular contrast media: Ionic versus nonionic: Current status. Radiol Clin North Am 29:437, 1991

100. MENA E, BOOKSTEIN JJ, MCDONALD FD, ET AL: Angiographic findings in renal medullary cystic disease. Radiology 110:277, 1974

101. MENG C-H, ELKIN M: Venous impressions on the calyceal system. Radiology 87:878, 1966

102. MILLER SS, WINSTON MC: Nephrogenic diabetes insipidus. Radiology 87:893, 1966

103. MINEAU DE, KOEHLER PR: Ultrasound diagnosis of neonatal adrenal hemorrhage. Am J Roentgenol 132:443, 1979

104. MITNICK JS, BOSNIAK MA, ROTHBERG M, ET AL: Metastatic neoplasm to the kidney studied by computed tomography and sonography. J Comput Assist Tomogr 9:43, 1985

105. MOONEY JK, BERDON WE, LATTIMER JK: A new dimension in the diagnosis of posterior urethral valves in children. J Urol 113:272, 1975

106. MOORE RD, STEINBERG EP, POWE NR: Frequency and determinants of adverse reactions induced by high-osmolarity contrast media. Radiology 170:727, 732, 1989

107. MOSS AA: Milk of calcium of the adrenal gland. Br J Radiol 49:186, 1976

108. MULLIGAN SA, HOLLEY HC, KOEHLER RE, ET AL: CT and MR imaging in the evaluation of retroperitoneal fibrosis. J Comput Assist Tomogr 13:277, 1989

109. MUNDTH ED, SHINE K, AUSTEN WG: Correction of malignant hypertension and return of renal function following late renal artery embolectomy. Am J Med 46:985, 1969

110. MURRAY RL: Milk of calcium in the kidney: Diagnostic features on vertical beam roentgenograms. Am J Roentgenol 113:455, 1971

111. NEBESAR RA, POLLARD JJ, FRALEY EE: Renal vascular impressions: Incidence and clinical significance. Am J Roentgenol 101:719, 1967

112. NEEDLEMAN L, KURTZ AB: Doppler evaluation of the renal transplant. J Clin Ultrasound 15:661, 1987

113. NEIFELD JP, WALSH JW, LAWRENCE W JR: Computed tomography in the management of soft tissue tumors. Surg Gynecol Obstet 155:535, 1982

114. NEWHOUSE JH: Clinical use of urinary tract magnetic resonance imaging. Radiol Clin North Am 29:455, 1991

115. OSATHANONDH V, POTTER EL: Pathogenesis of polycystic kidneys: Type III due to multiple abnormalities of development. Arch Pathol 77:485, 1964

116. PALMER FJ: Renal cortical calcification. Clin Radiol 21:175, 1970

117. PALUBINSKAS AJ: Renal pyramidal structure opacification in excretory urography and its relation to medullary sponge kidney. Radiology 81:963, 1963

118. PEAKE SL, ROXBURGH HB, LANGLOIS SLP: Ultrasonic assessment of hydronephrosis of pregnancy. Radiology 146:167, 1983

119. PFISTER RC, MCLAUGHLIN AP III, LEADBETTER WF: Radiological evaluation of primary megaloureter. Radiology 99:503, 1971

120. PFISTER RC, NEWHOUSE JH: Interventional percutaneous pyeloureteral techniques: I and II. Radiol Clin North Am 17:341, 1979

121. PLATT JF, RUBIN JM, BOWERMAN RA, ET AL: The inability to detect kidney disease on the basis of echogenicity. Am J Roentgenol 151:317, 1988

122. POLLACK HM, ARGER PH, BANNER MP, ET AL: Computed tomography of renal pelvis filling defects. Radiology 138:645, 1981

123. POLLACK HM, BANNER MP, ARGER PH: The accuracy of gray-scale renal ultrasonography in differentiating cystic neoplasms from benign cysts. Radiology 143:741, 1982

124. POYNTER JD, HARE WSC: Necrosis in situ: A form of renal papillary necrosis seen in analgesic nephropathy. Radiology 111:69, 1974

125. POZNIAK MA, KELCZ F, D'ALESSANDRO A, ET AL: Sonography of renal transplants in dogs: The effect of acute tubular necrosis, cyclosporine nephrotoxicity, and acute rejection on resistive index and renal length. Am J Roentgenol 158:791, 1992

126. POZNIAK MA, KELCZ F, STRATTA RJ, ET AL: Extraneous factors affecting resistive index. Invest Radiol 169:367, 1988

127. RESNICK MI, SANDERS RC: Ultrasound in urology, 2nd ed. Baltimore/London, Williams & Wilkins, 1984

128. REYNOLDS L, FULTON H, SNIDER JJ: Roentgen analysis of renal mass lesions (cysts and tumors). Am J Roentgenol 82:840, 1959

129. RIFKIN MD, McGLYNN ET, CHOI H: Echogenicity of prostate cancer correlated with histologic grade and stromal fibrosis: Endorectal US studies. Radiology 170:549, 1989

130. RIFKIN MD, NEEDLEMAN L, PASTO ME, ET AL: Evaluation of renal transplant rejection by duplex Doppler examination: Value of the resistive index. Am J Roentgenol 148:759, 1987

131. RUZAL-SHAPIRO C, NEWHOUSE JH: Imaging of scrotal contents, in Taveras JM, Ferrucci JT (eds): Radiology—diagnosis, imaging, intervention, vol 4. Philadelphia, JB Lippincott, 1988, pp 1–10, 134

132. SANDLER CM, PHILLIPS JM, HARRIS JD, ET AL: Radiology of the bladder and urethra in blunt pelvic trauma. Radiol Clin North Am 19:195, 1981

133. SANDLER CM, TOOMBS BD: Computed tomographic evaluation of blunt renal injuries. Radiology 141:461, 1981

134. SARTI DA,: Diagnostic ultrasound text and cases, 2nd ed. Chicago. Year Book Medical Publishers, 1987

135. SCOTT WW, McDONALD DF: Tumors of the ureter. In Campbell MF, Harrison JH (eds): Urology, vol 2, 3rd ed. Philadelphia, WB Saunders, 1970, pp 977–1002.

136. SEGAL AJ, SPATARO FR, LINKE CA, ET AL: Diagnosis of nonopaque calculi by computed tomography. Radiology 129:447, 1978

137. SEMELKA RC, SHOENUT JP, KROEKER MA, ET AL: Renal lesions: Controlled comparison between CT and 1.5-T MR imaging with nonenhanced and gadolinium-enhanced fat-suppressed spin-echo and breath hold FLASH techniques. Radiology 182:425, 1992

138. SNIDER JF, HUNTER DW, MORADIAN GA, ET AL: Transplant renal artery stenosis: Evaluation with duplex sonography. Radiology 172:1027, 1989

139. SPATARO RF: Newer contrast agents for urography. Radiol Clin North Am 22:365, 1984

140. STANLEY JC, FRY WJ: Pediatric renal artery occlusive disease and renovascular hypertension: Etiology, diagnosis and operative treatment. Arch Surg 116:669, 1981

141. STANLEY JC, RHODES EL, GEWERTZ BL, ET AL: Renal artery aneurysms: Significance of macroaneurysms exclusive of dissections and fibrodysplasic mural dilations. Arch Surg 110:1327, 1975

142. SUBRAMANYAM BR, BOSNIAK MA, HORII SC, ET AL: Replacement lipomatosis of the kidney: Diagnosis by computed tomography and sonography. Radiology 148:791, 1983

143. TALNER LB: Urographic contrast media in uremia? Physiology and pharmacology. Radiol Clin North Am 10:421, 1972

144. TALNER LB, GITTIS RF: Megacalyces. Clin Radiol 23:355, 1972

145. TAYLOR A JR, ZIFFER JA, ESHIMA D: Comparison of Tc-99m-MAG$_3$ and Tc-99m-DTPA in renal transplant patients with impaired renal function. Clin Nucl Med 15:371, 1990

146. TAYLOR KJW, MORSE SS, RIGSBY CM, ET AL: Vascular complications in renal allografts: Detection with duplex Doppler ultrasound. Radiology 162:31, 1987

147. THORNBURY JR: Acute renal infections. Urol Radiol 12:209, 1991

148. THORNBURY JR: The roentgen diagnosis of ureterocele in children. Am J Roentgenol 90:15, 1963

149. THORNBURY JR, McCORMICK TL, SILVER TM: Anatomic/radiologic classification of renal cortical nodules. Am J Roentgenol 134:1, 1980

150. THORNBURY JR, PARKER TW: Ureteral calculi. Semin Roentgenol 17:133, 1982

151. THORNBURY JR, SILVER TM, VINSON RK: Ureteroceles vs pseudoureteroceles in adults. Radiology 122:81, 1977

152. THORNBURY JR, STANLEY JC, FRYBACK DG: Optimizing work-up of adult hypertensive patients for renal artery stenosis. Radiol Clin North Am 22:333, 1984

153. THRALL JH, KOFF SA, KEYES JR: Diuretic radionuclide renography and scintigraphy in the differential diagnosis of hydroureteronephrosis. Semin Nucl Med 11:89, 1981

154. TUITE MJ, WEISS SL: Ultrasound and computed tomographic appearance of extramedullary hematopoiesis encasing the renal pelvis. J Clin Ultrasound 19:238, 1991

155. TWERSKY J, LEVIN DC: Metastatic melanoma of the adrenal. Radiology 116:627, 1975

156. WELCH TJ, SHEEDY PF II, VAN HEERDEN JA, ET AL: Pheochromocytoma: Value of computed tomography. Radiology 148:501, 1983

157. WEYMAN PJ, McCLENNAN BL, STANLEY RJ, ET AL: Comparison of computed tomography and angiography in the evaluation of renal cell carcinoma. Radiology 137:417, 1980

158. WHITE EA, SCHAMBELAN M, ROST CR, ET AL: Use of computed tomography in diagnosing the cause of primary aldosteronism. N Engl J Med 303:1503, 1980

159. WICKS JD, THORNBURY JR: Acute renal infections in adults. Radiol Clin North Am 17:245, 1979

160. WINOGRAD J, SCHIMMEL DH, PALUBINSKAS AJ: The spotted nephrogram of renal scleroderma. Am J Roentgenol 126:734, 1976

161. WITTEN DM, MYERS GH, UTZ DC: Emmett's Clinical Urography, 4th ed. Philadelphia, WB Saunders, 1977

162. WOLFMAN MG, THORNBURY JR, BRAUNSTEIN EM: Nonobstructing radiopaque ureteral calculi. Urol Radiol 1:97, 1979

*Paul and Juhl's Essentials of Radiologic Imaging,
Sixth Edition*, edited by John H. Juhl and
Andrew B. Crummy. J.B. Lippincott Company,
Philadelphia, © 1993.

CHAPTER *21*

Obstetric and Gynecologic Imaging

Jeffrey D. Wicks

Obstetric and gynecologic imaging has undergone marked changes in the past 15 years, primarily because of the influence of new imaging modalities. The single modality that has most significantly changed the diagnostic approach to obstetric and gynecologic problems is diagnostic ultrasonography. The remarkable ability of this technique to display the anatomy of the gravid and nongravid female pelvis without the use of ionizing radiation motivated the development of techniques and instrumentation that have supplanted but not totally replaced many x-ray–based examinations. The use of diagnostic ultrasonography for the evaluation of obstetric and gynecologic problems is the dominant theme of this chapter. Areas of patient diagnosis and management in which additional imaging techniques, x-rays, or magnetic resonance imaging (MRI) are presented where appropriate. The role of MRI in obstetric and gynecologic imaging is still being assessed.

It is beyond the scope of this chapter to discuss the physical principles of ultrasound,[191] x-ray,[107] and MRI[147] examinations. Both ultrasonography and MRI are nonionizing imaging techniques that offer a lower potential risk to the developing fetus. The relative newness of MRI has not permitted a thorough investigation of its potential biologic effects on the developing fetus. Ultrasonography has been used to image the developing fetus for two decades, and no harmful effects in humans have been identified. However, much investigation on the potential biologic hazards of ultrasonography is yet to be done. The National Institutes of Health (NIH) consensus on the use of diagnostic ultrasonography in pregnancy does not recommend the indiscriminate use of ultrasonography; readers are referred to the NIH report, which provides guidelines for appropriate use.[57]

OBSTETRIC IMAGING

THE FIRST TRIMESTER

The first trimester of pregnancy begins with fertilization and implantation and extends through the 12th menstrual week. It is the embryonic stage of pregnancy in which the fertilized ovum develops into an embryo with major organogenesis occurring. When one discusses the various stages of development, a specific number of weeks of gestation usually serves as a reference. Embryology texts usually identify weeks of gestation from the time of fertilization, which in a normal 28-day menstrual cycle usually occurs on day 14 or at 2 menstrual weeks. In the sonographic literature, gestational age is equated with menstrual age. For example, if a patient is found to have an intrauterine pregnancy of a gestational age of 10 weeks, it means that 10 weeks have passed since the first day of the patient's last normal menstrual period; presuming she had a 28-day menstrual cycle, it is 8 weeks since fertilization. Therefore, the dates referred to in this chapter as gestational age are in fact menstrual age.

The introduction of endovaginal transducers has permitted earlier and more precise visualization of intrauterine pregnancies. The earliest sonographic finding of an intrauterine pregnancy is the identifica-

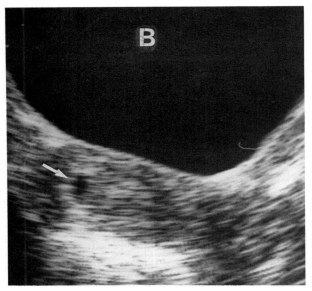

Figure 21–1. Pregnancy of 5½ weeks. Sagittal view of the uterus shows an early gestational sac (*arrow*) located in the fundus. *B* indicates the bladder.

tion of a gestational sac in the endometrial cavity (Fig. 21-1). The sac can be identified in 4.5 menstrual weeks by endovaginal ultrasonography and in the fifth menstrual week by transabdominal scanning.[89] A normal gestational sac has a well-defined, thick, echogenic rim, which is called the decidual reaction. The decidual reaction is actually composed of the cyto- and syncytotrophoblastic tissue surrounded by decidua. Implantation usually occurs in the fundus but has been reported in other intrauterine and extrauterine locations as well. The sac usually measures approximately 1 cm at 5 weeks' gestation and gradually enlarges with increasing gestational age. The sac size can be used as a rough estimate of gestational age.[161]

Depending on the type of equipment used, a small fetal pole may be identified as early as 6 menstrual weeks by transabdominal scanning and in the fifth menstrual week by transvaginal scanning (Fig. 21-2). With most modern transvaginal ultrasound equipment, fetal cardiac activity is seen in the sixth menstrual week and should be documented in all studies thereafter.[121] At 8 menstrual weeks, a thickened area in the decidual reaction denotes the early formation of the placenta. It is easily visible by 10 menstrual weeks (Fig. 21-3). With transvaginal scanning, it is frequently possible to identify a small cystlike structure, which represents the fetal yolk sac. It should always be visualized by a mean sac diameter of 8 mm.[120] By 12 menstrual weeks (Fig. 21-4), the fetal calvarium should be well formed and easily identified. At 7 to 8 weeks, gross movement of the fetal pole is also easy to identify. As the extremities develop, the activity of the fetal extremity can be seen in the later stages of the first trimester. In addition to evaluation of the gestational sac and embryo, all ultrasound examinations in the first trimester should comment on the uterus and adnexal structures. Any uterine or adnexal mass should be recorded.

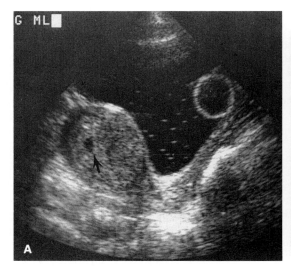
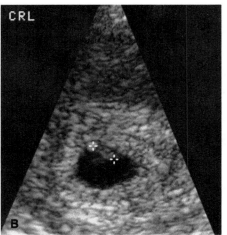

Figure 21–2. Forty-day intrauterine pregnancy. **(A)** Sagittal transabdominal sonogram shows a gestational sac (*arrow*) in the uterus. A fetal pole was not visualized. Foley catheter balloon is seen within the bladder. **(B)** Transvaginal ultrasonography revealed a fetal pole (*cursors*) within the gestational sac. A yolk sac was visualized on other images.

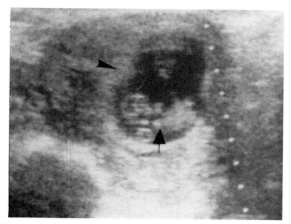

Figure 21–3. Ten-week pregnancy. Transverse view of the pelvis shows the gestational sac with the fetal pole (*arrow*) located dependently and the thickened area of decidual reaction (*arrowhead*) denoting the margin of the early placenta.

COMPLICATIONS OF EARLY PREGNANCY

One of the most common indications for ultrasound examination in the first trimester is vaginal bleeding. Ultrasonography is the most useful diagnostic test in making a differential diagnosis, which usually consists of missed or incomplete abortion, threatened abortion, spontaneous abortion, ectopic pregnancy, or gestational trophoblastic disease.

A woman with a missed or incomplete abortion usually has a malformed gestational sac with or without some internal echoes. No fetal cardiac activity or fetal pole motion is identified. A completely empty gestational sac is called a blighted ovum or anembryonic gestation (Fig. 21-5). It is sometimes difficult to distinguish a very early intrauterine pregnancy without an easily identified fetal pole from a blighted ovum. In most cases of blighted ovum, the decidual reaction is incomplete or lacking and the sac is larger than one would expect for a normal 6-week gestation period.[142] In addition, the patient's dates would suggest a more advanced gestational age. Visualization of a gestational sac with a mean diameter of 2.5 cm by transabdominal scanning or 17 mm by transvaginal scanning without an embryo is indicative of a nonviable pregnancy.[120, 142] If a patient is unsure of her dates, a follow-up examination in 1 to 2 weeks may be necessary to document whether there has been any interval growth in the sac or identification of a fetal pole. In some instances, solid, echogenic material is identified within the endometrial cavity, possibly indicating an incomplete abortion, with the echogenic material representing clotted blood and retained products of conception. This also could represent early gestational trophoblastic disease. A quantitative serum β-hCG level is helpful in distinguishing between these two entities, the level being elevated in gestational trophoblastic disease and low in an incomplete abortion.

The gestational sac normally implants in the fundus

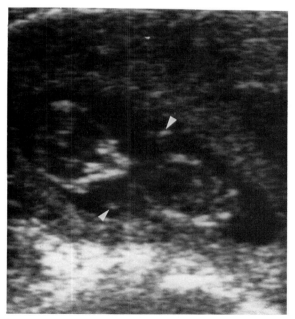

Figure 21–4. Twelve-week pregnancy. Sagittal sonogram of the uterus shows a 12-week fetus with the head on the left and upper trunk on the right. Part of the upper extremities (*arrowheads*) is seen.

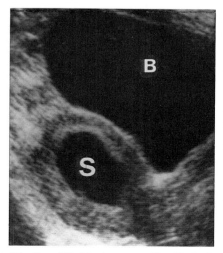

Figure 21–5. Blighted ovum. Sagittal view of the pelvis shows an enlarged uterus with an empty gestational sac (*S*). *B* indicates the bladder.

of the uterus. Some believe that low implantation is associated with an increased risk of spontaneous abortion. One sonographic finding that may be associated with increased risk for spontaneous abortion is extensive elevation of the chorioamniotic membrane (Fig. 21-6). This results in the appearance of a triangular-shaped or lenticular sonolucent fluid collection within the endometrial cavity, representing endometrial blood from exuberant implantation bleeding.[78] Statistically, the documentation of fetal cardiac activity in a patient with vaginal bleeding can be correlated with an approximately 90% chance of the pregnancy going to term.[62]

Ectopic Pregnancy

An ectopic pregnancy is a potentially life-threatening complication of early pregnancy that, unlike the previously mentioned clinical entities, almost always causes varying degrees of abdominal pain in addition to vaginal bleeding. Transvaginal scanning is superior to transabdominal scanning for evaluation of ectopic pregnancy,[178] although both examinations may be necessary for complete evaluation. The pathognomonic sonographic finding of ectopic pregnancy is the identification of an extrauterine gestational sac that contains a fetal pole. This finding is seen in approximately 30% of cases with transvaginal scans and 10% with transabdominal scans.[178] Additional sonographic findings include uterine enlargement, an adnexal mass, fluid in the posterior cul-de-sac, and the presence of a pseudogestational sac in the endometrial cavity (Fig. 21-7).[115]

It may be difficult to distinguish between a normal early intrauterine pregnancy as identified by the presence of a gestational sac and a pseudogestational sac, which forms from the sloughed decidual cast in association with an ectopic pregnancy (Fig. 21-7B).[137] In a normal intrauterine gestation, there is the appearance of a double gestational sac created by the apposition of the decidua capsularis and the decidua parietalis to the endometrial surface opposite the side of implantation (decidua basalis).[22] With the pseudogestational sac of an ectopic pregnancy, only a single layer of decidual reaction lines the entire endometrial cavity. The presence of a normal intrauterine gestational sac with a viable fetal pole essentially excludes the possibility of ectopic pregnancy.[14]

Adnexal masses in association with ectopic pregnancy have a variety of appearances and unfortunately do not individually add much to the ability to make a specific pathologic diagnosis. Adnexal hematomas secondary to bleeding from an ectopic pregnancy are usually sonographically complex or solid in appearance (Fig. 21-7C). Hemorrhagic corpus luteum cysts can be seen with both ectopic and intrauterine pregnancies and can mimic the ectopic gestation. Patients with preexisting masses, especially those due to previous pelvic inflammatory disease that predisposes patients to ectopic pregnancy, may simulate the ectopic gestation as well. Bleeding from an ectopic pregnancy may be identified sonographically as fluid in the posterior cul-de-sac (Fig. 21-7D). Clotted blood can have substantial internal echoes and appear solid on the ultrasound images (Fig. 21-7E). Although these additional findings taken individually are not specific, the presence of an enlarged uterus without a gestational sac, an adnexal mass, and fluid in the cul-de-sac in a patient with a positive pregnancy test is highly suggestive of ectopic pregnancy.

An extremely helpful adjunct to the diagnosis of ectopic pregnancy is the quantitative serum β-hCG determination.[164] This test, when performed as a radioimmunoassay, becomes positive approximately 10 days after conception. In normal intrauterine pregnancies, the β-hCG level doubles every 2 days in the mid–first trimester. In ectopic pregnancy, the β-hCG level is lower than one would find in a normal intrauterine pregnancy and plateaus or does not rise with time. By the time the β-hCG reaches 1000 mIU/L (Second International Standard), in a normal pregnancy a gestational sac should be visualized in the uterus using transvaginal scanning.[144] If no intrauterine gestational sac is identified and the β-hCG level is below the discriminating zone, there still may be an ectopic pregnancy; however, it could also be an early intrauterine pregnancy before the sonographic identification of a gestational sac. In this situation, serial quantitative β-hCG levels and follow-up sonograms are advised.

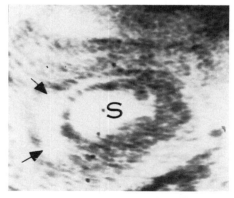

Figure 21–6.   Threatened abortion. Transverse view of the pelvis and uterus shows the gestational sac (*S*) and an adjacent fluid collection (*arrows*) presumed to be blood. Other images documented a viable fetal pole.

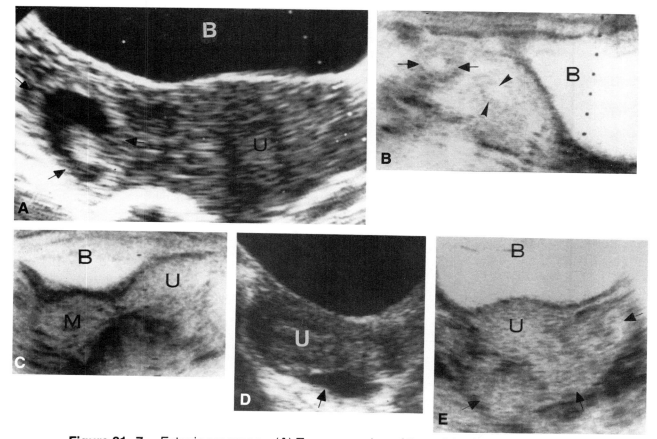

Figure 21–7. Ectopic pregnancy. (**A**) Transverse view of the pelvis shows an enlarged empty uterus (*U*). In the right adnexal region a gestational sac (*arrows*) with a viable fetal pole is identified. (**B**) Sagittal view of the pelvis in another patient shows an enlargement of the uterus, which contains a pseudo-gestational sac (*arrowheads*). The extrauterine gestational sac (*arrows*) is located near the fundus. (**C**) Transverse view of the pelvis of the patient in **B** 1 year after a left salpingo-oophorectomy for the previous ectopic pregnancy. The uterus (*U*) is displaced to the left by a solid-appearing right adnexal mass (*M*), which at surgery was a broad ligament hematoma secondary to a right ectopic pregnancy. (**D**) Ruptured ectopic pregnancy. Sagittal sonogram displays fluid (*arrow*) posterior to the uterus (*U*). (**E**) Ruptured ectopic pregnancy. Transverse image of the pelvis shows the posterior cul-de-sac and adnexal regions filled with echogenic clotted blood (*arrows*). *U* indicates the uterus; *B* indicates the bladder.

ESTIMATING GESTATIONAL AGE

Gestational age is determined by monitoring menstrual age, that is, the number of weeks since the first day of the last normal menstrual period. This convention is useful because there is significant variability in the time of ovulation and it is frequently difficult to ascertain exactly when fertilization occurred. From a practical standpoint, the patient can often recall the first day of the last normal menstrual period. However, as many as 30% to 40% of women cannot document a specific date.[56]

Several sonographic and radiologic parameters can be used to determine gestational age. In general, the earlier in pregnancy that an attempt is made to establish gestational age, the more accurate is its determination. This is because of increasing normal variability in the size of the fetus as pregnancy advances.

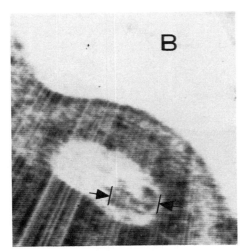

Figure 21–8. Crown-rump length (CRL). Sagittal scan of the pelvis shows a small fetal pole within a well-formed gestational sac. The arrows indicate the CRL measurement; *B* indicates the bladder.

In the first trimester, the size of the gestational sac can be used to estimate gestational age.[161] A much more accurate method is to measure the greatest length of the fetal pole and determine the crown-rump length (CRL) (Fig. 21-8). This measurement is most accurately determined using real-time ultrasound equipment and is accurate in establishing the gestational age to plus or minus 5 days (Table 21-1).[162] This measurement is useful between 5 and 12 weeks of gestation.

After the 12th menstrual week, several other fetal physical parameters can be measured to estimate gestational age. The fetal biparietal diameter (BPD) is the measurement that has undergone the most extensive study. This measurement is made on an image that displays a transaxial section through the fetal calvarium at the level of the thalamus and cavum septi pellucidi (Fig. 21-9). The measurement is made from the outer table of the calvarium closest to the transducer to the inner table of the far side of the calvarium. Extreme care must be taken to obtain the appropriate image and

Table 21–1. Menstrual Age Based on Crown-Rump Length

MENSTRUAL (weeks + days)	CRL		MENSTRUAL (weeks + days)	CRL	
	MEAN (mm)	2 SD		MEAN (mm)	2 SD
6 + 2	6.7	2.9	10 + 2	35.5	6.9
6 + 3	7.4	3.1	10 + 3	36.9	7.0
6 + 4	8.0	3.2	10 + 4	38.4	7.2
6 + 5	8.7	3.4	10 + 5	39.9	7.3
6 + 6	9.5	3.5	10 + 6	41.4	7.4
7 + 0	10.2	3.7	11 + 0	43.0	7.6
7 + 1	11.0	3.8	11 + 1	44.6	7.7
7 + 2	11.8	3.9	11 + 2	46.2	7.9
7 + 3	12.6	4.1	11 + 3	47.8	8.0
7 + 4	13.5	4.2	11 + 4	49.5	8.1
7 + 5	14.4	4.4	11 + 5	51.2	8.3
7 + 6	15.3	4.5	11 + 6	52.9	8.4
8 + 0	16.3	4.6	12 + 0	54.7	8.6
8 + 1	17.3	4.8	12 + 1	56.5	8.7
8 + 2	18.3	4.9	12 + 2	58.3	8.8
8 + 3	19.3	5.1	12 + 3	60.1	9.0
8 + 4	20.4	5.2	12 + 4	62.0	9.1
8 + 5	21.5	5.3	12 + 5	63.9	9.3
8 + 6	22.6	5.5	12 + 6	65.9	9.4
9 + 0	23.8	5.6	13 + 0	67.8	9.5
9 + 1	25.0	5.8	13 + 1	69.8	9.7
9 + 2	26.2	5.9	13 + 2	71.8	9.8
9 + 3	27.4	6.0	13 + 3	73.9	10.0
9 + 4	28.7	6.2	13 + 4	76.0	10.1
9 + 5	30.0	6.3	13 + 5	78.1	10.2
9 + 6	31.3	6.5	13 + 6	80.2	10.4
10 + 0	32.7	6.6	14 + 0	82.4	10.5
10 + 1	34.0	6.7			

Robinson HP, Fleming JEE: A critical evaluation of sonar "crown-rump length" measurements. Br J Obstet Gynaecol 82:702, 1975

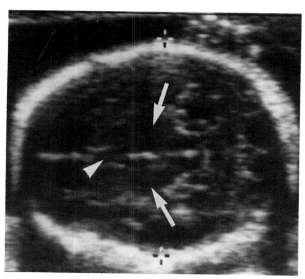

Figure 21–9. Biparietal diameter (BPD). Transaxial image through the fetal calvarium at the level of the thalami (*arrows*) and cavum septi pellucidi (*arrowhead*). BPD measurement is made from the outer table of the upper portion of the calvarium to the inner aspect of the dependent portion (see *cursors*).

Table 21–2. Menstrual Age Based on Biparietal Diameter

MENSTRUAL AGE (weeks)	KURTZ ET AL >1974	HADLOCK ET AL 1982	SHEPARD AND FILLY 1982
14	26	27	28
15	29	30	31
16	33	33	34
17	36	37	37
18	40	40	40
19	43	43	43
20	46	46	46
21	50	50	49
22	53	53	52
23	56	56	55
24	59	58	57
25	61	61	60
26	64	64	63
27	67	67	65
28	70	70	68
29	72	72	71
30	75	75	73
31	77	77	76
32	79	79	78
33	82	82	80
34	84	84	83
35	86	86	85
36	88	88	88
37	90	90	90
38	92	91	92
39	94	93	95
40	95	95	97

Kurtz AB, Wapner RJ, Kurtz RJ, et al: Analysis of biparietal diameter as an accurate indicator of gestational age. J Clin Ultrasound 8:319, 1980; Hadlock FP, Deter RL, Harrist RB, et al: Fetal biparietal diameter: A critical reevaluation of the relation to menstrual age by means of real-time ultrasound. J Ultrasound Med 1:97, 1982; Shepard M, Filly RA: A standardized plane for biparietal diameter measurement. J Ultrasound Med 1:145, 1982

to ensure that the midline echoes are equidistant between the inner tables of the skull. When gestational age based on the BPD is reported (Table 21-2), a mean gestational age should be stated plus the range of normal based on two standard deviations from normal or a 95% confidence level. The range of normal variation increases with gestational age.[51] From 13 to 19 weeks the range is plus or minus 1 week, from 20 to 26 weeks plus or minus 10 days, from 26 to 30 weeks plus or minus 2 to 2.5 weeks, and after 30 weeks plus or minus 3 to 4 weeks.[20]

Other fetal cranial measurements can be used as adjuncts to biparietal diameter in estimating gestational age. Most often used is the head circumference, which is measured on the same image as that used for the BPD.[88] Inner and outer orbital diameters can be roughly correlated with gestational age as well.[129]

Fetal femur length has been established as another accurate parameter for estimating gestational age (Table 21-3). This measurement is useful in the second and third trimesters with a 95% confidence limit of plus or minus 1 week between 14 and 22 weeks.[146] This measurement is most easily obtained using a real-time scanner, preferably a linear array configuration (Fig. 21-10). The iliac bone is the easiest to find. After this bone is found, the transducer should be rotated ante-riorly until the long bright echo of the femur is identified. Multiple images for measurements should be obtained until a confident estimate of the greatest femur length is achieved. With some high-resolution real-time scanners, the distal femoral and proximal tibial epiphyses can be identified later in pregnancy.[35] The distal femoral epiphysis and the proximal tibial epiphysis are the most widely used radiographic standards for estimation of gestational age. The distal femoral epiphysis is usually visible by the 36th to 37th weeks and the proximal tibial epiphysis by the 38th week. However, there is wide normal variation, ranging from 32 to 38 weeks for the distal femoral epiphysis and 33 to 41 weeks for proximal tibial epiphysis.[168] Charts that correlate the sonographic length of the humerus, ulna,

Table 21–3. Menstrual Age Based on Femur Length

MENSTRUAL AGE (weeks)	FEMUR LENGTH (mm)	
	JEANTY AND ROMERO	HADLOCK ET AL
12	8	08
13	11	11
14	14	15
15	17	18
16	20	21
17	23	24
18	25	27
19	28	30
20	31	33
21	34	36
22	36	39
23	39	42
24	42	44
25	44	47
26	47	49
27	49	52
28	52	54
29	54	56
30	56	58
31	59	61
32	61	63
33	63	65
34	65	66
35	67	68
36	68	70
37	70	72
38	71	73
39	73	75
40	74	76

Jeanty P, Romero R: Obstetrical Ultrasound, p 233, New York, McGraw Hill, 1984; Hadlock FP, Harrist RB, Deter RL, et al: Femur length as a prediction of menstrual age: Sonographically measured. AJR Am J Roentgenol 138: 875, 1982

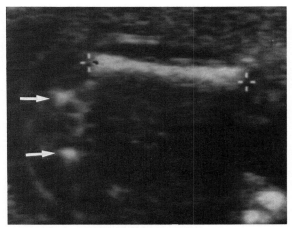

Figure 21–10. Fetal femur. Longitudinal image of the fetal thigh with cursors measuring the femur length. Arrows indicate the ischia.

tional age were obtained on the appropriately oriented images and that the measurements were accurately determined. Measurements of different physical parameters that correspond to within a 1 to 2 weeks, depending on the gestational age, increase one's level of confidence.

ASSESSMENT OF THE FETUS

The technical improvements and proliferation of ultrasound equipment in the past decade have greatly enhanced the assessment of fetal development and have allowed the identification of many fetal morphologic abnormalities. Ultrasonography can provide detailed analysis of fetal anatomy beginning early in pregnancy, and with real-time ultrasonography, fetal activities such as breathing, swallowing, coarse and fine motor movements, and cardiac activity can be closely monitored.

Consider the following aspects of normal fetal development. As previously mentioned, using transvaginal ultrasonography at the earliest time that a fetal pole can be identified is about 5 menstrual weeks. The flickering motion of fetal cardiac activity should be seen on real-time transvaginal ultrasound examination in all embryos with a CRL of 5 mm or more.[121] Between 5 and 10 weeks, a small cystic structure often can be identified in the amniotic fluid separate from the fetal pole (Fig. 21-11). This is the yolk sac, the site of early blood formation, and it contributes to the development of the gastrointestinal tract. This is a normal structure and should not be mistaken for a second fetal pole.

By the late first trimester, some intracranial anatomy is visible. Most of the calvarium is filled with large fluid-filled ventricles surrounded by a small amount of smooth primitive brain. As the brain develops through-

and tibia with gestational age[101] are useful when it is difficult to obtain an accurate femur length. They are also helpful in the evaluation of fetal skeletal dysplasias.

Assignment of a gestational age is not always straightforward. The radiologist must be technically competent in obtaining the appropriate image and in making the appropriate measurement. Sometimes the fetal position compromises the ability to obtain the optimum image, and this must be considered when one has to judge the value of a single parameter. The following guidelines should be used: (1) the normal variation of any biologic parameter that is measured generally increases with gestational age, (2) the CRL in the first trimester provides the most accurate estimation of gestational age, and (3) the BPD measurement between 16 and 20 weeks and the fetal femur length between 14 and 22 weeks are accurate to plus or minus 1 week. However, one must be comfortable with the fact that the measurements used to estimate gesta-

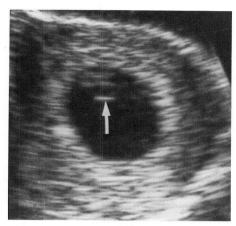

Figure 21–11. Yolk sac. Transverse view of the uterus shows the fetal pole (transverse section) and a small adjacent cystic structure, the yolk sac (*arrow*).

out pregnancy, there is a progressive increase in the relative volume of brain tissue and a relative decrease in the size of the ventricles. The echogenic choroid plexus are prominent structures early in fetal brain development and gradually decrease in relative size with increasing gestational age. One measure of the size of the ventricles (Fig. 21-12A) is the ventricular ratio (the ratio of the distance from the midline to the lateral ventricular wall at the level of the body of the lateral ventricle to the width of the hemisphere), with a normal range as high as 0.7 in the early second trimester, decreasing to less than 0.3 at term.[103] The lateral ventricular atrium should measure 10 mm or less throughout pregnancy (Fig. 21-12B).[66]

By the early second trimester, the fetal heart is recognizable as a distinct, contracting fluid-filled structure. By the mid–second trimester, the cardiac chambers (Fig. 21-13) and valves can be identified and studied with two-dimensional and m-mode fetal echocardiography. Fetal lungs appear as solid structures in the thorax with an echogenicity greater than that of the liver or spleen until late in pregnancy.

As the fetus begins to swallow amniotic fluid, the fetal stomach becomes visible as a cystic structure in the left upper quadrant (Fig. 21-14). It can be seen as early as 14 weeks and should be seen consistently after 16 to 18 weeks. The remainder of the fetal bowel is relatively echogenic and looks solid. Near term, the meconium-filled colon becomes more sonolucent, containing fine, low-level internal echoes. An important landmark to identify in the fetal abdomen is the course of the umbilical vein where it enters the portal sinus (see Fig. 21-14). The transverse image of the fetal

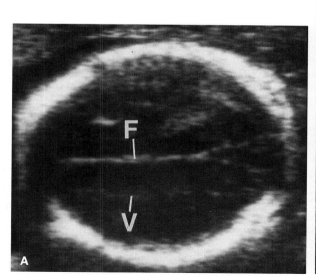
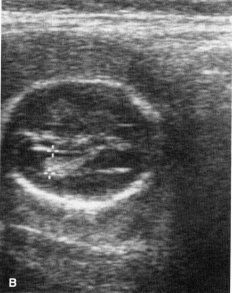

Figure 21–12. Ventricles. **(A)** Transaxial view of the fetal calvarium at the level of the bodies of the lateral ventricles. The dependent ventricle is usually imaged the best, since reverberation artifacts frequently obscure the upper half of the brain. *F* indicates the falx; *V* indicates lateral wall of the body of the lateral ventricle. **(B)** Transaxial view of a different fetus showing measurement of the lateral ventricle at the level of the trigone. Note the echogenic choroid plexus.

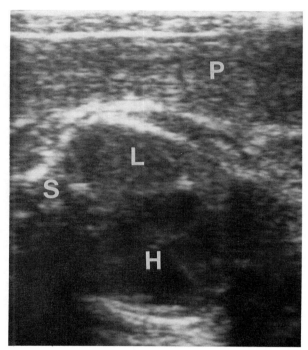

Figure 21–13. Fetal heart. Transverse view of the fetal thorax shows the cardiac chambers (*H*). Note the echogenic lung (*L*). *S* indicates the spine; *P* indicates the placenta.

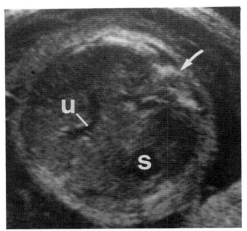

Figure 21–14. Fetal abdomen. Transverse section of the fetal abdomen shows the stomach (*s*), umbilical vein (*u*), and spine (*arrow*). The abdominal circumference is measured on this image.

abdomen is important in the assessment of fetal somatic growth, which is discussed later. The umbilical vein should not be mistaken for the fetal gallbladder, which can be seen later in the second trimester.

The fetal kidneys can be identified at as early as 15 weeks' gestation.[118] It is more important to document renal function by the identification of the fluid-filled fetal urinary bladder in the pelvis. The bladder can be seen at as early as 14 weeks' gestation and should always be identified after 18 weeks' gestation (Fig. 21-15). The fetal bladder may empty over a 30-minute to 2-hour period; if it is not visualized on the initial examination, the fetus should be rescanned every 30 to 45 minutes until the bladder is identified.

The discussion of the ultrasound diagnosis of fetal anomalies is beyond the scope of this chapter. Table 21-4 lists some anomalies that have been diagnosed and provides references to papers describing them. Amniotic fluid volume is an important indicator of the presence of a possible fetal anomaly. Open neural tube abnormalities, obstructive gastrointestinal tract defects proximal to the distal small bowel, some fetal skeletal dysplasias, and some cardiac defects are fetal abnormalities associated with polyhydramnios, or increased amounts of amniotic fluid. Obstructive genitourinary anomalies and agenesis of the kidneys are associated

with oligohydramnios, or markedly reduced amniotic fluid. The presence of polyhydramnios or oligohydramnios is not a definite indication of a fetal anomaly, because polyhydramnios can be idiopathic or associated with maternal diabetes, Rh incompatibility, and multiple gestations.[2] Oligohydramnios of varying degrees can result from premature rupture of the membranes or can be associated with a growth-retarded fetus that is structurally intact.

Ultrasound examination is extremely useful in assessing fetal growth.[96] Growth-retarded fetuses exhibit a much higher neonatal morbidity and mortality. Intrauterine growth retardation (IUGR) may be due to maternal causes, such as severe diabetes, renal disease, hypertension, or drug abuse, or to primary fetal abnormalities, such as congenital anomalies, chromosomal abnormalities, or congenital infection. Primary placental abnormalities can result in IUGR as well. Generally, maternal causes and primary placental abnormalities result in placental insufficiency leading to asymmetrical IUGR. Primary fetal abnormalities usually result in symmetrical IUGR. Symmetrical IUGR can be distinguished from asymmetrical IUGR by the head-to-abdomen circumference ratio. The head circumference measurement is obtained on the same image used for the BPD. Abdominal circumference is measured on a transverse image of the upper abdomen through the liver at the level of the umbilical vein. This ratio is normally greater than 1 until approximately 34 to 36 weeks, when the abdominal circumference becomes larger than the head circumference because of the deposition of increased amounts of subcutaneous fat. In the most common form of IUGR (asymmetrical IUGR), there is preservation of central nervous system

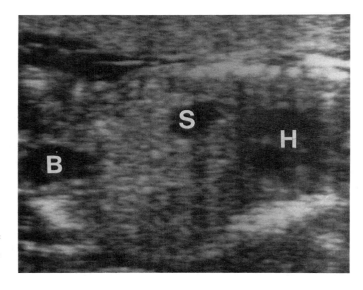

Figure 21–15.   Fetal bladder. Coronal view of the fetal trunk shows the bladder (*B*), the stomach (*S*), and the heart (*H*).

Table 21–4. Fetal Anomalies[11, 61, 93, 145, 166]

CENTRAL NERVOUS SYSTEM	*HEART*	*GASTROINTESTINAL*	*SKELETAL*
Hydrocephalus[27, 38, 143, 154]	Congenital heart block[170]	Esophageal atresia[155]	Thanatophoric dwarf[94]
Microcephaly[34, 114]	Single ventricle[112, 150]	Duodenal atresia[21]	Sirenomelus[156]
Anencephaly[27, 46]	Holoacardius[119]	Anal atresia[9]	Chondroectodermal dysplasia[125]
Encephalocele[140]	Ectopia cordis[192, 197]	Meconium ileus[49]	
Holoprosencephaly[27, 29, 67]	Pericardial effusion[53]	Volvulus[8]	Diastrophic dwarfism[128]
Hydranencephaly[40, 82]	Supraventricular tachycardia[91]	Meconium pseudocyst[117]	Camptomelic dysplasia[94]
Dandy-Walker syndrome[48]	Coarctation of the aorta[197]	Annular pancreas[18]	Osteogenesis imperfecta[5]
Teratoma[95]	Congestive heart failure[110]	Jejunal atresia[175]	Thrombocytopenia Absent Radius syndrome[122]
Meckel-Gruber syndrome[83]	Septal defects[110, 197]		Achondroplasia[68]
Intracranial hemorrhage[132]	Tetralogy of Fallot[110, 197]	*GENITOURINARY*	Achondrogenesis[68]
Spina bifida[25, 41, 66, 77]	Valvular disease[110, 112]	Renal agenesis[60]	Jeune's syndrome[167]
Diastematomyelia[196]	Hypoplastic right heart[111]	Hydronephrosis[4]	Arthrogryposis[76]
Agenesis of the corpus callosum[16]	Intracardiac tumor[54]	Posterior urethral valves[4, 10]	
Porencephaly[183]	Hydrops fetalis[70]	Urethral stenosis[105]	*CHROMOSOMAL*
Schizencephaly[113]	Echocardiography[150]	Renal dysplasia[4, 63]	Down's syndrome[6]
Arachnoid cyst[58]	Structural defects[3]	Infantile polycystic kidney disease[86]	Turner's syndrome[160]
Choroid plexus cyst[38]		Hydrocele[59]	Triploidy[31]
Intracranial hemorrhage[133]	*ABDOMEN*	Adult polycystic kidney disease[126]	Trisomy 19[32]
	Choledochal cyst[55]	Meckel-Gruber syndrome[83]	Trisomy 18[17, 92]
NECK	Ovarian cyst[100]	Primary megaureter[50]	Trisomy 13[81]
Cystic hygroma[151]	Ascites[87]	Sirenomelus[156]	
Teratoma[148]	Omphalocele[74, 159]	Prune-belly syndrome[39]	
Goiter[7]	Gastroschisis[85]	Cysts[72]	
Hemangioma[84]	Cholelithiasis[13]		
	Beckwith-Wiedemann syndrome[83, 188]		
CHEST	Cystic fibrosis[138]		
Cystic adenomatoid malformation[102]	Meconium peritonitis[73]		
Diaphragmatic hernia[36]	Limb–body wall complex[149]		
Pleural effusion[19]			
Chylothorax[47]			
Bronchogenic cyst[1]			
Sequestration[163]			

growth (head circumference) at the expense of somatic growth (abdominal circumference). In symmetrical IUGR, there is proportional growth reduction of both the fetal head and body. Normal ranges for the head-to-abdomen ratio have been compiled for various stages of gestation.[26]

In addition to the head-to-abdomen circumference ratio, fetal weight can be estimated. A variety of complicated formulas have been devised using BPD, femur length, abdominal circumference, and other factors. A useful chart compiled by Shepard and colleagues estimates fetal weight from the BPD and abdominal circumference.[169] The previously described measurements of physical parameters to estimate gestational age can also be used to quantify fetal growth rate. Serial examinations at 2- to 3-week intervals permit one to plot a growth curve for an individual fetus when necessary. MRI may be useful in identifying IUGR. A growth-retarded fetus has markedly reduced body fat, which can be identified on MR images.[172]

Real-time ultrasonography enables one to assess fetal well-being by documenting fetal activity. This sonographic biophysical profile includes the assessment of variations of fetal heart rate; of fetal breathing activities, coarse and fine motor activity, fetal tone, and amniotic fluid volume; and, sometimes, of the appearance of the placenta.[127, 182] Several scoring schemes provide useful information to the obstetrician, who must decide whether the intrauterine environment of the fetus has become hostile rather than protective.

Doppler ultrasonography is being increasingly used to aid in the assessment of fetal well-being by noninvasive evaluation of fetoplacental and uteroplacental blood flow.[42] Whereas direct velocity measurements can be made from fetal vessels such as the carotid arteries and aorta, analysis of the Doppler waveform is the most commonly used technique. A variety of indices (resistive index, pulsatile index, systolic to diastolic [S/D] ratio) are used to quantify the Doppler waveform.[28] The most common measurement currently obtained is the ratio of the velocity at peak systole to the velocity at end diastole (S/D ratio) in the midportion of the umbilical artery. Ranges of normal for various stages of pregnancy have been developed. Abnormally elevated umbilical artery S/D ratios have been associated with IUGR, preeclampsia, Rh incompatibility, placental abruption, and severe maternal illness.[28] Absent or reversed blood flow in diastole is associated with an increased risk of fetal morbidity and mortality.

FETAL DEATH

Radiographic signs have been described in association with intrauterine fetal death. Overlapping of the bones of the skull (Spalding's sign), marked curvature of the fetal spine, and gas in the fetal circulatory system are the most easily recognized. Ultrasound examination has replaced radiographic examinations for suspected fetal death.[152] The documentation of absent fetal cardiac activity and fetal extremity motion is now the most sensitive way of detecting fetal death. One must be confident of a technically satisfactory examination with the ability to view the fetal thorax in an unobstructed fashion. The real-time ultrasound equipment must have a frame rate that is adequate to see fetal cardiac activity if present. Fetuses have periods of relative inactivity in which there is no motion of the extremities or the trunk. However, repeated examination over an hour without documented fetal extremity or fetal cardiac activity is indicative of fetal death. Within days of the death of a fetus, the fetal skin becomes edematous and alterations in the fetal anatomy become obvious. Flattening and overlapping of the fetal skull bones with dissolution of the intracranial anatomy are seen. The internal anatomy of the trunk is difficult to define. After a few weeks, the fetal anatomy is markedly distorted and the fetus may appear as an ill-defined echogenic structure with no easily identifiable anatomy except for a deformed fetal skull.

THE PLACENTA

A thickening in the decidual reaction can be identified by 7 to 8 menstrual weeks as the site of early placenta formation. By 10 weeks this location is clearly defined, and by the end of the first trimester the placenta is identified as a discrete structure. In the beginning of the second trimester, the amnion and chorion fuse to form the smooth fetal surface of the placenta called the chorionic plate, which is identified as a specular echo at the interface of placental tissue and the amniotic fluid. The interface of the placenta and the myometrium is much less well defined. This basilar plate region of the placenta blends into the slightly more hypoechoic myometrium. The draining basilar veins usually can be seen as lacy structures near the interface of the placenta and myometrium (Fig. 21-16).

The appearance of the placenta changes as the pregnancy progresses. It begins as a smoothly marginated structure with a homogeneous, fine echo pattern that is more echogenic than the adjacent myometrium. As the placenta matures, the fetal surface of the placenta develops undulations and the internal echo pattern becomes more heterogeneous. Hypoechoic areas representing mucoid degeneration, intervillous thrombosis, or infarction can be identified. Bright echoes with and without associated acoustic shadowing can be seen with calcium deposition. Grannum and Hobbins have proposed a grading system of placental maturity using the sonographic findings.[80] Correlations that have been made with placental grade and gestational age can

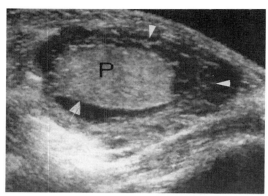

Figure 21–16. Placenta. Sagittal view through the margin of an anterior placenta (*P*) shows the chorionic plate (*arrow*) and the basilar veins (*arrowheads*).

provide helpful information in patient management. Advanced placental grade correlates well with fetal pulmonary maturity in some circumstances, and premature maturation of the placenta has been identified in maternal disease such as toxemia, hypertensive renal disease, and narcotics addiction.[79, 80] Delayed maturation has been correlated with gestational diabetes and fetal hydrops, as has a placental thickness of 5 cm or more.[80]

The most common cause of vaginal bleeding in the second and third trimesters is placenta previa (Fig. 21-17). Ultrasound examination has replaced all other imaging techniques in the assessment of possible pla-

centa previa. The relationship of the placenta to the region of the internal cervical os can be identified through a distended maternal urinary bladder. It is important to study patients before and after voiding because an overdistended bladder can alter the anatomy by distorting the uterus and by creating a false sense of the location of the internal cervical os by compressing the anterior and posterior walls of the uterus against the sacral promontory. Scans performed in the second trimester frequently show apparent placenta previa, but the incidence of placenta previa at term is much lower (0.5%).[30, 45] This phenomenon of apparent change in position of the placenta with advancing gestational age is frequently called placental migration. This most likely represents differential growth rate of the lower uterine segment later in pregnancy.[109] Patients with suspected placenta previa identified early in pregnancy should be observed before the time of anticipated delivery to document placental location. A placenta that appears to cross the internal cervical os from the posterior direction in the second trimester is more likely to persist at term than an anteriorly located placenta.[135]

A patient with placental abruption typically has painful vaginal bleeding. Placental abruption is less common than placenta previa and can be identified on sonograms as a retroplacental lucency representing blood clot between the placenta and myometrium or as an echogenic structure in the amniotic fluid representing an extramembranous clot.[171] Acute hemorrhage is hyperechoic to isoechoic compared with the placenta, and 1- to 2-week-old hemorrhages are sonolucent (Fig. 21-18).[141]

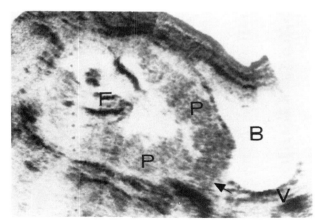

Figure 21–17. Placenta previa. Sagittal scan of the uterus shows the placenta (*P*) completely covering the region of the internal cervical os (*arrow*). The vagina (*V*), the bladder (*B*), and the fetus (*F*) are also indicated.

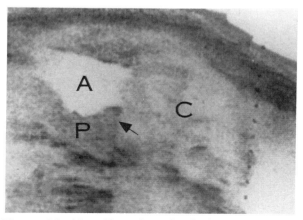

Figure 21–18. Abruption. Sagittal section of the uterus shows the placenta (*P*), amniotic fluid (*A*), and an intra-amniotic clot (*C*). The margin of the placenta is elevated from the myometrium (*arrow*).

LARGE FOR DATES

Ultrasound examination can be extremely helpful in evaluating patients with the clinical finding of the uterus being larger on physical examination than is expected for the estimated gestational age. Probably the most frequent finding in this clinical setting is a single fetus that is normal but of advanced gestational age as compared to the patient's recollection of her menstrual history. The discrepancy usually occurs at 4-week intervals and reflects an inaccurate menstrual history.

Multiple gestation is another frequent finding when a patient is large for dates. Ultrasonography can easily identify multiple fetuses. It is important to correlate the individual size parameters (BPD, head circumference, femur length, abdominal circumference) for each fetus because twins are at increased risk for IUGR. Discordant growth may also be associated with the twin-to-twin transfusion syndrome.[37] This syndrome is seen in approximately 15% to 20% of monozygotic twin pregnancies and can result in a growth-retarded donor twin and a hydropic recipient twin.[23] The fetal growth charts used for singleton pregnancies are accurate in twin pregnancies only to about 26 to 28 weeks; thereafter, twin fetuses are generally smaller than singleton fetuses. It is not always possible to reliably distinguish between monozygotic and dizygotic twins. If a chorion and amnion with a single placenta are confidently seen (that is, no intervening membrane between the fetuses), then the pregnancy is monozygotic. However, monozygotic pregnancies can also be associated with two amniotic or chorionic cavities depending on the time of division of the fertilized ovum. It is important to identify the presence or absence of an intervening membrane because there is a higher fetal mortality rate associated with monochorionic, monoamniotic twin gestations. It is also important if amniocentesis is to be performed so that the amniotic fluid from each amniotic sac is sampled.

The presence of a pelvic mass may also create the impression that a patient is large for dates. This mass may be of ovarian or uterine origin. The most common ovarian mass in pregnancy is a persistent corpus luteum cyst. It is generally a unilocular cystic structure that gradually diminishes in size but may persist beyond 16 menstrual weeks. On occasion it can be large, measuring up to 10 cm. The most common uterine mass is a myoma, which may enlarge during pregnancy and can undergo painful infarction. Documentation of the size and position of a myoma is important, especially if it is located in the lower uterine segment, and it may interfere with a normal vaginal delivery.

Polyhydramnios is another possible cause of a uterus larger than expected for menstrual dates. Polyhydramnios may be idiopathic but can be associated with maternal disorders such as diabetes mellitus. Careful attention must be paid to the fetal anatomy to exclude the presence of a morphologic defect such as an open neural tube defect or an obstructive anomaly of the gastrointestinal tract.

PELVIMETRY

Pelvimetry is the radiographic examination of the female bony pelvis to measure the size of the various bony structures. Anteroposterior (AP) and lateral radiographs with a known x-ray source to film distance and a strip of radiopaque material marked at 1-cm intervals placed on the patient permit measurements of the AP and transverse diameters of the inlet, midpelvis, and outlet of the pelvis.[104] There is significant controversy about whether this information is useful in assessing potential for difficulty with a vaginal delivery. It is generally agreed that these measurements are of little value in predicting progression of labor with the fetus in the vertex position.[106] The size of the bony pelvis represents only one of many factors that may affect the progression of labor and provides no useful information regarding the size and moldability of the fetal head and the contribution of maternal pelvic soft-tissue structures to cephalopelvic disproportion as a cause of arrest of labor.

Pelvimetry is a major source of ionizing radiation to the fetus. The United Nations Scientific Committee's report on the effects of atomic radiation estimated the mean fetal body dose to be about 620 mrad.[180] Data obtained in both the United States and England show an increased incidence of leukemia and other malignant diseases in children exposed in utero to diagnostic x-rays. For this reason, x-ray pelvimetry should be restricted to those patients in whom it will provide information not available from clinical examination or sonography. Lower dose digital x-ray techniques[65] have been described for pelvimetry, and early reports using nonionizing MRI[173] to assess pelvic size have been reported.

POSTPARTUM SONOGRAPHY

After delivery there is a relatively rapid decrease in uterine size. Within 1 day of delivery, the fundus of the uterus can be palpated just above the umbilicus as compared to its subxiphoid location at term. In most cases, physical examination is adequate in following the size of the uterus. However, in cases of postpartum hemorrhage, infection, and pain, sonography is the most useful imaging examination in patient management.

Sonography is an accurate method of documenting normal reduction in uterine size after delivery. In 1 day

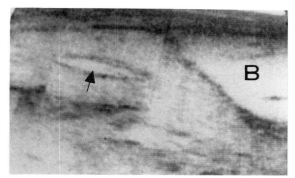

Figure 21–19. Postpartum uterus. Sagittal scan of the pelvis reveals an enlarged uterus with fluid in the endometrial cavity (*arrow*). The bladder is at *B*.

it is near the level of the umbilicus and by 2 weeks can be palpated in the suprapubic region. By 6 weeks postpartum its size should be normal. For patients with postpartum bleeding that does not respond to usual clinical measures, sonography is helpful in excluding the presence of retained placental tissue.[198] Normally, the endometrial cavity is collapsed in the postpartum state. The retained placenta appears as a somewhat globular, echogenic structure that separates the wall of the endometrial cavity. Retained clot usually has a more linear configuration, conforming to the configuration of the endometrial cavity, but may appear as echogenic as retained placenta. Liquefied blood or lochia in the endometrial cavity appears more sonolucent (Fig. 21-19).

Postpartum or puerperal infection is defined as a temperature above 38° C on two consecutive days, not including the first day of fever. The most common route of infection in the endometrial cavity is through the vagina. Puerperal infections are caused by a mixture of anaerobic and aerobic bacteria. Most patients respond to appropriate antibiotic treatment. In those patients

who fail to respond, retained clot or products of conception may be a nidus for the infection. In these cases sonography is useful in documenting the presence of material or fluid within the endometrial cavity. An unusual finding is gas artifacts within the endometrial cavity secondary to infections by gas-producing organisms such as *Clostridium welchii, Bacteroides,* or *Escherichia coli.* It should be kept in mind that air can be introduced into the endometrial cavity by a procedure, such as curettage, when attempting to remove retained products of conception.

Postpartum pelvic pain can also be evaluated by ultrasound examination. Some patients have a palpable mass. In the nongravid state, the broad ligaments usually are not visualized sonographically. However, as they enlarge to accommodate the growing uterus and its increased vascular requirements in pregnancy, they become visible. In the postpartum state, they appear as sonolucent structures located lateral to the uterus (Fig. 21-20). With some difficult deliveries, patients develop broad ligament hematomas that appear sonographically as symmetrical sonolucent or complex masses in an adnexal location. In patients who have undergone a cesarean section, the area of hysterotomy and postoperative hematoma can be defined sonographically (Fig. 21-21). The hematoma usually appears beneath the patient's abdominal incision in a preperitoneal location between the superficial layers of the abdominal wall and the anterior wall of the uterus. It is not possible sonographically to distinguish absolutely between a postoperative hematoma and an abscess.

GYNECOLOGIC IMAGING

NORMAL ANATOMY

The uterus is an elongated, pear-shaped, hollow, muscular organ. It is usually located in the midline and anteverted in position. The myometrium exhibits a

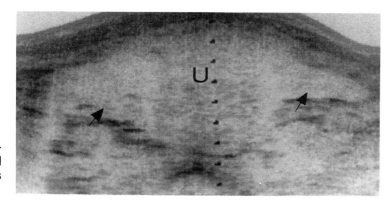

Figure 21–20. Postpartum uterus. Transverse scan of the pelvis shows the enlarged uterus (*U*) and prominent broad ligaments (*arrows*).

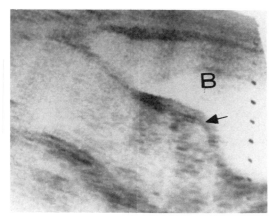

Figure 21–21. Post–cesarean section. Sagittal scan of the pelvis in a patient 2 weeks after cesarean section shows deformity (*arrow*) in the anterior lower uterine segment from the surgery and resolving hematoma. The bladder is at *B*.

homogeneous, medium-level amplitude echo pattern with a linear, bright echo representing the endometrial cavity (Fig. 21-22). The most common normal variation in position is the retroverted uterus. Not only does the tip of the fundus appear to point more posteriorly than anteriorly, but also there frequently is an associated globular deformity of the fundus that can mimic the presence of a uterine mass (Fig. 21-23). A more hypoechoic area often is identified surrounding the endo-

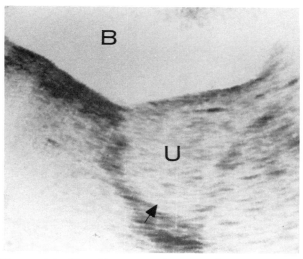

Figure 21–23. Retroverted uterus. Sagittal scan of the pelvis shows a posteriorly angulated uterus (*U*). Note the globular configuration of the fundus (*arrow*), which should not be mistaken for a mass. The bladder is at *B*.

metrial canal. Its appearance changes throughout the menstrual cycle, and this area is most prominent just before menstruation.[90] On computed tomography (CT), the uterus is usually a homogeneous soft-tissue density with variable degrees of enhancement after administration of intravenous contrast material (Fig. 21-24).

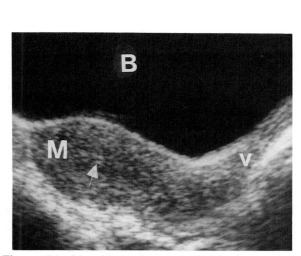

Figure 21–22. Normal uterus. Sagittal sonogram of the pelvis shows a normal uterus with homogeneous echoes from the myometrium (*M*) and bright echoes from the endometrial cavity (*arrow*). The vaginal canal (*V*) appears as the linear echoes posterior to the bladder (*B*).

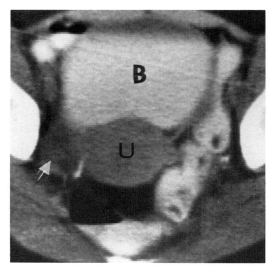

Figure 21–24. Normal uterus. Transverse CT of the pelvis shows the normal uterus (*U*), right ovary (*arrow*), contrast-filled bladder (*B*), and bowel.

When sufficient fluid or blood is within the endometrial cavity, it appears as a low-density area in the center of the uterus. The apparent shape of the uterus on CT is variable because only transverse sections are obtained, and the contour of the uterus varies depending on the amount of bladder distention and degree of anteflexion. On MRI, the appearance of the uterus changes depending on the pulse sequence used. Different layers of tissue display different signal intensities (Fig. 21-25).

The region of the cervix can be identified sonographically by its contiguity with the vagina (see Fig. 21-22). The vagina is normally a midline structure with a bright, linear echo representing the collapsed vaginal canal. On CT the vagina is more easily identified if a vaginal tampon is in place, in which case the vaginal canal is identified as a circular air-filled structure.

The ovaries are identified lateral to the uterus (Fig. 21-26). The ovaries normally measure up to 10 cc ($0.523 \times L \times W \times H$) in volume in women of reproductive age.[190] Small cystic structures representing developing follicles can be identified in the ovaries. The remainder of the adnexal structures, the fallopian tubes, the broad ligaments, and the mesosalpinx are not frequently visualized sonographically. The serpiginous, 7 to 14-cm-long fallopian tubes are best visualized by hysterosalpingography (Fig. 21-27).

Pelvic musculature is best demonstrated with CT or MRI (Fig. 21-28). The iliopsoas muscles are visualized during routine pelvic ultrasound examination and should not be mistaken for the ovaries. The air-containing rectum is identified by its reverberation artifacts on ultrasonography and is more clearly defined on CT. Unopacified bowel on CT and fluid-filled bowel on

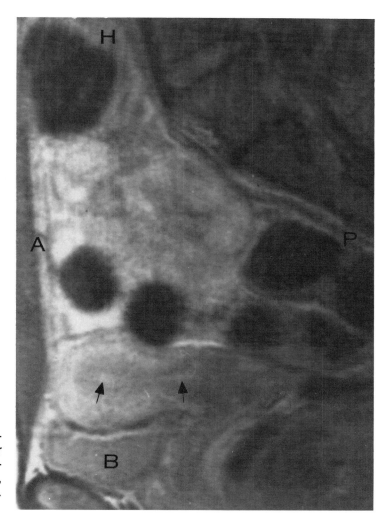

Figure 21–25. Normal uterus. Sagittal T2-weighted MRI of the pelvis shows a brighter signal from the endometrium (*arrow*) compared with the adjacent myometrium. *B*, bladder; *H*, head; *A*, anterior; *P*, posterior. (Courtesy of J.R. Thornbury, M.D.)

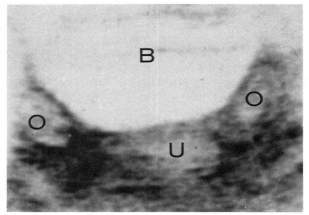

Figure 21–26. Normal ovaries. Transverse sonogram of the pelvis shows the uterus (*U*) and both ovaries (*O*). The bladder is at *B*.

ultrasonography may mimic pelvic pathology. Repeat CT scanning with adequate bowel opacification and observation of peristaltic activity using real-time ultrasonography are helpful in differentiating normal bowel from masses.

CONGENITAL ANOMALIES

Congenital malformations of the female genital tract occur in 1% to 2% of cases. Some are detected on physical examination, and others are identified using

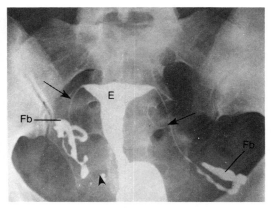

Figure 21–27. Normal hysterosalpingogram. The thin normal lumen of the midportion (*arrows*) and the larger fimbriated ends (*Fb*) of the fallopian tubes are best displayed with this technique. The endometrial cavity (*E*) and a small amount of intraperitoneal spill of contrast material on the right (*arrowhead*) are also seen.

ultrasonography often for an unrelated condition.[181] The müllerian ducts fuse to form the uterus and the vagina, and the unfused cranial portions become the fallopian tubes. Failure to fuse or incomplete fusion results in the most common types of congenital anomalies. Anomalies of the genital tract frequently are associated with urinary tract anomalies, and serendipitous identification of uterine or vaginal anomalies should trigger a thorough evaluation of the urinary tract.

Hysterosalpingography consists of opacification of the uterine cavity and fallopian tubes by injecting opaque contrast material into the uterus. A cannula or catheter is placed through the cervical os and usually a water-soluble iodinated contrast material instilled. Three to 10 ml of contrast material is usually sufficient to opacify the endometrial cavity and fallopian tubes (see Fig. 21-27). This study is useful for evaluating the configuration and shape of the endometrial canal and also the patency of the fallopian tubes.

Hysterosalpingography is contraindicated in the presence of an active infection of the genital tract, recent or active bleeding, or suspected intrauterine pregnancy. The examination is usually performed under fluoroscopic observation with appropriate films obtained to document the anatomy and the spill of contrast material into the peritoneal cavity.

Transabdominal pelvic ultrasonography should always be performed with a distended urinary bladder. This serves as an acoustic window to visualize the deeper structures in the pelvis and displaces air-filled bowel out of the lower pelvis. Failure to have an adequately distended urinary bladder results in inadequate visualization of the pelvic structures and unsatisfactory examinations. Longitudinal and transverse images should be obtained to completely display the normal and abnormal anatomy. Examination is usually performed with a real-time scanner.

Transvaginal ultrasound examination permits improved visualization of the uterus, ovaries, and adnexal structures. A specifically designed transducer is placed in the vagina. It typically has a higher frequency and shorter focal zone than a transabdominal transducer, and this allows higher resolution images of the uterus and ovaries.

An imperforate hymen or partial atresia of the vagina may lead to distention of the vagina. This is called hydrocolpos or hematocolpos and may be accompanied by pain and a palpable pelvic or lower abdominal mass. This is most easily diagnosed sonographically as a primarily cystic mass, which is located immediately posterior to the bladder (Fig. 21-29). A small uterus may be identified near the most cephalad portion of the mass. The most caudal aspect of the mass is difficult to define because of its location on the perineum. If the perineal membrane is perforated, con-

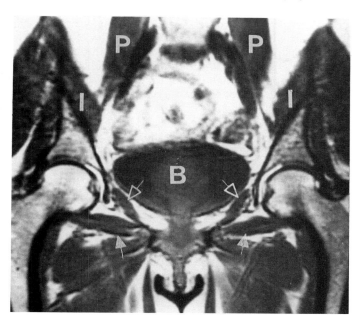

Figure 21–28. Pelvic musculature. Coronal MRI of the pelvis at the level of the femoral heads. The lower-intensity muscles are contrasted to the high-intensity fat. The psoas muscle (*P*), iliacus muscle (*I*), obturator internus muscles (*open arrows*), obturator externus muscle (*closed arrows*), and bladder (*B*) are also seen.

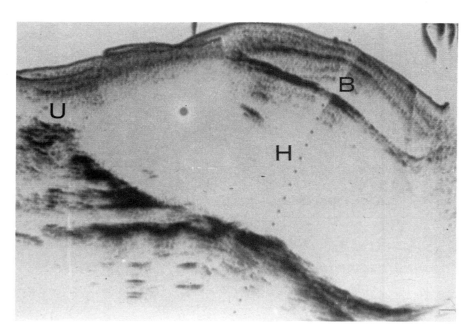

Figure 21–29. Hematocolpos. Sagittal sonogram of the pelvis reveals a large primarily cystic mass (*H*), which is the blood-filled, distended vagina posterior to the bladder (*B*). The small uterus (*U*) can also be seen. (Courtesy of R. Bree, MD)

trast material can be injected to display the distended vaginal and uterine cavities. Sonography or excretory urography is useful in evaluating the possibility of associated hydronephrosis.

Hematometra results from an obstructing lesion in the cervix or is secondary to agenesis of the vagina. Its clinical presentation is similar to that of hematocolpos. It is most easily identified sonographically as a some-

what bilobed, thick-walled pelvic mass that contains internal echoes caused by hemorrhagic material (Fig. 21-30). This condition may be associated with hematocolpos, in which case the overall size of the distended uterus is generally smaller.

Fusion anomalies of the uterus result in a spectrum of findings. Complete lack of fusion of the müllerian ducts results in uterine didelphia, which is complete duplication of the uterus, cervix, and vagina. Partial duplication with varying degrees of septation of the endometrial cavity is much more common. These abnormalities sometimes are identified sonographically as a wide transverse diameter of the uterus, and two endometrial canals occasionally can be seen (Fig. 21-31). Hysterosalpingography provides a more definitive depiction of the configuration of the endometrial cavities (Fig. 21-32). Correlation between sonographic and hysterosalpingographic findings is especially important in those patients who have an associated obstructive lesion (hematometra) and a duplication anomaly.

UTERINE MASSES

Leiomyoma is the most common benign neoplasm of the uterus. Commonly asymptomatic, leiomyomas may be multiple; when they are symptomatic, pain and abnormal uterine bleeding are present.

When large enough, they can be identified on plain films as a soft-tissue mass. However, they frequently contain calcification in a characteristic "popcorn" configuration (Fig. 21-33). Lesser degrees of calcification are more easily identified on CT. Typical sonographic appearance is that of a hypoechoic mass (Fig. 21-34). The typical MRI appearance of a nondegenerated myoma is a well-circumscribed mass that has low signal intensity on both T1- and T2-weighted images (Fig. 21-34).[98] The degree of deformity of the uterine contour depends on the size and location of the leiomyoma. Subserosal leiomyomas may be pedunculated and may project in an exophytic manner from the uterine surface. Intramural myomas are more common and may result in a more diffuse enlargement of the uterus with or without displacement of the endometrial canal. Calcification is identified as a very bright echo with distal acoustical shadowing.

Carcinoma of the endometrium is the most common malignant neoplasm of the uterine body. The patient typically has abnormal postmenopausal bleeding. The

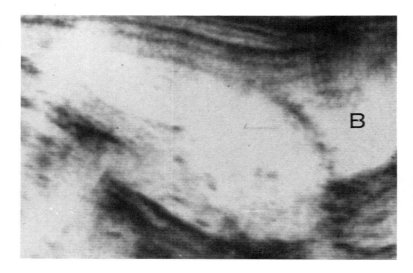

Figure 21–30. Hematometra. Sagittal view of the pelvis shows a thick-walled, fluid-filled structure with some internal debris, which is a distended, blood-filled uterus in a patient with vaginal agenesis. *B* indicates the bladder.

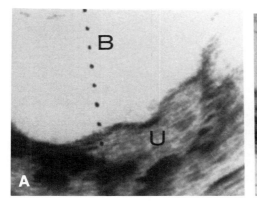 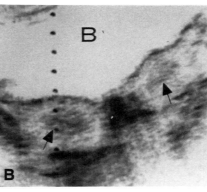

Figure 21–31. Uterine fusion anomaly. **(A)** Transverse sonogram of the lower uterus (*U*) shows broad bilobed appearance. **(B)** Transverse section 2 cm more cephalad demonstrates separation of the two uterine cornua, each with a endometrial cavity (*arrows*). The bladder is at *B*.

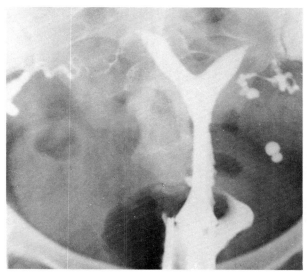

Figure 21–32. Uterine fusion anomaly. Hysterosalpingogram of a patient other than that in Figure 21-31 shows a bicornuate uterine configuration.

diagnosis is usually made by direct examination of the endometrial tissue obtained by endometrial curettage or biopsy. Generally, no changes are evident on plain x-ray studies of the pelvis. The diagnosis may be suggested sonographically when an enlarged uterus with distorted endometrial echoes is visualized. Other find-

ings include an inhomogeneous or hypoechoic pattern of the myometrium, a hypoechic ring surrounding a widened endometrial cavity, or a widened fluid-filled endometrial cavity due to the presence of hematometra.

Ultrasonography,[158] CT (Fig. 21-35),[185] and MRI[24, 97, 153] are helpful in staging endometrial cancer. Table 21-5 lists a commonly used staging classification system for carcinoma of the uterus. CT and probably MRI are useful in detecting disease that extends to the lateral pelvic sidewall and adjacent organs. Metastatic adenopathy can be identified only as nodal enlargement. The images that are obtained as an aid in staging known uterine neoplasm are also helpful for planning radiation therapy.

Carcinoma of the cervix is the second most common uterine neoplasm. It is usually diagnosed by direct observation of the cervix and sampling of the cervical epithelium for histologic analysis. Imaging examinations do not play a significant role in the de novo diagnosis of carcinoma of the cervix. Once a diagnosis is made, imaging of the pelvis is helpful in staging carcinoma of the cervix. Table 21-6 lists the staging criteria for invasive carcinoma of the cervix. CT (Fig. 21-36) and probably MRI are the best imaging examinations to aid in clinical staging.[165, 177, 189] In an adult, if a hematometrium or pyometrium is identified sonographically, it should raise suspicion of carcinoma of the cervix as the cause of the cervical obstruction. Imaging examinations for staging are probably not indicated for carcinoma in situ. MRI is more sensitive than CT in

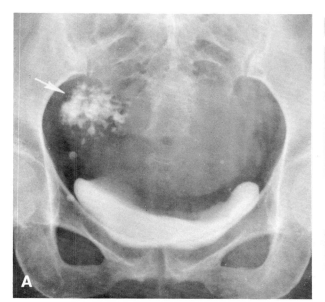
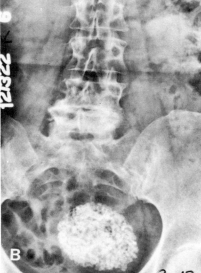

Figure 21–33. Uterine leiomyoma. (**A**) Mottled calcification characteristic of a leiomyoma of the uterus (*arrow*). The soft-tissue mass above the bladder is the enlarged uterus. This film was obtained during excretory urography. (**B**) Large, densely calcified uterine leiomyoma.

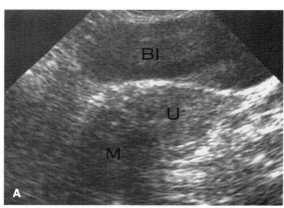

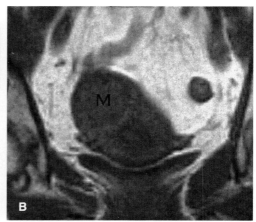

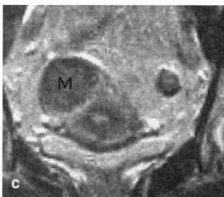

Figure 21–34. Leiomyoma (**A**) Transverse sonogram shows a hypoechoic mass (*M*) projecting from the right side of the uterus (*U*). *Bl* indicates the bladder. Coronal T1-weighted (**B**) and T2-weighted (**C**) MR images show the mass (*M*) is of low signal intensity on both pulse sequences.

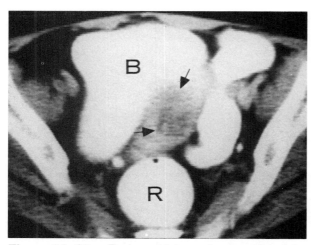

Figure 21–35. Endometrial carcinoma. CT of the pelvis demonstrates an irregular, low-attenuation region within the central uterus (*arrows*) in a patient with biopsy-proven adenocarcinoma of the endometrium. This appearance is not necessarily pathognomonic for cancer. The bladder is at *B*, and the rectum is at *R*.

distinguishing the exact degree of extension of cervical neoplasm beyond the confines of the cervix (Fig. 21-37).[108] Extension to the contiguous organs and to the pelvic sidewalls can be identified with both modalities, and the presence of enlarged lymph nodes is indicative of lymphatic spread. As with carcinoma of the endometrium, the staging examinations can be used for planning radiation therapy and are useful for

Table 21–5. Classification for Staging of Uterine Carcinoma

Stage 0	Histologic findings suggestive of malignancy but not proved (complex forms of atypia)
Stage I	Carcinoma confined to the body of the uterus
Stage II	Carcinoma involving the body and cervix
Stage III	Carcinoma extending outside the uterus but not outside the true pelvis
Stage IV	Carcinoma extending outside the true pelvis or involving the mucosa of the bladder or rectum

International Federation of Gynecology and Obstetrics: Classification and staging of malignant tumors of the female pelvis. J Int Fed Gynecol Obstet 3:204, 1965

Table 21–6. Classification for Staging of Cervical Carcinoma

Stage 0	Carcinoma in situ
Stage I	Carcinoma strictly confined to cervix IA: lesions less than 2 cm IB: lesions greater than 2 cm
Stage II	Carcinoma extends beyond cervix but has not reached pelvic wall or involves vagina but not lower third IIA: medial parametrial extension IIB: lateral parametrial involvement
Stage III	Carcinoma has extended onto pelvic wall or lower third of vagina
Stage IV	Carcinoma involves mucosa of bladder or rectum or has extended beyond limits of true pelvis

International Federation of Gynecology and Obstetrics: Classification and staging of malignant tumors of the female pelvis. J Int Fed Gynecol Obstet 3:204, 1965

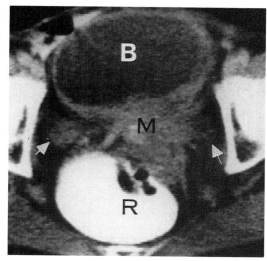

Figure 21–36. Carcinoma of the cervix. CT of the pelvis demonstrates an irregular soft-tissue mass (*M*) originating from the cervix. It invades the posterior wall of the bladder (*B*), extends to both pelvic sidewalls (*arrows*), and involves the rectum (*R*).

observing patients for progression or recurrence of disease.

Leiomyosarcoma is an uncommon malignant uterine neoplasm representing only 3% of uterine tumors.[184] Sonographically, these tumors demonstrate a heterogeneous echo pattern and may contain areas of calcification that exhibit acoustical shadowing. In most cases, the appearance is not sufficiently dissimilar from that of a leiomyoma to distinguish the two. The uterine mass, central calcification, and areas of low density representing hemorrhage and necrosis can be identified using CT as well.

OVARIAN MASSES

Ultrasonography is the best screening examination for a woman suspected of having an ovarian mass. The most common indication is a palpable abnormality at the time of routine physical examination. Unexplained

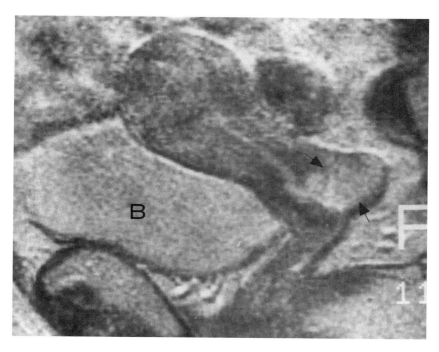

Figure 21–37. Carcinoma of the cervix. Sagittal MRI of the pelvis reveals an area of increased signal intensity (*arrows*), which pathologically corresponded to the limits of the carcinoma. *B* indicates the bladder; *F* indicates the foot. (Courtesy of J.R. Thornbury, MD)

pelvic pain and endocrine disorders are less common symptoms. Sonography is very sensitive for detecting ovarian masses; however, it is frequently not possible to make a specific pathologic diagnosis based on sonographic appearance alone. To narrow the sonographic differential diagnosis, it is extremely important to correlate with the clinical symptoms and signs. MRI is being used increasingly to evaluate pelvic masses. It is helpful in differentiating large uterine and ovarian masses,[187] and specific signal characteristics are associated with blood-containing masses, such as endometriomas, hemorrhagic cysts, some abscesses, and neoplasm.[134]

A useful method to separate various pathologic entities based on the ultrasound findings is studying the internal character of the mass.[71, 186] Cystic masses are fluid-filled structures that exhibit no internal echoes, have smooth walls, and display enhanced distal transmission of the sound (Fig. 21-38). Complex masses exhibit both cystic and solid characteristics (Fig. 21-39). They should be classed as primarily cystic with some solid elements, such as septa or internal debris, or as primarily solid complex masses with less dominant fluid-filled components. Solid masses that exhibit varying degrees of internal echoes in homogeneous or heterogeneous patterns constitute the last group (Fig. 21-40). Transvaginal ultrasonography can be used to

provide improved anatomic detail regarding the internal character of pelvic masses in ambiguous cases. Table 21-7 lists some common ovarian masses based on their sonographic characteristics. The same pathologic entity may be present in more than one group because of a variety of gross pathologic presentations. As mentioned, the clinical signs and symptoms are often helpful in the differential diagnosis.

Generally, cystic masses are benign. They can be followed conservatively if small enough. As the amount of solid tissue increases in complex masses and with heterogeneous-appearing solid masses, the potential for malignancy increases.[136, 157] The presence of ascites is not an absolute indication that an ovarian mass is malignant, although it is more commonly seen with malignant than benign ovarian masses.

Plain x-ray films of the abdomen are sometimes helpful in the diagnosis of ovarian masses. Dermoids frequently contain calcification that can be visualized radiographically. It can be curvilinear when located in the wall. Larger calcifications and areas of ossification can be seen as well, at times resembling teeth (Fig. 21-41). Fine, sandlike psammomatous calcification can be seen in papillary cystadenoma, papillary cystadenocarcinoma, and ovarian thecomas. Gonadoblastoma may contain a small circumscribed, mottled pattern of calcification. Mucinous cystadenocarcinomas may be

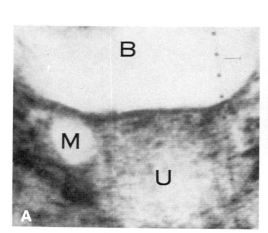

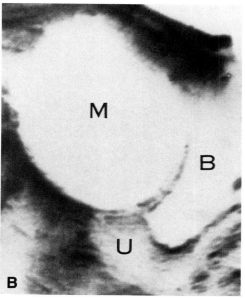

Figure 21–38. Cystic ovarian masses. **(A)** Follicular cyst. Transverse sonogram of the pelvis shows an anechoic, smooth-walled structure (*M*) with enhanced transmission of sound. The uterus (*U*) and the bladder (*B*) are also seen. **(B)** Cystic dermoid. Sagittal sonogram of the pelvis reveals a large cystic mass (*M*) separate from the uterus (*U*). The bladder is at *B*.

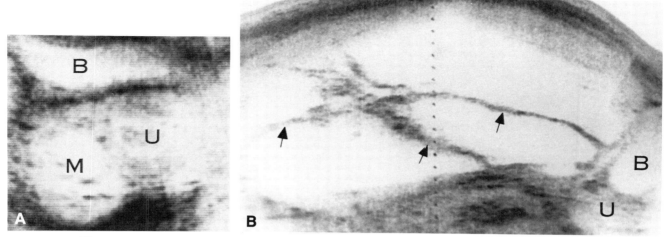

Figure 21–39. Complex masses. **(A)** Tubo-ovarian abscess. Transverse sonogram of the pelvis shows a primarily cystic complex mass (*M*) with internal septa and debris attached to the right side of the uterus (*U*). *B* indicates the bladder. **(B)** Mucinous cystadenoma. Sagittal sonogram of the abdomen shows a large complex mass that fills most of the abdomen. The multiple internal septa (*arrows*) characterize this as a complex mass. The bladder (*B*) and uterus (*U*) are at the lower right.

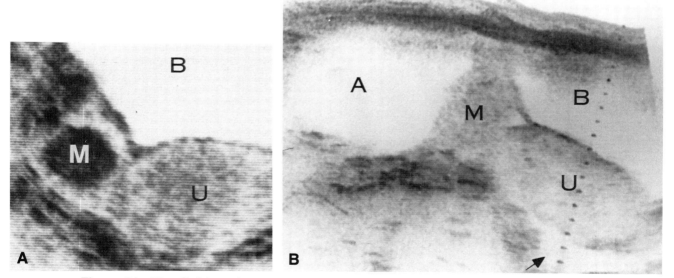

Figure 21–40. Solid ovarian masses. **(A)** Dermoid. Transverse sonogram of the pelvis shows a hyperechoic mass (*M*) in the right adnexal region. This is a common appearance of solid ovarian dermoids. The bladder (*B*) and uterus (*U*) are indicated. **(B)** Adenocarcinoma of the ovary. Sagittal sonogram shows a solid mass (*M*) near the fundus of the uterus (*U*). Ascites (*A*) is present in the lower abdomen and posterior cul-de-sac (*arrow*). The bladder is at *B*.

Table 21–7. Ovarian (Adnexal*) Masses Based on Ultrasound Appearance

CYSTIC	COMPLEX (PRIMARILY CYSTIC)
Functional ovarian cyst	Cystic teratoma
Corpus luteum cyst	Hemorrhagic cyst
Paraovarian cyst*	Infarcted cyst
Serous cystadenoma	Cystadenocarcinoma
Endometrioma	Endometrioma
Hydrosalpinx*	Theca lutein cysts
Dermoid cyst	Tubo-ovarian abscess*
	Ectopic pregnancy*
COMPLEX (PRIMARILY SOLID)	Bowel*
Cystadenocarcinoma	SOLID
Germ cell tumor	Fibroma
Teratoma	Brenner tumor
Endometrioma	Teratoma
Ectopic pregnancy*	Granulosa–theca cell tumor
Tubo-ovarian abscess*	Arrhenoblastoma
Bowel*	Adenocarcinoma
	Clear cell carcinoma
	Dysgerminoma
	Endodermal sinus tumor
	Lymphoma
	Metastatic tumor
	Bowel*

*Not a primary ovarian mass, but may simulate one sonographically.

calcified as well. However, the small calcified metastatic tumor deposits are better seen with CT.

In patients suspected of having an ovarian malignancy, further evaluation by ultrasonography or CT is indicated. Malignant ovarian neoplasm tends to spread throughout the abdomen by direct growth or perito-neal seeding. Table 21-8 lists a commonly used classification system for malignant ovarian neoplasm. Large masses of metastatic tumor involving the omentum, bowel, or other peritoneal surfaces can be diagnosed by CT,[190] ultrasonography,[193] and MRI. However, these techniques are insensitive for detecting small peritoneal implants of tumor, which require direct visualization by laparotomy. The finding of ascites by ultrasonography is the most sensitive and reliable indicator of recurrent disease in a patient with known carcinoma of the ovary. Barium gastrointestinal studies may be helpful in delineating serosal involvement or invasion by directly contiguous tumor growth or metastatic peritoneal implants.

GESTATIONAL TROPHOBLASTIC DISEASE

Gestational trophoblastic disease affects 1 of every 1500 to 2000 pregnancies. It represents a spectrum of disease, including complete or classic hydatidiform mole, partial hydatidiform mole, hydatidiform mole with coexistent live fetus, invasive mole, and metastatic gestational trophoblastic disease (choriocarcinoma). All of these entities are accompanied by an elevated serum β-hCG level, which is a reliable marker for the bulk of the mass. The clinical hallmark is vaginal bleeding in the first trimester or early second trimester. The uterus may be appropriate, large, or small for dates depending on the class of trophoblastic disease. Patients may also exhibit symptoms of hyperemesis gravidarum or preeclamptic toxemia.

Complete or classic hydatidiform mole can be distinguished pathologically from partial or incomplete hydatidiform mole.[176] Histologically, a complete mole shows no fetal tissue or amniotic membranes, whereas

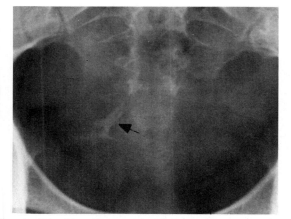

Figure 21–41.   Dermoid. Plain radiograph of the pelvis reveals a calcified structure (*arrow*) resembling a tooth.

Table 21–8. Classification for Staging of Carcinoma of the Ovary

Stage I	Growth limited to the ovaries IA: one ovary; no ascites IB: both ovaries; no ascites IC: one or both ovaries; ascites present with malignant cells in the fluid
Stage II	Growth involving one or both ovaries with pelvic extension IIA: extension and/or metastases to the uterus and/or tubes only IIB: extension to other pelvic tissues
Stage III	Growth involving one or both ovaries with widespread intraperitoneal metastases (the omentum, the small intestine, and its mesentery), limited to the abdomen
Stage IV	Growth involving one or both ovaries with distant metastases outside the peritoneal cavity

International Federation of Gynecology and Obstetrics: Classification and staging of malignant tumors of the female pelvis. J Int Fed Gynecol Obstet 3:204, 1965

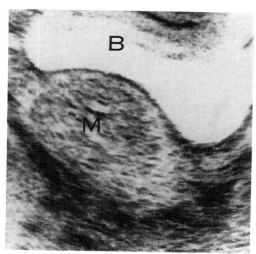

Figure 21–42. Hydatidiform mole. Sagittal pelvic sonogram shows enlargement of the uterus by a large, echogenic mass (*M*) located in the endometrial cavity. Some of the vesicles are large enough to be resolved. *B* indicates the bladder.

an incomplete or partial mole does. The classic mole most commonly has a 46, XX genotype, and partial moles have a polyploidy genotype. The gross pathology may be similar in both with vesicles of varying size, 2 mm early in the first trimester and up to 2 cm in the second trimester.

Sonography is the imaging modality of choice to confirm the presence of a hydatidiform mole.[139] The mole typically presents as an echogenic, solid-appearing mass that completely fills the endometrial cavity (Fig. 21-42). In the first trimester, when the vesicles are very small, they may not be individually resolved, but by the second trimester the appearance is more complex, with the vesicles reaching 2 cm. Larger hypoechoic areas represent areas of hemorrhage. Theca

lutein cysts of the ovaries are present in 20% to 50% of cases and are usually bilateral and multiseptated in appearance (Fig. 21-43). It is not possible at the time of the initial diagnosis to distinguish the various types of gestational trophoblastic disease reliably by the sonographic appearance. Sometimes an irregular, thickwalled gestational sac can be seen with a partial mole. At the time of initial ultrasound examination, the liver should be scanned for possible metastatic disease and a chest radiograph should be obtained before removal.

After evacuation of the mole, the most sensitive marker for residual disease is the serum β-hCG level. Sonography can be used to follow the decrease in uterine size and decrease in the size of the theca lutein cysts. Persistent or invasive disease can be identified sonographically as an area of increased echogenicity within the myometrium. CT and color-flow ultrasonography can also be useful in identifying the vascular myometrial lesions. In patients whose β-hCG level fails to return to normal within 8 to 12 weeks after evacuation, further imaging evaluation with a chest radiograph, cranial CT scan, liver CT scan, and pelvic sonography is indicated. These represent the most common sites of metastatic disease and will help to classify the patient as high or low risk.[195]

A mole with a coexistent live fetus is very uncommon. It may originate from a primary twin gestation in which one fetus developed from one fertilized ovum and the other developed into molar disease. This type of mole most commonly is a classic type. Others may have started as a single pregnancy with portions of the placenta undergoing molar degeneration. This most commonly is a partial mole.

INFERTILITY

Infertility is usually defined as a failure to achieve conception during the 1-year period in which no contraception is used. With increasing use of modern techniques of tubal reimplantation, pharmacologically in-

Figure 21–43. Theca lutein cysts. Transverse sonogram of the lower abdomen cephalad to the uterus reveals bilateral, septated ovarian masses with a typical "spoke-wheel" pattern.

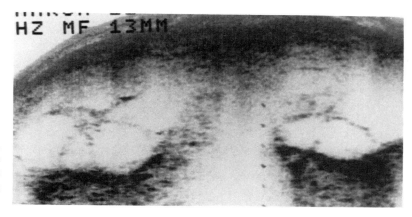

duced follicular development and ovulation, and in vitro fertilization, the role of diagnostic imaging in the diagnosis and management of patients with infertility has become increasingly important.[131]

Hysterosalpingography is the imaging modality of choice to exclude anatomic causes of infertility. Tubular obstruction secondary to previous pelvic inflammatory disease, surgery, or other causes can be identified as failure to confirm peritoneal spill of adequate amounts of contrast material. Uterine anomalies and intra-uterine synechiae as causes of infertility can also be diagnosed. Although initially performed as a diagnostic procedure, hysterosalpingography may also be therapeutic. Increased fertility rates have been reported after diagnostic hysterosalpingography in previously infertile couples with possible mechanisms of therapeutic action being mechanical release of small intra-tubal obstruction, release of peritubal adhesions, stimulation of the mucosal cilia, and an effect on the cervical mucus. This therapeutic effect occurs with both oil-based and water-soluble types of contrast material.[44, 124] Recently, direct transcervical catheterization of the fallopian tubes for selective salpingography and catheter dilatation of proximal obstructions have been performed with good results.[116, 179]

Diagnostic ultrasonography is used in the management of those patients undergoing pharmacologically induced follicular development.[69, 130] The number and size of the follicles are monitored on a daily basis (Fig. 21-44). Follicles are generally considered mature when they reach 18 to 20 mm. Ovulation is identified as a decrease in size of the follicle and the development of internal echoes secondary to hemorrhage. Ultrasonography can also be used to identify follicles suitable for percutaneous, transvaginal, or laparoscopic aspiration for in vitro fertilization.

PELVIC INFLAMMATORY DISEASE

Pelvic inflammatory disease refers to a spectrum of clinical entities affecting women of childbearing age. These entities usually arise from ascending infections first affecting the endometrium and then the fallopian tubes and adnexa. *Neisseria gonorrhoeae* is a common infecting organism; however, polymicrobial infections caused by both aerobes and anaerobes also occur. Untreated infections can spread from the endometrium out through the fallopian tubes and into the pelvic peritoneal cavity. If the fallopian tube becomes obstructed, a pyosalpinx may develop. In the pelvis, localized areas of inflammation can develop into tubo-ovarian or cul-de-sac pelvic abscesses. More extensive pelvic infections can spread along the pericolic gutters and involve the upper peritoneal cavity. Peritonitis localized to the right upper quadrant, which causes a perihepatitis leading to fever and abdominal pain, is the Fitz-Hugh-Curtis syndrome.

Sonography can be an important aid to the clinician in the diagnosis and management of pelvic inflammatory disease.[15] Early in the disease, no abnormality may be identified. With progression of the disease, the uterus becomes inhomogeneous, with patchy sonolu-

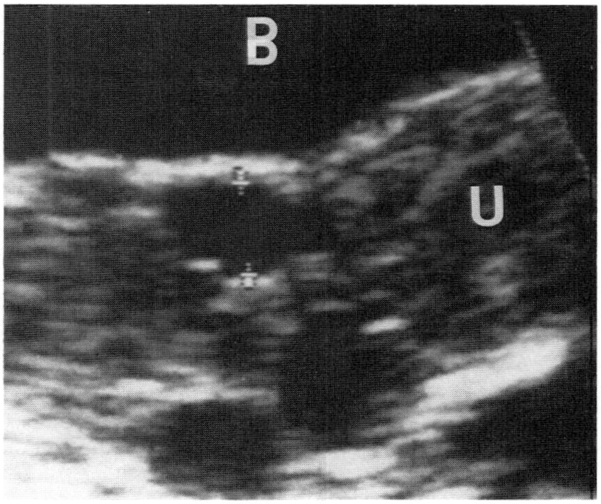

Figure 21–44. Follicles. Transverse sonogram of the right ovary shows three developing follicles in a patient undergoing Pergonal therapy for infertility. The cursors on the upper follicle are 10 mm apart. The bladder (*B*) and the uterus (*U*) are indicated.

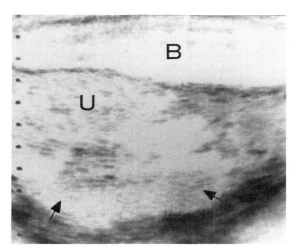

Figure 21–45. Pelvic inflammatory disease. Transverse sonogram of the pelvis shows an inhomogeneous, hypoechoic uterus (*U*) and a large, complex fluid collection with dependent debris (*arrows*). In this patient, multiple pelvic abscesses eventually formed. The bladder is at *B*.

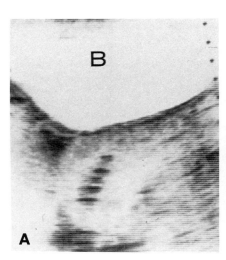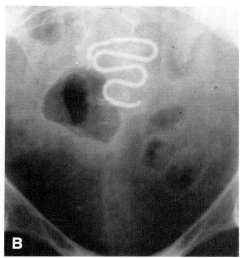

Figure 21–46. Intrauterine device. (**A**) Sagittal pelvic sonogram of a patient with a normally positioned Lippes Loop IUD. The uterus is retroverted in position. The bladder is at *B*. (**B**) Pelvic x-ray demonstrates the radiographic appearance of a Lippes Loop IUD. Note that the radiograph alone cannot confirm an intrauterine location.

cent areas. As infections spread into the pelvic peritoneal cavity, complex fluid may be identified in the posterior cul-de-sac (Fig. 21-45). When the infected fluid becomes localized to form an abscess, it generally appears as a complex mass with thick, irregular walls (see Fig. 21-39). This sequela of previous pelvic inflammatory disease can be identified sonographically as well. Hydrosalpinx appears as tubular or elliptical cystic mass located in the adnexal regions. Adhesions secondary to previous pelvic inflammatory disease are not easily identified sonographically. These inflammatory adhesions may cause loops of bowel to be attached to the uterus or adnexal structures and may simulate an abnormal pelvic mass. As mentioned, hysterosalpinography is the diagnostic test of choice to assess for tubal patency in patients who have had previous pelvic inflammatory disease. Ultrasonography is also useful in the management of patients who are undergoing treatment for pelvic inflammatory disease with antibiotics. The size of tubo-ovarian abscesses can be followed and used for guidance if percutaneous aspiration of abscess contents is desired.

LOCALIZATION OF INTRAUTERINE DEVICES

Intrauterine devices (IUDs) are a commonly used form of contraception. Most have an attached string or thread that extends through the cervical as into the vagina and is used to verify an intrauterine location of the device. When the thread is not palpated, the IUD is presumed to be "lost." The potential causes are unnoticed expulsion, misplacement within the uterus, perforation, or detachment of the thread. In these cases of lost IUD, some noninvasive method of localization is needed.

Sonography is the best method of confirming an intrauterine location of the IUD. IUDs appear as bright echoes in the endometrial cavity and have varying appearances depending on the type. Lippes Loop IUDs appear as a series of bright dashes on sagittal view (Fig. 21-46), whereas others, such as the Copper-7, have a more linear appearance. Careful scanning with a high-frequency transducer often demonstrates acoustic shadowing behind the IUD, which aids in differentiating it from the normally echogenic endometrial cavity.

If the IUD is not located within the uterus on ultrasound examination, a plain x-ray film of the pelvis is usually recommended if the patient is not pregnant. (There is a small but finite incidence of pregnancy with normally positioned IUDs.) Ultrasonography is not very useful for the detection of an IUD outside the uterus because of inability to distinguish the bright echoes of the IUD from pelvic soft tissues and bowel. If the IUD is not seen on the x-ray film, then it was inadvertently expelled from the uterus. If it is seen on the x-ray film, then perforation is likely. Further localization, if necessary, could be obtained with CT.

REFERENCES AND SELECTED READINGS

1. ALBRIGHT CB, CRANE JP, SHACKLEFORD GD: Prenatal diagnosis of bronchogenic cyst. J Ultrasound Med 7:91, 1988
2. ALEXANDER ES, SPITZ HB, CLARK RA: Sonography of polyhydramnios. Am J Roentgenol 138:343, 1982
3. ALLAN LD: Manual of Fetal Echocardiography. Lancaster, England, MTP Press, 1986

4. ARGER PH, COLEMAN BG, MINTZ MC, ET AL: Routine fetal genitourinary tract screening. Radiology 156:485, 1985

5. AYLSWORTH AS, SEEDS JW, GUILFORD WB, ET AL: Prenatal diagnosis of a severe deforming type of osteogenesis imperfecta. Am J Med Genet 19:707, 1984

6. BALCAR I, GRANT DC, MILLER WA, ET AL: Antenatal detection of Down syndrome by sonography. Am J Roentgenol 143:29, 1984

7. BARONE CM, VAN NOLTA FC, KOURIDES IA, ET AL: Sonographic detection of fetal goiter, an unusual cause of hydramnios. J Ultrasound Med 4:625–627, 1985

8. BAXI LV, YEH MN, BLARC WA, ET AL: Antepartum diagnosis and management of in utero intestinal volvulus with perforation. N Engl J Med 308:1519, 1983

9. BEAN WJ, CALONJE MA, APRILL CN, ET AL: Anal atresia: A prenatal ultrasound diagnosis. J Clin Ultrasound 6:111, 1978

10. BELLINGER MF, COMSTOCK CH, GROSSO D, ET AL: Fetal posterior urethral valves and renal dysplasia at 15 weeks gestational age. J Urol 129:1238, 1983

11. BENACERRAF BR, ET AL: Fetal ultrasound. Radiol Clin North Am 28:1, 1990

12. BENSON CB, DOUBILET PM: Doppler criteria for intrauterine growth retardation, predictive values. J Ultrasound Med 7:655, 1988

13. BERETSKY I, LANKIN DH: Diagnosis of fetal cholelithiasis using real-time high-resolution imaging employing digital detection. J Ultrasound Med 2:381 1983

14. BERGER MJ, TAYMOR ML: Simultaneous intrauterine and tubal pregnancies following ovulation induction. Am J Obstet Gynecol 113:812, 1972

15. BERLAND LL, LAWSON TL, FOLEY WD, ET AL: Ultrasound evaluation of pelvic infections. Radiol Clin North Am 20:367, 1982

16. BERTINO RE, NYBERG DA, CYR DR, ET AL: Prenatal diagnosis of agenesis of the corpus callosum. J Ultrasound Med 7:251, 1988

17. BOCIAN M, PATEL J: Ultrasonographic detection of fetal soft tissue swelling in the midtrimester: Correlation with trisomy 18. Birth Defects 18:165, 1982

18. BOOMSMA JHB, WEARNHOFF RA, POLMAN HA: Sonographic appearance of annular pancreas in utero. Diagn Imaging 51:288, 1982

19. BOVICELLI L, RIZZO N, ONSINI LF, ET AL: Ultrasonic real-time diagnosis of fetal hydrothorax and lung hypoplasia. J Clin Ultrasound 9:253, 1981

20. BOWIE JD, ANDREOTTI RF: Estimating gestational age in utero. In Callen PW (ed): Ultrasonography in Obstetrics and Gynecology, pp. 325–334 Philadelphia, W. B. Saunders, 1983

21. BOYCHUK RB, LYONS EA, GOODHAND TK: Duodenal atresia diagnosed by ultrasound. Radiology 127:500, 1978

22. BRADLEY WG, FISKE CE, FILLY RA: Double sac sign of an early intrauterine pregnancy: Use in exclusion of ecoptic pregnancy. Radiology 143:223, 1982

23. BRENNAN JN, DIWAN RV, ROSEN MG, ET AL: Fetofetal transfusion syndrome: Prenatal ultrasonographic diagnosis. Radiology 143:535, 1982

24. BRYAN PJ, BUTLER HE, LIPUMA JP: Magnetic resonance imaging of the pelvis. Radiol Clin North Am 22:896, 1984

25. CAMPBELL S, PYRSE DAVIES J, COLTART TM, ET AL: Ultrasound in the diagnosis of spina bifida. Lancet 1:1065, 1975

26. CAMPBELL S, THORNS A: Ultrasound measurement of fetal head to abdomen circumference in the assessment of growth retardation. Br J Obstet Gynecol 84:165, 1977

27. CARRASCO CR, STIERMAN ED, HARNSBERGER HR, ET AL: An algorithm for prenatal diagnosis of congenital CNS abnormalities. J Ultrasound Med 4:163, 1985

28. CARROLL B: Duplex Doppler systems in obstetric ultrasound. Radiol Clin North Am 28:189, 1990

29. CAYEA PD, BALCAR I, ALBERTI O, ET AL: Prenatal diagnosis of semilobar holoprosencephaly. Am J Roentgenol 142:401, 1984

30. CHAPMAN MG, FURNESS ET, JONES WR: Significance of the ultrasound location of placental site in early pregnancy. Br J Obstet Gynaecol 86:846, 1979

31. CHATTERJEE MS, TEJANI NA, VERMA UL, ET AL: Prenatal diagnosis of triploidy. Int J Gynecol Obstet 21:155, 1983

32. CHEN H, HY CW, WOOD WJ, ET AL: Mosaic trisomy 19 syndrome. Ann Genet 24:32, 1981

33. CHERVENAK FA, BERKOWITZ RL, TORTORA M, ET AL: Diagnosis of ventriculomegaly before fetal viability. Obstet Gynecol 64:652, 1984

34. CHERVENAK FA, JEANTY P, CANTRAINE F, ET AL: The diagnosis of fetal microcephaly. Am J Obstet Gynecol 149:512, 1984

35. CHINN DH, BOLDING DB, CALLEN PW, ET AL: Ultrasonographic demonstration of fetal lower extremity ossification center. Radiology 147:815, 1983

36. CHINN DH, FILLY RA, CALLEN PW, ET AL: Congenital diaphragmatic hernia diagnosed prenatally by ultrasound. Radiology 148:119, 1983

37. CHITKARA U, BERKOWITZ GS, LEVINE R, ET AL: Twin pregnancy: Routine use of ultrasound examinations in the prenatal diagnosis of intrauterine growth retardation and discordant growth. Am J Perinatol 2:49, 1985

38. CHITKARA U, COGSWELL C, NORTON K, ET AL: Choroid plexus cysts in the fetus—a benign anatomic variant or pathologic entity? Report of 41 cases and review of the literature. Obstet Gynecol 72:185, 1988

39. CHRISTOPHER CR, SPINELLI A, SEVERT D: Ultrasonic diagnosis of prune-belly syndrome. Obstet Gynecol 59:393, 1982

40. COADY DJ, SYNDER JR, LUSTIG-GILLMAN I, ET AL: Hydranencephaly: Prenatal and neonatal ultrasonographic appearance. Am J Perinatol 2:228, 1985

41. COCHLIN DL: Ultrasound of the fetal spine. Clin Radiol 33:641, 1982

42. COHEN-OVERBECK T, PEARCE JM, CAMPBELL S: The antenatal assessment of uteroplacental and fetoplacental blood flow using Doppler ultrasound. Ultrasound Med Biol 11:329, 1985

43. COHEN HL, TICE HM, MARIDEL FS: Ovarian volumes measured by US: Bigger than we think. Radiology 177:189, 1990

44. COOPER RA, JABOMONI R, PIETERS CH, ET AL: Fertility rate after hysterosalpingography with Sinografin. Am J Roentgenol 141:105, 1983

45. CRENSHAW C, JONES DED, PARKER PT: Placenta previa: A survey of twenty years experience with improved perinatal survival by expectant therapy and cesarean section. Obstet Gynecol Surv 28:461, 1973

46. CUNNINGHAM ME, WALLS WI: Ultrasound evaluation of anencephaly. Radiology 11:165, 1976

47. DEFOORT P, THIERY M: Antenatal diagnosis of congenital chylothorax by grayscale sonography. J Clin Ultrasound 6:47, 1978

48. DEMPSEY PJ, HOBB HJ: In utero diagnosis of Dandy-Walker syndrome: Differentiation from extra-axial posterior fossa cyst. J Clin Ultrasound 9:403, 1981

49. DENHOLM TA, CROW HC, EDWARDS WH, ET AL: Prenatal sonographic appearance of meconium ileus in twins. Am J Roentgenol 143:371, 1984

50. DETER RL, HADLOCK FP, GONZALES ET, ET AL: Prenatal detection of primary megaureter using dynamic image ultrasonography. Obstet Gynecol 56:759, 1980

51. DETER RL, HARRIST RB, HADLOCK FP, ET AL: Longitudinal studies of fetal growth with the use of dynamic image ultrasonography. Am J Obstet Gynecol 143:545, 1982

52. DEVORE GR: The prenatal diagnosis of congenital heart disease—a practical approach for the fetal sonographer. J Clin Ultrasound 13:229, 1985

53. DEVORE GR, DONNERSTEIN RL, KLEINMAN CS, ET AL: Fetal echocardiography. Am J Obstet Gynecol 144:693, 1982

54. DEVORE GR, HAKIN S, KLEINMAN CS, ET AL: The in utero diagnosis of an interventricular systal cardial rhabdomyoma by means of a real-time directed M-mode echocardiography. Am J Obstet Gynecol 143:967, 1982

55. DEWBURY KC, ALURVIHARE APR, BIRCH SJ, ET AL: Prenatal ultrasound demonstration of choledochal cyst. Br J Radiol 53:906, 1980

56. DEWHURST DJ, BERGLEY JM, CAMPBELL S: Assessment of fetal maturity and dysmaturity. Am J Obstet Gynecol 113:14, 1972

57. DIAGNOSTIC ULTRASOUND IMAGING IN PREGNANCY: NIH Publication No. 84–667. Washington DC, US Department of Health and Human Services, 1984

58. DIAKOWMAKIS EE, WEINBERG B, MOULIN J: Prenatal sonographic diagnosis of a suprasellar arachnoid cyst. J Ultrasound Med 5:529–530, 1986

59. DIGIACINTO TM, WILLSCHER MK, CONWAY JC: Bilateral fetal hydroceles in ureter. Urology 5:532, 1980

60. DUBBINS PA, KURTZ AB, WAPNER RJ, ET AL: Renal agenesis: Spectrum of in utero findings. J Clin Ultrasound 9:189, 1982

61. DUNNE MG, JOHNSON ML: The ultrasonic demonstration of fetal anomalies in utero. J Reprod Med 23:195, 1979

62. ERIKSEN PS, PHILIPSEN T: Prognosis in threatened abortion evaluated by hormone assays and ultrasound scanning. Obstet Gynecol 55:435, 1980

63. FADEL HE, MARTIN S: Real-time sonographic diagnosis of fetal dysplastic kidney. Int J Gynecol Obstet 18:140, 1980

64. FARRANT P: The antenatal diagnosis of oesophageal atresia by ultrasound. Br J Radiol 533:1202, 1980

65. FEDERLE MP, COHEN HA, ROSENWEIN MF, ET AL: Pelvimetry by digital radiography: A low dose examination. Radiology 143:733, 1982

66. FILLY RA, CARDOZAS JD, GOLDSTEIN RB, ET AL: Detection of fetal central nervous system anomalies: A practical level of effort for a routine sonogram. Radiology 172:403, 1989

67. FILLY RA, CHINN DH, CALLEN PW: Alobar holoprosencephaly: Ultrasonographic prenatal diagnosis. Radiology 151:455, 1984

68. FILLY RA, GOLBUS MS, CAREY JC, ET AL: Short-limbed dwarfism: Ultrasonographic diagnosis by mensuration of fetal femoral length. Radiology 138:653, 1981

69. FLEISCHER AC, DANIELL JF, RODIER J, ET AL: Sonographic monitoring of ovarian follicular development. J Clin Ultrasound 9:275, 1981

70. FLEISCHER AC, KILLAM AP, BOEHM FH, ET AL: Hydrops fetalis: Sonographic evaluation and clinical implications. Radiology 141:163, 1981

71. FLEISCHER AC, WALSH J, JONES H, ET AL: Sonographic evaluation of pelvic masses: Method of examination and role of sonography relative to other imaging modalities. Radiol Clin North Am 20:397, 1982

72. FONG KW, ROHMANI MR, ROSE TH, ET AL: Fetal renal cystic disease. Am J Roentgenol 146:767, 1986

73. FOSTER MA, NYBERG DA, MAHONY BS, ET AL: Meconium peritonitis: Prenatal sonographic findings and clinical significance. Radiology 165:661, 1987

74. FRIED AM, WOODRING JH, SKIER RW, ET AL: Omphalocele in limb/body wall deficiency syndrome: Atypical sonographic appearance. J Clin Ultrasound 10:400, 1982

75. GLAZER GM, FILLY RA, CALLEN PW: The varied sonographic appearance of the urinary tract in the fetus and newborn with urethral obstruction. Radiology 144:563, 1982

76. GOLDBERT JD, CHERVENAK FA, LIPMAN RA, ET AL: Antenatal diagnosis of arthrogryposis multiplex congenita. Prenat Diagn 6:45, 1986

77. GOLDSTEIN RB, PODIASKY AE, FILLY RA, ET AL: Effacement of the fetal cisterna magna in association with myelomeningocele. Radiology 172:409, 1989

78. GOLDSTEIN SR, SUBRAMANYAM BR, RAGHAVENDRA BN,

ET AL: Subchorionic bleeding in threatened abortion: Sonographic findings and significance. Am J Roentgenol 141:975, 1983

79. GRANNUM PAT, BERKOWITZ RL, HOBBINS JC: The ultrasonic changes in the maturing placenta and their relation to fetal lung maturity. Am J Obstet Gynecol 133: 915, 1979

80. GRANNUM PAT, HOBBINS JC: The placenta. In Callen PW (ed): Ultrasonography in Obstetrics and Gynecology, pp 141–157. Philadelphia, WB Saunders, 1983

81. GREENBERG F, CARPENTER RJ, LEDBETTER DH: Cystic hydroma and hydrops fetalis in a fetus with trisomy 13. Clin Genet 24:389, 1983

82. GREENE MF, BENACERRAF BR, CRAWFORD JM: Hydranencephaly: US appearance during in utero evolution. Radiology 156:779, 1985

83. GRUENEWALD SM, CROCKER EF, WALKER AG, ET AL: Antenatal diagnosis of urinary tract abnormalities: Correlation with ultrasound appearance with postnatal diagnosis. Am J Obstet Gynecol 148:278, 1984

84. GRUNDY H, GLASMAN A, BURLBAW J, ET AL: Hemangiomas presenting as a cystic neck mass in the fetal neck. J Ultrasound Med 4:147, 1985

85. GUILIAN BB, ALVCAR DT: Prenatal ultrasonographic diagnosis of fetal gastroschisis. Radiology 129:473, 1978

86. HABIF DV, BERDON WE, YEH MN: Infantile polycystic kidney disease: In utero sonographic diagnosis. Radiology 142:475, 1982

87. HADLOCK FP, DETER RL, GARCIA-PRATT J, ET AL: Fetal ascites not associated with Rh incompatibility. Am J Roentgenol 134:1225, 1980

88. HADLOCK FP, DETER RL, HARRIST RB, ET AL: Fetal head circumference. Relation to menstrual age. Am J Roentgenol 138:649, 1982

89. HADLOCK FP, DETER RL, HARRIST RB, ET AL: The use of ultrasound to determine gestational age: A review. Med Ultrasound 7:95, 1983

90. HALL DA, HANN LE, FERNUCCI JT, ET AL: Sonographic morphology of the normal menstrual cycle. Radiology 133:185, 1979

91. HEATON FC, VAUGHN R: Intrauterine supraventricular tachycardia. Obstet Gynecol 60:749, 1982

92. HELLER RH, ADAMS JE, HIRSCHFIELD RL, ET AL: Ultrasonic detection of an abnormal mass in a fetus later shown to have trisomy 18. Prenat Diagn 1:223, 1981

93. HILL LM, BRECKLE R, CEHRKING WC: The prenatal detection of congenital malformations by ultrasonography. Mayo Clin Proc 58:805, 1983

94. HOBBINS JC, MAHONEY MJ: The diagnosis of skeletal dysplasias with ultrasound. In Sanders RC, James AE (eds): The Principles and Practice of Ultrasonography in Obstetrics and Gynecology, 2nd ed, pp 191–203 New York, Appleton-Century-Crofts, 1980

95. HOFF NR, MACKAY IM: Prenatal ultrasound diagnosis of intracranial teratoma. J Clin Ultrasound 8:247, 1980

96. HOHLER CW: Ultrasound diagnosis of intrauterine growth retardation. In Sanders RC, James AE (eds): The Principles and Practice of Ultrasonography in Obstetrics and Gynecology. Norwalk, CT, Appleton-Century-Crofts, 1984, pp 157–173

97. HRIAK H, STERN JL, FISHER MR, ET AL: Endometrial carcinoma staging by MR imaging. Radiology 162:297, 1987

98. HRIAK H, TSCHOLAKOFF D, HEINRICHS L, ET AL: Uterine leiomyomas: Correlation with MR, histopathologic findings and symptoms. Radiology 158:385, 1986

99. INTERNATIONAL FEDERATION OF GYNECOLOGY AND OBSTETRICS: Classification and staging of malignant tumors of the female pelvis. J Int Fed Gynecol Obstet 3:204, 1965

100. JAFRI SZH, BREE RC, SILVER TM, ET AL: Fetal ovarian cysts: Sonographic detection and association with hypothyroidism. Radiology 150:809, 1984

101. JEANTY P, ROMERO P: Obstetrical Ultrasound, p 233. New York, McGraw-Hill, 1984

102. JOHNSON JA, RUMACK CM, JOHNSON ML, ET AL: Cystic adenomatoid malformation: Antenatal diagnosis. Am J Roentgenol 142:483, 1984

103. JOHNSON ML, DUNNE MG, MACK LA, ET AL: Evaluation of fetal intracranial anatomy by static and real-time ultrasound. J Clin Ultrasound 8:311, 1980

104. JUHL JH: Obstetrical and gynecologic roentgenology. In Essentials of Roentgen Interpretation, 4th ed. Hagerstown, Harper & Row, 1981, pp 776–782

105. KATZ Z, LANCET M, KASSIF R, ET AL: Antenatal ultrasonic diagnosis of complete urethral obstruction in the fetus. Acta Obstet Gynecol Scand 59:463, 1980

106. KELLEY KM, MADDEN DA, ARCARESE JS, ET AL: The utilization and efficacy of pelvimetry. Am J Roentgenol 125:66, 1975

107. KELSEY CA: Essentials of Radiology Physics. St Louis, Warren H Green, 1985

108. KIM SH, CHOI BI, LEC HP, ET AL: Uterine cervical carcinoma: Comparison of CT and MR findings. Radiology 175:45, 1990

109. KING DL: Placental migration demonstrated by ultrasonography. Radiology 109:167, 1973

110. KLEINMAN CS, DONNERSTEIN RL, DEVORE GR, ET AL: Fetal echocardiography for evaluation of in utero heart failure—a technique for study of nonimmune fetal hydrops. N Engl J Med 306:568, 1982

111. KLEINMAN CS, HOBBINS JC, JAFFE CC, ET AL: Echocardiographic studies of the human fetus: Prenatal diagnosis of congenital heart disease and cardiac dysrhythmias. Pediatrics 65:1059, 1980

112. KLEINMAN CS, HOBBINS JC, LYNCH DC, ET AL: Prenatal echocardiography. Hosp Pract 15:81, 1980

113. KLINGERSMITH W, CIOFFI-RAGAN D: Schizencephaly: Diagnosis and progression in utero. Radiology 159:617, 1986

114. KURTZ AB, WAPNER RI, RUBIN CE: Ultrasound criteria for in utero diagnosis of microcephaly. J Clin Ultrasound 8:11, 1980

115. LAING FC, JEFFREY RB: Ultrasound of ectopic pregnancy. Radiol Clin North Am 20:383, 1982

116. LANG EK, DUNAWAY HE, RONIGER WE: Selective osteal

salpingography and transvaginal catheter dilation in the diagnosis and treatment of fallopian tube obstruction. Am J Roentgenol 154:735, 1990

117. LAUER JD, CRADOCK TV: Meconium pseudocyst: Prenatal sonographic and antenatal radiologic correlation. J Ultrasound Med 1:333, 1982

118. LAWSON TL, FOLEY WD, BERLAND LL, ET AL: Ultrasonic evaluation of fetal kidneys: Analysis of normal size and frequency of visualization as related to stage of pregnancy. Radiology 138:153, 1981

119. LEHR C, DIRE J: Rare occurrence of holoacardius acephalic monster: Sonographic and pathologic findings. J Clin Ultrasound 6:259, 1978

120. LEVI CS, LYONS EA, LINDSAY DJ: Early diagnosis of nonviable pregnancy with endovaginal US. Radiology 167:383, 1988

121. LEVI CS, LYONS EA, ZHENG XH, ET AL: Endovaginal US: Demonstration of cardiac activity in embryos of less than 5.0 mm in crown-rump length. Radiology 176:71, 1990

122. LUTHY DA, HALL JG, GRAHAM CB: Prenatal diagnosis of thrombocytopenia with absent radii. Clin Genet 15:495, 1979

123. LYONS EA, LEVI CS, GREENBERG CR: The abnormal fetus. Semin Roentgenol 27:198, 1982

124. MACKEY BA, GLASS RH, OLSON LE, ET AL: Pregnancy following hysterosalpingography with oil and water soluble dye. Fertil Steril 22:504, 1971

125. MAHONEY MJ, HOBBINS JC: Prenatal diagnosis of chondroectodermal dysplasia (Ellis-van Creveld syndrome) with fetoscopy and ultrasound. N Engl J Med 297:258, 1977

126. MAIN D, MENNUTI MT, CORNFIELD D, ET AL: Prenatal diagnosis of adult polycystic kidney disease. Lancet 2:337, 1983

127. MANNING FA, BASKET TF, MORRISON I, ET AL: Fetal biophysical profile scoring: A prospective study 1,184 high-risk patients. Am J Obstet Gynecol 140:289, 1981

128. MANTAGOS S, WEISS BR, MAHONEY MJ, ET AL: Prenatal diagnosis of diastrophic dwarfism. Am J Obstet Gynecol 139:111, 1981

129. MAYDEN KL, TORTORA M, BERKOWITZ RL, ET AL: Orbital diameters: A new parameter for prenatal diagnosis and dating. Am J Obstet Gynecol 144:292, 1982

130. MCARDLE CR, SEIBEL M, WEINSTEIN F, ET AL: Induction of ovulation monitored by ultrasound. Radiology 148:809, 1983

131. MENDELSON EB, FRIEDMAN H, NEIMAN HL, ET AL: The role of imaging in infertility management. Am J Roentgenol 144:415, 1985

132. MINHOFF H, SCHAEFFER RM, DELKE I, ET AL: Diagnosis of intracranial hemorrhage in utero after maternal seizure. Obstet Gynecol 65:225, 1985

133. MINTZ MC, ARGER PH, COLEMAN BG: In utero sonographic diagnosis of intracranial hemorrhage. J Ultrasound Med 4:375, 1985

134. MITCHELL DG, MINTZ MC, SPRITZER CE, ET AL: Adnexal masses: MR imaging observations at 1.5 T1

weight US and CT correlation. Radiology 162:319, 1987

135. MITTLESTAEDT CA, PARTAIN CL, BOYCE II, ET AL: Placenta previa: Significance in the second trimester. Radiology 131:465, 1979

136. MOYLE JW, ROCHESTER D, SIDER L, ET AL: Sonography of ovarian tumors: Predictability of tumor type. Am J Roentgenol 141:985, 1983

137. MUELLER CE: Intrauterine pseudogestational sac in ectopic pregnancy. J Clin Ultrasound 7:133, 1979

138. MUELLER F, AUBRY MC, GANER B, ET AL: Prenatal diagnosis of cystic fibrosis. Prenat Diagn 5:109, 1986

139. MUNYEAR TP, CALLEN PW, FILLY RA, ET AL: Further observations on the sonographic spectrum of gestational trophoblastic disease. J Clin Ultrasound 9:349, 1981

140. NICOLINI U, FERRAZI E, MINONZIO M, ET AL: Prenatal diagnosis of cranial masses by ultrasound: Report of five cases. J Clin Ultrasound 11:70, 1983

141. NYBERG DA, CYR DR, KACK LA, ET AL: Sonographic appearance of placental abruption. Am J Roentgenol 148:161, 1987

142. NYBERG DA, LAING FC, FILLY RA: Threatened abortion: Sonographic distinction of normal and abnormal gestational sacs. Radiology 158:397, 1986

143. NYBERG DN, MACK LA, HIRSCH J, ET AL: Fetal hydrocephalus: Sonographic detection and clinical significance of associated anomalies. Radiology 163:187, 1987

144. NYBERG DA, MACK LA, LAING FC, ET AL: Early pregnancy complications: Endovaginal sonographic findings correlated in human chorionic gonadotropin levels. Radiology 167:619, 1988

145. NYBERG DA, MAHONEY BS, PRETORIUS DH (EDS): Diagnostic Ultrasound and Fetal Anomalies—Text and Atlas. Chicago, Year Book Medical Publishers, 1990

146. O'BRIEN GD, QUEENAN JT, CAMPBELL S: Assessment of gestational age in the second trimester by real-time ultrasound measurement of femur length. Am J Obstet Gynecol 139:540, 1981

147. PARTAIN CL, JAMES AE, ROLLO FD, ET AL: Nuclear Magnetic Resonance Imaging. Philadelphia, WB Saunders, 1983

148. PATEL RB, GIBSON JY, D'CRUZ CA, ET AL: Sonographic diagnosis of cervical teratoma in utero. Am J Roentgenol 139:1220, 1982

149. PATTEN RM, VAN ALLEN M, MACK LA, ET AL: Limb–body wall complex: In utero sonographic diagnosis of a complicated fetal malformation. Am J Roentgenol 146:1019, 1986

150. PERONE N: A practical guide to fetal echocardiography. Contemp Ob Gynecol 1:55, 1988

151. PHILLIPS HE, MCHAHAM JP: Intrauterine fetal cystic hygromas: Sonographic detection. Am J Roentgenol 136:799, 1981

152. PLATT LD, MANNING FA, MURATA Y, ET AL: Diagnosis of fetal death in utero by real-time ultrasound. Obstet Gynecol 55:191, 1980

153. POSNIAK HV, OLSON MC, DUDIAK CM, ET AL: MR

imaging of uterine carcinoma: Correlation with clinical and pathologic findings. Radiographics 10:15, 1990

154. PRETORIUS DH, DAVIS K, MANCO-JOHNSON ML, ET AL: Clinical course of fetal hydrocephalus: 40 cases. AJNR 6:23, 1985

155. PRETORIUS DH, MEIER PM, JOHNSON ML: Diagnosis of esophageal atresia in utero. J Ultrasound Med 2:475, 1983

156. RAABE RD, HARNOBERGER HR, LEE TG, ET AL: Ultrasonographic antenatal diagnosis of "mermaid syndrome:" Fusion of fetal lower extremities. J Ultrasound Med 2:463, 1983

157. REQUARD C, METTLER FA, WICKS JD: Preoperative sonography of malignant ovarian neoplasms. Am J Roentgenol 137:79, 1981

158. REQUARD C, WICKS JD, METTLER FA: Ultrasonography in the staging of endometrial adenocarcinoma. Radiology 140:781, 1981

159. ROBERTS C: Intrauterine diagnosis of omphalocele. Radiology 127:762, 1978

160. ROBINOW M, SPISSO R, BUSHI AJ, ET AL: Turner syndrome: Sonography showing fetal hydrops simulating hydramnios. Am J Roentgenol 135:846, 1980

161. ROBINSON HP: Gestational sac volume as determined by sonar in the first trimester of pregnancy. Br J Obstet Gynaecol 82:100, 1975

162. ROBINSON HP, FLEMING JEE: A critical evaluation of sonar "crown-rump length" measurements. Br J Obstet Gynaecol 82:702, 1975

163. ROMERO R, CHERVENAK FA, KOTZEN J, ET AL: Antenatal sonographic findings of extralobar pulmonary sequestration. J Ultrasound Med 1:131, 1982

164. ROMERO R, KADAR N, JEANTY P, ET AL: Diagnosis of ectopic pregnancy: Value of the discriminatory human chorionic gonadotropin zone. Obstet Gynecol 66:357, 1985

165. RUBENS D, THORNBURY JR, ANGEL C, ET AL: Stage IB cervical carcinoma: Comparison of clinical, MR, and pathologic staging. Am J Roentgenol 150:135, 1988

166. SABBAGHA RE, SKOLNIK A: Ultrasound of fetal abnormalities. Semin Perinatol 4:213, 1980

167. SCHINZEL A, SAVODELLI G, BRINER J, ET AL: Prenatal sonographic diagnosis of Juene syndrome. Radiology 154:777, 1985

168. SCHREIBER MH, MORETTIN LB: Antepartum prediction of fetal maturity. Radiol Clin North Am 5:21, 1967

169. SHEPARD MJ, RICHARDS VA, BERKOWITZ RC, ET AL: An evaluation of two equations for predicting fetal weight by ultrasound. Am J Obstet Gynecol 147:47, 1982

170. SILVER TM, WICKS JD, SPOONER WE, ET AL: Prenatal detection of congenital heart disease. Am J Roentgenol 133:546, 1979

171. SPIRT BA, KAGAN EH, ROZANSKI RM: Abruptio placenta: Sonographic and pathologic correlation. Am J Roentgenol 133:877, 1979

172. STARK DD, MCCARTHY SM, FILLY RA, ET AL: Intrauterine growth retardation: Evaluation by magnetic resonance. Work in progress. Radiology 155:425, 1985

173. STARK DD, MCCARTHY SM, FILLY RA, ET AL: Pelvimetry by magnetic resonance imaging. Am J Roentgenol 144:947, 1985

174. STEWART PA, WLADIMIROFF JW, GUSSENHOVEN WJ: Antenatal real-time diagnosis of a congenital cardiac malformation. Eur J Obstet Gynecol Reprod Biol 14:233, 1983

175. STRINGEL G, GILLIESON M, MURAM D, ET AL: Perinatal management of major gastrointestinal anomalies diagnosed by maternal ultrasound. Clin Pediatr (Phila) 22:564, 1983

176. SZULMAN AG, SURTI U: The syndromes of hydatidiform mole I. Cytogenic and morphologic correlations. Am J Obstet Gynecol 131:655, 1978

177. THICKMAN D, KRESSEL H, GUSSMAN D, ET AL: Nuclear magnetic resonance imaging in gynecology. Am J Obstet Gynecol 149:835, 1984

178. THORSEN MK, LAWSON TL, AIMAN EJ, ET AL: Diagnosis of ectopic pregnancy: Endovaginal versus transabdominal sonography. Am J Roentgenol 155:307, 1990

179. THURMOND AS, NOVY M, UCHIDA BT, ROSCH J: Fallopian tube obstruction: Selective salpingography and recanalization. Radiology 163:511, 1987

180. UNITED NATIONS SCIENTIFIC COMMITTEE ON THE EFFECTS OF ATOMIC RADIATION 1977 REPORT TO THE GENERAL ASSEMBLY. Sources and Effects of Ionizing Radiation. New York, United Nations, 1977

181. VALDES C, MALINI S, MALINAK LR: Ultrasound evaluation of female genital tract anomalies: A review of 64 cases. Am J Obstet Gynecol 149:285, 1984

182. VINTZILEOS AM, CAMPBELL WA, INGARDIA CJ, ET AL: The fetal biophysical profile and its predictive value. Obstet Gynecol 62:271, 1983

183. VINTZILEOS AM, HOVICK TS, ESCOTO DT, ET AL: Congenital midline porencephaly—prenatal sonographic findings and review of the literature. Am J Perinatol 4:125, 1987

184. WALSH JW, BREWER WH, SCHNEIDER V: Ultrasound diagnosis in diseases of the uterine corpus and cervix. Semin Ultrasound CT MR 1:30, 1980

185. WALSH JW, GOPLERUD DR: Computed tomography of primary, persistent, and recurrent endometrial malignancy. Am J Roentgenol 1339:1149, 1982

186. WALSH J, TAYLOR K, WASSON J, ET AL: Gray scale ultrasound in 204 proved gynecologic masses: Accuracy and specific diagnosis criteria. Radiology 130:391, 1979

187. WEIMEB JC, BARKOFF ND, MEGIBOW A, ET AL: The value of MR imaging in distinguishing leiomyomas from other solid pelvic masses when sonography is indeterminate. Am J Roentgenol 154:295, 1990

188. WEINSTEIN L, ANDERSON O: In utero diagnosis of Beckwith-Wiedemann syndrome by ultrasound. Radiology 134:474, 1980

189. WHITLEY ND, BRENNER DE, FRANCIS A, ET AL: Computed tomography of carcinoma of the cervix. Radiology 142:439, 1982

190. WHITLEY N, BRENNER D, FRANCIS A, ET AL: Use of computed tomographic whole body scanner to stage

and follow patients with advanced ovarian carcinoma. Invest Radiol 16:479, 1981

191. WICKS JD, HOWE KS: Fundamentals of Ultrasonographic Technique. Chicago, Year Book Medical Publishers, 1983

192. WICKS JD, LEVINE MD, METLER FA: Intrauterine diagnosis of ectopia cordia. Am J Roentgenol 137:619, 1981

193. WICKS JD, METTLER FA, HILGERS RD, ET AL: Correlation of ultrasound and laparotomy in patients with epithelial carcinoma of the ovary. J Clin Ultrasound 12:397, 1984

194. WIKLAND M, NILSSON L, HANSSON R, ET AL: Collection of human oocytes by use of sonography. Fertil Steril 5:603, 1983

195. WILLIAMS AG, METTLER FA, WICKS JD: Utility of diag-

nostic imaging in the staging of gestational trophoblastic disease. Diagn Gynecol Obstet 4:159, 1985

196. WILLIAMS RA, BARTH RA: In utero sonographic recognition of diastematomyelia. Am J Roentgenol 144:87, 1985

197. WLADIMIROFF JW, STEWART PA, VOSTERO RPL: Fetal cardiac structure and function as studied by ultrasound. Clin Cardiol 7:239, 1984

198. YEC CY, MEDRAZO B, DRUKKER BH: Ultrasonic evaluation of the postpartum uterus in the management of postpartum bleeding. Obstet Gynecol 58:227, 1981

199. ZIMMERMAN HB: Prenatal demonstration of gastric and duodenal obstruction by ultrasound. J Can Assoc Radiol 29:1338, 1978

The Chest

Paul and Juhl's Essentials of Radiologic Imaging, Sixth Edition, edited by John H. Juhl and Andrew B. Crummy. J.B. Lippincott Company, Philadelphia, © 1993.

CHAPTER **22**

Methods of Examination, Anatomy, and Congenital Malformations of the Chest

John H. Juhl

METHODS OF EXAMINATION

It is generally agreed that the radiographic examination of the chest is extremely important in the diagnosis of pulmonary disease. Its value is equally great in the diagnosis of diseases of the mediastinum and bony thorax. It is a very cost-effective study and the most frequently performed procedure in most departments. The chest roentgenogram serves as a record of the presence or absence of disease on the date it was taken, and follow-up examinations can determine progress or development of disease. On the other hand, the chest roentgenogram should not supplant routine physical examination and clinical history even though it is well established that this method will demonstrate lesions that cannot be found in any other manner. It is possible to make positive diagnoses of several conditions on the basis of chest roentgenograms alone, while in other instances a lesion is disclosed, the nature of which must be ultimately determined by bacteriologic, cytologic, or other laboratory studies. Cardiovascular disease can also be studied by radiographic and other imaging methods and is discussed in Chapter 32.

RADIOGRAPHY

Standard roentgen examination of the chest varies in different institutions but should consist of at least a posteroanterior and possibly a lateral projection. Most departments include a lateral film in the standard chest examination of patients with suspected thoracic disease, although some studies suggest that its value is limited, particularly in patients under 40 years of age.[12] It is not cost-effective in routine follow-up or screening studies. The chest radiographs are obtained at a tube-film distance of at least 6 feet to minimize divergent distortion and magnification as much as possible and are secured in full inspiration. Most radiologists prefer a high-voltage technique (120 to 150 kVp). This permits good penetration and visualization of retrocardiac and mediastinal structures. Chest radiographs taken at a higher voltage (350 kVp) have been used in some institutions. However, there is a difference of opinion as to the advantages of this method,[26, 53] and it is not generally employed. It is desirable to visualize the upper thoracic vertebral interspaces and to define clearly the vascular markings behind the heart (Fig. 22-1). It is also imperative to obtain films of sufficient penetration to permit identification of retrocardiac disease. Slight overexposure is preferable to underexposure since viewing in bright light may compensate for overexposure, but there is no way to compensate for underexposure. A stationary grid and ionization chamber timing are helpful in obtaining quality films. Fine-line grids do not detract appreciably from film quality but are not necessary when an air-gap technique is used.[63] It is advantageous to use copper wedge filtration of the x-ray beam to secure good mediastinal pene-

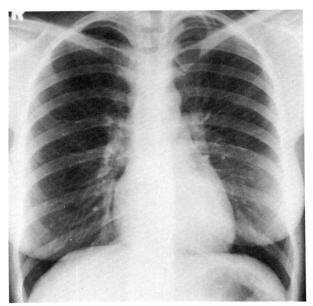

Figure 22–1. Normal chest. This frontal radiograph was obtained with a high-voltage technique. Note that the vascular markings at the left base are visible through the cardiac shadow. The upper thoracic intervertebral spaces are also visible.

tration. Some departments use a tunnel or trough filter for this purpose.

Several other views are used in special circumstances to outline local lesions or to visualize areas that are not well seen on the routine roentgenograms. Oblique projections are obtained at approximately 45° angles and are named according to the side of the chest nearest the film and away from the roentgen-ray tube. For example, the designation *right anterior oblique* indicates that the patient is standing with the right anterior chest wall in contact with the cassette holder at an angle of 45° so that the left posterior chest wall is nearest the tube; the rays then traverse the thorax from posterior to anterior in an oblique direction. Greater or lesser degrees of obliquity may be used as desired. When small nodules below the level of the dome of the diaphragm are poorly seen on routine examination, the tube may be angled upward or downward as necessary. Special views may also be obtained tangential to lesions of the thoracic wall to define them clearly.

The apical lordotic view is used to see disease in the pulmonary apices, which may be obscured by the clavicle and first rib. This roentgenogram is taken in an anteroposterior direction with the patient leaning backward on the cassette holder. An anteroposterior upright projection with the tube angled cephalad 15°

may be used when it is difficult or impossible to obtain a standard apical lordotic view. This is somewhat easier for the patient and is more readily reproducible. This projection results in clear visualization of the lung apices because the clavicle and first rib are projected above the pulmonary apex (Fig. 22-2).

The lordotic projection does cause difficulty in interpreting basal abnormalities because there is an apparent elevation of the diaphragm and poor visualization of basal disease. Also, the aortic arch may be poorly defined, an apparent superior mediastinal widening may be present, the left heart border may be indistinct, and the left hilum is projected caudally and may be hidden by the heart.[27] The anteroposterior supine view used for taking many portable films may also be taken inadvertently in a somewhat lordotic position. Many of the patients are in intensive care facilities for some severe problems and are candidates for basal pneumonia or atelectasis. When the tube is angled in a cephalad direction in these patients, the loss of left diaphragmatic definition may simulate these basal conditions. Therefore, care must be taken not to overlook this possibility.[70]

Lateral decubitus views are sometimes indicated to outline fluid levels in cavities or in the pleural space and to determine the presence of free pleural fluid. The films are exposed with the roentgen-ray beam directed in a horizontal plane with the patient lying on either the right or left side as indicated by the posteroanterior and/or lateral views. When there is any question of obstructive emphysema (overinflation) involving a lung, lobe, or segment, a film in complete expiration in addition to a film in inspiration is indicated. This combination can also be used to record diaphragmatic motion in conditions affecting the diaphragm on one or both sides.

Stereoscopic roentgenograms are used by some radiologists and are particularly helpful in localizing small solitary nodular lesions and in studying chronic pulmonary granulomatous diseases in which pulmonary opacities and cavities at varying depths can more readily be identified. Since there are two films, this method of examination also tends to eliminate the danger of misinterpreting an artifact. An automatic film changer is used and two films are exposed in quick succession. The patient remains stationary and the tube is shifted approximately one-tenth of the distance between the anode of the roentgen-ray tube and the film. There is some question as to whether this extra film is necessary and cost-effective, however, and routine stereoscopic radiographs have been discontinued in most radiology departments. It may be that stereoscopic radiographs are cost-effective in very high-risk patients for the detection of lung nodules.[33]

In the air-gap technique described by Jackson a 10-

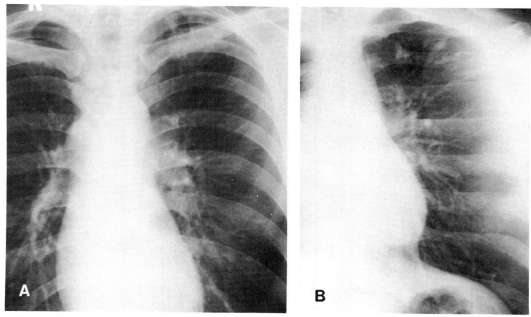

Figure 22–2. The value of the lordotic view is demonstrated. **(A)** In the routine frontal projection the disease at the left apex is partially hidden by the clavicle and first rib. **(B)** The lordotic view shows several irregular nodules in this patient with pulmonary tuberculosis.

foot distance from the focal spot of the tube to the film is used.[31] The patient is separated from the film cassette a distance of 15 cm by a suitable frame. Moderately high voltages are employed (average of 120 kVp for adults). There is no need for a grid. Jackson prefers to use the anteroposterior position. The outstanding advantage is the clarity of vascular markings in the lung.[63] Patient exposure to radiation is comparable to that of nongrid techniques and is less than that of grid techniques. The major disadvantage is the additional space required by the longer focal film distance. Direct magnification is another type of examination. Although used infrequently, it is of particular value in the examination of the chest of the newborn.[1] The object (chest)–film distance is increased in this technique, but focal spot size must be very small (0.3 mm or less) to avoid unacceptable lack of sharpness of the image.

The prone chest film is useful in patients in whom the lung bases are obscured by fluid. Simultaneous frontal and lateral views may be useful in evaluating heart size and lung volumes in infants with respiratory distress.[23] An anteroposterior view with the tube angled caudad about 30° may be used to define posterior pulmonary lesions obscured by the dome of the diaphragm on standard chest films, but it is seldom used since oblique and lateral films usually suffice. The angle may be altered to fit the situation if this method is

used. Supine radiographs are used extensively, especially in intensive care units, which have increased considerably in size and number in recent years. Technique is a problem, since patients often cannot cooperate very well. Therefore, shorter focal film distances are used; also, optimal equipment may not be available. High kilovoltage equipment is necessary to obtain good-quality films.

Newer techniques such as digitization and processing of x-ray exposures on a special cassette or digital processing of radiographs using a laser scanner show promise and may turn out to be very helpful in manipulating suboptimal supine films taken with portable equipment.[60] There is now a considerable interest in scanning systems and in production of digital images, directly and indirectly, in order to improve the diagnostic usefulness of chest images.[17, 52, 60] Slit radiography is also being studied, since decreasing scatter improves the image by improving contrast.[17, 61] Unsharp masking techniques also show promise when used with the digital chest scanning devices now being developed.[2] In these systems for chest imaging, the patient is exposed to an x-ray beam; the image is captured by a detector and digitized by an analog-to-digital converter. This processes the image, which can then be viewed on a video display terminal or recorded on film. Among the most promising are (1) film digitization; (2)

an image intensifier–based system; (3) phosphor plates, which are photostimulable[16]; and (4) a scanned projection system.[17] Advanced Multiple Beam Radiography (AMBER) uses an (effectively) patient-specific filter. Higher contrast film can be used.[64] The ultimate place of these and other new systems in chest radiography remains to be determined. None of them appears to be generally accepted now. However, many workers in the field believe that a cost-effective system will evolve and be generally accepted in the next two decades or so.

FLUOROSCOPY

There are several indications for fluoroscopy of the chest; they are discussed under the various conditions for which fluoroscopy is used. The dynamics of the cardiovascular system and respiration can be studied by this method. Fluoroscopy is also particularly useful in acute obstructive overinflation secondary to aspiration of a foreign body. Air trapping, regardless of cause, may produce mediastinal motion on respiration, which may be more readily apparent fluoroscopically than on films, particularly in children. Conditions affecting diaphragmatic motion are also indications for fluoroscopy of the thorax. Loculated effusions can be localized, if necessary, for thoracentesis. However, ultrasonography is now being used extensively for this purpose and carries no radiation hazard.

Since there are radiation hazards to both patient and physician in the use of fluoroscopy, it is important to reduce radiation to a practical minimum. Image intensification is used to improve visualization and to decrease radiation. It is necessary to have chest roentgenograms available for study and to know as much as possible about the patient's problem before beginning fluoroscopy. This avoids unnecessary search for a lesion that is much better examined by radiographic methods. It is necessary to use the smallest possible aperture and to limit the total fluoroscopic time in order to reduce radiation exposure. A built-in timer that indicates the duration of radiation exposure is the best method for timing fluoroscopy. We attempt to keep the total fluoroscopic time as low as possible and always less than 5 minutes.

The actual procedure used in fluoroscopy varies with the indication for it and with the examiner, but the examination should be systematic. For example, diaphragmatic motion is observed during normal and deep inspiration in the oblique as well as in the anteroposterior positions; slight weaknesses can often be detected by having the patient sniff. It is sometimes helpful to observe diaphragmatic motion in both lateral decubitus positions to detect small variations in motion on the two sides. Valsalva's maneuver (forced expira-

tion with the glottis closed) can be used to increase the intrathoracic pressure to empty or decrease the size of veins, cardiac atria, and arteriovenous malformations. Müller's experiment (forced inspiration with the glottis closed) can be used to decrease intrathoracic pressure and thereby increase the size of these thin-walled vascular structures. At times it is necessary for the patient to be examined while in the supine position, particularly when pleural effusion tends to obscure the diaphragm on one or both sides. Fluoroscopy of the chest is often useful but should be undertaken only when roentgenographic studies do not or cannot answer the question raised by the clinical problem at hand.

BRONCHOGRAPHY

Bronchography is the study of the bronchial tree by means of the introduction of opaque material into the desired bronchus or bronchi, usually under fluoroscopic control (Fig. 22-3).

INDICATIONS

At present, bronchography is used much less frequently than in the past, mainly because direct methods such as fiberoptic bronchoscopy with biopsy, brush biopsy, and percutaneous biopsy permit a tissue or bacteriologic diagnosis that is not obtained with bronchography. The procedure is rarely used at the institutions with which I have been associated in the last few years. According to some clinicians and radiologists, however, a few indications for its use remain and are described in the following paragraphs.

Bronchiectasis. Bronchography was used to map the entire bronchial tree of both lungs in patients with known bronchiectasis before surgical removal of involved lobes or segments since it might demonstrate unsuspected disease. Unless surgical resection is contemplated, there is no need to use this examination. Most patients are now treated medically so there is no need to know the exact extent of disease.

Suspected Bronchogenic Tumor. When clinical findings, computed tomography (CT), bronchoscopy, aspiration, and bronchial brushing fail to reveal the site of tumor in a patient with positive cytologic findings, bronchography may demonstrate enough abnormality to establish the site of the lesion and suggest the diagnosis.

Anomalies of the Bronchial Tree. Bronchography is the only method short of surgical exploration to determine the presence of various anomalies of bron-

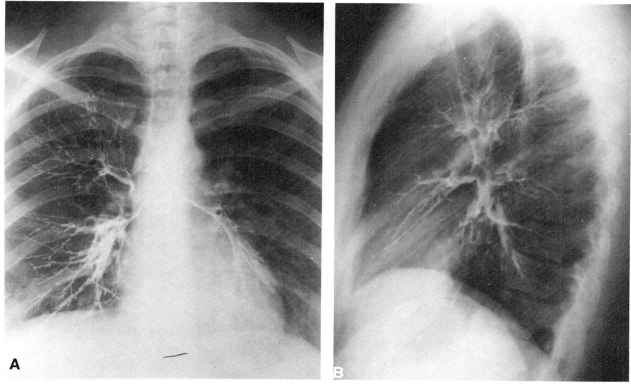

Figure 22–3. Normal bronchographic findings. Note that the iodized oil has coated the trachea and outlines the bronchi, which branch in a treelike manner into the lungs. The peripheral bronchi are somewhat better filled in the frontal (**A**) than in the lateral (**B**) projection.

chopulmonary segmentation, but it should be performed only if surgery is contemplated.

Selective Bronchography. Combined with Fiberoptic Bronchoscopy. This may be useful for the study of lesions beyond the subsegmental level.[41] Small stenotic lesions, bronchiectasis, and bronchial anomalies may be detected.[34]

CONTRAINDICATIONS

Respiratory Insufficiency. This is a contraindication to a degree related to its severity; eg, severe forms completely rule out the possibility of doing bronchography.

Allergy. Patients with bronchial asthma often tolerate bronchography poorly, and highly allergic individuals without asthmatic manifestations are also poor risks. The examination should not be performed on these patients unless it is essential. Known iodine sensitivity and sensitivity to local anesthetic agents are also contraindications.

Recent Hemoptysis. Hemoptysis of 2 ounces or more contraindicates bronchography for a time, but after the bleeding has stopped for 7 to 14 days it is usually possible to examine the patient. Minimal hemoptysis, even though repeated, is probably not a contraindication.

Infections. Acute pulmonary parenchymal infections, including acute lung abscess and chronic active infections, contraindicate bronchography.

TECHNIQUE

Numerous methods of performing this procedure have been described, and most of them are satisfactory in the hands of those who use them long enough to gain proficiency.

Dionosil (3,5-diiodo-4-pyridone-N-acetic acid) is the

contrast medium used most extensively. It contains 34% iodine and is available as an aqueous and an oily suspension. Since aqueous Dionosil is more irritating than Dionosil oily, the latter is used in most departments in the United States.

COMPLICATIONS

Anesthetic Reactions. The danger of anesthetic reactions can be minimized by proper premedication and by keeping the total amount of lidocaine (Xylocaine) used to less than 200 mg. The examination should be avoided in patients who have had previous reactions to local anesthetics.

Iodized Oil Reactions. Reactions to iodized oil are infrequent and relatively mild. Manifestations consist of bronchial asthma and urticaria; when these reactions are immediate, they can be treated by the use of antihistaminic drugs.

TOMOGRAPHY

Tomography has been largely replaced by CT but is still used occasionally by some in the study of hilar abnormalities. This is a method of radiographic examination by which it is possible to examine a single layer of tissue and to blur the tissues above and below the level by motion. This is accomplished by simultaneous motion of the roentgen-ray tube and the film cassette during the exposure by means of a connecting rod or bar. The tube and film move in opposite directions, and the fulcrum of the bar or rod connecting the tube and film carrier is placed at the level to be examined (Fig. 22-4). The amount of blurring depends on the distance of the object or tissue from the level of the fulcrum. The thickness of the plane of tissue examined is determined within certain limits by the distance traveled by the tube and film during the radiographic exposure. Zonography is a variation in which the thickness of the plane of tissue examined is increased by shortening the excursion of the tube. By raising or lowering the fulcrum, one can then examine planes of tissue within the chest at various levels as desired. Some manufacturers of radiographic equipment also make or distribute attachments for linear tomography. Special tomographic units allowing circular, elliptical, and hypocycloidal motion are also available. These pluridirectional units are preferred to the linear tomographic units,[40] since linear tomography does not represent planar anatomy as accurately as pluridirectional tomography. When whole-lung tomography is used, the anteroposterior projection is employed. Posterior oblique tomography at a 55° angle is preferred when the hilum is being studied.

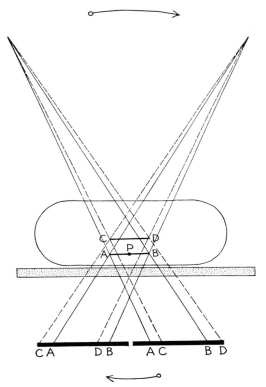

Figure 22–4. Diagram illustrating the principles of tomography. The upper arrow indicates the direction of the tube shift. The fulcrum is at the level *P* on line *AB*. Note that the relationship of the projected image of *AB* remains the same on the initial and final positions of the cassette, whereas the image of the line *CD* at some distance from the fulcrum has moved from right to left. Therefore, the tissues at the level of the fulcrum are clearly defined and those above and below it are blurred by motion.

There were many indications for tomography of the chest, but standard tomography has been replaced for most of them by CT. Some observers still believe that tomography remains superior to CT in the study of the hila in patients with suspected masses or other abnormalities. It is also a relatively inexpensive and effective way to study cavitary lesions of the lung.

COMPUTED TOMOGRAPHY

Although the ultimate place of CT scanning in all conditions involving the chest is not yet determined, many applications have been found for the use of this modality.[32, 59] In the *lung* it is of value in the detection of (1) *occult pulmonary neoplasms* in patients with positive cytologic or histologic findings and a normal chest film; (2) *pulmonary metastases* when surgery is contemplated for a primary nonpulmonary tumor, which often metastasizes to the lung; (3) *pulmonary metastases* in patients with a solitary nodular metastasis; and (4) *detection of calcium* in nodules when tumor is a possibility. It is helpful in guidance for needle biopsy when fluoroscopy is inadequate. It may also be helpful in the study of cavitary masses, peripheral lung tumors, and pulmonary collapse. In the *mediastinum*, it is useful in the study of causes for mediastinal widening and in differentiating cysts from solid tumors and fatty from nonfatty masses. In patients with myasthenia gravis, it can be used to evaluate possible thymic masses; in hyperparathyroidism it may be helpful in finding adenomas, particularly if they are ectopic and have not been located at surgery. In the *pleura*, plaques, masses, loculated fluid and occult calcification can be localized and the extent determined. In the *chest wall*, masses involving soft tissue, bone, spinal canal, and adjacent lung can be studied advantageously.

Additional uses include the study of trauma involving the pleura, chest wall, mediastinum, and lung. Diffuse pulmonary disease such as emphysema and bronchiectasis has been studied, but the ultimate place of CT in such conditions has not been determined. Since CT is not tissue specific, it is not adequate to stage mediastinal node involvement in patients with lung cancer but is very useful in mapping the nodes for biopsy guidance. In masses adjacent to the mediastinum and chest wall, invasion can be simulated because of lack of tissue specificity.

High-resolution thin-section CT is being used and studied in patients with chronic diffuse interstitial disease of the lung by Naidich (Radiology 171:22, 1989) and Müller and colleagues (Am Rev Respir Dis 142:1206 and 1440, 1990) among others. The findings are promising, but the ultimate place of this modality in clinical pulmonology is yet to be determined.

ULTRASONOGRAPHY OF THE THORAX

Ultrasonography, particularly real-time scanning, is noninvasive and may be very useful in certain conditions. There is no radiation exposure of the patient. It is used in patients with pleural disease. Fluid can be detected, localized, and differentiated from solid pleural masses and can be removed if necessary using ultrasound guidance. Fluid can also be detected in peripheral lung lesions in contact with the chest wall. Mediastinal cysts in contact with the chest wall can be differentiated from solid masses. Several conditions in and near the diaphragm can be detected, localized, and often diagnosed; these include loculated effusion (intrathoracic or subphrenic), or he-

patic abscess or cyst; and in some instances diaphragmatic rupture and hernia.

MAGNETIC RESONANCE IMAGING

The place of magnetic resonance imaging (MRI) in diseases of the chest has not yet been determined. Several obvious advantages of this modality include the following: (1) There is no radiation hazard or other known biologic risk at imaging levels now in use. (2) The images may be obtained without the use of mechanical motion devices and reconstructed in several planes as needed. (3) Intravenous contrast agents are not necessary to identify intrathoracic vascular structures.

Several disadvantages include the following: (1) Motion artifacts due to respiration and blood flow in the heart and major vessels cause degradation of the image. (2) Patients requiring cardiac monitoring and those with pacemakers, metal implants, or metal clips cannot be examined. (3) Biopsy and other interventional techniques are not possible with current equipment. (4) The time required is much greater than that for CT scanning. (5) Cost is currently higher than for CT scans.

It is possible and quite likely that some of these disadvantages will be overcome as technology and instrumentation improve, however. Currently, the major use of this modality appears to be in the examination of the mediastinum since no intravenous contrast material is necessary to differentiate vessels from other structures in the mediastinum. Flow patterns in the heart and great vessels can be studied using cardiac gating. MRI is also useful in the study of chest wall lesions, in part because of multiplanar capability. There is great potential, and the use of MRI in the study of intrathoracic disease, particularly in vascular structures and vascular anomalies, will very likely expand greatly in the future.

PULMONARY ANGIOGRAPHY

TECHNIQUE

The purpose of this examination is to outline the pulmonary arterial system (Fig. 22-5). This can be accomplished in several ways: (1) injection of contrast material into the superior vena cava using digital subtraction angiography (DSA); (2) injection of contrast material into the right atrium using DSA; (3) direct injection of contrast medium through a catheter placed in a main pulmonary artery; and (4) selective injection of contrast material into a pulmonary artery branch using DSA or balloon-occlusion cineangiography or serial filming.[15, 21]

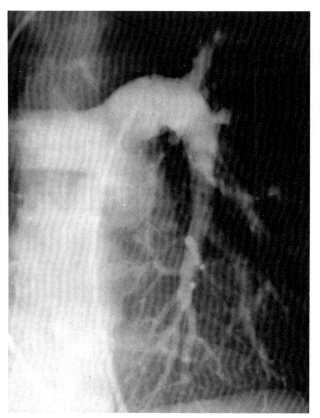

Figure 22–5.   Pulmonary arteriogram showing normal findings. This is an example of selective pulmonary arteriography. The catheter is seen to lie in the left pulmonary artery near its origin.

The nature of the process for which the procedure is performed tends to determine the method used. The advantage of DSA is that a very small amount of iodinated contrast material is necessary. The major disadvantages are artifacts produced by motion and the limited field of view. These may be overcome with the use of dual energy rather than temporal subtraction and a large field image intensifier.

INDICATIONS

Pulmonary angiography is used in the study of patients with suspected pulmonary arterial or venous anomalies or diseases. Most important is the study of thromboembolic disease of the lungs by means of pulmonary arteriography. The procedure is not used routinely but may be needed when the diagnosis remains in doubt following roentgen and scintiscan studies and when the patient is not responding to treatment for presumed pulmonary embolism.

BRONCHIAL ARTERIOGRAPHY

Bronchial arteriography requires selective catheterization of bronchial arteries. Its use in pulmonary disease is very limited.

PERCUTANEOUS TRANSTHORACIC NEEDLE BIOPSY

This method of examination is used extensively to obtain material for histologic and bacteriologic study. Indications include peripheral lung masses beyond the reach of fiberoptic bronchoscopy[5, 35] and focal or general pulmonary infections in the immunocompromised host.[65] In the hands of experienced operators, there is a high diagnostic yield and a low incidence of complications. The major complications are pneumothorax and hemorrhage. Pneumothorax is usually easily managed, but hemorrhage occurring after any of the percutaneous procedures can be difficult to manage and has been fatal in rare instances.[51] Therefore, these percutaneous procedures are contraindicated in patients with bleeding diathesis or thrombocytopenia, a suspected vascular lesion, recent severe hemoptysis, or severe dyspnea at rest as well as in those who cannot cooperate.

THE NORMAL CHEST

GENERAL CONSIDERATIONS IN CHEST INTERPRETATION

Interpretation of chest roentgenograms requires that the viewer first find the abnormality. It is useful to develop a method of studying the film to make certain that all areas are searched. The mediastinum, including the heart and great vessels, trachea and central bronchi, lungs, diaphragm, bony thorax, soft tissues of the thorax and neck, and subdiaphragmatic upper abdominal structures, should be inspected. It is helpful for the student or trainee to compare the two lungs interspace by interspace until the normal chest is thoroughly understood and variations and abnormalities can be recognized. Once an abnormality is observed, interpretation of the changes follows. We find it valuable to make the initial examination of the film without knowledge of the clinical findings. Before a decision is reached, however, roentgen observations must be correlated with all of the available clinical information. This requires a second study of the film, which has been found valuable in reducing errors. Specific questions may arise, the answers to which may not be available on the chart. Additional information must then be sought from the referring physician or from the patient.

In the chapters on chest roentgenology to follow, the presentation is disease oriented. Patterns of pulmonary opacities of various types are observed. The terms *interstitial* and *alveolar* are used to describe the predominant pattern of pulmonary involvement. The terms are not intended to indicate that the pathologic process is necessarily interstitial or alveolar in each instance. *Alveolar* or air-space pattern is characterized by homogeneous opacity, which may vary from a small area, just large enough to be recognizable, to consolidation of an entire lobe or more. The alveoli are filled with exudate, transudate, blood, or tissue, which replaces the air. When the lung parenchyma is opacified by some type of fluid, the *acinus* may be observed as the anatomic unit that initially appears as a rosette measuring 6 to 10 mm in diameter; later, when filling is more complete, it appears to be spherical. The acinus may be defined as the lung parenchyma distal to a terminal bronchiole. As parenchymal disease progresses, individual acini are obscured by the overlapping of many opaque acini; this results in uniform density of the lung affected. Classic *Streptococcus pneumoniae* pneumonia is a good example of the alveolar pattern. Bronchi may become visible when such consolidation occurs; the *air bronchogram* is then observed, which indicates adjacent alveolar disease.

Genereaux has analyzed diffuse lung disease, which he defines as an acute or chronic increase in radiographic density of lungs caused by fluid, cells, or other tissue elements in the small air spaces, interstitium, or both.[18] When distal air spaces are involved to a relatively minimal extent, acinar involvement causes a small nodule 4 to 10 mm in diameter with poor margination in which small radiolucencies are observed. The subacinar nodule is about the same size and configuration but contains many more radiolucencies than the acinar nodule. The subacinar nodule is interspersed against a background of tiny opacities, which cause a stippled, granular, or ground-glass appearance. The spoke-wheel nodule is infrequent, is difficult to define clearly, and consists of a central lucent area from which small linear radiolucencies radiate into the periphery. When these findings are minimal, it may be very difficult to differentiate the alveolar from the interstitial pattern.

Interstitial pattern is characterized by an increased prominence of the perivascular, interlobular, and parenchymal interstitial spaces. Alveolar aeration is maintained and the interstitial tissues increase in volume. The process may be localized, as in viral pneumonia, or general, as in extensive interstitial fibrosis. The pattern may range from reticular or latticelike to reticulonodular, nodular, linear, or various combinations of these findings. Genereaux subdivides reticular pattern into fine (such as in berylliosis) or micronodular, medium (3- to 10-mm cystic spaces), and coarse (large cystic spaces such as histiocytosis X) types.[18]

Combinations of interstitial and alveolar patterns may also occur. A common example of this is the patient with combined interstitial and alveolar pulmonary edema. Mycoplasmal and viral pneumonia are also sometimes observed to have a combined pattern.

The localization and at times the recognition of pulmonary disease depend in many instances on the *silhouette sign*. The term was coined by Felson, who credited Dr. H. Kennon Dunham with making the initial observations. Felson and Felson defined this sign as follows: "An intrathoracic lesion touching a border of the heart, aorta or diaphragm will obliterate that border on the roentgenogram. An intrathoracic lesion not anatomically contiguous with a border of one of these structures will not obliterate that border."[14] This principle is very useful in a variety of chest conditions. Relative density is also a factor, since juxtaposed borders of similar opacity will produce the sign. The borders of opacities that are markedly dissimilar may not be obscured. Furthermore, there must be sufficient exposure to penetrate the margins of the structures in question.

In addition to air flow into alveoli through the bronchial system, there is peripheral communication, which may explain normal aeration or sometimes hyperaeration that may be observed distal to an endobronchial obstruction. The pores of Kohn are small (3 to 13 microns in diameter) openings in alveolar walls, lined with alveolar epithelium. Collateral air drift probably occurs through these pores. Some collateral ventilation may also occur through the canals of Lambert, which are accessory epithelium-lined tubular communications between bronchioles larger than the terminal bronchiole, and the alveoli. They range up to 30 microns in diameter. There is some evidence to indicate that there are larger collateral channels, but their anatomic nature is not certain.[25]

THE ADULT CHEST

The roentgenogram of the adult chest outlines the heart, lungs, bony thorax, including the ribs and thoracic vertebrae, the diaphragm, all or part of the clavicles, and all or part of the scapulae. The soft tissues making up the chest wall also are included. The thorax is divided by the mediastinum into right and left compartments, each containing an air-filled lung that is recognized by its relative radiolucency as compared with the mediastinum, chest wall, and upper abdominal viscera. The greater part of the trachea is also included so that most of the lower respiratory tract is visible.

BONY THORAX

Roentgenography of the chest is undertaken primarily for visualization of intrathoracic structures, but the shoulder girdles, ribs, cervical and thoracic vertebral bodies, and sternum are often well enough outlined so that disease or anatomic variation can readily be recognized. Therefore, these structures should be studied on all chest roentgenograms. The shape of the thorax varies with age and with body habitus so that the range of normal is wide. The angulation of the ribs varies considerably with body type; downward angulation is minimal in short hypersthenic individuals and maximal in asthenic patients. The intercostal spaces are numbered according to the rib above them. In describing disease in relation to intercostal spaces, the interspace must be designated as either anterior or posterior because there is considerable difference in position of these interspaces in relation to the horizontal plane of the lung. The costal cartilages are not visible unless there is calcification within them. When calcification is present, it assumes a rather characteristic mottled appearance (Fig. 22-6). In males, it tends to be peripheral, in females, central. The diaphragm in a normal adult is very slightly higher on the right than on the left and is at approximately the level of the posterior arc of the tenth rib or the fifth anterior rib or interspace in deep inspiration. The ribs below the level of the diaphragm are usually not as clearly seen as those above it because of the greater opacity of the contents of the abdomen. The rhomboid fossa is an irregularly rounded indentation on the inferior surface of the clavicle near its sternal end. It marks the attachment of the costoclavicular (rhomboid) ligament and varies from slight roughening to a deep, irregular indentation. It should be recognized on the chest roentgenogram as an anatomic variant of no clinical significance (Fig. 22-7). Such abnormalities as inferior rib notching in coarctation and superior erosions of the fourth and fifth ribs in quadriplegia and poliomyelitis can be outlined readily on the chest roentgenogram.

SOFT TISSUES

The soft-tissue structures covering the bony thorax also produce shadows on the chest roentgenogram; they can project over the lung and pleura in a manner that simulates disease. Skin folds in patients who have lost weight can produce linear shadows running in any direction. Breast shadows are usually not difficult to identify but do result in increased opacity over the lower thorax bilaterally. Nipple shadows may appear as round opacities in the fourth anterior interspace or lower (Fig. 22-8). They are usually bilaterally symmetrical, but a film with metallic nipple markers may occasionally be necessary to differentiate them from intrapulmonary lesions. The skin and subcutaneous tissues

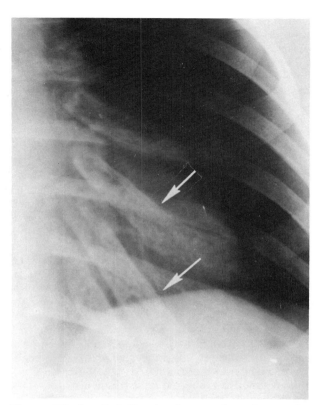

Figure 22–6. Calcification in costal cartilages. An unusually large amount of calcification is noted in several of the costal cartilages, two of which are indicated by the arrows. The mottled appearance of the calcium is characteristic.

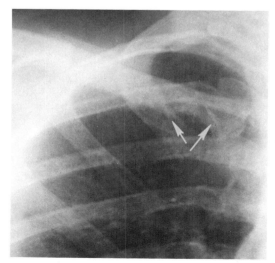

Figure 22–7. Rhomboid fossa. Arrows indicate the irregular, round indentation on the inferior aspect of the clavicle.

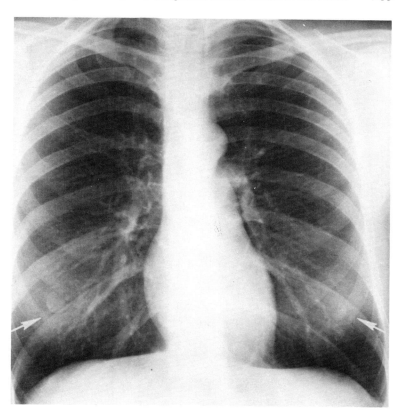

Figure 22–8. Nipple shadows. Female with a small amount of breast tissue in whom nipple shadows appear as small rounded opacities (*arrows*) in the sixth anterior interspace.

over the clavicles produce a faint, soft-tissue shadow paralleling the clavicles, the clavicular companion shadow. This measures from 2 or 3 mm to 1 cm in thickness but projects beyond the lung so that it can be identified. Soft-tissue masses or nodules projected over the lungs can simulate pulmonary nodules. These nodules in the subcutaneous or deeper structures of the thoracic wall are usually more sharply defined than intrapulmonary lesions of comparable size and shape. Therefore, an extrapulmonary nodule can be suspected and examination of the patient will confirm its presence. At times, lateral, oblique, or other projections must be employed to localize some nodules observed on only one projection of the initial frontal and lateral roentgenograms. If a question remains regarding the location of a nodule, CT may be required.

MEDIASTINUM

Anatomic Division and Contents

The mediastinum is the space lying between the right and left pleurae in and near the median sagittal plane of the chest. It extends from the posterior aspect of the sternum to the anterior surface of the thoracic vertebrae and contains all of the thoracic viscera except the lungs. It is divided into three major parts—anterior, middle, and posterior (see Fig. 22-12). The superior mediastinum has also been described and lies between the manubrium sterni and the upper four thoracic vertebrae. It contains structures of the anterior, middle, and posterior mediastinum that extend into it from below and above as well as those that traverse it and the mediastinum below it. Therefore, the designations anterior, middle, and posterior mediastinum are most frequently used to include the length of the thorax without specific designation of superior, which contains the aortic arch and its branches as well as the brachiocephalic veins, upper half of the superior vena cava, trachea, esophagus, thoracic duct, thymus, lymph nodes, and various nerves, some of which traverse the length of the mediastinum. If the three compartments are used to include their portion of the superior mediastinum, the *anterior mediastinum* is bound above by the thoracic inlet, laterally by the pleura, anteriorly by the sternum, and posteriorly by the pericardium and great vessels. It contains loose areolar tissue, lymph nodes, some lymphatic vessels that ascend from the convex surface of the liver, thymus, thyroid, parathyroids, and internal mammary arteries and veins. It is termed "prevascular space" by Zylak and colleagues.[71] The *middle mediastinum*, the "vascular space,"[71] contains the heart and pericardium, the ascending and transverse arch of the aorta, the superior vena cava and the azygos vein that empties into it, the brachiocephalic arteries and veins, the phrenic nerves, the upper vagus nerves, the trachea and its bifurcation, the main bronchi (Fig. 22-9), the pulmonary artery and its two branches, the pulmonary veins, and adjacent lymph nodes (see Fig. 22-11). It is bound in front by the anterior mediastinum and posteriorly by the posterior mediastinum. The *posterior mediastinum*, the "postvascular space,"[71] lies behind the heart and pericardium and extends from the level of the thoracic inlet to the twelfth thoracic vertebra. It contains the thoracic portion of the descending aorta, esophagus, thoracic duct, azygos and hemiazygos veins, lymph nodes, sympathetic chains, and inferior vagus nerves. There is some difference of opinion regarding the limits of the mediastinal divisions and the contents of each, but the preceding description is used extensively.

There are several other classifications of medistinal anatomy. Woodring and Daniel[69] as well as Chasen and associates[9] have described the anatomy using CT analysis.

Mediastinal Pleural Reflections

1. Anterior Junction Line. This is a thin vertical line anterior to the trachea and behind the sternum in the sagittal plane. It extends from the level of the sternal

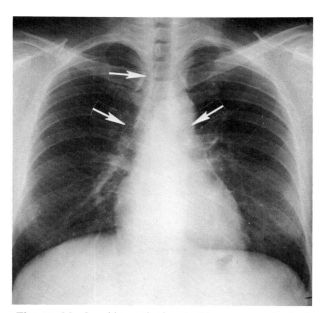

Figure 22–9. Normal chest. The arrows indicate the trachea and main bronchi.

angle (junction of manubrium and body of the sternum) downward and to the left for several centimeters. It represents the apposition of the visceral and parietal pleura of the upper lobes anteriorly and a little areolar tissue and is 1 to 2 mm wide. It usually is projected over the trachea as a thin linear shadow, convex to the left.[10]

2. Posterior Junction Line. This is a thin vertical line posterior to the trachea and esophagus. It extends from the thoracic inlet downward to the level of the azygos and aortic arches. It represents the approximation of visceral and parietal pleura of the upper lobes posteriorly, is thicker and begins higher than the anterior junction line (above the sternal angle), projects over the tracheal air shadow, and is convex to the left.

3. Azygoesophageal Recess. This recess extends from the inferior surface of the azygos arch (vein) downward and to the left to the level of the diaphragm anterior to the thoracic spine. It outlines the medial aspect of the right lower lobe and the right lateral aspect of the esophagus. The recess is usually concave on its right side.

4. The Right Paratracheal Stripe. This is a vertical stripe consisting of the right lateral tracheal wall and adjacent parietal and visceral pleura of the right upper lobe. It measures 1 to 4 mm in width at a level 2 cm above the azygos vein and is widened or altered by tracheal mediastinal and pleural disease.

5. Paraspinal Interface (Pleural Reflection). On the right side posteriorly, the parietal pleura is closely applied to the lateral aspect of the thoracic vertebrae. This creates a vertical linear interface between these structures. Abnormalities causing soft-tissue thickening or widening are readily seen, providing that there is a normal pleura, pleural space, and adjacent lung. On the left side, the left lateral wall of the descending aorta creates an interface with the lung and often results in slight lateral but usually uniform displacement of the paraspinal interface when the aorta is normal.

Lymph Nodes

The mediastinal nodes are divided into two major groups: anterior mediastinal and paratracheobronchial.[57] The *anterior mediastinal* (prevascular) nodes lie anterior to the superior vena cava and the right innominate vein on the right side. On the left, they lie anterior to the aorta and carotid artery. One or two nodes lie anterior to the ligamentum arteriosum, the ductus node(s) in the region of the *aortopulmonary window*, which is a concave area between the inferior aspect of the transverse aortic arch and the pulmonary artery. When these nodes are enlarged, the concavity is effaced or a convexity is produced. The anterior group of nodes cannot be reached by mediastinoscopy, but a biopsy can be done via an anterior parasternal approach.

The *paratracheobronchial* nodes can be subdivided into paratracheal, bifurcation, and pulmonary root nodes. The *right paratracheal* nodes lie behind the superior vena cava and innominate vein, anterolateral to the trachea. The lowermost node in this chain, the azygos node, lies medial to the azygos arch. The drainage to the azygos node comes not only from the right lung and other nodes on the right but also from the left lung and nodes, so it is very important clinically. A biopsy of these nodes can be done by mediastinoscopy. The *left paratracheal* nodes are more posterior than those on the right, and they lie posterolateral to the trachea and posterior to the left subclavian artery and the adjacent portion of the aortic arch. The *subcarinal (bifurcation)* nodes lie below the tracheal bifurcation, and a few small nodes extend along the undersurface of the main bronchi. There may also be a few small nodes in the pretracheal and posttracheal areas at the level of the carina. The *pulmonary root nodes,*[57] now termed hilar nodes, extend in a variable manner along the central portions of the major bronchi and pulmonary vessels. They can be divided into anterior, posterior, superior and inferior groups according to their relationship to the bronchi and vessels. A few inconstant nodes may be found more peripherally, the interlobar and the lobar or intrapulmonary nodes. The interlobar group lies at the division of the lobar bronchi and the lobar group at the division of the segmental bronchi. Radiographic differentiation of the pulmonary root (hilar) nodes from the more central interlobar nodes is virtually impossible.

In addition to the node groups described in the mediastinum, there are three more peripheral groups termed *parietal or extrapleural.* The *posterior* group is variable and lies along the intercostal vessels and nerves and along the thoracic vertebral surfaces. The paravertebral nodes are more numerous along the lower half of the thoracic spine. The *internal mammary* nodes lie adjacent to the internal mammary arteries and posterior to the ribs and interspaces. They are more numerous superiorly. The *diaphragmatic nodes* lie anterior to the pericardium, usually lateral to the midline on both sides.

As indicated, a biopsy can be done of the right paratracheal nodes but not of the anterior (prevascular) nodes at mediastinoscopy. The left paratracheal nodes are infrequently involved by lung tumors, but right paratracheal nodes are involved by right-sided and occasionally by left-sided lung tumors. Tumors of the left lung tend to metastasize to the anterior (prevascular) nodes such as the aortopulmonary window (ductus) nodes, which are visible on chest radiographs when enlarged. Subcarinal nodes are more commonly involved by lower lobe than by upper lobe tumors. Normal nodes are small and cannot be identified on chest radiographs. Some small normal nodes are sometimes observed on CT, however. The American Joint Committee on Cancer uses a numbering system and presents it in the Manual for Staging of Cancer.[4]

Other Roentgen Features of the Mediastinum

The trachea and main bronchi are usually visible in a chest roentgenogram of good quality. These structures lie within the mediastinum, and the trachea is situated in the midline except for very slight deviation to the right at the level of the aortic arch. In infants, moderate tracheal deviation away from the side of the aortic arch (usually to the right) is common, but this is not usually observed in children after the age of 5 years. In older persons the trachea may curve slightly to the left above the arch and then to the right as it passes the arch. As a rule, the angle formed by the bronchi with the sagittal plane is equal bilaterally until age 15 or so. Then the tracheal deviation to the right causes an increase in the angle on the left, the normal adult configuration. The sum of the two angles, the *subcarinal angle,* averages about 60°, but there is a wide variation in normal subjects. The trachea extends from the level of the sixth cervical vertebra downward to the level of the fifth thoracic vertebra or slightly lower, where it divides into the right and left main bronchi. It is identified on the roentgenogram as a band of radiolucency in the midline that extends from the lower cervical region downward to the point of bifurcation.

The main bronchi are somewhat smaller in diameter (see Fig. 22-9). The right main bronchus continues downward more vertically than the left in the adult and divides into two main branches. On the right the first branch is the upper lobe bronchus, which curves sharply upward above the right pulmonary artery (the *eparterial bronchus*). The continuation downward is termed the *hyparterial* or *bronchus intermedius,* which continues as the *right lower lobe bronchus.* The *middle lobe bronchus* arises from and marks the lower end of the bronchus intermedius. It extends downward and laterally from its point of origin. On the left side the main bronchus is somewhat longer, deviates laterally more than on the right, and forms a greater portion of the subcarinal angle. In addition to the lateral angulation, it curves outward in its distal portion and divides into a lower lobe bronchus and a left upper lobe bronchus that courses horizontally for a short distance before dividing. A continuation of the left main bronchus downward and laterally forms the lower lobe bronchus. It is usually possible to outline the main bronchi and portions of the upper and lower lobe bronchi in the normal patient. These structures have an appearance similar to that of the trachea, namely, a band of radiolucency, but are smaller in diameter.

In the frontal projection of the chest, the mediastinum along with the sternum and thoracic spine forms the dense central shadow observed on the normal roentgenogram. On the right side the superior border is formed by the brachiocephalic artery or vein, below which lies the superior vena cava. The ascending aortic arch is usually not border forming, but in cardiac diseases or aortic diseases that produce aortic dilatation it may form the right border (usually convex) for a short distance. Immediately below the ascending aortic arch is the hilum. The smooth convex border of the right atrium forms the lower right mediastinal border. On the left side the left subclavian artery forms the superior border of the mediastinum. Below this, the rounded convexity of the aortic arch is outlined. The aortopulmonary window is a local concavity or notch between the aortic arch and the pulmonary artery. The pulmonary artery and the hilum of the left lung lie immediately below the aortic arch, and the left ventricle forms most of the left lower mediastinal border, although a short segment of the pulmonary outflow tract may be visible below the hilum.

In infants the thymus is often a large structure that lies in the superior portion of the anterior mediastinum. When visible, it produces widening of the mediastinum superiorly; this widening is often asymmetrical. The thymus then forms the lateral border of the upper mediastinum on both sides. At times, the inferior aspect of the enlarged thymus forms an acute angle on one or both sides, a configuration (sail sign) likened to a sail (see Fig. 22-24). It is not unusual to note some lobulation of the thymus. When such superior mediastinal widening is present, it may be necessary to obtain a lateral projection to prove that the shadow is in the anterior mediastinum and thus represents the thymus. Moderate widening of the superior mediastinal shadow is not considered abnormal in infancy; this portion of the mediastinum usually assumes its normal width during the first year of life.

The left superior intercostal vein arises from the second, third, and fourth intercostal veins posteriorly, courses downward in the lateral vertebral gutter, and turns anteriorly at the level of the aortic arch. It empties into the posterior aspect of the left innominate vein. In 75% of patients, this vein communicates with the accessory hemiazygos vein at its lower end. The course of this vein around the aortic arch is somewhat variable,[3] and when it is lateral, inferolateral, or superolateral to the aorta, a small protuberance, *the aortic nipple*, is observed (Fig. 22-10). This represents the vein, seen in cross section, as it courses around the aorta. It was observed on 1.4% of normal chest films by Friedman and colleagues,[19] who found that it measured up to 4.5 mm in diameter in normal patients.

The lungs approach the midline in the anterior mediastinum. As a result, the air in the lung on either side defines a vertical linear shadow called the anterior junction line described earlier. It extends from a point near the level of the sternal angle superiorly to a point 3 or 4 inches below it. The line is visible on most roentgenograms of good quality. When one lung herniates across the midline, the line is displaced accordingly. The line thickens or diverges on either end.

The lungs also outline a pleural interface in the paraspinal area on both sides. This is usually 2 to 5 mm thick when measured from the lung to the lateral vertebral margin and is often most clearly defined on overexposed high-voltage films. As indicated, the soft tissue between the vertebrae and the lung is usually thicker on the left than on the right. A pleural interface is also observed on the right in the lower thorax outlining the lateral esophageal wall (the azygoesophageal recess); this is medial to the right paraspinal interface in the normal individual.

The hilum of the lung contains the pulmonary arteries, the pulmonary veins, the bronchi, the bronchial arteries and veins, as well as the lymph nodes. In the

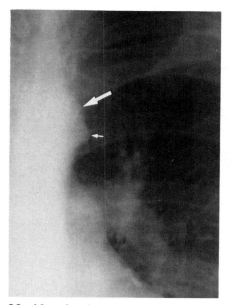

Figure 22–10. Aortic nipple. The superior intercostal vein (*small arrow*) as it courses around the transverse aortic arch (*large arrow*).

normal chest the pulmonary arteries and veins produce most of the opacity outlined on the roentgenogram (Fig. 22-11). The left hilum is higher in position than the right because the left pulmonary artery extends above the left main bronchus, and the right pulmonary artery crosses below the right upper lobe bronchus. The *hilar height ratio* may be useful in determining relative volume gain or loss in lower versus upper lobes.[28] It can be altered by intra-abdominal disease and by diaphragmatic abnormalities also. The vertical diameter of the chest is measured by a line drawn parallel to the thoracic spine from the highest point of the lung apex to the diaphragm on each side. On the right side, the hilar level is measured at the angle between the right upper lobe artery coursing upward and the right upper lobe pulmonary vein as it courses toward the left atrium. On the left, the hilar level is measured at the midpoint between the superior border of the pulmonary artery and the superior border of the left main bronchus. The ratio is then calculated by dividing the length of the vertical line above the hilum by the length of the line below the hilum, so the ratio on the left is below 1.0 and on the right above

1.0. Measurements are made on standard full inspiration films taken at 72 inches. Inspiratory effort is adequate if the dome of the right hemidiaphragm is between the anterior fifth and sixth ribs. The ratio on the right (mean) is 1.31 (standard deviation 0.21); the ratio on the left (mean) is 0.84 (standard deviation 0.09).[28] This ratio permits the assessment of the height of each hilum without needing to compare it with the other. Normal-sized lymph nodes in the region of the hilum do not contribute enough to the hilar opacity to be identified, but when enlarged or when these nodes contain calcium, they can be recognized. The size of the hilum varies in the normal so that it is difficult to set a standard beyond which hilar size is abnormal. Since the size of the pulmonary vessels is related to pulmonary blood flow, the vessels that make up the hila are increased when the blood flow is increased and decreased in diseases that produce a diminution in pulmonary blood flow. In addition to the variation in hilar size produced by the variability of caliber of the blood vessels, enlargement of hilar nodes may cause hilar enlargement. It is often difficult if not impossible to distinguish the cause of slight hilar enlargement.

In the *lateral* view of the chest the anatomic divisions of the mediastinum are well demonstrated (Fig. 22-12). The superior mediastinum lies above the horizontal line and is included because of many references to it in the literature. The anterior mediastinum is seen as an area of relative radiolucency between the sternum and the heart. It is roughly triangular in shape, with the apex pointing downward. The large thymus is noted as an area of opacity in the anterior mediastinum in infants. The middle mediastinum is clearly defined in a lateral roentgenogram, since it contains the heart and aorta. The posterior mediastinum is the area lying between the heart and the spine. It is visualized as a radiolucency approximating that of aerated lungs in normal subjects because it contains no opaque structures such as the heart and great vessels, which occupy the middle mediastinum. The trachea is visible in the lateral roentgenogram of the chest as a radiolucent structure that angles slightly posteriorly as it extends into the chest. The posterior tracheal stripe (wall), about 2 to 4 mm thick, is outlined by tracheal air anterior to it and air in the lung posterior to it. When there is sufficient air in the esophagus, a tracheoesophageal stripe may be seen, a vertical shadow composed of the adjacent tracheal and esophageal walls. The tracheal bifurcation is sometimes visible along with short segments of one or both upper lobe bronchi if the patient is not in a true lateral position. The left upper lobe bronchus is lower than the right and is usually clearly outlined against the opacity of the left pulmonary artery, which lies immediately above it. In contrast, the right upper lobe bronchus, which is above

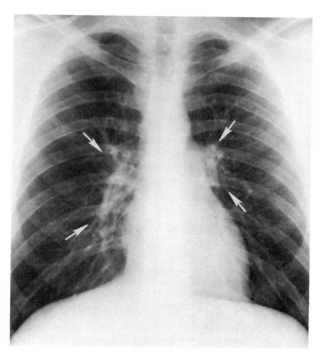

Figure 22–11. Normal chest. The hila are well outlined and indicated by arrows. The difference in height is noted. Continuation of the hilar opacities can be followed in the lung, and these are noted to branch in a treelike fashion. They represent pulmonary arteries.

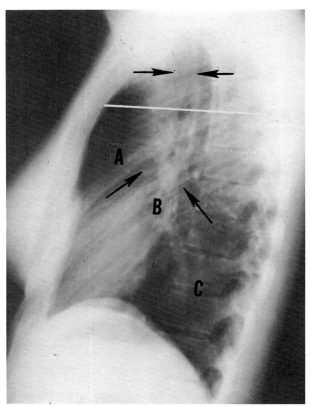

Figure 22–12. Lateral view of chest showing divisions of the mediastinum. The superior mediastinum lies above the line extending from the sternal angle to the fourth dorsal vertebra. **(A)** The anterior mediastinum; **(B)** the middle mediastinum; and **(C)** the posterior mediastinum. In the superior mediastinum the trachea is indicated by arrows. Arrows (*lower*) also indicate the region of the superimposed hila. Compartment margins on the film are not clear, because the mediastinum is a conglomeration of the structures.

the artery, is difficult to see in most instances. It lies about 1 to 2 cm above the left upper lobe bronchus. In this region an irregular, somewhat stellate shadow is noted that represents the vascular structures which produce the hila. The left pulmonary artery courses posterolaterally and lies above and posterior to the right pulmonary artery as viewed on the lateral film. If the patient is in a slight (5° to 10°) right anterior oblique position, the pulmonary arteries are separated and, with no overlapping, are each clearly defined. On the right, the bronchus intermedius is slightly anterior to the left lower bronchus, so the posterior wall of the bronchus intermedius is clearly outlined within the

radiolucent band produced by the left bronchus in more than 50% of patients. Thickening of the wall of this bronchus can then be demonstrated if present. In the examination of the mediastinum it may be useful to opacify the esophagus by having the patient ingest thick barium paste. Then the relationship of the esophagus to the other structures in the mediastinum can be determined and abnormalities clearly defined that would otherwise be very difficult to outline. The relationship of the esophagus to the trachea as well as to the heart can also be determined.

Computed Tomography of the Normal Mediastinum

The images of the mediastinum obtained by CT depict cross-sectional anatomy that is quite different from the anatomy depicted in sagittal and coronal planes on chest radiographs. Individual structures can be recognized and the site of an enlargement can be determined.

At the level of the sternoclavicular junction, which is at about the thoracic inlet, five vessels can usually be identified (Fig. 22-13)—right (from anterior to posterior): brachiocephalic vein, brachiocephalic artery (usually medial to vein); left (from anterior to posterior): left brachiocephalic vein, left carotid artery, and left subclavian artery. The left brachiocephalic vein may be seen longitudinally as it crosses the midline. At a level slightly above the sternoclavicular junction, the paired jugular veins, carotid arteries, and subclavian arteries may be visible. The trachea and esophagus are recognized at both levels. The veins are usually anterior to the arteries and the carotids anterior to the subclavian. At the level of the aortic arch, only the superior vena cava and aorta are seen in addition to the trachea and esophagus. When the aorta is dilated and tortuous, the left brachiocephalic vein may lie anterior to the arch. At the level of the aortopulmonary window, immediately below the aortic arch and just cephalad to the carina, the ascending and descending aorta, the superior vena cava as well as the trachea and esophagus are seen in cross section. In about this area, the azygos arch may be included as the vein courses anteriorly from the prevertebral area to enter the superior vena cava. At a level just below the carina, the aorta, superior vena cava, and esophagus are seen along with the left pulmonary artery, the left main bronchus, the right upper lobe bronchus, the right upper lobe artery (truncus anterior) just anterior to the bronchus, and the prevertebral portion of the azygos vein. A short segment of the distal azygos vein may also be seen as it enters the superior vena cava. Just below this level, the right pulmonary artery is seen as it bifurcates from the main pulmonary artery and courses from anterior to posterior in an oblique position behind the ascending

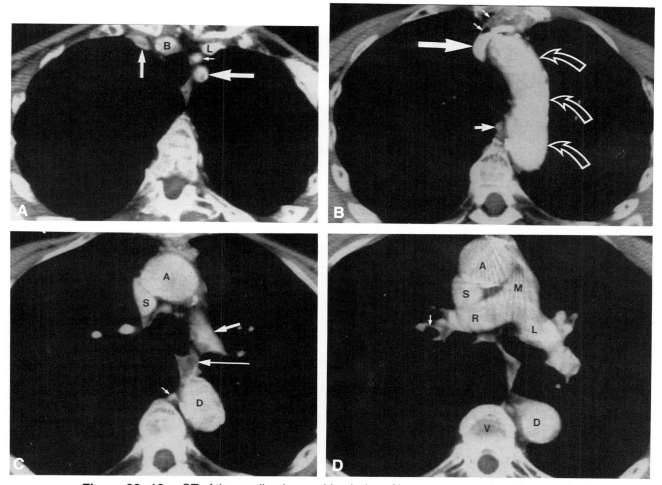

Figure 22–13. CT of the mediastinum with a bolus of intravenous contrast (mediastinal window) demonstrating normal anatomy in the mediastinum. (**A**) *L*, Left brachiocephalic vein; *B*, brachiocephalic artery; left subclavian artery (*large arrow*), right brachiocephalic vein (*medium arrow*); left common carotid artery (*small arrow*). (**B**) CT at the level of the aortic arch. Transverse aortic arch (*open arrows*), superior vena cava at junction with brachiocephalic vein (*large arrow*), esophagus (*medium arrow*), gas (abscess) in anterior mediastinum (*small arrows*). (**C**) CT at the level of aortopulmonary window. *A*, Ascending aorta; *D*, descending aorta; *S*, superior vena cava; left pulmonary artery (*medium arrow*), esophagus (*large arrow*); azygos vein (*small arrow*). (**D**) CT at pulmonary artery bifurcation. *A*, Ascending aorta; *D*, descending aorta; *M*, main pulmonary artery; *L*, left pulmonary artery; *R*, right pulmonary artery; *S*, superior vena cava; right upper lobe bronchus (*arrow*); *V*, vertebral body. (All photos courtesy of Robert Rosenberg, MD)

aorta and superior vena cava. The descending aorta, bronchus intermedius, and left upper lobe bronchus are usually visible at this level. The hilar vessels and bronchi are discussed in greater detail in paragraphs to follow.

At a level about a centimeter below the left upper lobe bronchus, the left and right atria, the aortic root,

descending aorta, and main pulmonary artery are visible along with the esophagus and azygos vein. One or more pulmonary veins may be observed draining into the left atrium. The esophagus is just posterior to the left atrium at this level. Lower, at the level of the ventricles, the anterior pericardium is usually identified as a thin, dense, retrosternal structure with fat anterior and posterior to it. The inferior vena cava lies lateral to a narrow venous structure extending forward to the right atrium, the coronary sinus. The esophagus and descending aorta are also seen on this section. The septal groove is often identified anteriorly. When a bolus of intravenous contrast medium opacifies the ventricles, the septum is visible. Below the heart, the diaphragmatic crura are observed, with lung anterior to them and the esophagus, descending aorta, azygos and hemiazygos veins, and thoracic duct noted in the retrocrural space. This marks the lower extent of the posterior mediastinum. The superior aspect of the liver is observed on the right and sometimes on the left, where stomach and spleen may also be visible.

Intravenous contrast enhancement can be accomplished by dynamic scanning, which consists of injecting a bolus of contrast material followed quickly by a series of rapid sequence scans at the same or different levels. This method is used to identify suspected vascular structures or lesions. Continuous drip of additional contrast material may be added as more scans are obtained. In many departments, CT of the mediastinum is usually performed after and during infusion of intravenous contrast material in doses ranging from 125 to 150 ml of 60% contrast agent.

Comprehensive review of CT of the normal mediastinum and hila, including anatomic variations, is beyond the scope of this book. Several texts and papers on this subject are available, including those by Kieffer and Heitzman (anatomy), Lee and colleagues, Naidich and associates, and Zylak and coworkers.[36, 39, 49, 71] Normal hilar anatomy is discussed in papers by Webb and Naidich and their coworkers.[48, 49, 67]

PULMONARY HILA

The pulmonary hila consist of arteries, veins, and bronchi that have a fairly constant relationship to each other. Scans 1 cm thick obtained at 1-cm intervals are usually obtained. They are monitored and additional scans can be done if indicated. Dynamic scans are usually not necessary. The arteries and veins are best studied in relation to the bronchi, since bronchi are readily recognized. Scans must be studied in relation to each other to avoid misinterpretation (Figs. 22-14 and 22-15).

RIGHT HILUM

The superior hilar scan is obtained at the level of the distal trachea just above the carina. The apical segmental bronchus of the right upper lobe is visible, with the artery medial and the vein lateral to it. Although other vascular shadows may be seen in this region, normally

they are smaller than the vessels adjacent to the bronchus. At the next section, 1 cm lower, the carina is usually visible along with the apical segmental bronchus and the artery and vein, medial and lateral to it respectively. The next section is through the right upper lobe bronchus. The posterior wall of this bronchus is in direct contact with lung parenchyma. The pulmonary artery of the right upper lobe (truncus anterior), the first large branch of the pulmonary artery, is anterior to the bronchus and the superior pulmonary vein lateral to it between the anterior and posterior segmental bronchi. The apical anterior vein from the upper lobe may also be seen as a small convexity anterior and medial to the truncus anterior. About 1 cm below this, the next section is through the bronchus intermedius, seen in cross section, the posterior wall of which is in contact with lung parenchyma, which extends posteromedially into the azygoesophageal recess. The right main pulmonary artery crosses anterior to, and then courses downward as the interlobar artery, and lateral to the bronchus intermedius. The superior pulmonary veins are lateral to the artery. When the pulmonary artery reaches the lateral border of the bronchus intermedius, it courses downward and its lateral border may appear somewhat irregular and triangular. The next section is at the level of the middle lobe bronchus seen in longitudinal section; the lower lobe bronchus is seen in cross section at about the level or slightly below it. The interlobar artery is lateral and adjacent to these bronchi in an angle formed by the bronchi. The superior pulmonary vein is medial to the middle lobe bronchus as it enters the left atrium. In the section below this, the medial and lateral segmental branches of the middle lobe bronchus may be seen at about the bifurcation. The middle lobe artery is anterolateral to the bronchi, and the interlobar pulmonary artery has divided into its basal segmental branches, which lie posterolateral to the lower lobe bronchus. This relationship is maintained when the bronchi divide into the basal segmental branches. The inferior pulmonary veins lie below the hilum but lower sections identify pulmonary veins, which can be seen entering the left atrium; they are more horizontal than the arteries.

LEFT HILUM

The first section in the upper hilum is usually obtained at or slightly above the carina. The relationship of vessels to the bronchi is not as constant as on the right side. At this level, the apical posterior bronchus of the upper lobe is seen in cross section separated from the left main bronchus by the left main pulmonary artery as it crosses over the upper lobe bronchus. The superior pulmonary vein is medial to the upper lobe artery,

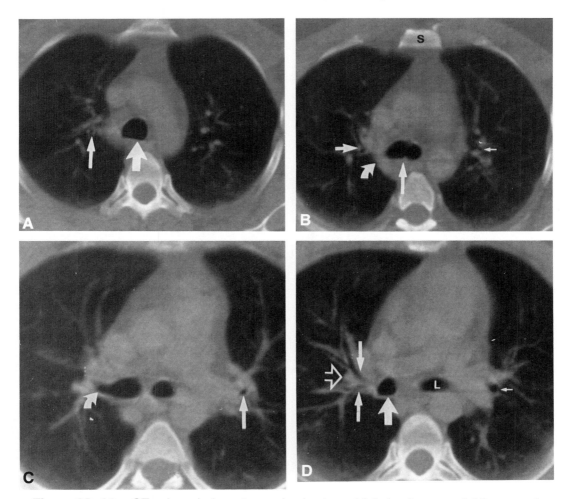

Figure 22–14. CT using windows to emphasize bronchial structures; serial 8 mm × 8 mm sections. (**A**) CT above tracheal bifurcation. Trachea (*large arrow*), right apical segmental bronchus (*small arrow*). (**B**) CT at carinal level. Carina (*large arrow*), left apical segmental bronchus (*small arrow*), right apical segmental bronchus (*medium arrow*), azygous arch (*curved arrow*). (**C**) CT below carina. Origin of right upper lobe bronchus (*curved arrow*), left apical segmental bronchus (*straight arrow*). (**D**) CT at level of bronchus intermedius. Left main bronchus (*L*), left apical superior segmental bronchus (*small arrow*), bronchus intermedius (*large arrow*), anterior and posterior segmental right upper lobe bronchi (*medium arrows*), right superior pulmonary vein (*open arrow*). (**E**) CT at level of lingular bronchus (*curved arrow*), left upper lobe bronchus (*large arrow*), bronchus intermedius (*small arrow*). (**F**) CT at level of right middle lobe bronchus (*large arrow*), superior segment bronchus of right lower lobe (*medium arrow*), right interlobar artery (*small arrow*). (**G**) CT at bifurcation of right middle lobe bronchus into medial and lateral segments (*small arrow*), right lower lobe basal bronchi (*long arrow*). (**H**) CT at level of inferior pulmonary veins (*curved arrows*), azygos vein (*long arrow*), basal segmental bronchi (*small arrows*). *M*, medial; *A*, anterior; *L*, lateral; *P*, posterior. (All photos courtesy of Robert Rosenberg, MD) (*continued*)

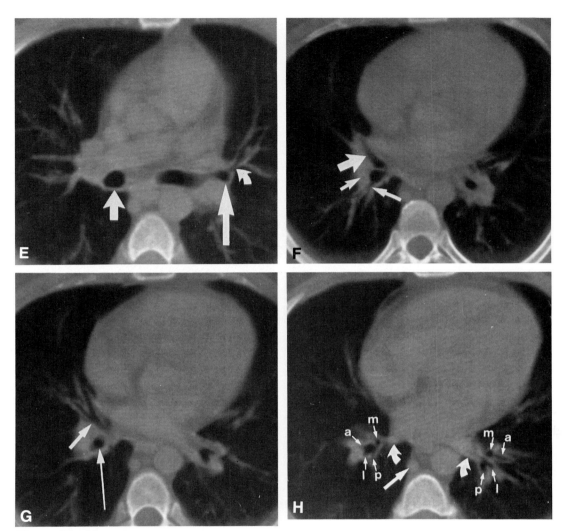

Figure 22–14. (Continued)

and both vessels are anterior to the apical posterior bronchus. The next section is through the upper lobe bronchus as it courses horizontally. The pulmonary artery crosses above the bronchus, turns downward and posteriorly, and becomes the interlobar artery. The superior pulmonary vein lies anterior to the upper lobe bronchus opposite the posterior position of the interlobar artery. The next lower section is through the inferior aspect of the upper lobe bronchus. An upper lobe spur divides the upper and lower lobe bronchi, and the interlobar artery lies in the angle lateral to the spur while the superior vein remains anterior to the upper lobe bronchus. If the lingular bronchus is included, the lingular artery may be observed lateral to its origin. Pulmonary parenchyma extends between the aorta and pulmonary artery at the level of the upper lobe bronchus, and aerated lung is adjacent to the posteromedial wall of the left upper and lower lobe bronchi. Any thickening or density in the retrobronchial area indicates abnormality. Below the left upper lobe bronchus, the next section shows the lower lobe bronchus and often the origin of the superior segmental bronchus. The interlobar artery lies lateral to this bifurcation and posterior to the lingular bronchus. At lower sections, the left hilum is similar to the right. The arterial branches to the lower lobe lie lateral and posterior to the lower lobe bronchus, and the inferior pulmonary vein courses horizontally into the left atrium just anterior to the aorta. Minor hilar variations are often observed, as indicated earlier.

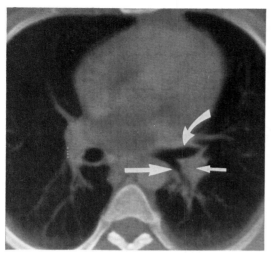

Figure 22–15. CT (between Fig. 22-14*E* and *F*) at the level of the superior segmental bronchus of the left lower lobe (*large arrow*), left upper lobe bronchus (*curved arrow*), and left interlobar artery (*small arrow*).

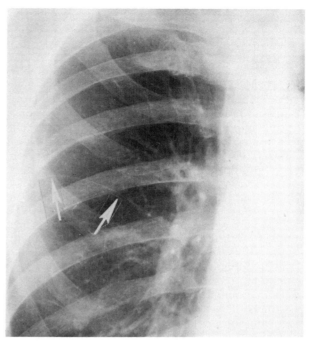

Figure 22–16. The minor interlobar fissure is indicated by arrows. It is slightly less horizontal in this patient than in the average person and its lateral aspect is higher in position than normal.

LUNGS

Lobar and Segmental Anatomy

The right lung is divided into three lobes, the upper, middle, and lower, by two fissures. The major or primary interlobar fissure separates the lower lobe from the upper and middle, and the secondary (minor) fissure separates the middle from the upper lobe. On the left side two lobes are separated by the major interlobar fissure. The major fissures are sometimes visible in the lateral roentgenogram in the normal person and are readily seen in this projection when there is a small amount of thickening of the interlobar pleura or a small amount of fluid in the fissure. These fissures are visible in the frontal projection only when there is pleural disease, fluid, or pleural thickening. The minor interlobar fissure on the right is often visible in the frontal projection in the normal individual (Fig. 22-16) and when pleural thickening is present can be easily identified in this projection as well as in the lateral view. It is generally horizontal and lies at the level of the anterior arc of the fourth rib or interspace. The major fissure on the right extends from the level of the fifth posterior rib downward and forward to the level of the sixth rib anteriorly, whereas the left major fissure is slightly more vertical and extends from the level of the third to fifth posterior ribs down to the level of the seventh rib anteriorly. The levels are somewhat variable in the normal person, and in those with dis-

ease, there may be marked variation in position. Occasionally, the major fissure on the right is directed slightly anteriorly into the sagittal plane in its lateral portion. It may then be visible as a vertical fissure line roughly paralleling the curve of the lower lateral chest wall.[11] This is observed frequently in adults with small amounts of pleural fluid and has also been described in infants, particularly those with cardiac enlargement. Occasionally, the anterior minor fissure may assume a sagittal position as well. It appears as an oblique linear shadow inferomedially.[22]

When the major fissures are both seen in the lateral view, the left usually intersects the diaphragm more posteriorly and more vertically than the right fissure. Not infrequently, the major fissures do not extend to the mediastinal surface of the lungs, so that lobar division is incomplete medially.

The *pulmonary ligament* (inferior pulmonary ligament) is a sheath of parietal pleura that extends from the pleural investment of the inferior pulmonary vein downward and somewhat posteriorly to the diaphragm. It is attached to the mediastinum medially, to the lower lobe laterally, and usually to the diaphragm inferiorly and stabilizes the lower lobes medially. It is triangular when the lung is pulled laterally.[54] The apex of the triangle is at the level of the inferior pulmonary vein. Normally it is not visible on chest radiographs. However, it partially separates the anterior from the posterior hemithorax inferomedially so that fluid can be trapped anteriorly or posteriorly to simulate atelectasis or other abnormality. It also anchors the lower lobe to the mediastinum and diaphragm when collapse or a large pneumothorax is present. Any process extending into it from the mediastinum may simulate an intrapulmonary mass. The ligament is frequently observed on CT.[56] It appears as a thin linear opacity extending posterolaterally at or slightly above the diaphragm. In a CT study of 129 patients,[56] the ligament was seen on the left in 67.4%, on the right in 37.2%, on both sides in 27.1%, and on neither side in 22.4% of patients. It extended posteriorly from its mediastinal attachment in 92%.

The importance of bronchopulmonary segmental anatomy has increased now that segmental resection and subsegmental pulmonary resection are common procedures. These segments have been classified by several investigators[6, 7]; the classification by Jackson and Huber[30] will be used here. The segments and subsegments are not strictly morphologic units, since arteries may cross from one segment to another and the segments contain veins that drain adjacent segments. The bronchi to the lobes and segments are not outlined on the chest roentgenogram unless they are diseased. When an opacity is present in a lung, CT is sometimes helpful in localization; if not, it may be necessary to use bronchography if accurate localization of a small lesion to a segment is required. However, using lateral and oblique roentgenograms along with frontal film, it is often possible to be moderately accurate in localization of pulmonary parenchymal disease without bronchography. In chronic inflammations, however, it is common to have sufficient fibrosis and contraction to distort the involved segment as well as the adjacent segments to the point that localization is not accurate. There are few situations in which such accurate location is needed, so bronchography is seldom necessary. The positions and names of the bronchopulmonary segments are given in the accompanying roentgenograms and drawings (Figs. 22-17A through F).

Roentgen Features

The normal lungs contain a considerable amount of air, and since chest roentgenograms are obtained in inspiration, they appear much more radiolucent than other structures making up the thorax and its contents. There is a distinct radiographic pattern that is produced largely by the blood vessels as they extend from the hilum into the lungs. The right midlung window is an area of decreased vascularity and therefore increased radiolucency adjacent to the minor fissure. It has been described on CT[20] and has been observed on plain films as well. The large bronchi can often be seen as radiolucent tubes in the hilum, adjacent to which are dense, smooth-walled tubes that represent the pulmonary arterial branches. These arteries branch in a tree-like manner and decrease in caliber rapidly as they extend into pulmonary parenchyma. This pattern is readily visible on the roentgenogram. The pulmonary arteries lie in close relationship to the bronchi. They branch and subdivide the same as the bronchi. Therefore, they lie within the pulmonary lobules. The pulmonary veins, on the other hand, have an anatomic distribution entirely separate from the bronchi. They begin at the periphery of the lobules in the pleura or interlobular septa and course to the left atrium between the lobules.

The vessels can be identified to within about 1.5 cm of the pleural surfaces of the lungs except at the apices, where the distance may be 3 cm from the pleura. In the upright position, the upper lobe vessels are smaller than those at the bases. The difference in size tends to reflect distribution of blood flow, which is greater in the lower lungs in the upright position, but tends to be nearly equal in the recumbent position. The lungs are often divided arbitrarily into zones, depending on the size of the vessels. The inner zone or inner one-third adjacent to the hilum contains the large main trunks. The middle zone contains intermediate-sized vessels, and the peripheral one-third of the lung or peripheral zone usually contains vessels that are less than 1 mm in diameter. The pulmonary veins cannot be differentiated from the arteries in the peripheral or middle zones, but in the central zone the veins do not course near the arteries. They lie below the comparable arteries and empty into the left atrium at the lower margin of the hila. They rarely fuse into a single common trunk, so that there are usually two or more veins entering the atrium on either side. It is often difficult to outline them distinctly and differentiate them from arteries, but on tomograms or CT, they are seen as smooth, elongated opacities extending into the left atrium in the lower hilum on either side (Figs. 22-18 and 22-19). Occasionally, they are clearly defined on a routine frontal chest roentgenogram. This is particularly true in patients with congenital cardiac defects resulting in high-volume, left-to-right shunts. In patients with venous congestion, the upper lobe vessels can often be seen as hornlike structures extending into the lower hila from the medial aspects of the upper lobes.

As indicated, the pulmonary vessels at the bases are generally larger than the upper lung vessels, and since the right medial base is better visualized than the left,

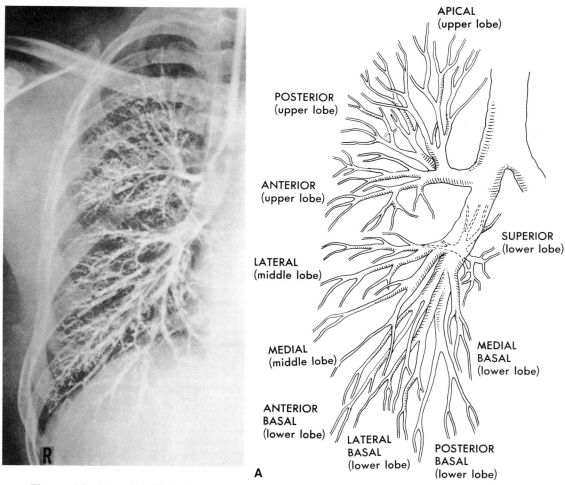

Figure 22–17. (**A**) Right lung. Bronchogram with diagram of the normal bronchopulmonary segments in the frontal projection. (*continued*)

the trunks stand out more clearly in this region than elsewhere in the lungs. The anteroposterior diameter of the chest is greater inferiorly than it is superiorly, and this means that more vessels are superimposed at the bases. This factor also adds to the apparent difference in size and number of vessels between the upper and lower lung. The branched vascular markings tend to increase slightly in prominence with an increase in age of a given individual, but there is marked variation in their size in the normal lung. Care is needed to avoid interpreting the chest roentgenogram as abnormal in a patient in whom these vessels are slightly more prominent than usual. The vessels can be identified by their smooth margins, decreasing caliber, and typical branching pattern as they leave the hilum.

In addition to the vascular markings in the lungs,

there are interstitial markings that are much less prominent. They produce a fine lacy or reticular pattern throughout the lung that is visible in some patients and may become more prominent with advancing age. These interstitial markings may stand out clearly in patients with emphysema and may be greatly increased in diseases that produce diffuse interstitial disease in the lungs.

Pulmonary Apex

The lung apices (radiographic) occupy the portion of the thoracic cavity above the level of the clavicles as seen on the posteroanterior roentgenogram. Since inflammatory disease or tumors may arise there, it is important to be able to differentiate pulmonary disease

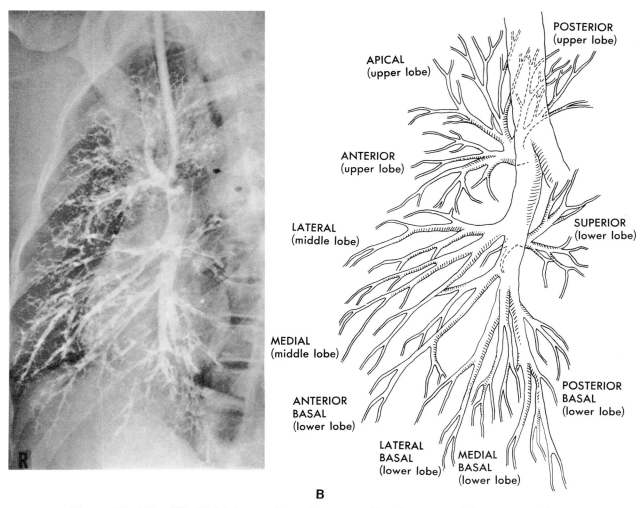

B

Figure 22–17. (B) Right lung. Bronchogram with diagram of the normal bronchopulmonary segments in the left anterior oblique projection. (*continued*)

from the various shadows representing normal soft-tissue structures that overlie the pulmonary apex. This portion of the lung is in the peripheral zone so that the markings due to vessels are very small and are often difficult to outline. Several soft-tissue structures can be demonstrated on most chest roentgenograms in normal persons. The supraclavicular border or companion shadow is a linear band of soft-tissue density that parallels the clavicle and extends for 2 or 3 mm to 1 cm above it, depending on the amount of subcutaneous tissue in the individual. It represents the skin and subcutaneous tissue observed tangentially as they cover the superior clavicular margin. This shadow can be followed laterally beyond the pulmonary apex and can therefore be

identified as being outside of the lung. It often fades off medially, or it may be apparent as far as the clavicular attachment of the sternocleidomastoid muscle. This muscle produces another soft-tissue density, which is a vertical shadow clearly defined laterally. It can be traced upward into the neck above the pulmonary apex and can thus be identified (Fig. 22-20). The muscle is not visible in all patients but is particularly well outlined in those who are old or emaciated. The medial borders of the pulmonary apices are formed by the mediastinum. The soft-tissue margin of the left mediastinal border is smooth and slightly concave owing to the curve of the left subclavian artery that forms it. On the right side the medial soft-tissue mediastinal de-

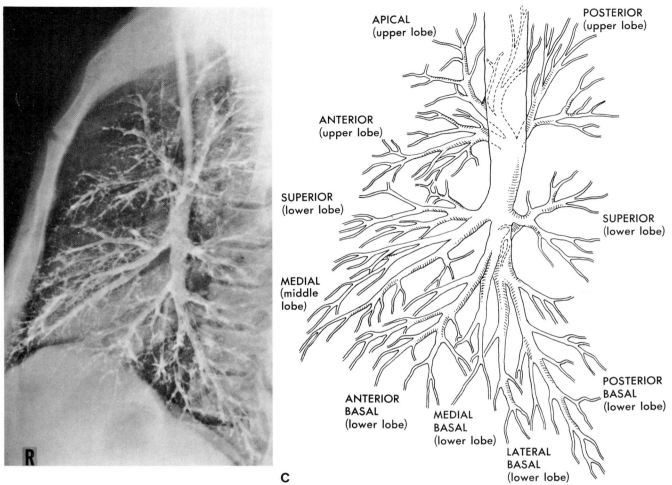

C

Figure 22–17. **(C)** Right lung. Bronchogram with diagram of the normal bronchopulmonary segments in the lateral projection. (*continued*)

marcation is produced by the brachiocephalic artery or superior vena cava and is often slightly less distinct than on the left side, particularly in young individuals. When this artery becomes tortuous and dilated in patients with arteriosclerotic disease, this margin may become more distinct and often convex.

The posterior portions of the upper three ribs and sometimes the fourth rib lie above the clavicle and are readily identified. Companion or border shadows are sometimes visible along the inferior aspects of the upper two ribs and are identified as smooth linear bands from 1 to 3 mm in thickness. The densities are parallel to the inferior rib margins (Fig. 22-21). Occasionally, a very thin border shadow is noted in the same relation-

ship to the posterior arc of the third rib. These findings are produced by the soft tissues beneath these ribs, which are at a tangent to the roentgen-ray beam. There is enough soft tissue made up of pleura, subpleural connective tissue, and intercostal arteries and veins to produce them.

The pleura at the extreme lung apex often appears thickened and is recognized on the roentgenogram as a soft-tissue opacity. These shadows are termed apical pleural caps by some, may be unilateral or bilateral, and usually represent subpleural scarring, often the result of inflammatory disease, including tuberculosis. Several other causes have been reported, including postradiation change, trauma, fat, vascular abnormal-

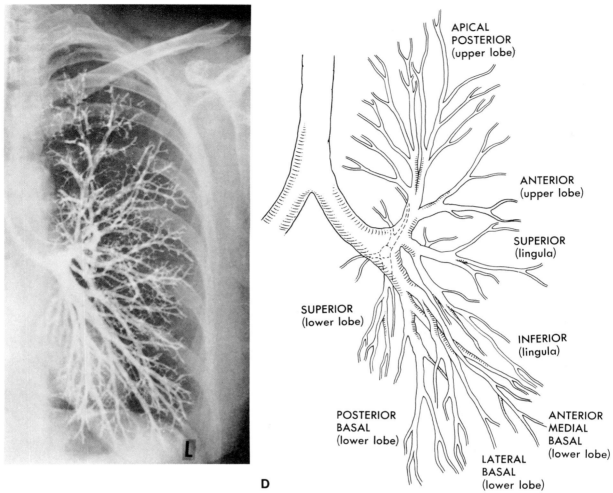

Figure 22–17.   (D) Left lung. Bronchogram with diagram of the normal bronchopulmonary segments in the frontal projection. (*continued*)

ities, and tumor, particularly the superior pulmonary sulcus (Pancoast) tumor. Most of them are benign and of no significance. Any change in the absence of specific cause should alert the observer to the possibility of malignancy, although the vast majority of these shadows are not significant. Although this shadow often presents as a soft-tissue opacity below the inferior aspect of the second rib, there are certain characteristics that differentiate it from the companion shadow of this rib. In pleural or subpleural scarring, the density is likely to vary somewhat and the thickness is often asymmetrical on the two sides in contrast to the symmetry and homogeneous density of the companion shadows. Furthermore, the inferior surface of the scar is likely to be somewhat irregular and that of the com-

panion shadow is perfectly smooth in outline (Fig. 22-22). Although apical scars may be bilateral, they are not necessarily symmetrical.

DIAPHRAGM

The diaphragm is a muscular structure that separates the thorax from the abdomen. Its superior surface is covered by parietal pleura. There is a central membranous portion, called the central tendon, in which there is no muscle. The diaphragm arches upward toward the central tendon to form a smooth, dome-shaped appearance on both sides. It is attached to the xiphoid process and lower costal cartilages anteriorly, the ribs laterally, and the ribs and upper three lumbar

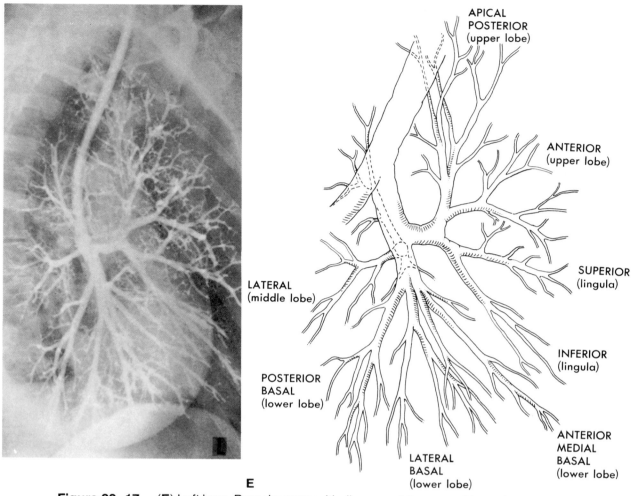

E

Figure 22–17.   **(E)** Left lung. Bronchogram with diagram of the normal bronchopulmonary segments in the right anterior oblique projection. (*continued*)

vertebrae posteriorly. In the roentgenogram, the upper surface of the diaphragm is clearly defined as a smooth, dome-shaped structure that stands out in sharp contrast to the radiolucent aerated lung above it. In the frontal projection the most inferior visible portion of the diaphragm meets the lateral chest wall at an acute angle. This is called the costophrenic angle or sulcus. It is sharply and clearly defined in the normal individual but may be obliterated in patients with diseases that produce pleural effusion, thickening, or adhesions. The position of the diaphragm varies considerably with the body habitus of the individual, with respiration, and with the position of the patient when the roentgenogram is obtained. These factors should be known to interpret correctly alterations in height of

the diaphragm. It is apparent, therefore, that there can be no accurate standard for position of the diaphragm, but in the average adult during moderately deep inspiration, the dome of the diaphragm on the right lies in the region of the fifth anterior interspace or at the level of the rib above or below it, while that on the left is slightly lower in position. The position of the diaphragm in children and young adults is somewhat higher, and in the aged the diaphragm is usually lower. In the supine and prone positions the diaphragm is higher than in the upright position.

In the lateral roentgenogram the right and left hemidiaphragmatic domes are outlined as separate structures, since they are usually not at the same level. The dome (or highest part) of the diaphragm is slightly

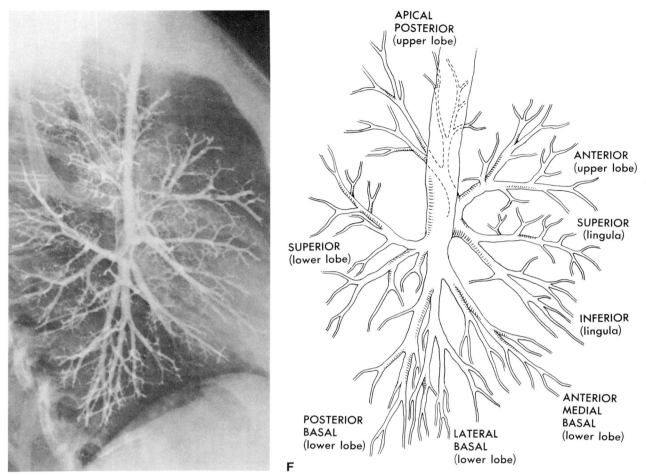

APICAL
POSTERIOR
(upper lobe)

ANTERIOR
(upper lobe)

SUPERIOR
(lingula)

SUPERIOR
(lower lobe)

INFERIOR
(lingula)

ANTERIOR
MEDIAL
BASAL
(lower lobe)

POSTERIOR
BASAL
(lower lobe)

LATERAL
BASAL
(lower lobe)

F

Figure 22–17.   (*F*) Left lung. Bronchogram with diagram of the normal bronchopulmon-ary segments in the lateral projection. (*F*, courtesy of Dr. J. Stauffer Lehman, Dr. Antrim Crellin, and Eastman Kodak Company.)

anterior to the midpoint between the anterior and posterior chest walls. On the average, the anterior aspect of the diaphragm is at the level of the anterior arc of the sixth rib or interspace, whereas the posterior sulcus is at or slightly below the level of the twelfth rib. It is usually possible to identify the diaphragm on each side in the lateral roentgenogram even though it may be at or very near the same level, because the anterior aspect of the left dome is obscured by the heart above it while the anterior portion of the right side stands out clearly. In addition, there is often gas in the stomach or colon immediately beneath the left hemidiaphragm, which aids in its identification in this projection. Also, the left major pulmonary fissure is more vertical near the diaphragm than the right fissure, and its diaphrag-

matic end is posterior to that of the right fissure. Fur-thermore, the ribs on the side away from the film are large. For example, in a left lateral radiograph the right ribs are larger than the left ribs; this may be of help in differentiating right from left.

The several normal openings in the diaphragm as well as the several weak areas are indicated in Figure 31-29. Diaphragmatic hernia may present through these openings.

PLEURA

The pleura is a thin, serous membrane that is visible roentgenographically only when it is seen in contrast to adjacent structures that are more or less dense. Thus,

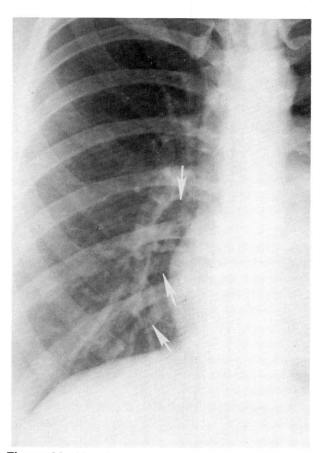

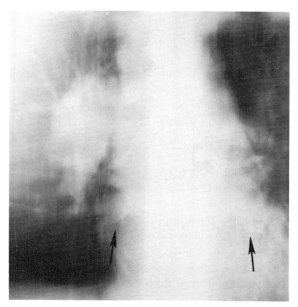

Figure 22–19. Tomogram, obtained to outline the mass involving the right hilum, shows the pulmonary veins on the right and also on the left, but not as clearly as on the right. The arrows indicate the veins.

Figure 22–18. Right pulmonary veins, which are unusually clearly defined in this patient, are indicated by arrows.

the visceral pleura is not often definitely outlined in the normal individual. When pneumothorax is present, it is seen as the thin outer wall or covering of the lung. It is also occasionally visible when a sufficient part of it is parallel to the roentgen-ray beam; for example, the secondary interlobar fissure on the right, made up of the visceral pleura covering the inferior aspect of the upper lobe and the superior aspect of the middle lobe, is visible in approximately 20% of individuals as a thin, straight, horizontal line. The major fissures are occasionally visible on a lateral roentgenogram in the absence of disease. The parietal pleura covers the diaphragm and lines the thorax, but it blends with the other structures of the chest wall and is not identified separately on roentgenograms. The relationships of visceral pleura to the bony thorax are shown in Figure 22-23.

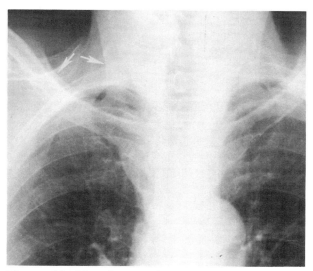

Figure 22–20. Companion shadows of the clavicle and sternocleidomastoid muscle are indicated by arrows.

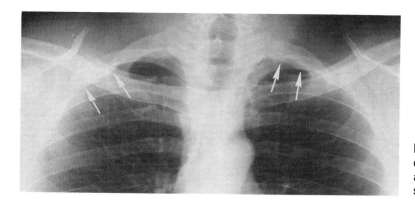

Figure 22–21. Companion shadows of the second (*right*) and first (*left*) ribs are indicated by arrows on respective sides.

THE CHEST IN INFANCY AND CHILDHOOD

In the newborn infant the thorax in the anteroposterior diameter is greater as compared to the transverse diameter than in adults. The diaphragm is higher, and this makes the vertical diameter of the thoracic cavity relatively less than in the adult. With growth the chest becomes narrower in its anteroposterior diameter, and the vertical and transverse diameters gradually increase. The ribs are nearly horizontal in position and gradually angulate downward as the child grows. The sternum is incompletely ossified at birth; this structure ossifies in a segmental manner. There are two ossification centers lying side by side in each segment. The centers for the manubrium are united at birth, but the remainder may not fuse for several years. The centers are of radiographic importance because they appear as small rounded opacities that may overlie the lungs in oblique or semioblique projections. They should be recognized as ossification centers and not be mistaken for lesions within the pulmonary parenchyma.

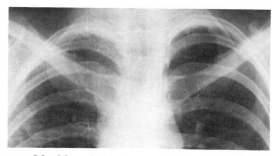

Figure 22–22. Apical pleural thickening in a patient with minimal tuberculosis of the right upper lobe. Note the irregularity of the soft tissue at both apices. Note also the irregular nodular disease in the right second anterior interspace representing the tuberculous disease.

The thymus gland is often large enough in the newborn period or early infancy to produce widening of the superior mediastinum. The roentgen appearance has been described earlier (Fig. 22-24). The appearance of the heart in the infant and child differs from that in the adult. The heart in the newborn is globular and relatively large in comparison to the diameter of the chest than in adults. The left ventricle becomes more prominent with increase in age, resulting in downward displacement of the apex, and the relative heart size gradually decreases. These changes are discussed more fully in Chapter 32.

The lungs in the infant and child tend to be slightly more radiolucent than in the adult, since the pulmonary interstitium is usually not visible, but the relative size of the visible vascular trunks is comparable. The root of the lung making up the hilar shadow is relatively high and is usually situated at the level of the third thoracic vertebra. The tracheal bifurcation gradually descends and reaches the adult level (fifth thoracic vertebra) at about 10 years of age.

The diaphragm tends to be higher in infancy and childhood than in adult life, and in the newborn it is not unusual to note a reversal of the adult situation with regard to relative height. The left hemidiaphragm is slightly higher than the right, probably because the stomach is frequently distended with air. There is considerable variation in position of the diaphragm in infancy and childhood, and the same factors of position of the patient as well as habitus are involved as have been noted in the discussion of the adult diaphragm (Fig. 22-25).

THE CHEST IN ADVANCING AGE

There is gradual alteration in the shape of the bony thorax with advancing age. The amount of alteration varies widely, and there is also a great individual variation in the age at which these changes appear and become severe. The tendency is for a gradual increase

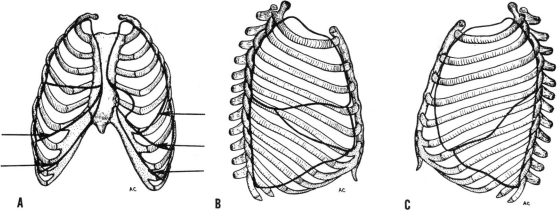

Figure 22–23. **(A)** Relationship of the visceral pleural to the bony thorax in the frontal plane. On the right, the upper arrow indicates the anteroinferior border and the lower arrow the posteroinferior border of the visceral pleura. In the left hemithorax, the anterior aspect is indicated by the upper and middle arrows and the posterior border by the lower arrow. **(B)** Visceral pleural on the right as visualized in the left lateral projection. Note the primary and secondary interlobar fissures separating the three lobes. **(C)** Pleural outlines on the left as visualized in the right lateral position.

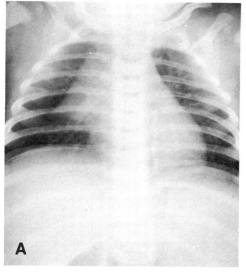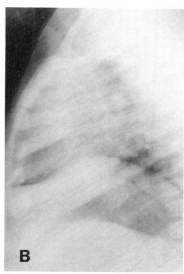

Figure 22–24. Infant with enlargement of the right lobe of the thymus. **(A)** Note the angulation on the right, which represents the sail sign. **(B)** In this lateral view, an anterosuperior mediastinal density produced by the thymus is noted. This is also an example of an infant's chest.

in the dorsal kyphotic curve, resulting in an increased anteroposterior diameter of the chest; it may approach or even exceed the transverse diameter in some instances. Varying amounts of osteopenia may be noted in the bones included in the chest roentgenogram, particularly in women. Rib irregularities caused by healed fractures are commonly noted and calcification may be seen in costal cartilages. This calcification varies greatly in amount and tends to appear earlier

and be more extensive in women than men. Its roentgen appearance is that of increased opacity caused by calcium outlining the cartilage extending from the anterior rib edge toward the sternum, often peripheral in males and central in females.

The changes in the mediastinum with advancing age are largely caused by alteration in the aorta and its branches, which tend to become elongated, dilated, and tortuous. As a result, the right superior mediasti-

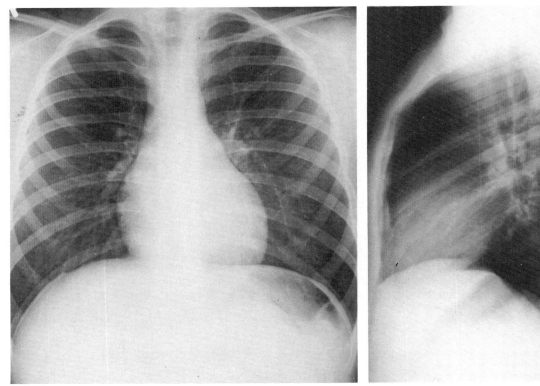

Figure 22–25. Normal chest in a 10-year-old child. Note that the heart is somewhat globular and that the anteroposterior diameter of the chest is relatively large in comparison to the transverse diameter.

nal border may become more prominent and clearly defined, because of increasing visibility of the brachiocephalic artery. The ascending arch of the aorta projects farther to the right and causes a convex shadow of soft-tissue density, the lower half of which overlies the right hilum. Similar prominence of the left upper mediastinum may be apparent with sclerotic changes in the left subclavian artery, and the aortic arch tends to become increasingly prominent (Fig. 22-26). The presence of calcification in the aortic arch is common, and calcification in the brachiocephalic and subclavian arteries is not rare.

Alteration in appearance of the lungs varies widely with advancing age, but there is a general tendency for the vessels in the mid- and peripheral zones to be separated by overinflation of alveoli and loss of alveolar walls representing emphysema. An associated decrease in perfusion results in a decrease in size of the peripheral vessels. Pulmonary hypertension may develop. This is associated with increased size of the arteries in the hila. In addition, linear shadows produced by residues of previous inflammatory disease in one or both bases are often observed, and there is a

tendency for the pulmonary interstitial pattern to become more pronounced. Small pulmonary parenchymal calcific foci are common along with calcification in hilar nodes. Apical scarring producing irregular soft-tissue opacities at the extreme apices is also found commonly in the aged, as indicated earlier. One or both costophrenic sulci may be at least partially obliterated by previous basal pleural disease. The diaphragm tends to become lower and flatter, with alteration in the shape of the bony thorax and the appearance of "senile emphysema." Irregularities of the diaphragm resulting from pleural inflammatory residuals are not uncommon. As the diaphragm becomes lower, the dome becomes more horizontal and the costophrenic angles less acute (Fig. 22-26).

CONGENITAL MALFORMATIONS

THE BONY THORAX

Minor developmental abnormalities are common in the ribs and are usually of no clinical significance, but they should be noted and recognized as such on the

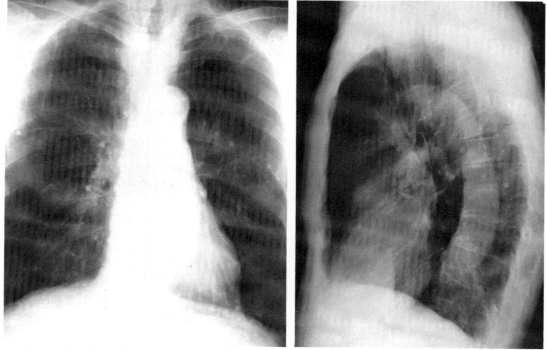

Figure 22–26. The chest in the aged. The patient is a 71-year-old man with a considerable amount of calcification in the aortic wall, aortic dilatation, and elongation. The lungs are slightly hyperlucent. There is a little increase in the thoracic curve, resulting in an increase in the anteroposterior diameter of the chest. The scattered parenchymal calcifications represent residues of previous histoplasmosis.

roentgenogram. Cervical ribs are not unusual and may be very small and difficult to outline, or they may be long and easily recognized as they project downward to overlie the pulmonary apex. They are usually asymptomatic. Occasionally, the transverse processes of the seventh cervical vertebra are unusually long and simulate short cervical ribs. One or both first ribs are often rudimentary. The most common anomaly of the remaining ribs is an anterior bifurcation, usually resulting in a broad, thin rib anteriorly that bifurcates near the costochondral junction. Complete fusion along the arcs of the ribs and pseudarthrosis between the ribs are other common anomalies. More severe rib anomalies may be associated with segmentation anomalies of the spine.[68] *Intrathoracic rib* is extremely rare. The anomalous rib usually arises from the posterior inferior margin of an otherwise normal rib or from a vertebral body, most often on the right side. The rib is sometimes attached to the diaphragm by a fibrous band. It projects into the pleural space and may be surrounded by lung even though its location is extrapleural. Diagnosis is suspected on viewing the chest roentgenogram and confirmed by tomography or CT.

Anterior protrusion deformities of the sternum resulting in the so-called pigeon breast, or pectus carinatum, are usually so mild that no significant abnormality is noted on the frontal projection and only in the lateral view can the diagnosis be made. In these patients the sternum protrudes anteriorly to a greater or lesser degree. The amount of protrusion is readily apparent on the lateral roentgenogram. This anomaly may be associated with right-to-left cardiac shunts.

Funnel-chest deformity, or *pectus excavatum*, produces changes that can usually be recognized on a posteroanterior roentgenogram. There may be displacement of the heart to the left, often with a bulge below the pulmonary artery suggesting left atrial enlargement. In others, the heart is compressed between the spine and the sternum, resulting in pseudo-enlargement in this projection. Often there is increased opacity in the right medial lung base, probably caused by a combination of crowded vessels and compressed lung in this area. In the lateral projection the posterior displacement of the sternum is readily discerned. Congenital midline defect or fissure in the sternum is a rare anomaly.[38] The sternum is divided into equal halves by the fissure, which is easily recognized on the roentgenograms. Rarely, small accessory ossicles are noted immediately above the manubrium in the region of the suprasternal notch. They are termed episternal or suprasternal bones; they may be single or paired and range from a few millimeters to more than a centimeter in diameter.[8] They may be fused to the manubrium or articulate with it, or there may be no contact with the sternum. Oversegmentation of the sternum may be associated with trisomy 21, and undersegmentation with trisomy 18.

Scoliosis is a common abnormality in the thoracic spine and may be congenital. Hemivertebrae and other vertebral anomalies occur in conjunction with scoliosis and often produce it. In many instances, however, no definite anomaly is noted involving the vertebral bodies in patients with scoliosis. The deformity of the thorax is proportional to the severity of the scoliosis, and when marked, the anatomic alteration produced in the heart and lungs may result in altered cardiac and pulmonary function. Kyphosis often accompanies scoliosis and adds to the thoracic deformity. Kyphosis of the thoracic spine may also occur as an isolated deformity. It results in an increase in the anteroposterior diameter and a decrease in the vertical diameter of the thorax.

ANOMALIES OF THE LUNG

ACCESSORY LOBES, FISSURES, AND BRONCHI

Azygos Lobe (Fissure)

The azygos lobe is not a true accessory lobe or fissure but is commonly observed on the chest radiograph. It is formed when the arch of the azygos vein fails to migrate medially to lie in its normal position just above the right upper lobe bronchus. Since this vein remains in a lateral position, the small portion of the apex of the lung that lies medial to it early in development is deeply invaginated. The vessel carries two layers of visceral pleura and two layers of parietal pleura with it, since it lies peripheral to the parietal pleura. As a result, the "azygos fissure" is visible as a thin curvilinear line extending upward toward the apex to end at the parietal pleura of the apex. This line is usually bowed outward, and its base, formed by the vein itself, is comma shaped with the tail of the comma pointing upward to the fissure. The upper end of the fissure usually ends in a small triangle of soft-tissue opacity with its base superiorly and its apex pointing downward continuous with the fissure (Fig. 22-27). The azygos lobe varies in size, but it is seldom very large. It is a common anomaly, occurs in about 0.5% of the population, and is usually of no significance.

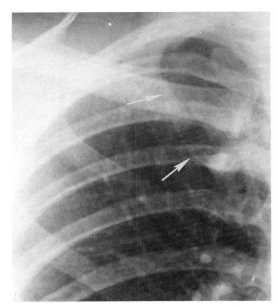

Figure 22–27. Azygos lobe. Note the vein below the sternal end of the clavicle and the fissure (*arrows*) extending in an arc up to the pleural surface of the apex.

Inferior Accessory Lobe

The inferior accessory or cardiac lobe is the most common accessory lobe (in about 25% to 40% of humans). The fissure may be complete or incomplete and is seen on the posteroanterior roentgenogram as a faint line at the right medial base beginning at the diaphragm and extending upward toward the hilum. There is often a very small triangular upward projection of soft-tissue density at the diaphragmatic end of the fissure. This accessory lobe is usually supplied by a bronchus branching off the medial basal segment of the lower lobe. The anomaly is probably less common on the left than on the right but is more difficult to see because it is often hidden by the cardiac shadow. Therefore, it may be more common on the left than is generally realized. It is of no particular significance but occasionally becomes involved by disease, may limit the process, and is then more readily identified (Fig. 22-28).

Other Accessory Lobes

The left upper lobe may be divided by a horizontal fissure in a manner similar to the division on the right producing an accessory middle lobe. In these instances the interlobar fissure that divides the upper and accessory lobes is in approximately the same position as the

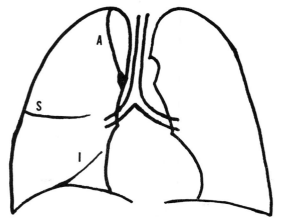

Figure 22–28. Sketch showing position of the two most common accessory fissures: *A*, Azygos; *I*, inferior accessory lobe fissure. The secondary interlobar fissure is also indicated as *S*.

minor fissure on the right. This is a rare anomaly and of no clinical significance.

The posterior or dorsal lobe is produced when the superior segment of the lower lobe is separated from the basal segments by a horizontal fissure, the *superior accessory fissure*. This accessory lobe is rarely identified radiographically unless it is involved by disease sufficient to outline the smooth fissure separating it from the base of the lower lobe. It is somewhat more common anatomically, however, than radiographic examination would indicate (see Fig. 22-28).

Supernumerary Bronchi

Supernumerary bronchi are uncommon and can be recognized roentgenographically on bronchography and sometimes on CT, since they result in supernumerary segments rather than lobes. The most common site is the right upper lobe, where the anomalous bronchus arises from the lateral aspect of the right main bronchus above the upper lobe bronchus; usually no symptoms are produced by this anomaly. Occasionally, an accessory bronchus arises from the lower right trachea, a right *tracheal bronchus*.[44] It is less common on the left. It usually arises within 2 cm of the carina but may arise higher, and it usually supplies the apical segment of the upper lobe but may supply the entire upper lobe. Although usually asymptomatic, occasionally a tracheal bronchus may be of clinical significance because it may be associated with a cyst, obstructive emphysema, or bronchiectasis leading to infection, so there is an increased incidence of pneumonia in these patients. Other anomalies associated with tracheal bronchus are fairly common. A *bridging bronchus*[34] is extremely rare and is usually associated with multiple anomalies resulting in death in infancy. In this anomaly, a bronchus arises on the left side and extends across the mediastinum to supply the lower lobe on the opposite side, the right lower lobe. Minor variation in origin of segmental bronchi is not uncommon, and displacement of a bronchus is often difficult or impossible to differentiate from a supernumerary bronchus. Numerous minor variations of bronchial segmentation have been found in all lobes and are not uncommonly demonstrated on bronchographic examination, which is necessary to identify these bronchial variations. An entire lobe may be affected, or one or more segments may be involved (Fig. 22-29).

Bronchial Atresia and Stenosis

Bronchial atresia and stenosis is an uncommon anomaly that usually involves the apical posterior segment of the left upper lobe. Such a stenosis may also be acquired. Usually the segmental bronchus is involved, but occasionally a lobar bronchus or a subsegmental bronchus may be affected. There is usually a mucus plug (impaction) at the point of atresia, which is observed as an elongated tubular shadow on the film. The lung distal to the atresia is usually overinflated, presumably a result of collateral air drift. The involved segment may be opaque at birth, since fetal lung fluid clears slowly. This anomaly is usually asymptomatic, so no treatment is necessary.[34]

Absence of Fissures

Variations of interlobar fissures are relatively common, but since they occur without alteration in bronchopulmonary segmentation, they produce no roentgenographic findings. In a study of 1200 lungs in cases of sudden death, Medlar[43] found the interlobar fissure on the left complete in 82%, the major fissure on the right was complete in 69% and the minor fissure complete in only 37.7%. In the remainder the fissures were absent or incomplete.

PULMONARY AGENESIS, APLASIA, AND HYPOPLASIA

Agenesis of a lobe indicates complete absence of the lobe, including the bronchus and blood supply. In aplasia, there is absence of lung tissue, but a rudimentary lobar bronchus is present.[58] These anomalies are very rare, usually unilateral, and often associated with other anomalies. Agenesis of the right lung carries a higher mortality than the same anomaly on the left. In

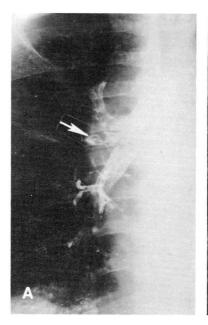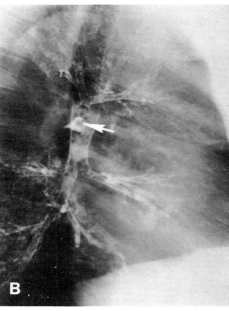

Figure 22–29. Accessory lobe arising below the right upper lobe bronchus. This is outlined on the bronchogram, but its branches are not filled because of the presence of an intraluminal lipoma obstructing it. Arrows indicate the bronchus on the frontal (**A**) and lateral (**B**) projections.

hypoplasia, there is incomplete development of a lobe or lung. There is the normal number of lobes and bronchi, but parenchyma is incompletely developed. In some instances, the hypoplasia is secondary to compression of the developing lung by abdominal viscera in congenital diaphragmatic hernia, congenital eventration, and several other conditions that encroach on the intrathoracic space. Also, a decrease in blood supply or pulmonary artery agenesis may cause hypoplasia. Roentgen findings on routine examination include a marked shift of the heart and other mediastinal structures to the involved side, with a decrease in size of that hemithorax. There is herniation of the normal lung across the midline and evidence of increased volume of the normal lung, which is very likely due to a combination of hyperplasia and compensatory overinflation. The cardiac border may be indistinct on the ipsilateral side if the remaining lung fails to fill the hemithorax to the anterior chest wall. The anterior space is then occupied by loose areolar tissue that blurs the heart border. Bronchoscopy is necessary to visualize the bronchial tree, and on this examination, either a small bronchial stump or no bronchus at all is visualized. When an entire lung is absent, no lung is noted on the involved side except that which has herniated across the midline from the normal side. Angiography can be used to outline the vascular system. It demonstrates the pulmonary arterial supply and thus helps to differentiate agenesis and aplasia from hypoplasia.

Pulmonary hypogenesis indicates incomplete development of the lung or a part of it and is also uncommon.

All gradations from minor to severe degrees may occur. Unless the anomaly is severe, there is usually very little alteration in the size of the affected hemithorax because some normal lung tissue remains; mediastinal shift along with elevation of the diaphragm on the involved side and compensatory overinflation on the opposite side all help to fill the hemithorax. This condition must be differentiated from previous inflammatory disease resulting in fibrosis and contraction of a lobe or portion of a lobe. The evidence of previous disease may be apparent, but if not, bronchoscopy and sometimes bronchography can be used to show the bronchial distribution.

Lobar hypoplasia, aplasia, or agenesis may be associated with other anomalies, including accessory diaphragm, partial anomalous pulmonary venous return below the diaphragm, as well as skeletal gastrointestinal and genitourinary defects.

Horseshoe lung consists of an isthmus of lung joining the lower lobes behind the heart. The isthmus is usually supplied by the right pulmonary arterial and bronchial systems, is often hypovascular and therefore radiolucent, and is usually associated with right lung hypoplasia and dextrocardia. Other arteriovenous anomalies may also be present.[34]

BRONCHOPULMONARY SEQUESTRATION

Pulmonary sequestration is a congenital anomaly in which a portion of pulmonary tissue supplied by an arterial branch of the systemic circulation is sequestered from normal bronchial communication within a lobe or outside of the normal lung. Occasionally, there is a communication with the esophagus or stomach, so a more inclusive term, *bronchopulmonary foregut malformation*, may be used to describe a spectrum of anomalies that includes sequestration. These anomalies include a wide range of defects; tracheoesophageal fistula, bronchopulmonary sequestration, aberrant systemic arterial supply to the lung, bronchogenic cyst, bronchial mucosal rests in the esophageal wall, and bronchoesophageal and bronchogastric communications.

Bronchopulmonary sequestration may be intralobar or extralobar, depending on the relationship of the sequestered tissue to the lung. As indicated, it is likely that they have a common embryologic origin. The intralobar form occurs on the left side in about 60% of patients, and extralobar sequestration is left sided in 90%. *Intralobar sequestration*[47] is an anomaly in which a systemic artery arising from the lower thoracic or upper abdominal aorta extends into the lung on either side, where it supplies a portion of pulmonary tissue that is not connected with the normal bronchial tree and is therefore termed "sequestered." It is drained usually by the pulmonary venous system. If it is uninfected, the lesion produces no symptoms. If it becomes infected and communicates with the bronchial tree, signs and symptoms of pulmonary infection are produced. Therefore, the diagnosis is usually made in adults. Rarely, in children, there may be enough arterial shunting through the sequestration to the pulmonary venous system to cause congestive failure. It is almost entirely a lower lobe lesion and usually involves the posterior basal segment (60%). The anomaly has been found somewhat more frequently in males than in females; the ratio is approximately two to one. Occasionally, the arterial supply arises from the ascending aorta, the subclavian artery, the intercostal arteries, and, rarely, the celiac or innominate artery, and occasionally the venous drainage is into the inferior vena cava or azygos system and, rarely, into the portal system.

Roentgen findings depend on the presence or absence of infection. In the patients in whom there is no infection, the condition is usually an incidental finding and presents as a round or oval mass in the posterior lung base on either side that may range up to 10 cm or more in diameter. It is usually found in the medial aspect of the lung base, and occasionally, a poorly defined, fingerlike projection extends toward the mediastinum from the medial aspect of the mass representing the artery supplying the tissue. When infection is present, there is enough bronchial communication so that fluid levels and air are often visible in a single cyst or in several adjacent or multilocular cysts,

the walls of which are usually thin. Even though there is evidence of bronchial communication manifested by the presence of air within the cysts, bronchography does not ordinarily demonstrate the communication. Normal bronchial branches are usually draped around the mass. This may be demonstrated on CT or on conventional tomography at times. The lesion must be differentiated from lung abscess, acquired infected cysts, and chronic pulmonary inflammatory disease with cavitation. The asymptomatic type with no apparent connection with the bronchi must be differentiated from tumors and cysts of other origin. The location of these lesions is rather characteristic, however, and when a soft-tissue mass or an infected cyst is noted in the lung base, intralobar sequestration should be considered (Fig. 22-30). If this lesion is suspected, aortography is indicated. The diagnosis is established when the anomalous artery is opacified. However, CT and MRI are now being used, and one or the other may supplant angiography in the future.[47]

Extralobar sequestration results when the sequestered tissue is contained in its own pleural covering between the lower lobe and the diaphragm, within the diaphragm, in the mediastinum, or beneath the diaphragm. The arterial supply is similar to that of intralobar sequestration. It is drained usually by the vena cava or azygos venous system and occasionally by the portal system in contrast to the intralobar form, which usually drains into the pulmonary venous system. The sequestration is on the left side in 90% of cases. The diagnosis is usually made in infancy.[24] Associated anomalies of the diaphragm are common, eventration being a frequent finding. In addition to an abnormal diaphragm, a mass representing the sequestered lung may be visible. Rarely, hemorrhage into an extralobar sequestration will cause a mass to appear or to enlarge in the vicinity of the posteromedial aspect of the left hemidiaphragm.[55] Aortography can be used for confirmation when sequestration is suspected and must be differentiated from other masses such as malignancy, which may require surgical removal (Fig. 22-31).

Other pulmonary anomalies involving blood vessels, such as the *scimitar syndrome*, which indicates partial anomalous venous return, and *arteriovenous malformations* are discussed in Chapter 32.

BRONCHOGENIC (BRONCHOPULMONARY) CYSTS

Most cystic lesions of the lung are now believed to be acquired, but it is likely that the cysts occurring within the lung, lined by bronchial epithelium and resembling the bronchogenic cysts found in the mediastinum, represent congenital rather than acquired lesions. They are usually solitary and may occur anywhere within the

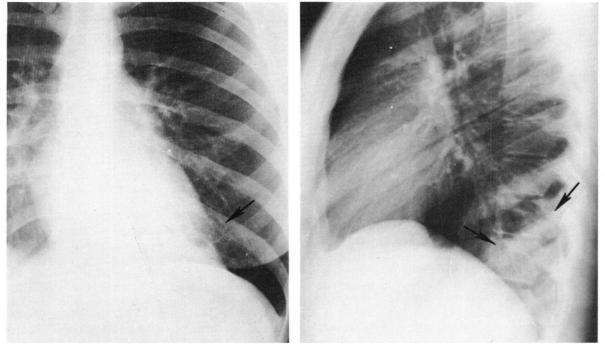

Figure 22–30.   Intralobar sequestration. The poorly defined mass at the left postero-medial base is indicated by arrows.

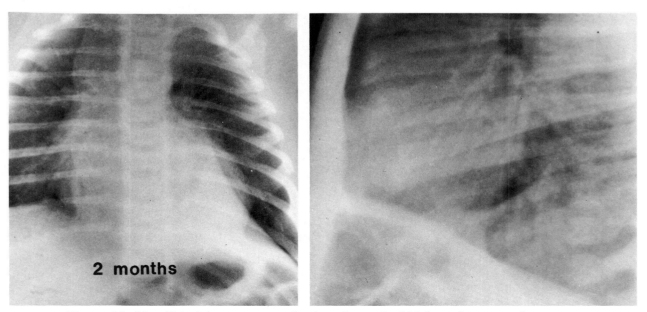

Figure 22–31.   Extralobar sequestration in a 2-month-old infant. A retrocardiac mass rests on the diaphragm posteriorly as visualized in the lateral view.

lung. They present as round, clearly defined, intrapulmonary, soft-tissue masses. Since the lining may contain mucus-secreting glands, the cysts may become large. If this occurs in infancy, atelectasis, local hyperinflation, and/or infection may result from compression of adjacent lung. This lesion usually produces no symptoms, however, and may be found on routine chest roentgenograms. If the cyst becomes infected and communicates with the bronchus, the roentgen findings are those of a thin-walled cavity containing gas and fluid that may be considerably obscured by inflammatory disease in the adjacent lung. In this situation, it may be very difficult or impossible to differentiate congenital from acquired cyst even on histologic study.

CONGENITAL CYSTIC ADENOMATOID MALFORMATION OF THE LUNG

This is a rare form of congenital cystic disease of the lung in which neonatal respiratory distress is often present. It usually involves a single lobe that is greatly enlarged and consists of a mass of disorganized tissue that probably represents a pulmonary hamartoma.[42, 50] The lobe is firm and rubbery. One type consists of multiple large cysts of varying size, with no normal bronchial or lobular pulmonary pattern. This type occurs in 50% of cases and is the most common pattern. The cysts usually expand gradually and may fill with air. The prognosis is usually good after resection of the large mass, which often compresses the normal lung. In 40%, the cysts are small, multiple, and evenly spaced throughout the lobe. In this type, there is a high incidence of associated severe anomalies, so the prognosis is generally poor. In some cases, the anomaly takes the form of a large solid mass containing fluid-filled cysts. This mass is usually bulky, displaces normal lung, and carries a poor prognosis.

About 25% of infants with this anomaly are stillborn and many are premature. Polyhydramnios is common, as are associated fetal anomalies. Occasionally, the anomaly has been reported in adults when it involves a relatively small amount of lung, so that pulmonary function is not compromised. Radiologic findings are those of a pulmonary mass that displaces the mediastinum and heart and often herniates into the opposite hemithorax. The multiple cysts result in a coarse, honey-combed appearance. Air–fluid levels may be observed. Irregular areas of opacity often outline some of the cysts and form part of the enlarged lobe. All cysts may be filled with fluid, presenting a roentgen picture of a large, solid mass. In some instances a single large cyst may be the predominant feature. CT is useful to define the cysts within the mass. Ultrasonography is also helpful in defining the fluid-filled cysts, and a prenatal diagnosis can be made using this modality.

The clinical symptoms appear to be related to the size of the involved lobe and to infection within the cysts. Surgical removal is necessary to allow the remaining lung to expand.

IMMOTILE CILIA SYNDROME

Immotile cilia syndrome is a genetically determined (presumably an autosomal recessive) defect of cilia in which electron microscopic examination reveals a heterogeneous group of defects in nasal and bronchial cilia. The defects result in impaired motility and defective mucociliary clearance. Situs inversus is present in 50% of patients. Clinical findings include upper respiratory infections with sinusitis appearing as early as 6 months and recurrent otitis media in nearly all patients. Bronchiectasis causing cough with sputum is found in 75% of adults with the condition.

The radiographic findings, which are present in all symptomatic patients, are similar to those found in cystic fibrosis but tend to be less severe and less progressive. Bronchial wall thickening and hyperinflation are followed by segmental bronchiectasis, often in the middle lobe. Segmental consolidation and atelectasis may appear with exacerbations of infectious disease.[45]

CONGENITAL PULMONARY LYMPHANGIECTASIA

Congenital pulmonary lymphangiectasia is a rare congenital disease[34] that causes neonatal respiratory distress. The lungs are large and lobulated with prominent subpleural lymphatics, which are cystic. Interlobular septa are enlarged by the cystic lymphatics. Most affected infants survive for only a short time. When this disease occurs as a primary developmental defect, it is usually evident in the neonatal period. Associated congenital cardiac anomalies are common. Also, the disease may occur as a part of general lymphangiectasia. In some instances, it appears to be secondary to venous obstruction. Occasionally, only a single lobe is involved. The lobe is large and dense and may compress the remaining ipsilateral lung and displace the mediastinum. Some unilobar cases have been reported in adults. Resection of the involved lobe may be necessary. A milder form is also found in older persons in whom the major roentgen findings are related to lymphatic enlargement. Roentgen findings in this form are those of bilateral increase in pulmonary opacity with a reticulonodular pattern. Kerley's A and B lines are observed on the chest film, probably representing enlarged lymphatics. The lines may become very large and coarse. In other patients, the lung or lobe may be uniformly dense. Both the severe and milder forms may be associated with peripheral lymphangiomas.

INFANTILE (CONGENITAL) LOBAR EMPHYSEMA

Lobar emphysema in infants may not be manifest until some weeks or months after birth. Therefore, the term *infantile* or *neonatal* is probably more accurate than *congenital* in referring to this condition. Obstructive emphysema (obstructive overinflation) appears to be caused by bronchial obstruction, which may be produced by extrabronchial pressure, caused by a vessel, abnormality of bronchial cartilages, or redundant bronchial mucosa. In nonobstructive lobar "emphysema" (polyalveolar), there are three to five times the normal number of alveoli[34] and an increase in the size of alveoli. In some patients no definite cause can be found. Associated cardiac anomalies are common. There is a male predominance with a ratio of about 3:1. The left upper and right middle lobes are most commonly involved. The lower lobes are rarely affected. The involved lobe is greatly overexpanded and usually contains air, rendering it radiolucent. Occasionally, the involved lobe is opaque, presumably caused by intrapulmonary fluid accumulation distal to the bronchial obstruction. The fluid usually drains spontaneously, leaving the overexpanded lobe radiolucent.[13]

The roentgen findings consist of marked radiolucency in the region of the involved lobe. The volume is markedly increased, resulting in depression of the hemidiaphragm on the side of involvement and displacement of the mediastinum away from it. There may be compression atelectasis of the remaining lobe or lobes. Vascular markings in the affected lobe are widely separated and small, adding to the radiolucency produced by the air trapping. Respiratory distress in affected infants usually occurs during the first few days or weeks of life, and the diagnosis is usually not difficult to make. In some instances, emergency surgery is necessary to remove the overexpanded lobe. In others, symptoms may be mild, and surgery is not required.

PULMONARY ISOMERISM

Pulmonary isomerism is an anomaly in which both lungs are similar in that both may have either two lobes or three lobes. Sometimes the anomalies are described as bilateral pulmonary right- or left-sidedness. In most instances there are associated splenic and congenital cardiac anomalies. In Ivemark's syndrome, there are bilateral three-lobed lungs and abnormal visceral situs associated with asplenia. There may also be congenital heart disease such as transposition, pulmonary stenosis or atresia, atrial septal defect, common ventricle, and total anomalous pulmonary venous return. In males, three-lobed lungs may also be associated with anisosplenia (multiple accessory spleens) and congenital heart disease. Bilateral two-lobed lungs in males are associated with polysplenia, a lower incidence of con-

genital heart disease, and normal visceral situs. In females, there may be anisosplenia and congenital heart disease sometimes associated with abnormal visceral situs in conjunction with bilateral two-lobed lungs.

Corrected transposition, ventricular septal defects, common atrium, anomalous pulmonary venous connections, and bilateral superior vena cava are the cardiovascular anomalies associated with asplenia; pulmonary stenosis or atresia may also occur. Polysplenia is often associated with azygos or hemiazygos continuation of the inferior vena cava, septal defects, anomalous pulmonary connections, and bilateral superior vena cava.[37] These complicated anomalies often cause abnormalities observed on chest films. Accurate diagnosis often depends on extensive clinical and cardiovascular studies using ultrasonography and sometimes angiography.

APICAL HERNIATION OF THE LUNG

Herniation of the lung into the soft tissues of the neck is more common on the right than on the left. It is a rare anomaly, probably representing a congenital defect in the costovertebral fascia, which permits the upward extension of pulmonary tissue. Unless the mass increases or becomes incarcerated, no treatment is necessary, but surgical repair can be done if there are complications.[62]

REFERENCES AND SELECTED READINGS

1. ABLOW RC, GREENSPAN RH, GLUCK L: The advantages of direct magnification technic in the newborn chest. Radiology 92:745, 1969

2. ARMSTRONG JD II, SORENSON JA, NELSON JA: Clinical evaluation of unsharp masking and slit scanning techniques in chest radiography. Radiology 147:351, 1983

3. BALL JB JR, PROTO AV: The variable appearance of the left superior intercostal vein. Radiology 144:445, 1982

4. BEAHRS OH, HENSON DE, HUTTER RVP, ET AL: Manual for Staging of Cancer. American Joint Committee on Cancer, 3rd ed. pp 120–121, Philadelphia, JB Lippincott.

5. BERQUIST TH, BAILEY PB, CORTESE DA, ET AL: Transthoracic needle biopsy—accuracy and complications in relation to location and type of lesion. Mayo Clin Proc 55:475, 1980

6. BOYDEN EA: A synthesis of the prevailing pattern of the bronchopulmonary segments in the light of their variations. Dis Chest 15:657, 1949

7. BOYDEN EA: The distribution of bronchi in gross anomalies of the right upper lobe, particularly lobes subdivided by the azygos vein and those containing preeparterial bronchi. Radiology 58:797, 1952

8. BROWN WH: Episternal bones. Radiology 75:116, 1960

9. CHASEN MH, MCCARTHY MJ, GILLILAND JD, ET AL: Concepts in computed tomography of the thorax. Radiographics 6:793, 1986

10. CIMMINO CV: The anterior mediastinal line on chest roentgenograms. Radiology 82:459, 1964

11. DAVIS LA: The vertical fissure line. Am J Roentgenol 84:451, 1960

12. EISENBERG RL, HEDGCOCK MW, WILLIAMS EA, ET AL: Optimum radiographic examination for consideration of compensation awards: 1. General methodology and application to chest examination. Am J Roentgenol 135:1065, 1980

13. FAGAN CJ, SWISCHUK LE: The opaque lung in lobar emphysema. Am J Roentgenol 114:300, 1972

14. FELSON B, FELSON H: Localization of intrathoracic lesions by means of the posteroanterior roentgenogram. Radiology 55:363, 1950

15. FERRIS EJ, HOLDER JC, LIM WN, ET AL: Angiography of pulmonary emboli: Digital studies and balloon-occlusion cineangiography. Am J Roentgenol 142:369, 1984

16. FLOYD CE, CHOTES HG, DOBBINS JT, ET AL: Quantitative radiographic imaging using a photostimulable phosphor system. Med Phys 17:454, 1990

17. FRASER RG, BREATNACH E, BARNES GT: Digital radiography of the chest: Clinical experience with a prototype unit. Radiology 148:1, 1983

18. FRASER RG, PARE JAP, PARE PO, ET AL: Diagnosis of the Diseases of the Chest, Vols 1–4, 3rd ed., Philadelphia, WB Saunders, 1988

19. FRIEDMAN AC, CHAMBERS E, SPRAYREGEN S: The normal and abnormal left superior intercostal vein. Am J Roentgenol 131:599, 1978

20. GOODMAN LR, GOLKOW RS, STEINER RM, ET AL: The right midlung window. Radiology 143:135, 1982

21. GOODMAN PC, BROUT-ZAWALZKI M: Digital subtraction pulmonary angiography. Am J Roentgenol 139:305, 1982

22. GROSS BH, SPIZARNY DL, GRANKE DS: Sagittal orientation of the anterior minor fissure. Radiography and CT. Radiology 166:717, 1988

23. GROSSMAN H, WINCHESTER PH, AULD PA: Simultaneous frontal and lateral chest roentgenograms on low birth weight infants. Am J Roentgenol 108:550, 1970

24. HADDON MJ, BOWEN AD: Bronchopulmonary and neurenteric forms of foregut anomalies: Imaging for diagnosis and management. Radiol Clin North Am 29:241, 1991

25. HEITZMAN ER: The Lung Radiologic-Pathologic Correlations. St. Louis, CV Mosby, 1973

26. HERMAN PG, GOLDSTEIN J, BALIKIAN J, ET AL: Visibility and sharpness of lung structure at 90, 140 and 350 kV. Radiology 134:591, 1980

27. HOLLMAN AS, ADAMS FG: The influence of the lordotic projection on the interpretation of the chest radiograph. Clin Radiol 40:36, 1989

28. HOMER MJ: The hilar height ratio. Radiology 129:11, 1978

29. HUNTER TB, KUHNS LR, ROLOFF MA, ET AL: Tracheobronchiomegaly in an 18-month-old child. Am J Roentgenol 123:687, 1975

30. JACKSON CL, HUBER JF: Correlated applied anatomy of the bronchial tree and lungs with a system of nomenclature. Dis Chest 9:319, 1943

31. JACKSON FI: The air-gap technique and an improvement by anteroposterior positioning for chest roentgenography. Am J Roentgenol 92:688, 1964

32. JOST RG, SAGEL SS, STANLEY RJ, ET AL: Computed tomography of the thorax. Radiology 126:125, 1978

33. KELSEY CA, MOSELEY RD JR, METTLER FA JR, ET AL: Cost-effectiveness of stereoscopic radiographs in detection of lung nodules. Radiology 142:611, 1982

34. KESLAR P, NEWMAN B, OH KS: Radiographic manifestations of anomalies of the lung. Radiol Clin North Am 29:255, 1991

35. KHOURI NF, STITIK FP, EROZAN YS, ET AL: Transthoracic needle aspiration biopsy of benign and malignant lung lesions. Am J Roentgenol 144:281, 1985

36. KIEFFER SA, HEITZMAN ER: An Atlas of Cross-Sectional Anatomy: Computed Tomography, Ultrasound, Radiography, Gross Anatomy. Hagerstown, Maryland, Harper & Row, 1979

37. LANDING BH, LAWRENCE T-WK, PAYNE VC JR, ET AL: Bronchial anatomy and syndromes with abnormal visceral situs, abnormal spleen and congenital heart disease. Am J Cardiol 28:456, 1971

38. LARSEN LL, IBACH HF: Complete congenital fissure of the sternum. Am J Roentgenol 87:1062, 1962

39. LEE JKT, SAGEL SS, STANLEY RJ: Computed Body Tomography. New York, Raven Press, 1983

40. LITTLETON JT, DURIZCH ML, CALLAHAN WP: Linear vs. pluridirectional tomography of the chest: Correlative radiographic anatomic study. Am J Roentgenol 134:241, 1980

41. LUNDGREN R, HEITALA S-O, ADELROTH E: Diagnosis of bronchial lesions by fiberoptic bronchoscopy combined with bronchography. Acta Radiol 23:231, 1982

42. MADEWELL JE, STOCKER JT, KORSOWER JM: Cystic adenomatoid malformation of the lung: Morphologic analysis. Am J Roentgenol 124:436, 1975

43. MEDLAR EM: Variations in interlobar fissure. Am J Roentgenol 57:723, 1947

44. MORRISON SC: Case report: Demonstration of a tracheal bronchus by computed tomography. Clin Radiol 39:208, 1988

45. NADEL HR, STRINGER DA, LEVISON H, ET AL: The immotile cilia syndrome. Radiological manifestations. Radiology 154:651, 1985

46. NAIDICH DP, RUMANCIK WM, ETTINGER NA, ET AL: Congenital anomalies of the lungs in adults: MR diagnosis. Am J Roentgenol 151:13, 1988

47. NAIDICH DP, RUMANCIK WM, LEFLEUR RS, ET AL: Intralobar pulmonary sequestration: MR evaluation. J Comput Assist Tomogr 11:531, 1987

48. NAIDICH DP, KHOURI NF, SCOTT WW JR, ET AL: Com-

puted tomography of the pulmonary hila: 1. Normal anatomy. J Comput Assist Tomogr 5:459, 1981

49. NAIDICH DP, ZERHOUNI EA, SIEGELMAN SS: Computed Tomography of the Thorax. New York, Raven Press, 1984

50. NEWMAN B, OH KS: Abnormal pulmonary aeration in infants and children. Radiol Clin North Am 26:323, 1988

51. PEARCE JG, PATT NL: Fatal pulmonary hemorrhage after percutaneous aspiration lung biopsy. Am Rev Respir Dis 110:346, 1974

52. PLEWES DB, WANDTKE JC: A scanning equalization system for improved chest radiography. Radiology 142:765, 1982

53. PROTO AV, LANE EJ: 350 kVp chest radiography: Review and comparison with 120 kVp. Am J Roentgenol 130:859, 1978

54. RABINOWITZ JG, COHEN BA, MENDLESON DS: The pulmonary ligament. Radiol Clin North Am 22:659, 1984

55. REICHERT JR, WINKLER SS: Spontaneous hemorrhage into an extralobar bronchopulmonary sequestration. Radiology 110:359, 1974

56. ROST RC JR, PROTO AV: Inferior pulmonary ligament: Computed tomographic appearance. Radiology 148:479, 1983

57. ROUVIERE H: Anatomy of the Human Lymphatic System. Ann Arbor, Edwards Bros, 1938

58. SINGLETON EB, DUTTON RV, WAGNER ML: Radiographic evaluation of lung abnormalities. Radiol Clin North Am 10:333, 1972

59. SOCIETY FOR COMPUTED BODY TOMOGRAPHY: Special report. New indications for computed body tomography. Am J Roentgenol 133:115, 1979

60. SOMMER FG, SMOTHERS RL, WHEAT RL, ET AL: Digital processing of film radiographs. Am J Roentgenol 144:191, 1985

61. SORENSON JA, NELSON LT, NIKLASON LT, ET AL: Rotating disc device for slit radiography of the chest. Radiology 134:227, 1980

62. THOMPSON JS: Cervical herniation of the lung: Report of a case and review of the literature. Pediatr Radiol 4:190, 1976

63. TROUT ED, KELLEY JP, LARSON VL: A comparison of air gap and a grid in roentgenography of the chest. Am J Roentgenol 124:404, 1975

64. VLASBLOEM H, SCHULTZE KOOL LJ: AMBER: A scanning multiple-beam equalization system for chest radiography. Radiology 169:29, 1988

65. WALLACE JM, BATRA P, GONG H JR: Percutaneous needle lung aspiration for diagnosing pneumonitis in patients with acquired immunodeficiency syndrome (AIDS). Am Rev Respir Dis 131:389, 1985

66. WEBB WR, GAMSU G, STARCK DD, ET AL: Evaluation of magnetic resonance sequences in imaging mediastinal tumors. Am J Roentgenol 143:723, 1984

67. WEBB WR, GLAZER G, GAMSU G: Computed tomography of the normal pulmonary hilum. J Comp Assist Tomogr 5:476, 1981

68. WEINSTEIN AS, MUELLER CF: Intrathoracic rib. Am J Roentgenol 94:587, 1965

69. WOODRING JH, DANIEL TL: Medical analysis emphasizing plain radiographs and computed tomograms. Med Radiog Photog 62:1, 1986

70. ZYLAK CJ, LITTLETON JT, DURIZCH ML: Illusory consolidation of the left lower lobe: A pitfall of portable radiography. Radiology 167:653, 1988

71. ZYLAK CJ, PALLIE W, JACKSON R: Correlative anatomy and computed tomography: A module on the mediastinum. Radiographics 2:555, 1982

Paul and Juhl's Essentials of Radiologic Imaging,
Sixth Edition, edited by John H. Juhl and
Andrew B. Crummy. J.B. Lippincott Company,
Philadelphia, © 1993.

CHAPTER **23**

Acute Pulmonary Infections

John H. Juhl

Acute pulmonary infection may be caused by a variety of organisms. In some instances they produce a reasonably characteristic, gross pathologic pattern and therefore a recognizable roentgen pattern. The findings can be classified as follows:

1. Lobar (alveolar, air-space) pneumonia. This is exemplified by Streptococcus pneumoniae pneumonia. The organism reaches the periphery of the lung via the airways. Alveolar transudation (edema) is followed by migration of leukocytes into the alveolar fluid. As the disease progresses, peripheral homogeneous (consolidation) opacity spreads toward the hilum and tends to cross segmental lines. Alveolar (air-space) pneumonia is not necessarily confined to a lobe, nor does it involve an entire lobe in many instances. Therefore, the term *lobar* is a misnomer in most cases, but is still used by many.
2. Bronchopneumonia (lobular). This is often observed in staphylococcal infection of the lung. The disease originates in the airways and spreads to peribronchial alveoli. The process tends to be confined by interlobular septa, so the appearance is one of patchy disease causing poorly defined opacities. However, a variety of roentgen patterns may result, including a confluent consolidation resembling lobar (alveolar) pneumonia.
3. Acute interstitial pneumonia. This is usually caused by a virus or a mycoplasma. Often the interstitial involvement is masked by alveolar exudate. A variety of roentgen patterns are observed, but alveolar consolidation, if present, is not usually as confluent or dense as in lobar or lobular pneumonia.

4. Mixed. This is a combination of lobar, bronchopneumonia, and interstitial pneumonia.

In the subsequent discussions, the most common gross anatomic findings in the pneumonias of various causes as reflected in chest roentgenograms are described. The roentgenographic manifestations of pulmonary infections are so varied that the pattern observed often gives us little, if any, information regarding the causative organism. Therefore, in each instance it should be remembered that roentgen findings must be correlated with clinical, bacteriologic, and laboratory data to ascertain the correct etiologic diagnosis on which treatment is based. The role of the radiologist is to locate and define the extent of the disease and any complications such as lung abscess and pleural effusion or empyema. An opinion as to whether the pattern is indicative of pneumonia should also be given. Serial films may be very useful in differentiating pulmonary edema from infection and are also used to follow the course of the pneumonia, particularly when clinical problems arise.

BACTERIAL PNEUMONIAS

PNEUMOCOCCAL PNEUMONIA

The acute pulmonary infection caused by *Streptococcus pneumoniae* is commonly termed lobar pneumonia. However, the infection does not usually involve an entire lobe and may be termed alveolar pneumonia. *S. pneumoniae* causes about 70% of bacterial pneumonia in the United States, often in otherwise healthy individuals, but the disease is generally more severe in those with alcoholism, neoplasms, chronic pulmonary disease, or altered immunity. There are more than 82 serotypes of *S. pneumoniae*, but most of the pneumonias are caused by types 1, 3, 4, 5, 7, 8, 9, or 12. Type 8 is the most common. Type 14 causes pneumonia in children but rarely in adults. Mortality from pneumonia caused by type 3 is higher than that caused by the others.

The organisms causing pneumococcal pneumonia are aspirated in droplets of saliva or mucus, so the lower lobes and posterior segments of upper lobes are most commonly involved. The onset is sudden and the gross pathologic changes are evident early in the disease, so that roentgen findings can be observed within 6 to 12 hours after onset of symptoms. In some instances, dehydration may decrease the pulmonary manifestations of pneumonia, so that there may be a delay in roentgenographic appearance of the disease. Then hydration might result in apparent rapid development of visible roentgen signs. There is conflicting evidence of this phenomenon, however. Involvement usually begins peripherally and spreads centripetally with homogeneous involvement that may cross segmental boundaries. The consolidation produced by the disease is manifested on the roentgenogram by homogeneous density. An entire lobe may be affected; more commonly only one or more segments are involved. The density usually extends to the pleural surface.

A peripheral, nonsegmental, sublobar consolidation is seen when peripheral spread across segmental boundaries occurs.[10] This tends to separate the acute pneumococcal pneumonia from the pneumonias of segmental distribution, such as those caused by bronchial obstruction by tumor. The latter disease does not ordinarily cross the barrier formed by interlobar fissures and is therefore clearly defined by the fissure on either the frontal or lateral projection, depending on the lobe or segment infected (Fig. 23-1).

In pneumococcal pneumonia, all of the elements in the diseased lobe except the larger bronchi may be affected, resulting in almost complete airlessness. The larger bronchi can often be seen as air-containing, radiolucent tubes within the otherwise homogeneous density, the "air bronchogram." There is often enough pleural involvement to result in elevation of the hemidiaphragm on the affected side because of pain. A small amount of pleural fluid sufficient to obscure the depth of the costophrenic sulcus is not uncommon. The volume of the lobe or segment is not decreased significantly, so that the opacity caused by this disease can be differentiated from that produced by atelectasis (Fig. 23-2).

Variations in the distribution of pulmonary consolidation may occur. The spherical pattern (round pneumonia) often reported in children is a form in which the well-circumscribed spherical consolidation may simulate a pulmonary or paramediastinal mass.[28] In patients with emphysema, radiolucent blebs surrounded by

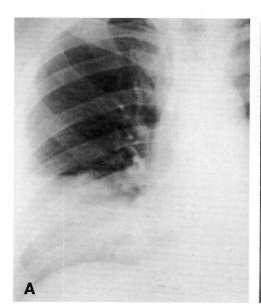
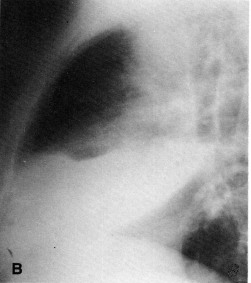

Figure 23–1.   Lobar pneumonia in the right middle lobe. Note the homogeneous opacity clearly defined by the secondary fissure in the frontal projection (**A**) and by the major fissure as well as the secondary fissure in the lateral view (**B**).

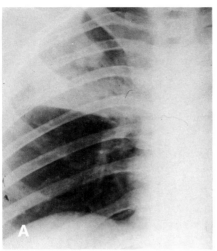 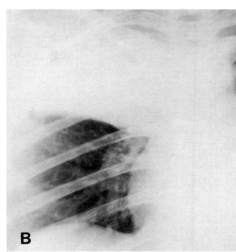

Figure 23–2. Right upper lobe pneumococcal pneumonia. **(A)** Roentgenogram obtained the day after onset of symptoms shows the disease clearly defined by the minor fissure. Consolidation is not complete. **(B)** Three days later, there is complete consolidation of the right upper lobe. The upper lobe volume is slightly reduced, but there is no significant collapse.

consolidation may simulate cavities. In some patients, the distribution of the disease is somewhat patchy or lobular, simulating the distribution in bronchopneumonia.[10, 15] Occasionally, an interstitial pattern may be observed, and sometimes a mixed alveolar and interstitial pattern is present. Therefore, the roentgen findings are not diagnostic of pneumococcal pneumonia as indicated earlier.

The bronchopneumonic pattern is common in hospitalized patients who frequently have underlying diseases. Resolution is fairly rapid if there are no complications and tends to start at the hilum and progress peripherally in the lobe or segment. The opacity becomes more irregular and patchy during resolution in contrast to its homogeneous character earlier in the disease. Focal atelectasis often develops.

Complications are few in otherwise healthy persons since the disease responds well to antibiotics, which are often given at the first sign of respiratory infection. Complications include delayed resolution or non-resolution, empyema, and lung abscess. The roentgen finding in delayed resolution is persistence of density in the area, which becomes rather irregular and patchy but eventually clears. Very rarely the process clears incompletely, leaving some irregular fibrosis manifested by irregular strands of density in the segment or lobe, often with decrease in volume of the affected lung. The findings in empyema and lung abscess are discussed later.

BRONCHOPNEUMONIA

Bronchopneumonia (lobular pneumonia) is an acute pulmonary infection, bacterial in origin, that usually occurs as a complication of various debilitating diseases, often at the extremes of life. Therefore, it is most commonly found in the very young or very old who are afflicted with another disease. The infection is often mixed, so that several pathogenic bacteria can be isolated from the sputum. The disease originates in numerous adjacent areas of the lung, resulting in scattered foci of inflammation that vary in size and shape but produce enough density to be visible on the film. The inflammatory disease does not cross septal boundaries. Therefore, the pattern of disease is discontinuous or patchy.

The roentgen findings in bronchopneumonia are varied, since the disease may be localized to a single lobe or segment or may involve all lobes. The pneumonic consolidation causes densities of varying sizes that are usually rather small and poorly defined and may be described as mottled. The disease may progress so that these small areas may coalesce to form large, irregular opacities. The location is usually basal, but the disease may occur anywhere in the lung (Fig. 23-3). It often occurs as a complication of another pulmonary disease, which may obscure the pneumonia or vice versa. It is particularly difficult to define and diagnose when it occurs as a complication in cardiac failure with pulmonary congestion and edema, which also cause basal opacity. It is also difficult to differentiate from other acute or subacute pulmonary disease such as adult respiratory distress syndrome (ARDS). Occasionally, the process is extremely widespread and simulates miliary pulmonary disease, with small, poorly defined nodules scattered uniformly throughout both lungs. Since bronchopneumonia produces a variety of roentgen patterns and is caused by a number of organisms, its designation is now used as a descriptive term rather than a definitive one as far as etiology is concerned. In contrast to alveolar pneumonia, it originates in bronchial airways and involves the surround-

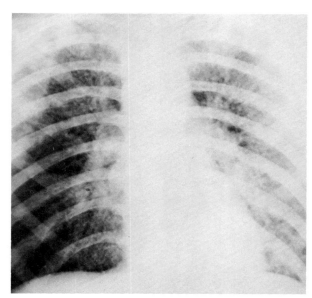

Figure 23–3. Bronchopneumonia. Note the widespread, mottled opacity is more severe on the left than on the right. The disease is very extensive.

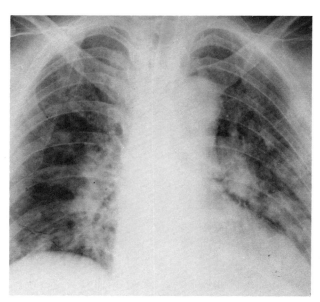

Figure 23–4. Aspiration pneumonia. Note the scattered patchy opacities in the lower half of the left lung and a similar but less extensive change at the right base. This was an acute process, which cleared quickly on treatment.

ing parenchyma. As indicated, it may become confluent and then resemble alveolar pneumonia. It should be remembered that neoplasms can be masked by patchy focal pneumonia, and if clinical symptoms persist unduly, progress roentgenograms as well as cytologic studies should be recommended.

ASPIRATION PNEUMONIA

Aspiration pneumonia is usually a mixed bacterial infection caused by aspiration of foreign material into the bronchial tree. The causes are numerous and range from aspiration of vomitus by a postsurgical or semicomatose patient to aspiration as a result of paresis or paralysis of the pharyngeal muscles. Tracheoesophageal fistula, gastroesophageal reflux, and various other esophageal lesions may also cause aspiration pneumonitis. Gram-negative organisms included in the aspirate may produce pneumonia followed by necrosis and abscess formation.[32] This complication is discussed in the section on lung abscess.

The radiographic findings vary with the extent of the disease and its location. The right lower and middle lobes are the most frequently affected, but left lower lobe involvement is not unusual. Irregular, poorly defined areas of increased density are seen and may be extensive (Fig. 23-4). Early in the disease these densities are focal, but later they may become conglomerate. In some instances the disease is acute and clears rap-

idly as the patient recovers from the condition that produced the aspiration. In other instances the pneumonia results from a chronic disease and repeated aspiration leads to chronic basal pneumonitis, which causes patchy or linear basal opacity (Fig. 23-5). Aspiration of acid-containing gastric contents (Mendelson's syndrome), can produce a chemical pneumonitis causing pulmonary edema, often in a dependent portion of one or both lungs. The appearance is similar to basal pulmonary edema of other etiologies. The roentgen findings are therefore varied, and it may not be possible to differentiate this basal inflammatory disease from other nonspecific basal pneumonia and from the chronic pneumonia associated with bronchiectasis. However, correlation of the history with clinical and roentgen findings usually leads to the proper diagnosis.

PNEUMONIA IN CHILDREN

Differences in response to pulmonary infection in infants and young children as compared with older children and adults are probably based on anatomic and immunologic factors.[2, 18] Airways are small, soft, and easily collapsible; resultant air trapping with overinflation can be found in a variety of infections in the first 12 to 18 months of life. In the newborn period, B strep-

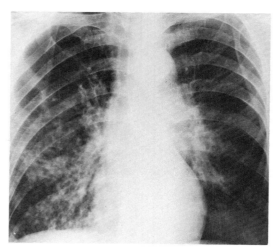

Figure 23–5. Chronic aspiration pneumonia. The pneumonia in the parahilar areas and at the right base is somewhat more clearly defined and stringy than the acute process noted in Figure 23-4. This patient had partial esophageal obstruction and had aspirated intermittently for several months.

tococcal pneumonia causes an appearance similar to that in hyaline membrane disease. In fetal aspiration syndrome, rapid roentgenographic changes result as the aspirated material is cleared and overinflation disappears.

Staphylococcal pneumonia has a very rapid course, with early development (within hours) of effusion, empyema, and bronchopleural fistula with pyopneumothorax or lung abscess.[21] Pneumatoceles are very common as the pneumonia clears.

Upper airway infection may be associated with pulmonary disease, so a chest roentgenogram may be the initial study. When lungs are hypoaerated or edematous, obstruction due to epiglottitis should be suspected.

It is very important to correlate the roentgen findings with clinical signs and symptoms. For example, *Chlamydia trachomatis* causes conjunctivitis in neonates and may produce pneumonia, which is interstitial, scattered, and bilateral and is associated with overinflation of the lungs. Cough is often the only symptom, so a chest film showing the preceding findings in a neonate with conjunctivitis should suggest the diagnosis.[27]

KLEBSIELLA PNEUMONIA (FRIEDLÄNDER'S)

Klebsiella pneumonia is a confluent alveolar type of pneumonia caused by *Klebsiella pneumoniae*. The disease occurs most frequently in elderly and debilitated

patients. The onset is usually sudden, and the illness is often fatal within a few days. It may begin as bronchopneumonia manifested by patchy areas of opacity, usually in one or both upper lobes, but spreads rapidly to become confluent. It may involve an entire lobe. The involved lobe tends to increase in volume, resulting in convexity of the adjacent interlobar fissure. Extensive destruction of tissues leads to abscess formation in many of these patients, and the abscess cavities are typically thin walled, if a wall can be demonstrated (Fig. 23-6). Often, the confluent pneumonia surrounding the cavity obscures its actual wall. At times the necrosis is extensive and extremely large cavitation results when the necrotic material sloughs out. Pleural effusion is common, and empyema often follows the effusion. In the more chronic form, the disease tends to be patchier, the cavitation is smaller, and the lesions may closely simulate those of tuberculosis. Pneumatoceles may occasionally occur during resolution of Klebsiella pneumonia.

The diagnosis should be suspected when a rapidly progressing confluent pneumonia is observed in one or both upper lobes, resulting in increased lung volume, in which cavitation forms quickly. When the disease progresses more slowly, it is often less confluent and its distribution in one or both upper lobes plus the presence of cavities often leads to a mistaken diagnosis of tuberculosis. Bacteriologic studies are then needed for differentiation. In patients who survive, a considerable amount of fibrosis may result, leading to contraction of the lobe with secondary changes in the thorax resulting from the loss of lung volume. In this respect, the disease may resemble chronic tuberculosis.

Enterobacter and *Serratia* are similar gram-negative bacteria that cause pneumonia infrequently. The most common of these is *Serratia marcescens*, which usually causes either a focal pneumonia or a diffuse process that may involve several lobes. Pleural effusion is common. Both *Enterobacter* and *Serratia* are usually found in debilitated hospitalized patients and are often associated with other organisms as a cause for pulmonary infection. As an opportunistic pathogen in immunosuppressed patients, *Serratia* may produce a necrotizing bronchopneumonia but usually does not cause a frank lung abscess.

STAPHYLOCOCCAL PNEUMONIA

Pneumonia caused by *Staphylococcus aureus* may be primary in the lungs or secondary to a primary staphylococcal infection elsewhere in the body. In the secondary type, there is hematogenous spread of the organism, whereas in the primary type, the pulmonary spread is usually bronchogenic. The disease usually occurs in debilitated adults and in infants during the

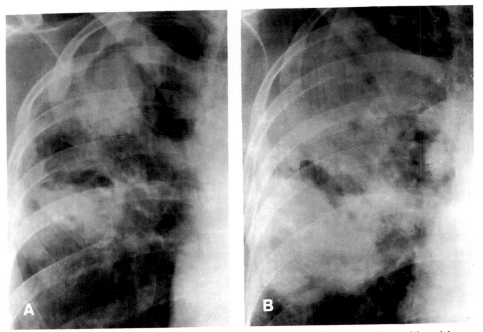

Figure 23–6.   Klebsiella pneumonia. **(A)** The disease is extensive, with evidence of cavitation in which there are masses of dense necrotic material. **(B)** Ten days later, considerable advance of the disease is evident.

first year of life. The onset of the illness is usually abrupt, with severe prostration. Death may occur within 24 to 48 hours. Because some of the many areas of involvement occur adjacent to the pleura, it is common to have pleural infection with empyema and bronchopleural fistula.

In children, the roentgen findings are rather characteristic and consist of dense areas of pulmonary involvement that may be segmental and local or diffuse.[21] Consolidation rapidly spreads to involve a whole lobe (confluent bronchopneumonia); bronchi are usually obscured by exudate, so an air bronchogram is not ordinarily seen. Pleural effusion, empyema, and pneumothorax are common, and pneumatoceles are often noted. Abscess formation may also occur, and coalescence of small abscesses is frequent. A pneumatocele is distinguished from an abscess by its thin wall and rapid change in size. It is caused by a check-valve obstruction between the lumen of a small bronchus and adjacent interstitium and possibly a check-valve obstruction of a small bronchus in some instances. Multiple pneumatoceles may develop, usually in the first week of the disease, and may become very large. Accumulation of fluid with air–fluid levels is common during the active phase of pneumonia. Pneumatoceles may persist for months but usually disappear completely (Fig. 23-7). In adults the findings are not as characteristic. Pneu-

mothorax and pneumatocele are rare, and pleural effusion and empyema are not as common as in children. Abscesses are slightly more common than in children and tend to coalesce (Fig. 23-8). The disease is usually bilateral, may be diffuse and somewhat nodular, but is seldom lobar in distribution.

Pleural effusion, often resulting in empyema, occurs in about one-half of the patients. Rapid change and lack of correlation between severity of clinical symptoms and roentgen findings are often observed. Resolution is usually slow in both children and adults. When the disease is hematogenous, septic emboli may cause multiple small abscesses and widespread, small foci of pneumonia.

STREPTOCOCCUS PYOGENES PNEUMONIA

Pneumonia caused by *S. pyogenes* (Lancefield group A, hemolytic streptococcus) usually occurs after such acute infectious diseases as measles and influenza. This disease is now rare and is roentgenographically similar to staphylococcal pneumonia in the frequency of pleural involvement, including empyema if antibiotic therapy is not initiated promptly. The pulmonary involvement has a tendency to be more diffuse and interstitial in type than in staphylococcal pneumonia, with fine opacities radiating outward to the periphery from the

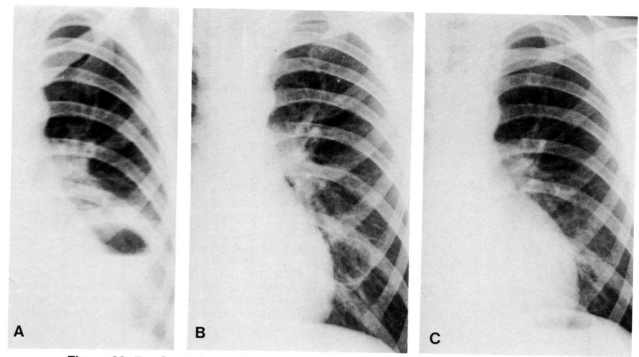

Figure 23-7. Staphylococcal pneumonia in the left lower lobe resulting in the formation of a pneumatocele. (**A**) Note the homogeneous opacity at the left base, indicating rather extensive pneumonia. There is a radiolucent area surmounting a fluid level. The pulmonary alveolar disease surrounding the pneumatocele makes it impossible to determine the thickness of the wall. (**B**) Note that the inflammatory disease has cleared nearly completely, leaving the thin-walled, cystlike pneumatocele. This film was obtained 1 month after that shown in A. (**C**) The pneumatocele is no longer visible on this film obtained 3 months after the initial examination.

hila. The combination of rapidly developing, hazy, nodular opacities in an acutely ill patient with subsequent cavitation in many of the areas is highly characteristic of either staphylococcal or streptococcal pneumonia, with the former more likely. *S. pyogenes* infections usually do not cause pneumatoceles.

TULAREMIC PNEUMONIA

Tularemia is an infectious disease caused by *Francisella tularensis*, a small gram-negative bacillus. It is a disease of small animals and may spread to humans directly from the animals.[31] The most common mode of infection of this type is through the skin of hunters who dress small game. The infection may also be transmitted by means of tick bites as well as the bites of horse and deer flies. Pulmonary involvement in the form of pneumonia resulting from this organism is present in approximately 50% of humans affected. The roentgen findings are not characteristic, but some authors have

reported a high incidence of oval lesions resembling an abscess without cavitation. However, others have indicated a great variability in pulmonary findings.[22] The infection may produce unilateral or bilateral pulmonary inflammatory disease, which is usually poorly circumscribed. Occasionally, the distribution is lobar, resulting in consolidation of an entire lobe. The infection is commonly a basal one, and there is usually more disease on one side than the other so that it is asymmetrical when bilateral. A small amount of pleural effusion is not uncommon,[6] and hilar lymph-node enlargement is also present in many instances. The time required for resolution varies widely. In some patients complete clearing may occur within a week or 10 days, and in others the disease may persist for 6 weeks. Since the roentgen picture is not characteristic, the diagnosis must be confirmed by laboratory methods. The organisms are difficult to isolate from the sputum, but if the disease is suspected, its presence can be proved by means of agglutination tests.

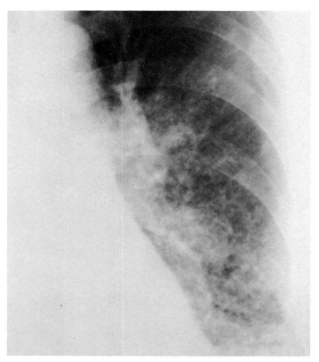

Figure 23–8. Staphylococcal pneumonia. There is extensive disease in the left lower lobe, in which numerous small, rounded, lucent areas represent small pneumatoceles or abscesses.

BRUCELLOSIS PNEUMONIA

Brucellosis in humans in the United States is usually caused by *Brucella suis*. Pulmonary involvement is rare and symptoms are usually mild.[14, 24] The roentgen findings are varied. Strands of opacity that radiate outward from the hila are often associated with hilar adenopathy and may be bilateral. Pleural involvement with effusion is occasionally encountered. In other instances, widespread miliary disease that resembles miliary bronchopneumonia is found. Solitary, circumscribed pulmonary nodules have also been described. The pulmonary roentgen changes appear quickly but tend to persist for long periods with very slow resolution. The diagnosis cannot be made on roentgen examination but must depend on the results of bacteriologic studies, agglutination, and skin tests.

PERTUSSIS PNEUMONIA

Whooping cough is usually caused by *Bordetella pertussis*. The organism may also cause pneumonia, an unusual but not rare complication. The pulmonary disease begins in the paroxysmal stage of whooping cough and extends into the resolution phase. It is usually found in children but may occur in adolescents and adults.

The pulmonary disease tends to be central, with radiating parabronchial strands of opacity. The radiographic findings resulting from this distribution of disease consist of blurring of the cardiac margins and an irregular appearance termed the shaggy heart pattern. There may also be some subsegmental areas of consolidation as well as scattered areas of atelectasis presumably caused by mucus plugs, particularly in older children and adults. In some instances, the pneumonia may be caused by other organisms complicating whooping cough, a widespread bronchopneumonia.

PSEUDOMONAS PNEUMONIA

There is an increasing incidence of pneumonia caused by *Pseudomonas aeruginosa*, a gram-negative bacillus, usually found in hospitalized patients and often related to the use of antibiotics, steroids, and immunosuppressive and cytotoxic drugs. There is evidence that positive-pressure breathing apparatus,[16] suction and nebulizing devices, and tracheostomies are major factors in the development of this disease. The causative organism is extremely difficult to eradicate once pulmonary disease is established.

Several roentgen patterns of pulmonary involvement have been described: (1) bilateral pneumonic consolidation, with early patchy, scattered disease progressing and coalescing to involvement of the major portions of both lungs; (2) extensive bilateral pneumonic consolidation with abscess formation (abscesses may be multiple and small or few and large); (3) diffuse nodular or patchy densities with or without abscess formation; and (4) unilateral pneumonia, similar to the coalescent bilateral pneumonia. Therefore, almost any pattern may occur, so the radiographic findings are not diagnostic (Fig. 23-9). Pleural effusion may occur, but it is not a prominent feature of the disease. There is evidence that the presence of *P. aeruginosa* in the sputum of patients with chronic lung disease indicates underlying bronchiectasis.

Melioidosis, which is due to infection with *P. pseudomallei*, is endemic in the tropics, chiefly in India, Burma, Sri Lanka, and South America. Since the Vietnam War, sporadic cases have been reported in the United States, chiefly in Vietnam veterans.[4] The infection may be acute or chronic. The acute form is more common and is characterized by indistinct nodular disease that is often widely scattered but tends to involve the upper lobes. The nodules coalesce and cavitate in a high percentage of cases. The chronic form simulates pulmonary tuberculosis since the nodules

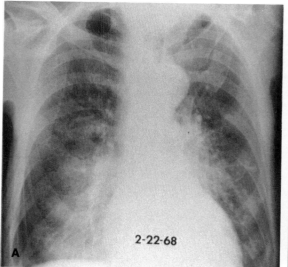
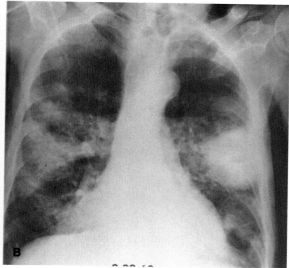

2-22-68

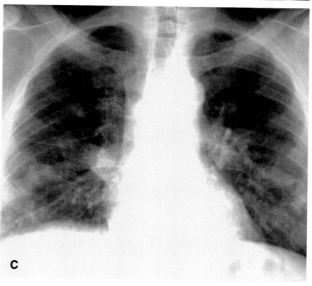

Figure 23–9. Pseudomonas pneumonia in a patient with chronic debilitating disease. **(A)** Initial examination reveals bilateral diffuse disease at the right medial base and in the left parahilar area. **(B)** One week later, note the masslike opacity in the left midlung and more patchy disease in the right midlung and medial base. There is nothing characteristic about the disease pattern, as is often the case. **(C)** Diffuse hematogenous dissemination in another patient. Note scattered, poorly defined disease, largely basal.

often involve the upper lobes and frequently cavitate. Hilar adenopathy is uncommon and pleural effusion is rare.

Occasionally, pulmonary cavitation may appear acutely years after the initial infection, so it should be suspected when a parenchymal cavity appears in an apparently healthy patient who had been in an endemic area some years earlier.

ANAEROBIC BACTERIAL PNEUMONIAS

Several anaerobic organisms may cause pulmonary infection. They include, among others, *Bacteroides fragilis*, *B. melaninogenicus*, and *B. oralis*; members of

the genera *Fusobacterium*, *Clostridium*, and *Eubacterium*; and the gram-positive cocci of the genera *Peptostreptococcus* and *Peptococcus*. Most of the infections are caused by several organisms, since many are caused by aspiration of oral secretions, particularly in patients with poor oral hygiene. They may also occur in diabetic patients, those with malignant disease, or immunosuppressed patients. An alveolar type of pneumonia, which may be extensive, is usually produced. The right lower lobe is the most common site, but frequently more than one lobe is involved. About one-half of patients have pulmonary disease only, about one-fourth have pleural and parenchymal disease, and the remainder have only the pleura involved, usually with empyema. Abscess formation and necrotizing pneumonia are common complications. Abscess occurs in more than 50% of patients with pulmonary disease. Bronchopleural fistula may also complicate the disease. Anaerobic bacteria thus are a prominent cause of aspiration pneumonia, lung abscess, necrotizing pneumonia, and empyema. The mortality is high in these patients, many of whom have depressed immune responses or leukopenia.[3]

OTHER BACTERIAL PNEUMONIAS

Pneumonia due to infection with *Proteus vulgaris* is largely basal, may be alveolar or lobular in distribution, and tends to produce cavitation. It may cause a decrease in volume of the involved lung. Rarely, *Escherichia coli* may cause pneumonia, which is usually multilobar and basal. Pneumatoceles are occasionally seen in this infection, and the alveolar pneumonia caused by this organism rarely may result in massive cavitation. Pleural effusion is common. Pneumonic involvement may occur in *typhoid fever*, usually as a bronchopneumonia with cavitation, pleural effusion, or empyema. *Salmonella* organisms other than *S. typhosa* may produce a similar pattern in the lung. An acute miliary pattern has also been described in salmonella bacteremia.[13] *Hemophilus influenzae*, type B, is a rare cause of pneumonia.[2]

In adults, these infections appear as acute lobular lower lobe pneumonia or as a more confluent lobar alveolar process. The latter is somewhat more common. Pneumatoceles are rare but have been reported. Patients with alcoholism, who are immunocompromised, or who are undergoing chemotherapy are at risk. In infants, pleural effusion and empyema are common in addition to extensive alveolar disease, which may be a patchy segmental type of density, but a variety of manifestations such as (1) reticular or linear, (2) nodular, (3) reticulonodular, (4) ground-glass, and (5) honeycomb patterns have been described. Pleural effusion is fairly common and may be complicated by empyema. Cavitation is rare; roentgenographic findings clear slowly.

Pulmonary involvement also occurs in patients with *anthrax* and *bubonic plague*. In anthrax pneumonia, there is often substantial mediastinal lymph node enlargement, pleural effusion, and sometimes intrapulmonary hemorrhage in addition to extensive pulmonary disease. *Plague* can often involve the lung.[1] In secondary pneumonic plague, bilateral small densities are the most common early manifestation. The disease may spread to involve much of the lungs with a dense alveolar process, which is often fatal. Rarely, the pattern is that of bilateral extensive mottled densities, which resemble the pattern of ARDS. This pattern reflects intravascular coagulopathy in some instances.

LEGIONNAIRES' DISEASE

Legionnaires' disease, which affected nearly 200 persons at the Legionnaires' Convention in Philadelphia in July 1976, is caused by the gram-negative bacillus *Legionella pneumophila*.[7] Clinically, the acute disease is characterized by a high fever, chills, and a nonproductive cough, often associated with chest pain, malaise, muscle and abdominal pain, headaches, and gastrointestinal symptoms. Since the outbreak in Philadelphia, many sporadic as well as local outbreaks of the disease in several areas throughout the United States have been reported. Predisposing factors include smoking, alcoholism, diabetes, heart disease, and immunosuppression. Roentgen findings are largely those of an alveolar pneumonic process that is bilateral in about one-half of the reported cases. There tends to be lower lobe predominance. The alveolar disease may have a lobar or lobular distribution. At times, the alveolar process appears as a large, very poorly marginated, generally round or oval opacity. Some of these are central and some peripheral; they may be unilateral or bilateral. The round lesions appear to be somewhat more common than any other roentgen manifestation. The round masslike lesions often progress rapidly to involve an entire lobe. Early in the disease, there may be patchy, ill-defined opacities that in many cases progress to a lobar pattern. One patient has been reported in whom there was virtually universal involvement of both lungs by an alveolar process in which air bronchograms were very prominent. Cavitation, presumably a result of necrotizing pneumonia, has been reported in several patients, most of whom were immunosuppressed. One patient has been reported in whom pneumatocele formation and spontaneous pneumothorax were manifest. Pleural effusion may occur, but its incidence is difficult to evaluate since many of the patients have complicating renal or cardiovascular disease. Resolution is usually slow and lags behind clinical improvement. An interstitial pattern may appear during resolution.

It is evident that there is a wide variety of roentgen patterns in this disease so that the diagnosis cannot be made on the basis of chest roentgenograms. However, the disease should be suspected in a patient with atypical pneumonia in whom roentgenograms show unilateral or bilateral large, poorly marginated, rounded aveolar opacities that may progress rapidly to involve one or more entire lobes.

The Pittsburgh pneumonia agent (*Tatlockia micdadei*, *Legionella micdadei*) was described in 1979. It is a gram-negative, weakly acid-fast bacillus that appears to be identical to the Tatlock organism isolated 37 years earlier. It has been recognized as a disease seen mainly in renal transplant patients and others treated with high-dose corticosteroid therapy. However, it has also been reported[23] in patients who were not immunosuppressed. Radiographic findings are those of an alveolar type of pneumonia, usually in one lobe, either segmental or subsegmental and nodular in appearance. In the compromised patient, it spreads very rapidly and occasionally cavitates. Pleural effusion is found in about 30% of patients. The organism is similar to *Legionella pneumophila*, and the two diseases are found simultaneously in a few patients. The diagnosis is made by lung biopsy.

PULMONARY INFECTION IN THE COMPROMISED HOST (OPPORTUNISTIC INFECTIONS)

Several conditions alter the defense mechanisms in a given patient, leading to susceptibility to one or more organisms that may or may not be pathogens in normal individuals. Diseases and organisms often associated with them include (1) acute myelocytic leukemia and leukopenia—*Pseudomonas, Staphylococcus, Aspergillus,* and *Mucor;* (2) chronic lymphocytic leukemia and lymphosarcoma—*S. pneumoniae, Staphylococcus, Cryptococcus, Pneumocystis,* and herpes viruses; (3) Hodgkin's disease—*Cryptococcus, Listeria, Pneumocystis,* and organisms causing tuberculosis and toxoplasmosis; (4) myeloma and chronic myelocytic leukemia—*S. pneumoniae,* gram-negative bacilli, *Pneumocystis,* and the tubercle bacillus; (5) renal transplants—many bacteria, *Cryptococcus, Pneumocystis,* cytomegalovirus, and

organisms causing toxoplasmosis, nocardiosis, and histoplasmosis; (6) cystic fibrosis—*Staphylococcus* and *Pseudomonas;* (7) sickle cell disease—*S. pneumoniae* and *Salmonella;* (8) drug addiction—*Staphylococcus,* mixed anaerobes, *Pseudomonas,* and *Candida;* (9) hypogammaglobulinemia—gram-positive bacteria, *Pneumocystis,* and viruses; (10) chronic granulomatous disease of childhood—*Serratia, Salmonella,* and *Staphylococcus;* (11) bone marrow transplant—cytomegalovirus, herpes simplex virus, gram-negative bacteria, fungi, *Pneumocystis,* and combinations of organisms such as cytomegalovirus and *Aspergillus* or *Pneumocystis.*

There may be early (during the first 2 weeks after transplant) roentgen findings consisting of transient nonspecific interstitial disease resembling the interstitial edema caused by direct lung injury secondary to radiation or chemotherapy. Infection caused by the preceding organisms occurs later, usually from 2 weeks to several months after transplant. Nearly all of the preceding infections may also occur in acquired immunodeficiency syndrome (AIDS) (Fig. 23-10). In immunosuppressed patients, Pneumocystis pneumonia is the most common, aspergillosis is uncommon, and viral and Mycoplasma pneumonia are rare.

The preceding list is not complete, and many of the organisms listed can cause pneumonia in several of the conditions mentioned. The organism listed first tends to be most common in the diseases noted previously. Several other organisms have been implicated as the

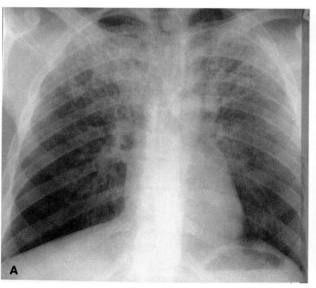
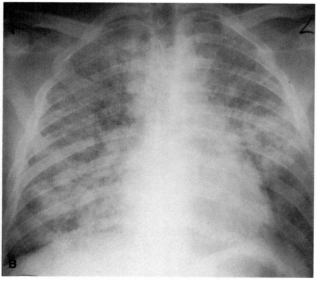

Figure 23-10. Legionella pneumonia in an AIDS patient. **(A)** Initial film shows bilateral upper lobe disease, which appears to present a mixed interstitial and alveolar pattern. **(B)** Two and one-half weeks later. There is now extensive bilateral disease, which appears to be in a largely alveolar pattern. This disease is more diffuse and less masslike than the original descriptions.

cause of pneumonia in these patients. Many of them are unusual or rare, and some are not ordinarily pathogens. Mortality is high and treatment may be very difficult, since multiple organisms are often found in these patients. Therefore, an aggressive approach, with percutaneous needle aspiration or transbronchial or at times open lung biopsy, may be necessary to obtain material for specific bacteriologic diagnosis. The pulmonary findings in most of these pneumonias are described elsewhere. Chest roentgenology is more useful in identifying the pneumonic process and following its course than it is in suggesting the organism responsible for the disease. When a patient with one of the preceding diseases develops fever, an opportunistic pneumonia may be developing. Any opacity that was not present on an earlier chest radiograph should arouse the suspicion of pneumonia.

HOSPITAL-ACQUIRED (NOSOCOMIAL) PNEUMONIAS

Hospital-acquired pneumonias are important because the impaired resistance of the hospital patients renders them very susceptible to several gram-negative bacilli such as *Pseudomonas aeruginosa*, *E. coli*, and other *Enterobacter* species. Outbreaks of Staphylococcus, Klebsiella, Proteus, and other pneumonias have also been reported. Furthermore, the wide use of antibiotics has resulted in resistant pathogens that may also cause pneumonia. The lungs are involved in 10% to 30% of infections acquired in hospitals. In this patient population, mortality may be very high and every precaution must be taken to avoid contamination of respiratory therapy equipment, anesthesia machines, air-conditioners, and other devices used in patient care. *Pseudomonas* infection is particularly common in this group of patients, is very difficult to treat, and has a high mortality despite various combinations of antibiotics. Nosocomial pneumonia should be considered when a hospitalized patient develops leukocytosis, cough, or fever. Then any new or increasing pulmonary opacity may represent pneumonia. There are no specific patterns for the various organisms involved, so the radiologist's role is to note the disease and suggest the possibility of pneumonia.

VIRAL, MYCOPLASMAL, AND RICKETTSIAL PNEUMONIAS

MYCOPLASMAL PNEUMONIA

Mycoplasma pneumoniae (the Eaton agent) pneumonia is responsible for a significant percentage of primary atypical pneumonia in children and young adults, in the range of 15% to 20% or more. It probably accounts for nearly 50% of pneumonia found in children under age 16. The remainder of patients with primary pneumonia have disease caused by adenovirus, parainfluenza virus, respiratory syncytial virus, and probably other viruses. In many patients, the etiology is not determined. Cold agglutinins are found in the serum of 50% to 60% of patients with Mycoplasma pneumonia. A titer of 1:32 or higher is considered positive and is usually found 10 to 14 days after onset of the symptoms. A high titer is usually present. Mycoplasmal pneumonia tends to occur in epidemics, as well as sporadically, so it is difficult to obtain meaningful figures as to relative frequency. The disease usually occurs in young, healthy adults. It is acute, mild, and self-limited in most instances but may be severe with widespread pulmonary disease. Occasional fatalities have been reported. The inflammatory exudate is sometimes more interstitial than in the bacterial pneumonias, but alveolar exudate, which contains fewer cells and more fluid than in the bacterial type, is also present. The onset of symptoms is gradual and there is often a delay in the appearance of visible pulmonary density on roentgen examination for 2 or 3 days. Putman and colleagues described two groups of patients with different clinical and radiographic findings.[25] One group with acute chest pain, cough, and fever developed segmental or lobar air-space disease. The other group had a more chronic course, were afebrile, and had no cough or chest pain. They developed interstitial changes and a reticulonodular or mixed pattern of focal air-space and interstitial disease. Others have noted less relationship between symptoms and anatomic distribution.

Roentgen findings reflect the anatomic changes. Recognizable forms can be divided into several types:

1. Peribronchial or interstitial type. The findings in the peribronchial type consist of streaky densities extending outward from the hilum following the pattern of the vascular markings limited to a single segment or affecting one or several lobes. Alveolar exudate may produce scattered patchy density as well as the linear shadows (Fig. 23-11).
2. Bronchopneumonic type. The roentgen findings are similar to those described for bronchopneumonia and may be just as widespread. Opacities that are usually poorly defined and scattered may be noted in any lobe or segment and may be bilateral.
3. Segmental and lobar types. The findings are those of homogeneous density representing consolidation in a segment, several segments, or a lobe. Single lobe involvement occurs in nearly 50% of patients. Air bronchograms may be present. The appearance of the consolidation is simi-

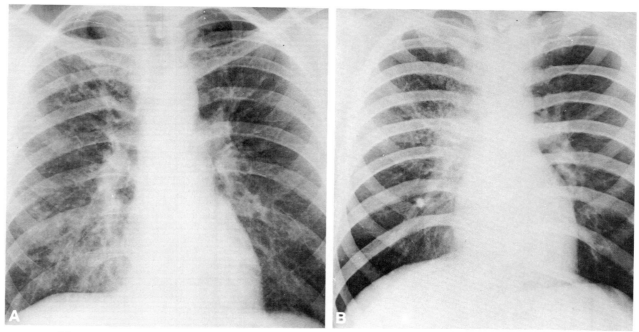

Figure 23–11. Viral pneumonia. **(A)** Extensive interstitial disease is seen throughout the entire right lung, with similar but much less marked change on the left. **(B)** There is diffuse involvement, which appears to be mainly interstitial, confined largely to the right upper lobe in another patient.

lar to that found in *S. pneumoniae* lobar pneumonia. Pleural effusion occurs in about 20% of patients with this type of disease and is rare in the interstitial type (Fig. 23-12).

4. Diffuse type. A bilateral reticulonodular pattern throughout both lungs. Pleural effusion is rare.

One or more of these gross anatomic types of the disease may be present in a single patient. There is a tendency for the disease to clear in one area and spread in another, often in the opposite lung. Atelectasis may be produced by bronchial obstruction and is frequently lobular and focal in type. Occasionally, a pneumatocele may result from check-valve obstruction and must be differentiated from lung abscess (see Fig. 23-7). Resolution is usually slow, and it is common to see persistent pulmonary lesions for a week or more after the clinical findings have disappeared. Occasionally, the delay is considerably greater. Mycoplasmal pneumonia cannot be differentiated from viral infections of the lung, and when the distribution is segmental or lobar, it is similar to bacterial pneumonia (Fig. 23-13).

Differential Diagnosis. There are findings that help to differentiate mycoplasmal from bacterial pneumonia. They consist of the lack of pleural involvement

manifested by absence of elevation of the diaphragm and absence of pleural fluid in most cases. The delay in appearance of pulmonary disease after clinical onset is also helpful. The tendency to clear in one area and spread in another is more common in this disease than in bacterial pneumonia. Bilateral involvement is probably more common than in bacterial pneumonias, with disease often in one lower lobe and the opposite upper or middle lobe. However, because the roentgen pattern may vary widely, the diagnosis must be substantiated by clinical and laboratory findings (Fig. 23-14).

ADENOVIRUS PNEUMONIA

There are 28 types of the adenovirus, which is a common cause of upper respiratory disease and may cause pneumonia, often in epidemics. The disease is usually more severe in infants and young children than in adults. The most common roentgenographic pattern is that of a widely scattered patchy or confluent disease, usually in a peribronchial distribution. Slow resolution is usually noted, with residual bronchiectasis in some children and obliterative bronchiolitis and other chronic lung disease in others. This virus also causes acute bronchiolitis with overinflation in infants

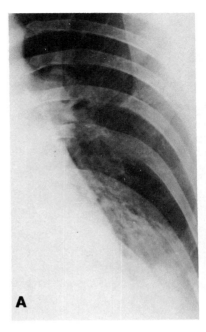
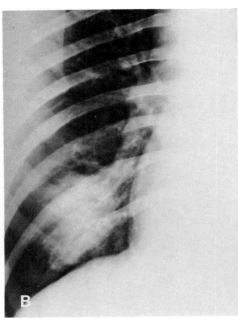

Figure 23–12. Viral pneumonia. In these two patients, the disease is largely alveolar in type, being rather diffuse in the patient shown in **A** and localized into an irregular masslike lesion in the patient shown in **B**.

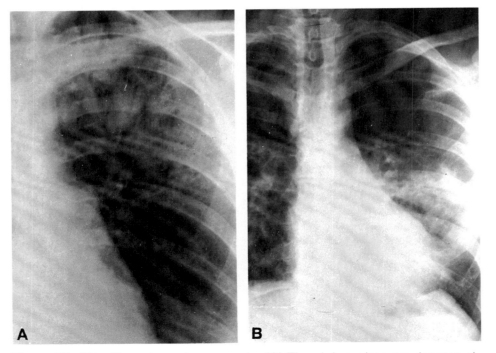

Figure 23–13. Mycoplasmal pneumonia. (**A**) The air bronchogram denotes alveolar disease, but there also appears to be some interstitial change in the upper central lung. (**B**) Alveolar pneumonia is noted in the left lower lobe, which is probably subsegmental.

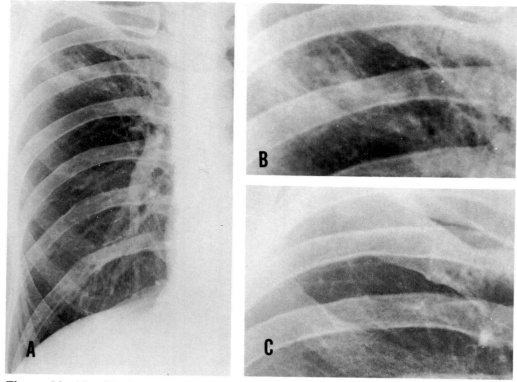

Figure 23–14. Viral pneumonia simulating minimal tuberculosis. **(A)** Note the disease in the right subclavicular area. **(B)** Close-up showing the disease in the first anterior interspace. **(C)** Roentgenogram of the same area shown in *B*, obtained 2 weeks later, showing complete clearing of the disease.

and can cause unilateral hyperlucent lung (Swyer-James syndrome). Bronchiolitis can also be caused by other viruses such as the respiratory syncytial virus, rhinovirus, influenza virus, and parainfluenza virus, usually in children. It is unusual in adults and is rarely diagnosed. Although pulmonary involvement may be extensive, the acute illness may not be severe, particularly in adults.

OTHER VIRAL PNEUMONIAS

Several viruses are capable of causing pneumonia, often in epidemics.[5] The roentgenographic findings are similar to those described in mycoplasmal pneumonia, so that the etiology cannot be established on the basis of disease patterns in the lung as shown on the chest film. In some epidemics, the pericardium is involved, leading to effusion, often associated with pleural effusion as well. Often the virus is not definitely identified in these patients and the diagnosis is based on clinical findings. The disease is usually not as prolonged or severe as mycoplasmal pneumonia.

Epidemic influenza, which is a virus disease, may be associated with virus infection of the pulmonary parenchyma in addition to involvement of the tracheobronchial tree. Roentgen signs are variable, with findings often bilateral and extensive. Especially in severe epidemics of the past, the pneumonia was often of the interstitial type with hazy, strandlike densities radiating outward from the hila. These result in a coarse appearance of the bronchovascular pattern and irregular hilar thickening. In other patients, segmental or lobar consolidation may be present; it may be bilateral. A diffuse patchy pattern resembling pulmonary edema has also been described. Pleural effusion is rare in uncomplicated influenza pneumonia. The diagnosis is often made from clinical findings during an epidemic. The roentgen changes are then largely confirmatory, but radiographic examination is useful to observe the course of the pulmonary parenchymal disease. A complicating staphylococcal pneumonia may also occur, particularly in epidemics in which influenza may be severe. Most fatalities are caused by this complication.

Herpes simplex pneumonia may occur in neonates

and in an immunocompromised host. It is a severe, often fatal disease in neonates in which there is an initial interstitial pattern, progressing to coalescent air-space densities and a diffuse alveolar "white-out" of both lungs in the fatal cases. Pathology is that of a necrotizing hemorrhagic pneumonia. The disease is usually widely disseminated in these neonates.

Pneumonia associated with *chickenpox (varicella)* is believed by some to be viral in origin and has been reported occasionally. It usually occurs in adults with severe chickenpox (up to 50%). Roentgen findings consist of widespread poorly defined patchy or nodular densities associated with an increase in parahilar markings and occasional enlargement of the hilar nodes. Densities are most marked in the parahilar areas and at the bases. Individual nodules are generally round but are poorly defined peripherally. There is often considerable change in the roentgen findings from day to day, since the densities are transitory. Clearing is generally slow, however. In patients with fatal disease, pulmonary involvement may be virtually total, with little if any visible aerated lung. In rare instances, scattered small calcifications will result from varicella pneumonia in adults. No hilar node calcification is observed. It is entirely possible for bacterial pneumonia to appear in patients with these various viral diseases and there is no way to differentiate the cause on chest radiographs.

Measles (rubeola) is occasionally associated with pneumonia caused by the virus.[26] Pneumonia caused by other organisms sometimes complicates measles, however, so roentgen differentiation is not possible. The measles virus causes reticuloendothelial involvement resulting in hilar and mediastinal adenopathy. The virus may also involve the lung to produce an interstitial process that is manifested as a widespread reticular type of reaction, with predilection for the bases. Consolidation of lung with varying degrees of atelectasis most probably represents a complicating bacterial pneumonia.

Atypical measles pneumonia occurs in adolescents and young adults after previous "incomplete" immunity conferred by killed rubeola virus vaccine. It is probably a hypersensitivity response in incompletely immunized patients. The pneumonia is usually segmental and bilateral but may involve most or all of a lobe. Other patterns include "round" pneumonia, diffuse perihilar opacity, and multiple nodules. Pleural effusion and hilar adenopathy occur in about one-third of patients. Usually the patients have the skin eruption of measles. The acute pneumonia usually clears promptly, but rarely a nodule persists for 1 to 2 years.[20]

Pneumonic involvement may occur with several other viral diseases, including smallpox, lymphocytic choriomeningitis, and cytoplasmic inclusion disease in infants and children. There is nothing characteristic about the roentgen appearance of the pneumonia asso-ciated with these diseases except that the pneumonia is usually bilateral and often extensive. *Cytomegalovirus* infection is the most common viral infection in immunosuppressed patients. In patients having cytomegalovirus disease, nodules have been reported involving the outer one-third of the lungs. Lung biopsy may be necessary to establish the diagnosis.

PSITTACOSIS (ORNITHOSIS)

Psittacosis, or ornithosis, caused by *Chlamydia psittaci*, is primarily a disease of birds and is transmitted to humans by members of the parrot family.[29] It is also found in other domesticated and wild birds and may be transmitted to humans by them. The disease may be unilateral or bilateral, focal or multifocal, resembling lobular pneumonia. This results in a roentgen pattern of patchy consolidation that may be relatively focal or bilateral and widely scattered. A reticular pattern (interstitial) has also been reported. Enlargement of hilar nodes may also be present. Pleural involvement is uncommon. The roentgen changes tend to persist for a long time (6 to 9 weeks) after the initial symptoms. The diagnosis is confirmed by serologic and bacteriologic studies but can be suspected when this type of disease is seen in a patient who has had contact with birds.

CHLAMYDIA TRACHOMATIS PNEUMONIA

In recent years there have been several reports on the radiographic findings in Chlamydia trachomatis pneumonia in infants under 6 months, since this organism has been reported as the causative one in a distinctive pneumonia in this group. Radkowski and associates[27] reported on 125 patients observed over three and one-half years. Although the x-ray findings are not diagnostic, most patients have hyperinflation plus a variety of patterns of bilateral disease, including relatively minimal interstitial disease, areas of atelectasis, patchy coalescent pneumonia involving small volumes of lung, and rare pleural effusion.[30] The clinical signs and symptoms are relatively few, so the chest findings on radiography are those of more disease than would be expected. The infants are afebrile but have a cough, conjunctivitis, and elevated serum immunoglobulins.

In adults there are streaky opacities, usually bilateral with associated atelectasis but rarely pneumonic consolidation.[8]

RICKETTSIAL PNEUMONIAS

Q Fever. Q fever is caused by a rickettsia, an intracellular parasite considered to be intermediate between the bacteria and virus. The causative organism is *Coxiella burnetii*. The roentgen findings consist of a subsegmental, segmental, or lobar consolidation varying from a patchy inhomogeneous shadow to frank air-space opacity in the area of involvement. Hilar node involvement and small focal lesions are uncommon. There appears to be a difference between sporadic and epidemic disease.[12] Round pneumonia, sometimes multiple, is common in the epidemic group and less so in sporadic cases. Pleural involvement is rare in epidemic disease and occurs in approximately one-third of the sporadic cases. This is manifested by a small amount of pleural fluid. The roentgen findings appear within 48 hours of the onset of the disease in the usual instance and resolve rather slowly so that the pulmonary consolidation persists longer than in pneumococcal pneumonia. This disease does not exhibit the migratory type of change often found in viral pneumonia. As in other pneumonias, the diagnosis depends on correlation of clinical, roentgen, and serologic findings.

Other Rickettsial Pneumonias. Pulmonary involvement has been reported occasionally in patients with other rickettsial diseases such as *Rocky Mountain spotted fever* and *typhus*, when severe. The roentgen findings are not characteristic in these diseases, but the opacities are usually scattered and produce disseminated shadows on the chest roentgenogram.

OTHER INFECTIONS

LUNG ABSCESS

When an acute suppurative pulmonary infectious process breaks down to form a cavity, regardless of size, it is termed lung abscess. Most lung abscesses are bronchogenic in origin and result from aspiration of foreign material after dental operations, surgery of the respiratory tract and elsewhere, and various conditions that produce unconsciousness. This type of abscess may also be secondary to stasis of secretions from various causes such as bronchogenic carcinoma or other endobronchial obstructions that result in incomplete drainage of a bronchus. As indicated, anaerobic organisms are often the cause of lung abscess. Hematogenous lung abscess, which is usually produced by staphylococcus and occasionally by streptococcus, has been discussed in a previous section. The abscess formation in pneumonia produced by *Klebsiella* has also been discussed earlier. Cavitation occurs in approximately 5% of patients with pulmonary infarction and, when infected, an abscess is formed.

Because lung abscess is, in many instances, the result of aspiration of foreign material, it is usually found in areas of the lung that are dependent at the time of aspiration. Therefore, the posterior segment of the upper lobe is the most common site, and the right side is affected more than the left. The next most common

sites are the superior segments of the lower lobes because these segments are dependent when the patient is supine. The basal segments of the lower lobes are also commonly involved, and abscess can occur in any segment of any lobe. The lesion is peripheral in relation to the bronchopulmonary segment involved but on the frontal roentgenogram it may project in a central position. The pleura adjacent to the abscess is usually involved, so there may be pleural effusion.

The early roentgen finding is consolidation that produces an opacity that is usually confined to one pulmonary segment. Characteristically, the lesion has an opaque center with a hazy and poorly defined periphery and is often roughly spherical in shape. When bronchial communication is established, the fluid contents of the cavity are replaced, at least in part, by air, and the radiolucent abscess cavity will appear within the area of disease. It is usually incompletely drained so that an air–fluid level can be outlined within it. In these cases the fluid produces, in the dependent portion, homogeneous opacity that blends with the wall of the cavity. Drainage of the abscess may vary so that at times it may contain more or less air. When the necrotic lung tissue has not sloughed completely, it is common to observe a crescent-shaped radiolucency due to air in the superior aspect of the partially formed cavity. In some patients, several small cavities may appear within the area and may remain as separate lesions or may coalesce to form one or more larger cavities. These may be well outlined on the routine frontal and lateral roentgenogram, but small cavities can be hidden by the surrounding pneumonic consolidation. When cavitation is suspected, computed tomography (CT) may be indicated because it may reveal lesions not seen on plain films. This examination as well as multidirectional tomography also aids in localizing and in defining the inner and outer walls of the abscess cavity (Fig. 23-15). Tomography or CT may also be of value in differentiating lung abscess from bronchogenic carcinoma in which the central portion of the carcinoma has become necrotic and has sloughed, leaving a central cavity. The wall of the lung abscess is usually relatively smooth on its inner aspect, whereas a carcinoma is usually irregular. In acute lung abscess the outer wall is poorly defined. As the abscess becomes more chronic, its wall thickens and the external surface is more sharply marginated. Complications are much less common now than before the use of antibacterial drugs, but empyema and spread of the infection locally or by aspiration of pus from the abscess into a more dependent portion of the lung may occur. CT occasionally may be necessary to differentiate lung abscess from empyema and may also be useful to guide percutaneous catheter drainage.

Differential diagnosis depends on the stage of disease when the roentgenogram is obtained. In the early

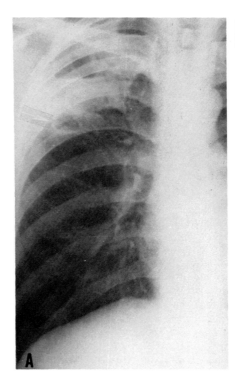

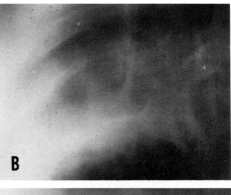

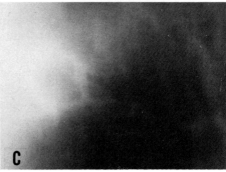

Figure 23–15. Acute lung abscess. (**A**) Note the irregular radiolucency in the right subclavicular area in which there is a fluid level. There is a smaller cavity in the plane of the third anterior rib. (**B**) Tomogram of the upper cavity, which lies posteriorly. The wall is difficult to define, and a considerable amount of inflammatory disease is adjacent to the cavity. (**C**) The smaller cavity is faintly defined on this tomogram. Its medial wall is visualized, whereas the inflammatory disease laterally produces homogeneous density, making the wall indistinct.

stage before excavation and communication with a bronchus have occurred, the process cannot be differentiated from that of a segmental pneumonia. However, excavation usually occurs early and the abscess cavity can then be seen on the roentgenogram if the examination is made with the patient upright. The clinical findings of cough with profuse, foul-smelling sputum shortly after the onset of the acute process strongly suggest lung abscess. If the cavity is not visible on a plain film, CT is indicated. Chronic lung abscess must be differentiated from cavitary tuberculosis, the fungal infections that produce cavitation, infected lung cyst, and bronchogenic carcinoma in which the central portion of the lesion has sloughed. This differentiation may be very difficult roentgenographically, and examination of the sputum for bacteria and fungi along with appropriate cultures is used to confirm the diagnosis. Cytologic study of the sputum and bronchial aspirates is also indicated in patients with these chronic abscesses, particularly in smokers over 40 years of age, because of the high incidence of bronchogenic carcinoma.

MIDDLE LOBE SYNDROME

The term *middle lobe syndrome*, commonly used in the past, is not used frequently now. It refers to recurrent pneumonitis and atelectasis in the middle lobe caused by present or previous obstruction of the bronchus to this lobe.[9] The middle lobe bronchus arises approximately 2 cm below the origin of the upper lobe bronchus and is relatively pliable, and there are nodes adjacent to it that may produce compression of the bronchus when they become enlarged. When compression is sufficient to cause partial obstruction, infection may result. The obstruction may persist or decrease, leading to atelectasis, bronchiectasis, and chronic pneumonitis or to temporary resolution of the process. Endobronchial disease at the site of the lymph node compression may result in gradually increasing stenosis of the middle lobe bronchus. The roentgen findings in the lung are somewhat varied, depending on the relative amount of pneumonitis and atelectasis. The lobe is usually decreased in size. This results in downward displacement of the secondary interlobar fissure and an increase in opacity below and lateral to the right hilum. The opacity is sometimes difficult to see in the posteroanterior roentgenogram, although it may cause blurring of the right cardiac margin. It can usually be readily outlined on the lateral film. Then the middle lobe is clearly defined as a wedge-shaped or triangular area of opacity sharply bounded above and below by normally aerated lung. The apex of the triangle is at the hilum and the base at the anterior inferior thoracic wall. When the lobe is not clearly defined in either projection, it may be seen in an anteroposterior lordotic view. When bronchiectasis is marked, the dilated bronchi may be visible as air-filled tubular structures within the consolidated lung. The hilar nodes producing the obstruction may contain calcium. The relationship of these nodes to the middle lobe bronchus can be accurately determined by means of CT. Collateral ventilation of the middle lobe appears to be relatively ineffective as compared with that of the other lobes. This may account for the persistent collapse of the middle lobe in this syndrome.

Because bronchogenic carcinoma may cause similar findings, bronchoscopy, with biopsy or even surgical exploration, may be required to make the diagnosis in this type of disease (Figs. 23-16 and 23-17).

Surgical removal is the usual treatment since the bronchial changes are generally irreversible by the time the syndrome is recognized. Furthermore, there is a high incidence of bronchogenic carcinoma in patients with recurrent or persistent middle lobe infection and atelectasis.

PULMONARY CYSTIC FIBROSIS (MUCOVISCIDOSIS)

Cystic fibrosis is the term used to describe the generalized process of which fibrocystic disease of the pancreas is the most commonly recognized finding. It is a congenital disease, transmitted as an autosomal recessive, in which there is an abnormality involving the salivary, mucus, and sweat glands. There also may be an abnormality of mucociliary transport. Sodium and chloride levels in the sweat are elevated, so the diagnosis can be confirmed by a positive sweat test—a finding of more than 50 mEq of chloride per liter of sweat—and by demonstration of decreased amounts of pancreatic enzymes in duodenal contents. This disease is discussed here because a major pulmonary manifestation is one of repeated airway and parenchymal infections. Thick, tenacious mucus tends to obstruct the smaller airways. Pulmonary manifestations vary in degree but are almost invariably present if the child lives long enough to develop them.

The earliest roentgen change in fibrocystic disease is overinflation (emphysema), which is diffuse and symmetrical.[17] This is often difficult to recognize in children, but films exposed in inspiration and expiration may indicate the distended state of the lungs. The degree of obstruction tends to increase to a different extent in various segments so that small areas of opacity resulting from focal atelectasis are visible as the disease progresses. These patients develop repeated pulmonary infection so that findings of pneumonia are superimposed. The infection is usually widespread and peribronchial in distribution, which leads to a rather irregular, stringy accentuation of peribronchial markings extending outward from the hila on both sides. This is often associated with areas of poorly defined, hazy opacity caused by focal areas of pneumonitis. Segmental or lobar collapse may also occur, and the repeated infection leads to a considerable amount of fibrosis and often to bronchiectasis. Bronchial walls are thickened. This is manifested by the presence of parallel lines, which represent bronchial walls seen in pro-

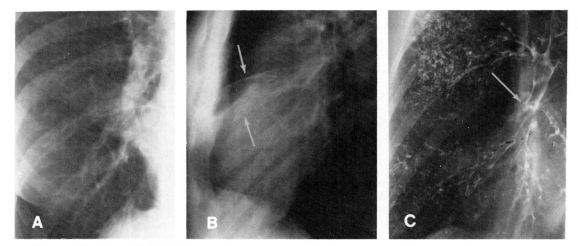

Figure 23–16.   Middle lobe syndrome. (**A**) Note the contracted middle lobe below the right hilum, which obscures the central portion of the right atrial silhouette. (**B**) The lateral view shows the contracted middle lobe (*arrows*). (**C**) The bronchogram shows obstruction (*arrow*) of the middle lobe bronchus. The upper lobe and lower lobe bronchi are partially filled.

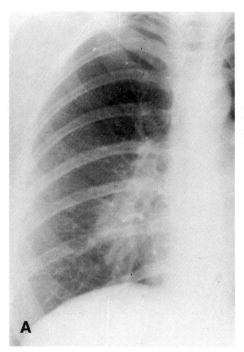
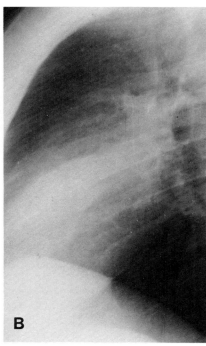

Figure 23–17. Acute pneumonia in the right middle lobe. **(A)** Note the hazy alveolar disease below the right hilum at the medial base, which blurs the right cardiac margin in this area. **(B)** In the lateral view, the disease is clearly defined. It lies in the right middle lobe.

file, or thick circles when the thickened bronchial walls are viewed in cross section. When bronchiectasis is severe, cystlike structures are visible, usually in the central and upper lungs. The fibrosis and inflammatory disease produce irregular stringy and patchy shadows. The lung between the consolidated areas is emphysematous, giving a characteristic roentgenographic picture in far advanced disease (Fig. 23-18). It is often possible to suspect the presence of cystic fibrosis early in the disease when emphysema, which may often be associated with small areas of focal atelectasis that are somewhat irregular in distribution, is noted in these infants. Bronchopulmonary aspergillosis (allergic bronchopulmonary aspergillosis, or ABPA), to which patients with cystic fibrosis are susceptible,[19] may be a complicating factor and is said to be present in 10% of patients. It is probably an important factor in clinical deterioration when it complicates cystic fibrosis. ABPA is discussed in Chapter 26.

An increasing number of patients live into adult life, and in these young adults, there is often a rather characteristic radiographic appearance. The disease usually involves the upper lobes with a combination of patchy, linear, and nodular densities interspersed with radiolucent areas. In one study bronchiectasis was observed in 90%; hyperinflation in 76%, particularly in the lower lobes; and cystlike air spaces in 24%.[11] There was an increase in hilar size in 74%. Parenchymal disease was more prominent in the upper and central

lung in 70% (Fig. 23-19); in the remainder, involvement was general. Mucus plugs with atelectasis were observed mainly in the upper lobes. In this study, 30 of 39 patients observed for 1 year or more showed progression of the pulmonary disease on chest films. Rarely, lung abscess may develop. Hypertrophic pulmonary osteoarthropathy has been reported in adults with cystic fibrosis. Chronic obstructive pulmonary disease is a major cause of disability in adults with cystic fibrosis. Infections with *Staphylococcus aureus* or *Pseudomonas aeruginosa* plus cor pulmonale are common causes of death.

CHRONIC GRANULOMATOUS DISEASE OF CHILDHOOD

Chronic granulomatous disease of childhood is another genetically determined disorder in which pulmonary infections begin early in life and persist or recur at intervals.[33] Their leukocytes phagocytize bacteria normally but do not destroy them properly. Lobar and lobular pneumonia may occur in these patients, complicated by lung abscess and empyema. The organisms usually involved are staphylococci, *Klebsiella*, *E. coli*, *Serratia marcescens*, and fungi.

The major features of the infections are hilar adenopathy and recurrent pneumonia, which often does not clear completely and may go on to abscess formation. In some patients, the pneumonia resolves slowly

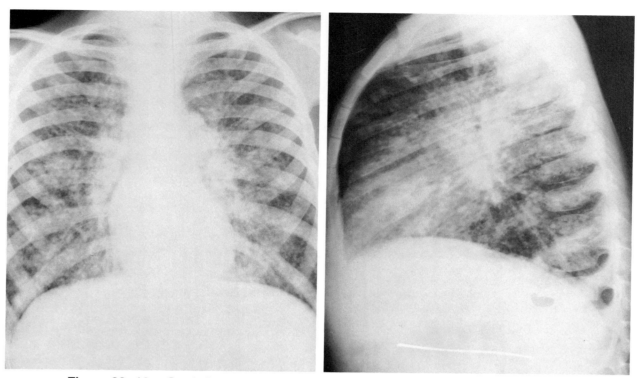

Figure 23–18. Cystic fibrosis of the pancreas with chronic pulmonary disease. There is extensive involvement throughout both lungs. Rounded and oval radiolucencies indicate thick-walled bronchi, some of which are dilated, indicating bronchiectasis. There also is evidence of some overinflation, bilateral hilar adenopathy, and patchy alveolar disease.

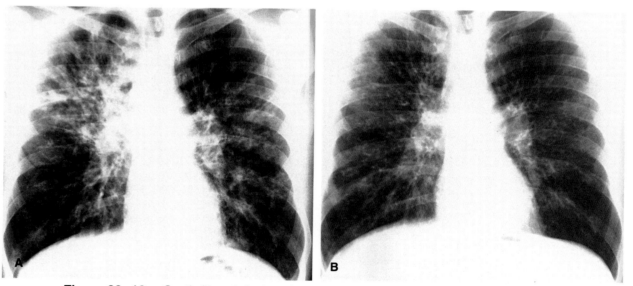

Figure 23–19. Cystic fibrosis in the adult. **(A)** Woman, age 28, with cystic fibrosis who is not acutely ill. Note upper lobe predominance, particularly on the right, but disease is rather general. **(B)** Nine months later, much of the acute disease has cleared, but thick-walled dilated bronchi are more clearly defined; upper and central predominance is again noted.

and may become clearly defined with sharp borders and homogeneous density. It is then termed *encapsulated pneumonia*.

REFERENCES AND SELECTED READINGS

1. Alsofrom DJ, Mettler FA Jr, Mann JM: Radiographic manifestations of plague in New Mexico. 1975–1980. Radiology 139:561, 1981

2. Asmar BI, Slovis TL, Reed JO, et al: Hemophilus influenza type B pneumonia in 43 children. J Pediatr 93:389, 1978

3. Bartlett JG, Finegold SM: Anaerobic infections of the lung and pleural space. State of the art. Am Rev Respir Dis 110:56, 1974

4. Carruthers MM: Recrudescent melioidosis mimicking lung abscess. Am Rev Respir Dis 124:756, 1981

5. Conte P, Heitzman ER, Markarian B: Viral pneumonia. Roentgen pathological correlations. Radiology 95:267, 1970

6. Dennis JM, Boudreau RP: Pleuropulmonary tularemia. Radiology 68:25, 1957

7. Dietrich PA, Johnson RD, Fairbank JT, et al: The chest radiograph in Legionnaires' disease. Radiology 127:577, 1978

8. Edelman RR, Hann LE, Simon M: Chlamydia trachomatosis pneumonia in adults: Radiographic appearance. Radiology 152:279, 1984

9. Effler DB, Ervin JR: The middle lobe syndrome. A review of the anatomic and clinical features. Am Rev Tuberc 71:775, 1955

10. Fraser RG, Wortzman G: Acute pneumococcal lobar pneumonia: The significance of non-segmental distribution. J Can Assoc Radiol 10:37, 1959

11. Friedman PJ, Harwood IR, Ellenbogen PH: Pulmonary cystic fibrosis in the adult: Early and late radiologic findings with pathologic correlation. Am J Roentgenol 136:1131, 1981

12. Gordon JD, Mackeen AD, Marrie TJ, et al: The radiographic features of epidemic and sporadic Q fever pneumonia. J Can Assoc Radiol 35:293, 1984

13. Greenspan RH, Feinberg SB: Salmonella bacteremia: A case with miliary lung lesions and spondylitis. Radiology 68:860, 1957

14. Harvey WA: Pulmonary brucellosis. Ann Intern Med 28:768, 1948

15. Heitzman ER: The radiological diagnosis of pneumonia in the adult: A commentary. Semin Roentgenol 24:212, 1989

16. Joffe N: Roentgenologic aspects of primary Pseudomonas aeruginosa pneumonia in mechanically ventilated patients. Am J Roentgenol 107:305, 1955

17. Keats TE: Generalized pulmonary emphysema as an isolated manifestation of early cystic fibrosis of the pancreas. Radiology 65:223, 1955

18. Kirkpatrick JA: Pneumonia in children as it differs from adult pneumonia. Semin Radiol 15:96, 1980

19. Laufer P, Fink JN, Bruns WT, et al: Allergic bronchopulmonary aspergillosis in cystic fibrosis. J Allergy Clin Immunol 73:44, 1984

20. Margolin FR, Gandy TK: Pneumonia of atypical measles. Radiology 131:653, 1979

21. Meyers HI, Jacobson G: Staphylococcal pneumonia in children and adults. Radiology 72:665, 1959

22. Miller RP, Bates JH: Pleural pulmonary tularemia. A review of 29 patients. Am Rev Respir Dis 99:31, 1969

23. Muder RR, Reddy SC, Yu VL, et al: Pneumonia caused by Pittsburgh pneumonia agent: Radiologic manifestations. Radiology 150:633, 1984

24. Patel PJ, Al-Sukaikani H, Al-Aska AK, et al: The chest radiograph in brucellosis. Clin Radiol 39:39, 1988

25. Putman CE, Curtis AM, Simeone J, et al: Mycoplasma pneumonia—clinical and roentgenographic patterns. Am J Roentgenol 124:417, 1975

26. Quinn JL III: Measles pneumonia in an adult. Am J Roentgenol 91:560, 1964

27. Radkowski JG, Kranzler JK, Beem MO, et al: Chlamydia pneumonia in infants: Radiography in 125 cases. Am J Roentgenol 137:703, 1981

28. Rose RW, Ward BH: Spherical pneumonias in children simulating pulmonary and mediastinal masses. Radiology 106:179, 1973

29. Stenstrom R, Jansson E, Wager O: Ornithosis pneumonia with special reference to roentgenological lung findings. Acta Med Scand 171:349, 1962

30. Strutman HR, Rettig PJ, Reyes S: *Chlamydia trachomatis* as a cause of pneumonitis and pleural effusion. J Pediatr 104:588, 1984

31. Stuart BM, Pullen RL: Tularemic pneumonia: Review of American literature and report of 15 cases. Am J Med Sci 210:223, 1945

32. Unger JD, Rose HD, Unger GF: Gram-negative pneumonia. Radiology 107:283, 1973

33. Wolfson JJ, Quie PG, Laxdal SD, et al: Roentgenologic manifestations in children with a genetic defect of polymorphonuclear leukocyte function. Radiology 91:37, 1968

Paul and Juhl's Essentials of Radiologic Imaging, Sixth Edition, edited by John H. Juhl and Andrew B. Crummy. J.B. Lippincott Company, Philadelphia, © 1993.

CHAPTER **24**

Airway Diseases

John H. Juhl

DISEASES OF THE UPPER AIRWAY

ACUTE OBSTRUCTIVE DISEASES

The division of the diseases of the upper airway into acute and chronic is somewhat artificial, since some masses may grow slowly to cause a chronic obstruction and other slowly developing lesions may be traumatized or become infected and cause an acute obstruction.

Pharynx

Acute Infections of the Tonsils and Adenoids
These inflammatory diseases can develop rapidly and in children may cause severe acute obstruction. In more gradual enlargement of these structures, whatever the cause, chronic airway obstruction may result. In children, it is a known cause of obstructive sleep apnea. When tonsils and adenoids are enlarged and sleep apnea is present, a videofluoroscopic examination of the pharynx in the lateral projection will show inspiratory collapse of the pharynx in the region of the tonsils and/or adenoids. In the acute infectious obstructions, the enlargement of these structures is readily observed on a lateral roentgenogram.

Acute Retropharyngeal Abscess or Cellulitis
The masses produced by these infections may also cause acute obstruction, particularly in children. There is a characteristic swelling of the prevertebral soft tissues posterior to the pharynx. When the swelling is large enough to cause obstruction, the pharynx above it tends to be distended on inspiration. Other causes of acute thickening of the retropharyngeal tissues include

infections within the pharynx caused by foreign bodies, hemorrhage, and the edema and hemorrhage secondary to trauma of the cervical spine. Lymphadenopathy, which may occur in association with lymphoma, chronic granulomatous disease, or histiocytosis X, and retropharyngeal tumors, such as cystic hygroma, neurofibroma, neuroblastoma, hemangioma, and retropharyngeal thyroid, may produce varying degrees of obstruction. In some instances the obstruction is acute, and in others it is chronic. The lungs are usually normal in volume in patients with acute upper airway obstructive conditions. When acute upper airway obstruction is suspected, a lateral soft-tissue view of the neck provides an expeditious means of imaging the hypopharynx (Fig. 24-1). In infants and young children, it is particularly important that the patient's neck be extended when the lateral film is exposed, since the flexibility of the upper airway is so great that a pseudomass or pseudostenosis may be produced if the patient's neck is flexed or incompletely extended. Large foreign bodies may lodge above the glottis and cause acute obstruction and may be a cause of sudden death in adults as well as children. There is no time for roentgen examination in this situation, since it is life-threatening from the moment of aspiration.

Epiglottitis

Epiglottitis commonly affects infants and young children and is usually caused by *Haemophilus influenzae.* It may also be the result of infection with other organisms such as *Streptococcus pneumoniae* (pneumococcus), hemolytic streptococci, and *Staphylococcus aureus* type B. Occasionally, it occurs in adults.[38] The radiographic findings consist of swelling of the epi-

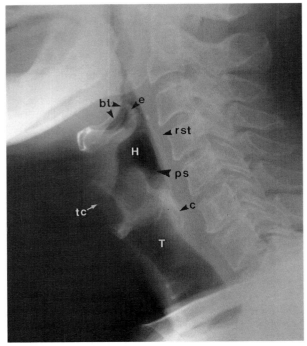

Figure 24–1. Normal lateral soft-tissue view of the neck. The base of tongue (*bt*), epiglottis (*e*), pyriform sinuses (*ps*), and subglottic and cervical portions of the trachea (*T*) are clearly identifiable. Note the normal anteroposterior diameter of the hypopharyngeal airway (*H*) and retropharyngeal soft tissues (*rst*). Portions of the thyroid (*tc*) and cricoid (*c*) cartilages are calcified.

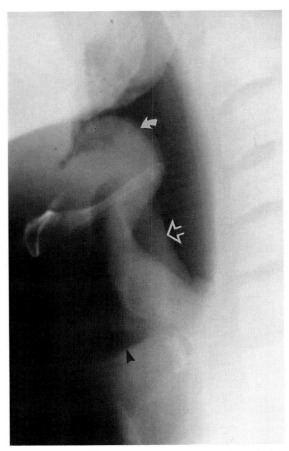

Figure 24–2. Acute epiglottitis. Lateral soft-tissue view of neck. There is marked swelling of the epiglottis (*curved arrow*) and aryepiglottic folds (*open arrow*). The hypopharyngeal airway is distended, and the laryngeal ventricles are dilated (*arrowhead*). Compare with Figure 24-1. (Case courtesy of K. A. Shaffer, M.D.)

glottis and the structures around it, including the aryepiglottic folds, the arytenoids, the uvula, and the prevertebral or retropharyngeal soft tissues. The valleculae and pyriform sinuses may be obliterated. The amount of swelling of the surrounding structures may vary from one patient to another, but enlargement of the epiglottis is present in all. There is often some ballooning of the hypopharynx, but there is no abnormality of the glottis. The subglottic region is usually normal, but in some children infected with *H. influenzae* type B, localized subglottic edema is observed,[40] similar to that found in croup. The lungs are not overinflated. A single lateral radiograph of the neck usually suffices to make the diagnosis in an individual with acute upper respiratory obstruction (Fig. 24-2). Since this condition may be life-threatening, manipulation required for laryngoscopy is often contraindicated and the lateral roentgenogram becomes the key examination.

Acute pulmonary edema has been reported in adults and children in this and other types of acute upper airway obstruction. Presumably the edema is caused by the sudden high negative intrathoracic pressure secondary to the obstruction.

Acute Laryngotracheobronchitis (Croup)

Croup is usually caused by a virus and most commonly occurs in children from 6 months to 3 years of age. The major finding on the roentgenogram is narrowing of the trachea in the subglottic area on inspiration, thickening and fuzziness of the vocal cords, and overdistention of the hypopharynx on inspiration. The appearance of the hypopharynx is variable on expiration, and there tends to be some ballooning of the cervical trachea below the subglottic region. These roentgen findings on lateral views of the neck are very characteristic[30]; however, good technique is essential. The subglottic narrowing may change on expiration but does not ordinarily disappear. In some patients the only abnormalities are the fuzzy appearance of the thickened cords and poor definition of the larynx and subglottic area. In the anteroposterior projection the glottic and subglottic areas show a somewhat fusiform or funnel-shaped narrowing on inspiration. The epiglottis and aryepiglottic folds are normal. Unlike in epiglottitis, which may require tracheostomy, in croup this procedure is not ordinarily needed.

Membranous Croup

Membranous or pseudomembranous croup is a severe form of laryngotracheobronchitis probably caused by superimposed bacterial infection on the viral disease or by bacterial infection alone; hemolytic *Staphylococcus aureus* is the usual cause.[17] The disease is more severe than viral croup and tends to affect slightly older age groups. Radiographically, the subglottic obstruction may be severe, upper tracheal mucosa is thick and irregular, and the detached or partially detached membranes may project into the tracheal airway, sometimes resembling foreign bodies, for which they may be mistaken. The mucosa may appear irregular in the subglottic area. An artificial airway may be necessary in some patients.

Sleep Apnea

Sleep apnea is a form of repetitive periodic apnea during sleep. It may be obstructive, central (absent inspiratory effort), or a mixture of the two. Radiologic examination may be useful in the diagnosis of the obstructive type. Obstructive sleep apnea is presumably caused in part by a narrow pharyngeal airway. Computed tomographic (CT) examination of nine patients with documented sleep apnea showed that the region posterior to the soft palate was the smallest part of the upper airway. The cross-sectional area of this region was significantly less in patients with sleep apnea than in normal individuals.[43] Fluoroscopy in six sleeping patients showed that the obstruction always began when the soft palate touched the tongue and posterior pharyngeal wall during inspiration. Therefore, CT and fluoroscopy may be useful in documenting the pharyngeal narrowing in patients with obstructive sleep apnea.

Anomalies and Diseases of the Larynx

The conditions in this category cause a varying amount of obstruction, which may be acute or chronic, depending on the severity and the circumstances in an individual patient. The true vocal cords and the space between them are termed the glottis. The conditions to be described involve the glottis and adjacent structures. Landing and Dixon have presented an extensive classification of malformations of the respiratory tract.[25] Some are described here, but space limitations make it impossible to include all of them.

Congenital Laryngeal Stenosis. This is the most common anomaly of the larynx. It is usually caused by an anterior web, which may be supraglottic, glottic, or subglottic. The amount of obstruction varies with the severity of the stenosis. Roentgenographic findings are usually observed on the lateral projection, where the web may be outlined and its thickness and extent noted. The subglottic area can also be examined on the same film. *Laryngeal atresia* is usually accompanied by other anomalies.

Laryngotracheoesophageal Cleft. This rare anomaly consists of failure of differentiation of the larynx and upper trachea from the esophagus. A common channel is observed on contrast study, with propyliodone (Dionosil) or barium as the medium, which may be performed after laryngoscopy and placement of an endotracheal tube. In addition to aphonia and other voice abnormalities, there may be signs of upper airway obstruction, resulting in respiratory distress in the neonatal period. The cleft is minimal in some infants and extensive in others.

Congenital Laryngeal Cyst. This is another rare cause of respiratory tract obstruction in infants.[39] Roentgen findings are those of a soft-tissue laryngeal mass occurring anywhere from the superior surface of the aryepiglottic fold to the laryngeal ventricle. This soft-tissue mass cannot be differentiated from other congenital masses such as hemangioma.

Laryngomalacia. This is caused by congenital aryepiglottic laxity and results in supraglottic obstruction and stridor at rest, which decreases or disappears when the child is excited. The obstructive soft tissue may be visible on the lateral roentgenogram of the upper airway.

Benign Laryngeal Mass-Producing Lesions

Numerous mass-producing lesions may involve the larynx. Singer's nodules (nodes), polyps, and papilloma are fairly common but are small and not usually visible, even on CT. Chondroma arising from laryngeal cartilages is outlined on CT and often contain calcium. Most chondromas arise in the cricoid cartilage. Hemangioma, neurofibroma, fibroma, adenoma, lipoma, hamartoma, and tumorlike mass caused by amyloid are all very unusual. Detection is best done radiographically by CT, but if small, they may be missed. Inflammatory masses produced by sarcoidosis, tuberculosis, and other infectious granulomas cannot be differentiated from tumors on CT.

Malignant Laryngeal Tumors

Nearly all malignant tumors are squamous cell in type (95%). Adenocarcinoma and connective tissue tumors such as fibrosarcoma and rhabdomyosarcoma are rare, as are lymphoma and plasmacytoma. The tumors may be limited to the true cords (glottic), but supraglottic tumors involving the false cords, aryepiglottic folds, posterior inferior surface of the epiglottis, and arytenoid and subglottic tumors are usually included in the classification and staging of laryngeal tumors.[21]

The tumor, nodes, and metastases (TNM) classification of laryngeal tumors modified from the American Joint Committee on Cancer is outlined by Horowitz and colleagues.[18] The continuing controversy regarding therapy for these tumors is beyond the scope of this text. In the past, tomography and contrast laryngography were used in the diagnostic work-up of malignant tumors of the larynx. These studies were primarily useful in assessing the degree of mucosal abnormality and determining the presence of subglottic extension. Because it permitted imaging of the submucosal tissues, CT became the imaging method of choice in the 1980s (Figs. 24-3 and 24-4). Current magnetic resonance imaging (MRI) is considered to be a valuable adjunct to CT, even replacing it in some centers because of more tissue specificity, high contrast resolution, and multiplanar imaging capabilities of MRI. Despite the improvement in imaging modalities, however, cartilage invasion may not always be apparent, and there continues to be difficulty in the identification of small mucosal tumors such as those confined to a true cord. Cartilage invasion can be detected only when it is definite, not microscopic. False-positive diagnoses may be caused by edema, which may appear as a tumorlike mass, or edema may add to the apparent size of a tumor.

Laryngeal Trauma

Fractures of laryngeal cartilages, hematomas caused by soft-tissue injury, and areas of edema are best examined by CT, which is the only imaging method that can reliably detect cartilage fractures.

Laryngocele

This abnormality consists of abnormal dilation and elongation of the appendix of the laryngeal ventricle. It arises from the anterior end of the ventricle and extends upward into the soft tissues lateral to the false

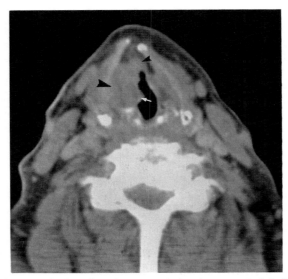

Figure 24–3.   Carcinoma of the larynx. Axial CT scan. There is enlargement and irregularity of the right true cord (*white arrow*), invasion of the paralaryngeal space (*large arrowhead*), and involvement of the anterior commissure (*small arrowhead*).

cord and aryepiglottic fold. It usually communicates with the ventricle via a narrow stalk. There are three types[12]: (1) internal, confined to the larynx; (2) external, with the sac extending through the thyrohyoid membrane laterally to produce a local bulge in the soft tissue of the neck; and (3) mixed, a combination of internal and external types.

Roentgenographically, laryngoceles present as clearly defined air spaces near the pre-epiglottic space and/or extending laterally into the soft tissue of the neck. CT can be used to define their extent. CT is particularly useful in complicated or atypical laryngoceles.

Thyroglossal Duct Cyst

A thyroglossal cyst of the base of the tongue may cause respiratory obstruction as well as difficulty in swallowing. It is outlined as a soft-tissue mass on the lateral film, exhibits water density on CT, and has a high signal on T1-weighted MR images.

CHRONIC OBSTRUCTIVE DISEASES

Tracheal Agenesis

Absence of the trachea is a rare anomaly in which air reaches the bronchi through an esophageal communication. The anomaly is readily noted on frontal and lateral roentgenograms. It is uniformly fatal.

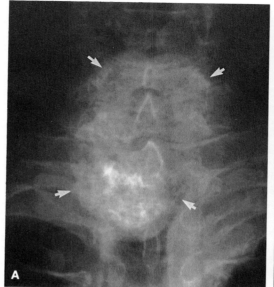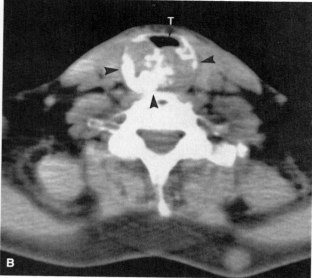

Figure 24–4. Chondrosarcoma arising in the cricoid cartilage. **(A)** Anteroposterior view of the cervicothoracic junction. A large calcified mass extends from the subglottic trachea to the proximal portion of the intrathoracic trachea (*arrows*). **(B)** Axial CT scan, level of cricoid cartilage. The densely calcified mass (*arrowheads*) almost totally occludes the tracheal lumen (*T*). (Case courtesy of R. Rosenberg, M.D.)

Tracheal Tumors

Benign tumors of the trachea are uncommon lesions and include papillomatosis, fibrolipoma, lipoma, and angioma in the pediatric population.[10] With the exception of papilloma, which is usually multiple, most benign tumors appear as well-circumscribed, noninvasive endotracheal masses.

Papilloma may occur in the trachea and may also involve the pharynx or larynx. This lesion is probably caused by a virus, but its etiology is not entirely clear. Since lesions are usually multiple, *papillomatosis* is a better term. Although common in children, these masses are also found in adults in whom the disease has a high mortality. Radiographic findings are often characteristic and consist of numerous tracheal nodules of varying sizes. There are usually associated laryngeal lesions and, later in the disease, nodules in the larger bronchi. They may extend far out into the lungs. As the nodules enlarge, they may excavate to form cystlike lesions in the lung that do not fill on bronchography. When the lesions become cystic, distal parenchyma is destroyed, so the prognosis is poor. Papillomatosis may evolve into squamous cell carcinomatosis in adults, and 10% of children with this condition die of bronchogenic carcinoma in early adult life.

Primary malignant neoplasms of the trachea are rela-

tively rare. Approximately 50% are squamous cell carcinomas, and 20% to 25% are adenoid cystic carcinomas, which exceed the occasional adenocarcinoma in frequency by 2:1. The remainder include mixed tumor, mucoepidermoid tumor, and certain types of sarcoma. In general, adenoid cystic carcinomas more frequently involve the proximal trachea, and the remaining neoplasms involve the distal portion. The prognosis with all tracheal tumors is poor, but survival tends to be somewhat longer with adenoid cystic carcinomas.[2]

Chronic granulomatous infectious diseases such as coccidioidomycosis or inflammatory pseudotumors caused by other infections may arise in the trachea and become large enough to cause stridor.

Tracheal Stenosis

Tracheal stenosis may result from external trauma or be secondary to intubation or tracheostomy.[20] Rarely it is congenital, usually in children with other congenital anomalies. Congenital tracheal occlusion, a rare anomaly, also may occur. Several vascular anomalies may cause varying degrees of tracheal stenosis. They include right aortic arch, with or without a vascular ring; anomalous right subclavian, innominate, or left carotid artery; pulmonary sling; or anomalous left pulmonary artery in which the tracheal narrowing is much longer than its contact with the left pulmonary artery. Extrinsic masses of various kinds may compress the trachea. They include mediastinal fibrosis and granuloma, amyloidosis and sarcoidosis, tuberculosis, and other chronic infectious diseases that may produce local disease as well as adenopathy. Several mediastinal neoplasms may also narrow and distort the trachea. Radiographic findings depend to some extent on the cause, so they may vary considerably. Good plain films may outline the lesions, but tomograms and sometimes CT may be necessary for optimum imaging of the stenosis and its cause. Angiography is useful in vascular anomalies. Roentgen findings of tracheal stenosis are those of persistent tracheal narrowing of varying length and severity that does not change or changes very little from the inspiratory to the expiratory phase of respiration.

Tracheomalacia

Tracheomalacia is another rare cause of obstruction. This abnormality should be suspected if the tracheal diameter decreases by more than 50% during expiration. There is a wide range of normal variation, however, and the diagnosis should be made with caution. Tracheomalacia is presumably caused by weakness of the tracheal wall, including the supporting cartilage, and is usually associated with deficiency of cartilage plates in the rare primary form. It is also seen in osseous dysplasias such as the Ellis–van Creveld syndrome. More often, it is secondary to some other abnormality of the upper respiratory tract. It may be acquired—for example, secondary to overdistention of an endotracheal tube cuff, which results in atrophy of cartilage with local tracheomalacia.

Relapsing Polychondritis[4]

This is probably an autoimmune disease. When it involves the trachea, it can cause tracheal stenosis, which may be severe. It usually begins in the subglottic area and extends distally. As the name implies, cartilage may be involved at other sites, namely the ear, nose, larynx, and joints. Destroyed cartilage is replaced by fibrous tissue. The narrowing is visible on frontal and lateral films of the trachea or on tomograms.

Tracheobronchomegaly (Mounier-Kuhn Syndrome)

Tracheobronchomegaly is another rare condition that may result in chronic obstruction. Although occasionally found in children, it usually involves men in the fourth and fifth decades and appears to be familial. There is atrophy of elastic tissue and thinning of mus-

cularis mucosa, leading to weakness of the tracheal walls. This condition has been described in some patients with the Ehlers-Danlos syndrome and may be a part of the syndrome or only coincidental.

On roentgenographic study the trachea and major bronchi are noted to be increased in caliber; a diameter of more than 3 cm is required for diagnosis. The trachea has an irregular, corrugated appearance caused by protrusion of the tracheal and bronchial walls between the cartilaginous rings, which is sometimes termed diverticulosis. CT is very useful if the diagnosis is in question or if no cause for chronic cough and/or repeated lower respiratory infection is apparent. The enlarged trachea is readily seen, along with any bronchiectasis that may be present. The obstructive symptoms appear to be secondary to an inefficient cough mechanism. Most patients having this condition develop infection with associated bronchiectasis, and many succumb to infection associated with respiratory failure. The tracheal width in children with this anomaly is equal to or greater than the thoracic vertebral body width, a distinct increase in diameter. On expiration or coughing, marked tracheobronchial collapse is observed.

Tracheopathia Osteoplastica (Tracheobronchopathia Osteochondroplastica)

This rare condition usually occurs in older men (over 50). It is characterized by osseous and cartilaginous masses on the inner surface of the trachea between the cartilage rings. It usually involves the lower two-thirds of the trachea and may extend into the bronchi. These submucosal nodules are visible in long segments of the trachea as small masses projecting into the tracheal lumen. Calcification may be present and can be demonstrated on tomography. The cause is unknown.

Saber-Sheath Trachea

In this condition, the coronal diameter of the trachea is narrow in relation to the sagittal diameter. The coronal diameter is decreased and the sagittal diameter is increased. The coronal narrowing may be severe, the diameter being less than two-thirds of the normal. The trachea is involved from the thoracic inlet to the level of the carina or a few centimeters above it. It usually occurs in males with chronic obstructive pulmonary disease (COPD), about 50% of whom do not have other roentgen signs of chronic obstructive disease. Chronic bronchitis is also common in patients with saber-sheath trachea. Tracheal rings have been found to be densely ossified at autopsy, so the tracheal alteration may be secondary to cartilage injury caused by coughing.[14]

BRONCHIAL DISEASES

BRONCHITIS

Acute Bronchitis

The term *acute bronchitis* usually refers to acute bronchial inflammation associated with upper respiratory infection, which is not usually a severe illness when uncomplicated. There are no positive roentgen findings in this condition, but roentgenograms are useful to indicate that there is no complicating pneumonia in patients with acute respiratory infections in whom symptoms are unusually severe.

Chronic Bronchitis

Chronic bronchial inflammatory disease may occur in patients with chronic specific pulmonary inflammatory disease. This is not considered here. We include chronic nonspecific bronchial inflammation, which results in chronic cough with sputum, often of several years' duration. If etiologic factors persist, this disease progresses to pulmonary insufficiency, emphysema, and cor pulmonale. Several etiologic possibilities exist, with one or more or a combination of several operating in an individual patient. They include air pollution, cigarette smoking in an estimated 82%,[45] and infection, with hereditary weakness of bronchial walls in a few patients. Recurrent obstructive bronchitis also may be a result of gastroesophageal reflux in children.[6]

It is common to see no roentgen findings in patients with chronic bronchial disease. In these patients, the chest roentgenogram excludes the possibility of other diseases that could cause the same symptoms. When the bronchitis results in thickening of bronchial walls and in peribronchial inflammation, these thick-walled structures may be seen extending well into the parenchyma, whereas the normal bronchi within the lungs are not outlined on the plain roentgenogram. The visibility of these bronchi, therefore, indicates thickening of bronchial walls and peribronchial disease, which is often associated with chronic bronchitis regardless of its etiology. These findings are often best outlined on CT. Hyperinflation of the lung may also be manifested by increased lucency of the lungs and increased thoracic volume. Roentgen changes must be correlated with clinical findings. The presence of prominent basal markings does not necessarily indicate chronic bronchial disease, since there is a wide variation in the normal. The roentgen diagnosis of chronic bronchitis, based on plain film study, is therefore made infrequently and with great caution.

Although there are no reliable plain film findings in chronic bronchitis, bronchographic signs have been described in this disease. Small diverticulum-like projections are often observed along the inferior surfaces of the large bronchi. They represent dilated ducts of mucus glands. Distal bronchial or bronchiolar occlusions have also been described. Some of them are tapering occlusions, whereas in others there is a bulbous expansion distally (bronchiolectasia). Irregularity or "beading" of the bronchial lumen may also be present. Dilation of small bronchi on inspiration, with return to normal caliber on expiration, has been described, but we have not observed this alteration with respiration. In the absence of bronchiectasis, the presence of dilated bronchial glands, bronchiolectasia, and irregularity or beading of the bronchial lumen may justify the diagnosis of chronic bronchitis. However, studies a decade ago using tantalum bronchography on 13 normal asymptomatic males who had never smoked revealed findings previously described in chronic bronchitis.[11] (*Tantalum* is no longer used for bronchography.) Eight subjects had filling of mucus gland ducts, 9 had airway irregularity, 12 had visible secretions in bronchi, and 10 had stagnation of secretions in intermediate-sized bronchi. Two of these men had recent respiratory infections; in both there was marked delay in clearance of the tantalum from peripheral airways as compared with the others. Bronchography is not ordinarily used in patients with suspected chronic bronchitis in our department. The signs described previously have been observed in patients who were studied for suspected bronchiectasis or for other reasons.

Acute Bronchiolitis (Infectious)

The term *acute bronchiolitis* refers to the acute disease usually observed in small infants or occasionally in debilitated elderly persons in whom a widespread involvement of small bronchi and bronchioles is manifested by roentgen signs of air trapping with hyperaeration and low, flat diaphragm (Fig. 24-5).[23] The lungs appear clearer than normal and there is very little change on expiration. This is produced by a check-valve type of obstruction of the bronchioles. As the disease progresses, focal areas of alveolar involvement are manifested by scattered small opacities, which may eventually resemble a very widespread, acute, miliary type of disease. These opacities appear to be caused by small areas of pneumonia around the bronchioles and by small foci of atelectasis. At times, extensive alveolar pneumonia may develop, so that there is a broad spectrum of radiographic findings.

The most frequent cause appears to be respiratory syncytial virus, but other viruses including adenovirus, rhinovirus, parainfluenza virus, and, occa-

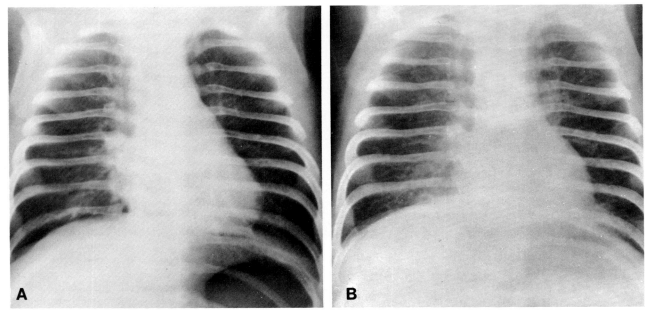

Figure 24–5.   Acute bronchiolitis. **(A)** Note the relatively low diaphragm with hyper-aerated lung and a small amount of opacity at the right medial base representing early associated pneumonia. **(B)** In this film, exposed 24 hours after that shown in *A*, emphysema is shown to be slightly less marked, but the pneumonia, particularly on the right side, has increased. The patient was acutely ill at the time of the examination.

sionally, mumps and influenza may be involved. In infants, *Mycoplasma pneumoniae* occasionally causes bronchiolitis. Adenovirus types 3, 7, and 21 may cause serious pulmonary infection in young children, with destruction and necrosis of bronchiolar and alveolar tissue and permanent lung damage. It is probably the cause of the Swyer-James (MacLeod) syndrome in some instances. In addition to hyperinflation, areas of air-space pneumonic consolidation and atelectasis may be observed on the chest roentgenogram.[48] Follow-up studies of 23 children who had been symptom-free for 10 years after bronchiolitis in infancy revealed abnormalities in blood gases and pulmonary function tests in most.[22] This suggests that persistent pulmonary abnormality is not unusual after bronchiolitis, even though there are no symptoms or radiographic signs. However, the question of whether these childhood infections eventually lead to chronic air-flow obstruction has not yet been determined.

Bronchiolitis Obliterans

Bronchiolitis obliterans results from lower respiratory tract damage, which may be caused by inhalation of toxic substance such as fumes from nitric, hydrochloric, or sulfuric acid, zinc stearate, and hot gases. It

may also be caused by viral infections of the respiratory tract, including influenza, measles, and infections due to adenovirus.[13] In some instances, no definite etiology can be established. The bronchioles become obstructed by masses of granulation tissue and organizing exudate. When fat-filled phagocytes accumulate behind the obstructed bronchioles, a "cholesterol" pneumonitis is produced. The clinical findings include cough, dyspnea, sputum production, fever, and malaise. Roentgenologic findings have been divided into three main categories[13]: (1) *Nodular densities* in the form of micronodular, discrete nodular, confluent nodular, or lineonodular densities. (2) *Alveolar opacities*, which may be diffuse or edemalike, linear (atelectatic), or a mixed or honey-comb pattern. These patterns are usually bibasilar. In other locations the alveolar opacities take the form of lobar or segmental consolidation and atelectasis; diffuse edemalike or multiple, irregular opacities may also occur. (3) *Hyperinflation*, which occurred in only 2 of 52 patients. The most distinctive appear to be the micronodular and lineonodular patterns similar to those in diffuse infectious granulomatous disease, occupational lung disease, or, possibly, sarcoidosis. The nodules tend to be less distinct in bronchiolitis obliterans than in the other conditions. The discrete and confluent nodular densities suggest such conditions as diffuse or localized vasculitis, multiple abscesses, or disseminated bronchioloalveolar cell carcinoma or metastases. The basilar opacities are suggestive of chronic interstitial pneumonia, which may coexist in some instances. This wide variation in roentgen findings makes roentgenographic diagnosis very difficult, although it can be suspected in patients with a suggestive past history and the clinical symptoms of cough, dyspnea, sputum, fever, and malaise. The relationship to diffuse interstitial pneumonia and bronchiolitis obliterans is not clear.

Occasionally, obliteration of the smaller airways without a recognized cause may be demonstrated on bronchography. Plain film findings consist of minimal overinflation and a decrease in mid- and lower-zone vasculature. The bronchographic findings consist of pruning of fifth- and sixth-generation bronchi, with no filling of smaller bronchi or alveoli and no evidence of other airway disease.[3]

Bronchiolitis Obliterans Organizing Pneumonia (BOOP)

This disease has been classified by Epler and coworkers according to etiology into the following groups[9]:

1. Caused by toxic fumes
2. Postinfectious
3. Associated with connective tissue disease
4. Associated with a localized lung lesion
5. Idiopathic

It is also a major complication of heart-lung transplantation,[28] and it is entirely possible that there are other causes.

In the group of 50 patients with the idiopathic form reported by Epler and colleagues, the age range was 40 to 60 years, there was no difference in number of males and females, and 50% occurred in nonsmokers. Symptoms consist of persistent, often severe, nonproductive cough in a patient with flulike symptoms of sore throat, fever, and malaise. Not all patients exhibit all symptoms; for example, mild dyspnea in 50% and flulike symptoms in one-third appeared in this series.

Radiographic findings consist of bilateral patchy, poorly defined areas of "ground-glass" opacities that may begin as focal lesions and progress. Diffuse small linear and nodular opacities occur in about 10%. CT is helpful in some instances because it reveals more extensive disease, particularly the small linear and nodular foci,[32, 44] in addition to the patchy alveolar process. The idiopathic form of BOOP responds to corticosteroids, often with complete remission. Therefore, the prognosis is better than that in patients with usual interstitial pneumonia and idiopathic pulmonary fibrosis, diseases from which BOOP must be differentiated.

Bronchiectasis

Bronchiectasis refers to persistent dilation of bronchi, which may vary widely in extent. It results from destruction of the elastic and muscle tissue of the bronchial walls. Descriptive adjectives such as cylindrical (tubular), varicose, and saccular (cystic) are used to distinguish the various forms of dilation. The cylindrical form of the disease is sometimes difficult to recognize, particularly when it is minimal. With progression, the bronchi tend to dilate further, making the diagnosis relatively easy on CT or bronchography. The varicose and saccular forms are readily recognized. The varicose form is dilated and irregular because of local constrictions, and the termination is somewhat bulbous in many instances. The saccular, or cystic form represents a more marked dilation. The disease may be local or general and is usually caused by obstruction and infection, but there is probably a congenital factor or a number of congenital factors in some instances. For example, the incidence of bronchiectasis associated with situs inversus is much greater than in the general population. The triad of situs inversus, paranasal sinus disease, and bronchiectasis is termed Kartagener's triad or syndrome. In this condition, the respiratory cilia are immotile. This ciliary dysmotility results in impaired transport of mucus and other secretions in the bronchi and in the paranasal sinuses as well. Bronchiectasis is also common in patients with cystic fibrosis. Immunologic defects such as agammaglobulinemia and dysgammaglobulinemia are also associated with bronchiectasis. The usual symptom of bronchiectasis is chronic productive cough, often associated with recurrent episodes of acute pneumonitis and hemoptysis.

It is often possible to make a presumptive diagnosis of bronchiectasis on plain film study, but it must be remembered that a roentgenogram of the chest showing no abnormality does not exclude bronchiectasis. The findings that indicate this disease are accentuation of markings in the area of disease, often with associated patchy pneumonic opacities in which parallel linear or circular ringlike shadows can be outlined (Fig. 24-6). Bandlike Y- or V-shaped opacities representing dilated bronchi filled with exudate or mucus may also be observed. It is sometimes possible to trace a thick-walled dilated bronchus well out into the periphery when there is enough peribronchial inflammatory disease so that the air-filled bronchus is visible. When severe saccular bronchiectasis is present, oval or circular opacities may be outlined and it is not uncommon to see fluid levels in some of the larger cystlike dilations. There is often decrease in volume of the lobe or segment associated with the chronic inflammation that produces fibrosis and atelectasis.

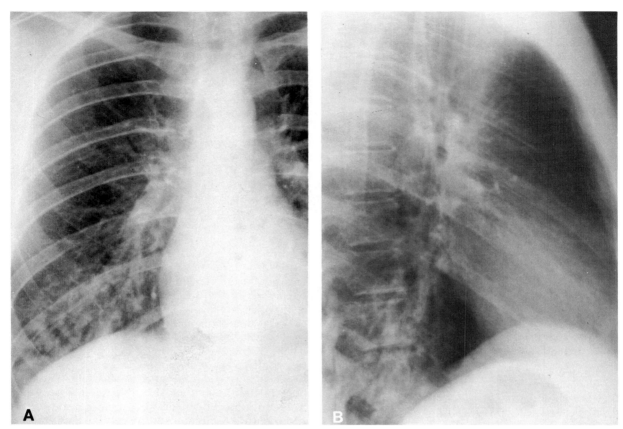

Figure 24–6.   Bronchiectasis of the basal segments of the right lower lobe. (**A**) Note the inflammatory disease represented by basal opacities in which there are some elongated radiolucencies representing dilated bronchi. (**B**) Lateral view of the same patient shown in *A*. Some of the elongated dilated bronchi are observed overlying the lower thoracic vertebrae in the posterior basal lung. A bronchogram obtained later confirmed the findings. The bronchiectasis was largely of the cylindrical type.

The fact that the presence of bronchiectasis can be determined on plain film study in some cases and can be suspected in others does not mean that CT or bronchography is unnecessary in these patients. Whenever surgical intervention is planned, complete bronchographic or CT mapping of the bronchial tree is necessary so that the surgery can be planned intelligently. In most instances the dilation is either saccular or varicose or a combination of the two (Figs. 24-7 through 24-9). Saccular bronchiectasis is not difficult to define, but unless there is good filling outlining the entire length of a bronchus, the presence of cylindrical bronchiectasis or the absence of it is sometimes difficult to ascertain and there is often some difference of opinion as to the presence or absence of dilation. It is often possible to define small amounts of dilation, however, by comparing the bronchus in question with an

adjacent bronchus of similar order.[16] Local bronchiectasis may follow obstruction by tumor, foreign body, or a constrictive bronchial process (Fig. 24-10).

There is still some difference of opinion as to the relative value of CT and bronchography in the diagnosis of bronchiectasis when its severity and extent must be determined as accurately as possible before surgery.[15, 34, 41] However, the use of bronchography appears to continue to decline.

Reversible bronchiectasis occurs in children and young adults, usually after acute pneumonia or atelectasis. In the postpneumonic group, the dilation clears after complete resolution of the pulmonary disease. In the atelectatic group the bronchi decrease in caliber with reexpansion of the lung. Evidently, the dilation is reversible if the mucosa and musculoelastic elements of the bronchial wall are intact. The reversible disease

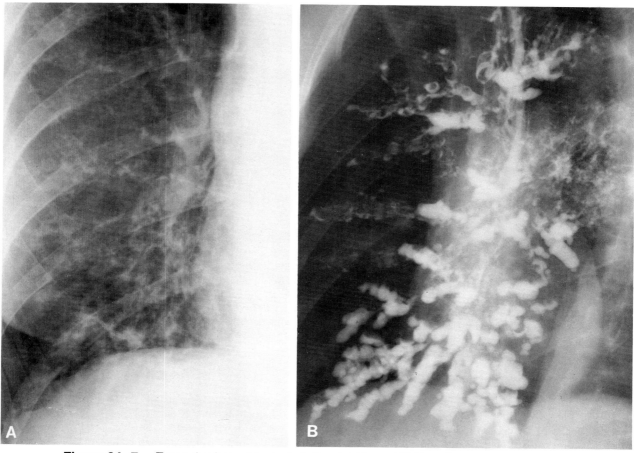

Figure 24–7. Extensive bronchiectasis in the right lung. (**A**) Note the extensive disease, producing linear densities with some suggestion of small rounded and oval radiolucencies at the base. (**B**) Bronchogram demonstrating the extensive bronchiectasis in this patient, which is a combination of saccular and varicose in type.

is usually cylindrical in type, and there may be slight narrowing proximal to the dilation caused by spasm secondary to inflammatory disease. The possibility of reversibility must be considered if surgical treatment is contemplated; a repeat bronchogram is the only accurate method of making a positive diagnosis of a return to normal. CT is a useful noninvasive method of making the diagnosis of cystic bronchiectasis but may be unreliable in the less severe varicose and cylindrical forms of the disease. Selective bronchography in conjunction with fiberoptic examination is helpful in the diagnosis of segmental post-stenotic bronchiectasis. A catheter can be passed through the area of stenosis, secretions aspirated, and the contrast agent injected.

The greatest dilation of bronchi in nonspecific bronchiectasis is usually peripheral. In the bronchiectasis associated with pulmonary tuberculosis, there is a somewhat different appearance since the peripheral portion of the involved bronchus is often obstructed and the dilation is more central. This is not invariably true, however, and there are patients with pulmonary tuberculosis in whom upper lobe bronchiectasis extends far peripherally. There are differences in the appearance of bronchiectasis associated with other conditions such as the Swyer-James syndrome, which are described in the appropriate sections.

PULMONARY CYSTS AND CYSTIC DISEASE

There is considerable confusion in the literature as to the origin and classification of pulmonary cysts. It is now recognized that several lesions that were formerly

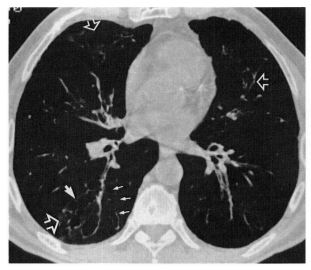

Figure 24–8. Cystic bronchiectasis, posterior basal segment, right lower lobe, middle lobe, and lingula (*open arrows*). A "cluster of grapes" appearance due to adjacent dilated cystic bronchi is present (*large arrow*), as well as the characteristic beaded appearance produced by consecutive areas of cystic dilation in a single bronchus (*small arrows*). High-resolution CT scan, 2-mm collimation, bone algorithm. (Case courtesy of Julie K. Mitby, M.D.)

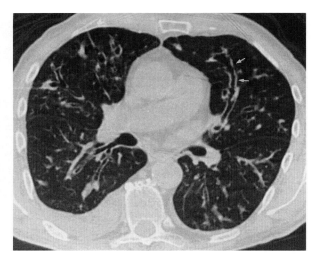

Figure 24–9. Cylindrical and varicose bronchiectasis. Dilated, thick-walled bronchi are present bilaterally. A lingular bronchus exhibits the "accordion" or pleated appearance of varicose bronchiectasis (*arrows*). High-resolution CT scan, 2-mm collimation, bone algorithm. (Case courtesy of Julie K. Mitby, M.D.)

thought to represent congenital cysts are actually acquired lesions, resulting from inflammatory disease. The size may vary considerably, and these acquired cysts may be single or multiple.

CONGENITAL PULMONARY CYSTS

It is generally recognized that the differentiation between congenital and acquired pulmonary cysts is not possible in many instances even when histopathologic studies are available. The cysts may contain fluid or air and vary considerably in size. The roentgen findings depend on the presence or absence of fluid. The air-filled cyst is visualized as a rounded radiolucency, which varies considerably in size. Unless infected, its wall is rather thin. In some instances a small amount of fluid may be present, and this produces an air–fluid level. The solitary cysts that contain only fluid are seen on roentgenograms as rounded masses that are usually very clearly circumscribed unless there is parenchymal infection in the area. When a cyst is acquired, there may be evidence of the inflammatory disease that initiated the lesion, but it is also possible that inflammatory disease may appear surrounding a congenital cyst or the latter may become secondarily infected. Whether

the congenital cysts are all originally fluid-filled or air-filled has not been settled, and it is possible that there are both types (Figs. 24-11 and 24-12). Some of these cysts are lined by bronchial mucosa; in others the lining is made up of mesothelium or fibrous tissue.

Transient fluid-filled cysts have been reported in Ehlers-Danlos syndrome. They may be related to subpleural vesicles, which have also been reported in this condition. Cystlike lesions have also been reported as a rare finding in the apices of patients with ankylosing spondylitis. They usually contain air but may contain fungus balls. Some pulmonary cysts may represent hamartomatous malformations.

PNEUMATOCELE

A pneumatocele is produced when a check-valve type of obstruction occurs either in a small branch bronchus or between a small peribronchial abscess and the lumen of a bronchus, resulting in marked overinflation of the lung distal to the obstruction in patients with pneumonia. The air may therefore be interstitial or within the bronchial system. The valve mechanism allows air to enter the lesion on inspiration but does not allow the air to get out during expiration. The marked overexpansion produces disruption of alveolar septa, and the pneumatocele may become large enough to cause res-

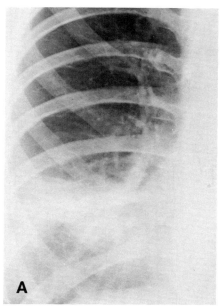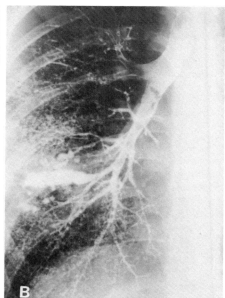

Figure 24–10. Localized bronchiectasis. (**A**) Note inflammatory disease at the right lateral base. (**B**) Bronchogram demonstrates the localized cylindrical bronchiectasis involving a subsegment in the right lower lobe. Several small saccular dilations are also observed.

piratory embarrassment because of its size. Presumably, the pneumatocele enlarges as long as the check-valve obstruction persists and may become very large. The terms *regional obstructive emphysema* and *air cyst* have been applied to this lesion. A pneumatocele is usually the result of inflammatory disease, most often staphylococcal infection, and may be found in

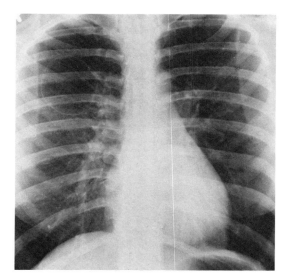

Figure 24–11. Air-filled cyst in the right upper lobe. The patient was asymptomatic. Note that the cyst is very thin walled and there is no sign of infection in the adjacent lung.

children and adults. It is not uncommon to see this type of lesion appear when a pneumonic process is resolving. It is not unusual to see a small amount of fluid within the otherwise thin-walled, rounded, radiolucent defect, and rapid change in size is common. These lesions usually clear if given enough time; therefore, surgery is not often indicated. The term is usually applied to large, thin-walled cystic lesions, but many of the smaller, acquired pulmonary cysts are also of similar origin and could therefore be termed pneumatoceles. This condition must be differentiated from lung abscess and from cavitation produced by suppurative or caseating types of pulmonary disease in which there is considerable destruction of pulmonary tissue. Serial roentgenograms along with bacteriologic studies and correlation with history and clinical findings are necessary (Fig. 24-13). The diagnosis is made on the roentgen findings of a thin-walled, air-filled cyst in the lung of a patient with a history of a recent acute pneumonic episode. Rapid change in size is a characteristic finding.

POST-TRAUMATIC CYSTS (PNEUMATOCELE)

Traumatic lung cysts probably result from laceration of small bronchi, bronchioles, or alveoli, with dissection of air into interstitial tissues. They might better be termed *traumatic pneumatoceles*. They are found most frequently in children and young adults with elastic thoracic cages, often immediately after trauma. Although they may occur in any area, the lower lungs are most commonly involved, often in a retrocardiac posi-

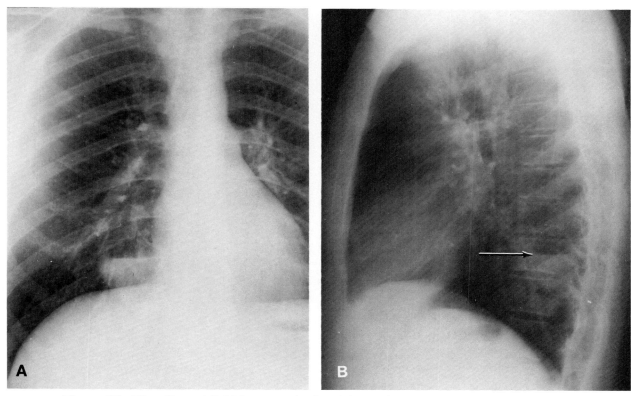

Figure 24–12.   Air and fluid in a cyst in the right medial base. **(A)** Frontal projection showing the cyst, just above the diaphragm, which contains air and fluid. **(B)** The arrow indicates the fluid level in the cyst, which is located posteriorly in this lateral projection.

tion or at the right medial base. A contrecoup effect may result in a cyst developing away from the site of chest wall trauma. These cysts are not secondary to hematoma or infection. Roentgen findings consist of a cystlike, thin-walled, air-filled space that may contain an air–fluid level. There may be opacity of the surrounding lung if there has been contusion with hemorrhage into the parenchyma. This may obscure the cyst for several days after the initiating trauma. Multiple cysts have been reported. The appearance of the cysts tends to change in the first few post-traumatic days, and most of them resolve slowly over a few weeks. Occasionally, the cysts are filled with fluid; when this occurs, they appear as a pulmonary mass.

CONGENITAL BRONCHIAL CYSTS

Intrapulmonary congenital bronchial cyst is a rare anomaly that is usually found in the lower lobes. It is produced by an anomalous bud or branch of the tracheobronchial tree during pulmonary development. When supplied by an arterial branch from the systemic

circulation, it represents bronchopulmonary sequestration. Roentgen findings are those of a sharply circumscribed, thin-walled, air-containing cyst that ordinarily does not change much in size on serial examinations. Infection is common, resulting in bronchial communication, loss of the clear definition of the wall, thickening of the wall, and an air-fluid level. When noninfected, this cyst may resemble other cystlike lesions such as pneumatocele, congenital pulmonary cyst, or bulla.

CYSTIC DISEASE

A considerable difference of opinion is noted in the literature relating to cystic disease of the lung. Many authors believe that there is no such thing as congenital cystic disease, and others disagree. Various terms are also used that apparently apply to the same condition; these include *cystic disease, congenital cystic disease, cystic bronchiectasis,* and *polycystic lung.* It is likely that this multicystic disease is not related to the solitary bronchopulmonary cyst. There are differences on bron-

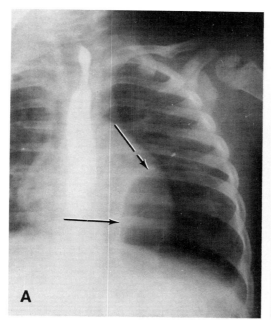
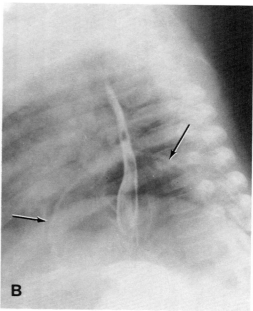

Figure 24–13. Pneumatocele. Note the large rounded radiolucent area at the left posterior base indicated by arrows in the frontal (**A**) and lateral (**B**) projections. This lesion resulted from an earlier staphylococcal pneumonia. It cleared completely in 3 months.

chography in patients who have similar findings on routine roentgenograms. Multiple cysts are usually bilateral and cause numerous rounded radiolucencies with walls that are usually thin. Infection is common, so that small fluid levels are often noted in some of these cysts and varying amounts of associated bronchial and parenchymal infection produce pneumonic changes in addition to the rounded air-filled spaces. There are no roentgen criteria to distinguish acquired from congenital types of cystic disease. Some authors would distinguish between cystic bronchiectasis and cystic disease by the bronchographic findings. In the latter disease there is very little filling of the cysts when iodized oil is introduced into the bronchial tree; in cystic bronchiectasis there is much more filling of the lesions, indicating more definite bronchial communication. Others point out that not all the cysts in cystic bronchiectasis fill with iodized oil and, conversely, some of those in cystic disease do fill. Furthermore, Di Rienzo describes a patient in whom the bronchographic findings were those of cystic bronchiectasis on one side and cystic disease on the other.[7] The cysts appeared similar on the two sides on routine chest roentgenograms. It is therefore likely that the two conditions are the same or represent different aspects of the same disease. Certainly, there is no positive differentiation on roentgen examination (Figs. 24-14 and 24-15).

Emphysematous bullae and blebs are also cystic spaces that are outlined as thin-walled areas of radiolucency on the roentgenogram. They are described in the section on bullous emphysema.

TRACHEOBRONCHIAL TRAUMA

Most injuries of the trachea below the thoracic inlet and of the bronchi are the result of blunt or crush injury of the chest caused by automobile accidents—the "steering wheel" injury. Upper tracheal injury is caused by sudden hyperextension of the neck. A variety of injuries may occur[8]; these include (1) complete rupture of the trachea or bronchus with separation; (2) incomplete rupture of the trachea or bronchus with partial separation of cartilaginous rings; and (3) incomplete rupture with communication to adjacent structures such as the esophagus.

Roentgen signs of tracheobronchial fracture include pneumothorax, which does not respond to aspiration, and mediastinal, deep cervical, and subcutaneous emphysema. In chest trauma, atelectasis of a lung indicates bronchial rupture until proved otherwise. When

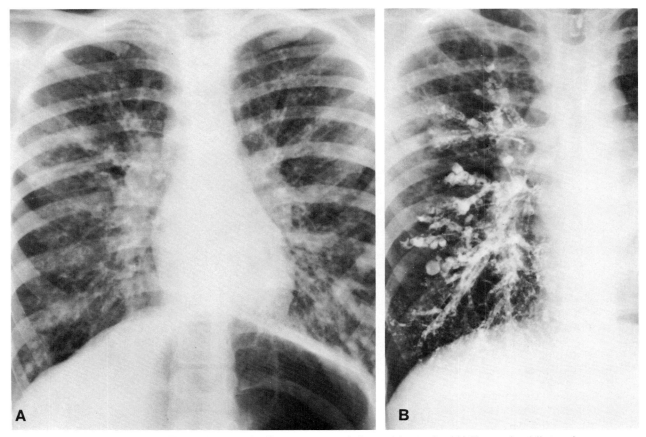

Figure 24–14.   Extensive cystic disease or cystic bronchiectasis. (**A**) Extensive bilateral inflammatory disease in which some rounded radiolucencies can be outlined. (**B**) Right bronchogram showing extensive bronchiectasis, which is cystic and cylindrical.

the atelectatic lung drops to the dependent lower or lateral thorax with the patient in the upright or lateral decubitus position respectively; this is pathognomonic of complete bronchial rupture. Suggestive signs are pulmonary contusion, angulation of an air-filled bronchus, and fracture of one or all of the upper three ribs, clavicle, scapula, or sternum, particularly if associated with mediastinal or cervical emphysema.[47] Some patients have no positive roentgen findings, so a chest film showing no abnormality does not exclude the possibility of this injury. Tomography may be helpful in revealing tracheobronchial defects, but bronchoscopy is needed to confirm the diagnosis. When the lesion is not detected after the initial injury, stenosis, which often results in obstruction, may occur, often with permanent loss of pulmonary tissue and function. Therefore, it is important to make the diagnosis in the immediate post-traumatic period, when appropriate surgery can restore anatomic continuity and preserve pulmonary function.

BRONCHOLITHIASIS

A calcified bronchopulmonary lymph node may erode into a bronchus to become a broncholith. This may be expectorated, causing only minor symptoms such as a temporary cough and minimal hemoptysis. However, it may become lodged in the bronchus, causing obstruction with atelectasis and infection distal to it. The term *broncholith* is also used to describe a calcification that impinges on and distorts a bronchus. Obstruction may or may not be significant in such patients. CT is useful in demonstrating the relationship of the calcification to a bronchus. Histoplasmosis is the most common cause.

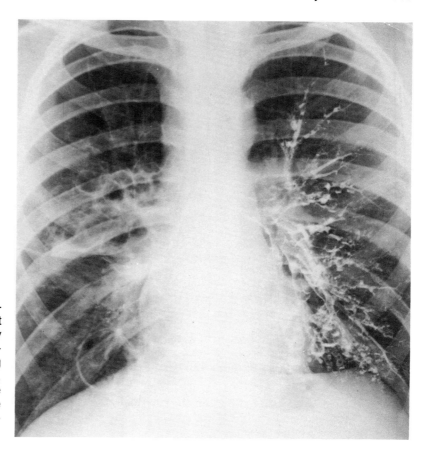

Figure 24–15. Extensive cystic disease. Note the large cysts on the right with evidence of some inflammatory disease. The upper lobe is overexpanded. On the initial film, the left lung appeared much less severely involved, but the bronchogram shows extensive cystic bronchiectasis in the lower lobe and scattered bronchiectasis elsewhere in the lung.

BRONCHIAL ATRESIA (MUCOCELE) (BRONCHOCELE)

A bronchial mucocele consists of a dilated mucus-filled bronchus distal to an area of occlusion in a segmental bronchus. It appears to be congenital atresia, but some authors believe that the thin septum or membrane producing the occlusion is secondary to infection.[46] Bronchocele may also occur in patients with neoplastic bronchial obstruction. If the occlusion is distal to the cartilage rings, dilation of the involved bronchus or bronchi may be extreme, producing a large, ovoid pulmonary mass with or without fingerlike branching. Despite the obstruction, there is no atelectasis, and emphysema is the usual finding distal to the mass. This is presumably the result of interalveolar air drift through the pores of Kohn. One hypothesis is that the air trapping occurs in these areas because the interalveolar air drift occurs more readily during expansion of the lung than during contraction, so that the pores of Kohn tend to close, producing a check-valve phenomenon on expiration. There may also be some air drift at the respiratory bronchiole level. Obstruction of a lobar bronchus causes atelectasis because the communications do not extend across intact lobar boundaries.

Roentgen findings consist of a mass that may be oval or lobulated. It is clearly defined and sometimes has fingerlike projections extending peripherally, resembling those observed in mucoid impaction. The overinflation is distal to the mass (Fig. 24-16). It may be observed best on an expiratory film. About 80% of these lesions occur in the upper lobes, predominately on the left. Local hyperinflation is not a feature in mucoid impaction, which aids in the differentiation. Also, the masses observed in bronchocele are larger than the bronchial cast observed in mucoid impaction.

CHRONIC OBSTRUCTIVE PULMONARY DISEASE[19, 31]

The common abnormality in all types of obstructive pulmonary disease is obstruction to air flow on expiration. The term *chronic obstructive pulmonary disease*

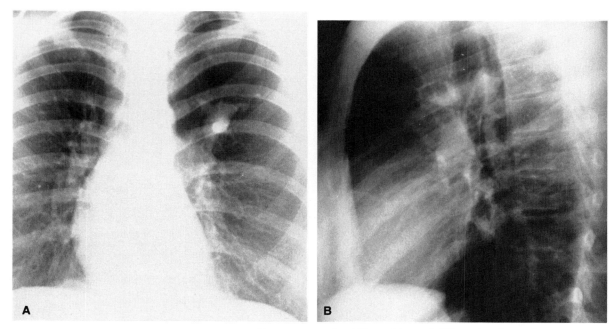

Figure 24–16. Bronchial atresia. Posteroanterior (**A**) and lateral (**B**) projections showing the opaque fingerlike mucocele distal to bronchial atresia of the left upper lobe. The lobe is overinflated and underperfused; therefore, it is relatively radiolucent.

(COPD) was coined because of the difficulty in differentiating the abnormalities caused by chronic bronchitis from those of emphysema or a combination of the two. COPD (COLD: Chronic Obstructive Lung Disease: COAD: Chronic Obstructive Airway Disease) is classified clinically and pathologically into five types:

Type I—Emphysema is predominant.

Type II—Chronic bronchitis is predominant (it may or may not be associated with chronic bronchiectasis); emphysema is minimal or absent.

Type III—Chronic asthma. In this group there is a high degree of reversibility when bronchodilators are used.

Type IV—Any combination of the first three types that do not fulfill the criteria for any single one of them. There is evidence of either partially reversible or irreversible airway obstruction in this, the largest group of patients.

Type V—Small airway disease, in patients who may or may not be symptomatic.

The radiologic manifestations of COPD are multiple, varied, and often nonspecific. Hyperinflation is the primary feature. In advanced COPD, the radiologic changes are often diagnostic, but in early disease, there is often poor correlation between pulmonary function studies and radiographic findings. The incidence of COPD is reported as 5% to 20% in American males.

EMPHYSEMA

The term *emphysema* is used to designate a variety of conditions in which overinflation occurs. This may involve the lungs and other tissues. Because the definition of *chronic pulmonary emphysema* is based on anatomic changes, it can be defined accurately only in morphologic terms. Nonpulmonary emphysema may occur anywhere in the body and is usually designated by its anatomic position. In the present discussion, nonpulmonary emphysema will be mentioned only in relation to the thorax, where it is usually either mediastinal or in the chest wall.

CHRONIC PULMONARY EMPHYSEMA

Chronic pulmonary emphysema is defined by the American Thoracic Society as follows[1]: "Emphysema is an anatomic alteration of the lung characterized by an abnormal permanent enlargement of the air spaces distal to the terminal nonrespiratory bronchiole, accompanied by destructive changes of the alveolar walls, and without obvious fibrosis."

The term *destructive* was later defined as follows:[42] "Destruction in emphysema is defined as nonuniformity in the pattern of respiratory airspace enlargement so that the orderly appearance of the acinus and its components is disturbed and may be lost." Such terms as *essential, substantial, alveolar, vesicular, irreversible*, and *obstructive* have been applied to this disease. Pathogenesis is somewhat controversial, but the disease seems to be the result of two basic mechanisms, namely, airway obstruction and elastolysis, which lead to destruction of alveolar walls. Chronic bronchial infection is found in a large majority of these patients, and infection probably predisposes to emphysema if it is not its cause. *Alpha₁-antitrypsin deficiency* is associated with an increased susceptibility to emphysema. Often this condition is manifest in several members of a family. It is more common in females than in males and usually occurs early in life (third or fourth decade). In patients with the heterozygous form of the disease, emphysema occurs only in those who smoke, and emphysema is more common in smokers than in nonsmokers with the homozygous form. Basal predominance of the emphysema is observed radiographically, often with bullae. Since this is an uncommon condition, it is not a factor in most cases of COPD. Emphysema also is observed in patients with bronchiectasis, severe pulmonary infections, silicosis, or other pneumoconioses.

Emphysema can be classified into selective and nonselective types[36] on the basis of morphology. The most important selective form is the *centrilobular (centriacinar)*, in which the destruction of parenchyma predominates in the central portion of the secondary lobule. This is the type most frequently associated with cigarette smoking. It usually begins and is most severe in the upper lung, and in the superior segments of the lower lobes, but may become general as severity increases. *Panlobular (panacinar)* is the term used for the diffuse nonselective form of the disease in which the acinus and secondary lobule are diffusely involved without particular relationship to the respiratory bronchioles. It tends to be more diffuse than the centriacinar type, but there is preferential involvement of the lower lobes. This form of emphysema may also be found associated with the centriacinar type in cigarette smokers. When either type becomes severe and extensive, it cannot be differentiated, and some pathologists believe that centrilobular emphysema progresses to the panlobular form. Panacinar emphysema is associated with *alpha₁-antitrypsin deficiency*.

Distal acinar (paraseptal) emphysema usually involves the alveolar ducts and sacs associated with the secondary interlobular septa. It tends to involve the lung periphery and usually does not produce symptoms. *Pericicatricial (scar)* emphysema is usually local and irregular and is associated with parenchymal scars.

There is general agreement that early mild manifestations of emphysema produce no roentgen findings in most instances. Roentgen signs are related to overinflation, vascular changes, and irregular involvement or bullae. They are as follows.

A. Changes in the Chest Wall and Diaphragm
   1. Low, flat diaphragm with blunting of the costophrenic angles. The diaphragm is at or below the level of the seventh rib anteriorly in deep inspiration. Reich and colleagues found that a height of the arc of the right hemidiaphragm (as measured perpendicular to a line drawn between the anterior and posterior costophrenic angles in the lateral view) of 2.6 cm or less identifies 67.7% of patients with abnormal pulmonary function tests and 78.3% of those with moderate to severe abnormality caused by emphysema.[35] They also found that a right lung height of 29.9 cm or more (measured from the tubercle of the first rib to the top of the dome of the right hemidiaphragm) on the posteroanterior film on inspiration identifies 69.8% of all patients with abnormal function tests and 79.7% of those with moderate to severe abnormality of function tests.
   2. Diminished diaphragmatic motion with excursion limited to 2 or 3 cm instead of a more normal 3 to 5 cm.
   3. Abnormal enlargement of the retrosternal space—between the posterior sternum and the anterior wall of the ascending aorta (greater than 3.5 cm from sternum to aorta). Separation of the aorta from the sternum extends more inferiorly than in the normal subject.
   4. Obtuse lung/sternodiaphragmatic angle (over 90°).
   5. Increase in length of retrosternal space.
   6. Anterior bowing of the sternum.
   7. Diaphragmatic contours scalloped.
B. Lung Parenchymal Changes
   1. Irregular increase in lucency of lungs. This is often detected most readily on CT. Clearly defined bullae may be present.
   2. Decrease in size of peripheral vessels in the lung, observed very well on CT where asymmetry may be observed; the vascular diminution coinciding with areas of increased radiolucency of lungs. Large bullae devoid of vessels may be present.[5]

3. Large central pulmonary arteries in severe disease indicating pulmonary hypertension (cor pulmonale).

C. Cardiac Changes

1. A narrow, vertical heart with a large pulmonary artery. The hilar arteries are also large secondary to pulmonary hypertension. In some instances, increase in heart size indicating right ventricular hypertrophy is evident (cor pulmonale) (Fig. 24-17).

An increase in vascular and interstitial markings has been described by several writers, presumably related to the chronic infection that so frequently accompanies emphysema. *Saber-sheath trachea*, in which the anteroposterior diameter of the trachea is increased and the transverse diameter decreased, is another finding that can be demonstrated radiographically. It is found in patients with emphysema usually associated with chronic bronchitis ("blue bloaters"). Cause of the tracheal change is not certain, but degeneration of cartilage associated with chronic

cough may play a part. "Pink puffers," also patients with emphysema, do not have chronic cough and probably no significant bronchitis.

CT is a sensitive method of evaluating the presence and distribution of pulmonary emphysema. The distribution and severity of the disease can be evaluated and the findings correlate well with pulmonary function studies. However, CT appears to be insensitive in detecting the very early manifestations of emphysema,[29] even though it may detect changes when they are functionally significant as indicated previously.

Small airway disease[27] is not associated with alveolar destruction. Therefore, it is an obstructive process that does not cause emphysema as anatomically defined. Rather, it is an obstruction caused by inflammatory narrowing and fibrous obliteration of the small airways of the lungs, plus obstruction of bronchioles by mucus plugs. Roentgen findings are those of widespread reticular density that varies from medium to coarse, suggesting restrictive disease such as sarcoidosis rather than an obstructive pattern. Evidence of pulmonary arterial hypertension may be present.

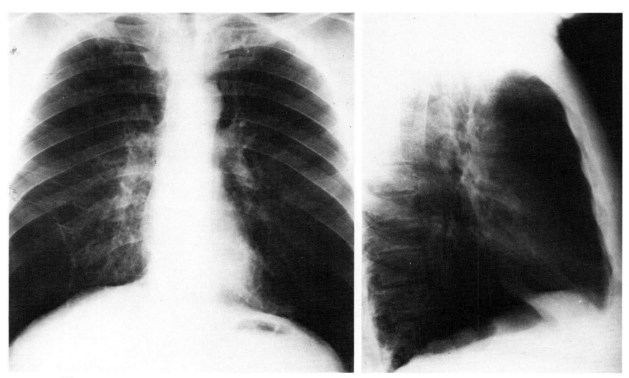

Figure 24–17. Chronic pulmonary emphysema (COPD). The diaphragm is flat, particularly as noted in the lateral projection. The retrosternal space is prominent. The lungs are hyperlucent, particularly at the bases, and the pulmonary artery and its main branches are somewhat enlarged.

BULLOUS EMPHYSEMA

William Snow Miller defined a bulla as a localized vesicular emphysema within the lung substance, which may project above the surface but leaves the pleura intact. Bullae are usually subpleural in location. Presumably, they may be secondary to severe local panacinar or paraseptal emphysema. When bullae constitute the major feature of the disease, the lesion is termed *bullous emphysema*. The size of the bulla varies from 1 or 2 cm to that of the lobe or even larger. A single lesion may become so large that differentiation between it and pneumothorax is difficult and sometimes impossible. CT may be very helpful and usually makes differentiation possible. As in chronic obstructive emphysema, the cause is often obscure. There is an obstructive component that may be peripheral in type, such as that produced by any disease in which bronchiolitis is a factor. This may range from acute infections to the inhalation of various irritating gases. The causative factor usually recedes and the bullous emphysema remains as the only evidence of previous disease.

Roentgen findings are characteristic. Large radiolucent, air-filled sacs appear at the periphery, either predominantly at the apices or at the bases (Fig. 24-18). The disease may be mainly unilateral but is usually present on both sides. When one lobe or a portion of it is involved, the lobe or segment may be inflated to the point that severe respiratory embarrassment is produced by compression of the remaining, relatively normal lung. In these instances, surgical removal of an affected lobe or segment may be indicated. Bronchography has been used to define the position of the bronchi and thus indicate the amount of compression and the lobe or segments that are compressed (Fig. 24-19) but has been largely replaced by CT, which is also used in the study of the pulmonary vessels in bullous emphysema (Fig. 24-20). It is of particular value if surgical resection of bullous disease is contemplated. The bullae are readily identified, and areas of relative avascularity indicating diffuse emphysema are also clearly outlined. Angiography can be used to study the pulmonary vascularity before surgical treatment if necessary, however. Films exposed at intervals often show progression of the disease; the term vanishing lung is used when the disease is severe and progressive. Basal bullous emphysema occurs commonly in patients with alpha$_1$-antitrypsin deficiency.

BLEBS

Emphysematous blebs are distinctly different anatomically from bullae and are much less common. A bleb is an interstitial collection of gas enclosed by visceral pleura. Blebs are relatively uncommon and are caused

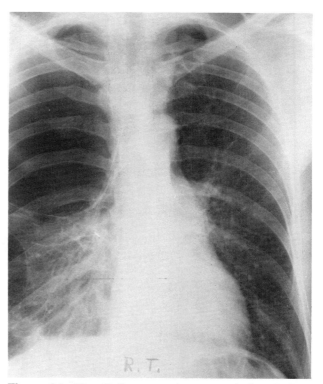

Figure 24–18. Bullous emphysema. A few bullae are in the left upper lung. On the right there is a very large bulla superiorly and at least one inferolaterally. The remaining right lung is considerably compressed.

by dissection of air from the lung into the interstitium, then along septal lines to the pleural surface of the lung. They are caused by barotrauma and may also be found in asthma, usually in infants and children. Rarely, they may cause spontaneous pneumothorax. Roentgen differentiation of a bleb and bulla is usually not possible, and the terms are used interchangeably by many.

ACUTE OBSTRUCTIVE EMPHYSEMA (OVERINFLATION)

The designation *acute obstructive emphysema (overinflation)* refers to the temporary condition, observed most frequently in children, in which there is a check-valve type of obstruction caused by a foreign body, usually in a main bronchus. Occasionally, the obstruction is lobar or segmental, however. The size of the foreign body and its situation are such that the foreign body does not completely obstruct the bronchus in which it is lodged. The normal bronchus enlarges in diameter during inspiration and narrows during expi-

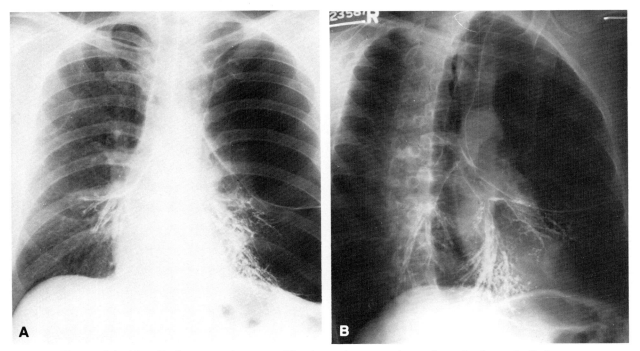

Figure 24–19. Bullous emphysema. The bronchogram shows how the large bulla has compressed much of the left upper and lower lobes.

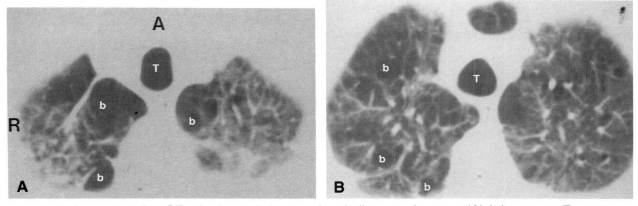

Figure 24–20. CT using lung windows to show bullous emphysema. (**A**) At lung apex. *T*, Trachea; *b*, bullae; *R*, right; *A*, anterior. (**B**) Two centimeters lower than *A*. *T*, Trachea; *b*, bullae.

ration. Inspiration also is an active phase of respiration in which muscular contraction is required. Expiration is a passive phase; therefore, a foreign body that does not completely obstruct a bronchus on inspiration may do so during expiration. When this happens, air can enter the lung distal to the foreign body but cannot

escape, or at least the ingress is less hampered than the egress. This situation will cause the lung, lobe, or segment distal to the foreign body to become increasingly distended until the pressure within it prevents more air from entering. This is known as a check-valve type of obstructive emphysema or overinflation. In children it usually results from the aspiration of a food particle; substances such as nuts, popcorn, or other hard and small particles are the common offenders. Because most of the objects are nonopaque to roentgen rays, diagnosis depends on the secondary changes caused by bronchial obstruction. If the obstruction is complete so that no air can pass in either direction, there is absorption of gas from the lung distal to the obstruction, the alveoli collapse, and the lung becomes decreased in volume and atelectatic. It is also possible for a foreign body to cause complete obstruction of one lobar bronchus and a check-valve type of obstruction of another, resulting in a combination of atelectasis in one lobe and overinflation in the other.

Rarely in adults, this type of overinflation in either a lobe, a segment, or an entire lung may be the earliest sign of carcinoma or other type of endobronchial tumor. In these instances the overinflation is more or less chronic, but as the tumor grows, complete obstruction occurs, leading to atelectasis.

Roentgen Observations. The roentgen diagnosis of acute obstructive overinflation is difficult to make on the findings evident on a single roentgenogram since there may be little change from normal if the film is exposed when the patient is in complete inspiration. Therefore, it is essential that films be exposed with the patient in inspiration and in expiration. Fluoroscopy may be extremely valuable when bronchial obstruction is suspected in small children who cannot cooperate for inspiratory and expiratory films. On inspiration the mediastinum moves toward the affected side in patients with obstructing foreign bodies, whether atelectasis or obstructive emphysema is produced. On expiration the mediastinum shifts away from the involved side, and the hemidiaphragm on the normal side tends to rise in a normal manner while the hemidiaphragm on the affected side remains more or less stationary or is limited in its motion. This is because the involved lung

remains fully aerated or hyperaerated, and the normal lung deflates normally to become smaller and more dense. In small children, in whom the mediastinum is usually movable, it tends to swing widely, away from the obstructing lesion on expiration and toward it on inspiration. The same findings are observed on inspiratory and expiratory films, but they may be difficult to obtain (Fig. 24-21). Occasionally, the obstructing foreign body may be opaque to roentgen rays and thus readily identified. When the obstructive emphysema involves a single lobe, the signs are similar but less marked; in these instances films exposed on inspiration and expiration as well as fluoroscopy may be necessary to make the diagnosis. Rarely, a foreign body becomes lodged in the trachea without causing sudden death and results in symmetrical, bilateral obstructive emphysema.

Congenital (infantile) lobar emphysema is described in Chapter 22.

UNILATERAL HYPERLUCENT LUNG

This syndrome (Swyer-James or MacLeod syndrome) is characterized by unilateral emphysema, hypoplasia of the pulmonary artery, and a widespread peculiar form of bronchiectasis manifested by extensive, irregular dilation of segmental bronchi that terminate in squared or tapered ends.[24] There is absence of filling of peripheral bronchioles. This is confined to the involved lung or lobe. There is diffuse, chronic expiratory obstruction with air trapping. The roentgen findings consist of (1) unilateral radiolucency of the lung or a lobe with no increase in volume of the lung; (2) failure of the involved lung to expand and contract normally on respiration; (3) usually a decrease in size of the involved lung; (4) limited excursion of the diaphragm and thoracic wall; and (5) shifting of the mediastinum away from the affected side on expiration and toward it on inspiration. The small size of the pulmonary artery and

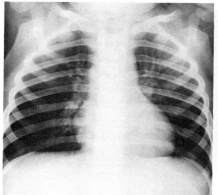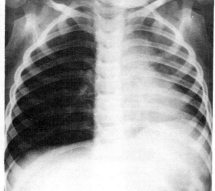

Figure 24–21. Acute obstructive emphysema (overinflation) caused by a peanut in the right main bronchus. **(A)** In complete inspiration, there is only a slight increase in radiability of the right lung. **(B)** In expiration, the mediastinum has moved to the left, the left diaphragm has moved upward normally, but the right diaphragm has remained in a position comparable to that noted in *A* and the difference in the amount of air in the lungs is now apparent.

its branches on the affected side causing the increased radiolucency is readily visible on plain films (Fig. 24-22). Bronchography shows no evidence of obstruction of major bronchi.

A strikingly constant type of bronchiectasis consists of moderate bronchial dilation in an irregular beaded pattern with clubbed or tapered ends accompanied by absence of alveolar filling. The bronchogram is of particular value in differentiating this condition from other causes of radiolucent lung. The cause is not established, but most cases are thought to be a result of pulmonary infection, usually by an adenovirus. Peters and associates reported an adenovirus A pulmonary infection in a 20-month-old girl with a baseline normal chest roentgenogram, who developed typical clinical and radiographic findings of Swyer-James syndrome after the pneumonia.[33]

Obliterative bronchiolitis is produced that causes distal air-space distention. Perfusion of the involved lobe or lung is then decreased, resulting in the vascular findings that have been described. Some authors believe that this radiographic syndrome may be the result of several conditions in addition to adenovirus pneumonia.

Clinically, there may be no symptoms, but often there is a history of repeated pulmonary infections. The disease may be recognized in children or adults, and there may or may not be a history of an initiating pulmonary infection. The diagnosis can be made on chest radiography, but the condition must be differentiated from other causes of unilateral hyperlucent lung such as unilateral pulmonary hypoplasia, bronchial obstruction, and chest-wall abnormalities. The evidence of air trapping usually confirms the diagnosis[24]; this can be confirmed by inspiratory and expiratory films.

NONOBSTRUCTIVE EMPHYSEMA (OVERINFLATION)

Compensatory Emphysema

Compensatory overinflation is a physiologic alteration of a lung or portion of it in response to loss of lung tissue elsewhere. There are many causes since there are many pulmonary lesions that lead to a decrease in volume of the involved areas. Whenever atelectasis occurs, there is compensatory emphysema in the adjacent lung. The same is true after removal of lung tissue

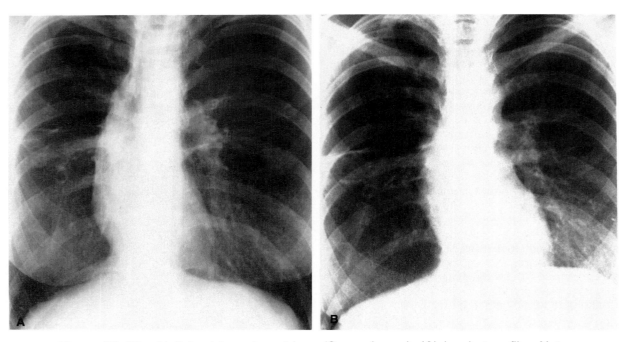

Figure 24–22. Unilateral hyperlucent lung (Swyer-James). (**A**) Inspiratory film. Note that the right lung is more radiolucent than the left and fewer pulmonary vessels are visible. The left lung is larger and the hemidiaphragms are almost equal in height. (**B**) Expiratory film. Note that the heart has shifted to the left because of air trapping on the right, which results in some expansion of this lobe. The left hemidiaphragm is now slightly higher than the right.

surgically. As in other forms of emphysema the affected area is more radiolucent than the uninvolved lung. This sign is important in detecting lobar atelectasis in patients in whom the volume of the atelectatic lobe has diminished so much that it is difficult to define it as an area of density. When pneumonectomy is performed, the normal lung undergoes compensatory emphysema and there is often a shift of mediastinal structures and a herniation of the lung into the opposite hemithorax that may be extreme. Focal compensatory emphysema occurs in relation to focal atelectasis, and it accentuates the opacity produced by the small atelectatic area. There is considerable variation in the amount of compensatory emphysema in patients with lobar atelectasis, depending on the chronicity of the disease producing it and the mobility of the diaphragm and mediastinum.

"Senile" Emphysema

Because an early theory regarding the role of aging in production of a defect in collagen or elastic tissue has not been substantiated, the term *senile emphysema* should probably be abandoned. However, there is an increased incidence of emphysema with age, particularly of the panlobular type in men. There is also an increase in alveolar duct diameter with aging, which probably represents simple dilation. It may be that there is some failure of protective mechanisms with advancing age, leading to some emphysema. Often, the emphysema is minimal and not symptomatic.

The designation is also sometimes used to indicate a nonobstructive type of overinflation secondary to the degenerative changes in the thoracic spine that lead to kyphosis. There is often an increase in the angulation between the body and manubrium of the sternum. The vertical diameter of the chest is often decreased, but the increase in the anteroposterior diameter is greater, resulting in an increased thoracic volume (barrel chest). This results in distention of the lungs that is usually uniform. The diaphragm is usually normally rounded, and diaphragmatic motion is not impaired to any great extent. In addition to the alterations in the thorax, the roentgen findings of increased radiability of the lungs are present along with a relative prominence of vascular and interstitial markings, which may not necessarily indicate chronic obstructive (panlobular type) emphysema in these elderly patients.

Interstitial Emphysema

The term *interstitial emphysema* refers to the presence of air or gas in the interstitial tissues of the lungs, resulting from rupture of one or more air spaces into the pulmonary interstitium, usually associated with increased intra-alveolar pressure. The air may then dissect to the mediastinum or to the periphery or pleural surface of the lung. Roentgen diagnosis may be very difficult, since small amounts of interstitial air are obscured by the air in the lungs. When the air dissects to the visceral pleura to form a round or oval radiolucency, a *bleb* is formed.

Pneumomediastinum (Mediastinal Emphysema)

Pulmonary interstitial emphysema leads to mediastinal emphysema (pneumomediastinum). There are three other ways in which air may reach the mediastinum, but they are less common: (1) along the fascial planes of the neck; (2) as a result of perforation of the trachea, esophagus, or main bronchus; and (3) by dissection along the retroperitoneal spaces. Pulmonary interstitial emphysema usually results from an increase in intra-alveolar pressure that is often acute and can be produced by anything that results in overinflation of the lungs. In the newborn, positive-pressure respiratory support is apparently a frequent cause. When the rupture of an alveolus occurs adjacent to a vessel, air dissects along vascular or interstitial channels to the mediastinum. From there it may extend into the soft tissue of the neck or into the retroperitoneal space, or it may rupture into the pleural space, producing pneumothorax. There may be so much pneumomediastinum in newborns that the heart is displaced to the right, because the potential space is largely anterior and on the left in these infants.

Mediastinal air may also be observed in patients with esophageal rupture. It is therefore advisable to examine the esophagus by means of contrast studies in patients with pneumomediastinum and chest pain.[37] Because pneumomediastinum is also associated with renal agenesis or cystic dysplasia, examination of the urinary tract of infants with unexplained pneumomediastinum or pneumothorax is suggested by some authors. Occasionally, tension pneumomediastinum may occur, particularly in patients who are receiving positive-pressure respiratory support. This is particularly dangerous in infants, because the air under pressure may compromise venous return to the heart and compress major bronchi. The roentgen diagnosis is usually not difficult to make, but roentgenograms in both frontal and lateral projections are necessary. In the frontal view, streaks of radiolucency representing air are noted outlining the pericardium and extending into the neck (Fig. 24-23). In the lateral view, the air collects retrosternally and extends in streaks anterior to the heart. Very small amounts are difficult to visualize, whereas a large pneumomediastinum is easily identified in either frontal or lateral projections. Both

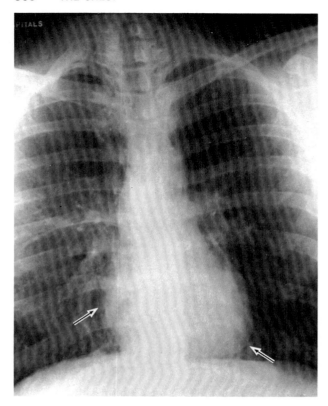

Figure 24–23. Mediastinal and interstitial emphysema. Arrows indicate streaks of gas along the cardiac borders. There is also a considerable amount of streaky lucency in the superior mediastinum and lower portion of the neck. This film was obtained during an acute asthmatic attack.

views should be obtained when pneumomediastinum is suspected, however.

In the newborn, air may dissect from the mediastinum into the extrapleural space between the parietal pleura and diaphragm. The resultant accumulation may simulate pneumoperitoneum because the air is confined to the space over the diaphragm. However, the pleural line above it is not as thick as the normal diaphragm, and the air remains in the same place on supine, decubitus, and upright projections. At times, the air is interposed between the heart and diaphragm; this results in a continuous horizontal radiolucency extending across the midline between the diaphragm and the heart.[26]

Interstitial Emphysema of Thoracic Walls

Thoracic interstitial emphysema is most commonly due to chest surgery but may also result from trauma and other causes. The amount varies considerably and,

when small, the gas is limited to the side of the surgical procedure or trauma. As the amount of gas increases, the gas extends downward into the soft tissues of the abdomen and upward into the neck, and from there into the mediastinum, producing pneumomediastinum. Occasionally, the amount of emphysema may be so great that tracheostomy is necessary to relieve tracheobronchial compression. Roentgen findings are similar to those in mediastinal emphysema secondary to pulmonary interstitial emphysema, but in addition, there is gas in the soft tissues of the neck and thoracic wall, producing linear streaks of radiolucency. There is also evidence of thoracotomy or of trauma, which usually is sufficient to indicate the cause.

REFERENCES AND SELECTED READINGS

1. AMERICAN THORACIC SOCIETY: Chronic bronchitis, asthma, and pulmonary emphysema. A statement by the Committee on Diagnostic Standards for Non-Tuberculous Respiratory Diseases. Am Rev Respir Dis 85:762, 1962
2. BATSAKIS JG: Tumors of the Head and Neck, 2nd ed. Baltimore, Williams & Wilkins, 1979
3. BREATNACH E, KERR I: The radiology of cryptogenic obliterative bronchiolitis. Clin Radiol 33:657, 1982
4. CHOPLIN RH, WEHUNT WD, THEROS EG: Diffuse lesions of the trachea. Semin Roentgenol 18:38, 1983
5. CHRISTENSEN EE, DIETZ GW: Subpulmonic pneumothorax in patients with chronic obstructive pulmonary disease. Radiology 121:33, 1976
6. DANUS O, CASAR C, LARRAIN A, ET AL: Esophageal reflux—an unrecognized cause of recurrent obstructive bronchitis in children. J Pediatr 89:220, 1976
7. DI RIENZO S: The Radiologic Exploration of the Bronchus. Springfield, Illinois, Charles C Thomas, 1949
8. EASTRIDGE CE, HUGHES FA JR, PATE JW, ET AL: Tracheobronchial injury caused by blunt trauma. Am Rev Respir Dis 101:230, 1970
9. EPLER GR, COLBY TV, MCLOUD TC, ET AL: Bronchiolitis obliterans organizing pneumonia. N Engl J Med 31:152, 1985
10. FELSON B: Neoplasms of the trachea and main stem bronchi. Semin Roentgenol 18:23, 1983
11. GAMSU G, FORBES AR, OVENFORS C-O: Bronchographic features of chronic bronchitis in normal men. Am J Roentgenol 136:317, 1981
12. GLAZER HS, MAURO MA, ARONBERG DJ, ET AL: Computed tomography of laryngoceles. Am J Roentgenol 140:549, 1983
13. GOSINK BB, FRIEDMAN PJ, LIEBOW AA: Bronchiolitis obliterans. Roentgenologic-pathologic correlation. Am J Roentgenol 117:816, 1973
14. GREENE R: "Saber-sheath" trachea: Relation to chronic obstructive pulmonary disease. Am J Roentgenol 130:441, 1978

15. GRENIER P, MAURICE F, MUSSET D, ET AL: Bronchiectasis: Assessment by thin-section CT. Radiology 161:95, 1986

16. GUDBJERG CE: Roentgenologic diagnosis of bronchiectasis. Acta Radiol [Diagn] (Stockh) 34:209, 1955

17. HAN B, DUNBAR JS, STRIKER TW: Membranous laryngotracheobronchitis (membranous croup). Am J Roentgenol 132:306, 1979

18. HOROWITZ BL, WOODSON GE, BRYAN RN: CT of laryngeal tumors. Radiol Clin North Am 22:265, 1984

19. HODGKIN JE, BALCHUM OJ, KASS I, ET AL: Chronic obstructive airway diseases. Current concepts in diagnosis and comprehensive care. JAMA 232:1243, 1975

20. JAMES AE JR, MACMILLAN AS JR, EATON SB, ET AL: Roentgenology of tracheal stenosis resulting from cuffed tracheostomy tubes. Am J Roentgenol 109:455, 1970

21. JING B-S: Malignant tumors of the larynx. Radiol Clin North Am 16:247, 1978

22. KATTAN M, KEENS TG, LAPIERRE J, ET AL: Pulmonary function abnormalities in symptom-free children after bronchiolitis. Pediatrics 59:683, 1977

23. KOCH DA: Roentgenologic considerations of capillary bronchiolitis. Am J Roentgenol 82:433, 1959

24. KOGUTT MS, SWISCHUK LE, GOLDBLUM R: Swyer-James syndrome (unilateral hyperlucent lung in children). Am J Dis Child 125:614, 1973

25. LANDING BH, DIXON LG: Congenital malformations and genetic disorders of the respiratory tract (larynx, trachea, bronchi and lungs). Am Rev Respir Dis 120:151, 1979

26. LEVIN B: The continuous diaphragm sign. A newly-recognized sign of pneumomediastinum. Clin Radiol 24:337, 1973

27. MACKLEM PT, THURLBECK WM, FRASER RG: Chronic obstructive disease of small airways. Ann Intern Med 74:167, 1971

28. MCLOUD TC, EPLER GR, COLBY TV, ET AL: Bronchiolitis obliterans: State of the art. Radiology 159:1, 1986

29. MILLER RR, MULLER NL, VEDAL S, ET AL: Limitations of computed tomography in the assessment of emphysema. Am Rev Respir Dis 139:980, 1989

30. MILLS JL, SPACKMAN TJ, BORNS P, ET AL: The usefulness of lateral neck roentgenograms in laryngotracheobronchitis. Am J Dis Child 133:1140, 1979

31. MILNE ENC, BASS H: The roentgenoglogic diagnosis of early chronic obstructive pulmonary disease. J Can Assoc Radiol 20:3, 1969

32. MÜLLER NL, STAPLES CA, MILLER RR: Bronchiolitis obliterans organizing pneumonia: CT features in 14 patients. Am J Roentgenol 154:983, 1990

33. PETERS ME, DICKIE HA, CRUMMY AB: Swyer-James-Macleod syndrome: A case with a baseline normal chest radiograph. J Pediatr Radiol 12:211, 1982

34. PHILLIPS MS, WILLIAMS MP, FLOWER CDR: How useful is computed tomography in the diagnosis and assessment of bronchiectasis? Clin Radiol 37:321, 1986

35. REICH SB, WEINSHELBAUM A, YEE J: Correlation of radiographic measurements and pulmonary function tests in chronic obstructive pulmonary disease. Am J Roentgenol 144:695, 1985

36. REPORT OF THE CONCLUSIONS OF A CIBA GUEST SYMPOSIUM: Terminology, definitions and classification of chronic pulmonary emphysema and related conditions. Thorax 14:186, 1959

37. ROGERS LF, PUIG AW, DOOLEY BN, ET AL: Diagnostic considerations in mediastinal emphysema. A pathophysiologic-roentgenologic approach to Boerhaave's syndrome and spontaneous pneumomediastinum. Am J Roentgenol 115:495, 1972

38. SCHABEL SI, KATZBERG RW, BURGENER FA: Acute inflammation of epiglottis and supraglottic structures in adults. Radiology 122:601, 1977

39. SHACKELFORD GD, MCALISTER WH: Congenital laryngeal cyst. Am J Roentgenol 114:289, 1972

40. SHACKELFORD GD, SIEGEL MJ, MCALISTER WH: Subglottic edema in acute epiglottitis in children. Am J Roentgenol 131:603, 1978

41. SILVERMAN PM, GODWIN JD: CT/bronchographic correlations in bronchiectasis. J Comput Assist Tomogr 11:52, 1987

42. SNIDER GL, CHAIRMAN: The definition of emphysema. Report of a National Heart, Lung and Blood Institute, Division of Lung Diseases Workshop. Am Rev Respir Dis 132:182, 1985

43. SURVATT PM, PAUL D, ATKINSON RL, ET AL: Fluoroscopic and computed tomographic features of the pharyngeal airway in obstructive sleep apnea. Am Rev Respir Dis 127:487, 1983

44. SWEATMAN MC, MILLAR AB, STRICKLAND B, ET AL: Computed tomography in adult obliterative bronchiolitis. Clin Radiol 41:116, 1990

45. TAGER IB, SPEIZER FE: Risk estimates for chronic bronchitis in smokers: A study of male-female differences. Am Rev Respir Dis 113:619, 1976

46. TALNER LB, GMELICH JT, LIEBOW AA, ET AL: The syndrome of bronchial mucocele and regional hyperinflation of the lung. Am J Roentgenol 110:675, 1970

47. UNGER JM, SCHUCHMANN GG, GROSSMAN JE, ET AL: Tears of the trachea and main bronchi caused by blunt trauma: Radiologic findings. Am J Roentgenol 153:1175, 1989

48. WOHL MEB, CHERNICK V: Bronchiolitis—State of the art. Am Rev Respir Dis 118:759, 1978

Paul and Juhl's Essentials of Radiologic Imaging,
Sixth Edition, edited by John H. Juhl and
Andrew B. Crummy. J.B. Lippincott Company,
Philadelphia, © 1993.

CHAPTER **25**

Pulmonary Tuberculosis

John H. Juhl

GENERAL CONSIDERATIONS

The incidence of pulmonary tuberculosis in the United States decreased from 53 cases per 100,000 in 1953 to 9 cases per 100,000 in 1985. However, in recent years, this steady decline in the incidence of the disease has stopped, and in 1986 there was a 2.6% increase in reported cases that has persisted through 1988. This upward trend seems to persist to the present. Most new cases have occurred among minority groups such as blacks and Hispanics. Other groups to be included now are the homeless, who sometimes use shelters, intravenous drug abusers, residents of prisons and nursing homes, immigrants and others from high-prevalence countries, as well as persons testing positive for the human immunodeficiency virus (HIV).[2] Therefore, the disease is still of considerable social and economic importance.

Most tuberculous infection is caused by inhalation of airborne tubercle bacilli, usually in droplets resulting from coughing by a person with active pulmonary disease. The tubercle bacillus *Mycobacterium tuberculosis* injures the tissues, resulting in an alveolar exudate termed *tuberculous pneumonia*. The disease may advance rapidly and cause a poorly defined pulmonary shadow of varying size and density. This is usually homogeneous when the lesion is small. If the process is halted by means of antibacterial drugs before caseation necrosis occurs, complete clearing of the process can occur. A chest roentgenogram does not permit a positive diagnosis of exudative tuberculosis, but the findings may be typical enough that the diagnosis of an exudative type of lesion can be suggested. Subsequent complete clearing then tends to substantiate the im-

pression. In other patients or in other areas the lesion may be productive in type with formation of tubercles consisting of epithelioid cells, lymphocytes, and Langhans' giant cells. The tubercles may coalesce to form large nodules that are visible as oval or rounded shadows on the roentgenogram. They are usually more clearly defined than the exudative type of lesion. Caseation necrosis may occur in these areas, or there may be gradual fibrous tissue replacement without necrosis. When liquefaction occurs in the necrotic area, the material is extruded via a bronchus, leaving a tuberculous cavity; these cavities may vary considerably in size.

Dissemination of the tubercle bacillus is of three types: bronchogenic, hematogenous, and lymphangitic. Bronchogenic dissemination occurs when exudate from a cavity or small area of caseation drains into a bronchus and is aspirated into previously uninfected areas either on the same or on the opposite side. This type of spread occurs frequently after bleeding and when there is a cavity emptying into a bronchus. Hematogenous dissemination leads to miliary tuberculosis and to extrapulmonary lesions throughout the body. Acute massive hematogenous spread causes miliary tuberculosis, whereas chronic spread in smaller amounts usually results in the chronic extrapulmonary foci. Lymphangitic dissemination is common in primary infection. It is responsible for involvement with subsequent enlargement of hilar and mediastinal nodes that is often seen in children and in young adult blacks.

The reaction to *M. tuberculosis* depends on the presence or absence of immunity to tuberculoprotein. In individuals having no tissue hypersensitivity or immunity, primary tuberculosis results. In those with immunity produced by previous infection or BCG vaccination, the reactivation (reinfection) disease may develop.*

PRIMARY PULMONARY TUBERCULOSIS

Primary, or first-infection, tuberculosis occurs when the living tubercle bacilli produce a local inflammatory process in the lung in a patient who has not been previously infected and therefore is not sensitized to the tuberculoprotein. This form usually occurs in children.[13] The disease is often undetected since there are few clinical symptoms. If a roentgenogram is obtained in the early phase, the disease resembles that noted in any other segmental pneumonic process in that it is a poorly defined opacity, usually limited to a relatively small subsegment. In some patients, the diseased area is larger, with one or several segments or an entire lobe involved. In susceptible individuals, such as blacks and poorly nourished children, the disease may be more widespread and may occasionally cavitate; pneumatoceles may occur.[13] The lymphangitic spread of the disease to the hilar and paratracheal nodes results in enlargement, which may be recognizable roentgenographically. At times adenopathy may be massive. The changes produced in the lymphatics may occasionally be sufficient to appear as streaks of increased opacity between the primary pneumonic disease and the hilum. If serial films are obtained, slow resolution will be noted over 6 months to a year. At times the original lesion disappears so completely that it cannot be recognized on later roentgenograms, but there is often a small nodule that later may become calcified. The calcification within the hilar nodes and the parenchymal calcification then remain as the only residues of primary tuberculosis. This combination of primary parenchymal opacity plus regional node calcification is termed a primary complex or primary *Ranke complex*, and the parenchymal nodule is called a *Ghon tubercle*. The diagnosis cannot be made on roentgen study alone, but in many patients the appearance is so typical that the diagnosis is relatively certain. Progress roentgenograms tend to substantiate the conclusion, and the tuberculin skin test can be used to confirm it (Fig. 25-1). As a rule, the calcifications secondary to histoplasmosis are larger than those in tuberculosis.

The primary pulmonary parenchymal focus is usually solitary but may be multiple. There are several variations from the typical findings described. In some patients the primary parenchymal opacity is so small as to be invisible on a roentgenogram, whereas lymph node enlargement in the hilum in the same patient may be considerable. Distribution in the lungs is random, so that lower lobe disease is at least as common as upper lobe disease. The lower lobe lesions usually do not cause atelectasis in children, so they often escape notice. In some cases, no visible hilar node enlargement is demonstrated. Occasionally, the first manifestations are pleural effusion and pleural disease, which may hide the parenchymal disease. As a part of the primary disease, pleural effusion is more common in adults than in children. The figures vary, but about 10% of children and 30% of adults with primary tuberculosis have pleural effusion, usually unilateral and on the side of the parenchymal disease. In some reports, the incidence of effusion is considerably higher. Many patients in whom primary tuberculosis develops have an uncomplicated course, which accounts for the relatively high incidence of tuberculin sensitivity in the general population, most of whom cannot recall any illness that could be interpreted as previous tuberculosis. When active primary pulmonary disease along with lymphadenopathy is found, however, treatment with antibacterial drugs is indicated.

COMPLICATIONS
Atelectasis

A major cause of the opacity that is sometimes associated with primary tuberculosis in children is now known to be atelectasis, which usually results from compression of an upper lobe bronchus by the large hilar nodes. Complete occlusion may occur when there is an added factor of bronchial infection or edema. The atelectasis may appear and disappear from time to time, producing opacity and decrease in volume of the involved lobe or segment when present. If the atelectasis persists despite treatment with antituberculous drugs, it usually indicates bronchostenosis. Surgical removal of the involved lobe may then become necessary. The more usual course, however, is for the atelectasis to clear as the inflammatory process subsides in the nodes and in the bronchial wall. Thus roentgen findings may vary from time to time in these patients. They consist of the hilar node enlargement plus varying amounts of opacity in the involved lobe depending on the amount of atelectasis present in addition to the actual tuberculous disease. The parenchymal opacity often remains when the atelectasis clears (Fig. 25-2). Bronchiectasis may also result as a complication of this type of disease.

---

* The classification of pulmonary tuberculosis has been revised by the American Lung Association and appears in *Diagnostic Standards and Classification of Tuberculosis and Other Mycobacterial Diseases*, published in 1974. The publication can be obtained from the American Lung Association at 1740 Broadway, New York, NY 10019.

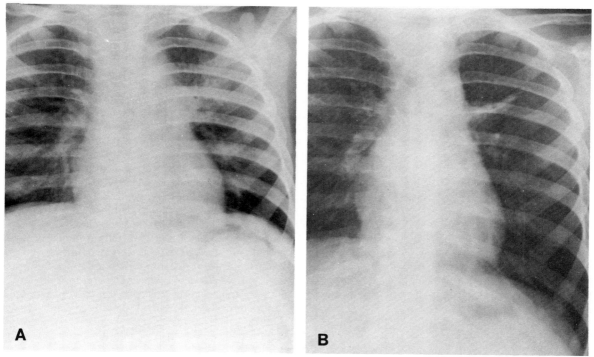

Figure 25–1. Primary tuberculosis. (**A**) The primary disease is noted in the left upper lung, largely in the plane of the second anterior interspace. It consists of poorly defined opacity in the parenchyma accompanied by enlarged hilar nodes. (**B**) Roentgenogram obtained 1 month later. There is now a clearly defined strand of opacity extending into the area of the previous disease. The enlarged nodes have regressed.

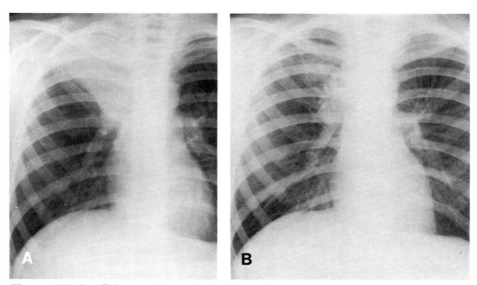

Figure 25–2. Primary tuberculosis with atelectasis. (**A**) Note the homogeneous opacity in the right upper lobe. The minor fissure is greatly elevated, indicating a considerable amount of atelectasis. (**B**) Roentgenogram obtained 5 weeks later. The upper lobe has expanded. Residual pulmonary disease is present above the right hilum; right upper hilar nodes are enlarged.

Progression

The usual course of primary tuberculosis is slow resolution, which may occur in 3 to 9 months. Progressive primary tuberculosis may occur in several situations. It is most common in infants less than 1 year old, in patients using corticosteroids, and in other susceptible patients, often with other chronic illness. The pulmonary involvement increases; often cavitation occurs, with subsequent bronchogenic spread or pleural involvement with effusion and/or empyema and with bronchopleural fistula occasionally.

Tuberculous Pericarditis

Tuberculous pericarditis usually is caused by rupture of a caseous mediastinal node into the pericardium. This may cause acute tamponade, making immediate pericardiocentesis imperative. In other cases, a more gradual accumulation of pericardial fluid is associated with tuberculous pericarditis. The size of the cardiac shadow increases and the presence of fluid can usually be determined by ultrasonography.

Hematogenous Dissemination

Widespread hematogenous dissemination of tuberculosis as the result of primary infection is uncommon but is a very serious complication because it may lead to miliary tuberculosis and to involvement of many extrapulmonary structures, including the meninges. This complication usually occurs in infants less than 2 years of age and is much less common in older children. It usually develops within 6 months of the initial primary infection. The pulmonary manifestations are discussed later in the section Hematogenous Tuberculosis.

Other Complications

Occasionally the hilar or paratracheal lymph nodes may become so large that they extend into the adjacent pulmonary parenchyma and may require surgical removal. Bronchoesophageal fistula has also been reported, when caseating nodal disease extends into the esophagus and into a bronchus.

Pleural effusions in primary tuberculosis usually clear completely in a month or two without treatment. Occasionally, the effusion persists, leaving a residual sac of fluid often encased in thickened pleura. Eventually, some of these pleural residues may calcify peripherally or centrally.

Primary Tuberculosis in the Adult

Unusual pulmonary manifestations of tuberculosis have been reported in recent years because there has been decreased exposure in childhood and the primary form of the disease develops in many adults.[3, 9] There is more lower lobe disease in adults. Equal incidence or slight predominance of lower and middle lobe disease has been reported.[16] Choyke and associates[4] reported a 40% incidence of lower lobe disease and a 58% incidence of upper lobe disease in one series of 103 adults. Cavitation was present in 8%, which is higher than that reported in children. Pleural effusion was present in about 30%, also more common than in children. On the other hand, adenopathy occurred in only about 10%, nearly half in the right paratracheal nodes. Others have reported a higher incidence of adenopathy. All of the patients with adenopathy had parenchymal disease demonstrated on chest roentgenogram. In this series, about 15% of the patients were immunocompromised, so that tuberculosis can be an opportunistic infection. Adult respiratory distress syndrome (ARDS) occurred as a complication of miliary tuberculosis in four patients. This is a particularly difficult situation, and prompt antituberculous drug therapy may be life saving.

POSTPRIMARY (REINFECTION, REACTIVATION) TUBERCULOSIS

Reinfection or reactivation tuberculosis occurs when tubercle bacilli produce pulmonary inflammatory disease in an individual who has been previously sensitized to tuberculin. Unlike primary tuberculosis, this condition tends to be progressive, leading to symptomatic pulmonary disease unless treated. Lymph node involvement is much less common than in primary disease. The disease has a considerable tendency to localize in the upper lobes. There is no certain way to distinguish between the two types on roentgen study, however.

EARLY REINFECTION TUBERCULOSIS

The upper lobes are the most common site, and the parenchymal disease is most often found in the apical and posterior segments of the upper lobe. The right side is affected somewhat more frequently than the left. However, it is not uncommon to see the initial opacity in the superior segment of the lower lobe on either side. The basal segments of the lower lobe are not often the site of the original disease in reactivation pulmonary tuberculosis. The disease is asymptomatic in its early stages, and a chest roentgenogram often indicates a lesion before the onset of subjective symptoms and before physical findings can be elicited on examination of the chest. As far as the roentgen findings are concerned, there is nothing characteristic about early tuberculous disease except its location in

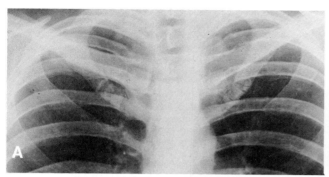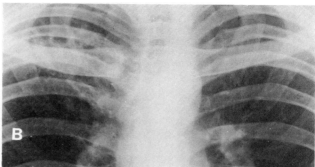

Figure 25–3. Minimal pulmonary tuberculosis in the right upper lobe. Note the hazy, poorly defined opacity in the first anterior interspace laterally, immediately below the clavicle. Some disease was also concealed by the clavicle. Compare this area with the same area on the patient's left side, which is normal. **(B)** Somewhat more extensive disease is in the right upper lobe in the supraclavicular area, in the first anterior interspace, as well as medial to the first rib. Some of the disease is obscured by the clavicle. The left side is normal.

the upper lobe, which is usually fairly peripheral in relation to the hilum. Characteristically, the disease appears as an area of mottled opacity that varies considerably in size and the limits of the lesion are usually poorly circumscribed. The hazy character and poor definition of the lesions suggest a pneumonic or exudative process in contrast to the more clearly defined, strandlike character of chronic fibrotic disease. It is not uncommon for this disease to be obscured to a greater or lesser extent by the clavicle or by one of the upper ribs and thus escape attention unless the roentgenogram is examined carefully (Figs. 25-3 through 25-5). In other patients the disease may be undetected until it is well advanced, so it is not unusual to find extensive disease with cavitation and bronchogenic spread to the opposite lung or the lower lobe of the same lung. In others the initial chest roentgenogram reveals a large area of segmental or lobar consolidation representing tuberculous pneumonia.

At times the disease appears as a relatively clearly defined linear opacity, resembling a fibrotic scar. However, it must be remembered that tuberculosis cannot be classified as inactive on the basis of a single study. Because there is a wide variation in the susceptibility of individuals, the virulence and number of organisms, and the gross pathologic response to the disease, it is not surprising that roentgen study of tuberculosis should demonstrate a wide variation in the appearance of the disease.[16] In some patients the location and appearance of the initial tuberculous process are characteristic enough for the radiologist to make a presumptive diagnosis of pulmonary tuberculosis, but this should always be confirmed by bacteriologic study of

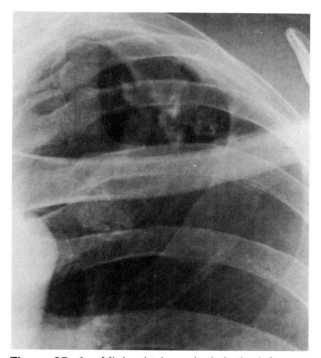

Figure 25–4. Minimal tuberculosis in the left apex. The disease is clearly defined in the supraclavicular area. It contains some calcium. There were also several calcified nodes in the left hilum, some of which are shown on this illustration. Note the minimal amount of pleural thickening lateral to the pulmonary disease.

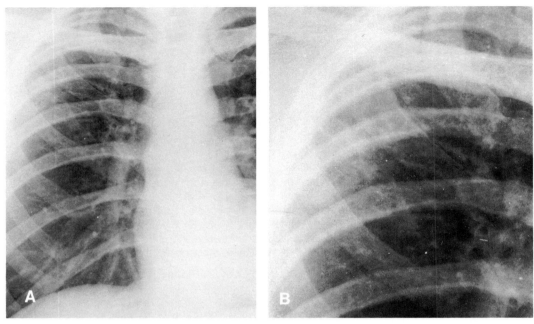

Figure 25–5.   Minimal tuberculosis. **(A)** The disease is rather poorly defined, largely in the lateral aspect of the second anterior interspace. **(B)** Close-up of the upper right lung shows the hazy opacity to better advantage. Its haziness and poor definition are compatible with active disease.

sputum or of specimens obtained during fiberoptic bronchoscopy.

BRONCHOGENIC SPREAD OF TUBERCULOSIS

When enough necrosis is produced by the action of the tubercle bacillus, a cavity is formed and the necrotic material is extruded through a bronchus. The cavity appears on the roentgenogram as a rounded or oval area of radiolucency, usually surrounded by a moderately thick wall and often by a considerable amount of disease in the same area. Exudate from this cavity can be expectorated, or it may be aspirated, resulting in bronchogenic spread of infection to other parts of the same lung or to the opposite lung. New foci of infection are then set up that in turn may undergo eventual cavitation. Small foci of tuberculous pneumonia are started by these bronchogenic aspirates. All of these lesions may heal, go on to caseation and cavitation, or become productive lesions resulting in the formation of a considerable amount of granulation tissue and eventual fibrosis. The fibrosis may be extensive, leading to a considerable loss in lung volume and tracheobronchial distortion.

CAVITATION

The presence of cavitation in a patient with pulmonary tuberculosis is common and is often readily detected roentgenographically since the cavity is large enough to produce a distinct round or oval radiolucency with a moderately thick wall. It is often necessary to use several methods of roentgen examination to ascertain the presence of cavity and to localize it. Stereoscopic views are often of considerable value, and films in lateral and oblique projections sometimes outline cavities not clearly defined in frontal projection. Computed tomography (CT) is very valuable in detection of cavitary disease and is more reliable than chest radiography.

There is wide variation in the appearance of tuberculous excavation just as there is considerable variation in the appearance of other tuberculous disease from one patient to the next. The cavitations appear as radiolucent areas that vary widely in size but are generally round or oval. The inner wall of a cavity may be smooth or irregular (Fig. 25-6). The walls are usually moderately thick except in tension cavities, which become fairly large and may exhibit thin walls. A tension cavity develops because of a check-valve type of obstruction of the bronchus leading to it, allowing air to enter the cavity more freely than it can escape. This type of cavity

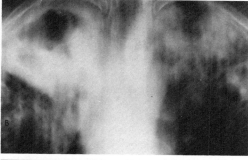

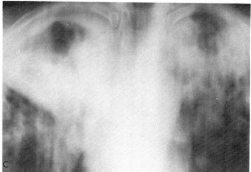

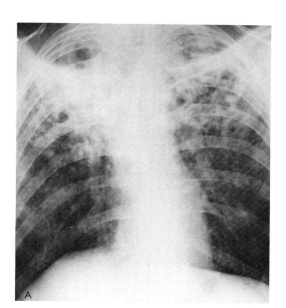

Figure 25–6. Advanced bilateral pulmonary tuberculosis. **(A)** Note the large apical cavity on the right in the supraclavicular area. The disease is extensive in the upper half of both lungs, and several suspicious radiolucent areas are noted on the left. **(B and C)** These are tomograms of the patient shown in *A*. The apical cavity on the right, some shift of the trachea to the right, and several small cavities on the left are evident.

may disappear very quickly when treatment is instituted because the bronchial obstruction that contributed to its size may be relieved quickly and permit the cavity to collapse. Thick-walled cavities, on the other hand, often show little tendency to close or may close or decrease in size very slowly when treated. Although not as common as in lung abscess, fluid can occasionally be present in a tuberculous cavity, so fluid levels can be demonstrated on horizontal-beam roentgenograms. In general, the walls of the cavities are noted to decrease in thickness and become less distinct as the disease regresses under treatment. Fibrosis, with contraction of the previously involved lung, and emphysema may result in production of irregular or oval radiolucencies that may simulate cavities very closely. In these instances it is often difficult and sometimes impossible to differentiate a thin-walled cavity from an area of emphysema unless the disease has been well documented by repeated roentgenograms during its course. In these patients, computed tomography is often of considerable value.

If there has been cavitation or extensive disease in a lobe or segment, fibrosis is a part of the healing process

and results in volume loss, often with bronchial, hilar, and mediastinal distortion.

BRONCHIECTASIS

Endobronchial involvement in pulmonary tuberculosis is very common and leads to bronchiectasis in some instances. The presence of bronchiectasis in patients with tuberculosis can often be diagnosed or at least suspected on routine roentgenograms because the thick-walled bronchi filled with air stand out in contrast to the diseased lung surrounding them. In other instances the diagnosis can be made with a high degree of certainty on CT, particularly in patients with far advanced disease. If the extent of bronchiectasis is to be determined before surgical removal, bronchography may occasionally be necessary. Bronchiectasis in patients with pulmonary tuberculosis may be saccular or cylindrical and is found in the lobe or segment involved by the disease. Occasionally, it is detected in an area where there is no obvious parenchymal involvement. Presumably, the bronchiectasis was caused by tuberculous disease, which has resolved to the point where no roentgen evidence of parenchymal involvement remains. Therefore, many investigators consider that CT or bronchography is indicated before segmental surgery is undertaken in patients with pulmonary tuberculosis. Since antituberculous drug therapy is very effective, surgery is now limited to the occasional patient with severe bronchiectasis, hemorrhage, or repeated infection localized to the site of earlier tuberculosis. There is some difference in the appearance of bronchiectasis in tuberculosis from that caused by other conditions. In tuberculosis there is often peripheral obliteration and more fibrosis with greater distortion of bronchi (Fig. 25-7).

UNUSUAL RADIOGRAPHIC MANIFESTATIONS OF PULMONARY TUBERCULOSIS

In addition to the unusual distribution and other differences described in adults with primary tuberculosis, several other findings should be mentioned:

1. Multiple bilateral large pulmonary nodules.
2. Multiple small scattered cavitary foci that resemble hematogenous staphylococcal abscesses. These lesions remain unchanged and can therefore be differentiated from acute staphylococcal disease, which changes rather rapidly.
3. Pulmonary gangrene can result from tuberculosis. The patients are very ill and this disease is often fatal. A large homogeneous lobar alveolar process is observed to increase in density; the lobe increases in volume, and cavitation appears with a large intracavity mass of necrotic tissue, similar to that sometimes observed in Klebsiella pneumonia.[7]
4. *Rasmussen aneurysm* is a rare pseudoaneurysm

caused by erosion of a peripheral pulmonary artery branch within a tuberculous cavity. It can simulate a mass within a cavity. Complications include formation of an arteriovenous fistula, rupture with hemoptysis, and sometimes exsanguination. These aneurysms can be treated by embolization to occlude the involved pulmonary artery branch.

5. A nonspecific severe widespread interstitial pattern throughout both lungs. This occurs in middle-aged and elderly patients with emphysema. The patients are not very ill and there is no radiologic change over many months. Diagnosis is usually made by open lung biopsy. Response to good antituberculous drug therapy is very slow. Pneumothorax may complicate this unusual form of tuberculosis.[9]

TUBERCULOSIS IN THE IMMUNOSUPPRESSED PATIENT

The cell-mediated immune response (T lymphocytes) is largely involved in the destruction of tubercle bacilli. There are several situations in which cell-mediated immunity is depressed.[8] They include acquired immunodeficiency syndrome (AIDS),[10] aging, starvation, chronic illness, alcoholism, cancer, sarcoidosis, silicosis, pregnancy, radiation, and drugs such as corticosteroids, immunosuppressive drugs, and cytotoxic drugs used in cancer chemotherapy. This group of patients is at risk if exposed to the organism. The highest incidence appears to be in elderly persons, debilitated persons, and patients with AIDS, chronic diseases, or malignancy. Although tuberculosis is difficult to manage in patients with silicosis, the incidence of tuberculosis in silicotic individuals is decreasing, so these patients no longer appear to be in the high-risk group,

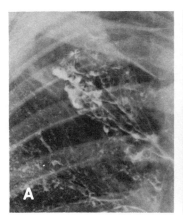 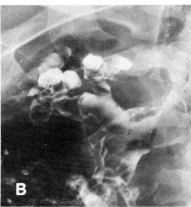

Figure 25-7. Bronchiectasis in tuberculosis. **(A)** Note the dilation of the upper lobe bronchi, which are also crowded in a patient who had previous extensive tuberculosis of the right upper lobe. There is very little alveolar filling, and the distal ends of the bronchi are obstructed. The latter finding is characteristic of tuberculosis. **(B)** Bronchogram of a patient with far advanced tuberculosis of long duration. The right upper lobe is contracted, and there is extensive saccular bronchiectasis, bronchial distortion, and failure of parenchymal filling.

probably because of better hygiene and tuberculosis control. Whether this will remain true in the future is not certain, since the incidence of tuberculosis may be increasing.

The radiographic appearance of tuberculosis is similar to that in others, except that in patients with T-cell depression, the disease is likely to progress more rapidly, to become far advanced, and to develop miliary spread. This can occur in primary as well as in reactivation tuberculosis.

TUBERCULOMA

The term *tuberculoma* refers to the round, focal, tuberculous lesion that may be solitary or multiple. There are many inflammatory nodules in which tubercle bacilli cannot be found. The histopathologic findings are nonspecific. They are termed chronic nonspecific granuloma and cannot be differentiated from tuberculoma by roentgenographic methods. The tuberculous nodules vary in size from a few millimeters to 5 or 6 cm but usually range from 1 to 3 cm. They may or may not contain calcium and usually contain caseous debris. Small flecks of calcium may be scattered in the lesion, and in some instances calcium may form a more or less complete shell or ring in or near the outer wall of the nodule. Several concentric rings of calcium or an eccentric or central nidus of calcium may be present. The pathogenesis is varied and the nodule may represent either the primary or reinfection type of disease. Sometimes the nodule results when a cavity is sealed by obstruction of its draining bronchus. It may also be a residual localized area of caseation that persists when the remainder of the primary disease clears. It is not unusual to see a few tiny satellite nodules or poorly defined areas of opacity in the vicinity of a tuberculoma. All of these lesions are potentially dangerous, since they may contain viable tubercle bacilli for long intervals and may break down at any time with resultant dissemination of the disease. They may remain constant in size or may grow very slowly over a period of years.

The roentgen finding is that of a round parenchymal nodule. If concentric rings of calcium are visible, the lesion is almost certainly a tuberculoma or other chronic inflammatory granuloma (Fig. 25-8). If no calcium is demonstrated on the routine roentgen study of the chest, computed tomography is indicated. Calcium can often be seen on CT when its presence is not detected on the preliminary film. If no calcification is found, there is no way to differentiate the tuberculoma or other infectious granuloma from bronchogenic carcinoma, other lung tumors, or solitary pulmonary metastasis. In the patient with a small, solitary nodule

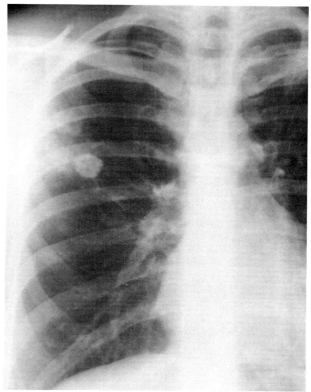

Figure 25–8. Tuberculoma. Note the dense calcified nodule in the right midlung. Some disease is also noted lateral to it and above it in the lateral aspect of the second anterior interspace. Some calcified hilar nodes are noted bilaterally.

the lesion is usually benign, but resection must be considered in all patients when no calcification is present unless previous films from 2 or 3 years ago indicate that the lesion has been present for a long time and is unchanged. Transbronchial or percutaneous needle biopsy may clearly demonstrate granulomatous disease. If there is doubt or if malignancy is found, resection is necessary.

HEALING OF PULMONARY TUBERCULOSIS

In general, pulmonary tuberculosis heals slowly, so that it is possible by means of serial roentgenograms to follow the gross anatomic changes in the disease. Differences can be noted in the manner of healing, which very likely depends on the type of involvement and the susceptibility of the tubercle bacilli to the antituberculous drugs as well as on the response of the patient.

Complete resolution often occurs in some areas. It is a common observation that complete resolution is likely to occur and be most striking in patients with relatively acute disease in which the process is presumed to be largely exudative (Fig. 25-9). This accounts for the decreased thickness of the walls of cavities often noted in patients undergoing treatment. The exudative portion of the process making up the cavitary wall resolves, resulting in a decrease in thickness. In patients in whom the disease has progressed to the point of necrosis, complete resolution is not possible. In these patients, fibrosis with contraction of the scars results in shrinkage in the volume of the involved lobe or segment and sometimes a decrease in the size of the hemithorax. The mediastinal structures are retracted to the side of involvement. The hilum is elevated in upper lobe disease and sometimes the hemidiaphragm is raised. The lesions that contain granulation tissue as well as caseation, and are often noted as poorly defined nodules, show gradual reduction in size. The individual nodules tend to become more clearly defined on the roentgenogram, evidently also because of contraction and fibrosis. This type of lesion often is the site of calcium deposition and in some instances becomes densely calcified with the passage of time. Many of the lesions contain central areas of necrosis in which viable organisms can be found after long periods of apparent inactivity. In summary, as visualized roentgenographically, there is considerable difference in the healing process from one patient to another, but it is unusual to see the disease disappear entirely (Fig. 25-10).

CT is very helpful in demonstrating nodular residuals that cannot be clearly defined on routine chest roentgenograms. Examination of surgical specimens has demonstrated that it is very difficult to be certain on roentgen examination that no residual disease is present.

Roentgenographic changes observed during the healing process have very little prognostic value. Studies have shown that it is not necessary to take routine follow-up roentgenograms when a patient undergoing treatment has no clinical signs to warrant concern. After treatment, chest radiographic study is necessary if symptoms recur. When examining a patient with residuals of tuberculosis, it is *imperative* to compare the earliest available chest film with the current one, since changes are subtle and gradual and may be overlooked if only the most recent film is used for comparison.

COMPLICATIONS OF REINFECTION PULMONARY TUBERCULOSIS

PLEURAL EFFUSION AND EMPYEMA

Because pulmonary tuberculosis is a peripheral lesion, pleural involvement is common (Fig. 25-11); effusion may be found in patients without an obvious pulmonary lesion. In some instances the opacity produced by the fluid obscures the parenchymal disease. In others, pleural effusion may be the only roentgen manifesta-

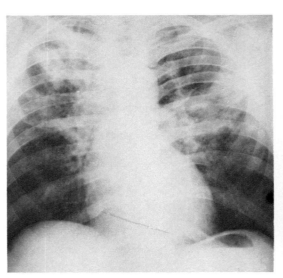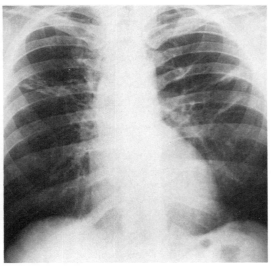

Figure 25–9.   Far-advanced bilateral pulmonary tuberculosis showing the regression resulting from treatment with antituberculous drugs. (**A**) Note the extensive bilateral disease. (**B**) Study made 9 months later shows great improvement. The remaining disease consists largely of fibrous strands with a few nodules in each lung.

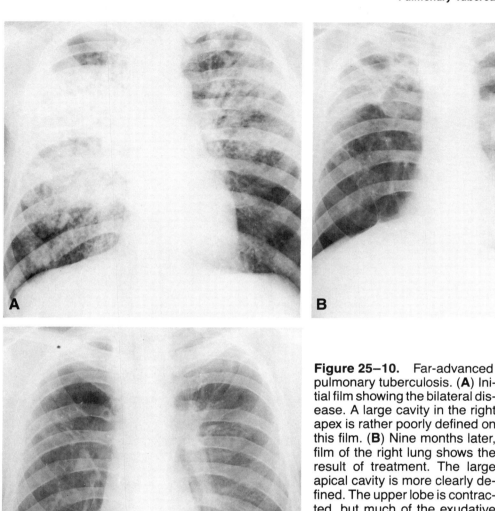

Figure 25–10. Far-advanced pulmonary tuberculosis. (**A**) Initial film showing the bilateral disease. A large cavity in the right apex is rather poorly defined on this film. (**B**) Nine months later, film of the right lung shows the result of treatment. The large apical cavity is more clearly defined. The upper lobe is contracted, but much of the exudative disease has cleared. (**C**) Sixteen months after the initial examination, most of the residual disease has been resected and now the findings are those of surgical scarring in the right second anterior interspace and in the left subclavicular area.

tion and, even when the fluid has been removed or absorbed, no definite pulmonary parenchymal focus is roentgenographically visible. In some patients the fluid disappears spontaneously or can be successfully aspirated, and in others, tuberculous empyema may result. Occasionally, the pleural space may be involved by secondary infection. The tuberculous empyema is similar to empyema of nonspecific origin in its roentgen appearance. It is usually loculated and may become very large. If it is present and undrained for a long time, calcification may occur, producing marked radiographic opacity outlining the wall. Bronchopleural fistula may also occur, with drainage of all or part of the contents of the empyema and entrance of air into it. Pleurocutaneous fistula is a rare complication. In some patients with tuberculous pleural disease, considerable fibrosis in the pleural space may result in marked pleural thickening and constriction of the adjacent lung or of the entire hemithorax if the disease is extensive. Calcification may then occur in or adjacent to either the

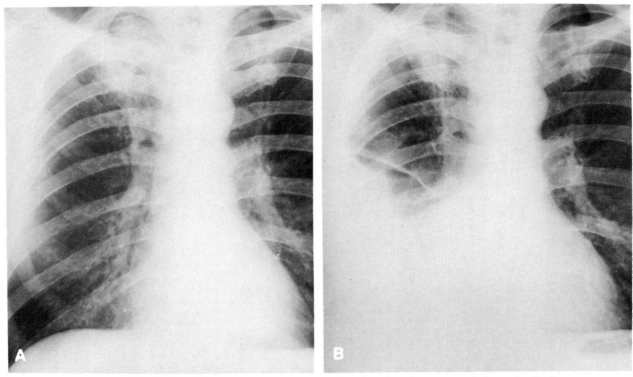

Figure 25–11.   Pulmonary tuberculosis showing the development of pleural effusion. **(A)** Bilateral tuberculosis of the upper lobe manifested by opacity that is rather homogeneous and more intense on the right than on the left. There is no evidence of pleural fluid on the right, and there was none on the left. **(B)** Four weeks later, a large pleural effusion on the right is evident. Note that the parenchymal disease has regressed slightly owing to treatment during the interval.

visceral or parietal pleura or both. Occasionally, an empyema develops years after the initial pleural infection and should be suspected if the volume of the fibrothorax increases. The presence of fluid within the pleural space or between the layers of fibrothorax can be detected by ultrasonography in most instances; CT may also be useful in this situation, particularly if ultrasonography is equivocal.

BRONCHOSTENOSIS

Narrowing of a bronchus may result from pressure of an enlarged lymph node that is involved by tuberculosis. This is usually found in children with primary tuberculosis. It is also caused by endobronchial inflammation and granuloma formation or fibrosis in the postprimary or reinfection form of the disease. Roentgen findings are not evident until the obstruction is sufficient to cause either atelectasis or obstructive overinflation, and the findings in these conditions are similar to those described in the appropriate sections of

Chapters 24 and 30. Bronchostenosis may also result in repeated nonspecific infections distal to the narrow bronchus. Complete bronchial occlusion as the result of tuberculous fibrosis rarely may be the cause of mucoid impaction.

BRONCHOLITHIASIS

Occasionally, a calcified node adjacent to a bronchus will erode into the bronchus and the calcified material from the node will be extruded into the bronchus, producing a broncholith. This may cause very few symptoms or rarely it may result in bronchogenic spread of tuberculous disease or hemorrhage. The calcification may also cause bronchial obstruction with overinflation or atelectasis. This complication may also occur in patients with calcified nodes secondary to lesions other than pulmonary tuberculosis. Radiographic findings vary with the situation. The calcified nodes are often visible and their relation to the bronchus can best be determined by CT.

TUBERCULOUS PNEUMOTHORAX

When pneumothorax complicates pulmonary tuberculosis, it creates the hazard of widespread pleural involvement leading to tuberculous empyema and bronchopleural fistula. This is because the pneumothorax often results from rupture of a caseous subpleural focus into the pleural space in advanced disease. It is also possible for a small subpleural bleb to rupture, leading to a simple pneumothorax that will resolve quickly without further complication. The roentgen appearance is similar to that noted in pneumothorax from other causes, but the tuberculous disease is visible and a considerable amount of adhesive pleuritis may result in irregular or loculated pneumothorax. This is an uncommon complication of tuberculosis.

DISSEMINATION TO OTHER ORGANS

Patients with pulmonary tuberculosis occasionally develop disease in other organs and systems such as the larynx, ileum and cecum, urogenital organs, and skeletal system. Gastrointestinal disease and laryngeal disease are frequently the result of contact with sputum and only rarely indicate a hematogenous spread. On the other hand, renal tuberculosis as well as skeletal involvement indicates hematogenous or lymphangitic spread. These lesions are discussed under the organ or system involved.

HEMATOGENOUS TUBERCULOSIS

Hematogenous pulmonary tuberculosis includes several types of disease. When the organisms enter the blood stream, it is possible to get hematogenous involvement of numerous other organs and systems. The actual mode of dissemination is difficult to determine in any specific instance, but dissemination may occur by way of the lymphatics and enter the blood stream through the thoracic duct, by direct rupture of a caseous focus into a vessel, or by formation of a subintimal tubercle that serves as a source of organisms. The invasion of the blood stream may occur in any stage of tuberculosis. When hematogenous dissemination develops, numerous factors have a bearing on the resultant disease. These factors include the following: the age of the patient, the number and virulence of the organisms entering the blood stream, the individual and racial susceptibility, and the general health of the patient, as well as the state of allergy and immunity at the time of the invasion. Prompt treatment with antibacterial drugs usually alters the disease considerably in a favorable manner.

MILIARY PULMONARY TUBERCULOSIS

Two clinical types of miliary tuberculosis are recognized—acute miliary tuberculosis and subacute or chronic miliary pulmonary dissemination. Acute miliary tuberculosis follows massive blood stream invasion, producing a severe acute illness, frequently with fatal termination before the use of antituberculous drugs. In infants and children it may result from a spread from a primary site and produces severe clinical manifestations. It usually occurs in malnourished or chronically ill infants, who are unusually susceptible. In most children, however, the number of organisms is small and the host resistance sufficient to prevent miliary spread of the disease, so there are no clinical manifestations. In adults, particularly in the older age group, the disease may be very insidious and extremely difficult to recognize. Findings on chest roentgenograms depend on the size and number of miliary tubercles. The actual nodules visualized on a roentgenogram are the result of superimposition of many small parenchymal lesions that create sufficient opacity to be recognized as a small nodule. In the typical patient the appearance is that of a fine granularity or tiny nodulation scattered uniformly throughout both lungs. At times the lesions are rather clearly defined as innumerable fine nodules, each sharply delineated; in other patients they are less sharply outlined, with hazy margins (Fig. 25-12 and 25-13). In some patients with miliary pulmonary tuberculosis, no lesions can be seen on the initial chest film, but in most instances, a classic miliary pattern de-

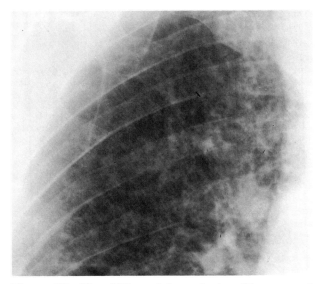

Figure 25–12. Miliary tuberculosis. Close-up of the right upper lung in a patient with miliary tuberculosis shows the numerous small opacities along with a small increase in interstitial markings.

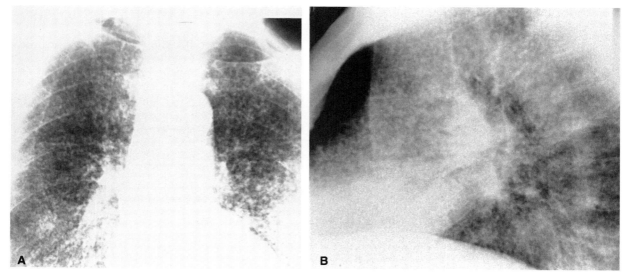

Figure 25–13. (**A**) Posteroanterior and (**B**) lateral views. Miliary tuberculosis. Note the extensive miliary nodules, more dense and clearly defined than those in Figure 25-12. Patient had weight loss, fever, and a cough.

velops during the course of the disease.[6] Usually, some findings suggest tuberculosis on the initial film in these patients, however. Pleural involvement is common, resulting in unilateral or bilateral pleural effusion that varies considerably in amount. Rarely, recurrent pneumothorax may complicate the disease. The cause is not certain, but subpleural caseating nodules may rupture into the pleural space in some instances. The individual lesions are largely exudative, and when treatment with antibacterial drugs is effective, the widely scattered foci usually disappear completely. They do not result in scattered pulmonary calcifications.

The differential diagnosis of miliary tuberculosis is often difficult from a roentgen standpoint because numerous other diseases produce widespread scattered and miliary type of nodulation in both lungs. Correlation of clinical and roentgen findings is very important in all instances. Several acute processes cannot be differentiated from miliary tuberculosis on a single chest roentgenogram. Miliary bronchopneumonia, which may be of viral or bacterial etiology, and bronchiolitis in children, resulting in widespread miliary nodulation, may closely resemble miliary tuberculosis. In other diseases such as sarcoidosis, the pneumoconioses, and miliary pulmonary carcinomatosis, the history and clinical course usually permit differentiation. Several conditions can produce acute, diffuse miliary lesions in the lung. They include, in addition to those mentioned, other bacterial infections such as staphylococcal and streptococcal pneumonia, viral and

rickettsial infections such as chickenpox and Q fever, mycotic infections such as histoplasmosis and blastomycosis, and parasitic infestations such as schistosomiasis. Also included are the noninfectious diseases, acute berylliosis, miliary hemorrhages, and acute, diffuse, interstitial fibrosis as described by Hamman and Rich. It is therefore evident that the roentgen findings must be correlated with the results of clinical and laboratory examinations. In some instances, serial roentgenograms, spaced over a period of days or weeks, are helpful in establishing the diagnosis.

In the immunocompromised patient and the infant with acute febrile illness and miliary pulmonary disease, and in difficult cases in the elderly, lung biopsy to get a prompt diagnosis may be indicated, since a delay in treatment may be fatal.

SUBACUTE AND CHRONIC HEMATOGENOUS PULMONARY DISSEMINATION

Subacute and chronic hematogenous pulmonary dissemination is a somewhat different clinical entity from acute miliary tuberculosis in that it is often asymptomatic. Repeated small episodes may occur so that lesions, although widespread and distributed rather uniformly throughout both lungs, are likely to be somewhat more variable in size than in the acute miliary process. When this type of dissemination is extensive, the roentgen findings are similar to those in the acute type of miliary tuberculosis, but there is considerable difference in the clinical course. In other instances the hematogenous pulmonary dissemination may be relatively localized, producing small, poorly defined, rounded or oval areas of density in a segment or lobe. Some of these nodules may regress, and others may coalesce to form larger nodules and they may heal in a manner similar to that described earlier in the discussion of reinfection type of tuberculosis. In patients with far advanced pulmonary tuberculosis and a considerable amount of cavitation there may be hematogenous spread to the lower lobes or to the opposite lung, resulting in scattered lesions that cannot be differentiated from the secondary lesions produced by bronchogenic spread of the disease.

ATYPICAL MYCOBACTERIA

There is a group of mycobacteria that can cause pulmonary disease that is similar to tuberculosis caused by *M. tuberculosis* but is slightly different from the standpoint of roentgen findings. These mycobacteria have been classified according to growth characteristics when exposed to light into four groups as follows:[15]

Group I. Photochromogens: *M. kansasii*, *M. marinum*, and *M. simiae*.

Group II. Scotochromogens: *M. scrofulaceum*, *M. szulgai*, and *M. gordonae*.

Group III. Nonphotochromogens: *M. avium-intracellulare*, *M. nonchromogenicum*, *M. terrae*, *M. novum*, *M. triviale*, *M. xenopi*, *M. malmoense*, and *M. ulcerans*.

Group IV. The rapid growers: *M. fortuitum*, and *M. chelonei*.

The clinical and radiologic aspects are discussed at length by Wolinsky,[14] Woodring and Vandiviere,[15] and others.[1, 5, 11, 12] The most important of these pulmonary pathogens are *M. intracellulare* (*M. avium-intracellulare*), *M. xenopi*, particularly in Ontario,[12] and *M. kansasii*. *M. avium-intracellulare* infections appear to be increasing, particularly in those with decreased cellular immunity or chronic lung disease, but also in those without predisposing cause. The radiologic features are slightly different from those of *M. tuberculosis* and show the following contrasts:

1. Increase in cavitation in relation to the amount of lung involved.
2. Thin-walled cavities without much surrounding disease; cavities may be small.
3. Spread is contiguous rather than bronchogenic.
4. Anterior segment of the upper lobe appears to be involved more frequently than in *M. tuberculosis*.
5. Marked pleural thickening over the involved areas of lung.
6. More involvement of apical and anterior segments of the upper lobes.
7. Clustered opacities around irregular translucent areas with radiating line shadows; opacities resembling tumors occasionally occur.
8. Usually unilateral even when far advanced.
9. Usually found in older age groups.
10. Pleural effusion is uncommon and small in amount.
11. Adenopathy is uncommon.
12. Disease is often extensive when first discovered.
13. Marked predominance of whites to blacks (10 to 1).

Although the preceding findings differ somewhat from those in tuberculosis, the variety of findings in *M. tuberculosis* infections is such that roentgenographic differentiation cannot be made. At times atypical mycobacterial infection can be suggested, however. These atypical organisms usually do not respond well to antituberculous drug therapy. *M. avium* complex appears to be particularly difficult to control, so surgical removal of residual disease may be necessary and should perhaps be considered after antituberculous therapy.

SURGICAL MEASURES IN PULMONARY TUBERCULOSIS

Despite the undoubted value of the various antibacterial drugs now available for the treatment of tuberculosis, in some patients cavities fail to close or tubercle bacilli continue to discharge in pulmonary secretions. Tuberculous bronchiectasis may cause repeated hemorrhage, may cause repeated nonspecific infections, or may harbor an aspergilloma, which may also cause bleeding and be difficult to eradicate. These patients then become possible candidates for surgery, which is usually a resection of the residual disease. The roentgen findings after pulmonary resection for tuberculosis are similar to those described in Chapter 30.

Before effective drugs were available, thoracoplasty and plombage were used in an attempt to close cavities and promote healing. Thoracoplasty is used very rarely and plombage is no longer used. Older patients who have had these procedures are examined by means of chest films, so examples of patients who have under-

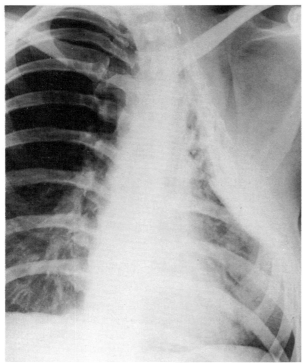

Figure 25–14. Left thoracoplasty. This surgical procedure, which was used extensively before the advent of antituberculous drugs, is employed rarely at present. There has been extensive resection of the upper seven ribs on the left, compressing the left upper lung. Regeneration of the ribs has formed a solid bony plate along the upper lateral chest wall. The scoliosis is a common result of thoracoplasty.

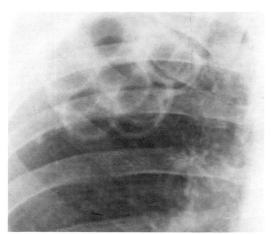

Figure 25–15. Lucite-ball plombage. Although this procedure has been abandoned, occasionally patients are observed with the rounded lucencies representing Lucite balls, usually at the apex of one hemithorax, as in this patient.

gone these procedures are included (Figs. 25-14 and 25-15).

REFERENCES AND SELECTED READINGS

1. ALBELDA SM, KERN JA, MARINELLI DL, MILLER WI: Expanding spectrum of pulmonary disease caused by non-tuberculous mycobacteria. Radiology 157:289, 1985
2. BUCKNER CB, LEITHISER RE, WALKER CW, ET AL: The changing epidemiology of tuberculosis and other mycobacterial infections in the United States: Implications for the radiologist. Am J Roentgenol 156:255, 1991
3. BUCKNER CB, WALKER CW: Radiologic manifestations of adult tuberculosis. J Thorac Imaging 5:28, 1990
4. CHOYKE PL, SOSTMAN HD, CURTIS AM, ET AL: Adult-onset pulmonary tuberculosis. Radiology 148:357, 1983
5. CONTRERAS MA, CHEUNG OT, SANDERS DE, ET AL: Pulmonary infection with nontuberculous mycobacteria. Am Rev Respir Dis 137:149, 1988
6. GELB AF, LEFFLER C, BREWIN A, ET AL: Miliary tuberculosis. Am Rev Respir Dis 108:1327, 1973
7. KHAN FA, REHMAN M, MARCUS P, ET AL: Pulmonary gangrene occurring as a complication of pulmonary tuberculosis. Chest 77:76, 1980
8. MILLER WT: Tuberculosis in the immunosuppressed patient. Semin Roentgenol 14:249, 1979
9. PALMER PES: Pulmonary tuberculosis—usual and unusual presentations. Semin Roentgenol 15:204, 1979
10. PITCHENIK AE, RUBINSON HA: The radiographic appearance of tuberculosis in patients with acquired immune deficiency syndrome (AIDS) and pre-AIDS. Am Rev Respir Dis 131:393, 1985
11. PRINCE DS, PETERSON DD, STEINER RM, ET AL: Infections with *Mycobacterium avium* complex in patients without predisposing conditions. N Engl J Med 321:863, 1989
12. SIMOR AE, SALIT IE, VELLEND H: The role of *Mycobacterium xenopi* in human disease. Am Rev Respir Dis 129:435, 1984
13. STANSBERRY SD: Tuberculosis in infants and children. J Thorac Imaging 5:17, 1990
14. WOLINSKY E: Non-tuberculous mycobacteria and associated diseases. Am Rev Respir Dis 119:107, 1979
15. WOODRING JH, VANDIVIERE HM: Pulmonary disease caused by non-tuberculous mycobacteria. J Thorac Imaging 5:64, 1990
16. WOODRING JH, VANDIVIERE HM, FRIED AM, ET AL: Update: The radiographic features of pulmonary tuberculosis. Am J Roentgenol 146:497, 1986

Paul and Juhl's Essentials of Radiologic Imaging, Sixth Edition, edited by John H. Juhl and Andrew B. Crummy. J.B. Lippincott Company, Philadelphia, © 1993.

CHAPTER 26

Mycotic and Other Nonbacterial Infectious Diseases

John H. Juhl

The infectious diseases discussed in this chapter are caused by a variety of organisms, many of which are capable of producing acute, fulminating, generalized disease in which there is associated involvement of the lungs. These organisms may also cause disease, usually chronic, limited primarily to the lungs. Some of them are saprophytes or are of very low virulence, but in compromised hosts they may produce life-threatening acute pneumonia. The diseases must be differentiated from each other as well as from pulmonary tuberculosis and occasionally from lung tumor. The ultimate diagnosis depends on demonstration of the causative agent in bronchial secretions or in sections of the lung. In some instances studies based on immunologic reactions are sufficient. These consist of skin tests, agglutination, complement fixation, and precipitation reactions.[47]

The gross anatomic changes in pulmonary disease produced by these varied organisms may be similar. On the basis of roentgen examination it is often possible to indicate only that the lesion is a chronic inflammatory disease of unknown etiology. At other times it is possible to make the diagnosis with a considerable degree of accuracy on the basis of clinical findings correlated with roentgen manifestations.

MYCOTIC DISEASES OF THE LUNG

ACTINOMYCOSIS

Actinomycosis is caused by an anaerobic organism, *Actinomyces bovis*, in cattle. In humans it is caused by *A. israelii*, a similar organism that occurs in rod-shaped bacterial form in the mouth and in mycelial form in infected tissues. Other actinomycetes may cause human infection; these include *A. bovis*, *A. naeslundii*, *A. ericksonii*, *A. meyeri*, and *A. propionicus*. The organisms are now established as bacteria, but roentgen and clinical findings similar to those of mycotic infections justify[49] the inclusion of actinomycosis here. The disease may affect any part of the body but is found most frequently in and about the jaw. Pulmonary infection is said to occur in approximately 15% of patients with the disease. However, in recent years, the incidence of pulmonary involvement has declined considerably and the classic empyema with chest wall sinus tracts and pulmonary parenchymal disease is rarely seen and is avoided by timely antibiotic therapy. This form of the disease is characterized by its tendency to produce suppurative sinus tracts and its ability to cross tissue planes that provide a barrier to the usual infections.

The roentgen findings vary greatly. The disease may be unilateral or bilateral but tends to be unilateral unless widely disseminated. It produces a dense, confluent opacity in the affected lung, usually in a lower lobe peripherally, in which cavitation may be present (Fig. 26-1). The cavity may persist after treatment as a thin-walled bullalike shadow. In the classic chest wall disease, pleural involvement results in varying amounts of pleural thickening and fluid. Infection of the chest wall causes soft-tissue swelling and may cause periosteal reaction and/or destruction of ribs with sinus tract formation. This is characteristic of advanced disease, which is now observed infrequently. The parenchymal involvement may resemble acute alveolar pneumonia in some instances. In other cases, the disease is manifested as a local masslike opacity resembling bronchogenic carcinoma. Another roentgen pattern is that of a fan-shaped consolidation near the hilum or radiating from the hilum into the superior segment of the lower lobe. Rarely, hematogenous spread from a focal area of disease results in a miliary pulmonary pattern. When the combination of pulmonary disease and chest wall involvement with empyema and sinus tracts is present, actinomycosis may be strongly suspected. However, it must be differentiated by bacteriologic examination from tuberculosis, from chronic fungal infections, and from tumors.

NOCARDIOSIS

Nocardia asteroides is the most common of several species of *Nocardia* that may cause disease. It is an aerobic, gram-positive, acid-fast bacterium, formerly classified as a fungus, with finely branched hyphae. It is recognized increasingly as an opportunistic infection in patients with underlying chronic debilitating disease, particularly in those who have undergone therapy with immunosuppressive or cytotoxic agents or steroids and in patients with liver transplants or chronic liver disease.[44] In nocardiosis, pulmonary roentgen findings are similar to those of actinomycosis and consist of homogeneous segmental or lobar airspace consolidation; cavitation is common.[15] Pleural involvement with empyema is not common, as has been reported in the past (Fig. 26-2). Single nodular lesions may also occur and may progress to cavitation. The disease is frequently bilateral. It crosses fissures and anatomic barriers if not properly treated but not as frequently as actinomycosis. Computed tomography (CT) is useful for localization when aspiration or biopsy is needed for diagnosis. The roentgen alterations in the lungs persist for long periods, frequently with little change unless the patient is treated with sulfonamides. *N. asteroides* is difficult to isolate in many instances, so that the diagnosis is often obscure until material for histologic study is obtained by aspiration lung biopsy, transbronchial aspiration, bronchial brushing, or open lung biopsy. It is not unusual for the disease to run a protracted course with very little variation in the appearance of the pulmonary lesions and very few symptoms. Pleural involvement with empyema and extension to involve the ribs with production of chest wall abscess is not as common as in actinomycosis and is not ordinarily observed in nocardiosis. Occasionally, *Nocardia* may involve the skin when inoculated in a traumatic event. Then, extremely rarely, it may spread via the blood stream to the lungs to produce disseminated pulmonary disease. Mediastinitis with adenopathy and obstruction of the superior vena cava has been reported, however. Nocardiosis is one of the few benign diseases that can cause obstruction of the superior vena cava.[40] In addition to differentiation of this disease from tuberculosis, the other chronic infectious lesions of the lungs must be included in the differential diagnosis. Identification of the causative agent is necessary to confirm the diagnosis.

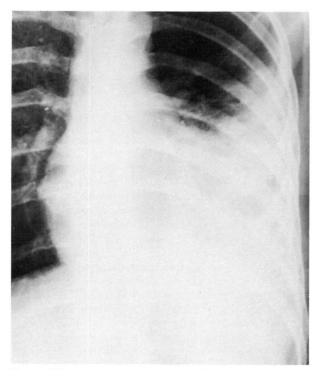

Figure 26–1. Actinomycosis. The dense, confluent consolidation in the left lower lung obscures the left hemidiaphragm and left lower cardiac border. The patient also had a chest wall mass and sinus tracts typical of this disease.

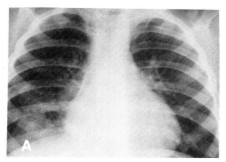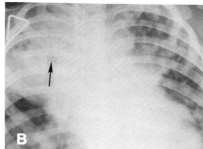

Figure 26–2. Nocardiosis. **(A)** This film shows a small amount of poorly defined opacity at the right base just above the diaphragm. **(B)** Roentgenogram obtained 9 months later shows extensive progression of the disease with large, poorly defined nodular and patchy opacity in both lungs. A large homogeneous consolidation in which there is a cavity (*arrow*) is seen in the right upper lobe. There has been open drainage of the plural space in the right upper anterolateral chest wall.

COCCIDIOIDOMYCOSIS

Coccidioidomycosis is caused by the fungus *Coccidioides immitis.*[7] It is an endemic pulmonary disease occurring in the arid southwestern part of the United States, particularly in the San Joaquin valley in California and in southern Arizona. The *primary* form is usually asymptomatic and is discovered incidentally on a chest film (60%). There may be calcified granulomas in the lung or hilar nodes; others have a focus of pulmonary fibrosis or pleural thickening and in some there may be no recognizable residual. If a chest film happens to be obtained during the asymptomatic acute phase, a focus of alveolar pneumonia may be observed. The primary or initial infection may also produce an acute pneumonia associated with symptoms of an acute pulmonary disease including fever, malaise, headache, and cough. Erythema nodosum is a frequent clinical manifestation during the acute febrile illness, and in the San Joaquin valley, this clinical syndrome is known as valley fever. Erythema nodosum is often associated with arthralgias and occurs at about the time the reaction to the coccidioidin skin test becomes positive. It may be the only symptom and indicates a good prognosis. Before this time, some patients (about 10%) develop a toxic erythema, usually in the first few days of illness. The rash is a diffuse, fine, macular erythematous reaction covering the trunk and extremities and usually occurs in children with the disease. Roentgen findings in the symptomatic primary disease are those of air-space pneumonia, which results in homogeneous opacity that is poorly circumscribed and may be segmental or lobar. It tends to involve the lower lobes and may be associated with some atelectasis. In other patients, there is patchy central disease that tends to resolve quickly (in 1 to 2 weeks). Pleural involvement is found in about 20%, usually manifested by a minimal effusion. The hilar nodes are enlarged in about 20% of these patients, usually on the side of the alveolar disease. The roentgen findings in this type of involvement simulate those of other acute, atypical pneumonias. The pneumonia of coccidioidomycosis may be localized to one segment, but wider dissemination has also been reported, with multiple areas of pneumonic consolidation. Occasionally, the adenopathy in the hilar and mediastinal nodes is the predominant feature, and in these patients there may or may not be evidence of pulmonary parenchymal involvement. Multiple nodular parenchymal lesions have also been reported but are not as common as the more localized pneumonitis. Cavitation within the area of disease is not uncommon. The cavities are usually small and may disappear quickly in the primary type of infection. Occasionally, small pleural effusion is the only evidence of the disease noted on the chest roentgenogram. Although effusion occurs in about 20% of patients with coccidioidomycosis, pleuritic chest pain has been reported in 70%. Massive effusion is rare and may result from direct spread of pulmonary disease across the pleural space.

Persistent pulmonary coccidioidomycosis is found in about 5% of patients. It is a much more significant type of disease and may be fatal. In these patients, coccidioidal pneumonia may persist for months, with large areas of dense consolidation clearing very slowly. The patients are often very sick with persistent fever, prostration, chest pain, productive cough, and occasional hemoptysis. This type of the disease usually occurs in susceptible patients and occasionally in immunosuppressed patients. Cavitation, either thick- or thin-walled, may also occur in this type of disease and may be very chronic. Bronchiectasis and bronchial stenosis are uncommon.[34]

A more benign type of residual or persistent pulmonary coccidioidomycosis results when the acute primary disease subsides without much dissemination. The primary disease may clear completely, but when there is residual disease, it usually assumes one of three general radiographic types: (1) cavitation; (2) nodules, which may be single or multiple; and (3) pulmonary opacity, which may be relatively focal and occur in a single area or in several areas. The residual type of cavitation in this form of coccidioidomycosis often is thin-walled and may remain unchanged in size and shape for years. There usually is some fibrotic disease in the area of cavitation, but this is not always true.

Studies of many patients have shown that the thin-walled cavity that was originally thought to be characteristic of the disease occurs in only 50% to 60% of patients, while the remaining cavities have relatively thick walls. Spontaneous closure of cavities occurs in about one-half of the patients. Most of the cavities are single and in the upper lung, and more than half are 4 cm in diameter or less. Cavitation may be complicated by secondary infection, including formation of *Aspergillus* fungus balls, pyopneumothorax when the cavity is subpleural in location, and pulmonary hemorrhage, which usually is not significant. These complications are uncommon. Cavitation in coccidioidomycosis must be differentiated from that in pulmonary tuberculosis and in other mycotic infections. This is usually not possible on roentgen examination alone, but as a general rule, the residual cavity in coccidioidomycosis has less pulmonary disease around it than is seen in untreated pulmonary tuberculosis, since bronchogenic spread is much less common in coccidioidomycosis than in tuberculosis. This finding is important in the differential diagnosis of untreated patients with chronic pulmonary disease in whom there is persistent cavitation (Fig. 26-3).

Rarely, a pulmonary mycetoma (fungus ball) may be caused by *Coccidioides immitis*.[42] Arthrospores and spherules may be present along with hyphae of the mycelial phase in a pulmonary cavity. The appearance is similar to that of an aspergilloma, a much more common cause of fungus ball.

The nodular residuals of coccidioidomycosis vary considerably in size and number. They may or may not contain calcium. When single, they must be differentiated from other diseases that cause solitary pulmonary nodulation, including primary bronchogenic tumor. When multiple, the lesions must be distinguished from other mycotic disease and from pulmonary tuberculosis. These differentiations are not possible on roentgen examination and must be based on skin tests with coccidioidin and by means of serologic studies. The infiltrative fibrotic type of residual disease is similar to the fibrotic residues of numerous other inflammations, so that there is nothing in the roentgenogram to indicate the nature of the original disease. Pleural thickening and effusion are occasionally noted as the end results of this disease, but there is nothing charac-

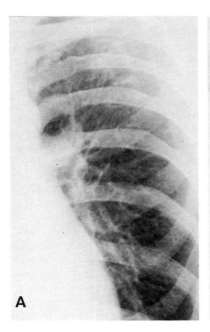
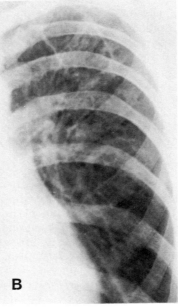

Figure 26–3. Coccidioidomycosis. (**A**) Note the cavity in the left subclavicular area. The elongated cavity has a moderately thick wall, but there is very little parenchymal disease around it. (**B**) One year later, the cavity is noted to be larger, the wall is thinner, and again very little other parenchymal disease is observed.

teristic about these findings. Cavities are often peripheral and tend to rupture into the pleural space, resulting in empyema. Occasionally, they cause spontaneous pneumothorax.

Dissemination occurs rarely when the initial infection fails to become localized. This is very uncommon in whites, but members of dark-skinned races are more susceptible. Clinically, dissemination is a continuation and progression of the primary infection, is often manifested by exacerbation of symptoms, and may result in acute respiratory failure. Occasionally, an acute form of the disease may progress rapidly and disseminate widely. Although the miliary spread usually occurs early in the disease, it is sometimes a late complication of chronic pulmonary or extrapulmonary forms. Radiographic findings vary considerably from universal hematogenous spread of disease resembling miliary tuberculosis to local spread confined to the lungs. There is often bronchogenic dissemination to the opposite lung or other lobes, which results in scattered involvement of varying extent. Large cavities may appear, along with pleural involvement leading to empyema. Associated with the extensive pulmonary opacities in this form of the disease, there is often spread to abdominal viscera, the skeletal system, lymph nodes, and sometimes the brain and meninges. The disseminated type of involvement is usually lethal.

HISTOPLASMOSIS

Histoplasmosis is caused by the fungus known as *Histoplasma capsulatum*.[13] It was originally thought to be a rare and fatal disease, but it is now known that the disseminated form, which may be fatal, is only one of several types of the disease. The *primary* form is much more common and is by far the most common fungal disease in the United States. It is endemic in the Mississippi and Ohio valleys and along the Appalachian Mountains. In many areas, histoplasmin skin sensitivity indicating previous infection is almost universal in young adult lifetime residents. The disease is less common elsewhere in the United States but is found in nearly all states, as well as in Mexico and Panama.

The primary form of histoplasmosis, a localized pneumonic disease, is usually relatively benign and passes unnoticed in most instances (95%). The roentgen changes found in the acute benign disease are varied with single or multiple areas of pneumonic consolidation. The disease cannot be distinguished from primary tuberculosis roentgenographically. It is often segmental in distribution and may be accompanied by hilar node enlargement. The hilar node involvement may be more prominent than the parenchymal disease in some subjects (Fig. 26-4), particularly children. In addition to the localized pneumonic consolidation,

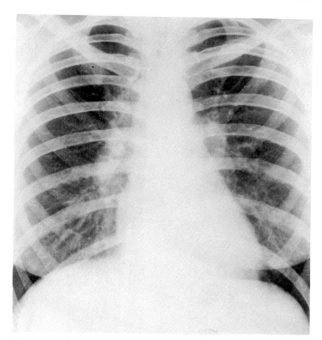

Figure 26–4. Histoplasmosis. The parenchymal disease is minor and consists of a small amount of patchy opacity above the right hilum; there is bilateral hilar node enlargement, more on the right than the left.

there is a more disseminated form, often occurring in local epidemics. Poorly defined, patchy or nodular lesions are scattered throughout both lungs (Fig. 26-5). Later they become more clearly defined, round nodules varying in size up to a centimeter. With healing, some of the nodules may disappear completely, whereas others may gradually decrease in size and become calcified (Fig. 26-6). Calcification often occurs in the involved hilar nodes as well.

Histoplasmosis is the most common cause of broncholithiasis, which is produced when a calcified node erodes into a bronchus. Studies of large groups of people in endemic areas have shown that, as a general rule, the amount of calcification in parenchymal nodules and in hilar nodes is greater in histoplasmosis than in tuberculosis. The primary form of the disease may clear and leave no pulmonary residuals that can be recognized on roentgenograms. However, in others, a solitary calcified parenchymal nodule with or without calcified hilar nodes may be present (Fig. 26-7). Caseous lymphadenitis is common during the primary infection (Fig. 26-8). Cystlike lesions may develop in the mediastinum and become very large when liquefaction occurs in enlarged coalescent nodes. These

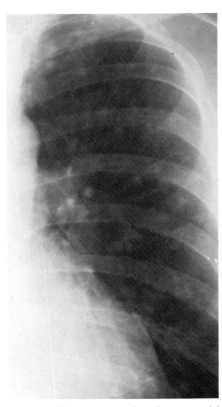

Figure 26–5. Disseminated pulmonary histoplasmosis. Note the small, poorly defined nodules scattered throughout the left lung. The patient had been ill for several weeks.

lesions may measure 10 cm or more in diameter and may be asymptomatic. Air–fluid levels may develop within them when there is communication with the bronchial tree or lung. Remnants of lymph node tissue may be observed in these cystlike lesions, which tend to confirm the impression that they represent excavated lymph nodes. Miliary parenchymal calcifications scattered throughout the lungs and large "mulberry" calcified hilar nodes are usually associated with histoplasmin sensitivity rather than tuberculin sensitivity.

Symptomatic primary infection is usually found in infants and young children. In contrast to those having the more benign common form, these patients usually have a cough and are often febrile for a few days, or occasionally for 2 to 3 weeks or longer. Roentgen findings consist of hilar and mediastinal adenopathy with a focal opacity representing air-space disease in the lung. Nodes may calcify and occasionally may obstruct a bronchus or rupture into it.

The *acute epidemic form* of histoplasmosis reported in several localities in the endemic regions probably represents a heavy exposure that results in more pulmonary parenchymal involvement than in the usual primary form of the disease. Extensive bilateral lobular or nodular air-space disease may involve both lungs, and sometimes a miliary spread throughout both lungs is observed. The residuals are similar to those of the benign primary form, except that there may be more scattered, calcific, parenchymal foci in the severe acute epidemic form. It appears that reinfection may produce the acute, chronic, or disseminated form of histoplasmosis.

Disseminated histoplasmosis is a progressive disease with dissemination not only to the lungs but also to other organs, including the bone marrow. The course may be extremely rapid and fulminating or slowly progressive, leading to cachexia and anemia. It usually occurs in infants, in patients with compromised cellular immunity, or in those who have been immunosuppressed. Marked variation has been found in the roentgen manifestations of disseminated pulmonary histoplasmosis, ranging from widespread granular nodulations throughout both lungs, which is the most common, to lobar type of pneumonic consolidation. Scattered involvement simulating other types of pneumonia is also noted, and occasionally there is massive pleural effusion. In infants under 1 year of age the acute disseminated form is often fatal; hepatosplenomegaly is common in addition to the extensive pulmonary involvement.

There is an *intermediate form* of histoplasmosis resulting in chronic active pulmonary disease and resembling reinfection tuberculosis clinically and radiographically. Cavitation along with local ill-defined opacities and nodulation similar to that noted in chronic pulmonary tuberculosis is often found. Pleural involvement, fibrosis, and contraction of the involved lobe or segment with alteration in the size of the thorax and mediastinal deviation may also be produced (Fig. 26-9). Histoplasmosis involving hilar nodes adjacent to bronchi may cause collapse of the middle lobe (middle lobe syndrome) or of other pulmonary segments. It may also be the cause of broncholithiasis. In patients with chronic active pulmonary histoplasmosis, the apical posterior segments are involved and cavitation is common, often persisting for long periods. These persistent cavities often enlarge gradually and may become very large. Disease in the adjacent lung is common and fibrosis may become extensive.

Mediastinal involvement resulting in a chronic fibrosing process leading to obstruction of the superior vena cava has also been reported in this disease.[27] The primary disease may have been asymptomatic, but the

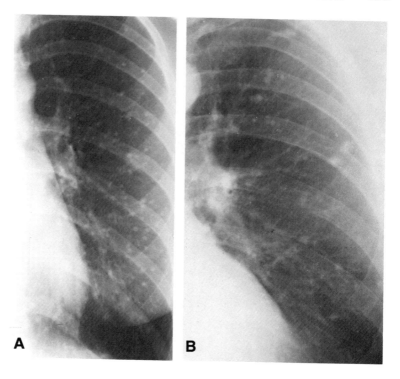

Figure 26–6. Histoplasmosis. Examples of calcified pulmonary nodules. (**A**) The nodules seen here are rather uniform in size and all are calcified. (**B**) Fewer nodules but less calcification and more variation in size are noted in this patient.

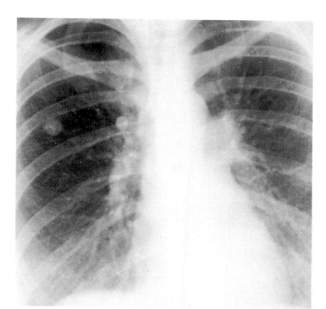

Figure 26–7. Histoplasmosis. There is a solitary, partially calcified parenchymal nodule in the right upper lung with several partially calcified right hilar nodes. The left hilum is also prominent; enlarged nodes appear there.

resultant fibrous mediastinitis may produce pulmonary arterial and venous obstruction and pericardial and esophageal involvement in addition to caval obstruction. Any or all of these findings may be present to a greater or lesser degree. Rarely, calcification of the pericardium may result from *Histoplasma* pericarditis.

The sole manifestation of the disease may be a solitary pulmonary nodule, the *histoplasmoma*. This lesion may be associated with calcified hilar nodes, and there may be a few satellite nodules in the lung. Calcification may or may not be present in the lesion, which may vary from 1 to 3 cm or more in diameter. The calcification may be laminated, annular, solid, or stippled and may be central with a laminated or annular peripheral ring. The vast majority remain stable for years, but occasionally a slow increase in size is observed, suggesting that an occasional histoplasmoma contains viable organisms in contrast to most lesions, which are quiescent. Skin testing, complement-fixation studies, and mycologic studies are required to differentiate this disease from pulmonary tuberculosis; occasionally, both diseases may be present in the same patient. When the nodule does not contain calcium, it cannot be differentiated from neoplasm on chest radiography, tomography, or CT. Then biopsy may be necessary.

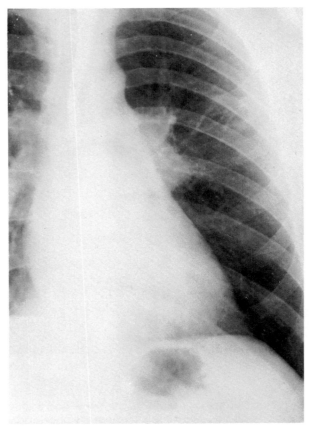

Figure 26–8.   Histoplasmosis. There are enlarged nodes in the left hilum and some parenchymal disease in the lung lateral to the hilum, which appears somewhat nodular. No other disease was observed.

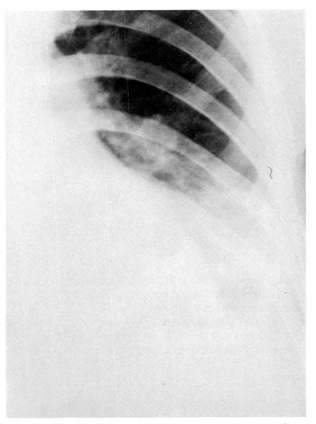

Figure 26–9.   Histoplasmosis. Note the conglomerate disease in the central and basal lung. There is also some pleural thickening and a small amount of fluid. No definite hilar enlargement is present. This is the same patient whose roentgenogram, obtained 5 years before this study, is shown in Figure 26-8. Slow progression of disease as illustrated here is unusual in our experience.

CRYPTOCOCCOSIS

Cryptococcosis (torulosis) is caused by *Cryptococcus neoformans*. Pulmonary lesions have been reported in increasing numbers of patients with and without involvement of the central nervous system. As in other chronic pulmonary infections, several forms of pulmonary involvement are found and the diagnosis cannot be made from roentgenograms alone.[8,19] Three general types of radiographic change have been described. The *first* is a fairly well circumscribed, round mass or nodule usually occurring in the lower half of either lung, which must be differentiated from neoplasm as well as from other chronic pulmonary granulomas. They tend to be peripheral and may become large (up to 10 cm in diameter). At times, multiple, closely grouped, mass-like densities may be observed. The *second* is a pneumonic type of lesion consisting of a somewhat irregular opacity more likely to appear in the lower than in the upper lobe. It represents granulomatous disease.[8] This type of disease may be extensive but usually is confined to one segment or lobe and often is associated with lymph node enlargement; cavitation is rare. This is the most common. The *third* type is a widespread miliary variety of nodulation often found in conjunction with severe central nervous system infection. This type of disease is frequently found as an opportunistic infection associated with such chronic processes as Hodgkin's disease, leukemia, and lymphoma or is found to occur after steroid or antibiotic therapy. Cavitation may occur in this form, and pleural involvement with effusion may be present but is uncommon. Often the diagnosis is not made until autopsy in the patients having disseminated disease.

In seven patients with acquired immunodeficiency syndrome (AIDS) complicated by cryptococcosis, Miller and associates found that hilar or mediastinal adenopathy and interstitial pulmonary disease alone or in combination were the most common findings on chest films.[35] They believe that the interstitial process is a manifestation of disseminated disease and its presence should indicate a search for silent cryptococcal meningitis. Although the diagnosis cannot be made on the basis of roentgenographic findings, the combination of signs of meningeal irritation and pulmonary lesions resembling those described is suggestive. When the disease is confined to the lung in a noncompromised host, spontaneous resolution without treatment occurs in most cases.

NORTH AMERICAN BLASTOMYCOSIS

North American blastomycosis is caused by the yeast-like fungus, *Blastomyces dermatitidis*. Although much less common than histoplasmosis, it occurs in approximately the same geographic areas of the United States but extends more eastward and northward. The two general types of the disease are cutaneous and disseminated. In the disseminated form, the portal of entry is usually the respiratory tract, and 95% of the patients have some form of pulmonary involvement. The roentgen findings in pulmonary disease produced by this organism are not diagnostic and are related to the clinical form of the disease.[43] In the acute form, there are four major roentgenographic patterns. (1) Air-space involvement causing a patchy segmental or lobar consolidation is present in most patients. There are often several foci of disease, and involvement may be multilobar. The disease is usually located in the upper lung. In this type, resolution usually takes place slowly and may require several months. Cavitation may complicate this acute form. (2) Large, round, tumorlike mass or masses that may also cavitate. (3) Extensive reticulonodular or miliary interstitial pattern. (4) A severe form of acute disease in which there is bilateral exudate with the distribution resembling pulmonary alveolar edema. The onset is rapid, and the condition is very toxic in patients. Several patients have developed adult respiratory distress syndrome (ARDS) as a result of this severe disease; this combination is usually fatal.

The chronic form of the blastomycosis in the upper lobe resembles pulmonary tuberculosis. In the most common form, there is a fibronodular appearance consisting of pulmonary nodules and linear fibrotic strands (Figs. 26-10 and 26-11). Only slightly less frequent is cavitary upper lobe disease in which the walls are moderately thick and smooth. Much less common is a masslike appearance, which can closely resemble bronchogenic carcinoma (Fig. 26-12). The disease may ex-

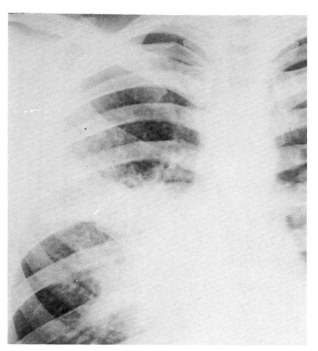

Figure 26–10. North American blastomycosis. Note the extensive disease in the right parahilar and medial basal areas as well as in the central and right lung laterally. Adjacent to the dense homogeneous involvement, several scattered, poorly defined nodules are observed. Roentgenographic findings in this disease are nonspecific.

tend to the pleura, cross interlobar fissures, invade the chest wall, and cause rib destruction but not as frequently as in actinomycosis.

Chest radiographic findings in 63 patients reported by Sheflin and colleagues showed single upper lobe involvement in 27 patients and multilobar disease in 21.[48] In nine, the major abnormality was a pulmonary mass. Pleural effusion and/or adenopathy (hilar or mediastinal) was present in 20%. Cavitation was found in 23 patients. Five patients had diffuse disease and only one had a miliary type of disease.

Blastomycosis is unusual in children except in small epidemics, which have been reported on several occasions. Children develop alveolar disease, with multiple small, thin-walled cavities in about 25% of cases. Hilar adenopathy may also be present, and pleural effusion is not unusual. If children develop the disseminated form, it may be fulminant with a high mortality. Since these changes are similar to those noted in pulmonary tuberculosis, mycotic infections, and other chronic inflammatory diseases as well as neoplasm, the diagnosis must be based on mycologic studies.

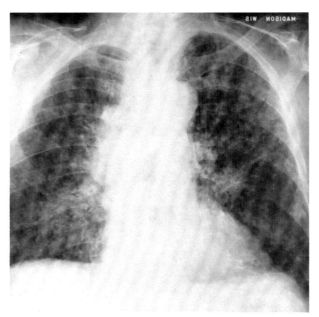

Figure 26–11. North American blastomycosis. Numerous disseminated nodules, ranging up to a centimeter or more in diameter, are observed. On the right, either dense disease overlies the hilum or adenopathy is present, but no adenopathy is noted on the left.

SOUTH AMERICAN BLASTOMYCOSIS (PARACOCCIDIOIDOMYCOSIS)

This disease, caused by *Blastomyces brasiliensis*, is found most commonly in Brazil but has also been reported in the other South American countries. Pulmonary involvement is said to occur in 80% of the patients with the visceral type of disease. The portal of entry may be the intestinal tract in this disease so that the pulmonary lesions are secondary and are widespread and nodular in type, often associated with hilar adenopathy. The disease may also present as a cavitary pulmonary mass.[1] Destructive bone lesions are common in the disseminated form.

PRIMARY ASPERGILLOSIS

Primary pulmonary aspergillosis is rare despite the fact that fungi of the genus *Aspergillus* are ubiquitous. More often it is a secondary process in patients who have been treated with antibiotics and in those with debilitating disease. It occurs rarely as a primary disease in otherwise healthy individuals, however. Two clinical and roentgen types of the primary disease have been described.

1. An acute bronchopneumonic form with scattered

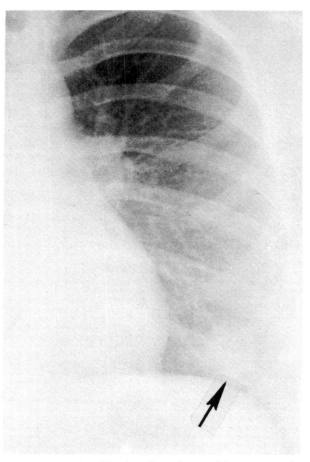

Figure 26–12. North American blastomycosis. The large round mass at the left base resembling a tumor (*arrow*) was the only evidence of pulmonary disease in this patient. Examination after resection proved the mass to be blastomycosis.

multiple areas of pneumonic consolidation, some of which break down to form cavities. This disease may progress with severe invasive destructive pulmonary disease eventually leading to death. The invasive form is usually seen in infants. There is often enough hilar node enlargement to be recognized as such on the roentgenograms.

2. A more chronic and milder form than the first type. Irregular and rounded nodular opacities closely resembling those seen in pulmonary tuberculosis are present. The clinical course of this disease is less severe than that of tuberculosis; the diagnosis must be made on the basis of identification of the organism in the sputum, often with some reservation because the organism is so commonly found there.

SECONDARY ASPERGILLOSIS

Secondary aspergillosis is found in three forms, the aspergilloma (mycetoma), allergic (hypersensitivity) bronchopulmonary aspergillosis, and a severe diffuse form (invasive aspergillosis) found in patients with debilitating disease, malignancies, or AIDS, and those on cytotoxic drugs, steroids, or immunosuppressive agents.

Invasive Aspergillosis

Immunocompromised patients and rarely immunocompetent patients develop invasive aspergillosis. Patients with acute leukemia and granulocytopenia are particularly susceptible. Occasionally, it occurs as a complication of influenza-like viral infections in the noncompromised host. It may be associated with other infections; mucormycosis appears to be the most common of these.[26]

The radiographic changes are quite variable. Airspace disease in the form of "round" pneumonia resembling a poorly defined mass, single or multiple, seems to be a common finding. Many of these lesions eventually cavitate, and some are probably hemorrhagic pulmonary infarcts (Fig. 26-13). The latter results when the organism invades and obstructs a branch of the pulmonary artery. Some of the cavitations exhibit an air crescent sign caused by a mass within the cavity that does not move with a change in the position of the patient and probably represents necrotic tissue in an area of infarction. In other cavities, mycetoma (fungus ball) may develop. A diffuse bronchopneumonia pattern may develop at any time. This may progress to an extensive bilateral pulmonary involvement. Chest wall invasion can occur, with bone destruction, but is not common. If this is complicated by empyema, the prognosis is poor. Rarely, a miliary spread throughout the lung is observed. In these patients, the prognosis is also poor and the immediate cause of death may be aspergillosis. Since the organism is difficult to demonstrate on sputum and blood cultures, procedures such as percutaneous transthoracic aspiration biopsy may be necessary to make the diagnosis.

Mycetoma (Aspergilloma)

The aspergilloma (mycetoma) or fungus ball consists of a localized round or ovoid mass made up of *Aspergillus* hyphae (the mycelial form), blood, cellular debris, fibrin, and mucus, which occupies a cavity slightly larger than the mass. It is usually found in the upper lobe, probably because the primary disease, commonly tuberculosis, occurs in the upper lobe. A thin, radiolucent rim is observed surrounding the mass. This is caused by air in the space between the thin cavity wall and the mass and is virtually pathognomonic. The mass usually moves within the cavity. This can be demonstrated on tomography or CT, which is often helpful in the diagnosis when mycetoma is suspected (Figs. 26-14 and 26-15). Calcification may occur within the mass and may be extensive. Hemorrhage is common

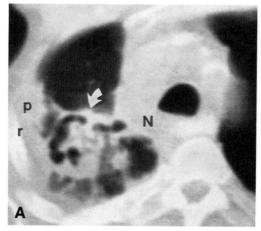
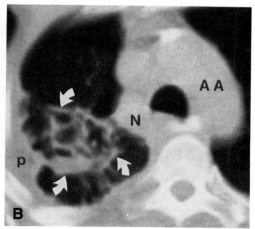

Figure 26–13. Invasive aspergillosis with extensive cavitation of right upper lobe (RUL). (**A**) CT using lung windows. Note extensive pulmonary destruction, cavitation, and loss of volume as compared with the left lung (*curved arrow*). *N*, Homogeneous density representing mediastinal node involvement; *p*, pleural thickening; *r*, rib. (**B**) Two centimeters lower than *A*. *AA*, Aortic arch; *N*, nodes; pulmonary involvement with cavitation (*arrows*), *p*, pleural thickening. (Courtesy of Richard Logan, MD)

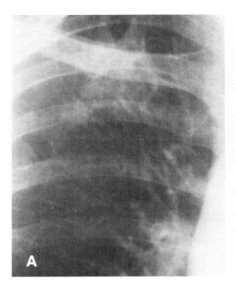

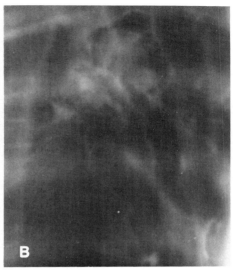

Figure 26–14. Fungus ball. (**A**) This film shows an irregular mass, somewhat obscured by the clavicle and first rib, with some disease below it and above it. (**B**) Tomogram shows a somewhat irregular cavity filled with a mass (fungus ball) separated from the wall by a radiolucent area that is wide superiorly and medially and rather narrow laterally.

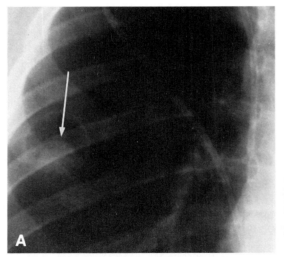

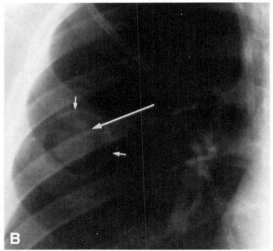

Figure 26–15. Mobile fungus ball (aspergilloma). (**A**) Upright chest film. Dense fungus ball dependent within cavitary area (*arrow*). (**B**) Fungus ball (*large arrow*) in central position in cavity (*small arrows*). (Courtesy of June Unger, MD)

and occasionally may be severe; there are usually no other symptoms.

Rarely, other organisms can form fungus balls. The following organisms, among others, have been implicated: *Candida* species, *Coccidioides immitis, Monosporium, Sporotrichum,* and *Trichophyton* species. The mycetomas usually do not undergo spontaneous lysis, but this occurs in about 10%.

Allergic (Hypersensitivity) Bronchopulmonary Aspergillosis

This form of aspergillosis is seen in patients with chronic bronchial asthma and is presumably caused by a hypersensitivity reaction to antigens of species of the genus *Aspergillus,* chiefly *Aspergillus fumigatus.*[29] Occasionally, the organism is found in the sputum during an initial asthmatic attack or early in the course of bronchial asthma. The patients usually have fever, cough, and mucopurulent sputum, often with expectoration of mucus plugs. Eosinophilia and leukocytosis are usually present. The roentgenographic findings have been divided into transient and permanent shadows.[21] Transient shadows are: (1) Homogeneous consolidation that may be large or small without loss of volume. They may be massive and often are multiple and tend to be central in location. (2) Nonhomogeneous shadow or patchy consolidation. (3) Small, circular, or nodular shadow. (4) Transient atelectasis of a segment lobe or lung. (5) Bandlike and gloved-finger shadow 2 to 3 cm long and 5 to 8 mm wide, at times having a rounded end, caused by mucoid impaction. (6) Two parallel hairline shadows, with a radiolucent zone between the lines representing a normal bronchus (tram line). (7) Well-outlined, circular (ring) shadow with a diameter of 2 to 3 cm, also representing a bronchus.

The permanent shadows include (1) parallel lines similar to tram lines but with a width larger than that of a normal bronchus; (2) hairline ring shadow 1 to 2 cm in diameter; (3) decreased volume but with aeration in the segment or lobe involved; (4) narrowing or loss of vascular shadows; (5) long-line shadows. Most patients progress to varying degrees of pulmonary overinflation, some develop areas of fibrosis, and others have small areas of atelectasis (segmental or less) that may persist. Pleural effusion is rare but may appear. Bronchocentric granulomatosis with severe bronchial necrosis and granuloma formation appears to be a variant. The toothpaste and gloved-finger shadows represent mucus plugs or impactions in most instances (Fig. 26-16). Occasionally, mucoid impaction may occur in asthmatics without aspergillosis. The tram-line shadows represent bronchi that are normal in diameter, whereas parallel-line shadows represent bronchi that are increased in diameter. The ring shadow represents a dilated bronchus observed on end. The latter two findings indicate bronchiectasis, which is usually central and becomes permanent if the patient is not treated promptly. Long-line shadows probably represent a wall of a bulla in some instances and pleura in others. The diagnosis is made on the basis of a history of bronchial asthma, the presence of eosinophilia, and the changing roentgenographic pattern of the lungs as described. This disease usually responds quickly to corticosteroids.

Patients with cystic fibrosis are susceptible, in addition to asthmatics. The complication of bronchopulmonary aspergillosis appears to be a major factor when these cystic fibrosis patients deteriorate rapidly, so prompt treatment is important. If it is important to outline the bronchi for detection of bronchiectasis as

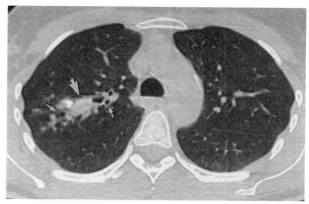

Figure 26-16. Allergic bronchopulmonary aspergillosis, posterior segment of right upper lobe. There is cylindrical bronchiectasis (*small arrows*) adjacent to an area of mucus plugging (*large arrow*). High-resolution CT scan, 2-mm collimation, bone algorithm. (Case courtesy of Julie K. Mitby, MD)

well as extent of the pulmonary involvement, CT is very helpful in evaluation of this disease. Bronchial wall thickening as well as bronchiectasis is usually clearly defined.

MONILIASIS (CANDIDIASIS)

Candida (Monilia) albicans is a yeastlike organism, frequently present in the normal mouth, usually saprophytic, but occasionally mildly pathogenic for humans. Since the organism is often present in the normal individual, it is difficult to document this disease. The literature is very confusing, and many reported cases are probably examples of other diseases. However, most investigators agree that *Monilia* can produce bronchopulmonary disease, particularly in elderly or debilitated persons, immunocompromised hosts, and infants. It is therefore an opportunistic organism that can produce disseminated fatal disease in susceptible subjects. Roentgen findings consist of a rather fine, mottled type of nodulation ranging from 2 mm to 1 cm in diameter associated with some prominence of pulmonary markings or, more commonly, segmental homogeneous consolidation. It may also produce a diffuse bronchopneumonia pattern that may be bilateral.

Segmental or lobar air-space pneumonia has also been described. In infants, it can be a fatal disease with progressive alveolar consolidation and occasional cavitation. It can also be widely disseminated to other organs as well as to the lungs. Cavitation, with or without a mycetoma, is rare but is simulated when the disease involves an area of lung in which there are preexisting emphysematous bullae. There may be some enlargement of the hilar nodes. As in the other fungal diseases, the diagnosis must rest on identification of the organism. The bronchial secretions rather than sputum should be examined since the organism is a normal inhabitant of the mouth.

GEOTRICHOSIS

Geotrichum candidum is a fungus frequently found in the mouth and gastrointestinal tract of healthy subjects, but it occasionally becomes pathogenic and causes pulmonary as well as skin and mucous membrane infection. Pulmonary manifestations of geotrichosis are not characteristic. Irregular patchy densities are noted, often in the upper lungs. Cavitation may develop, the cavities having rather thin walls. Enlargement of the hilar nodes is frequent. The disease may closely resemble pulmonary tuberculosis (Fig. 26-17). *Geotrichum* has a tendency to produce an opportunistic type of pulmonary disease in severely debilitated or immunosuppressed patients. In these patients, bronchopulmonary involvement is often extensive with airspace disease resembling extensive bronchopneumo-

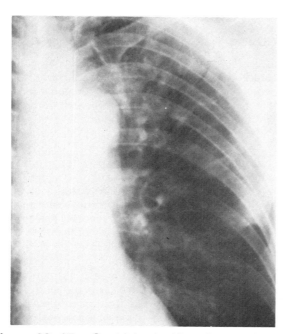

Figure 26–17.   Geotrichosis. Note the nodular disease in the left upper portion of the lung, which resembles pulmonary tuberculosis. Since the disease progressed slowly, resection was done, proving it to be geotrichosis.

nia; often the infection is fatal. Endobronchial disease, with positive sputum cultures and no pulmonary involvement visible on chest films, may also occur in these patients. The diagnosis is based on a positive skin test plus demonstration of the organism on repeated sputum examination. The possibility of other fungal infections, as well as of tuberculosis, must be excluded by appropriate studies, since, in this disease, as in moniliasis, the organism may be saprophytic rather than pathogenic.

OTHER MYCOSES

Sporotrichosis

Sporotrichosis, produced by *Sporotrichum schenckii*, usually involves the skin, mucous membranes, and lymphatics. Rarely, pulmonary infection may be the primary manifestation of the disease, presumably caused by inhalation of spores. Most reported cases have been in the Mississippi and Missouri river valleys.[41] Of all reported cases, 40% have been in alcoholics. There is nothing characteristic about the pneumonia it produces.[32] Cavitation, which may be bilateral, is often observed, however, usually in upper lobes. The pulmonary infection may be local, indolent, and granulomatous and resemble chronic pulmonary tuberculosis, or it may be suppurative and produce foci of bronchopneumonia. Scattered hematogenous small nodular disease is rare, but hilar adenopathy is common. *Sporotrichum schenckii* is sometimes found as a secondary invader in chronic pulmonary tuberculosis.

Penicilliosis

Fungi of the genus *Penicillium* are capable of producing pulmonary infection known as penicilliosis. This disease is very rare. The fungus can cause lung abscess that cannot be distinguished from cavitation produced by other organisms, so that there are no roentgen signs that would lead to the specific diagnosis.

Mucormycosis (Phycomycosis)

Mucor is a genus of fungus widely distributed in nature and is not usually pathogenic to humans. It is a member of the class *Phycomycetes* along with *Absidia* and *Rhizopus*. Several cases of severe disseminated infection due to this fungus have been reported in diabetics. This infection is also found in patients with other underlying debilitating disease, such as leukemia or lymphoma, and in immunosuppressed patients. It is therefore an opportunistic organism usually found most often in patients with hematologic disorders. In some of these, a widespread, rapidly fatal confluent pneumonia that may cavitate is present. The hyphae tend to invade and occlude vessels and the resultant infarction leads to the cavitation. In some instances, mucormycosis may be the cause of a solitary pulmonary nodule.

DISEASES OF SPIROCHETAL ORIGIN

SYPHILIS

Involvement of the lungs in syphilis is very rare, but when this does occur it may simulate other chronic pulmonary diseases symptomatically and radiographically. The diagnosis therefore depends on exclusion of other diseases and on laboratory studies as well as response to antiluetic therapy.

Roentgenographic Findings. Three radiographic types of pulmonary involvement have been described: (1) Interstitial fibrosis resulting in linear opacities radiating into the lungs from the hila. (2) A large solitary mass (gumma) that may be clearly circumscribed and resemble pulmonary tumor. There may be some irregular inflammatory disease surrounding it, so that the lesion may simulate other types of inflammatory disease.[17] (3) Chronic lobar pneumonia with fibrosis and decreased size of the diseased lobe. This type resembles chronic pulmonary tuberculosis. Radiographic findings are not diagnostic, so serologic and histologic studies are necessary.

LEPTOSPIROSIS

Leptospirosis is produced by a group of spirochetes called *Leptospira*. Four of more than 100 serogroups cause most of the disease in humans. Several clinical forms have been described, and pulmonary involvement (in 20%) is only a part of widespread disease in most instances. Occasionally, hemorrhagic pneumonitis is an early or striking manifestation.[23]

Roentgenographic Findings. Three general types have been described. The most common (57% of 58 patients)[18] consists of widely disseminated small areas of air-space consolidation representing hemorrhage and edema. The individual lesions are poorly defined with hazy nodules that resemble other acute, disseminated, pulmonary inflammations. A second type of leptospirosis (16%) is characterized by a large confluent area of consolidation similar to that found in lobar or segmental pneumonia. A third type (27%) consists of small patchy densities that resemble bronchopneumonia or a more linear interstitial type of disease, such as is noted in virus pneumonitis. Im and colleagues describe this type as having a diffuse ground-glass appearance.[18] Pleural effusion, often large, is common. Since the "pneumonia" is hemorrhage, it usually resolves within 2 weeks in patients who survive. The diagnosis cannot be made on the basis of roentgen findings and depends on bacteriologic studies.

PROTOZOAN DISEASES

AMEBIASIS

Amebic infection of the thorax is usually secondary to gastrointestinal involvement, which follows the ingestion of the cysts of *Entamoeba histolytica*. It often is associated with hepatic amebiasis. Rarely (less than 5%), amebic lung abscess or ameboma is found without other signs or symptoms of amebiasis.

The roentgen signs are somewhat different in the two types of disease. In the pulmonary disease without hepatic abscess, parenchymal consolidation often complicated by abscess develops well above the diaphragm. The abscess is similar to lung abscesses produced by other organisms. When an abscess evacuates into a bronchus, an air–fluid level can be demonstrated in upright views. The abscess cavity may become very large, and associate pleural effusion is not uncommon. When an ameboma without cavitation is present, it resembles any other lung mass and must be differentiated from other inflammatory masses and from tumor.

When the pulmonary disease or pleural disease is secondary to hepatic involvement, the appearance is somewhat more characteristic. The hepatic abscess causes elevation of the diaphragm, and fluid in the right pleural space is common. The lower and middle lobes adjacent to the diaphragm are involved by a confluent pneumonia in which cavitation may occur. In some instances the infection is confined to the pleural space, in which case an amebic empyema is formed; this is often loculated at the base. In other instances, there is a combination of pleural and pulmonary involvement with empyema and lung abscess. Amebic lung abscess may rupture into a bronchus and drain spontaneously. Empyema must be drained if it does not rupture into the lung and drain spontaneously. Rarely, hepatic amebic abscess may extend into the pericardium, resulting in amebic pericarditis. The diagnosis is confirmed by the presence of *Entamoeba histolytica* in the sputum or in the pleural fluid.

TOXOPLASMOSIS

Toxoplasmosis is caused by the protozoan parasite *Toxoplasma gondii*. The organism has an affinity for the central nervous system, the eyes, and the lungs. There is an infantile form of the disease in which it is not uncommon to find cerebral involvement, beginning in utero, resulting in scattered intracranial calcifications in the newborn. The disease behaves differently in the adult and involves the lungs primarily rather than the central nervous system. The roentgen findings in the lungs are similar to those noted in bronchopneumonia or viral pneumonia, namely, that of air-space disease often with some interstitial involvement. Enlargement of the hilar nodes is frequently associated with the pulmonary involvement. Miliary dissemination produces opacities not unlike those noted in other acute miliary infections. If the disease becomes chronic, it may result in scattered areas of fibrosis and in scattered nodules, some or all of which may become calcified.

Toxoplasmosis can also be an opportunistic disease involving the central nervous system and the lungs. Radiographic changes in the lung are variable. Widely scattered, small, nodular, or miliary densities have been described as the most common manifestation. In others, there is focal air-space disease bilaterally, and changes simulating interstitial pulmonary edema have also been described. The diagnosis can be made by serologic tests.

PNEUMOCYSTIS CARINII PNEUMONIA

Pneumocystis carinii pneumonia is caused by *Pneumocystis carinii*, a protozoan first observed in animals and thought to be a harmless saprophyte. However, epidemics and sporadic cases of the human disease have been reported in Europe since 1945. The disease has been apparently less frequent in the United States; the first case was reported in 1955. In recent years, it has become very common, particularly as an opportunistic organism. It usually occurs in premature or debilitated infants, in infants or children with agammaglobulinemia or low gamma globulin levels, and in debilitated adults who have been on antibiotic, long-term steroid, cytotoxic, or immunosuppressive therapy. It is most common in patients with acute lymphocytic leukemia, and it is not infrequent in renal transplant patients. Its role in AIDS is discussed in the next section.

The clinical onset may be either rapid or insidious, but there is usually a discrepancy between the physical findings in the chest, which are minimal, and the marked dyspnea and often extensive roentgen findings. Pathologic findings are those of interstitial pneumonia, with mononuclear cells infiltrating the interstitial tissues; very few polymorphonuclear cells are present. The alveoli and alveolar ducts tend to be compressed by the interstitial involvement; there is often enough obstruction to result in peripheral obstructive overinflation (emphysema). Interstitial and alveolar edema may be extensive in severe disease. Simultaneous cytomegalovirus infection is very common.

The roentgen findings are sometimes characteristic.

The disease begins in the hilum and spreads peripherally; ultimately, it may involve the entire lung. There is an element of linear opacity spreading out from the hilum; it often presents as a bilateral diffuse, reticular, interstitial type of pattern. The peripheral lungs are clear and may be "honey-combed" by local areas of emphysema and small areas of atelectasis producing linear opacities, usually basal. As the disease progresses, generalized involvement produces a rather homogeneous density spreading outward from the hila. This may progress to the point of nearly total involvement, the lungs appearing virtually airless. Cytomegalovirus pulmonary infection is often associated with *Pneumocystis* and can produce similar pulmonary radiographic findings. Hilar adenopathy does not usually occur but has been reported in several patients, and evidently nodes rarely calcify.[14] Pleural effusion is uncommon and tends to be minimal. Pneumothorax and pneumomediastinum may occur, usually associated with subpleural cysts or bullae,[10] which are relatively common.[22]

"Atypical" or unusual roentgenographic findings are very common in this disease, having been reported in about 50% of patients. Local segmental and lobar consolidation, which may be bilateral, symmetrical or asymmetrical, and at times mainly unilateral, has been reported. At times, the disease resembles miliary tuberculosis. A nodular pattern resembling hematogenous metastasis and cavitation are other atypical findings that are rare. The disease may also occur with no visible radiographic abnormalities of the chest in 5% to 10% of cases. Some of these patients later develop typical findings on the chest roentgenogram. Since the pattern may not be characteristic, the disease should always be considered when persistent and extensive pneumonic disease is found in immunosuppressed adults (Fig. 26-18), post-transplant patients, and debilitated infants. In the immunosuppressed patient with fever and hypoxemia and in the patient with AIDS, the disease should be suspected even though the plain chest roentgenogram shows no abnormality.[22]

Since *Pneumocystis carinii* cannot be cultured and the disease it causes is usually fatal if treatment is not given, transbronchial biopsy, bronchial brushing, percutaneous transthoracic biopsy, open lung biopsy, or bronchoalveolar lavage is often necessary to obtain material for microbiologic study. Because *Pneumocystis carinii* is present in most patients at some time during the course of AIDS, the latter condition is discussed here.

ACQUIRED IMMUNODEFICIENCY SYNDROME

This syndrome was first recognized in a few patients in 1979. Since then, the number of cases has increased rapidly, so that in 1984, more than 7500 cases were

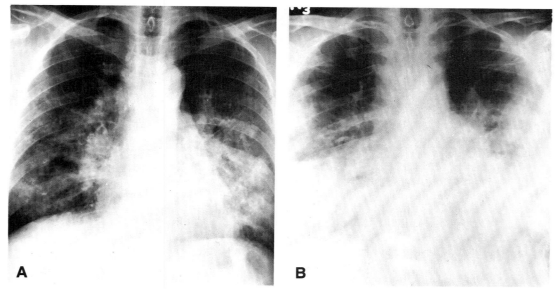

Figure 26–18. Pneumocystis carinii pneumonia. **(A)** Bilateral inflammatory disease with considerable consolidation in the left lower portion of the lung and more scattered disease at the right base. **(B)** Examination 1 month later showed that, although the disease had advanced extensively bilaterally, it was confined to the basal and central lung, sparing the upper lungs. This patient had lymphoma. We have observed wide variability in roentgenographic manifestations of this infestation.

reported to the Center for Disease Control. The incidence has increased rapidly since then. There is a severe deficiency of cell-mediated immunity in these patients, who present with either an opportunistic infection, an unusual neoplasm, or both. Risk groups are as follows: (1) male homosexuals—71%; (2) intravenous drug abusers—17%; (3) Haitians—5%; (4) hemophiliacs—1%; (5) miscellaneous and no known risk factor—6%.

Most patients with AIDS develop pulmonary infections, usually caused by *Pneumocystis carinii*. Percentages quoted vary somewhat, but nearly 80% have P. carinii pneumonia, 10% have both P. carinii pneumonia and Kaposi sarcoma, 15% have Kaposi sarcoma, and the remainder have pulmonary infections caused by a variety of opportunistic organisms that include cytomegalovirus, *Cryptococcus, Toxoplasma, Aspergillus, Candida, Legionella, Coccidioides,* and atypical mycobacteria. A combination of *Pneumocystis*, Kaposi sarcoma, and cytomegalovirus is not unusual.[11] Kaposi sarcoma is often unusually aggressive in these patients but does not always involve the lungs.

The chest radiographic pattern varies in P. carinii pneumonia, but the most common finding in patients with AIDS is a diffuse, reticular, interstitial or a ground-glass pattern starting in parahilar areas and progressing to a diffuse consolidation.[31] Asymmetrical focal opacities usually occur in patients with a second

infection, often fungal. When Kaposi sarcoma is present, a pattern of coarse central, linear, and nodular densities is present, at times associated with hilar adenopathy.[4] Pleural effusion has been reported in up to 50% of patients with Kaposi sarcoma. Differentiation of infection and Kaposi sarcoma in the lung must be made by open lung biopsy, since a satisfactory tumor specimen usually cannot be obtained on transbronchial bronchoscopic biopsy or other methods and the roentgen patterns are not diagnostic.[51]

Lymphoma (non-Hodgkin's) is the other tumor found in patients with AIDS. The tumor is not common but is manifested by adenopathy, pleural effusion in a few, and pulmonary parenchymal nodules, which may grow rapidly.

Clinically, the prodromal symptoms of Pneumocystis pneumonia are prolonged in patients with AIDS; a 3-week history of cough and dyspnea, often preceded by a fever for 6 or 7 weeks, is common. Response to therapy is also slower in these patients than in others. The reason for this is not clear.

Mycobacterium avium complex is also a common cause of infection in AIDS. It usually presents as a systemic infection, but organisms are found in the lungs. It usually causes adenopathy, but little pulmonary change may be recognizable on chest radiographs. Prognosis tends to be poor. Tuberculosis (*M. tuber-*

culosis)[12] is also common in AIDS. It may present as primary or progressive primary disease causing adenopathy, parenchymal disease, and pleural effusion. Miliary disease with unusual increase in size of the miliary nodules may also occur. Reactivation (post-primary) tuberculosis may also be found, usually early in the course of AIDS when the patients have some functioning T cells.

Numerous fungal diseases may also occur, including cryptococcus, histoplasmosis, and coccidioidomycosis, which are fairly common, as well as blastomycosis, candidiasis, sporotrichosis, and nocardiosis. Findings are varied, consisting of scattered alveolar disease, interstitial nodular disease, adenopathy, and pleural effusion. These granulomatous diseases cause nonspecific findings, so biopsy is usually indicated so that prompt, specific treatment can be instituted.

In some AIDS patients, chest radiographs reveal a diffuse linear or reticular pattern, which is nondiagnostic for any specific organism.[50] In some, repeated studies fail to find a causative organism. It is therefore possible that repeated infections with one or more organisms may produce this finding, but cause is not established in some instances.

PLATYHELMINTH (FLATWORM) INFESTATION

ECHINOCOCCOSIS (HYDATID DISEASE)

The small tapeworm, *Echinococcus granulosus*, is found in the intestinal tract of dogs. Its larval form is the cause of hydatid cysts. The ova are ingested by humans and migrate to the liver or lungs, where they produce a round or oval density that may become massive. Since the cyst is readily molded as it grows, the shape may be varied, depending on its relation to the bony thorax. Therefore, it appears on the roentgenogram as a round or oval, clearly defined, dense mass that may produce some adjacent atelectasis. A change in shape may be noted at fluoroscopy and with change in position of the patient. A wall, the pericyst, composed of an external capsule caused by the host tissue, is formed. The hydatid cyst itself has a double wall composed of an outer thick membrane (the exocyst) and a thin inner wall of germinal cells (the endocyst). The cyst may rupture into a bronchus and empty part of its contents, in which case an air–fluid level is noted. This indicates separation of the cyst from the host tissue capsule (pericyst). When this is observed, the roentgenographic diagnosis can be made with reasonable certainty. The collapsed cyst wall may float on the fluid surface and be outlined by air above it on an upright film. This is virtually pathognomonic of hy-

datid disease. Rarely, rupture of the pericyst or host capsule leaves air between it and the exocyst.

The crescent or meniscus sign representing the radiolucent air between the cyst and the host may then be observed, a distinctive roentgen sign of hydatid cyst. Pulmonary cyst walls rarely calcify in contrast to the hepatic lesions, in which calcification is common. When the cyst ruptures, there is a possibility of spread to other parts of the lung, giving rise to multiple, small daughter cysts. Occasionally, many small cysts are scattered throughout the lungs. Rarely, the cysts form in the pleural space or rupture into the pleural space and cause pleural effusion. When calcified hydatid cysts are present in the liver and a pulmonary cyst in the lung is detected, the diagnosis can be made with a considerable degree of accuracy.[45]

CYSTICERCOSIS

Occasionally, humans develop autoinfection when they ingest eggs of the pork tapeworm *Taenia solium*. The eggs emerge as oncospheres in the gastrointestinal tract of humans, enter the blood stream, and are carried to various organs and tissues where they metamorphose into cysticerci. In these individuals the cysticeri may be found scattered widely throughout the tissues, including the lungs, where they produce scattered soft-tissue nodular densities. When the tapeworms die, calcification occurs and multiple oval or spindle-shaped calcifications measuring about 3 by 10 mm can then be noted, scattered in the lungs and in other tissues as well. The disease, cysticercosis, is very rare in the United States but common in Africa, China, and India.

PARAGONIMIASIS

The lung fluke *Paragonimus westermani* is distributed widely in the Far East, particularly Korea, Taiwan, and Indonesia; in Africa; and in parts of South America.[2, 6, 39, 52] Humans are infested by eating undercooked crayfish or crabs or drinking infested water. The larval forms are liberated in the jejunum and migrate through the diaphragm and pleural space and into the lung, where they mature into adult flukes, usually in the lower lobes. The disease is mild and seldom fatal but does produce symptoms in some patients. Hemoptysis is a frequent symptom of infestation with this organism, along with cough productive of brown or rusty sputum and chest pain. In about one-third of those infested, the organism causes an ill-defined consolidation in the lower lung in the form of a hazy shadow of low, uneven density. In about another one-third, the density is more homogeneous, is more clearly defined, and may appear lobulated. Thin-walled cystlike cavitation may develop within the area of consolidation. Often the cavities are multiple and have a bubblelike appearance. In some patients, the disease may be manifested by linear streaks that may appear within a shadow of low-density consolidation. The involved area does not usually occupy a very large volume of the lung and may be unilateral or bilateral. The basal and peripheral midzone pulmonary disease is often not very conspicuous because of the small volume of lung involved and the low density of the disease that may disappear completely. Pleural thickening in the interlobar fissures is also observed, and fleeting densities thought to represent Löffler's pneumonia often accompany the disease. Dense linear opacities are caused by burrows of the organism, which can be demonstrated by bronchography to be independent of bronchi. The burrows probably communicate with the cavities. Pleural effusion is common (in about 50%) and may be the only manifestation of the disease in some patients.

Reports differ somewhat as to incidence of various findings. Suwanik and Harinsuta found the following:[52] (1) Ringlike cystic cavities with crescent-shaped opacity along one side ranging from 6 mm to 4 or 5 cm in 82%. (2) Poorly defined nodular opacities up to 3 or 4 cm, usually basal or peipheral, were found in 48%. (3) Linear shadows present at bases usually associated with ringlike shadows in 21%. (4) Pleural thickening in 21%.

Calcification may develop, probably in dead parasites. Complications include empyema, bronchopleural fistula, and pulmonary cavitation. Ova may be found in the pleural fluid and in the sputum during the periods of hemoptysis. The disease may persist for many years.

SCHISTOSOMIASIS

Schistosomiasis is caused by three blood flukes, *Schistosoma mansoni*, *S. japonicum*, or *S. haematobium*. It is common in many parts of the world, including Africa, Asia, and Puerto Rico, but is rarely, if ever, acquired in the United States. Pulmonary disease is usually caused by *S. mansoni* or *S. japonicum*. Several types of pulmonary reaction to the infestation may occur. As the larval forms pass through the lungs, an apparent allergic response produces transient mottled densities. Roentgen findings in this acute form consist of transient interstitial opacities, usually a fine nodular pattern that may resemble miliary tuberculosis but clears spontaneously without treatment.

Ova reach the lungs from the veins of the bladder, intestine, and liver. They may implant in or around pulmonary arterioles, producing a necrotizing arteritis and intra-arterial and peri-arterial granulomas, which

result in a chronic pulmonary disease. Either of these granulomas may obstruct the vessel. The organisms rarely cause multiple arteriovenous fistulas.

Roentgen findings in the chronic form consist of central enlargement of pulmonary arteries secondary to pulmonary hypertension and evidence of cor pulmonale, which occurs in only 5% of patients with pulmonary disease.[30] More commonly, a diffuse, fine, reticular pattern is observed. At times, the appearance is more nodular, as reaction to the ova produces local densities in the interstitial tissue of the lung. The multiple arteriovenous fistulas caused by the necrotizing arteritis result in cyanosis with very little change noted on roentgenograms; this is a rare phenomenon. Occasionally, a circumscribed nodule is produced by a granulomatous mass surrounding an adult worm.[5]

NEMATHELMINTH (ROUNDWORM) INFESTATION

Several roundworms cause pulmonary symptoms and transitory roentgen changes in the lungs as the larvae are carried to the lungs through the veins or lymphatics. As the larvae emerge from the alveolar capillaries into the bronchial tree, they produce an allergic response, usually accompanied by eosinophilia. A combination of edema and hemorrhage causes radiographic findings of patchy areas of poorly defined opacity scattered throughout the lungs. The changes are transitory, and their extent is related to the severity of the infestation. The following roundworms are among those causing such a reaction: *Ascaris lumbricoides*, *Strongyloides stercoralis*, *Ancylostoma duodenale*, and *Necator americanus* (hookworm disease). Ascariasis is often the cause of a Löffler's type pneumonia, which changes rapidly and usually clears in about 10 days.

Opportunistic pulmonary strongyloidiasis has been reported in compromised hosts, and it may be fatal.[16] However, it responds to treatment with antihelminthic agents if recognized soon enough. The usual pulmonary reaction to *Strongyloides* is similar to that of ascariasis. In the opportunistic form, a variety of lung manifestations have been described, including miliary, lobular, or lobar patterns. Cavitation or pleural effusion is rare. Filariasis due to infestation with *Filaria* or *Wuchereria bancrofti*, *Wuchereria malayi*, or *Loa loa* is probably the cause of tropical eosinophilia (see next section). *Dirofilaria immitis* (dog heartworm) may also cause pulmonary disease in humans.[24, 25] Typically, it produces a solitary pulmonary nodule, often peripheral, without calcification and with a slightly irregular appearance. At first the small area of consolidation may be poorly defined, but then it tends to decrease in size over a few weeks or months. Then the nodule becomes more clearly defined. Rarely, multiple nodules are observed that may resemble pulmonary metastases. They produce no symptoms. Histologic examination of tissue is required to differentiate the nodule from tumor. *Trichinella spiralis* larvae usually produce no pulmonary reaction as they pass through the pulmonary circulation. In the roundworm infestations, the diagnosis is made by discovery of the larvae or mature worm in a stool specimen.

TROPICAL EOSINOPHILIA

Tropical eosinophilia or pulmonary eosinophilosis is manifested by symptoms of cough, fever, lassitude, wheezing, chest pain, and sometimes dyspnea and weight loss associated with an elevation of the white blood cell count. Eosinophilia is extreme (usually more than 3000 eosinophils per cubic millimeter of blood) and persists for weeks. Most reported cases originate in India, Indonesia, Sri Lanka, Pakistan, Southeast Asia, North Africa, and some areas of South America. A few have been reported in the United States and elsewhere throughout the world, largely in persons who have been in an endemic area. Some cases have also been reported in persons who have lived in India but who have been away more than a year before the onset of symptoms. The disease is mild and self-limited, but relapses may occur. Most cases are definitely caused by filarial infestation, usually by *Wuchereria bancrofti*, and the disease usually responds well to diethylcarbamazine, a drug effective in filariasis.[38] In other cases, the cause cannot be established.

Roentgen findings are of several types. The most common appearance is that of increased pulmonary markings extending out from the hila, associated with mottled parenchymal disease that is rather general in distribution. The hilar nodes may be enlarged. Next in frequency is the addition of areas of patchy pneumonitis to the small mottled densities. Increased markings alone are nearly as frequent, and extensive scattered involvement by a pneumonia-like process is noted occasionally. The apices are usually spared.

SARCOIDOSIS

Sarcoidosis is discussed here because its histopathology is similar to that of several chronic inflammatory diseases, although the etiology is not definite.

Sarcoidosis, or Boeck's sarcoid, is a granulomatous disease that may affect many organs and tissues in the body. The etiology is not clear. Several theories have been advanced but none has been proved. It is probably the result of interaction between an infective agent (not necessarily the same in all patients) and an individual with unusual immunologic responses. On average, there are ten times more lymphocytes in the fluid from bronchoalveolar lavage of patients with sarcoidosis than in normal controls. Most are T lymphocytes, with a decrease in B lymphocytes. The ratio of T to B lymphocytes is reversed in the blood of patients with sarcoidosis, with an increase in T lymphocytes and a decrease in B lymphocytes. These changes in cell populations reflect the fact that pulmonary sarcoidosis is initially an alveolitis characterized by diffuse infiltration of monocytes, macrophages, and lymphocytes. As the alveolitis resolves, it is replaced by multinucleated giant cell granulomas. It is known that most patients show no reaction or only slightly positive reaction to tuberculin, and 10% to 20% of patients with sarcoidosis develop frank tuberculosis. The process resembles a tuberculous granuloma except that there is no central caseation necrosis. The lesions develop slowly and may resolve completely in some instances. They may also heal by a process of sclerosis leading to fibrosis and tissue distortion that may be extensive. Pulmonary involvement is common; the reported incidence ranges from 90% to 95%. These figures include enlargement of hilar and paratracheal nodes as well as pulmonary parenchymal lesions.

Roentgenographic Findings. Since sarcoidosis may be asymptomatic or nearly so for long periods, the roentgenographic changes produced by it are often noted for the first time in a survey film or on roentgenograms obtained as part of an examination performed before entrance into the armed services or industry. It is therefore somewhat difficult to be certain that the findings observed in these asymptomatic patients represent early disease.

Roentgen findings can be classified as follows:[20, 36]

Stage 0. No abnormality is defined.

Stage 1. Hilar and paratracheal adenopathy without parenchymal involvement (see Fig. 26-16). This occurs at some time during the course of the disease in more than 90% of patients with sarcoidosis. Although bilateral hilar and right paratracheal adenopathy has been reported as characteristic of the disease, a study of 62 patients with sarcoidosis[3] showed that bilateral hilar adenopathy was the most common, followed by adenopathy in the right paratracheal area or aortopulmonary window area on the left. More than a third had a combination of bilateral hilar adenopathy, right paratracheal adenopathy, and aortopulmonary window nodes. Anterior mediastinal nodes and para-aortic posterior mediastinal nodes are found only in patients with combinations of bilateral hilar nodes with or without right paratracheal and aortopulmonary window nodes.

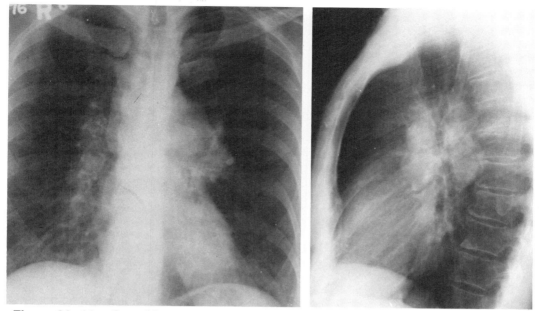

Figure 26–19. Sarcoidosis. Hilar and right paratracheal adenopathy, which is rather characteristic of sarcoidosis.

Stage 2. Adenopathy with parenchymal involvement. The parenchymal involvement includes a diffuse accentuation of interstitial markings resulting in a reticular pattern, a miliary nodular pattern, and a reticular pattern plus miliary nodules (reticulonodular) or somewhat larger nodules (Figs. 26-19 and 26-20). This combination of an increase in linear interstitial shadows plus nodules, the reticulonodular pattern, is more common than either of the changes occurring alone. An air-space or acinar type of disease may also occur in the lungs. It resembles an acute inflammatory process with poorly defined periphery and, at times, an air bronchogram. Although this is a matter of some controversy, "alveolar" sarcoidosis appears to be caused by collapse of the alveolar walls by a confluence of interstitial granulomas rather than by intra-alveolar fluid or cells (Fig. 26-21). The amount of general interstitial change may be varied when associated with nodularity. There is often an inverse relationship between the adenopathy and parenchymal disease, the latter increasing while the adenopathy regresses. This does not ordinarily occur in Hodgkin's disease from which sarcoidosis must be differentiated.[3]

Stage 3. Parenchymal involvement without adenopathy.

Stage 4. Fibrotic change progressing to pulmonary insufficiency, with cor pulmonale. There may be exten-

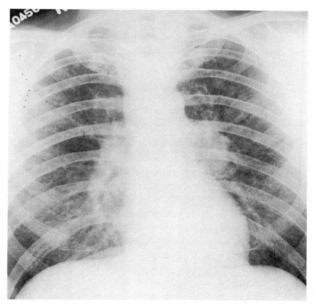

Figure 26–20. Sarcoidosis. In this patient there is bilateral hilar adenopathy, some paratracheal adenopathy (more on the right than on the left), and moderately extensive pulmonary parenchymal involvement manifested by small, widely scattered nodules and a small increase in interstitial opacities.

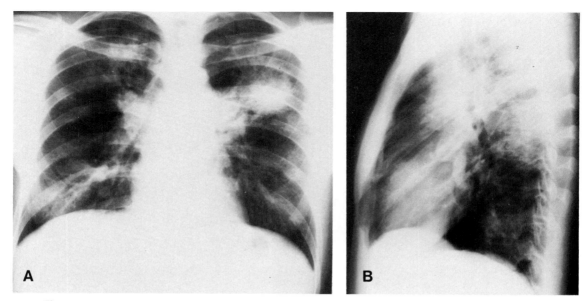

Figure 26–21. "Alveolar" sarcoidosis. Note the hilar adenopathy and the large poorly defined areas of parenchymal involvement lateral to the left hilum in the right clavicular area and at the right base in the frontal view (**A**). Basal disease is not very well outlined in the lateral view (**B**).

sive distortion with conglomerate areas of fibrosis and emphysema. This is the late irreversible form of the disease (Fig. 26-22). It occurs in 20% to 25% of patients with sarcoidosis. It is somewhat more common in patients with acinar form than in those having other forms of sarcoidosis.

UNUSUAL FORMS OF PULMONARY SARCOIDOSIS

Large nodular densities ranging up to 5 cm or more are occasionally found. They resemble hematogenous pulmonary metatases to some extent but are not as clearly defined, since the periphery of the individual nodules tends to be indistinct. They may become confluent. Occasionally, cavitation may be seen in large nodular or alveolar sarcoidosis.[46] The cavitations are probably caused by ischemic necrosis of conglomerate granulomas. They are usually round with thin, smooth walls and range from 3 to 5 cm in diameter; they may persist for months with little change. We have also observed a unilateral solitary nodular mass that resembled primary lung tumor. Unilateral interstitial disease may also occur. Calcification in mediastinal nodes is also observed in some patients. It usually occurs in those who have persistent long-term disease involving parenchyma and nodes and may be peripheral (eggshell)

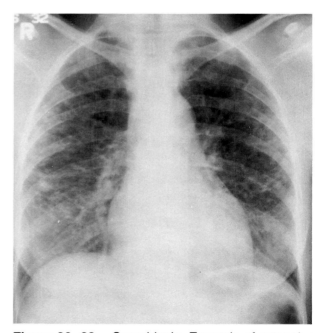

Figure 26–22. Sarcoidosis. Example of extensive parenchymal involvement that is somewhat reticulonodular. Some of the nodules appear rather large. No evidence of hilar adenopathy is observed.

in type. The calcification appears in the second or third decade after onset of the disease.

Late in the disease a somewhat cystic pattern may be observed, usually associated with extensive fibrosis (Fig. 26-23), which results in bullous emphysema. Pleural involvement is rare, but CT studies show that minor pleural changes may be present more frequently than earlier studies suggested. When present, pleural involvement may cause a small pleural effusion or pleural thickening. Mycetoma (fungus ball) is found occasionally in pulmonary sarcoidosis. Other occasional findings include spontaneous pneumothorax and atelectasis, the latter evidently secondary to endobronchial involvement. Since the roentgen findings in this disease are so varied, sarcoidosis must be considered in all asymptomatic patients with unusual pulmonary roentgenographic findings.

All of these manifestations can be seen at various times in a single patient, and the mediastinal adenopathy has been observed to regress and reappear in patients with disseminated pulmonary lesions. The node enlargement is often massive but is usually symmetrical in the hila, and the descriptive term *potato nodes* has been applied to the large masses. The enlarged nodes form slightly lobulated masses extending throughout the hilum. Characteristically, there is a relatively translucent space between the mass of nodes and the cardiovascular margin. This is more apparent on the right side, where the hilum normally is better seen than on the left. In contrast, Hodgkin's disease, which

is a frequent source of difficulty in differential diagnosis, is more likely to involve the more centrally situated nodes around the tracheal bifurcation in addition to those in the hila, and the mass of nodes tends to merge with the cardiovascular silhouette.

The radiographic findings are of some prognostic significance, since those patients in whom hilar and paratracheal adenopathy are observed without pulmonary parenchymal involvement often regress to complete disappearance of the large nodes over months or years. Miliary nodular or reticulonodular disease with or without adenopathy also regresses completely in most patients. Steroids are used effectively in some patients, but long-term studies show that the effect may not persist, so that the course of the disease probably is not altered.

High-resolution thin-section CT is being used in several institutions to study patients with sarcoidosis and other interstitial diseases. Parenchymal involvement is now recognized to be present in several stage 1 (by routine chest radiography) cases. This may be of value in determining the method of further diagnostic study (needle biopsy versus open lung biopsy) in this and other interstitial diseases. Also, it may be of value in determining whether treatment is instituted. The CT findings consist of small nodules and irregular linear opacities along the bronchovascular bundles, interlobular septa, major fissures, and subpleural areas.[37] Patchy focal increases in lung opacity appear to be related to active alveolitis.[28] Obstruction of the supe-

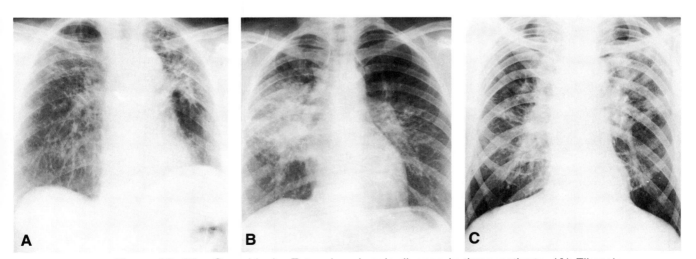

Figure 26–23. Sarcoidosis. Extensive chronic disease in three patients. **(A)** Fibrosis with elevation of the hila is evident in this patient. **(B)** In this patient unusual asymmetry is noted. **(C)** Hilar adenopathy persists along with extensive parenchymal involvement in the third patient.

rior vena cava, innominate vein, and pulmonary artery has also been reported. Occasionally, the disease is aggressive, progressing rapidly over a few years.

Prognosis, classification and physiologic correlation are discussed by McLoud and colleagues, using the ILO/UC classification for the pneumoconioses.[33] Bronchoalveolar lavage and gallium scanning appear to be very useful in staging the patients and predicting prognosis.

The roentgen diagnosis of sarcoidosis can often be made with a considerable degree of certainty. The symmetry of the bilateral hilar node enlargement along with the frequent associated enlargement of the right paratracheal and aortopulmonary window nodes is characteristic. The pulmonary parenchymal involvement is often symmetrical also, and this is of diagnostic importance. The discrepancy between the extensive roentgen changes and the mild symptoms is the third finding of diagnostic significance. Finally, when progress roentgenograms are available, the long and slowly progressing or regressing nature of the process can be observed. The diagnosis must be confirmed by the presence of the typical granuloma in involved nodes; therefore, it is necessary to perform scalene node biopsy or a lung biopsy to secure positive proof of the disease. The fibrotic stage of the disease is probably irreversible to a certain extent, but improvement has been obtained in some patients by the use of steroids, perhaps indicating that the observed findings did not actually represent fibrosis.

Differential Diagnosis. Pulmonary lesions of sarcoidosis can simulate those of pulmonary tuberculosis to such a degree that bacteriologic and histopathologic studies are required to make differentiation. It is often possible, however, to be fairly certain of the diagnosis because of the relative lack of symptoms in the patient with sarcoidosis. In differentiation between sarcoidosis and carcinomatosis, the wasting and weakness usually noted in patients with carcinomatosis and the presence of a known primary tumor along with clinical and roentgen findings make the diagnosis of carcinomatosis almost certain. Hodgkin's disease and lymphoma may result in mediastinal lymph node enlargement, which cannot be differentiated from that noted in sarcoidosis. However, these conditions usually produce more symptoms than sarcoidosis and the adenopathy is not as symmetrical as in sarcoidosis. The more benign types of Hodgkin's disease, however, may be relatively asymptomatic, and biopsy is necessary to differentiate the two diseases. In general, the nodes are larger in Hodgkin's disease than in sarcoidosis. Other chronic pulmonary lesions such as mycotic infections, the pneumoconioses, and several conditions producing interstitial pulmonary fibrosis may result in opacities in the lungs similar to those noted in sarcoidosis. In these patients all clinical data must be evaluated along with the history to make the differentiation. Even then it is often necessary to obtain biopsy specimens of available peripheral or scalene nodes or of the lung. In some patients with the characteristic lesions and clinical symptoms of erythema nodosum, roentgen examination of the chest reveals enlarged hilar nodes and, occasionally, linear and patchy opacities in the perihilar zones, resembling in all respects the changes of sarcoid disease. This does not necessarily indicate that the primary disease is sarcoidosis, but the combination of findings is very suggestive of this diagnosis.

REFERENCES AND SELECTED READINGS

1. AGIA GA, HURST DJ, ROGERS WA: Paracoccidioidomycosis presenting as a cavitating pulmonary mass. Chest 78:650, 1980

2. BARRETT-CONNOR E: Parasitic pulmonary disease. Am Rev Respir Dis 126:558, 1982

3. BEIN ME, PUTMAN CE, McLOUD TC, ET AL: A reevaluation of intrathoracic lymphadenopathy in sarcoidosis. Am J Roentgenol 131:409, 1978

4. BROWN RKJ, HUBERMAN RP, VANLEY G: Pulmonary features of Kaposi sarcoma. Am J Roentgenol 139:659, 1982

5. CHAIT A: Schistosomiasis mansoni: Roentgenologic observations in a nonendemic area. Am J Roentgenol 90:688, 1963

6. CHARTRES JC: Radiological manifestations of parasitism by the tongue worms, flat worms and the round worms more commonly seen in the tropics. Br J Radiol 38:503, 1965

7. DRUTZ DD, CATANZARO A: Coccidioidomycosis. State of the art, Part II. Am Rev Respir Dis 117:727, 1978

8. FEIGIN DS: Pulmonary cryptococcosis: Radiologic-pathologic correlates of its three forms. Am J Roentgenol 141:1263, 1983

9. FELSON B: Less familiar patterns of pulmonary granulomas. Am J Roentgenol 81:211, 1959

10. FEUERSTEIM IM, ARCHER A, PLUDA JM, ET AL: Thin-walled cavities, cysts and pneumothorax in Pneumocystis carinii pneumonia: Further observations with histopathologic correlation. Radiology 174:697, 1990

11. GAMSU G, HECHT ST, BIRNBERG FA, ET AL: Pneumocystis carinii pneumonia in homosexual men. Am J Roentgenol 139:647, 1982

12. GOODMAN PC: Pulmonary tuberculosis in patients with acquired immunodeficiency syndromes. J Thorac Imaging 5:38, 1990

13. GOODWIN RA JR, DES PREZ RM: Histoplasmosis. State of the art. Am Rev Respir Dis 117:929, 1978

14. GROSKIN SA, MASSI AF, RANDALL PA: Calcified hilar and

mediastinal lymph nodes in an AIDS patient with Pneumocystis carinii infection. Radiology 175:345, 1990

15. GROSSMAN CB, BRAGG DG, ARMSTRONG D: Roentgen manifestations of pulmonary nocardiosis. Radiology 96: 325, 1970

16. HIGENBOTTAM TW, HEARD BE: Opportunistic pulmonary strongyloidiasis complicating asthma treated with steroids. Thorax 31:226, 1976

17. HOLLINGSWORTH G: Gumma of lung. Br J Radiol 24:467, 1951

18. IM JG, YEON KM, HAN MC, ET AL: Leptospirosis of the lung: Radiographic findings in 58 patients. Am J Roentgenol 152:955, 1989

19. KERKERING TM, DUMA RJ, SHADOMY S: The evolution of pulmonary cryptococcosis. Ann Intern Med 94:611, 1981

20. KIRKS DR, GREENSPAN RH: Sarcoid. Radiol Clin North Am 11:279, 1973

21. KLEIN DL, GAMSU G: Thoracic manifestations of aspergillosis. Am J Roentgenol 134:543, 1980

22. KUHLMAN JE, KAVURN M, FISHMAN EK, ET AL: Pneumocystis carinii pneumonia: Spectrum of CT findings. Radiology 175:711, 1990

23. LEE REF, TERRY SI, WALKER TM, ET AL: The chest radiograph in leptospirosis in Jamaica. Br J Radiol 54:939, 1981

24. LEONARDI HK, LAPEY JD, ELLIS FH JR: Pulmonary dirofilariasis: Report of a human case. Thorax 32:612, 1977

25. LEVINSON ED, ZITER FMH, WESTCOTT JL: Pulmonary lesions due to dirofilaria immitis (dog heartworm). Radiology 131:305, 1979

26. LIBSHITZ HI, PAGANI J: Aspergillosis and mucormycosis: Two types of opportunistic fungal infection. Radiology 140:301, 1981

27. LLOYD JE, TILLMAN BF, ATKINSON JB: Mediastinal fibrosis complicating histoplasmosis. Medicine 67:295, 1988

28. LYNCH DA, WEBB WR, GAMSU G, ET AL: Computed tomography in pulmonary sarcoidosis. J Comput Assist Tomogr 13:405, 1989

29. MALO JL, PEPYS J, SIMON G: Studies in chronic allergic bronchopulmonary aspergillosis. 2. Radiological findings. Thorax 32:262, 1977

30. MARCHAND EJ, MARCIAL-ROJAS RA, RODRIGUEZ R, ET AL: The pulmonary obstruction syndrome in Schistosoma mansoni pulmonary endarteritis. Arch Intern Med 100: 965, 1957

31. MCCAULEY DI, NAIDICH DP, LEITMAN BS, ET AL: Radiographic patterns of opportunistic lung infections and Kaposi sarcoma in homosexual men. Am J Roentgenol 139:653, 1982

32. MCGAVRAN MH, KOBAYASHI G, NEWMARK L, ET AL: Pulmonary sporotrichosis. Dis Chest 56:547, 1969

33. MCLOUD TC, EPLER GR, GAENSLER EA, ET AL: A radiographic classification for sarcoidosis. Physiologic correlation. Invest Radiol 17:129, 1982

34. MCGAHAN JP, GRAVES DS, PALMER PES, ET AL: Classic and contemporary imaging of coccidioidomycosis. Am J Roentgenol 136:393, 1981

35. MILLER WT JR, EDELMAN JM, MILLER WT: Cryptococcal pulmonary infections in patients with AIDS: Radiographic appearance. Radiology 175:725, 1990

36. MITCHELL DN, SCADDING JG: Sarcoidosis. State of the art. Am Rev Respir Dis 110:774, 1974

37. MULLER WL, KULLNIG P, MILLER RR: The CT findings of pulmonary sarcoidosis: Analysis of 25 patients. Am J Roentgenol 152:1179, 1989

38. NEVA FA, OTTESEN EA: Tropical (filarial) eosinophilia. N Engl J Med 298:1129, 1978

39. OGAKWU M, NWOKOLO C: Radiological findings in pulmonary paragonimiasis as seen in Nigeria: A review based on 100 cases. Br J Radiol 46:699, 1973

40. PITCHENIK AE, ZAUNBRECHER F: Superior vena cava syndrome caused by *Nocardia asteroides*. Am Rev Respir Dis 117:795, 1978

41. PLUSS JL, OPAL SM: Pulmonary sporotrichosis: Review of treatment and outcome. Medicine 65:143, 1986

42. PUTNAM JS, HARPER WK, GREEN JF JR, ET AL: Coccidioides immitis. A rare cause of pulmonary mycetoma. Am Rev Respir Dis 112:733, 1975

43. RABINOWITZ JG, BUSCH J, BUTTRAM WR: Pulmonary manifestations of blastomycosis. Radiology 120:25, 1976

44. RABY N, FORBES G, WILLIAMS R: Nocardia infection in patients with liver transplants or chronic liver disease: Radiologic findings. Radiology 174:713, 1990

45. REEDER MM: RPC of the month from the AFIP (hydatid cyst). Radiology 95:429, 1970

46. ROCKHOFF SD, ROHATGI PK: Unusual manifestations of thoracic sarcoidosis. Am J Roentgenol 144:513, 1985

47. SCHWARZ J, BAUM GL: Fungus diseases of the lungs. Semin Roentgenol V:1, 1970

48. SHEFLIN JR, CAMPBELL JA, THOMPSON GP: Pulmonary blastomycosis: Findings on chest radiographs in 63 patients. Am J Roentgenol 154:1177, 1990

49. SLADE PR, SLESSER BV, SOUTHGATE J: Thoracic actinomycosis. Thorax 28:73, 1973

50. SUFFREDINI AF, OGNIBENE FP, LACK EE, ET AL: Nonspecific interstitial pneumonitis: A common cause of pulmonary disease in the acquired immunodeficiency syndrome. Ann Intern Med 107:7, 1987

51. SUSTER B, AKERMAN M, ORENSTEIN M, ET AL: Pulmonary manifestations of AIDS: Review of 106 episodes. Radiology 161:87, 1986

52. SUWANIK R, HARINSUTA C: Pulmonary paragonimiosis. Am J Roentgenol 81:236, 1959

Paul and Juhl's Essentials of Radiologic Imaging, Sixth Edition, edited by John H. Juhl and Andrew B. Crummy. J.B. Lippincott Company, Philadelphia, © 1993.

CHAPTER **27**

Diseases of Occupational, Chemical, and Physical Origin

John H. Juhl

The term "pneumoconiosis" refers to the group of conditions in which solid foreign substances, usually inorganic dusts of varying degrees of pathogenicity, are inhaled and stored in the lung.[26] These conditions form a group of occupational diseases of considerable economic importance. Some of them may cause enough atmospheric pollution to cause pulmonary disease in people who live near the source. Many foreign materials are capable of producing fibrosis leading to decrease in pulmonary function, while some substances included in this section do not cause significant fibrosis or alteration in pulmonary function. The latter include coal dust (anthracosis), iron oxide (siderosis), barium sulfate (baritosis), and tin (stannosis). Benign changes have also been reported with exposure to titanium oxide and tungsten carbide. Some of these dust diseases occur together, in which case terms such as "anthrasilicosis" and "siderosilicosis" are used to designate them. The ILO 1980 International Classification System should be consulted in the evaluation of pulmonary disability in patients with industrial or environmental exposure.[30] This system is also used to classify diseases for statistical or epidemiologic purposes because it provides a quantitative method using standard radiographs for comparison. It is the latest modification of a classification system that has been updated a number of times since 1930.[31]*

* The ILO 1980 Standard Radiographs may be purchased from the International Labor Office, 1750 New York Avenue, N.W., Washington, D.C. 20006.

SILICOSIS

Silicosis is caused by inhalation of silicon dioxide particles that are 0.5 to 5 microns or less in diameter. Most particles 5 to 10 microns in diameter are removed from the upper respiratory tract, probably by ciliary action.

According to the U.S. Public Health Service, concentrations below 5×10^6 particles less than 10 microns in size per cubic foot do not cause silicosis, while concentrations of 100×10^6 particles or more of similar diameter will cause silicosis in all exposed persons. The most active particles in producing the fibrotic reaction are those smaller than 3 microns. When these small particles are deposited in the alveoli, they are ingested by phagocytic cells—the alveolar macrophages. A number of macrophages are killed, stimulating the formation of collagen in the area. Relatively acellular silicotic nodules are then produced in alveoli, respiratory bronchioles, lymphatics, and lymphoid tissue. Some of them remain in the peripheral lymphoid follicles while others reach the intrapulmonary, bronchial, hilar, and paratracheal nodes. There is some evidence to suggest that an adsorbed protein on the silica particle acts as an antigen, which results eventually in an antibody reaction. This would explain the long latent period as well as progression of the disease long after the patient has been removed from exposure to silica.

Silicosis is found in a large number of industries including mining, foundries, and rock drilling, as well as grinding involving the production of silica dust. The development of fibrosis requires time. In most occupations, the average time for development of disease in workers exposed to moderate concentrations of silica is 20 years or more. Accelerated silicosis is said to occur when the exposure has occurred over 5 to 20 years. When dust counts are unusually high, exposure of less than 5 years may cause acute silicosis. This acute disease, produced by intense exposure over relatively short periods, may progress to severe respiratory failure and death within a year of the onset of symptoms. The patients are often acutely ill, with fever, cough, dyspnea, and weight loss. This type of disease may occur in tunnel workers, sandblasters, and in mining and milling of silica into a fine powder (silica flour). Roentgen findings are quite different than in simple silicosis. There is a perihilar alveolar process, with air bronchograms. The appearance is similar to alveolar proteinosis, except that it involves the suprahilar areas more than the lung bases. Silicotic nodular opacities are helpful in making the diagnosis, but may not be present.

RADIOGRAPHIC OBSERVATIONS

Since radiographic findings in silicosis early in its development are similar to those in a number of diseases, it is essential to obtain an adequate history of exposure to make or suggest the diagnosis. Scattered small, round nodular opacities are found in the upper and central portions of the lung as the initial roentgenographic change (Fig. 27-1). At first the opacities are discrete and small, on the order of 1 to 2 mm in diameter. At this stage, it is likely that an additive effect caused by overlapping nodules is necessary to make them visible. They are usually distributed symmetrically and widely, with a tendency to spare the lung bases. These opacities are usually clearly defined and uniform in density. They may be accompanied by small, irregular opacities, which are fewer in number than the round ones. The nodules gradually increase in size (Fig. 27-2). This may be termed "simple" or uncomplicated silicosis.

As the pulmonary nodules continue to increase in size, to 1 cm or more in diameter, they may coalesce and tend to become conglomerate (progressive massive fibrosis) (Fig. 27-3). The conglomeration and coalescence are usually accompanied by retraction toward the hilum, leaving the periphery of the lung overinflated and relatively free of nodules (complicated silicosis). By the time this stage is reached there is often enough emphysema present to cause downward displacement of the diaphragm and a decrease in diaphragmatic motion with respiration. There can be a considerable variation in the relative amounts of nodulation, hilar enlargement, and emphysema. Hilar node enlargement is common and may become appar-

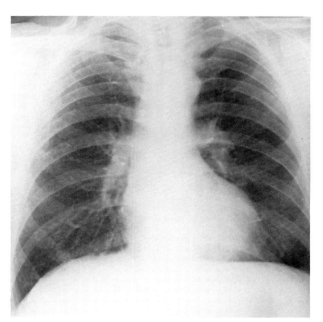

Figure 27–1. Silicosis. Scattered small nodules are associated with minimal prominence of interstitial markings representing early nodular silicosis. Category 1, ILO Classification, 1980.[31]

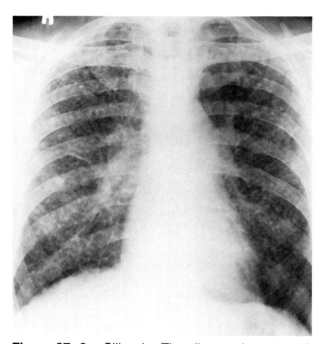

Figure 27–2. Silicosis. The disease is more advanced than in the patient shown in Figure 27-1. The nodules are larger, much more easily outlined, and probably more profuse. There is also hilar node enlargement. This type of silicosis is similar to category III of the ILO Classification.[30]

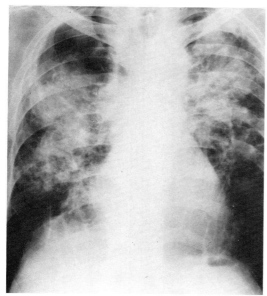

Figure 27–3. Category C silicosis. There is basal emphysema as well as conglomerate nodular disease (progressive massive fibrosis), which is extensive in both lungs.

ent at any time during the development of the pulmonary abnormalities. The hilar nodes may undergo fibrosis and decrease in size by the time the nodular parenchymal lesions are large enough to be detected readily. Occasionally there is calcification in the silicotic pulmonary nodules. This is a manifestation of long-standing disease. In complicated silicosis, progressive massive fibrosis may ultimately cause migration of the conglomerate nodules toward the hila, and often slightly above them. Large, dense masses are then observed slightly above and lateral to the hilum. Although this process is bilateral, it is not always symmetric. When this occurs, peripheral emphysema may become very severe. Very few nodules or pulmonary vessels are observed in this hyperlucent peripheral pulmonary tissue.

The hilar nodes are sometimes outlined because of the presence of a thin shell of calcium peripherally. This has been termed "eggshell calcification," and when present it is very suggestive of silicosis. However, this type of calcification has also been described in patients with no exposure to silica or silicates and has been described in sarcoidosis, postradiation Hodgkin's disease, blastomycosis, histoplasmosis, scleroderma, and amyloidosis (Fig. 27-4). Rarely, an "eggshell" node may erode a bronchial wall and become a broncholith.

The diagnosis of silicosis can often be suspected on roentgen examination, but the clinical history is of great importance, because the diagnosis cannot accurately be made unless there is a history of enough exposure to silica-containing dust to produce it. Because workers in "dusty" industries are often followed at intervals by means of chest roentgenograms, a review of these serial films will often lead to an accurate diagnosis. Extensive roentgen findings can be present without much alteration in pulmonary function; the reverse is also true in some instances; therefore, there may be lack of correlation between roentgen appearance and pulmonary function.

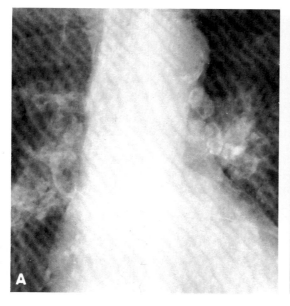
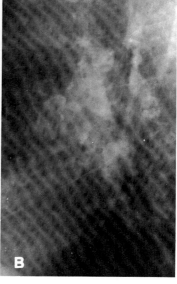

Figure 27–4. Eggshell node calcification in silicosis demonstrated in (**A**) frontal and (**B**) lateral projections.

CT has been correlated with plain films and pulmonary function tests in silicosis.[7] The amount of the emphysema correlated well with pulmonary function tests, but profusion of pulmonary nodules did not. High-resolution, thin-section CT has also been used in the study of silicosis. Nodules ranging from 1 to 10 mm in diameter in the posterior aspect of the upper lung zones appear to be characteristic. In severe disease the conglomerate nodules are defined.[46] The ultimate place of CT in management of patients with silicosis has yet to be determined.

SILICOTUBERCULOSIS

Tuberculosis is known to complicate silicosis. However, silicosis patients' immune systems are compromised, so they tend to be susceptible to other infectious diseases as well. Massive areas of density representing conglomerate fibrosis (progressive massive fibrosis) are seen late in the course of silicosis, and some believe infection is necessary to produce these large masses. The typical location for progressive massive conglomerate fibrosis with or without tuberculosis is above and lateral to the hilum in the infraclavicular part of the lung. The masses are usually bilateral and are often symmetric in size and location. Usually the mass does not reach to the periphery of the lung; rather, a zone of emphysematous lung is to be seen lateral to the area of fibrosis, the emphysema developing as the involved lung shrinks with increasing fibrosis.

Atypical forms of conglomerate fibrosis are not uncommon. Thus a mass of fibrous tissue may be present in one lung and not in the other; the lesions may occur in areas other than the subclavicular zones. Progressive massive fibrosis is often present with little or none of the characteristic nodulation of silicosis in the remainder of the lung, so when massive fibrosis is observed in the presence of nodular silicosis, pulmonary tuberculosis should be suspected (Fig. 27-5). Cavitation occurs in silicotuberculosis, but it is also observed in the absence of infection. Bacteriologic confirmation is necessary, but is sometimes very difficult to obtain. In the absence of positive bacteriologic findings, silicotuberculosis should be suspected when the roentgenograms reveal the large conglomerate masses in the upper lung and cavitation is present, when the disease is asymmetric, and when there is a considerable amount of pleural disease. Patients with such roentgenographic findings should be followed carefully by means of frequent chest roentgenograms and examination of sputum and bronchial aspirates to exclude tuberculosis. Cavitation in conglomerate nodular silicosis, as noted earlier, is not always indicative of tuberculosis. In one series of 182 patients with cavitation, 18% were found to be non-

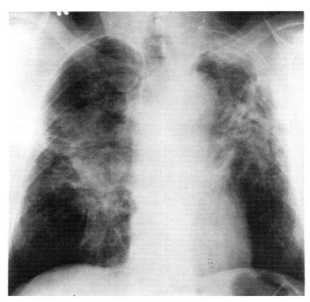

Figure 27–5.   Silicotuberculosis, with bilateral conglomerate disease. Several cavities are present in the left upper lobe, and tubercle bacilli were found in the sputum.

tuberculous. In these patients the cavity evidently results from ischemic necrosis within the conglomerate mass.

COAL WORKER'S PNEUMOCONIOSIS

Coal worker's pneumoconiosis occurs in coal miners and in those who work with coal elsewhere in extremely dusty conditions, such as in the holds of coal barges or ships. The condition is found chiefly in anthracite (hard coal) workers. The disabling pneumoconiosis is usually caused by silica and is, in reality, anthrasilicosis. There is a considerable variation in the amount of quartz (silica) in coal, so the disease varies somewhat in groups of miners who work in different mines. When most of the exposure is to coal dust with little silica, there is little tendency toward progressive massive fibrosis, and large nodules appear to represent the increasing size of small nodules, rather than the coalescence of small nodules. There is less diminution of pulmonary function and fewer symptoms. Roentgen findings consist of granular-appearing nodules in the uncomplicated benign form, since they are less dense than silicotic nodules. Progressive disease leading to massive fibrosis with nodules or masses that arise peripherally in the upper lungs and tend to migrate toward the hila is found in about one third of those with coal workers pneumoconiosis. The characteristic appearance consists of: (1) flat lateral border which is often elongated and parallels the rib cage; (2) thin mass in the sagittal plane; (3) thick-walled, eggshell calcifications within the mass; and (4) multiple satellite nodules.[67] Cavitation may develop as a result of necrosis or tuberculosis; however, the cause is not definitely known. In some instances there may be enough silica to be a factor; in others, it may be caused or accentuated by infection such as tuberculosis.

CAPLAN'S SYNDROME

Caplan's syndrome is the combination of coal worker's pneumoconiosis with rheumatoid arthritis.[44] Roentgen findings consist of rounded, peripheral nodules from 0.5 to 5.0 cm in diameter, which are clearly defined and may cavitate, on a background of nodular pneumoconiosis. This syndrome usually occurs in patients who have subcutaneous rheumatoid nodules but do not necessarily have arthritis. The pulmonary nodules may appear at intervals and often portend exacerbation of arthritis. They are similar to the necrobiotic nodules found in rheumatoid lung in patients without pneumoconiosis. This syndrome is uncommon, if not rare, in the United States but is evidently more common in coal miners in Wales.

ASBESTOSIS

Asbestos, a hydrated magnesium silicate, is a fibrous mineral used as an insulator against heat and cold and as a fireproofing material. The most important form, from the standpoint of pneumoconiosis, is the serpentine (wavy) mineral, *chrysotile* (white asbestos), which is magnesium silicate. This makes up 90% of the asbestos used in the United States and Canada. The other important forms (straight or amphibole) are *amosite* (brown asbestos), an iron magnesium silicate; *anthophyllite*, produced largely in Finland; and *crocidolite* (blue asbestos), an iron sodium silicate with very fine fibers that appears to have more carcinogenic properties than chrysotile, particularly in the causation of mesothelioma. In many industries, combinations of asbestos fibers are used, which creates problems in the study of relative carcinogenicity. Occupational exposure occurs in the mining industry, and in the manufacture and installation of insulating materials containing asbestos. Asbestos exposure also occurs in ship building, in the automotive industry (gaskets, brake linings, undercoating), and in the manufacture of certain "paper" products (roofing felt, flooring felt) and textiles.

Pulmonary asbestosis is defined as chronic interstitial pneumonia with diffuse interstitial fibrosis caused by inhaled asbestos fibers. This excludes pleural disease such as pleural plaques, diffuse pleural thickening, and pleural effusion—which may also be caused by asbestosis.

Although asbestos fibers can be detected in the lungs of many urban dwellers, in Houston the amount is very low and is below the limits of detectability in some.[16] In contrast, small numbers of ferruginous bodies (asbestos bodies) have been found in residents of San Francisco.[11] Usually there is no tissue reaction and only a minor amount of fibrosis, so this level of exposure probably poses no risk. However, in individuals exposed in the neighborhood of asbestos mines and mills, and in those who repeatedly handle the clothing of asbestos workers, there is some risk of developing asbestosis and asbestos pleural disease. The extent of this problem has not been completely assessed.

PATHOGENESIS

The mechanical irritation of the long, stiff fibers when they become lodged in the lungs is believed to account, at least in part, for the fibrosis that results. The autoimmune hypothesis has been proposed as the pathogenesis in this disease as in silicosis, and there is circumstantial evidence to support this. The silicates are more soluble than silica, so the fibrosis may be a response to the silicic acid and metallic ions released in solution. Bronchoalveolar lavage in pulmonary asbestosis reveals that first there is an alveolitis with an increase in alveolar macrophages, lymphocytes, and neutrophils. Fibroblast replication is accelerated, eventually leading to fibrosis, which is typical of asbestosis. The changes occur in the respiratory bronchioles and alveolar ducts, and the fibrosis is peribronchiolar in location. The cause of the pleural changes is not entirely clear. However, there is some evidence to show that the pleural reaction is at least in part caused by mechanical irritation by the fibers that penetrate the visceral pleura.

The disease does not develop unless there is a lengthy exposure, usually 10 years or more, to a fairly high concentration of dust. When the pulmonary lesion is established, it progresses even though exposure is not continued. The clinical findings are those of progressive dyspnea that is often out of proportion to the amount of change noted on the chest films. There is often cyanosis and cough with sputum in which asbestos bodies can be detected. However, many patients with asbestos fibers in the lungs are asymptomatic. The incidence of tuberculosis is not as high as in silicosis. There is an increased incidence of carcinoma of the lung in patients with asbestosis. In patients with asbestos exposure who smoke, lung cancer is 70 times more likely than in those non-smokers who have no asbestos exposure. The lung tumors often develop in areas of fibrosis and are therefore extremely difficult to detect at an early stage. Insulation workers in building trades are six to seven times more likely to develop cancer of the lung or pleura than those not exposed to asbestos. This high incidence is found despite the relatively light and intermittent asbestos exposure in this group. An increased incidence of gastrointestinal cancer and of pleural and peritoneal mesothelioma has also been established. However, in one report of 36 cases of mesothelioma, 19 were not associated with asbestosis.[27] This is an unusual figure, however, because other reports indicate that only 11% to 16% of patients with malignant mesothelioma do not have a history of exposure to asbestos.

ROENTGEN OBSERVATIONS

The fibrosis produced by the foreign material results in the appearance of small irregular opacities, primarily in the lung bases as the earliest finding (Fig. 27-6). As the number of these opacities increases, there may be an accentuation of interstitial markings extending into the perihilar regions and bases. Later there is an increase in the basal fibrotic changes, which usually appear stringy, irregular, and reticular. The cardiac borders assume a shaggy, poorly defined appearance as a result of a combination of interstitial fibrosis and small, irregular opacities. Increasing fibrosis may lead to large opacities, usually when interstitial fibrosis is extensive. This is not very common in asbestosis, however. Lung bases are usually involved and in some instances the disease may involve the central and upper lungs as well. As a result of extensive basal disease, the outline of the diaphragm may become poorly defined. Cavitation and peripheral emphysema with central conglomeration (as seen in silicosis) does not occur.

High-resolution CT is capable of detecting pulmonary parenchymal abnormality in 96% of patients with clinical asbestosis.[1, 2] An irregular linear pattern of increased opacity in the peripheral bases seems to be present in these patients. The opacities tend to extend to the pleural surface.[46] Round atelectasis is present in many patients with diffuse pleural thickening and is readily detected on high-resolution CT.[1] Another finding described in asbestosis is that of irregular pulmonary opacities, some of which appear to be related to the pleura, whereas others represent parenchymal lesions of various pathologic characteristics.[52] The combination of peripheral interstitial and honeycomb pattern is strongly suggestive of asbestosis; diagnostic criteria have not been worked out completely, so pulmonary asbestosis remains a pathologic diagnosis.

Other findings which have been reported on CT include fissural pleural plaques, dense fibrotic bands, thickened interlobular septa, and an increase in intralobular core structures.[40] Subpleural lines, particularly at the bases, seem characteristic.[39] Round atelectasis is common in patients who have pleural effusion. The CT findings include contiguity to an area of diffuse pleural thickening, lentiform or wedge-shaped outline, volume loss in adjacent lung, and the characteristic comet tail of vessels and bronchi. The need for biopsy may be obviated if these criteria are met in the diagnosis of round atelectasis versus tumor. The ultimate place of high-resolution CT in the management of patients with asbestosis has yet to be determined. However, it is clear that the pulmonary opacities can be detected earlier and the extent of pulmonary and pleural disease can be evaluated more accurately with CT than with chest radiography.

The pleural changes in asbestosis occur independently and are often observed when no parenchymal disease can be detected. The following pleural manifestations may occur alone or in combination with the others: diffuse pleural thickening, pleural plaque formation, calcification in pleural plaques, and pleural effusion. Diffuse pleural thickening, which may extend into the fissures, is a common roentgen finding; it is

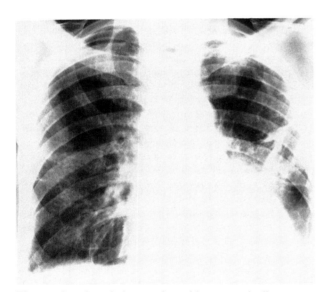

Figure 27–6. Asbestosis with mesothelioma on the left in a 61-year-old male with industrial asbestos exposure. Note scattered opacities in the right central and basal lung, and the large mass at the left base, extending into the interlobar fissure. Lung changes are obscured by the large left mesothelioma. Calcified pleural plaque at the right base and pleural plaques laterally indicate asbestos-related pleural disease as well as asbestosis.

usually bilateral and is more likely to be associated with interstitial fibrosis than the combination of pleural plaques and interstitial fibrosis. Diffuse pleural thickening involves the visceral pleura, and can be recognized as such only when it extends into the interlobar fissures, where there is no parietal pleura. It may encase the entire lung. In asymptomatic patients, the presence of bilateral pleural thickening has a high predictive value for previous asbestos exposure—about 80% when patients with known causes (other than asbestos) for pleural disease are excluded.

Parietal pleural plaques are often the only findings in asbestos-related pleural disease. The plaques vary in thickness (from 1 to 10 mm) and, because they often occur posterolaterally or anterolaterally in the mid-thorax, oblique films may be very useful in demonstrating them. However, oblique films also may be confusing and are more useful in demonstrating involvement of the major fissures in patients with diffuse pleural thickening. In problem cases CT is very useful, because it not only demonstrates the pleural plaques, but also differentiates them from fat, which may be confusing on plain films. CT is not very useful in demonstrating diaphragmatic plaques in the absence of calcification. Plaques appear early as thin, local areas of pleural thickening in the mid-thorax, and are often overlooked until they enlarge and become thicker. Fissural (visceral pleura) pleural thickening is common in asbestos exposure, and its presence may indicate pulmonary asbestosis even when the chest x-ray is normal.[54] As indicated previously, asbestos-related pleural thickening is more easily detected on CT than on chest radiography, and extrapleural fat can readily be differentiated from thick pleura. High-resolution CT has been shown to be more accurate in detecting pleural changes than CT. It can identify reduced lung function indicative of restrictive lung disease in patients with asbestos exposure and normal chest radiographs.[60]

Calcification also occurs in pleural plaques. It is noted most frequently over the diaphragm in the form of a thin, curvilinear opacity conforming to the upper surface of the diaphragm bilaterally and is virtually pathognomonic. Oblique and lateral projections are useful in its detection. Unilateral pleural calcification, particularly when it extends upward along the chest wall, usually indicates previous infection, not asbestos exposure.

Bilateral or unilateral pleural effusion may also occur, but the possibility of other causes must be excluded before effusion can be attributed to asbestosis. The effusion tends to be relatively small in amount (i.e., under 500 ml) and may be bloody or blood-tinged. It is often the earliest sign of asbestos-related disease and may be accompanied by pleural pain. In some instances, the effusion may contribute to or cause diffuse pleural thickening. Multiple recurrences appear to be rare, but a single recurrence of fluid is observed in nearly one third of patients.[41]

The relative incidence of pleural findings has been studied by McLoud and co-workers.[42] In a group of 1,373 exposed persons, 16.5% had pleural plaques and 13.5% diffuse pleural thickening. In those with diffuse thickening (185), the radiographic findings appeared to indicate that it was caused by the residuals of effusion in 31.4%, represented confluent plaques in 25.4%, and was accompanied by pulmonary fibrosis in 10.3%. Malignancy and infection accounted for 25% of pleural thickening, and in 5% it was caused by obesity. As in silicosis, the diagnosis is based on correlation of the roentgen findings with the clinical findings, plus an accurate occupational history of exposure to asbestos (see Fig. 27-6).[43]

TALCOSIS

Talc is a hydrous magnesium silicate in which there is no free silica. If no asbestos or silica is present, talc causes very little pulmonary dysfunction and minor radiographic changes. Widely scattered, small, poorly defined nodules have been reported in patients who inhaled cosmetic talcum powder, which contains no impurities. Other reports of changes in miners or milling operations involving pure talc indicate minimal basal radiographic findings consisting of small, irregular nodules.

When asbestos is present in talc, it causes pneumoconiosis in workers exposed to it in mining and milling operations. The roentgen findings are similar to those in asbestos workers. Pleural plaques, diffuse pleural thickening, pleural calcification, and pleural effusion may be observed. Pulmonary parenchymal findings similar to those in asbestosis may also be observed. When talc contains silica, the findings resemble those in silicosis, and may be simple, with small nodules, or complicated, with progressive massive pulmonary fibrosis. Emphysema is also a prominent feature of this disease.

A form of talcosis has been described in methadone abusers who inject oral methadone intravenously. Oral methadone contains talc, which appears to be the cause of diffuse interstitial micronodular process in the lungs. This may go on to conglomerate upper-lobe, mass-like opacities similar to those of progressive massive fibrosis in silicosis. The masses may develop rapidly and are associated with basal emphysema and upper-lobe volume loss.[56] The diagnosis, as in the other pneumoconioses, is based on correlation of historical, clinical, and radiographic findings.

RARE SILICATE PNEUMOCONIOSES

Mica, a silicate containing potassium, aluminum, magnesium, calcium, and fluorine, is a rare cause of pneumoconiosis. Although the findings may be similar to those of asbestosis, the patients may have no disability and only minimal pulmonary fibrotic changes. A few cases have been reported in which mica seems to be the cause of interstitial pulmonary disease leading to fibrosis and decrease in pulmonary function.[36]

Kaolin (China clay), a mixture of sand, mica, and aluminum silicate, is another rare cause of pneumoconiosis. It may cause a complicated pneumoconiosis, with large masses (progressive massive fibrosis?) in the upper lobes on a background of small, round opacities. The large masses are not always bilateral, however.[37]

Cement dust may cause a pneumoconiosis in persons exposed to high concentrations for long periods of time. Roentgen findings appear to be quite variable and not diagnostic. Usually there is very little pulmonary disability.

A mixed dust of iron ore containing silica and a form of asbestos (anthophyllite) can cause a pneumoconiosis known as *Labrador lung* after a brief exposure.[17] The latent period is short, but there is no abnormality of pulmonary function. Irregular, nodular opacities are noted on roentgenograms. Histopathologic study reveals various combinations of silicotic nodules, granulomatous reaction, large amounts of hemosiderin, and, in one specimen, a ferruginous body. Apparently this disease is localized to one geographic area and has not been studied extensively.

Nepheline rock, which is milled to a fine powder and used in glazing pottery, is also capable of producing a severe pneumoconiosis.

Bauxite fibrosis is a form of pneumoconiosis that occurs in workers exposed to fumes containing fine particles of aluminum oxide and silica used in the manufacture of synthetic abrasives. The ore, known as bauxite, is fused in furnaces.

The radiographic findings consist of fibrosis with a slight increase in interstitial markings progressing to extensive fibrotic change. Emphysematous blebs are commonly observed, and spontaneous pneumothorax is not infrequent. There is often a history of repeated spontaneous pneumothorax and, in some patients, there may be considerable pleural thickening. In severe disease the strands of reticulonodular opacities radiating from the hilum become coarse, conglomerate, and produce apparent mediastinal widening. In these late stages, emphysema is usually marked. The diagnosis depends on the history of exposure to the fumes of bauxite ore, along with the clinical and roentgen findings. The disease is believed to be caused by the silica, but it is known that aluminum oxide can also induce pneumoconiosis under some conditions. There may be a sensitivity factor in the latter disease.

Diatomaceous earth is used widely in filtration processes, as insulating material, as a catalyst carrier, and as an admixture for concrete. The crude diatomite contains amorphous silica. In certain types of processing, some of the amorphous silica is changed to crystalline silica in the form of cristobalite, which produces a pneumoconiosis not seen in crude diatomite workers. There is no increase in the incidence of tuberculosis in workers with this disease and there is no alteration of the course of tuberculosis.

The roentgen patterns are described as linear, nodular, or coalescent. The linear form results in accentuation of the bronchovascular pattern, increasing to a reticular network of density throughout the lungs. Nodulation is very fine and granular at first; this may progress to coarse nodulation and eventually to confluent or coalescent masses, usually appearing in the lung apices. Emphysema is often marked; bullae may rupture, leading to spontaneous pneumothorax. There is no constant progression from one stage to another as in silicosis. Hilar adenopathy is not present in this disease, and eggshell calcifications are not present in hilar nodes.

BERYLLIOSIS

Beryllium compounds are used in the manufacture of metal alloys in the aerospace industry, nuclear reactors, and in the manufacture of gyroscopes. Workers in industries concerned with these materials or products may be exposed to small amounts of beryllium and develop hypersensitivity leading to a chronic form of beryllium granulomatosis. Workers in the beryllium-extraction industries may be exposed to larger amounts, leading to an acute pneumonitis. Laboratory research workers who have been exposed have developed the pneumonitis. The disease has also been observed in people who live in the neighborhood of plants as a result of exposure to exhaust fumes that contain beryllium.

The disease produced by inhalation of dust containing beryllium might better be termed "beryllium granulomatosis" or "beryllium hypersensitivity" because (1) the pathologic lesion that follows is a granuloma resembling that found in sarcoidosis; and (2) relatively small exposure can produce extensive disease—in sharp contrast to the pneumoconioses produced by silica and the silicates, which require years of continued exposure in dusty occupations.[34] In addition to causing pulmonary disease, beryllium results in severe reaction in other organs and tissues wherever it is lodged. There is considerable variation in individual sensitivity to this metal. Two distinct types of pulmonary disease are observed: (1) an acute beryllium pneumonitis that develops within a few days of exposure and (2) a chronic beryllium granulomatosis that occurs after a latent period ranging from 3 months to 3 or more years after exposure.[15]

ACUTE BERYLLIUM PNEUMONITIS

Acute beryllium pneumonitis results in pulmonary edema and hemorrhage. It may be fulminating if exposure has been overwhelming. Acute pulmonary edema and hemorrhage may be rapidly fatal. Roentgen findings are those of massive alveolar edema. In the less acute form, the onset is more insidious than other types of chemical pneumonitis and tends to develop over a period of several days to 2 or 3 weeks or even months. Following the initial pulmonary edema, there is often an alveolar exudate made up largely of plasma cells leading to a severe organizing pneumonia. Hyaline membranes similar to those in viral or "uremic" pneumonitis may be present. If the disease does not terminate fatally in 2 or 3 weeks, gradual recovery tends to take place over a period of several months and may be complete. The roentgen findings in the acute process are similar to those noted in pulmonary edema. There is a diffuse, symmetric increase in density that is most marked in the mid-lung, with poorly defined, soft shadows noted peripherally. In other instances the densities may be smaller and more patchy and tend to simulate widespread bronchopneumonia. As the patient recovers there is gradual clearing, which may be irregular, resulting in a more patchy or conglomerate nodular appearance. Complete clearing usually is slow and requires 1 to 4 months. The history of exposure to beryllium is necessary to differentiate this disease from chemical pneumonitis and pulmonary edema secondary to other causes.

CHRONIC BERYLLIUM GRANULOMATOSIS

Chronic beryllium granulomatosis is characterized by a long latent period of 1 to 20 years after an initial exposure to beryllium of over 2 years' duration. Roentgen findings are somewhat variable and may be extensive before symptoms are marked. Fine, diffuse nodularity that resembles fine sand may be observed (Fig. 27-7). In other patients, a diffuse reticular pattern plus nodularity is noted.[3] The hila are fuzzy and indistinct. In some, the lesions are larger, and distinct nodules ranging from 1 to 5 mm in diameter, as well as linear scars, are present. Combinations may be observed. In addition, it is likely that earlier change consisting of slight increase in linear markings could be recognized if films were taken at frequent intervals following the initial exposure. Hilar enlargement indicating adenop-

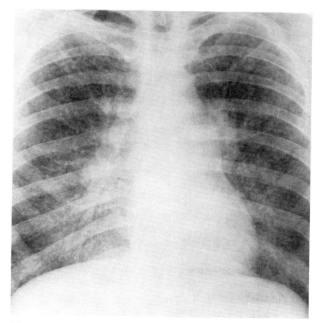

Figure 27–7. Chronic beryllium granulomatosis. Note the massive hilar-node enlargement and granuloma nodularity throughout both lungs. Some of the nodules range up to 3 or 4 mm in size.

athy is a common finding. There is also enlargement of pulmonary vessels secondary to pulmonary hypertension leading to cor pulmonale. As the fibrosis continues, in the late stages there is some tendency to confluence, but this is much less than is noted in silicosis. Emphysema is found and may be severe with lung distortion and bullae. Spontaneous pneumothorax is common. There is no evidence of calcification in nodes. Pleural reaction leading to pleural thickening with pulmonary restriction has been observed, but is not common. Tuberculosis is not ordinarily a complication; cavitation is not present and the large conglomerate masses noted in silicosis are not common in beryllium granulomatosis. The diagnosis may be suspected on the roentgen examination, but must be confirmed by adequate history of exposure. If history of exposure is lacking, or open to question, pulmonary biopsy and chemical determination of the presence of beryllium in the tissues are necessary.

HARD-METAL LUNG DISEASE (COBALT LUNG)

Hard metals such as tungsten carbide and the carbides of titanium, tantalum, or vanadium are bonded with cobalt and used as cutting or grinding tools or in diamond polishing. Cobalt seems to be the major, if not only, substance causing pulmonary disease in such workers.[13, 14] The signs and symptoms are those of a work-related allergic alveolitis, often accompanied by asthma. A diffuse interstitial fibrosis is eventually produced in the lungs that is perivascular and peribronchial. In bronchoalveolar lavage specimens early in the disease, multiple multinucleated giant cells are observed and open-lung biopsies have revealed a fibrosing alveolitis which evidently precedes the diffuse interstitial fibrosis. Early roentgen findings have the appearance of pulmonary edema of varying degrees of severity. This may clear rapidly if exposure is not repeated. Later, the chronic changes consist of small, irregular opacities with a tendency to central and basal distribution. The opacities increase and are accompanied by a thickening of interstitial structures, causing a reticular pattern that may increase with time as the pulmonary fibrosis increases. Workers in the hard-metal industry who have symptoms should probably have a chest radiograph, and if there are signs of disease, consideration should be given to removing them from exposure. Continued exposure to high concentrations of cobalt can be rapidly fatal.[47]

RADIOPAQUE DUST PNEUMOCONIOSES

A number of inorganic dusts are radiopaque, may be stored in the lungs following inhalation, and produce no fibrosis or other reaction. As a result they cause roentgen findings in patients with no clinical evidence of disease.

Siderosis is a benign pneumoconiosis secondary to accumulation of iron oxide in the lung. It is found in electric-arc and acetylene welders, silver polishers, boiler scalers, and in grinders and burners in foundries in which there is insufficient silica to produce silicosis. The iron is inhaled as small particles or in fumes containing iron oxide produced by welding. The roentgen findings are caused by the fact that the iron accumulates in the lymphatics and interstitial tissues of the lung in sufficient quantity to produce radiographic opacity. No fibrosis or decrease in pulmonary function is caused and there is no predisposition to tuberculosis in these individuals.

The roentgen findings consist of discrete, sharply defined, nodular opacities (1 to 3 mm in size) scattered uniformly and symmetrically throughout both lungs. The individual lesions are often more clearly defined than in silicosis and there is no tendency toward conglomeration. There is no reticular pattern extending from the hilum into the lung and no hilar adenopathy. There is no emphysema and no clinical symptoms are present. The opacities tend to regress and may disappear when the exposure is discontinued.

Baritosis is caused by deposition of barium sulfate in the lungs of workers in barium mines. The findings are similar to those in siderosis except that the density of the barium is greater and the individual lesions tend to be larger. When exposure is heavy, roentgen signs may appear after a relatively short time (1 to 2 years). The opacities disappear gradually after removal of the patient from exposure. The condition probably produces no alteration in pulmonary function. Fibrotic changes leading to diminished function have been reported, but the patients were also exposed to other dusts known to cause fibrosis, so uncomplicated baritosis is probably benign.

Stannosis is found in ore handlers and grinders, in tin-smelting workers, and in those who pack tin oxide into bags. It is caused by deposition of tin in the form of stannic oxide in pulmonary tissues. This results in a pneumoconiosis similar to baritosis and is relatively benign.

ANTIMONY PNEUMOCONIOSIS

Antimony when inhaled is sufficiently radiopaque to produce small opacities on roentgen study. It is a rare cause of pneumoconiosis. *Acrylic resin pneumoconiosis* can occur in dentists or dental students exposed to high levels of acrylic plastic in dental laboratories.[4] The interstitial pulmonary changes observed tend to clear when the patient is removed from the environment, so it is possible that it is a hypersensitivity reaction.

OCCUPATIONAL DISEASES RELATED TO PULMONARY HYPERSENSITIVITY

TRACHEOBRONCHIAL HYPERSENSITIVITY

In tracheobronchial hypersensitivity, the hypersensitivity response is in the form of the bronchospasm or asthma. Bronchial asthma, allergic aspergillosis (usually with mucoid impaction), bronchocentric granulomatosis, and byssinosis are manifestations of this type of response. The roentgenographic findings in bronchial asthma are described in Chapter 30 and those in allergic aspergillosis in Chapter 26.

BRONCHOCENTRIC GRANULOMATOSIS

Bronchocentric granulomatosis is a necrotizing granulomatous inflammatory lesion involving bronchial walls in which replacement of bronchial epithelium by palisaded granulation tissue is the major pathologic finding.[32] Some of the patients are asthmatics, and, in these, the granulomas contain many eosinophils and peripheral eosinophilia is present. Fungi are almost always present. The patients are usually young. In the patients who do not have bronchial asthma, the granulomas contain plasma cells and very few have eosinophilia. Fungi are not present. The patients are usually much older. The disease is evidently related to hypersensitivity and is very similar to allergic bronchopulmonary aspergillosis and mucoid impaction. The roentgen findings may be similar but are usually (about 75%) unilateral. There may be lobar or segmental alveolar disease or atelectasis; one or more large nodular or mass densities are observed more frequently than alveolar-type disease. In these instances, the appearance simulates that of tumor. Small nodular or mixed nodular and linear patterns may also be seen. In some patients, more than one roentgen pattern may be observed. Pleural disease and adenopathy are infrequent. Bronchography in four of twenty-two patients reviewed showed segmental bronchial obstruction in two, bronchiectasis in one, and atelectasis with no bronchial abnormality in the other.[32] In this series, the lesions were unilateral in three fourths of the patients, with upper-lobe predominance. Little radiographic difference was noted when comparing asthmatics with non-asthmatics.

BYSSINOSIS

Byssinosis is a pulmonary disease occurring in cotton-processing workers; it is sometimes called "cotton-mill fever." It appears to result from inhalation of cotton dust, but the substance causing it has not been definitely identified. Symptoms consisting of sneezing, coughing, and wheezing tend to come on in attacks related to exposure to the dust. When the patient is removed from the dusty atmosphere, the attacks subside. The symptoms are most severe on the first day of work after a short absence (eg, on Mondays following a weekend off), then tend to decrease on the following days. Many patients with symptoms have no detectable radiographic abnormality. When present, radiographic findings are nonspecific and consist of some accentuation of parahilar markings, along with relatively symmetric distribution of irregular opacities in the form of patchy, poorly defined densities in the central lung. They may not appear until after the patient has had a number of acute attacks, so there may be no radiographic findings early in the course of the disease. Emphysema and permanent fibrosis may result, particularly in smokers. There is some evidence that no significant alteration in pulmonary function occurs in non-smoking cotton workers.[28] Therefore, the public health significance of this disease remains open to question. The target tissue of the antigen–antibody reaction appears to be the respiratory airways

and not the alveoli, as in many of the other occupational diseases related to hypersensitivity.

ALVEOLAR HYPERSENSITIVITY

Alveolar hypersensitivity, sometimes termed "extrinsic allergic alveolitis" or "hypersensitivity pneumonitis," indicates a response of pulmonary tissue to antigens contained in a wide variety of organic dusts in which the particles are so small that they penetrate into the most distal lung parenchyma.[21] Most of the conditions caused by such dusts are associated with specific occupations. Although chest radiographic findings are similar, some of the more common causes of extrinsic allergic alveolitis are described in the sections that follow.

BAGASSOSIS

Bagasse is the product remaining after the juice has been extracted from sugar cane. Inhalation of this dust contaminated with *Thermoactinomyces sacchari* may cause symptomatic pulmonary disease. After an exposure of 2 to 4 months, the clinical manifestations appear in the form of an acute febrile illness with coughing and dyspnea that may become severe. The symptoms are believed to represent an antigen–antibody reaction with possible additional injury caused by the presence of foreign bodies in the lung tissue. The clinical findings usually disappear slowly when the patient leaves the dusty occupation.

Radiographic findings vary with the stage of the disease. Early in the acute stage, few, if any, abnormalities may be present. During severe acute attacks, findings are those of pulmonary acinar disease, probably caused by edema. A fine nodular or reticulonodular type of opacity is noted bilaterally in a more subacute stage; this is usually symmetric and fairly widespread. Regression is slow and the roentgen findings clear gradually in 6 to 12 months if the patient leaves the environment. The findings progress if exposure continues, leading to fibrosis and permanent decrease in pulmonary function. The history of adequate exposure to the dust, along with the clinical manifestations and radiographic findings, lead to the diagnosis. The illness causes fever along with the nonspecific radiographic findings and must be differentiated from other chronic pulmonary inflammatory diseases. Therefore it is necessary to examine and culture the sputum when there are questions as to the diagnosis.

FARMER'S LUNG

Farmer's lung, or thresher's lung, is a pulmonary disease that occurs in farm workers following exposure to moldy hay, grain, or silage, particularly in a closed area. It is the best understood of the conditions causing hypersensitivity pneumonitis (extrinsic allergic alveolitis). The clinical symptoms, pathology, and roentgen findings depend on the stage of the disease—acute, subacute, or chronic. The *acute stage* is characterized by the sudden onset of intense dyspnea, cyanosis, cough, slight fever, and night sweats that usually start a few hours after exposure to moldy material. Respirations are rapid and rales are often present, but there is no typical asthmatic type of breathing. If the patient leaves the working environment, the course is one of gradual improvement of clinical and roentgen findings in 6 to 8 weeks; this is the *subacute stage*. If the patient returns to the same working environment, symptoms recur. The disease varies in severity but eventually the patient is forced to stay away from the source of the dusty material that causes it. Permanent roentgen and pathologic changes are then present which represent the *chronic stage*. It has been demonstrated that this is an antigen–antibody reaction, with the principal antigen being *Micropolyspora faeni* and, to a lesser extent, other thermophilic actinomycetes. Histopathologic study shows a granulomatous interstitial and alveolar pneumonitis in early cases. Later, interstitial fibrosis may result when repeated exposure has resulted in chronic disease.

Radiographic Observations

There is a considerable variation in the radiographic pattern in patients with farmer's lung.[25] In the acute phase, the findings are those of pulmonary edema, acinar or alveolar, the extent of which varies with the severity of the pulmonary reaction. This is often superimposed on a fine nodular pattern of opacities, scattered in the central and basal portions of the lung, presumably representing granulomatous change in the lung resulting from earlier attacks (i.e., the subacute phase). The hila occasionally appear thickened and poorly marginated. The disease regresses over a period of 6 to 8 weeks, often in an irregular manner so that the lesions become mottled and patchy; there is often some accentuation of interstitial markings extending outward from the hila for some time after the major part of the opacity has disappeared (Fig. 27-8). Eventually this interstitial type of disease may also clear completely. Pulmonary function studies often indicate a definite decrease in function even after all roentgen signs have disappeared.

In patients in whom there have been several attacks, permanent changes indicating chronic disease are present. These consist of evidence of pulmonary emphysema and interstitial fibrosis. The latter is mani-

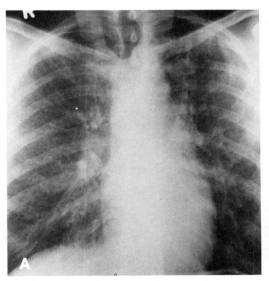
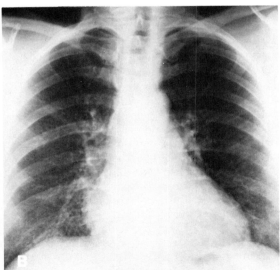

Figure 27–8.   Farmer's lung. (**A**) This patient had an acute episode of cough and fever. There are some poorly defined nodularities and an increase in interstitial markings, best seen in the central lung. (**B**) The disease in this patient is manifested by some small granular-appearing nodules at the bases, best observed on the right, along with a slight increase in interstitial markings.

fested by a general increase in interstitial markings extending from the hilum out to the periphery, often resulting in a rather coarse reticular or reticulonodular appearance of the peripheral lung (Fig. 27-9). As indicated earlier, there is a remarkable variety in pulmonary radiographic patterns in this disease, so an accurate history is of vital importance in making the diagnosis. These patients may become respiratory cripples if they persist in returning to the dusty environment.[20]

PIGEON BREEDER'S LUNG

The disease known as "pigeon breeder's lung" occurs in handlers of pigeons as well as other birds, so "bird breeder's lung" or "bird handler's lung" are actually the preferred terms to designate this condition. It appears to be caused by hypersensitivity to antigens in feathers, serum, and droppings. Radiographic findings include accentuation of interstitial markings with superimposed small nodulations. In acute or severe disease, scattered areas of poorly defined, patchy opacity indicating alveolar exudation are observed. On biopsy, a granulomatous interstitial pneumonitis is observed. Symptoms disappear and radiographic signs clear when the patient is removed from contact with the birds and their habitat.[64]

MAPLE-BARK DISEASE

Maple-bark disease occurs in sawmill or papermill workers exposed to the spores of the fungus *Cryptostroma corticale*, which lies deep in the bark of the maple tree. Radiographic findings are similar to those of other pulmonary hypersensitivity states—namely, an increase in interstitial lung markings and nodularity producing a reticulonodular pattern in parahilar areas and lower lungs. More severe involvement results in a scattered alveolar exudate progressing to a confluent alveolar pattern. Removal from the environment results in clearing of the process.[18]

OTHER OCCUPATIONAL HYPERSENSITIVITY STATES

In addition to the conditions already described, a number of others have been reported in which pulmonary disease is caused by inhalation of material that evidently contains antigens to which the lungs react as a result of hypersensitivity. The radiographic findings in the lungs and the histopathologic manifestations are quite similar. However, the mechanism of the pulmonary reaction is not clear in all of these conditions. Examples include: pituitary snuff-users lung—inhaled posterior pituitary extracts used in treating patients

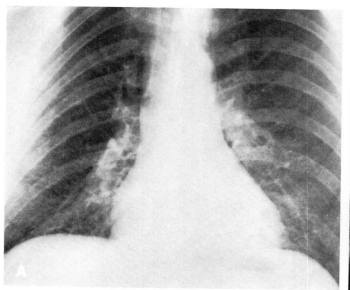
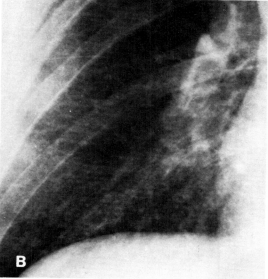

Figure 27–9. Farmer's lung. (**A**) In this patient, there was a fine granular nodularity in the lower lung, which is not very well seen. (**B**) In this enlargement, the nodular appearance is well defined on the right base.

with diabetes insipidus; mushroom-worker's lung; malt-worker's lung; sequoiosis; wood-pulp–worker's disease; grain-weevil hypersensitivity; suberosis (cork); cheese-worker's lung; fishmeal-worker's lung; coffee-worker's lung; lycoperdonosis; alveolitis from contaminated forced-air apparatus and contaminated humidifiers; Bakelite alveolitis; and hypersensitivity to synthetic materials of various kinds including nylon, polyurethane, acrylic fibers, and possibly polyvinyl chloride.

A number of other occupational diseases have also been reported, including sensitivity to organic chemicals such as isocynates including diphenylmethane diisocyanate and toluene diisocyanate used in the manufacture of synthetic foams, synthetic rubbers, paints, and adhesives.[10, 12]

DISEASES CAUSED BY CHEMICAL AGENTS

HYDROCARBON PNEUMONITIS

A number of products have been implicated in hydrocarbon ingestion or inhalation or both. They include kerosene, gasoline, furniture polish, lighter fluid, cleaning fluid, turpentine, insecticides, and some synthetics. Accidental hydrocarbon poisoning is common, especially in children. These products are usually ingested, but some of the irritant material is also aspirated or inhaled. The aspiration is generally the most important factor in the etiology of pneumonitis. The ingested hydrocarbon is absorbed and excreted into the lungs, adding to the pulmonary injury. If vomiting occurs, some additional hydrocarbon as well as particulate material may be aspirated. The petroleum distillates cause an acute alveolitis with exudation of leukocytes, fluid, and fibrin and a more chronic proliferative interstitial infiltration. The pathologic findings in patients who have succumbed are those of severe hemorrhagic pulmonary edema, bronchiolar necrosis, and alveolar exudation. There are sometimes few, if any, clinical signs of pulmonary involvement despite roentgen evidence of pulmonary disease.

Radiographic Observations

There is considerable variation in pulmonary roentgen findings, depending on the severity of the injury. The early changes probably represent edema, fibrin, and cells in the alveoli secondary to acute chemical alveolitis. Usually diffuse opacity—either homogeneous or somewhat flocculent and confined to the lower lobes—is present. In severe cases the diffuse opacity extends into the upper lung. When the involvement is less marked, mottled acinar opacities are noted in one or both lungs. The individual foci are hazy and poorly defined; there may be conglomeration in some areas (Fig. 27-10). These changes develop rapidly and can be seen as early as one-half hour following ingestion. Less frequently, the alveolar changes are confined to the parahilar areas, resembling pulmonary edema and very likely caused by edema resulting from alveolar and/or capillary injury. Clearing of roentgen signs usually lags behind clinical improvement. Pneumatocele formation has been reported in these patients and obstructive emphysema may also occur. Rarely, pleural

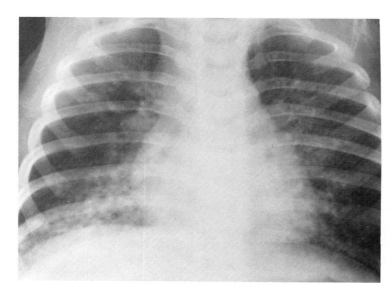

Figure 27–10. Hydrocarbon pneumonitis (kerosene). The disease is confined to the bases of the lungs and is more marked on the right than on the left. It is a poorly defined, diffuse alveolar chemical pneumonitis.

effusion, pneumothorax, and interstitial emphysema occur. The diagnosis is based on the history, along with the roentgen manifestations described. Some patients appear to respond quickly to corticosteroids.

INDUSTRIAL AND WAR GASES

A number of irritant gases are capable of producing pulmonary changes that can be visualized roentgenographically. They include nitric fumes (which consist of five oxides of nitrogen), hydrogen sulphide, chlorine, phosgene, and mustard gas, as well as a number of other irritating gases such as ammonia, manganese oxides, zinc chloride fumes, various insecticides, fluorocarbons, and chemicals found in glue. All of these gases produce pathologic changes in the lungs that vary with the intensity of exposure and the nature of the chemical. Inflammatory changes are found in the trachea and larger bronchi with minimal exposures. As the amount of exposure increases, the damage to these structures is intensified, with a tendency for the process to extend farther into the smaller bronchi and bronchioles. This results in pulmonary edema and congestion secondary to the chemical bronchitis and bronchiolitis. If the injury is severe enough, death may result. There is often a delay in onset of clinical symptoms following exposure—ranging from 1 to 2 hours to as long as 36 hours. Chest pain, cough, and dyspnea are the most common symptoms. Some of the gases are carried to the myocardium, liver, and kidneys following diffusion through the alveolocapillary membrane and may produce damage in these sites.

Radiographic Observations

Roentgen findings vary with the extent and severity of the injury. They consist of a patchy mottling, usually most marked in the perihilar areas, where the lesions may be confluent (Fig. 27-11). In the central and peripheral lungs, individual nodules may be visible that range up to 1 cm in size and are "fluffy" in appearance, with poorly defined edges. They resemble bronchopneumonia but probably represent alveolar edema. The periphery of the lung is usually spared unless the injury has been overwhelming. When the injury has not been severe, clearing occurs rather rapidly, with striking changes noted from day to day, and is often complete in 10 to 14 days. During this period the lesions become more irregular and asymmetric, because small areas of atelectasis and often some patchy bronchopneumonia develop. In some instances, complete recovery occurs. In others, the bronchiolar damage results in obliterative bronchiolitis, which may cause no roentgen findings but does cause decreased

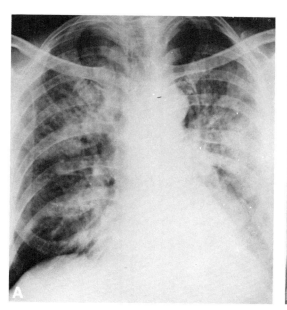
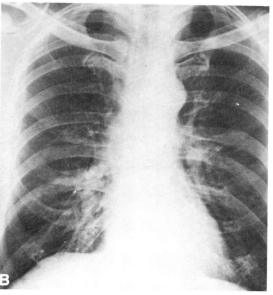

Figure 27–11. Chemical pneumonitis. (**A**) The widespread, mottled, poorly defined densities resemble, and most likely represent, pulmonary edema. Therefore, a history of exposure is necessary to differentiate this condition from others producing pulmonary edema. (**B**) The changes noted above cleared completely, as shown in this roentgenogram obtained 3 weeks later.

pulmonary function. If the bronchiolitis is severe enough, tiny nodules scattered in the area of damage are produced. These may gradually disappear, but some may persist. The diagnosis is based on the history of exposure to noxious gas followed by the symptoms of cough and dyspnea plus the roentgen findings of pulmonary edema as described.

SILO-FILLER'S DISEASE

It is known that nitrogen dioxide is produced in silos within a few hours of filling and reaches a maximum concentration about 2 days after a silo is filled. Dangerous concentrations of gas may remain in closed silos for 2 weeks. Any person entering such a confined space and remaining there is exposed to this irritating gas. Some persons succumb to the fumes and do not get out of the silo alive. Cough and dyspnea often occur immediately. Pulmonary edema in parahilar areas and at the bases may appear in a few hours. If the patient recovers, the edema usually clears rather rapidly. This may be followed by a period of relative freedom or remission of symptoms lasting 2 or 3 weeks. At this time a second phase occurs, which may be fatal or may lead to recovery. This phase is characterized by fever, progressive dyspnea, cyanosis, and cough. The roentgen findings on films obtained during this phase consist of widespread, scattered miliary opacities resembling the lesions of acute miliary tuberculosis. Later these

may become confluent, producing a more patchy and nodular type of appearance (Fig. 27-12). The diagnosis is based on a combination of clinical history and roentgen findings. At autopsy, patients who died a month or more following exposure were found to have bronchiolitis obliterans, with each of the small opacities apparently representing the typical silo-filler's lesion. In patients who die immediately or within a few hours following exposure, diffuse pulmonary edema has been found similar to that described in deaths secondary to nitric-fume inhalation in industry.

Therefore, exposure to nitric acid fumes and oxides of nitrogen can lead to pulmonary damage sufficient to cause death within a short time of exposure, or symptoms may be delayed for several weeks or months, followed by a second, more chronic disease phase. It is likely that some patients recover completely with no residual illness, while in others there is enough bronchiolar alteration to result in fibrosis and emphysema, which develop over a long period following the initial injury. It is also probable that other irritant gases are capable of producing similar pulmonary alterations, which may lead to varying amounts of chronic pulmonary insufficiency.

Toxic exposure to liquid manure can produce similar clinical and radiologic findings, presumably caused by inhalation of toxic gases including hydrogen sulfide and carbon monoxide. This rare occupational disease is appropriately called "dung lung."[49]

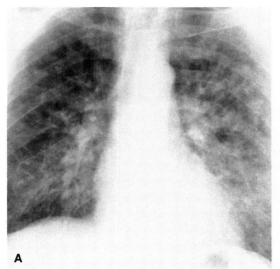
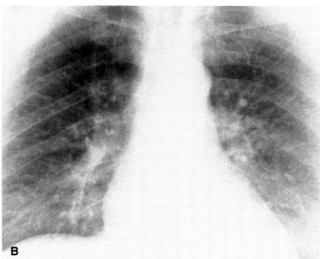

Figure 27–12.   Silo-filler's disease. A 49-year-old male was removed from a silo that had been filled 2 weeks earlier. (**A**) Immediate film shows extensive, poorly defined bilateral opacities, most likely representing alveolar edema. (**B**) Two days later the condition was much improved, although some residual linear opacities remain, and possibly some residual edema. This patient recovered completely.

CARBON MONOXIDE POISONING

Acute carbon monoxide poisoning is frequently fatal, but in a number of persons who receive sublethal doses, abnormalities may be demonstrated on chest roentgenograms. The following manifestations were found in 18 of 62 patients with acute carbon monoxide poisoning: A ground-glass appearance was observed in 11 patients; of these 11, a parahilar haze was noted in 2, 4 had a combination of parahilar haze and peribronchial and perivascular cuffing, while 3 had evidence of intra-alveolar edema. All of these findings are believed to represent pulmonary edema, probably caused by tissue hypoxia and/or the toxic effects of carbon monoxide on alveolar membranes. Cardiac enlargement occurred in 4 patients, and elevation of the right hemidiaphragm in 7—usually as a later manifestation indicating hepatic enlargement. Intra-alveolar edema and parahilar haze indicated a poor prognosis; the presence of any roentgen abnormality is an indication for intensive treatment with oxygen.[58]

PARAQUAT LUNG

The herbicide paraquat produces acute pulmonary edema and hemorrhage, causing rapid death when large doses are ingested.[57, 63] When smaller amounts are taken, patients may survive for a number of days. In addition to its known cytotoxic effects on alveolar cells, paraquat induces an alveolitis in which activated neutrophils and macrophages are produced. The macrophages recruit fibroblasts and release a growth factor that leads to the development of fibrosis. Roentgenographic findings consist of fine granular opacities in the lower lung, which may be discrete in some areas and confluent in others. There is usually rapid progression into a pattern resembling severe pulmonary edema. Positive radiographic findings in the chest usually indicate that a fatal amount of paraquat has been ingested. Patients who survive show a pattern of diffuse interstitial fibrosis. Pathologically the fibrosis is associated with pulmonary vascular disease in which there is muscularization of pulmonary arterioles; extensive fibrosis usually develops before these patients die.

VINYL AND POLYVINYL CHLORIDE EXPOSURE

Vinyl and polyvinyl, both used in the plastics industry, are known to cause angiosarcoma of the liver and a scleroderma-like syndrome. They can also cause pulmonary disease in workers. Symptoms include dry cough, an insidious onset of dyspnea, and exertional weakness. Pathologically there is alveolar hyperplasia and desquamation of alveolar cells. Also there is an interstitial infiltration of mononuclear cells leading to fibrosis. Radiographic changes of a diffuse reticulonodular pattern most likely are secondary to the interstitial fibrosis noted pathologically.[12]

SMOKE INHALATION

Because toxic effects of smoke inhalation on the lung depend on the content of chemicals present, a wide variety of potential injuries exists. Injury severe enough to cause pulmonary changes usually occurs within 24 hours. Most of the toxic materials inhaled cause pulmonary edema, so the radiographic pattern may be one of interstitial edema, including perivascular and peribronchial cuffing or blurring; a mixed pattern of interstitial and acinar edema; or alveolar edema, usually starting in the perihilar areas and progressing to involve greater volumes of pulmonary tissue. The edema may be asymmetric, but is usually bilateral. In addition to these changes, atelectasis occurs and can cause focal and/or widely scattered opacities with no consistent distribution. Lee and associates studied 45 patients from a major fire disaster, 33 of whom suffered acute smoke inhalation and had abnormal chest radiographs on admission. Bronchial-wall thickening was present in 29, pulmonary edema in 7, and subglottic edema in 13. The authors believed subglottic edema and probably bronchial-wall thickening indicate upper airway injury, which may herald parenchymal and bronchiolar damage requiring ventilatory support. However, the extent of pulmonary parenchymal, bronchiolar, and bronchial injury cannot be determined on chest radiographs, so the determination of blood carboxyhemoglobin levels and arterial blood gases is necessary in these patients.[38, 51]

DRUG-INDUCED LUNG DISEASE

Drug reactions are a major problem, because 5% of hospital admissions are a result of drug reactions and an estimated 10% to 18% of hospital patients have some form of drug reaction while in the hospital.[53, 55] Several types of drug reaction may occur; the major types are: hypersensitivity reactions; idiosyncrasies—genetically determined biochemical abnormalities; overdose; drug intolerance; and side-effects.

In this section, a brief discussion of the factors involved in hypersensitivity drug reaction, including the radiographic findings, will be followed by a listing of the major radiographic patterns and drugs most commonly involved. This means several drugs may be listed in more than one radiographic pattern. A list of drug categories and some of the drugs in each will be followed by a discussion of some of the major findings and problems.

Pulmonary reactions to drugs are characterized by the following:

The reactions need not be related directly to dosage.
A latent period is needed following initial exposure to some drugs, but not on readministration.
A minority of drug recipients are involved.
There is often no direct correlation between the reaction and the pharmacologic properties of the drug.
Other hypersensitivity reactions such as anaphylaxis, serum sickness, urticaria, contact dermatitis, or asthma may be present.
Readministration of the drug reproduces the symptoms.

The hypersensitivity reactions are usually accompanied by eosinophilia. In some, the onset is acute with sudden chills, fever, cough, and dyspnea; in others, it may be insidious with increasing dyspnea and cough.

The radiographic features consist of (1) a diffuse, acute alveolar type of disease resembling alveolar edema, which varies in extent and distribution but is usually bilateral; (2) an acute, diffuse interstitial pattern resembling interstitial edema; (3) a chronic interstitial pattern; (4) a pleuropulmonary or lupus-like pattern; and (5) hilar adenopathy which may be accompanied by pulmonary changes (Fig. 27-13). The drugs commonly involved are antibiotics, antimetabolites (antineoplastic agents), analgesics, anticonvulsants, and vasoactive agents (antiarrhythmics), neuroactive agents

(e.g., antidepressants), antirheumatics, and immunosuppressive agents.

Five major radiographic patterns in patients with drug reactions have been described by Morrison:[45]

1. Diffuse interstitial or reticulonodular pattern.
2. Diffuse air space disease (consolidation).
3. Pleural effusion or fibrosis.
4. Hilar or mediastinal widening.
5. Localized areas of consolidation.

Drugs associated with each of these findings are listed in Table 27-1. As indicated, several of them appear on more than one list and can have all or some of the findings in categories in which they are listed at any given time (Fig. 27-14).

The various categories of drugs are listed in Table 27-2. They include: (1) Cytotoxic drugs, used mainly in treatment of malignancies; (Note: New drugs are being added to this, as well as to some of the other categories at frequent intervals.) (2) Antibiotics; (3) Drugs acting on the central nervous system; and (4) Miscellaneous drugs. These lists are incomplete, since reactions to a number of other drugs have been reported. However, the major lung–disease-inducing agents are included.

As a rule, drug-related lung disease is diffuse and bilateral, but not necessarily symmetric. Pleural effusion may be the only radiographic sign and a normal chest roentgenogram doesn't exclude injury caused by drugs. Patients receiving cytotoxic drugs for malignancy pose a particularly difficult problem because,

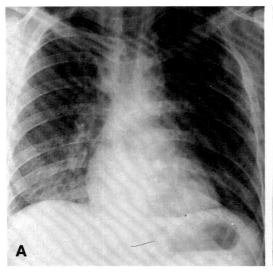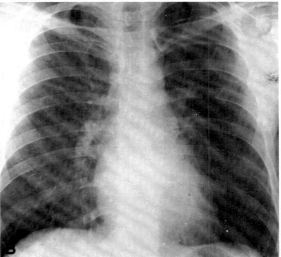

Figure 27–13. Mesantoin sensitivity. **(A)** The patient complained of cough and fever. Note the paratracheal and hilar adenopathy as well as some basal pulmonary involvement on the right. **(B)** Three weeks later, after use of the drug had been discontinued, the chest appears to be normal.

Table 27-1. Patterns of Drug-Induced Pulmonary Disease*

A. DIFFUSE INTERSTITIAL PATTERN (RETICULONODULAR)

busulfan	tetracycline
bleomycin	mitomycin
methotrexate	methysergide
BCNU (nitrosureas)	thiazides
visablastine	diphenylhydantoin
cyclophosphamide	gold
nitrofurantoin	

B. DIFFUSE AIRSPACE PATTERN

methotrexate	amitryptyline
heroin	propoxyphene
methadone	nitrofurantoin
bleomycin	thiazides
codeine	salicylates (aspirin)
Darvon	mineral oil
ethchorynol	

C. PLEURAL EFFUSION OR FIBROSIS

nitrofurantoin	methysergide
isoniazid	hydralizine
methotrexate	procainamide
tetracycline	

C-1. DRUG-INDUCED SYSTEMIC LUPUS ERYTHEMATOSIS

guanoxan	methylthiouracil
procainamide	propylthiouracil
hydralazine	nitrofurantoin
isoiazid	ethosuximide
diphenylhydantoin	oral contraceptives
phenylbutazone	streptomycin
methyldopa	penicillin
quinidine	aminosalicyclic acid
digitalis	griseofulvin
PAS	reserpine
mephenytoin	thiazides
trimethadione	lithium
sulfonamides	gold
tetracycline	

D. HILAR ENLARGEMENT AND/OR MEDIASTINAL WIDENING

diphenylhydantoin	methotrexate
mephanytoin	corticosteroids
trimethadione	

E. LOCALIZED AREAS OF CONSOLIDATION (AIRSPACE DISEASE)

pencillin	chlorpropamide
sulfonamides	nitrofurantoin
PAS	

* The list is incomplete, in part because new drugs are constantly being introduced. Drugs listed can cause patterns indicated.

depends on a history of drug administration plus the radiographic findings plus a high index of suspicion. The diagnosis of drug reactions is very often a difficult problem and in some instances, permanent pulmonary damage results.

Drug addiction is now very common, and overdoses of a number of drugs are an increasing problem.[62] Acute pulmonary edema is commonly observed in overdose of heroin and is not accompanied by cardiac enlargement. With successful treatment, the extensive alveolar edema may resolve very quickly, but the overdose is often fatal. Injection of the drug is nonsterile in many instances, leading to septic embolism, subsequent lung infarcts, and abscesses. Foreign-body granulomas caused by cotton fibers may cause small nodules visible on chest films which may progress to a varying amount of fibrosis manifested by linear opacities. Intravenous talc administration in addicts can cause vascular granulomas which may become confluent. As a result, nodules or conglomerate masses can be seen on the chest film, usually in the mid or upper lung. They may become very large, with peripheral and lower lung overinflation (See section on Talcosis). Intravenous drug abusers may also develop peripheral bullous disease, with sparing of central lungs.

Crack cocaine smoking, common at this time, can cause local pulmonary opacities, atelectasis, pulmonary edema, pneumothorax and pneumomediastinum. Therefore, chest radiography is often helpful, particularly in patients with chest pain following the smoking of cocaine.[19, 29]

Bleomycin is a cytotoxic antibiotic which has long been recognized as being capable of producing permanent pulmonary damage, chiefly in the form of interstitial fibrosis. If pulmonary injury is minimal or moderate, resolution of pulmonary changes is usually complete. Radiographic findings range from a reticular or nodular interstitial pattern (which is often basal) to more extensive involvement by similar changes, to more confluent, irregular opacities which may be large and can simulate metastasis.[6] Bleomycin appears to produce more pulmonary damage than the other cytotoxic antibiotics.

Of the antiarrhythmia agents, amidarone is the one that causes the most pulmonary damage. In some reports upper-lobe patchy consolidation was the major finding, usually in patients with symptoms.[8, 33] In other instances, combinations of alveolar and interstitial opacities have been reported, predominantly basal.[35] It is likely, therefore, that there is no specific pattern of pulmonary involvement. Pleural thickening has also been reported. Pulmonary changes may occur early (i.e., a month or two after initiation of therapy) or late (i.e., after a year or more of therapy). Steroid therapy is helpful in many of these patients. Tocainamide, an-

being immunocompromised, they are susceptible to numerous opportunistic organisms which can cause disease similar to changes observed in drug-related pulmonary disease.[59] In these patients, it is important to make an early diagnosis so appropriate treatment can be given. Furthermore, some of these drugs can increase the effect of radiation on the lung. Diagnosis

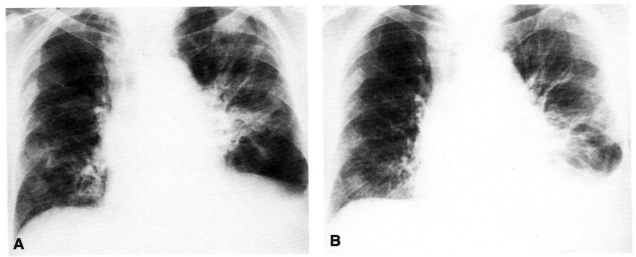

Figure 27–14. Drug hypersensitivity, in this case methotrexate toxicity. (**A**) This film shows a pleuropulmonary reaction with some pleural fluid on the left and interstitial pulmonary disease in the left lung field and at the right base. (**B**) Examination 4 days later shows a considerable increase in the amount of fluid and persistence of the pulmonary interstitial pattern on the left. There has been some improvement on the right. The changes cleared very slowly when the drug was discontinued.

Table 27-2. Major Drug Categories*

A. CYTOTOXIC DRUGS

bleomycin	chlorambucil
nitrosureas	mitomycin
busulfan	procordazine
methotrexate	phenylalanine mustard
cyclophosphamide	

B. ANTIBIOTICS

bleomycin	ethionamide
penicillin	isoniazid
griseofulvin	tetracycline
sulfonamides	erythromycin
PAS	neomycin
nitrofurantoin	streptomycin
cephaloridine	

C. DRUGS ACTING ON THE CENTRAL NERVOUS SYSTEM

heroin	diphenylhydantoin
methadone	mephantoin
propoxyphene	carbamazepine
marijuana	clonazepam

D. MISCELLANEOUS AGENTS

thiazides	pencillamine
gold	corticosteroids
methysergide	amiodarone
hexamethonium	imipramine
pentolinium	amitryptyline
mecamylamine	iodinated compounds

* This list is incomplete, in part because new drugs are constantly being introduced. All drugs listed can cause pulmonary disease.

other antiarrhythmic agent, can also produce a combination of interstitial and alveolar changes in the lung, which also responds to steroids.[61]

Tricyclic antidepressants are dangerous if an overdose is taken and may cause acute respiratory distress syndrome as well as pulmonary edema, which clears in patients in whom there appears to be less toxicity or perhaps a lower dose.[65]

L Tryptophan–induced eosinophilia-myalgia syndrome, caused presumably by self-medication, was reported in several states in 1989. It appears that certain lots of the material may have been contaminated, but the exact agent is not yet clear. In addition to eosinophilia and myalgia, many developed pulmonary symptoms. In a study of 18 patients, 9 had abnormal chest radiographs.[68] Six had irregular linear opacities, chiefly at the bases, three of whom also had pleural effusion. The remaining three patients had pleural effusion with no pulmonary lesions. Several deaths were reported in patients with this syndrome. Because this substance is rarely used now, this syndrome is not likely to be seen again.

Methotrexate-induced pneumonitis has long been known as a hazard when this drug was used in neoplastic and non-neoplastic diseases. The pulmonary findings are varied and consist of an initial interstitial reticular pattern, soon followed by alveolar consolidation which may be patchy, usually bilateral, but not always symmetric. Pleural effusion may also occur. Pulmonary disease is not strictly dose-related and may appear after some years of therapy; in some instances it may appear after treatment has been discontinued. Methotrexate is the most frequently used antimetabolite, so more cases of pulmonary toxicity have been reported than with other antimetabolites.

EXOGENOUS LIPID PNEUMONIA

Lipid (lipoid) pneumonia is the term used to designate the granulomatous and fibrotic changes resulting from aspiration of various organic or inorganic fatty materials. In adults, the most common cause is the use of mineral oil for the treatment of constipation. Frequent or continued use of oily nose drops can also cause this condition. Therefore, it is included in this section on drug-induced lung disease. In children it is caused by aspiration of cod liver oil, and, in some instances, milk fats probably produce the condition in infants. Lipid pneumonia also occurs in achalasia. Inhalation of burning animal fats has also been reported as a cause of lipid pneumonia.[48] As the result of aspiration of lipid materials, an inflammatory process is produced that results

in consolidation of pulmonary parenchyma. Large phagocytes containing lipid material are noted in the alveoli and in the interstitial tissues. Chronic inflammatory cells may also be present within the alveoli. As the disease progresses, a considerable amount of fibrosis develops that causes contraction of the involved lung, compression of the alveoli, and often compression and obliteration of the bronchi. These pathologic changes result in abnormalities that can be outlined on chest radiographs.

The radiographic findings are of two general types—diffuse and nodular.[22] In the diffuse type, there are scattered areas of increased density that are usually at the bases but may involve the right middle lobe and the superior segment of the lower lobe as well. Occasionally the condition involves the upper lobes. The individual lesions are usually poorly defined, with the opacity fading off into normal lung. The lesions are not unlike those found in other types of aspiration pneumonitis, but tend to be more linear with a fine nodular and linear pattern (Fig. 27-15A). There is also reduction in volume of the affected lobe. Serial films show that the opacity in this condition persists with little change over a long period, in contrast to the changes noted in bacterial and viral pneumonias which resolve

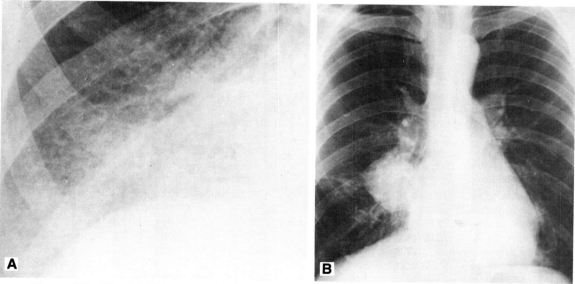

Figure 27–15. Lipid pneumonia. **(A)** Diffuse type of lipid pneumonia, in which there was a rather marked increase in density at both lung bases. This film is a close-up of the right base to show the strandlike increase in density, along with the somewhat nodular disease. **(B)** This film illustrates the nodular type of lipid pneumonia. Note the large mass in the right medial base. Another mass of similar size situated behind the heart was best noted on a tomogram.

leaving little, if any, residual opacity. In some of these patients, as lipid pneumonitis progresses the area involved may become fibrotic and decrease in size. At times, there may be persistent, irregular, patchy opacities scattered in one or both lungs which resemble chronic, nonspecific inflammatory disease. In the presence of a suggestive history, diagnosis can be suspected and can then be confirmed by MRI or CT.[9]

The nodular type of disease may also be unilateral or bilateral and probably results from a local conglomeration of the diffuse type. The area of opacity varies considerably in size, but may reach 8 to 10 cm in diameter. It appears as a mass, usually oval or round in shape. The periphery of the nodule is usually irregular but occasionally becomes very smooth, so the lesion may resemble a tumor or cyst (Fig. 27-15B). This lesion is also known as an *oil* or *lipid granuloma*. In some patients, the right middle lobe is involved. It is then contracted and completely airless with its bronchus obstructed by inflammatory reaction.

Lipid pneumonia usually produces fewer symptoms than comparable involvement by an infectious process. This is of help in differentiating it from infectious disease. Serial examinations also show more stability of the lesion than in most of the lesions it may simulate. The nodular type may resemble bronchogenic carcinoma or other intrapulmonary tumors, and in some instances biopsy is the only method of differentiation. There are a few reports of squamous cell and alveolar cell carcinoma occurring at the site of lipid pneumonia. However, it is not certain that the neoplasm is caused by the lipid material in the lung. If a history of ingestion of mineral oil or the use of oily nose drops can be obtained and the radiographic findings described are also associated with the presence of lipid-containing phagocytes in the sputum, the diagnosis can be made with a considerable degree of accuracy.

IRRADIATION CHANGES IN THE LUNG

When tumors of the breast, lung, and mediastinum are irradiated, the lung tissue in the beam receives radiation in varying amounts. This is capable of causing injury sufficient to be noted radiographically and pathologically. The reaction in the lung depends on a number of factors, such as variations in the rate of treatment, port size, the presence of arteriosclerosis, and individual sensitivity of the patient. These factors alter the relationship between the total dose of radiation to the lungs and the damage produced by it. Generally there is not a direct dose or dose–time relationship. There are some studies which suggest that postradiation pneumonitis may be a hypersensitivity reaction in addition to a direct effect of ionizing radia-

tion.[23] The changes respond to corticosteroid therapy, which tends to support this theory. Therefore, it may be a factor in some instances.

The clinical symptoms are often minor and there may be considerable pulmonary change with no symptoms. Cough and dyspnea may be present, however. During the acute phase there is damage to the pneumocytes, causing decrease in surfactant and a deposition of fibrinlike material in the alveoli to produce a hyaline membrane. There is damage to or destruction of capillary and alveolar walls, and edema. These acute changes are often delayed for 4 to 6 weeks, just as the severe acute skin reactions are delayed, even though the injury occurred at the time of irradiation. Occasionally the findings may occur many months following completion of irradiation. The late changes are those of fibrosis, resulting in thickening of the alveolar walls and a decrease in the caliber of the vessels. In some patients an acute reaction may be superimposed on the late fibrosis when multiple courses of radiation are given.

These pathologic alterations are reflected in the radiographic findings. During the early acute phase when edema is a prominent feature there is a hazy, poorly defined increase in density, usually confined to the area of radiation, but sometimes extending a short distance beyond it. This reaction may occur from 1 month to as long as 4 to 6 months following completion of irradiation. Most of the reaction is very likely caused by pulmonary edema, but there may also be some pleural reaction leading to a small amount of fluid and pleural thickening that very likely contributes to the findings. Pleural fluid in significant amounts is rare. After a time the opacity becomes somewhat more irregular and patchy. Strands of opacity develop that radiate from the hilum toward the periphery. These manifestations may clear gradually and disappear completely in a year or more, but if the original injury was severe enough there is sufficient fibrosis to cause permanent changes. These changes consist of contraction of the lung and a shift of hilar and mediastinal structures to the side or area of radiation (Fig. 27-16). Both hila may be elevated following irradiation of the upper mediastinum. Pleural thickening may appear, manifested by increased opacity and irregularity of the pleural surface involved. Elevation of the diaphragm and tenting of its summit may also occur. Severe thoracic and pulmonary distortion may result. Chronic dry, irritating, persistent cough may be a problem in the more severely involved patients. Rarely, a unilateral radiolucent lung has been reported after irradiation.[66] There may be a long latent period before this change becomes apparent. Etiology is uncertain, but pulmonary embolism secondary to obliterative vasculitis is a possibility. CT studies have indicated that

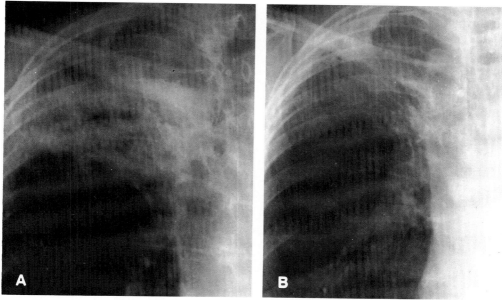

Figure 27–16. Radiation pneumonitis. (**A**) Roentgenogram 5 months after completion of irradiation of the right upper thorax in a patient with breast carcinoma. There is a shift of the trachea and upper mediastinal structures to the right, elevation of the right hilum, and a rather diffuse, poorly defined density above the level of the anterior arc of the second rib, representing a relatively acute alveolar process. (**B**) This film, made 2 years later, shows only a little strandlike density, largely confined to the clavicular and subclavicular areas. The elevation of the right hilum persists, but the tracheal shift is somewhat decreased.

pulmonary vessel size decreases, which may account, at least in part, for the radiolucency. These vascular changes have been shown to occur outside the area irradiated on CT, but do not appear to be detectable on chest radiographs. Maximum damage seems to be related to irradiation of the hilum or mediastinum.[5]

Cancer chemotherapy augments the effect of irradiation on the lung in some patients. Presumably this may be suppressed by corticosteroids, since irradiation pneumonitis has been reported in patients following withdrawal of the steroids as part of the chemotherapy program. Usually the signs of pneumonitis do not appear for several days, but they may be very severe. Reinstitution of corticosteroid therapy usually causes prompt remission of the irradiation changes.[50]

The diagnosis is made on the basis of the clinical history of previous radiation plus the roentgen manifestations described, which are confined to the irradiated area. There is often accompanying evidence of radiation osteitis of ribs, consisting of fractures with demineralization of ribs in the area of fracture. There is no evidence of fracture healing for long periods of time as far as can be detected on the roentgenogram. Radia-

tion pneumonitis must be differentiated from recurrent tumor. This differentiation is often difficult if the radiation has been given for treatment of a lung tumor. MRI has proved to be useful in differentiating fibrosis from recurrent tumor. In patients with breast cancer, the localization of the changes to the area of irradiation without lesions elsewhere is indicative of a radiation pneumonitis and not metastasis. The signs of decrease in lung volume are not found with metastases, and it is rare for metastatic carcinoma to involve one lung to any significant degree without evidence of disease on the other side. The problem of recurrence or residual disease after irradiation of the mediastinum for Hodgkin's disease offers a particularly difficult problem, because involvement of pulmonary parenchyma extending from the mediastinal tumor is found in this disease. These findings can simulate the fibrotic changes resulting from radiation after treatment of hilar and mediastinal nodes. In problem situations, MRI may be very helpful. All factors—including the clinical condition of the patient, the interval following radiation, and the progress of the lesions—must be considered in these instances. The acute pulmonary reaction must be differentiated from acute pneumonia resulting from irritants or bacterial infections. This can be done on the basis of clinical history plus the presence of the localized radiating strands that are common in postradiation pneumonitis.

REFERENCES AND SELECTED READINGS

1. ABERLE DR: High resolution computed tomography of asbestos-related diseases. Semin Roentgenol XXVI: 118, 1991
2. ABERLE DR, GAMSU G, RAY CS: Asbestos-related pleural and parenchymal fibrosis: Detection with high resolution CT. Radiol 166:729, 1988
3. ARONCHICK JM, ROSSMAN MD, MILLER WT: Chronic beryllium disease: Diagnosis, radiographic findings, and correlation with pulmonary function tests. Radiol 163:677, 1987
4. BARRETT TE, PIETRA GG, MAYCOCK RL, ET AL: Acrylic resin pneumoconiosis: Report of a case in a dental student. Am Rev Resp Dis 139:841, 1989
5. BELL J, MCGIVERN D, BULLIMORE J, ET AL: Diagnostic imaging of post-irradiation changes in the chest. Clin Radiol 39:109, 1988
6. BELLAMY EA, HUSBAND JE, BLAQUIERE RM, ET AL: Bleomycin-related lung damage: CT evidence. Radiol 156:155, 1985
7. BERGIN CJ, MULLER NL, VEDAL S, ET AL: CT in silicosis: Correlation with plain films and pulmonary function tests. Am J Roentgenol 146:477, 1986
8. BUTLER S, SMATHERS RL: Computed tomography of amiodarone pulmonary toxicity. J Comput Assist Tomogr 9:375, 1985
9. CARRILLON Y, TIXIER E, REVEL D, ET AL: MR diagnosis of lipoid pneumonia. J Comput Assist Tomogr 12:876, 1988
10. CHARLES J, BERNSTEIN A, JONES B, ET AL: Hypersensitivity pneumonitis after exposure to isocynates. Thorax 31:127, 1976
11. CHURG A, WARNOCK ML: Analysis of the cores of ferruginous (asbestos) bodies from the general population: Patients with and without cancer. Lab Invest 37:280, 1977
12. CORDOSCO EM, DEMETER SL, KERKAY J, ET AL: Pulmonary manifestations of vinyl and polyvinyl chloride (interstitial lung disease). Chest 78:828, 1980
13. DAVISON AG, HASLAM PL, CORRIN B II, ET AL: Interstitial lung disease and asthma in hard-metal workers. Thorax 38:119, 1983
14. DEMEDTS M, GHEYSENS B, NAGELS J, ET AL: Cobalt lung in diamond polishers. Am Rev Resp Dis 130:130, 1984
15. DENARDI JM, VAN ORDSTRAND HS, CURTIS GH: Berylliosis: Summary and survey of all clinical types in ten-year period. Cleve Clin Q 19:171, 1952
16. DODSON RF, GREENBERG D, WILLIAMS MG JR, ET AL: Asbestos content in lungs of occupationally and nonoccupationally exposed individuals. JAMA 252:68, 1984
17. EDSTROM HW, RICE DMD: "Labrador lung:" An unusual mixed dust pneumoconiosis. Can Med Assoc J 126: 27, 1982
18. EMANUEL DA, WENZEL FJ, LAWTON BR: Pneumonitis due to Cryptostroma corticale (maple-bark disease). N Engl J Med 274:1413, 1966
19. EURMAN DW, POTASH HL, EYLER WR, ET AL: Chest pain and dyspnea related to "crack" cocaine smoking: Value of chest radiography. Radiology 172:459, 1989
20. FRANK RC: Farmer's lung. Am J Roentgenol 79:189, 1957
21. FRASER RG, PARE JAP: Extrinsic allergic alveolitis. Semin Roentgenol 10:31, 1975
22. GENEREUX GP: Lipids in the lungs: Radiologic–pathologic correlation. J Can Assoc Radiol 21:2, 1970
23. GIBSON PG, BRYANT DH, MORGAN GW, ET AL: Radiation-induced lung injury: A hypersensitivity pneumonitis? Ann Intern Med 108:288, 1988
24. GURNEY JW, BATES FT: Pulmonary cystic disease: Comparison of Pneumocystis carinii pneumatoceles and bullous emphysema due to intravenous drug abuse. Radiology 173:27, 1989
25. GURNEY JW, UNGER JM, DOBRY CA, ET AL: Agricultural Disorders of the Lung. Radiographics 11:625, 1991
26. HARDY HL: Current concepts of occupational lung disease of interest to the radiologist. Semin Roentgenol 2: 225, 1967
27. HASAN FM, NASH G, KAZEMI H: The significance of asbestos exposure in the diagnosis of mesothelioma: A 28-year experience from a major urban hospital. Am Rev Resp Dis 115:761, 1977
28. HEYDEN S, PRATT P: Exposure to cotton dust and respiratory disease. JAMA 244:1797, 1980
29. HOFFMAN CK, GOODMAN PC: Pulmonary edema in cocaine smokers. Radiology 172:463, 1989
30. ILO INTERNATIONAL CLASSIFICATION OF RADIOGRAPHS OF PNEUMOCONIOSIS. Revised Edition, 1980, International Labour Office, Geneva, Switzerland.
31. JACOBSON G, LAINHART WS (EDS): ILO U/C International Classification of Radiographs of the Pneumoconioses. Med Radiog Photog 48:67, 1972
32. KATZENSTEIN A, LIEBOW AA, FRIEDMAN PJ: Bronchocentric granulomatosis, mucoid impaction, and hypersensitivity reactions to fungi. Am Rev Resp Dis 111:497, 1975
33. KOSLIN DB, CHAPMAN P, YOUKER JE, ET AL: Amiodarone-induced pulmonary toxicity. J Can Assoc Radiol 35:195, 1984
34. KRIEBEL D, BRAIN JD, SPRINCE NL, ET AL: The pulmonary toxicity of beryllium: State of the art. Am Rev Resp Dis 137:464, 1988
35. KUHLMAN JE, TEIGEN C, REN H, ET AL: Amiodarone pulmonary toxicity in symptomatic patients. Radiology 177:121, 1990
36. LANDAS SK, SCHWARTZ DA: Mica-associated pulmonary interstitial fibrosis. Am Rev Resp Dis 144:718, 1991

37. LAPENAS D, GALE P, KENNEDY T, ET AL: Kaolin pneumoconiosis. Am Rev Resp Dis 130:282, 1984

38. LEE MJ, O'CONNELL DJ: The plain chest radiograph after acute smoke inhalation. Clin Radiol 39:33, 1988

39. LYNCH DA, GAMSU G, ABERLE DR: Conventional and high resolution computed tomography in the diagnosis of asbestos-related disease. Radiographics 9:523, 1989

40. LYNCH DA, GAMSU G, RAY CS, ET AL: Asbestos-related focal lung masses: Manifestations on conventional and high-resolution CT scans. Radiology 169:603, 1988

41. MARTENSSON G, HAGBERG S, PETTERSSON K, ET AL: Asbestos pleural effusion: A clinical entity. Thorax 42:646, 1987

42. MCLOUD TC, WOODS BO, CARRINGTON CB, ET AL: Diffuse pleural thickening in an asbestos-exposed population. Am J Roentgenol 144:9, 1985

43. MINTZER RA, GORE RM, VOGELZANG RL: Rounded atelectasis and its association with asbestos-induced pleural disease. Radiology 139:567, 1981

44. MORGAN WKC, LAPP NL: Respiratory disease in coal miners: State of the art. Am Rev Resp Dis 113:531, 1976

45. MORRISON DA, GOLDMAN AL: Radiographic patterns of drug-induced lung disease. Radiology 131:299, 1979

46. MULLER NL: The differential diagnosis of chronic diffuse infiltrative lung disease on high-resolution computed tomography. Semin Radiol 26:132, 1991

47. NEMERY B, NAGELS J, VERBEKEN E, ET AL: Rapidly fatal progression of cobalt lung in a diamond polisher. Am Rev Resp Dis 141:1373, 1990

48. OLDENBERGER D, MAUERER WJ, BELTAOS E, ET AL: Inhalation lipoid pneumonia from burning fats. JAMA 222:1288, 1972.

49. OSBERN LN, CRAPO RO: Dung lung: A report of toxic exposure to liquid manure. Ann Intern Med 95:312, 1981

50. PARRIS TM, KNIGHT JG, HESS CE, ET AL: Severe radiation pneumonitis precipitated by withdrawal of corticosteroids: A diagnostic and therapeutic dilemma. Am J Roentgenol 132:284, 1979

51. PUTMAN CE, LOKE J, MATTHAY RA, ET AL: Radiographic manifestations of acute smoke inhalation. Am J Roentgenol 129:865, 1977

52. REMY-JARDIN M, BEUSCART R, SAULT MS, ET AL: Subpleural micronodules in diffuse infiltrative lung diseases: Evaluation with thin section CT scans. Radiology 177:133, 1990

53. RIGSBY CM, SOSTMAN HD, MATTHAY RA: Drug-induced lung disease. In: Recent Advances in Respiratory Medicine. Fleuley DB, Petty TL (eds). pp. 131–158 New York: Churchill Livingstone, 1983

54. ROCKOFF SD, KAGAN E, SCHWARTZ A, ET AL: Visceral pleural thickening in asbestos exposure: The occurrence and implications of thickened interlobar fissures. J Thoracic Imaging 2:58, 1987

55. ROSENOW EC III: The spectrum of drug-induced pulmonary disease. Ann Intern Med 77:977, 1972

56. SIENEWICZ DJ, NIDECKER AC: Conglomerate pulmonary disease: A form of talcosis in intravenous methadone abusers. Am J Roentgenol 135:697, 1980

57. SMITH P, HEATH D: Paraquat lung: A reappraisal. Thorax 29:643, 1974

58. SONE S, HIGASHIHARA T, KOTAKE T, ET AL: Pulmonary manifestations in acute carbon monoxide poisoning. Am J Roentgenol 120:865, 1974

59. SOSTMAN HD, PUTMAN CE, GAMSU G: Diagnosis of chemotherapy lung. Am J Roentgenol 136:33, 1981

60. STAPLES CA, GAMSU G, RAY CS, ET AL: High resolution computed tomography and lung function in asbestos-exposed workers with normal chest radiographs. Am Rev Resp Dis 139:1502, 1989

61. STEIN MG, DEMARCO T, GAMSU G, ET AL: Computed tomography: Pathologic correlation in lung disease due to tocainide. Am Rev Resp Dis 137:458, 1988

62. STERN WZ, SUBBARAA K: Pulmonary complications of drug addiction. Semin Roentgenol 18:193, 1983

63. THURLBECK WM, THURLBECK SM: Pulmonary effects of paraquat poisoning. Chest [Suppl] 69:276, 1976

64. UNGER J DEB, FINK JN, UNGER GF: Pigeon breeder's disease. Radiology 90:683, 1968

65. VARNELL RM, GODWIN JD, RICHARDSON ML, ET AL: Adult respiratory distress syndrome from overdose of tricyclic antidepressants. Radiology 170:667, 1989

66. WENCEL ML, SITRIN RG: Unilateral hyperlucency after mediastinal irradiation. Am Rev Resp Dis 137:955, 1988
mediastinal irradiation. Am Rev Resp Dis 137:955, 1988

67. WILLIAMS JL, MOLLER GA: Solitary mass in the lungs of coal miners. Am J Roentgenol 117:765, 1973

68. WILLIAMSON MR, EIDSON M, ROSENBERG RD, WILLIAMSON SL: Eosinophilia-myalgia syndrome: Findings on chest radiographs in 18 patients. Radiology 180:849, 1991

*Paul and Juhl's Essentials of Radiologic Imaging,
Sixth Edition*, edited by John H. Juhl and
Andrew B. Crummy. J.B. Lippincott Company,
Philadelphia, © 1993.

CHAPTER **28**

Circulatory Disturbances

John H. Juhl

PULMONARY EDEMA

Pulmonary edema is the term used to indicate an abnormal accumulation of fluid in the extravascular pulmonary tissues.[12] There is a constant flow of fluid and proteins from the microvascular spaces (arterioles, capillaries, and venules) in the lung into the interstitial space.[17] The interstitial space includes the alveolar wall interstitium and the interlobular, perivascular, peribronchial, and subpleural connective tissue spaces.

The flow can increase from an estimated 20 ml per hour to about eight to ten times that amount in the normal individual without causing pulmonary edema, or an appreciable increase in extravascular lung fluid. Respiratory pumping action appears to be an important factor in lymphatic flow. Direction of flow is determined by valves in the lymphatics.

The pulmonary lymphatic vessels begin in loose connective tissue spaces proximal to but not in the alveoli. There are five groups of lymphatics in the lungs:[18] (1) *Pleural*—common over the lower lobes (95% to 100%) and uncommon over the upper and middle lobes (14% to 31%). The flow is for a variable distance on the surface and then to the hilum via the interstitial spaces of the interlobular septa. (2) *Interlobular*—arise at the periphery of the acinus (not in the alveolar walls) and extend in the septa to join with the veins, where they become (3) the *perivenous* group, which extend to the hilum. (4) *Peribronchial*—arise at the junctions of the alveolar septa and accompany the pulmonary arteries and bronchi to the hilum. (5) *Anastomotic*—run in the deep interlobular septa.

The lymphatics in the juxta-alveolar spaces have a poorly developed discontinuous basement membrane and endothelium with partially open cell junctions so fluid can be cleared rapidly. The pulmonary lymphatics carry the excess microvascular filtrate into the systemic venous system. When the capacity of the lymphatics is exceeded, edema results. Endothelial cells form a continuous lining of the alveolar capillaries and the remainder of the pulmonary vascular system. Connective tissue fibers weave through the interstitium in such a way that one half of two thirds of the alveolar capillary walls have an interstitial space; elsewhere the capillary endothelium and the alveolar epithelium are fused. The endothelial cell junctions are not as tight as those in alveolar epithelium and are therefore more permeable. Fluid and sizeable protein molecules can escape through endothelial and epithelial junctions without causing permanent damage, which probably accounts for the rapid resolution of pulmonary edema in some patients when the inciting cause is removed.

The major causes of pulmonary edema and conditions associated with them are:

I. Hemodynamic Pulmonary Edema (Elevated Capillary Hydrostatic Pressure—(the most common form)
 1. Left heart failure
 2. Mitral valvular disease
 3. Left atrial tumor (myxoma)
 4. Pulmonary venous obstruction*
  a. mediastinal fibrosis
  b. mediastinal tumor
  c. veno-occlusive disease

*This has been reported in patients with postpulmonary lobectomy pulmonary venous thrombosis.

5. Neurogenic (hemodynamic in some, if not all, cases)
II. Permeability Pulmonary Edema
  1. Narcotic overdose?
  2. Salicylate poisoning
  3. Smoke inhalation
  4. Inhalation of chemical fumes including
     a. oxides of nitrogen
     b. oxides of sulfur
     c. organic chemical fumes
     d. carbon monoxide
  5. High altitude
  6. Near drowning
  7. Rapid re-expansion of lung (as in thoracentesis or removal of large pneumothorax)†
  8. Snake venom and other circulating toxins
  9. Aspirated hydrocarbons
  10. Posttraumatic fat embolism
  11. Irradiation
  12. Epiglottitis (acute upper airway obstruction)?
III. Combined Hemodynamic and Permeability Edema
  1. Shock lung, including septic shock
  2. Adult respiratory distress syndrome (ARDS)—a variety of causes
  3. Intravenous iodinated contrast media?
  4. Narcotic overdose?
IV. Renal Disease Edema?—combination of hypervolemia, hypoproteinemia and increased hydrostatic pressure; fluid overload is similar to renal disease.
V. Lymphatic Obstruction Edema—mechanical, anatomic, or neurogenic
VI. Edema of Unknown Etiology—The pathophysiology of several of the above are still controversial, and the list is incomplete, since new conditions causing pulmonary edema are being reported frequently.

Decompression sickness in divers and tunnel workers is recognized as a cause of non-cardiogenic pulmonary edema.[22] It occurs within 6 hours of rapid decompression, whatever the cause. Since it may be life-threatening, hyperbaric chamber recompression is recommended. Pathogenesis of edema in these cases is complex because nitrogen bubbles may obstruct and produce ischemia, leading to altered permeability distally and an increase in hydrostatic pressures proximally, leading to overperfusion. A release of vasoactive substances has also been considered as part of the process by some.

† Since this can be fatal, slow evacuation of a very large pneumothorax, massive pleural effusion, or hydropneumothorax is recommended by those who have written on the subject.

Clinical symptoms of pulmonary edema are varied and depend on the associated disease or injury. When the edema is extensive and acute there is usually severe respiratory distress, but when the onset is insidious, particularly in uremia, there may be very few respiratory symptoms. There is a notable discrepancy between roentgen and physical findings in chronic pulmonary edema and in some patients with acute or subacute interstitial edema. Therefore the radiographic examination of the chest is very important. Two major roentgen patterns of edema are observed, depending on the site of the transudate—namely, alveolar and interstitial. Fluid enters the interstitial spaces from the pulmonary capillaries to produce interstitial edema, and as the amount of extravascular fluid increases, a point is reached where it escapes into the alveoli. At first, the amount of alveolar filling may be minimal, but as the amount of fluid increases, the edema progresses and may become very extensive.

INTERSTITIAL EDEMA

As indicated, interstitial edema precedes alveolar edema; therefore, it is necessary to be able to recognize the interstitial fluid in order to determine the presence of congestive heart failure or other causes of edema early in the course of the disease.

There are several signs of interstitial edema which are reliable as a group, particularly when correlated with the clinical findings. They are:

1. Perivascular blurring or cuffing, in which the margins of the vessels become indistinct and widened in the parahilar area extending out to involve vessels in the lung parenchyma
2. Peribronchial blurring or cuffing with loss of the clear definition of the outer bronchial wall as seen in cross-section on the roentgenogram
3. "Hilar haze"—a loss of definition of large central pulmonary vessels with a slight general increase in opacity. This is very likely caused by interstitial edema anterior and posterior to the hilum, since the central vessels do not have perivascular interstitium until they enter the lung. This is probably the phase in which the alveolar wall interstitium contains excess fluid, is very difficult to evaluate, and is an accessory sign at best (see Fig. 28-2). It can often be best appreciated when an earlier film is available for comparison; when a film is obtained after successful treatment of the edema, it can be recognized in retrospect.
4. Appearance of septal lines
   a. Kerley's B lines are dense, horizontal lines that measure about 1.5 to 2.0 cm in length.

They are best seen in the lower lung on oblique projections on films of good quality. They represent secondary interlobular septa thickened by fluid (Figs. 28-1 and 28-2).

b. Kerley's A lines are longer and range in length from 5 to 10 cm. They tend to be straight or slightly curved and extend from the hila or parahilar area toward the periphery. They are seen in the upper lobes and tend to appear in acute interstitial edema. They represent fluid in the secondary interlobular septa, chiefly in the upper lobes (see Fig. 28-1).

5. A diffuse, reticular pattern may be observed associated with other findings noted in the signs already described. This is difficult to assess, but probably represents interstitial fluid in these patients with edema. A similar pattern may be seen in patients with widespread interstitial fibrosis, but Kerley's A lines are not usually present in these so the differentiation usually is not difficult.

In chronic congestive failure, interstitial edema may resemble chronic interstitial thickening associated with pulmonary disease. In some cases, only when treatment of the cardiac condition brings about regression can the true nature of the process be diagnosed with certainty.

Interstitial edema often occurs in combination with the alveolar type (Fig 28-3). Interstitial edema precedes alveolar edema in these instances, but often the onset is very rapid with massive alveolar edema overshadowing all subtle signs.

6. Subpleural edema may be observed best adjacent to the minor fissure on the right, but may also be observed along the major fissures in lateral projections. Peripherally there may be enough edema fluid to simulate pleural thickening.

The fluid accumulates first in peribronchial, perivascular, and interlobular interstitial spaces to produce the findings as noted. Edema (thickening) of the alveolar wall probably doesn't occur until later, after the other interstitial spaces are filled. Then alveolar flooding may occur if fluid continues to accumulate in the lungs.

ALVEOLAR EDEMA

The classic roentgen findings of alveolar pulmonary edema are those of bilateral opacities that extend outward in a fan-shaped manner from the hilum on both sides. The peripheral lungs are relatively clear. This includes the bases as well as the apices except in congestive failure, in which basal congestive changes and

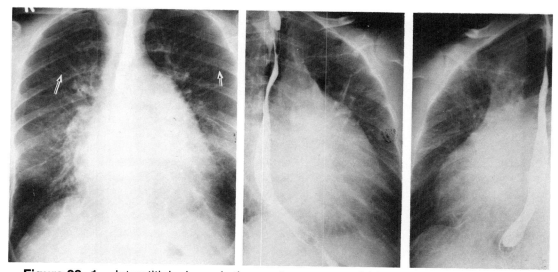

Figure 28–1. Interstitial edema. In the roentgenograms of this patient who had rheumatic mitral disease and a grossly enlarged heart, typical Kerley's B lines are evident at both lateral bases. Some longer, finer lines in the upper central lungs (*arrows*) probably represent Kerley's A lines. A little parahilar haze is seen, particularly on the right side. A general increase in interstitial markings resulting in a somewhat reticular pattern, noted best in the oblique projections, is apparent. Also, a small amount of pleural fluid is present on the left.

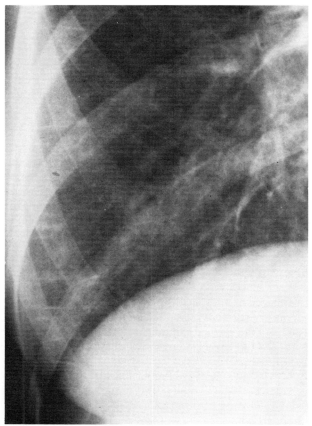

Figure 28–2. Kerley's B lines. Close-up of the right lateral lung base in a patient with mitral stenosis and interstitial edema. The numerous transverse, short, opaque lines at the periphery of the lung represent secondary interlobular septa thickened by edema fluid.

edema produce changes there. Because interstitial edema precedes the alveolar form, some or all of the signs of interstitial edema may be observed. However, the alveolar edema may be so extensive that other signs are obscured. When the edema is moderate, the opacity is somewhat patchy and mottled, but it may become quite homogeneous as the amount increases (Fig. 28-4). In the latter instance, the fluid-filled alveoli surrounding the bronchi produce contrast with the air-containing bronchi and, as a result, the bronchi are visible as linear radiolucent spaces (air bronchogram) traversing the opaque edematous area (Fig. 28-5). The opacity is often bilaterally symmetric, or nearly so. There are many exceptions to this rule and a number of cases have been reported in which the edema was unilateral.

Serial films often show rapid changes in the amount and distribution of the edema from day to day. When pulmonary edema is early and minor, it may produce scattered localized opacities that may simulate nodular disease (Fig. 28-6). The "nodules" are poorly defined, however, and probably represent acini (the portion of lung distal to a terminal bronchiole) filled with edema fluid. Bizarre forms may also be present with large, rather rounded areas of increased density that may simulate tumor. As a general rule, the alveolar opacity is hazy and poorly defined, so there is no difficulty in making the diagnosis. Pleural effusion is commonly associated with edema, particularly in congestive heart failure and in uremia.

Numerous reports of unusual and asymmetric distribution of edema have led to some experimental work and much speculation as to the factors involved in the distribution of edema fluid.[5] Gravity is undoubtedly a factor in many cases, but lateral views of patients who have been supine sometimes shows the fluid to be in anterior or lingular segments or in the middle lobe. Lack of peripheral edema is probably related to better peripheral drainage of lymphatics and to the increased respiratory motion of the peripheral lung acting to "pump" the fluid out. The relative lack of compliance in the central lung and in lung which has been previously diseased may also be involved. Defective lymphatic drainage favors accumulation of fluid in areas of pulmonary disease, which has resulted in scarring or decrease in compliance.

Gravity definitely plays a part in many patients with unilateral pulmonary edema. Other factors include differences in perfusion and in microvascular pressures in different areas. A gravitational shift test has been devised and studied to detect edema and to differentiate it from other causes of lung opacity.[21] The patient is kept in a supine or semi-erect position for 2 hours before a baseline bedside radiograph is obtained. Then the hemithorax with the lesser density is placed in a dependent position and the patient is kept in this lateral decubitus position for not less than 2, nor more than 3 hours. A second bedside radiograph is then obtained. In this study there was a recognizable shift of fluid opacity to the dependent side in 85% of patients with edema and in 86% of patients with edema and inflammatory disease. There was no shift in 78% of patients with inflammatory disease only. Therefore, this may be of help in differentiating edema from other pulmonary conditions in some cases.

There are no constantly reliable changes that will determine the cause, but in edema secondary to cardiac failure, the observations of cardiac enlargement, pulmonary vascular redistribution to the upper lobes, basal edema, and pleural effusion are strong indications that the edema is the result of heart disease. Excep-

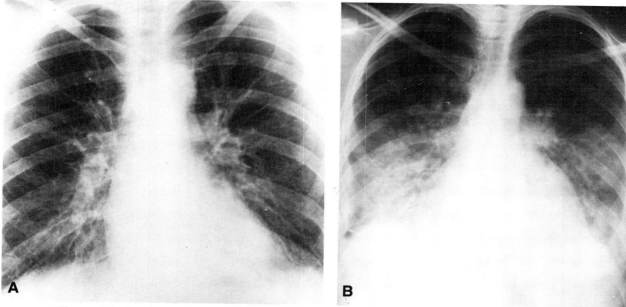

Figure 28–3. Interstitial and alveolar edema. (**A**) Interstitial edema. There is a general increase in interstitial markings, particularly in the parahilar areas and at the bases. The vessels are poorly defined, particularly at the bases, as a result of perivascular edema. Also, a little parahilar haze blurring the vessels is noted there, particularly on the right. (**B**) Alveolar edema. Same patient shown in *A*, with renal failure and evidence of extensive alveolar opacity in the parahilar areas and at the bases. There is now some pleural fluid bilaterally. The unequal distribution of the alveolar edema is not unusual.

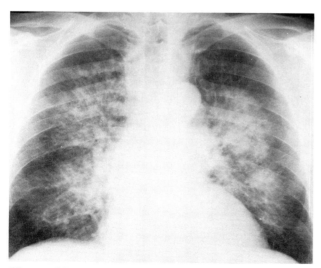

Figure 28–4. Pulmonary edema. This is a rather typical example of alveolar edema with a fan-shaped distribution in the parahilar and mid zones of the lungs. This patient had chronic renal failure.

tions include the absence of cardiac enlargement in some patients with pulmonary edema secondary to acute coronary thrombosis, and the absence of basal congestive changes in patients with edema secondary to acute left ventricular failure. As a general rule, pulmonary edema caused by uremia (azotemic edema) produces the classic central perihilar opacity of the lungs with or without evidence of cardiac enlargement and balanced pulmonary vascularity.

Pulmonary edema (injury edema, permeability edema) caused by inhalation of irritant gases tends to be somewhat more widespread than the other types and results in a mottled and patchy appearance extending farther to the periphery with slightly less central involvement than that seen in uremia; it also tends to be more basal. Roentgen distribution is not characteristic, however, and the history is of great importance in arriving at the diagnosis in these patients. Milne and co-workers have studied the problem of etiology of pulmonary edema and have shown that the cause can often be determined on plain chest radiographs.[10, 11] A remarkable degree of accuracy (91%) was obtained in differentiating capillary permeability edema from

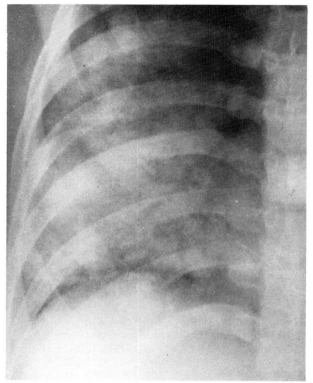

Figure 28–5. Alveolar pulmonary edema. Close-up of the right lower lung to show air-filled bronchi (air bronchogram) in the otherwise dense fluid-filled lung.

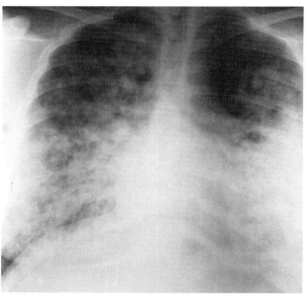

Figure 28–6. Alveolar edema. The rounded, poorly defined opacities noted best in the upper lung and in the right central and lower lung represent the acinar type of fluid distribution.

other varieties. The lowest (81%) accuracy was in distinguishing cardiac failure from renal failure and their overall accuracy ranged from 86% to 89%. The factors listed in Table 28-1 were evaluated by these authors in differentiating the etiology of pulmonary edema. Several studies have been done to evaluate Milner's method but to the present time none have conclusively disproved it (see Table 28-1).*

PULMONARY THROMBOEMBOLISM

Pulmonary embolism with or without infarction is a more common lesion than is generally realized. Since the majority of thromboembolic episodes cause no symptoms, they are not recognized. In addition to its occurrence as a postoperative complication and in patients with cardiac disease, pulmonary embolism occurs in a number of other conditions such as immobilization for any reason (e.g., sitting or standing for long periods, leg casts, stroke, pregnancy, oral contraceptives, and

* Personal communication

varicose veins). The most common sources of pulmonary emboli are thrombi in the deep veins of the thigh and pelvis, and to a lesser extent, the calf. When the embolus is very large and occludes almost the entire pulmonary arterial tree, death may occur very quickly. When the embolus is somewhat smaller it may or may not produce infarction, but will often cause immediate symptoms of chest pain and dyspnea. There may be no symptoms or signs with small emboli.[3]

In addition to thrombi, a number of other materials may act as emboli. Air embolism may follow trauma, surgical procedures, intravenous procedures of all types, thoracentesis, percutaneous lung biopsy, or any manipulation with the potential of exposing a vein to air. The air is not usually demonstrated radiographically; it disappears very quickly if the patient survives. If air embolism is not immediately lethal, air may be observed in the pulmonary artery and has been observed in the heart of a patient who subsequently died.[7] Pulmonary edema may result when the patient survives, because venous air embolism affects the lungs. If air embolism is suspected, the patient should be placed in the left lateral decubitus position, to keep the air in the right atrium, if possible, until it is absorbed.

Arterial air embolism results when air enters the pulmonary venous system; it affects the heart and brain. If it causes sudden death, the air can usually be demonstrated on postmortem films. Opaque contrast

Table 28-1. Radiographic Features of Pulmonary Edema*

	CARDIAC	RENAL	INJURY
Heart size	Enlarged	Enlarged	Not enlarged
Vascular pedicle	Normal or enlarged	Enlarged	Normal or reduced
Pulmonary blood flow distribution	Inverted	Balanced	Normal or balanced
Pulmonary blood volume	Normal or increased	Increased	Normal
Septal lines	Not common	Not common	Absent
Peribronchial cuffs	Very common	Very common	Not common
Air bronchogram	Not common	Not common	Very common
Lung edema, regional distribution (horizontal axis)	Even	Central	Peripheral
Pleural effusions	Very common	Very common	Not common

* Each factor listed has been shown to have statistical significance in determining which type of edema is present.

† Reproduced with permission of Milne and associates and the *American Journal of Roentgenology*.

materials used in lymphangiography, hysterosalpingography, and myelography occasionally enter the bloodstream and have been demonstrated in the lungs following these procedures. A few cases of barium in the pulmonary vessels following barium enema have been reported in which fatalities have occurred during the examination. Metallic mercury injected intravenously has been reported in a few instances. Dense, small globular and branching linear opacities may then be demonstrated on the chest radiograph.

PULMONARY INFARCTION

The incidence of infarction varies in different groups of patients with pulmonary thromboembolism. In patients with chronic heart disease and congestive failure, it approaches 100%, while in young, healthy individuals, infarct with necrosis is rare unless there are complicating factors such as severe trauma. In the elderly, or chronically ill who are bedridden, the incidence of infarct is in the range of 60% to 70% of those who have pulmonary emboli. The roentgenographic diagnosis is often difficult to make. Often no abnormalities are present on the chest film.[4] The major error is usually failure to suspect infarction as the cause for abnormal roentgen findings in the chest. The roentgen signs are: (1) elevation of the hemidiaphragm on the involved side indicating decrease in lung volume; (2) unilateral pleural effusion, usually small; (3) pulmonary parenchymal consolidation; (4) atelectasis; and (5) linear shadow(s). An infarct must be differentiated from pneumonia, edema, and atelectasis as well as other local conditions, including infected cysts and abscesses. The lower lobes are most frequently involved, but the lesion may occur in any lobe. Elevation of a hemidiaphragm or small unilateral pleural effusion or both may be the earliest signs of infarction. At times the shadow of the infarct may not be visible and the effusion is the only sign. It takes from 10 to 24 hours for an infarct to evolve to the point where it is visible roentgenographically. This is probably the hazy, poorly defined, edematous lesion that requires an additional 2 to 4 days and sometimes a week to form a well-defined complete infarct.

Infarction of a single secondary pulmonary lobule may occur, and since not all lobules have a pleural surface, it follows that not all infarcts have a pleural surface. Infarcts are usually aggregates of involved secondary lobules, however, so the lesion usually extends to a pleural surface. Since this may be the interlobar pleura, its shadow is not necessarily peripheral as visualized in the frontal projection. The shape of the infarct depends on the location. The visceral pleura usually forms one side of the lesion, and often two or three sides. The long axis of the infarct is in the plane of the longest pleural surface with which it is in contact. The actual shadow may be round, wedge-shaped, or roughly triangular. It may assume the shape of the lingula or of the right middle lobe or may fill and obliterate a costophrenic sulcus if the lateral segment of a lower lobe is involved. Oblique views aided by fluoroscopic positioning may be necessary to bring out the relationship of the lesion to the pleura in many cases. The hilar aspect of the infarct is usually described as rounded or hump-shaped, rather than resembling the apex of a triangle. The appearance of a typical hump is unusual, if not rare, and most any shape of opacity may be present. The amount of associated pleural effusion is usually not great and multiple lesions may be seen in one or both lungs (Fig. 28-7). At first, the periphery of the lesion is rather hazy and poorly defined, but as time goes on it becomes more sharply outlined and as it heals it gradually becomes smaller. The size of the infarct can vary greatly, from a small faint opacity to the greater part of a lobe. The average size is about 3 to 5 cm. The pulmonary changes resolve rather slowly. The complete hemorrhagic necrotic infarct requires 4 weeks or more for complete resolution. When infarction is incomplete and there is no necrosis, the local findings are caused by edema and hemorrhage. This process may clear quickly (i.e., within a week) and leave no residue.

When the initial opacity is noted, it is not possible to determine whether it represents an area of infarction with necrosis or an area of hemorrhage secondary to an embolus. When the opacity clears in a week or so, you can reasonably assume it represented an *incomplete infarct* (without significant necrosis). The *complete infarct* (with necrosis) slowly decreases in size over several weeks. About 50% of infarcts disappear completely without any scar or other residue. In the remainder, linear scars develop in about 50%, while in the others there is pleural change, either in the form of local pleural thickening or diaphragmatic adhesions.[9] Eventually only a linear band may remain to indicate

the site of a previous infarct.[4] It may be quite small and inconspicuous. It is not certain that all of the linear opacities represent the same pathologic process. Some may represent platelike or focal atelectasis caused by a combination of poor ventilation, narrowing of the bronchi, decreased compliance of the lung, and lack of surfactant, all of which occur in pulmonary embolism with infarction and eventually cause parenchymal fibrosis. Some probably represent linear shadows of pleural origin. Another possibility is that they represent thrombosed veins or arteries surrounded by fibrosis.

Diaphragmatic change secondary to the pleural involvement and loss of lung volume is represented by elevation of the diaphragm. This may be the only roentgen finding in some patients. If the possibility of pulmonary infarction is kept in mind in bedridden, debilitated, or cardiac patients with sudden pleuritic type of chest pain, the presence of one or all of the signs just described should lead to the diagnosis, or at least a suspicion of it, in most instances. The lack of a characteristic contour cannot be overemphasized because of the wide variety of shapes, depending on location; the size also varies greatly. It is also important to remember that infarction can occur in the absence of congestive heart disease. There may be enough fluid in the

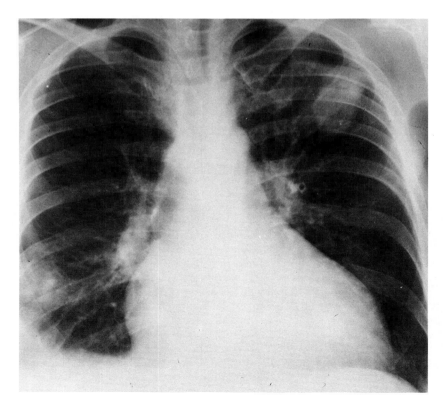

Figure 28–7. Pulmonary infarcts. The oval opacity at the left apex represents an old infarct. There is a little fluid remaining in the major fissure in the region of the infarct, which is now quite well circumscribed. There are two infarcts in the right base; one produces a humplike shadow obliterating the costophrenic angle and projecting above the level of the dome of the diaphragm; the other is somewhat rounded and lies above it. There is also some pleural effusion. The heart is greatly enlarged.

pleural space to hide the pulmonary lesion and decubitus films are of value to outline the basal lung when infarction is suspected.

Because plain chest radiographs are not specific, they are of limited utility in the diagnosis of thromboemboli; therefore other diagnostic methods are used. CT is not a primary diagnostic method but may be helpful in patients with undiagnosed pulmonary masses. Occasionally intraluminal arterial defects are observed on CT using contrast; they represent emboli. The use of CT is very limited; however, ultrafast CT may prove useful in the future.[6] The radionuclide perfusion scan is widely employed in patients with suspected pulmonary embolism. A negative perfusion scan excludes most embolisms and is therefore highly sensitive. However, a positive perfusion scan may be caused by a number of conditions other than embolism, so specificity is low. Ventilation–perfusion (V–Q) scans are also frequently used, and may add information. When an area of lung with a perfusion defect has normal ventilation, it is assumed to represent an embolus. However, abnormal ventilation in areas of abnormal perfusion have been reported in patients with pulmonary embolism, so matching ventilation–perfusion defects do not completely exclude embolism; therefore, pulmonary angiography may be indicated in those instances in which clinical suspicion is high.[13] Areas which are not perfused or ventilated have a low probability of representing emboli. The scintiscans must be compared with recent chest radiographs in these patients.

A retrospective analysis of ventilation–perfusion imaging and pulmonary angiography in 246 patients with suspected pulmonary embolism was done by Biello and associates[1] using ^{133}Xe for the ventilation study followed by an immediate perfusion scan using ^{99m}Tc macroaggregated albumin intravenously (250,000 to 500,000 particles). All had abnormal V–Q scans and 53 patients (36%) had pulmonary embolism documented by pulmonary angiography. Analysis of the scans revealed the following: (1) two moderate or one large V–Q mismatch—92% had embolism; (2) small V–Q mismatch—no emboli (19 patients); (3) matched V–Q abnormalities in radiographically normal areas—4.8% had embolism; (4) perfusion defect substantially larger than radiographic abnormality—87% had embolism; (5) perfusion defect substantially smaller than radiographic abnormality—7.7% had embolism; (6) matched perfusion and radiographic abnormality—27% had embolism. Thus, the patients could be classified into groups with high, intermediate, or low probability of pulmonary embolism (Table 28-2). The last group (6) is most inconclusive, so patients in this group are the most likely candidates for pulmonary angiography[19] (Fig. 28-8).

Pulmonary arteriography is the most accurate method for making the diagnosis, but selective segmental and subsegmental studies using oblique projections may be necessary to outline small-vessel involvement. The primary signs of embolism are a persistent intraluminal filling defect that may completely obstruct the involved artery and the abrupt cutoff of a vessel by the proximal end of a clot. Secondary signs, helpful but not diagnostic, are areas of avascularity, focal areas of prolonged arterial filling, and pruning or paucity of vessels. This method is used if a positive diagnosis of pulmonary embolism is imperative. Its use is usually limited to patients in whom surgical therapy of any type is contemplated, before thrombolytic therapy and, at least in some instances, before anticoagulants are used, particularly when the use of anticoagulants poses a threat to a specific patient for any reason.

Some studies have been done using magnetic resonance imaging (MRI) in patients with suspected pulmonary embolism, but there are a number of problems, so its ultimate usefulness has yet to be determined.

EMBOLISM WITHOUT INFARCTION

Pulmonary embolism without infarction may be massive and life-threatening and is more common than embolism with infarction. Prompt diagnosis is of utmost importance in these patients. Roentgen findings are often absent, in contrast to the clinical findings in a desperately ill patient. Roentgen findings do not include the pulmonary opacity which is observed in patients with infarction and are, at best, only suggestive of the diagnosis. The central pulmonary arteries may be increased in size. The descending branch of the right pulmonary artery measured at total lung capacity from the level of the bronchus intermedius to its outer border is a maximum of 16 mm in adult males and 15 mm in adult females.[2] Any measurement above this suggests the possibility of embolism. It is particularly useful when there is a change. If the patient happens to have had a roentgenogram of the chest in the recent past, comparison can be very helpful (Fig. 28-9). The increase in size is caused by the mass of the embolus, and there may be a bulge in the artery in its proximal portion, with sharp tapering to a smaller diameter immediately below it. Oligemia distal to the obstructing embolus manifested by a hyperlucent area (Westermark's sign) may be present, but is often difficult to assess. Loss of lung volume causing diaphragmatic elevation is the third sign. Occasionally a small pleural effusion may be present. Acute cor pulmonale, with secondary signs of dilatation of the superior vena cava

Table 28-2. Scheme for Interpretation of V/Q Imaging

INTERPRETATION*	PATTERN†	PULMONARY EMBOLISM (%)
Normal	Normal perfusion conforming to the shape of the lungs	0
PROBABILITY OF PULMONARY EMBOLISM		
Low	Small V/Q mismatches	<10
	Small focal V/Q matches with no corresponding radiographic abnormalities	
	Any perfusion defects substantially smaller than associated radiographic abnormalities	
Intermediate	Widespread severe COPD	<20 to 40
	Perfusion defects and radiographic abnormalities of same size and location	
	Single moderate or large V/Q mismatch without corresponding radiographic abnormality	
	Not falling into other categories	
High‡	Perfusion defects substantially larger than radiographic abnormalities in the same location	>85
	Two moderate and one large mismatches without corresponding radiographic abnormality in that area	
	Two large V/P mismatches without corresponding radiographic abnormalities	

* Highest applicable criteria apply. Thus, a patient with widespread diffuse COPD and two segmental mismatches should be interpreted as high probability.
† Small defects—less than 25% of a pulmonary segment (eg, a "rat bite"); moderate defect—between 25% and 75% of a segment; large defect—greater than 75% of a segment.
‡ Defects in this category are usually wedge-shaped and extend to the lung periphery.
Adapted from Biello DR, Mattar AG, Osei-Wusu A, et al: Interpretation of indeterminate lung scintigrams. Radiology 133:189, 1979; and Saltzman HA, et al: Value of ventilation/perfusion scan in acute pulmonary embolism: Results of the Prospective Investigation of Pulmonary Embolism Diagnosis (PIOPED). JAMA 263(20):2753, 1990. Courtesy of F.A. Mettler, Jr., with permission.

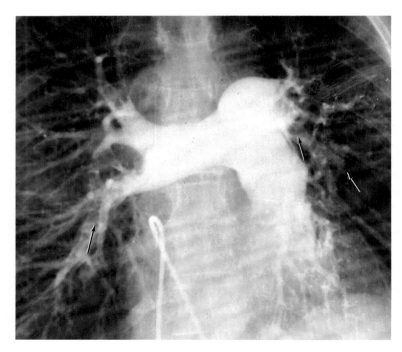

Figure 28–8. Pulmonary emboli. This arteriogram shows several small lucencies representing emboli obstructing the pulmonary arteries (*arrows*).

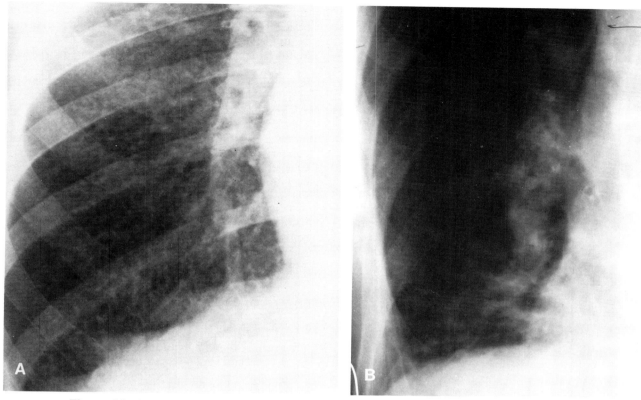

Figure 28–9. Pulmonary embolism. The patient developed chest pain while in the hospital. **(A)** Close-up of the right lower lung on admission. **(B)** One week later, on film exposed 1 day after the onset of chest pain, enlargement of the pulmonary artery, which was found to be the site of a large embolus, is demonstrated. The diaphragm is elevated. The horizontal linear opacities at the lung base most likely represent areas of subsegmental atelectasis. The patient did not develop infarction that could be recognized radiographically.

causing some superior mediastinal widening on the right, azygous vein enlargement, and cardiac enlargement may be helpful in diagnosis. At best, the diagnosis of massive pulmonary embolism can be suggested. Since embolectomy may be done when the patient is hypotensive and cyanotic, pulmonary arteriography may be indicated to confirm the presence of large central embolus, which can be removed surgically in such a patient.

As in embolism with infarction, the diagnosis can usually be made by employing the combination of a chest roentgenogram and lung scan. When serious doubt regarding the diagnosis arises following these procedures, pulmonary arteriography can be done. The angiographic signs of pulmonary embolism are the same as those listed in the section on embolism with infarction.

In embolism without infarction that is not life-threatening, plain film findings are often very subtle and the chest is often normal. The steps in imaging are the same as described for embolism with infarction.

SEPTIC INFARCTION

When the embolus producing infarction contains or is made up of bacteria, septic infarction results, which leads to tissue breakdown and formation of cavity. These lesions may occur in association with subacute bacterial endocarditis or in patients with septicemia. The lesions may be single but are usually multiple. There may be sequestration of the necrotic center of an infarct to produce cavity without infection. Usually infection supervenes, however, and when the infarcts become infected the pneumonia surrounding them causes further increase in opacity with a poorly circumscribed periphery. The appearance is that of a central cavity within a poorly defined area of increased opacity. When there is a typical history and other infarcts or cavities are present, the diagnosis is not difficult to make, but in single lesions the differentiation between infarct cavity and cavity secondary to primary inflammatory disease is difficult, if not impossible.

POSTTRAUMATIC FAT EMBOLISM

There is experimental and some clinical evidence to show that fat embolism is very common following bone and soft-tissue injury, particularly following fractures of the tibia and femur. However, despite the fact that many severely injured patients are observed, the clinical entity of posttraumatic fat embolism is relatively rare. As reported by Williams and associates, fat embolism occurs in from 0.5% to 2.0% of patients with long-bone fracture.[20] It is likely that small amounts of fat may form emboli without symptoms and signs. The fat embolism syndrome is probably caused by the entry of neutral fat into the venous system; from there it travels to the pulmonary vascular bed. A second theory which accounts for some instances of the syndrome is that the stress of trauma causes a release of catecholamines such as epinephrine, which causes mobilization of free fatty acids from adipose tissue and induces coalescence of serum lipid (e.g., in cases of pancreatitis, burns, or sepsis). In most instances, traumatic release of fat from sites of injury directly into the venous system is the most likely cause. The fat is converted into free fatty acids in the lung where they produce edema, hemorrhage, and leukocytic infiltration of interstitial spaces. Pathogenesis remains somewhat controversial, however.

Some of the fat or fatty acid or both get through the lungs into the systemic circulation. This accounts for the fat found in other organs, and for the central nervous system involvement that is sometimes present. The roentgen findings are varied, but are uniformly bilateral. They include: (1) Diffuse bilateral opacity, which resembles pulmonary edema except that there is more basal involvement than is usually observed in edema and the involvement is more peripheral, often with relatively little alveolar density centrally. (2) Bilateral, multiple small nodular opacities—often more in the lower lungs than elsewhere. At times the small opacities may be more linear than nodular. This probably represents a somewhat lesser involvement than the more confluent homogeneous edema pattern. (3) Usually there is no pleural effusion or cardiac enlargement. (4) Delayed onset, usually from 1 to 3 days following trauma. Clinical signs and symptoms occur within 24 hours of trauma in 60% and within 48 hours in 85% of patients who develop the syndrome.[20] Some patients do not manifest symptoms or signs for 72 hours or more. A high index of suspicion is necessary in patients with recent major fractures. It is likely that fat embolism is not recognized in many instances when symptoms are minimal.

The delay in the appearance of symptoms and of radiographic signs in fat embolism is in contrast to pulmonary contusion with hemorrhage and edema that appears as an abnormality on chest films taken very soon after injury. Also, contusion is usually unilateral or asymmetric in contrast to the bilateral symmetry of fat embolism. The diagnosis of fat embolism syndrome can usually be made on the basis of the history of chest pain, dyspnea, tachycardia, and cough 12 hours to several days following injury, along with chest findings as described. Resolution requires from 6 days to 2 weeks or more.

PULMONARY HYPERTENSION

Blood flow through the lungs and pulmonary artery pressure are dependent on a number of factors, including arterial and venous resistance, the amount of blood flow that may be altered by various shunts, and combinations of these factors. Pulmonary hypertension may be predominantly arterial (precapillary) or venous (postcapillary), or a combination of the two. Because the radiographic changes vary with the type and the site of the major causative factors, the classification of pulmonary hypertension by Simon and co-workers is useful:[16]

I. Precapillary (Arterial Hypertension)
   A. Increased resistance
     1. Obstructive—pulmonary embolism, idiopathic or primary pulmonary hypertension, pulmonary schistosomiasis, reverse shunts (ventricular septal defect, atrial septal defect, or patent ductus arteriosus)
     2. Obliterative—pulmonary emphysema, diffuse interstitial diseases (granulomatous, neoplastic, or infectious)
     3. Constrictive—anoxia
   B. Increased flow
     1. Large left-to-right shunts—PDA, VSD
II. Postcapillary (Venous Hypertension)
   A. Acute—Left ventricular failure regardless of cause
   B. Chronic—Mitral valvular disease, left atrial myxoma, anomalous pulmonary venous return, mediastinal fibrosis, idiopathic or primary veno-obstructive disease[8]

III. Combined Pre- and Postcapillary Hypertension
IV. Diffuse Pulmonary Arteriovenous Shunting Complicating Chronic Lung Disease[15]—Emphysema—shunt syndrome

Pulmonary hypertension is defined as elevation of pressure in the pulmonary circuit above certain limits at rest or during mild exercise. These limits are generally accepted as 30 mmHg systolic and 15 mmHg diastolic, with a mean of 18 mmHg on the arterial side. On the venous side, the upper limit is considered to be 12 mmHg; this is applied equally to the mean left atrial pressure and to the mean capillary-wedge pressure.

Most of the diseases causing pulmonary hypertension produce an increase in pulmonary vascular resistance. In the upright chest film of the normal person, the upper zone vessels are smaller than those in the lower zones. In recumbency, the difference disappears; this accounts in part for disparity between angiograms and routine films.

There are distinct radiographic differences in the precapillary and postcapillary groups. The roentgen changes in *pulmonary arterial (precapillary) hypertension* include dilatation of the pulmonary artery and its central branches on either side; narrowing of the peripheral pulmonary arteries, usually at the origin of the lobar artery branches, resulting in a rather sharp fall-off in size from central to peripheral arteries (Fig. 28-10); tortuosity of peripheral arteries, particularly in lower zones, observed along with a general decrease in caliber of pulmonary veins; and calcification observed in the pulmonary artery (Fig. 28-11). Cor pulmonale or heart disease secondary to pulmonary disease—with varying enlargement of the right ventricle caused by dilatation, hypertrophy, or both—is the eventual result. Signs of the underlying causative disease may be minimal, obvious, or absent. In general, increasing severity of the hypertension is accompanied by an increase in the radiographic signs, but there are exceptions, so caution should be observed in predict-

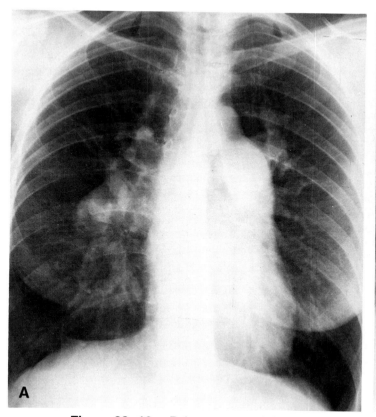
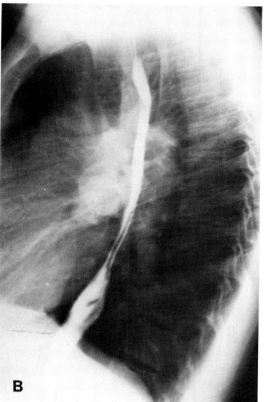

Figure 28–10. Pulmonary arterial hypertension. The pulmonary artery and its central branches are grossly enlarged, in contrast to the peripheral arteries, which are small. This patient had an atrial septal defect. She developed pulmonary hypertension, which resulted in reversal on the initial left-to-right shunt, and became cyanotic.

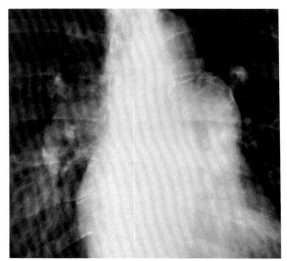

Figure 28–11. Pulmonary arterial hypertension. Note the dense calcification in the pulmonary artery and ductus in this patient with patent ductus. She had developed a reversal of the shunt as a result of the pulmonary hypertension.

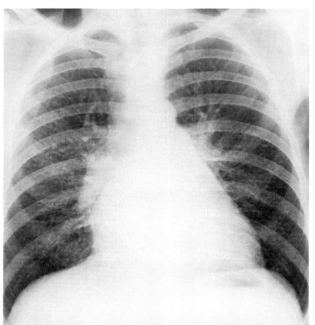

Figure 28–12. Pulmonary venous hypertension. This patient with mitral disease demonstrates some parahilar haze and distinct difference in vessel size, the upper-lobe vessels being definitely larger than those in the lower lobe. This represents redistribution of blood flow and indicates pulmonary venous hypertension.

ing pulmonary artery pressure ranges. The lungs are relatively clear unless the underlying pulmonary disease has produced considerable change.[14]

Another situation is one in which pulmonary arterial hypertension develops as systemic high pressures are transmitted across congenital defects with left-to-right shunts at the aortopulmonary (patent ductus) or ventricular (ventricular septal defect) level. A substantial high-pressure shunt at the aortic or ventricular level or a massive shunt at the atrial or great vein level will eventually cause a reactive sclerosis, intimal thickening, and medial hypertrophy in pulmonary arteries. This progresses to marked pulmonary arterial hypertension with resultant shunt reversal. The following roentgen signs are produced:

1. Marked enlargement of the pulmonary artery and its central branches extending out for a short distance along the lobar arteries. The central arteries are larger and the dilatation extends out farther than in pulmonary hypertension in the absence of a shunt. Calcification is occasionally observed in the pulmonary artery.
2. Constriction of segmental and peripheral arteries to normal or smaller than normal size
3. Normal or small pulmonary veins
4. The heart may show alteration consistent with the initial defect. However, eventually the right ventricle may enlarge to become the predominant chamber (cor pulmonale).

Postcapillary (venous) hypertension is often accompanied by changes that cause a considerable increase in pulmonary density (e.g., edema). Slight distention of all pulmonary veins is the earliest roentgen sign, but this is very difficult to evaluate unless comparison films are available. Constriction of the pulmonary arteries and veins in the lower zones and dilatation of the arteries and veins in the upper zones caused by redistribution of blood flow to the upper lobes are the most reliable early signs. These must be evaluated in the upright film, since there is normally some redistribution of flow to the upper lobes in films exposed with the patient recumbent. These findings may be striking when present, but are not well defined in every patient with venous hypertension. The signs may be obscured by pulmonary edema and congestion in left ventricular failure. The cause for the basal constriction, indicating a redistribution of blood flow, is most likely the increased amount of interstitial fluid in the lung bases as a result of the higher venous pressure. This restricts blood flow and the larger vessels respond by a reduction in diameter. Blood flow to the upper zones is increased and the arteries and veins dilate in these areas. Mild, venous hypertension shows only the basal vascular constriction, which may be difficult to assess (Fig. 28-12). As the venous pressure increases, additional findings of early interstitial edema can be observed; they include the appearance of Kerley's B lines and Kerley's A lines. A slight perihilar haze may be evident. Vascular margins are blurred and poorly defined in the lower zones, and there is a general increase in interstitial markings caused by an increased amount of interstitial fluid, which begins in the lower lungs (Figs. 28-13 and 28-14). Alveolar edema and pleural effusion appear when venous hypertension is marked and left ventricular failure occurs. Chronic postcapillary hypertension, such as that found in mitral stenosis, and left atrial myxoma may result in irreversible constriction of lower-zone pulmonary vessels.

When there is a *combined arterial (precapillary) and venous (postcapillary) hypertension*, the roentgen changes depend on the sequence of events. Mitral stenosis is a good example, with venous hypertension occurring for some time followed by arterial hypertension. The roentgen findings are then in combination and develop as the disease develops—a summation of changes.

The subject of the pulmonary blood flow, its quantitation, and the changes in arterial and venous hypertension are thoroughly discussed by Simon;[14] the reader is referred to his work for further information regarding these problems.

Chronic lung diseases such as pulmonary fibrosis and emphysema cause increased pulmonary arterial resistance, resulting in pulmonary arterial hypertension. Occasionally such a patient will develop general dilatation of pulmonary arteries and veins involving all of the lung zones. This is caused by diffuse arteriovenous shunting. There may be some interstitial edema and the patients are dyspneic and cyanotic. It is postulated by Simon and co-workers that a combination of increased pulmonary resistance and left ventricular decompensation probably caused by hypoxia results in this "emphysema-shunt syndrome."[16]

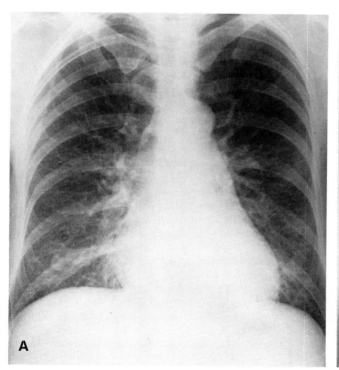 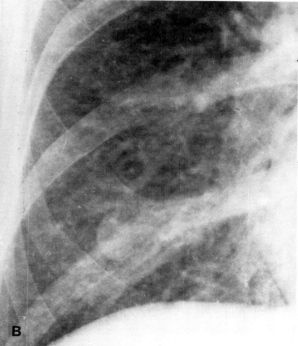

Figure 28–13. Congestive failure in a patient with arteriosclerotic cardiovascular disease. **(A)** Central and basal vessels are poorly defined, indicating perivascular edema. No Kerley's B lines are observed. Upper-lobe vessels are relatively prominent. Basal vessels are difficult to define because of the perivascular edema. **(B)** Close-up of the right base to show the poor definition of vessels in this patient.

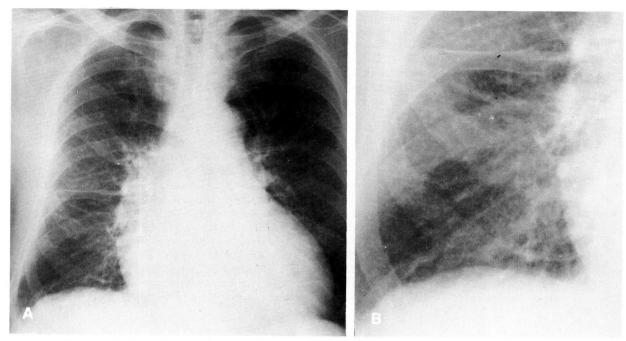

Figure 28–14.   Congestive heart failure. **(A)** The heart is distinctly enlarged. There is vascular redistribution and evidence of some parahilar haze and perivascular edema, noted best at the right base. **(B)** Close-up of area of involvement. The individual vessels are very poorly defined. There is a hint of a little interstitial edema peripherally, with short, horizontal linear densities that are poorly defined.

REFERENCES AND SELECTED READINGS

1. BIELLO DR, MATTAR AG, MCKNIGHT RC, ET AL: Ventilation-perfusion studies in suspected pulmonary embolism. Am J Roentgenol 133:1033, 1979

2. CHANG CH: The normal roentgenographic measurement of the right descending pulmonary artery in 1085 cases. Am J Roentgenol 87:929, 1962

3. FIGLEY MM, GERDES AJ, RICKETTS HJ: Radiographic aspects of pulmonary embolism. Semin Roentgenol 2:389, 1967

4. FLEISCHNER FG: Roentgenology of the pulmonary infarct. Semin Roentgenol 2:61, 1967

5. FLEISCHNER FG: The butterfly pattern of acute pulmonary edema. In Simon M, Potchen EJ, LeMay M (eds): Frontiers of Pulmonary Radiology, pp 360–379. New York, Grune & Stratton, 1967

6. GERAGHTY JJ, ET AL: Ultrafast Computed tomography in experimental pulmonary embolism. Invest Radiol 27:60, 1992

7. KIZER KW, GOODMAN PC: Radiographic manifestations of venous air embolism. Radiology 144:35, 1982

8. LIEBOW AA, MOSER KM, SOUTHGATE MT: Primary veno-obstructive disease of the lung: Clinical-pathologic conference. JAMA 223:1243, 1973

9. MCGOLDRICK PJ, RUDD TG, FIGLEY MM, ET AL: What becomes of pulmonary infarcts? Am J Roentgenol 133:1039, 1979

10. MILNE ENC: Some new concepts of pulmonary blood flow and volume. Radiol Clin North Am 14:515, 1978

11. MILNE ENC, PISTOLESI M, MINIATI M, ET AL: The radiologic distinction of cardiogenic and non-cardiogenic edema. Am J Roentgenol 144:879, 1985

12. RIGLER LG, SURPRENANT EL: Pulmonary edema. Semin Roentgenol 2:33, 1967

13. SANDLER MS, VELCHIK MG, ALAVI A: Ventilation abnormalities associated with pulmonary embolism. Clin Nucl Med 13:450, 1988

14. SIMON M: Physiologic considerations in radiology of pulmonary vasculature. In Abrams HL: Abrams Angiography, Vascular and Interventional Radiology, Vol 1, Chap 35, p 783. Boston, Little Brown, 1983

15. SIMON M, POTCHEN EJ, LEMAY M: Frontiers of Pulmonary Radiology. New York, Grune & Stratton, 1969

16. SIMON M, SASAHARA AA, CANNILLA JE: The radiology of

pulmonary hypertension. Semin Roentgenol 2:368, 1967

17. STAUB NC: Pathogenesis of pulmonary edema: State of the art review. Am Rev Resp Dis 109:358, 1974

18. TRAPNELL DH: Linear shadows in chest radiographs. In Potchen EJ (ed): Current Concepts in Radiology, p 282. St. Louis, C.V. Mosby, 1977

19. WELLMAN HN: Pulmonary thromboembolism: Current status report on the role of nuclear medicine. Sem Nucl Med 4:236, 1986

20. WILLIAMS AG, JR, METTLER FA JR, CHRISTIE JH, ET AL: Fat embolism syndrome. Clin Nucl Med 11:495, 1986

21. ZIMMERMAN JE, GOODMAN LR, ST ANDRE AC, ET AL: Radiographic detection of mobilizable lung water: The gravitational shift test. Am J Roentgenol 138:59, 1982

22. ZWIREWICH CV, MÜLLER NL, ABBOUD RT, ET AL: Non-cardiogenic pulmonary edema caused by decompression sickness: Rapid resolution following hyperbaric therapy. Radiology 163:81, 1987

*Paul and Juhl's Essentials of Radiologic Imaging,
Sixth Edition*, edited by John H. Juhl and
Andrew B. Crummy. J.B. Lippincott Company,
Philadelphia, © 1993.

CHAPTER 29

Tumors of the Lungs and Bronchi

John H. Juhl

MALIGNANT TUMORS

BRONCHOGENIC CARCINOMA

There has been an absolute as well as a relative increase in the incidence of carcinoma of the lung in the past 40 years that is reflected in the mortality rate. In white male smokers the reported incidence of cancer of the lung is 15 to 30 times higher than in non-smokers. Of all carcinomas this carries the highest mortality rate, but may have reached a plateau in males. The incidence and mortality rate in females is now rising, with one study showing a drop in male–female ratio from 15 to 1 in the years 1955 to 1959 to 6 to 1 in the years 1968 to 1971. By 1987, the ratio dropped to about 2 to 1, with an incidence of 20% of all cancers in males and 11% in females.[45] This appears to be related to an increase in the number of female smokers and probably to environmental exposure to cigarette smoke. An increase in all cell types of lung cancer occurs in cigarette smokers. There also appears to be an increase in lung cancer in persons exposed to asbestos, silica, lipids, hydrocarbons, arsenic, beryllium, chromate, nickel, vinyl chloride, radon gas, radiation, BCME (Bis [chloromethyl] ether), as well as a number of pulmonary conditions such as fibrosis, probably pulmonary tuberculosis, and other chronic bronchopulmonary infections. The number of individuals studied does not allow a final conclusion as to the cell type predominance in these groups. However, lung cancer is the leading cause of cancer-related death in the United States.

Classification of Malignant Lung Tumors

Numerous classifications of histologic types of lung tumors have been described and several are now used by various groups. This lack of agreement makes it difficult to compare the numerous studies regarding incidence or predominance of various cell types associated with various carcinogens. Classification of malignant tumors is excerpted from The World Health Organization Classification (1982) and is presented in Table 29-1.[57]

Various reports regarding the incidence of the cell types are available. The relative incidence (median) of cell types adapted from Modan[26] as reported by Ives are as follows[15]:

Squamous cell carcinoma—30% (41.3% in males, 18.6% in females)
Small-cell carcinoma—15.2% (19.4% in males, 11% in females)
Adenocarcinoma—31.5% (17.9% in males, 45.1% in females)
Large cell carcinoma—less than 1%

The numbers do not add up to 100% because all categories were not included in each of the studies reported.

A considerable difference in the incidence of the various cell types was found in a study of males in the Early Lung Cancer Cooperative Study done by Johns Hopkins, Mayo Clinic, and Memorial Sloan-Kettering Cancer Center.[49] A total of 31,360 men, all heavy cigarette smokers 45 years of age or older, have been fol-

Table 29-1. Classification of Histologic Types of Lung Cancer by the World Health Organization 1981[57]*

1. Squamous Cell Carcinoma
Variant:
   a. Spindle cell carcinoma
2. Small-Cell Carcinoma
   a. Oat cell carcinoma
   b. Intermediate cell type
   c. Combined oat cell carcinoma (multiple coding necessary) (eg, oat cell plus squamous cell carcinoma)
3. Adenocarcinoma
   a. Acinar adenocarcinoma
   b. Papillary adenocarcinoma
   c. Bronchioalveolar carcinoma
   d. Solid carcinoma with mucous formation
4. Large-Cell Carcinoma Variants:
   a. Giant-cell carcinoma
   b. Clear-cell carcinoma
5. Adenosquamous Carcinoma
6. Carcinoid Tumour
7. Bronchial Gland Carcinoma
   a. Adenoid cystic carcinoma
   b. Mucoepidermoid carcinoma
   c. Others
8. Others

* Malignant epithelial tumors of the lung. From Histological Classification of Lung Tumours, World Health Organization, Geneva, 1981. With permission.

lowed for at least 5 years. Of the 223 lung cancers detected in this group, cell types were as follows: squamous cell, 42%; adenocarcinoma, 32%; large cell, 15%; and small-cell, 10%. The differences in these two large studies emphasize the problem of obtaining accurate statistics on the relative incidence of the various cell types.[23]

Despite the advances in surgery, radiotherapy, and various combinations of chemotherapy, the overall 5-year survival rate remains very low, in the range of 5% to 12%. In contrast to this, the 5-year survival rate in one small series of patients with bronchogenic carcinoma discovered in a survey of asymptomatic patients was 30%. This suggests that there is an opportunity to decrease the high mortality rate in this type of cancer. Earlier diagnosis by means of radiographic examination is one way in which it may be accomplished. There are more than 100,000 new cases of lung cancer per year and 140,000 deaths per year.[46] The majority appear to be caused by cigarette smoking.

There are conflicting reports regarding the efficacy of screening the high-risk group (smokers older than 45 years of age) using chest roentgenograms, and there is not general agreement that earlier detection would result in decreased mortality. However, in the Cooperative Study, approximately 40% of radiologically visible cancers were Stage I, with a 5-year survival following resection of nearly 80%.[49] Therefore, it appears that screening warrants further study and consideration.[29]

However, there is no consensus that screening is of value, because mortality rates have not decreased. In patients in the high-risk group (smokers older than 45 years comprise the great majority) who desire a screening chest radiograph, there is very little reason to withhold the examination. Furthermore, the radiologist who interprets chest roentgenograms in patients with a long history of smoking should make certain that all roentgenograms are of good technical quality and should attempt to double-read each radiograph, because independent double reading appears to improve sensitivity.

The *epidermoid* or *squamous cell neoplasm* occurs predominantly in males, with a ratio of 2 or 3 males to 1 female. They make up about one third of all bronchogenic tumors and tend to occur in relatively old age groups, with the peak incidence at age 60. This tumor often arises in or immediately adjacent to lobar and segmental bronchi, but is occasionally peripheral. When a primary tumor is noted to invade the thoracic wall, it is more likely to be epidermoid than any other type. Necrosis with formation of cavity may also occur, and when a tumor with cavitation is found in an elderly male it is nearly always epidermoid in origin. The well-differentiated squamous cell tumor is more likely to remain confined to the bronchus of origin and adjacent nodes than the other cell types, and the rate of growth is often less rapid in this tumor than in the others. Invasion of veins with hematogenous metastasis does occur late in the course of the disease, however.

The *adenocarcinoma*, with an overall incidence of about 30%, is the most common of the bronchogenic tumors found in the female. It tends to be more peripheral than the other types, but in one study about 50% presented centrally, either as a hilar or mediastinal mass or as a combination of the two.[56] This is the tumor most often observed peripherally in relatively young females. The *small-cell carcinoma*, which makes up about 15% to 20% of bronchogenic tumors, often occurs centrally, with hilar enlargement and massive mediastinal lymph-node metastases. This type may resemble mediastinal lymphoma. It does not often arise as a peripheral tumor and does not undergo necrosis to form cavitation. The *large-cell carcinomas* are also anaplastic tumors and comprise about 5% to 15% of lung cancers. They tend to be large bulky tumors which usually occur peripherally. Pleural involvement with effusion is common.

The *bronchioloalveolar (bronchiolar) carcinoma*, a form of adenocarcinoma, is interesting because it is not related to smoking and appears to occur equally in males and females. It may sometimes be multifocal, but some investigators believe it begins as a single focus and spreads widely through the lymphatics or bronchi. Two general gross pathologic types are described: (1) the tumorlike or nodular form, and (2) the diffuse type, which may resemble pneumonic consolidation roentgenographically. There are also two histologic subtypes related to appearance of tumor cells—columnar cells (bronchiolar type) or cuboidal cells (alveolar type) that may predominate. Rarely a multicystic appearance occurs, which may or may not be associated with other solid lesions. There is a wide variation in the clinical course of the disease. Progression may be very slow or exceedingly rapid. Cough and dyspnea are prominent symptoms. Occasionally the cough may produce large amounts of mucoid sputum. In a review of 136 cases, Hill found a nodule less than 4 cm in 23%, a mass greater than 4 cm in 20%, diffuse nodules in 27%, consolidation in one lobe or less in 7%, and diffuse consolidation in 23%.[14] Bronchial dilatation and/or distortion, with air bronchogram best demonstrated by tomography or CT, appears to be characteristic in those with consolidation. Air bronchograms tend to be present in the bronchiolar cell type but not in the alveolar cell type.[39]

Roentgen Findings in Lung Cancer

The changes caused by bronchogenic carcinoma vary widely, depending on the site of the tumor and its relation to the bronchial tree.[37] The tumor itself may or may not be visible. When the tumor is not visible its presence can be detected by such findings as localized atelectasis and inflammatory disease, secondary to the tumor within or compressing a bronchus. Each radiologic sign of bronchogenic carcinoma may occur as the only evidence of tumor, or several of the signs may occur in a single patient. Any of the following may occur as the initial sign of bronchogenic carcinoma:

1. Atelectasis, which may be segmental or lobar
2. Unilateral hilar enlargement
3. Overinflation, obstructive in type, may be segmental or lobar; this is a very rare sign
4. Mediastinal mass, often simulating lymphoma; this is usually found in small-cell carcinoma
5. Apical pulmonary opacity with or without rib destruction—the superior pulmonary sulcus (Pancoast) tumor
6. Cavitation in a solitary mass; usually in squamous cell carcinoma in heavy smokers
7. Segmental consolidation resembling local pneumonitis, which does not clear or which clears incompletely
8. Parenchymal mass—a solitary mass or nodule larger than 4 cm in diameter is usually malignant. Rarely a hamartoma or granuloma may attain this size. The mass or nodule may be sharply defined but is more often poorly defined and irregular and may be surrounded by

abnormal thickened vessels or spiculation best demonstrated on tomography or CT.
9. Mucoid impaction distal to a small endobronchial tumor may be visible when a segmental bronchus is involved, because collateral ventilation may result in aeration of the distal lung. A persistent round or fusiform shadow, often with branching, is observed. It appears similar to mucoid impaction in allergic aspergillosis, but is local and persistent rather than transitory and multifocal.
10. Occasionally the initial sign may be a very poorly defined, irregular, nonhomogeneous density, which may be linear and resemble a fibrotic scar. Therefore, it is necessary to be suspicious of nearly every opacity in the lung that does not clear, or that appears in a patient with previously normal lungs, particularly if the patient is a male smoker older than 40 years of age.

In addition to those listed above, a number of other roentgen signs may result from metastasis or local invasion. These include pleural effusion; hematogenous or lymphangitic intrapulmonary metastasis; elevation of the diaphragm secondary to phrenic nerve paralysis; and pleural masses with or without rib destruction.

Atelectasis

Atelectasis is probably the most common single radiographic sign of bronchogenic carcinoma. It may be segmental, lobar, or massive atelectasis of one lung. The radiographic signs of atelectasis resulting from tumor are similar to those caused by any lesion producing endobronchial block. The amount of opacity produced varies with the size of the bronchus obstructed. It is not uncommon to find a combination of atelectasis and tumor (Figs. 29-1 through 29-4). This is most readily seen in the right upper lobe, where the atelectasis results in elevation and concavity of the secondary interlobar fissure laterally. A convexity medially with greater opacity there represents the tumor mass. In such patients the inferior margin of the lobe resembles the reversed letter "S" (Golden's sign). A combination of pneumonia and atelectasis may also occur, which may cause confusion. Persistence of the shadow in spite of antibiotic therapy or failure of complete disappearance is strong evidence of neoplasm. Occasionally a relatively central mass is visible associated with a more peripheral density representing atelectasis, infection, or infarction in various combinations distal to the central tumor.

Unilateral Enlargement of the Hilum

Unilateral enlargement of the hilum (Fig. 29-5) may be very difficult to evaluate when only a single roentgeno-

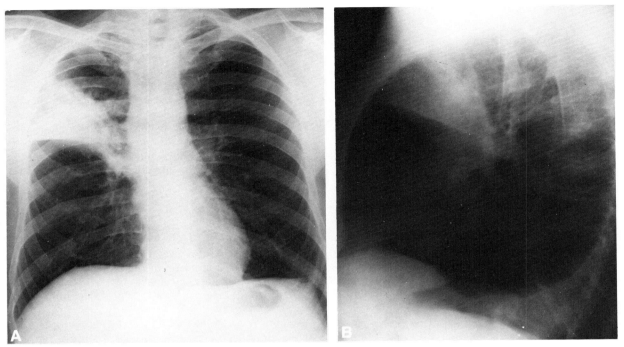

Figure 29–1. Bronchogenic carcinoma. (**A**) Frontal view shows a right hilar mass with an opacity in the anterior segment of the right upper lobe. The minor fissure is elevated, indicating that there is some atelectasis. (**B**) Increase in the hilar opacity is noted along with the opacity in the anterior segment of the upper lobe. There is also some fluid posteriorly, noted only on the lateral projection.

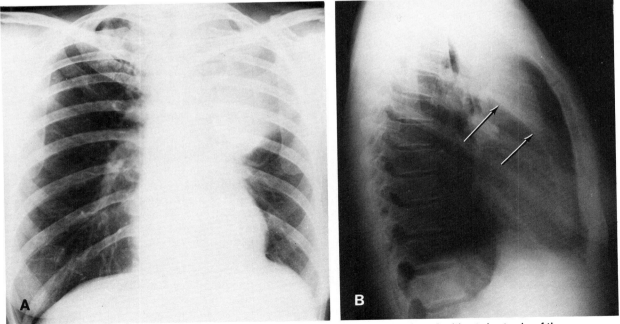

Figure 29–2. Bronchogenic carcinoma. This tumor is associated with atelectasis of the left upper lobe. (**A**) The mass obscures the upper cardiac border and aorta and fades off into the lung superiorly. There is some mediastinal shift to the left and elevation of the left hemidiaphragm. (**B**) Arrows point to the displaced fissure, with the partially atelectatic upper lobe anterior to it.

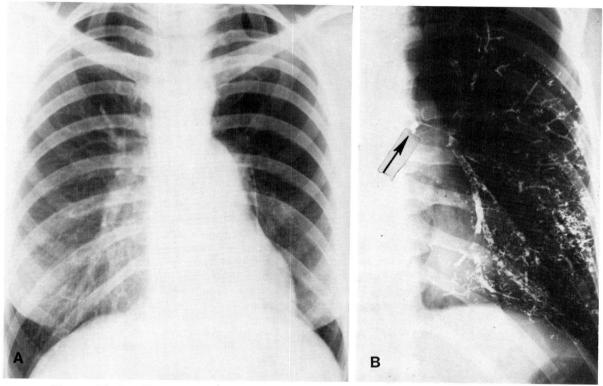

Figure 29–3. Endobronchial tumor. (**A**) Left lower-lobe atelectasis manifested by a shift of the mediastinal structures to the left and a retrocardiac opacity that obscures the paraspinal shadow, aorta, and medial left hemidiaphragm. (**B**) The bronchogram shows an endobronchial mass (*arrow*) within but not completely obstructing the upper-lobe bronchus. The lower-lobe bronchus is not visible and was completely obstructed by the bronchial adenoma.

gram is available. When there is a difference in the size of the hilum on the two sides, every effort should be made to obtain any previous roentgenograms of the patient that may be available. If a film of an earlier examination is obtained, any difference in hilar size between the two films is of particular significance. It is also of value to obtain tomograms or CT of the hilum in question in an attempt to outline the tumor or local bronchial narrowing produced by it. It is also helpful in detecting some loss of hilar vascular detail that may be caused by tumor. Roentgenograms in inspiration and expiration should also be obtained when there is a question as to the significance of unilateral hilar enlargement, because a small amount of obstructive overinflation may be determined by this examination. CT is not always useful when hilar mass or adenopathy is suspected.

Local Overinflation (Obstructive)

Bronchogenic carcinoma may not cause enough obstruction to interfere with air entering the segment, lobe, or lung supplied by the bronchus, but the slight decrease in bronchial size on expiration may result in partial obstruction to the egress of air. This causes overinflation, which may precede atelectasis by a considerable period of time. It is a rare sign of bronchogenic carcinoma. Films in inspiration and expiration and fluoroscopy accentuate the findings and may verify the presence of obstructive overinflation. These studies should be carried out when a wheeze is detected on auscultation or the presence of local overinflation is suggested on the chest roentgenogram. When obstructive overinflation is found in a patient past middle age, bronchogenic carcinoma should be suspected. Then further studies such as CT or tomography and bronchoscopy can be undertaken.

Mediastinal Widening

When the mediastinum is enlarged as a result of bronchogenic carcinoma, it often indicates the presence of a small-cell type of tumor. The primary tumor is usually in a stem bronchus and rarely beyond a lobar bronchus,

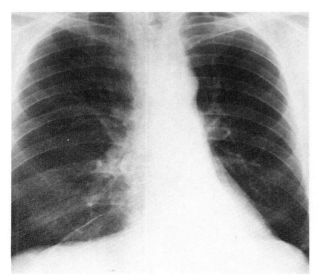

Figure 29–4. Left lower-lobe atelectasis secondary to bronchogenic carcinoma. Note the retrocardiac opacity, mediastinal shift to the left, and slight elevation of the left hemidiaphragm. The left upper lobe is overinflated and hyperlucent as compared with the right lung.

so the primary tumor mass is often obscured by a large mediastinal mass. Therefore this tumor cannot be differentiated from lymphoma in some patients. The tumor is nonresectable when there is mediastinal invasion, but may respond to irradiation and/or chemotherapy (Fig. 29-6).

Apical Density With or Without Rib Destruction

Apical density with or without rib destruction denotes the presence of a superior pulmonary sulcus tumor known as a *Pancoast tumor*. It is usually caused by either squamous cell carcinoma or adenocarcinoma, but other cell types may be found. The four cardinal signs of the Pancoast syndrome are: (1) mass in the pulmonary apex, (2) destruction of an adjacent rib or vertebra, (3) Horner's syndrome, and (4) pain radiating down the arm. In addition to bronchogenic carcinoma, other tumors, including metastatic carcinoma and malignant neurogenic tumor, may cause the Pancoast syndrome. When only a small amount of parenchymal density is visible representing the peripheral tumor, the diagnosis of malignancy is very difficult to make because this density simulates the minor amount of pleural thickening often seen in the apex in elderly patients. The presence of pain should lead to the strong

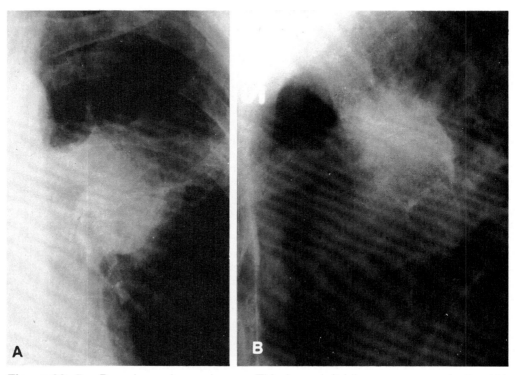

Figure 29–5. Bronchogenic carcinoma. This large left hilar mass, seen in the (**A**) frontal and (**B**) lateral projections, represents a tumor that surrounds the upper-lobe bronchus and narrows it somewhat. There is no difficulty in diagnosis when the mass reaches this size.

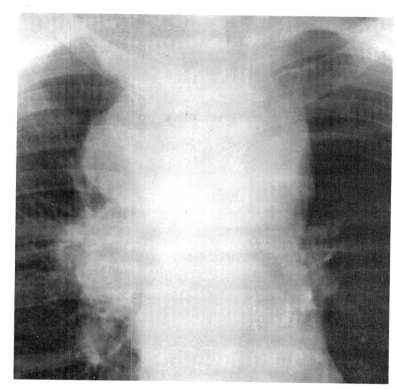

Figure 29–6. Small-cell bronchogenic carcinoma. A lobulated mass involving the right hilum and the superior mediastinum is noted to displace the trachea to the left. There is also tumor in the superior mediastinum on the left. This type of tumor cannot be differentiated from lymphoma on roentgenographic findings.

suspicion of tumor, and the other clinical findings of Horner's syndrome—loss of sensation in the forearm and atrophy of the hand muscles—make the diagnosis almost certain. The tumor may grow rapidly, with early destruction of the ribs (Fig. 29-7). O'Connell and associates reviewed 29 patients with this tumor.[33] An apical mass was found in 45%, while 55% had unilateral apical pleural thickening. CT was found to be the best method of demonstrating the extent of disease and presence of bone destruction, which was found in 34%. There now seems to be a consensus that MRI is the best imaging method to study the Pancoast tumor. It has the advantage of multiple projections and is better at delineating invasion of the brachial plexus, spinal canal, as well as cervical and thoracic soft tissues. The apical lordotic view was found to be misleading, but oblique projections were often helpful. Needle biopsy is the best non-surgical method of establishing the diagnosis.

Solitary Cavity

When a solitary cavity is found in an elderly man who has few if any signs of infection, the presence of bronchogenic carcinoma should be suspected. The cavity wall is usually thick and irregular, but may be very thin, at least in some areas. If tomograms or CT are obtained, almost invariably a local mass is seen projecting

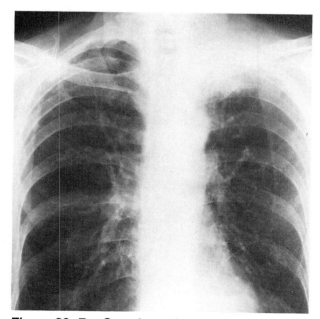

Figure 29–7. Superior pulmonary sulcus tumor. Note the homogeneous masslike opacity at the left apex, with absence of the posterior arc of the first rib, which is destroyed by this squamous cell carcinoma of the lung.

from the round or oval cavity wall into the cavity in one or more areas. Another helpful sign is the lack of evidence of inflammatory disease in the vicinity of the solitary cavity (Fig. 29-8). The epidermoid tumor is the usual type in which cavitation occurs; necrosis leads to the cavitation. Most of these tumors are found in the upper lobes. A long history of smoking is common in these patients. Rarely adenocarcinoma and large-cell carcinoma may cavitate, but small-cell carcinoma does not.

Pneumonitis That Does Not Clear

Partial obstruction of a bronchus by a tumor may cause inflammatory disease in the lobe or segment supplied by that bronchus. On radiographic study the findings simulate those of an ordinary pneumonia localized to the area. If the process fails to resolve or clears incompletely, bronchogenic carcinoma should be suspected (Fig. 29-9). Furthermore, if the pneumonitis clears and then reappears in the same area, endobronchial tumor should also be suspected and further studies including CT and bronchoscopy should be carried out to determine the cause. The opacity noted in these patients with disease that resembles pneumonia may be caused in part by tumor; CT may then outline tumor nodula-

tion within the area of pneumonic consolidation. Air bronchogram is occasionally observed in this situation. Alveolar (bronchiolar, bronchioloalveolar) cell carcinoma may simulate segmental or lobar pneumonia, as indicated earlier. This opacity does not clear (Fig. 29-10). Air bronchogram is commonly seen and CT often reveals dilated and/or distorted bronchi.

Smaller, poorly defined opacities resembling very small patches of inflammatory disease may actually represent the first sign of bronchogenic carcinoma. When such a lesion is found, particularly in a smoker, it is important to obtain follow-up roentgenograms and also to obtain previous roentgenograms, if available, for comparison. When such a lesion does not respond to antibiotic therapy and does not contain calcium, bronchogenic tumor is a distinct possibility.

Large Parenchymal Mass

Bronchogenic carcinoma that begins as a peripheral nodule may reach very large size before causing symptoms. These large lobulated but generally round or oval masses may lie far out in the periphery or adjacent to the hilum. They usually range from 4 to 12 cm in diameter, and sometimes are even larger. CT may show some areas of radiolucency, indicating necrosis within

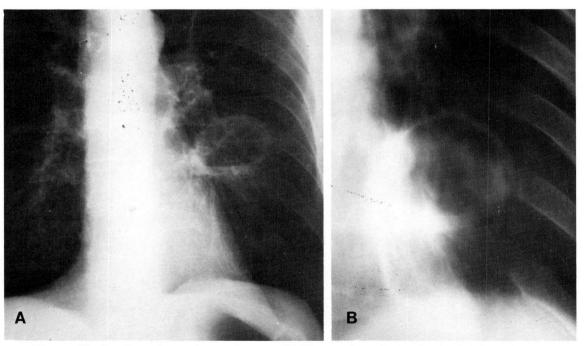

Figure 29–8. Bronchogenic carcinoma. (**A**) The cavitary lesion in the left lung is an excavating squamous cell carcinoma. (**B**) Tomogram shows a slightly irregular mass projecting into the cavity medially and variation in wall thickness laterally. These signs are very characteristic of cavitary bronchogenic carcinoma, usually the squamous cell type.

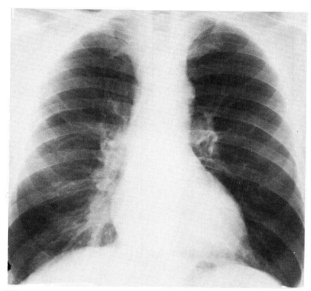

Figure 29–9. Bronchogenic carcinoma simulating inflammatory disease. The patient was febrile when the poorly defined disease in the right medial base was discovered. The acute symptoms subsided, but the pulmonary disease failed to clear. Thoracotomy revealed an infiltrating carcinoma.

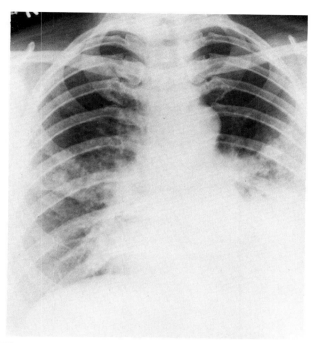

Figure 29–10. Bronchiolar (bronchioloalveolar cell) carcinoma. The disease is bilateral. The large areas of homogeneous opacity simulate those seen in alveolar pneumonia, but the patient was afebrile and the disease progressed.

the mass. There is usually very little difficulty in arriving at the diagnosis of pulmonary carcinoma in these patients because any solitary mass of large size in a patient in the age group at risk for carcinoma is most likely malignant and must be considered as such until disproved. There is often associated hilar-node involvement resulting in unilateral hilar enlargement (Fig. 29-11).

Solitary Pulmonary Nodule

The solitary peripheral pulmonary parenchymal nodule presents a diagnostic and therapeutic problem that has been extensively investigated and discussed in recent years.[11, 59, 60] When such a nodule is seen on a chest roentgenogram, the question of lung tumor always arises. These nodules may range from a few millimeters up to 4 cm or more in size. When they are larger than 2.5 cm and contain no calcium, it is highly probable that they are bronchogenic carcinomas. Surgical resection of the solitary nodular bronchogenic carcinoma results in a higher 5-year survival rate than in lung cancer, in which symptoms are present. The prognosis is better when the lesions are less than 2 cm in diameter and much better in patients younger than 55 years than in those who are older. Lillington, in a comprehensive review of solitary pulmonary nodules,

concluded that: (1) Most benign nodules are granulomas. (2) Most resected nodules are malignant. (3) Surgical mortality is low for resection of nodules. (4) Prognosis is better than in other types of lung cancer. (5) Resection of nodular metastasis results in prolonged survival in a significant number of cases.[18]

Detection of a solitary pulmonary nodule is therefore very important. As indicated earlier, double reading is very helpful in decreasing the number of false-negatives. Oblique films and fluoroscopy are useful when there is a question as to the location of a nodule seen on only one projection. Nodules can be seen when 3 mm in diameter, but true tumors can be separated from opacities, which mimic them only when they are 8 to 10 mm in diameter. Many methods have been tried to improve radiographic detection of pulmonary nodules. Most have showed promise but there is no consensus regarding the *one* best method at this time.[41, 50] Many other studies have been reported in addition to those cited here.[25]

Although mass screening of adults older than 45 to 50 is probably not cost-effective, the screening of heavy smokers older than 45—and particularly asbestos workers who are heavy smokers—may prove to be

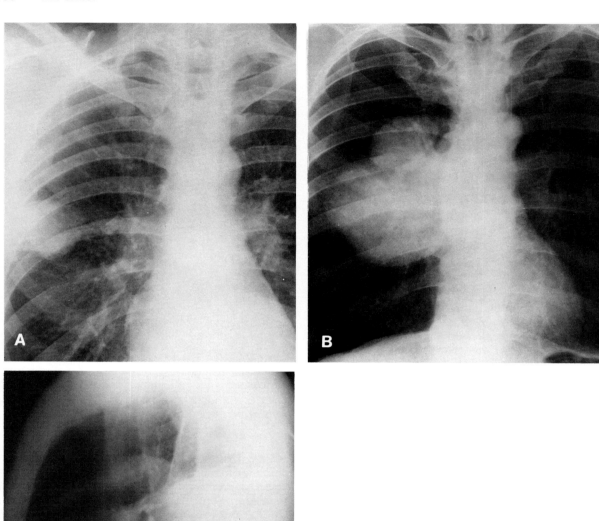

Figure 29–11. Bronchogenic carcinoma. **(A)** Small-cell bronchogenic carcinoma arising in the lower lobe as a large solitary mass in a patient who was asymptomatic. **(B)** Massive undifferentiated adenocarcinoma of the right lung in another patient who also was asymptomatic. **(C)** Lateral projection showing that the massive tumor seen in **B** is largely in the superior segment of the right lower lobe.

effective. When a small nodule is found, there are certain steps that should be taken to ascertain the nature of the lesion. If previous films are available they should be reviewed and if the lesion was not present on previous examination made within the preceding 1 or 2 years in a patient (particularly a smoker) older than 40, malignant tumor is the first consideration. Inflammatory granulomas occasionally appear in patients of middle age, but this is uncommon. If the nodule has undergone *no increase* in size for at least 2 years, it can be considered benign but should be followed at intervals for several more years. If the nodule is seen to have increased in size on review of films obtained several months or even years earlier, bronchogenic carcinoma is the first consideration in diagnosis, unless calcification can be demonstrated. CT should be used in the examination of patients with solitary pulmonary nodules to determine the presence or absence of calcification. When calcification is present the lesion is most likely benign, unless it is focal and eccentric, which may indicate a calcified granuloma engulfed by tumor.

The character of calcification is of significance. A central nidus, a laminated appearance, or both almost certainly indicate an inflammatory lesion. Curvilinear and popcorn-like calcifications are also benign, usually appearing in hamartomas. As indicated, calcium in a malignant nodule may (1) be coincidental—the tumor engulfs an old inflammatory granuloma; or (2) represent calcification in the tumor itself—this is very uncommon on plain film study, but may be observed on CT. Even when calcification is present the lesion should be kept under observation by means of follow-up roentgenograms. A few cases of bronchogenic carcinoma have been reported in nodules containing calcium, but by far the majority of calcified nodules are benign. Determination of density using CT numbers was described by Siegelman and co-workers in 1980.[44] Because of variation in Hounsfield numbers from one unit to another, Siegelman's colleague Zerhouni developed a phantom for standardization; this may make results reproducible and enable CT differentiation of calcium-containing granulomas from tumors, thus saving patients with high Hounsfield numbers from thoracotomy.[58] If the lesion containing calcium continues to grow, thoracotomy with removal should be considered because of the remote possibility of carcinoma; furthermore, if inflammatory, the growth indicates activity of the granulomatous process (Fig. 29-12).

When CT fails to show calcium within the nodule, this does not mean the nodule is malignant, but indicates that the possibility of malignancy cannot be excluded (Fig. 29-13). Active inflammatory nodules may be irregular, and small satellite nodules are often present; however, in the absence of calcium these signs cannot be taken to exclude the possibility of carcinoma,

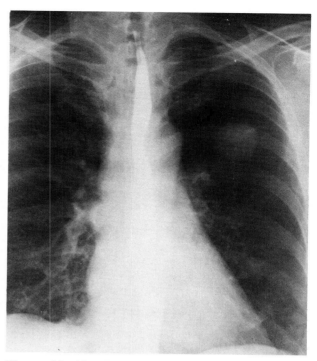

Figure 29–12. Benign pulmonary mass simulating a malignant tumor. Tomography revealed a small amount of calcification laterally, but the mass was removed because of its large size. It proved to be a tuberculoma.

because small satellite nodules may represent extensions of the tumor via the interstitium and lymphatics within it. There are several additional findings that are helpful in the roentgen differentiation of benign and malignant tumor nodules. The malignant tumors often have indefinite, irregular, or fuzzy borders—often with spiculation in contrast to the sharp borders of benign tumors. Linear opacities are more often associated with inflammatory nodules than with malignant tumors. They may extend from the hilum to the nodule or from the nodule to the pleura or both. The "tail" sign, a linear opacity from the nodule to or toward the pleura is found in both benign and malignant lesions, so it is not helpful in differentiation. Lobulation of the nodule is more suggestive of carcinoma than of inflammation.

If the above examinations have indicated the possibility of malignancy, further steps must be taken. If there are no symptoms of involvement of other organs, extensive investigation of other systems probably is not necessary. Transthoracic thin-needle aspiration biopsy may permit a definitive diagnosis in the hands of experienced, skilled operators. Guidelines for percutaneous transthoracic needle biopsy have been published

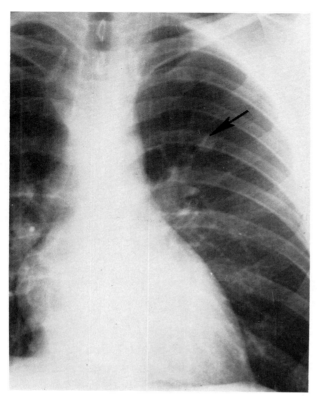

Figure 29–13. Solitary pulmonary nodule in the left upper lung (*arrow*). No calcium could be demonstrated within it on tomography, and it had not been present on earlier examinations. On biopsy, it proved to be small-cell bronchogenic carcinoma.

by the American Thoracic Society.[1] Their approach is conservative and worth study by anyone who does or contemplates doing this procedure.

Results in aspiration biopsy studies are widely varied.[10] There is very little morbidity and almost no mortality. When tumor is found, the results are nearly 100% accurate. The same is true when a benign nodule with specific evidence of a particular benign lesion, either inflammatory or neoplastic, is found. When a specific diagnosis of a benign cause of the nodule cannot be made, this method is not accurate and some recommend thoracotomy in this situation. Khouri and associates reported experience with 650 patients.[17] Malignant lesions were diagnosed in 95% and benign lesions in 88%. Diagnostic thoracotomies were necessary in fewer than 8% of patients with lung nodules. Of a total of 25% with pneumothorax, only 5% of biopsied patients had pneumothorax requiring chest tube placement. There were no deaths and minimal hemoptysis

occurred in 5% of the second group of 350 patients in this study. Lesions close to the hilum are accessible to transbronchial aspiration needle biopsy using the fiberoptic bronchoscope. Usually brushings and bronchial washings are obtained. Central tumors may be seen and biopsied directly. Unless there is satisfactory evidence that the nodule is benign, it should be resected.

Roentgen Signs Indicating Metastasis or Local Invasion

Pleural Effusion

The presence of pleural effusion in a patient with a visible pulmonary tumor mass usually indicates that there is involvement of the pleura by direct extension or as the result of metastasis. At times, clear fluid may indicate only that lymphatics are obstructed and is not a definite indication of spread of tumor to the pleura. In this situation, when no malignant cells are found in the fluid, the disease may be limited and should be staged as such. However, if the fluid is bloody, the pleura is almost invariably involved. Not infrequently, the effusion is massive and obscures the lung. When the fluid is removed, the tumor mass or secondary signs of tumor may be visible. Bronchopleural fistula may result in pyopneumothorax, and occasionally empyema occurs in patients with bronchogenic carcinoma.

Hematogenous and Lymphangitic Spread

Lymphangitic metastasis is the most common type of spread in bronchogenic carcinoma. The lymphatics drain toward the hilum; there are lymphatics on the pleural surface which extend to the adjacent interlobular septa, where they turn toward the hilum. If lymphatics in the vicinity of the tumor are obstructed, the increased pressure overcomes the valves and lymphatic flow is toward the periphery.[13] This produces tumor extension toward the pleura, causing line shadows called the "pleural tail." Line shadows may also extend from inflammatory masses to the pleura, so the finding does not necessarily indicate malignancy. When lymphatics are invaded without obstruction, malignant cells are carried to the hilar nodes. When obstruction occurs at or near the nodes, the lymph flow is also changed and is toward the periphery (centrifugal). As the disease progresses, linear opacities usually associated with lymphangitic metastases may appear. When the primary tumor is seen along with enlargement of the hilum or paratracheal nodes, it is most likely advanced and nonresectable (Figs. 29-14 and 29-15). It is not uncommon to observe strands of density extending from the peripheral or midzone type of tumor to the hilum, representing involvement of the lymphatics.

4. Search for distant metastases with appropriate imaging methods (e.g., bone and liver scans)—only if symptoms and signs suggest involvement

In those with small-cell carcinoma, always considered to be nonresectable, CT or MRI may be used as a guide for radiotherapy or as a baseline study when chemotherapy is used.[16] Mediastinal node size alone is not a reliable criterion for presence or absence of metastases. Therefore, accurate staging is not possible using current radiographic methods.[9,24] So routine use of CT for staging of mediastinal nodes may not be indicated in all patients with lung cancer. It should not be used to deny thoracotomy in a patient who shows no metastases except for possible lesions in enlarged nodes. Therefore, its major value may be in directing biopsy in possible surgical candidates or in treatment planning in inoperable patients. The same can be said for the use of tomography to evaluate the hila, although its use is declining rapidly.[36] A CT scan showing mediastinal abnormality may be an indication for mediastinoscopy or mediastinotomy before thoracotomy in some instances. When CT is used to study the mediastinum, direct mediastinal invasion indicates nonresectability and thoracotomy can be avoided. When the disease is confined to one lobe and the mediastinum is normal, thoracotomy can be done with no further study if there are no signs of distant metastases. However, it is difficult to differentiate tumor from surrounding infection and atelectasis in some instances. MRI has more potential than CT in resolving this problem. Furthermore, contiguity of a mass with the mediastinum or pleura is not necessarily equivalent to direct invasion.

OTHER MALIGNANT TUMORS

Bronchial Adenoma

Bronchial adenoma is included with the malignant lung lesions because metastases to lymph nodes are found in approximately 20% of these patients. It should be recognized, however, that this tumor is relatively benign even though hilar node involvement is present and its clinical course and prognosis are entirely different than those of bronchogenic carcinoma. The 10-year survival rate is 90% or better. There are two main relatively benign pathologic types: typical carcinoid, which is the most common (85% to 95%), and cylindroid, which resembles mixed salivary-gland tumors. Cylindromas (adenoid cystic carcinoma) tend to be more central in location and more invasive than the carcinoid type. The salivary gland types can be subdivided into mucoepidermoid and pleomorphic adenomas in addition to the cylindroma. Since very few of the carcinoid tumors of the bronchus secrete serotonin, the carcinoid syndrome is uncommon. Many believe the term "bronchial adenoma" should be dropped in favor of specific tumor-type designations. The tumors occur in females as frequently as in males and are found in younger age groups than bronchogenic carcinoma. They occur most often in persons between the ages of 20 and 50 years, with mean age in late 30s or early 40s; a number of cases have also been reported in children. Our youngest patient was 12 years of age. Because the adenoma tends to bleed rather easily, repeated hemoptysis may be the major clinical finding. Most of the tumors are central, grow slowly, and gradually produce progressing bronchial obstruction leading to repeated attacks of pneumonitis and eventually to atelectasis. An unusual case with diffuse miliary type of multifocal bronchial carcinoid in whom the roentgenographic appearance of diffuse miliary densities did not change during the 2-year period of observation has been described.[47] Metastases to bone are rare in bronchial carcinoid, and, when present, are usually osteoblastic.

Roentgen Findings

Occasionally the round or oval tumor may be visible as a solitary mass in the lung periphery. It usually arises in a large bronchus and is therefore near the hilum. More frequently, however, the tumor is not visible because of its small size. The diagnosis then rests on the manifestations of bronchial obstruction. The findings range from complete atelectasis (Fig. 29-16), to lobar or segmental obstructive overinflation when check-valve stenosis is produced. The latter is not very common in our experience, but there may be decreased perfusion which results in a decrease in radiographic density of the involved lung that may resemble the radiolucency found in obstructive overinflation. Signs of pulmonary infection and bronchiectasis are not infrequent in the lobe distal to the tumor. CT is useful when a lesion is suspected. The round tumor mass may then be seen within a bronchus. If it is ossified or calcified, it may resemble a broncholith.[42] Bronchography will almost invariably outline the endobronchial tumor, which produces a smoothly rounded mass resulting in partial or complete obstruction (see Fig. 29-3). Bronchography is not ordinarily needed, however, because fiberoptic endoscopy provides the opportunity to see and biopsy the tumor.

Atypical carcinoid is a neuroendocrine tumor with cellular features intermediate between carcinoid and small-cell carcinoma.[4] About one third of patients develop lymph-node invasion. In patients with atypical carcinoid, mortality is in the range of 50%. Radiographic features differ from those of typical carcinoid.

Table 29-2. Staging of Cancer of the Lung*

ANATOMY

PRIMARY SITE
The mucosa lining the bronchus is the usual site of origin of cancer of the lung. The trachea, which lies in the anterior mediastinum, divides into a right and a left main bronchus that extend into the right and left lungs, respectively, and then divides into lobar bronchi for the upper, middle, and lower lobes on the right and the upper and lower lobes on the left. The lungs are encased in membranes called visceral pleura and the chest cavity is lined by a similar membrane called parietal pleura. The potential space between these two membranes is the pleural space.

NODAL STATIONS
The first-station lymph nodes are the intrapulmonary, peribronchial, and hilar lymph nodes, which are contained within the visceral pleura reflections. Second-station lymph nodes are those in the mediastinum and may be paraesophageal, subcarinal, paratracheal, aortic, and pretracheal or retrotracheal. Involvement of scalene and more distant nodes is considered distant metastasis.

METASTATIC SITES
Lung cancer may metastasize to any distant site, the more common being scalene, supraclavicular, and other cervical lymph nodes, liver, brain, bones, adrenals, kidney, and contralateral lung, including contralateral hilar lymph nodes.

* Manual for Staging of Cancer, 1978 American Joint Committee for Cancer Staging and End-Results Reporting, Chicago, Illinois. Am Rev Resp Dis 127: 659, 1983. With permission. (See also Glazer GM, Grass BH, Quint LE, et al: Normal mediastinal lymph nodes: Number and size according to American Thoracic Society Mapping. Am J Roentgenol 144: 261, 1985).

Table 29-3. Definitions of T, N, AND M Categories for Carcinoma of the Lung*

PRIMARY TUMOR (T)

TX	Tumor proved by the presence of malignant cells in bronchopulmonary secretions but not visualized roentgenographically or bronchoscopically, or any tumor that cannot be assessed as in the retreatment staging
T0	No evidence of primary tumor
TIS	Carcinoma in situ
T1	A tumor 3 cm or less in greatest diameter, surrounded by lung or visceral pleura, and without evidence of invasion proximal to a lobar bronchus at bronchoscopy
T2	A tumor more than 3 cm in greatest diameter, or a tumor of any size that either invades the visceral pleura or has associated atelectasis or obstructive pneumonitis extending to the hilar region. At bronchoscopy, the proximal extent of demonstrable tumor must be within a lobar bronchus or at least 2 cm distal to the carina. Any associated atelectasis or obstructive pneumonitis must involve less than an entire lung, and there must be no pleural effusion.
T3	A tumor of any size with direct extension into an adjacent structure such as the parietal pleura or chest wall, the diaphragm, or the mediastinum and its contents; or a tumor demonstrable bronchoscopically to involve a main bronchus less than 2 cm distal to the carina; or any tumor associated with atelectasis or obstructive pneumonitis of an entire lung or pleural effusion

NODAL INVOLVEMENT (N)

N0	No demonstrable metastasis to regional lymph nodes
N1	Metastasis to lymph nodes in the bronchial or the ipsilateral hilar region, both including direct extension
N2	Metastasis to lymph nodes in the mediastinum

DISTANT METASTASIS (M)

MX	Not assessed
M0	No (known distant metastasis)
M1	Distant metastasis present; specific site

* Each case must be assigned the highest category of T, N, and M, which describes the full extent of the disease in that case. From Clinical staging of primary lung cancer. American Thoracic Society Node Mapping Scheme. Am Rev Resp Dis 127: 659, 1983. With permission.

occur in the lymphangitic type. CT is very useful in detecting pleural involvement but may be misleading at times. Bone destruction is usually readily detected by CT.

Diaphragmatic Elevation

Elevation with evidence of paresis, or paralysis, of the hemidiaphragm on the side of the tumor is another late sign and indicates involvement of the phrenic nerve. Fluoroscopy or inspiratory–expiratory films can be used to demonstrate the findings.

General Considerations

Various combinations of the findings described may occur in any individual patient. Occasionally none of the characteristic findings will appear, so some pulmonary malignancies cannot be identified by roentgen signs. An additional factor that makes the diagnosis difficult is the association of bronchogenic carcinoma with chronic inflammatory disease. Tuberculosis is estimated to be associated with bronchogenic carcinoma in 10% of patients with this chronic infection. In these patients the association makes the diagnosis of carcinoma extremely difficult, since a tumor nodule may appear in or near the nodular tuberculosis or may arise in the wall of a tuberculous cavity and thus escape recognition for a long time. It is therefore important to keep the possibility of bronchogenic carcinoma in mind, particularly in elderly men with tuberculosis. There are several roentgen signs that are suggestive of tumor: (1) an increase in hilar size during treatment with antituberculous drugs; (2) the failure of a local lesion to respond to treatment, while in other areas the disease is regressing; and (3) an increase in size of a lesion despite treatment. The same difficulty may also occur in smokers with asbestosis or silicosis.

The roentgen diagnosis of bronchogenic carcinoma is based on the finding of one or more of the signs described in the previous sections. In order to make this diagnosis, it is necessary to obtain good films in frontal and lateral projections—and in oblique or other projections when indicated. Examination in different phases of respiration using films and fluoroscopy must also be employed in some instances. CT is of particular value in the examination of solitary parenchymal nodules. Linear or pluridirectional tomography appears to be most valuable in the examination of the hila and is still used by some. Bronchography may be of value in patients with segmental involvement in whom bronchoscopy fails to demonstrate the lesion, but is rarely used, having replaced almost completely by fiberoptic bronchoscopy. Bronchography is of no value in the differential diagnosis of small peripheral pulmonary nodules. Many of the tumors are more indolent than is commonly realized, so the importance of comparison of all available chest roentgenograms cannot be overemphasized, particularly when a small parenchymal shadow is present or when one hilum is questionably enlarged.

Staging of Pulmonary Tumors

Clinical staging of pulmonary tumors is important in determining the potential for surgical cure. The TNM Classification,* with modifications, was revised in 1983.[6,22] There are difficulties in identification of nodes when preoperative images are compared with surgical findings, so further modifications will probably be made in the future. Tables 29-2 and 29-3 indicate anatomy and category definitions, respectively. Those interested in a complete review of lung cancer staging should refer to the original.[6] Glazer and co-workers discuss this method of staging; their paper should be reviewed by those interested.[8] As a rule, CT is used to determine tumor spread to the chest wall and mediastinum. Tomography appears to be preferable to CT in the evaluation of hilar node enlargement, although dynamic CT scanning is used by some. Magnetic resonance imaging is believed to have a definite potential for scanning the hila, and in the mediastinum it is nearly as useful as CT. It may be the modality of the future in staging pulmonary tumors.[5,51] In a study of 170 patients, there was no statistical difference between CT and MRI in staging non–small-cell bronchogenic carcinoma.[5,52] However, MRI was more accurate than CT in the diagnosis of mediastinal invasion.[53] MRI seems to be the method of choice for staging small-cell lung cancer.[16] Some doubt that CT and/or MRI are necessary for preoperative assessment of $T_1N_0M_0$ bronchogenic carcinoma, but this is still controversial.

An orderly approach to diagnosis and staging in patients with lung cancer might include the following:

1. Chest roentgenography using as many projections as necessary.
2. Biopsy using an appropriate method depending on site and extent of the lesion (e.g., peripheral nodule-transthoracic needle aspiration; central tumor—endoscopy and biopsy and/or bronchial washings; mediastinal nodes or masses—mediastinoscopy or mediastinotomy; at times open lung or mediastinal biopsy may be necessary)
3. Staging CT or MRI of the thorax including the diaphragm and upper abdomen in patients considered for surgical resection.

* Clinical Staging of Primary Lung Cancer. American Thoracic Society Node-Mapping Scheme. Am Rev Resp Dis 127:659, 1983

Rarely, lymphangitic metastasis is widespread and results in irregular strandlike opacities extending into the lung from both hila. Hematogenous pulmonary metastasis occurs occasionally in bronchogenic carcinoma. There are then signs of the original tumor plus scattered parenchymal lesions that appear as rounded or oval masses of varying size, usually smaller than the primary lesion. Massive mediastinal involvement, which is observed in small-cell carcinoma, was discussed earlier.

CT is useful and may be diagnostic at times in patients with lymphangitic metastases. Findings include irregular thickening of bronchovascular bundles and interlobular septa, local or diffuse reticular opacities, polygonal lines, and an increase in thickness of peripheral lines. The process is focal in about 50% of patients, so CT is helpful in selection of open-lung biopsy sites. The findings suggest the diagnosis and may be diagnostic in certain settings.[31]

Pleural Mass With or Without Rib Destruction

The visceral pleura may be involved as a result of lymphangitic metastasis, as implied above. Direct invasion of the parietal pleura and chest wall may result in a mass with or without destruction of the adjacent rib. This occurs in the superior pulmonary sulcus tumor and to a lesser extent with peripheral tumors elsewhere. The pleural mass is often obscured by effusion. Hematogenous metastasis to ribs may occur with destruction of bone and production of soft-tissue mass that may extend into the thorax. The roentgen findings are similar except that pleural effusion is more likely to

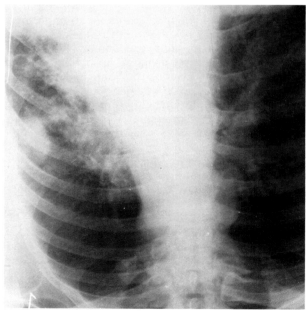

Figure 29–14. Bronchogenic carcinoma with metastases. The large hilar tumor on the left produced some lower-lobe atelectasis, a pleural metastasis in the left lateral thorax, some pleural effusion on the left, and metastases to the right paratracheal nodes.

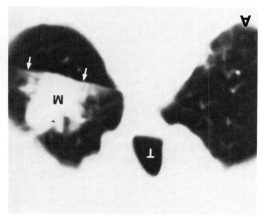

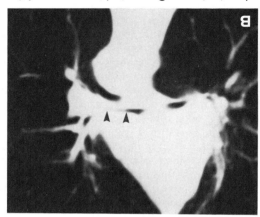

Figure 29–15. Lung cancer with mediastinal metastases. Computed tomogram of the chest using lung windows. **(A)** Tumor in the left upper lobe near the apex (*M*), elevated fissure (*arrows*), indicating partial volume loss in the left upper lobe, trachea (*T*). **(B)** This CT is about 1 cm below the carina. The left upper-lobe bronchus (*arrowheads*) is narrowed by tumor invading the mediastinum. (Courtesy of Richard Logan, MD)

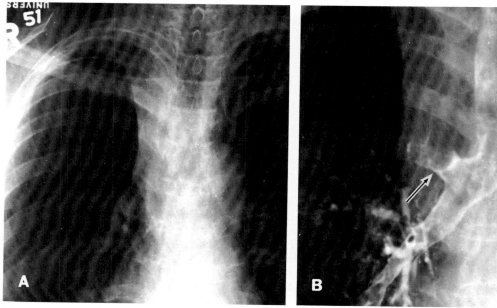

Figure 29–16.   Bronchial adenoma. **(A)** Atelectasis of the right upper lobe in a young woman who was asymptomatic. **(B)** Bronchogram of the same patient. The arrow indicates the endobronchial tumor obstructing the upper-lobe bronchus.

The tumor presents as an ovoid lobulated peripheral mass, small thin-walled cavity, ill-defined opacity sometimes resembling infection or mediastinal mass. Nearly one third of the patients have lymph-node invasion at the time of discovery.

Pulmonary Sarcoma

Primary sarcoma occurring in the lung is very rare, but leiomyosarcoma, neurogenic sarcoma, angiosarcoma, carcinosarcoma, chondrosarcoma, fibrosarcoma, and rarely, rhabdomyosarcoma have been reported. In some instances the cells are undifferentiated and difficult to classify. Occasionally they appear to be mixed, with some sarcomatous elements and some elements that resemble carcinoma. Leiomyosarcoma is more frequent in males (3 to 1 ratio) than in females. Although the lesion usually produces large masses, about 10% arise endobronchially. Chondrosarcoma may also arise endobronchially. Very rarely, teratoid tumor may arise in an endobronchial location. As in mediastinal teratoma, calcification may be present. Hemangiosarcoma may also arise in the chest wall, project into the thorax, and simulate a large peripheral bronchogenic sarcoma. Since these tumors usually arise peripherally and reach large size before producing symptoms, they may be found on routine roentgen examination of the chest.

Roentgen Findings

The roentgen findings often are not characteristic, but a large, sharply defined and somewhat lobulated mass is the usual presentation. When the lesion arises in the wall of a bronchus, obstructive signs similar to those described earlier in other tumors are found, including recurrent pneumonia and atelectasis. In the rare primary pulmonary-artery sarcoma, the characteristic finding of a lobulated hilar mass projecting into the lung in a lobar or segmental arterial distribution has been reported.[27] Obstructing pulmonary arterial sarcoma with roentgen findings simulating those of acute pulmonary embolism also has been reported.[35] Usually there is no lymph node involvement in sarcoma of the lung and pleural effusion is unusual. Since the various pulmonary sarcomas present as large masses, biopsy is necessary to make the histopathologic diagnosis.

Kaposi's Sarcoma

Although pulmonary involvement may be metastatic, Kaposi's sarcoma will be considered here in view of its increasing frequency in patients with AIDS. Furthermore, the lung may be the first and possibly the only site of disease recognized in some patients. The most common findings are hilar and mediastinal adenopathy, and there may be direct extension into the lung from the nodes. The tumor can also occur in the lung, presenting as poorly defined nodules or as in interstitial-type process causing irregular, poorly defined linear densities. Many patients have concurrent opportunistic infections, so biopsy is necessary to confirm the presence of Kaposi's idiopathic hemorrhagic angiosarcoma.

Pulmonary Blastoma

Pulmonary blastoma is a rare mixed tumor having malignant epithelial and connective-tissue components.[34, 54] Its histogenesis is controversial; some consider it to be a type of carcinoma, while others believe it arises from a multipotential mesenchymal blastoma, so it is sometimes called carcinosarcoma. The peak incidence is in the third and fourth decades. The tumor may be solid or multicystic, is usually peripheral, predominantly in the upper lung, and commonly appears as a large pulmonary parenchymal mass that cannot be differentiated radiographically from other large masses in the lung. The prognosis is generally poor, particularly if the mass is more than 5 cm in diameter. It may cause pneumothorax.

There is a tumor of childhood resembling blastoma, but presumably somewhat different.[21] The tumor is made up of small primitive cells with blastomatous qualities with focal areas of rhabdomyosarcomatous, chondrosarcomatous, and liposarcomatous cells. Prognosis is poor. Since this tumor differs somewhat from the adult form, the authors suggest that it be designated "pleuropulmonary blastoma" to distinguish it as a different tumor. It appears to be designated as blastoma by most authors, however.[54]

Leukemia and Lymphoma of the Lung

The leukemias primarily involve the hilar and mediastinal nodes, but pulmonary parenchymal involvement may occur, usually late in the course of the disease. Pulmonary involvement is most common in monocytic (46%) and least common in chronic myelocytic leukemia (15%).[3] Often the involvement that is visible histologically is not seen on the radiograph. Adenopathy is more frequent in lymphocytic leukemia than in the myelocytic type. When the lung is involved by leukemia, there is extension of the tumor cells into the peribronchial and perivascular connective tissues. This results in strands of increased density radiating outward from the hilum on one or both sides, resembling diffuse lymphangitic spread of carcinoma. This is usually accompanied by recognizable enlargement of the hilar lymph nodes.

Infection, edema, and hemorrhage are much more common than leukemic infiltration. Pleural effusion is also fairly common. Since infection is the most frequent pulmonary complication of leukemia, pneumonia should be the first consideration in the treatment of these patients.[20] Biopsy is sometimes indicated in late stages of the disease, however, when pulmonary opacities are observed and there are no clinical signs of infection. The roentgen findings are not characteristic and must be correlated with the known presence of leukemia in the patient. Local leukemic lesions, including nodules and focal densities that are poorly defined, may occur, but are rare and usually represent pneumonia or infarction with hemorrhage in the patients in whom they are present. Since infections are common in leukemia, they usually account for pulmonic involvement noted in this disease. Hemorrhage may also produce pulmonary opacities. Pleural involvement, resulting in effusion, is somewhat more common than pulmonary leukemic involvement. It tends to be unilateral and is often secondary to infection, heart failure, or lymphatic obstruction rather than to actual leukemic involvement of the pleura.

Hodgkin's Disease and Non-Hodgkin's Lymphoma*

Primary pulmonary involvement (about 10%) without hilar or mediastinal involvement is unusual. In recurrent Hodgkin's disease, however, parenchymal lung disease may appear in the absence of adenopathy in the hila or the mediastinum, particularly in the nodular sclerosis type, and is more common than pulmonary involvement in non-Hodgkin's lymphoma (about 11.6% versus 3.7%) (Figs. 29-17 and 29-18).[7] The non-Hodgkin's lymphomas may involve the lung along with mediastinal nodes and rarely may be primary in the lung. The primary pulmonary parenchymal form tends to be more benign than the secondary type and is usually lymphocytic.[2] Roentgen findings are those of a large mass, which is usually clearly defined, but slight haziness and irregularity of the edges are often observed. The mass grows slowly and, unlike bronchogenic carcinoma, does not ordinarily invade the bronchi and cause obstruction. Therefore, an air bronchogram can often be identified. When a segment or lobe is completely consolidated, the lesion resembles pneumonia. The tumor may cross interlobar fissures and invade the pleura peripherally. The rare primary histiocytic type may progress very rapidly early in the disease and resemble acute pneumonia. Mediastinal adenopathy is not a feature of this disease but hilar adneopathy may be present. Pleural effusion is rare, even though the tumor extends to a pleural surface.

---

* See Radiological Clinics of North America 28:4, July, 1990, for a series of papers regarding lymphoma.

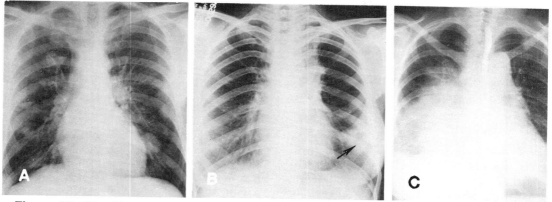

Figure 29–17. Hodgkin's disease. **(A)** Parenchymal nodules ranging up to 3 cm in diameter, plus some enlargement of the hilar nodes. **(B)** Mediastinal node involvement, most marked on the left. The rounded parenchymal mass at the left base (*arrow*) was noted on tomography to contain a central cavity. **(C)** Massive involvement of mediastinal nodes with direct invasion of adjacent pulmonary parenchyma and pleura, with some pleural effusion on the right.

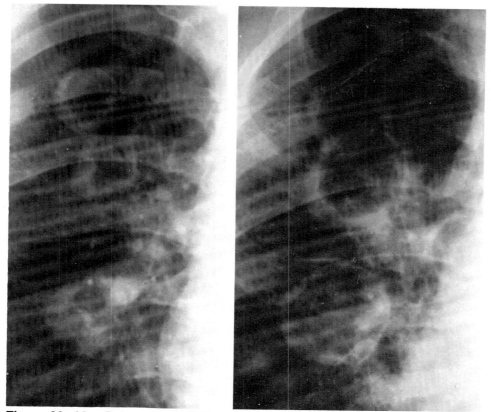

Figure 29–18. Pulmonary Hodgkin's disease with multiple excavating nodules. In the 2-month period of observation, the nodules increased in size, but there was a loss of soft-tissue tumor in their walls.

Secondary involvement of the lung in patients with mediastinal Hodgkin's and non-Hodgkin's lymphoma is usually a late feature of the disease. This occurs in a variety of forms, resulting in a number of different roentgen manifestations: (1) direct invasion of the lung in the presence of visible mediastinal mass, resulting in the sharp margins of the mediastinal mass becoming irregular and shaggy, a finding best outlined on CT; (2) large lobar opacities associated with mediastinal mass, or (3) smaller pulmonary parenchymal opacities, either solitary or multiple, that may be well circumscribed and discrete or irregular and poorly defined. At times, clusters of these lesions cause subsegmental or segmental opacities. Occasionally inhomogeneous involvement of large areas may progress to uniform density resembling pneumonia. Air bronchograms may be visible within the area of disease. If bronchi are compressed, atelectasis may occur, adding to the opacity; (4) a miliary pattern; and (5) pleural effusion. These manifestations are usually associated with hilar or mediastinal adenopathy or with disease elsewhere, so the diagnosis is not difficult to make on roentgen examination. Cavitation may occur in either the primary or secondary forms, but is less common in non-Hodgkin's lymphoma than in Hodgkin's disease. Endobronchial mass with secondary atelectasis has been reported as the only finding in non-Hodgkin's lymphoma. It is evident that roentgen manifestations are extremely variable, but the presence of associated adenopathy usually suggests that the disease is caused by one of the lymphoma group.

In some patients with secondary histiocytic lymphoma, however, there may be rapid development of pulmonary disease. When the lesion is bilateral and extensive, the symptoms may resemble those of pneumonia with fever, chills, and purulent sputum. Biopsy may be necessary to make the differentiation. In patients with Hodgkin's disease, interstitial opacities involving the parenchyma producing a coarse reticulonodular appearance is fairly common. Poorly defined nodules and direct extension from a mediastinal mass are less common. When the parenchymal involvement is a direct extension of the mediastinal disease, the tumor advances in a compact manner and tends to destroy the tissue that it invades. Pleural effusion is often present, usually the result of lymphatic obstruction. Parenchymal masses may be single or multiple and may be the only finding on the chest film; the other sites of the disease may be in nodes outside the thorax. Note that patients with Hodgkin's disease show a tendency to develop tuberculosis or fungal infections during terminal stages.

Peripheral T-cell lymphoma may present with diffuse pulmonary disease and angioedema. Pulmonary disease in the form of diffuse basal alveolar and perihilar hazy opacity are found at the time of diagnosis in 20% of patients and develop during the course of the disease in another 20%. Massive adenopathy usually develops later.[12]

Malignant Histiocytosis

Malignant histiocytosis is characterized by a systemic proliferation of atypical histiocytes resulting in hepatosplenomegaly, adenopathy, and systemic symptoms of fever and cachexia.[48] About two thirds of patients exhibit intrathoracic disease that can be identified radiographically. The most common manifestation is a combination of hilar and mediastinal adenopathy associated with coarse interstitial pulmonary opacities, which tend to radiate from hila into the lungs. Pleural effusion is observed occasionally. Differentiation from non-Hodgkin's lymphoma is made by histologic study.

Plasma Cell Diseases

Plasmacytoma may involve the thorax and lungs. Usually it involves the lung as part of a generalized disease—multiple myeloma. Rarely, in the absence of multiple myeloma, a solitary plasmacytoma may originate in the lung parenchyma where it resembles a peripheral type of bronchogenic carcinoma, often a lobulated nodule.[38] This lesion may also arise in the trachea or in a major bronchus, producing signs of obstruction including atelectasis or recurrent pneumonia. It is also a rare manifestation of plasma cell myeloma. More commonly, direct extension into the thorax from a mass associated with an osteolytic rib lesion in patients with multiple myeloma produces a pleural or peripheral pulmonary lesion which may vary considerably in size.

Waldenstrom's macroglobulinemia is a rare disorder that occasionally involves the lungs, usually producing a diffuse reticulonodular pattern. Rarely, a solitary parenchymal mass may be present in the lung in this disease. Pleural effusion is present in about one half of the patients affected.[55]

METASTATIC TUMORS

Hematogenous Metastasis

Hematogenous pulmonary metastases are usually multiple and consist of smoothly rounded nodules scattered throughout both lungs. They may be uniform or may vary considerably in size. The nodules range up to 10 cm or more in diameter, while others in the same lung will be less than 1 cm in diameter. Occasionally a solitary metastasis is present and cannot be differentiated from solitary primary tumor on the basis of plain film findings; CT may reveal other lesions (Fig. 29-19). The source of metastasis can be a malignant lesion anywhere in the body, but there are some tumors that show a marked tendency to metastasize to the lung. All of the sarcomas, including osteosarcoma and chondrosarcoma, as well as the various soft-tissue sarcomas and malignant melanoma frequently metastasize to the lung. Carcinoma of the breast, kidney, ovary, testis, colon, and thyroid also commonly metastasize to the lung, while tumors of the stomach, respiratory tract, and prostate do so infrequently. A solitary metastasis may also appear as a solitary round or lobulated pulmonary mass. Solitary lesions may originate from any tumor, but are slightly more common in tumors of the rectosigmoid, bone sarcomas, and occasionally from kidney, testes, or breast.

Roentgen Findings

The roentgen findings are those of multiple nodules that may be few or many in number. They may be uniform or vary considerably in size. Occasionally a solitary metastasis may be observed as a solitary parenchymal nodule that may become large without producing symptoms. A solitary metastasis may arise from any organ. There are some differences in the roentgen findings in pulmonary metastases from different organs, but these are variable and not reliable in differential diagnosis. Renal and thyroid tumors result in metastases that are few in number and often large in size. There are exceptions, however. Carcinoma of the thyroid occasionally produces very numerous (uncountable) small nodular metastases that remain unchanged for some time. Patients often have very few, if any, symptoms for many years, and the small nodules remain unchanged. We have observed a few thyroid carcinoma patients with solitary lytic bone metastasis or with a few lytic bone metastases whose bone and multiple pulmonary metastases changed very slowly over several years, indicating a low degree of malignancy. Osteosarcoma metastasizing to the lungs may cause formation of tumor bone in the metastases that may be characteristic. Calcification may occur in metastases from osteosarcoma, chondrosarcoma, synovial sarcoma, giant-cell tumor, and from papillary and mucinous adenocarcinoma of the thyroid, ovary, and gastrointestinal tract; and rarely in metastases from tumors of other organs. Dystrophic calcification can also be seen after treatment of nodular hematogenous metastases from a variety of primary tumors. Ovarian and testicular tumors and chorioepithelioma often result in widespread, rapidly growing, metastatic lesions (Fig. 29-20). Rarely endobronchial metastases may occur and in about one third of the patients, the diagnosis can be made by bronchial biopsy.[40]

Cavitation in Metastases

Occasionally central necrosis with cavitation is found in metastatic nodules (see Fig. 29-18). Cavitation occurs in metastases from bone sarcoma, colon carcinoma,

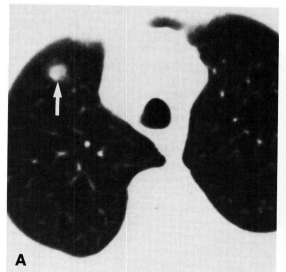
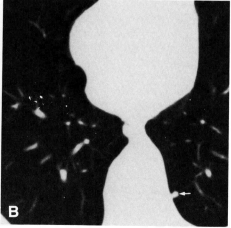

Figure 29–19. Solitary lung nodule (1 cm) was seen on initial chest film of this patient with pharyngeal carcinoma. **(A)** Original nodule (*arrow*) on the right on this computed chest tomogram using lung windows. **(B)** One of several small additional nodules (*arrow*) in a characteristic subpleural location in the left lung. (Courtesy of Robert Rosenberg, MD)

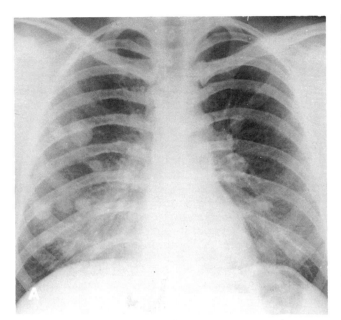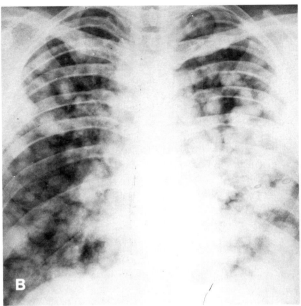

Figure 29–20. Hematogenous pulmonary metastases. **(A)** Scattered nodules, mainly on the right side. **(B)** Extensive nodular metastases. Despite the massive involvement, there was very little dyspnea. Primary tumor in both **A** and **B** was testicular seminoma.

and metastases from squamous cell tumors of the head and neck as well as tumors of the genital tract in females. Cavitation is uncommon in metastases but is much more common when metastatic pulmonary tumors respond to treatment with cytotoxic drugs.

Computed tomography of the lungs is important in the search for nodular metastases. In patients with a solitary nodule on plain film study, nearly 30% will have additional masses demonstrated on CT.

Muhm and colleagues compared whole-lung tomography with computed tomography in 91 patients.[28] In 35%, more nodules were detected on CT than on whole-lung tomography. Of 31 who had resection of nodules, 27 patients were found to have malignancy, either primary or metastatic. The authors believe that CT is the method of choice for detecting pulmonary metastases. In other studies, however, specificity on CT examination for nodules was relatively low. This matter, although still being debated, has largely been settled, since much additional information may be obtained from chest CT in patients with solitary pulmonary nodules.

Lymphangitic Metastasis

In contrast to the nodular hematogenous type of pulmonary metastasis, lymphangitic metastasis tends to cause respiratory dysfunction leading to dyspnea, which may be severe. This type of metastasis is usually

caused by primary tumors of the stomach, breast, thyroid, pancreas, larynx, cervix, or lung. It is generally agreed that they usually result from hematogenous spread to pulmonary capillaries, with subsequent invasion of the lymphatics and extension along the lymphatics toward the hila. Retrograde spread from central nodes to the lymphatics appears to be less common.

Roentgen Findings

The appearance of the chest in this type of metastasis is different than that of hematogenous metastases, although both may occur in a single patient. Sometimes there is enough hilar node enlargement to be recognized as such. This is particularly true if earlier roentgenograms are available for comparison. Massive mediastinal lymph-node involvement is not a prerequisite, and most patients have vascular tumor embolization as noted above, which may account for the pulmonary insufficiency. Tumor cells extend into the connective tissue adjacent to the lymphatics, sometimes producing nodularity that can be detected roentgenographically. There is an irregular strandlike network of interstitial-type density extending outward from the hila well into the parenchyma. When this change is early, findings are often minimal and comparison with an earlier examination is necessary to be certain of the diagnosis. Later the findings become more characteristic (Fig. 29-21). In some patients, there may be nodules ranging from a few widely scattered densities to exten-

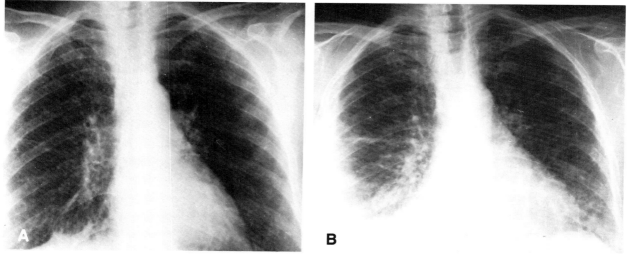

Figure 29–21. Lymphangitic metastases. (**A**) There is little general increase in interstitial markings, chiefly in the parahilar areas and bases. (**B**) Five weeks later, considerable advance in the disease process is noted and there is a sizable right pleural effusion in this patient with carcinoma of the pancreas.

sive gross parenchymal nodularity associated with the linear lymphatic accentuation. Unilateral or bilateral pleural effusions may also be present. Occasionally there are small granular opacities associated with the reticular network of increased density extending into the parenchyma that may resemble sarcoidosis, hematogenous tuberculosis, or other inflammatory disease. Correlation of the roentgen and the clinical findings usually permits a correct diagnosis in these instances.

Thin-section, high-resolution CT (HRCT) is useful in detection of lymphangitic pulmonary metastases when the chest radiograph is normal or equivocal. The HRCT findings consist of thickening of the interlobular septa. The septa have smooth margins.[30] There is also thickening of the bronchovascular bundles.[32] Interlobar fissures may also be thickened (Fig. 29-22).

BENIGN TUMORS

Benign tumors are much less common than malignant tumors of the lung. Unless they arise in an endobronchial location, they are usually found as solitary nodules in asymptomatic patients.[19]

HAMARTOMA

Hamartoma, the most common benign lung tumor, consists of a mass of tissue containing the elements of the organ within which it develops but without organization and without function. Hamartoma of the lung

may contain cartilage, muscle, fibrous connective tissue, fat, and epithelial elements. Often cartilage and fibrous connective tissue predominate. The tumor is usually peripheral in type and is found near a pleural surface. It may occur near the hilum, however, and 10% are endobronchial. It is usually relatively small in

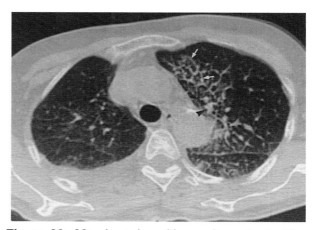

Figure 29–22. Lymphangitic carcinomatosis. The interlobular septa are markedly thickened (*white arrows*). The black arrowhead indicates thickening of a bronchovascular bundle. Note also the thickened interlobar fissure on the left. High-resolution CT scan, 2-mm collimation, bone algorithm. (Courtesy of Julie K. Mitby, MD)

size and grows very slowly. The peak incidence is in the sixth decade.

Roentgen Findings

Roentgenographic findings are those of a well-circumscribed, pulmonary parenchymal nodule, usually small in size (less than 4 cm in diameter). It is clearly defined and smoothly rounded or oval, but may be lobulated. No satellite nodules are demonstrated in the area. Calcification is present in 25% to 30% of cases and occasionally ossification is noted within the tumor. When calcification is present, it is scattered within the lesion; the distribution in some has been likened to the appearance of a popcorn ball. (In our experience this is exceedingly uncommon.) In others, the calcification is curvilinear or stippled. When such a mass is found within a lung, it is necessary to determine whether or not calcification is present. Computed tomography is indicated. If evidence of calcium is not visible on the routine roentgenogram it may be visible on CT. This has proved very reliable in the diagnosis of hamartoma.[43] If no calcification or fat is present, the mass cannot be differentiated from the peripheral type of primary bronchogenic carcinoma or from solitary metastasis, so some type of biopsy is indicated. When calcification is present, it usually indicates that the lesion is benign and the distribution of calcium may be characteristic enough to make a definite diagnosis. There may be enough fat in the nodule so the diagnosis can be made on CT. Occasionally, multiple hamartomas are present. This tumor has been observed to enlarge and, if no calcification is present, it may become impossible to differentiate it from malignant tumor, so biopsy or removal is indicated. When endobronchial hamartoma occurs, resultant obstruction of the bronchus may cause atelectasis or pneumonia.

LIPOMA

Most pulmonary lipomas are endobronchial and may cause bronchial obstruction, leading to atelectasis and infection. This type of lipoma is almost always found in males. Parenchymal lipoma presents as an asymptomatic pulmonary nodule, usually in a subpleural location. These masses may become very large. The low attenuation values of these tumors makes the CT diagnosis conclusive.

FIBROMA

Fibroma is another rare pulmonary tumor that may arise in an endobronchial location. Those in the lung tend to be peripheral, so findings are similar to lipoma except for the difference in attenuation on CT.

LEIOMYOMA

Leiomyoma is a rare tumor that usually occurs in women older than 40 years of age. It presents as a peripheral nodule, usually round or oval, in an asymptomatic patient. There is a considerable variation in size. Occasionally, multiple tumors are present in the lungs. The tumor may also arise centrally in a bronchus, producing obstruction with atelectasis or infection distal to it. Pulmonary metastases from uterine leiomyosarcoma may resemble leiomyoma histologically, so this possibility must be considered when multiple lung tumors are found in a patient with uterine leiomyosarcoma.

OTHER BENIGN TUMORS

A wide variety of tumors have been found within the lung. These include neurofibroma, chondroma, hemangioma, hemangiopericytoma, papilloma, endometrioma, chemodectoma, and the focal or nodular form of amyloidosis, which may be single or multiple and may be endobronchial. Granular cell myoblastoma usually arises in a major bronchus, produces hemoptysis and bronchial obstruction, and may become very large. These tumors occur most frequently in middle age, often in black females. They are usually asymptomatic when they occur peripherally and in some cases may reach large size before being discovered because of the absence of symptoms. If calcification is present within the tumor it is likely benign, but if there is no calcification the possibility of malignancy cannot be excluded. Occasionally a lymph node is observed as a small nodular mass in the pulmonary parenchyma, usually in a lower lobe.

Roentgen Findings

Findings are similar to those described in hamartoma, except that the tumors usually contain no calcium. Because they are clearly defined and appear as solitary pulmonary nodules, there are no differential characteristics on roentgen examination. Occasionally these benign tumors may reach massive proportions and fill most of the thorax on one side. They then appear as rounded, oval, or lobulated masses of considerable size. CT should be used to define them clearly and, if calcification is not present, biopsy is indicated to differentiate them from carcinoma. Rarely, one of the benign tumors mentioned may arise in a bronchus. Then the major findings are related to obstruction and consist of recurrent pneumonia and atelectasis.

REFERENCES AND SELECTED READINGS

1. AMERICAN THORACIC SOCIETY POSITION PAPER: Adopted by ATS Board of Directors, June, 1988. Guidelines for percutaneous transthoracic needle biopsy. Am Rev Resp Dis 140:255, 1989

2. BARON MG, WHITEHOUSE WM: Primary lymphosarcoma of the lung. Am J Roentgenol 85:294, 1961

3. BLANK N, CASTELLINO RA: The intrathoracic manifestations of the malignant lymphomas and the leukemias. Semin Roentgenol 15:227, 1980

4. CHAPLIN RH, KAWAMOTO EH, DYER RB, ET AL: Atypical carcinoid of the lung: Radiographic features. Am J Roentgenol 146:665, 1986

5. COHEN AM: Magnetic resonance imaging of the thorax. Radiol Clin North Am 22:829, 1984

6. CLINICAL STAGING OF PRIMARY LUNG CANCER. American Thoracic Society Node Mapping Scheme. Am Rev Resp Dis 127:659, 1983

7. FILLY R, BLANK N, CASTELLINO RA: Radiographic distribution of intrathoracic disease in previously untreated patients with Hodgkin's disease and non-Hodgkin's lymphoma. Radiology 120:277, 1976

8. GLAZER GM, GROSS BH, QUINT LE, ET AL: Normal mediastinal lymph nodes: Number and size according to American Thoracic Society Mapping. Am J Roentgenol 144:261, 1985

9. GLAZER HS, ARONBERG J, SAGEL SS: Pitfalls in CT recognition of mediastinal lymphadenopathy. Am J Roentgenol 144:267, 1985

10. GOBIEN RP, VALICENTI JF, PARIS BS, ET AL: Thin-needle aspiration biopsy: Methods of increasing the accuracy of a negative prediction. Radiology 145:603, 1982

11. GODWIN JD: The solitary pulmonary nodule. Radiol Clin North Am 21:709, 1983

12. HARRISON NK, TWELVES C, ADDIS BJ, ET AL: Peripheral T-cell lymphoma presenting with angioedema and diffuse pulmonary infiltrates. Am Rev Resp Dis 138:976, 1988

13. HEITZMAN ER, MARKARIAN B, RAASCH BN, ET AL: Pathways of tumor spread through the lung: Radiologic correlations with anatomy and pathology. Radiology 144:3, 1982

14. HILL CA: Bronchioloalveolar carcinoma: A review. Radiology 150:15, 1984

15. IVES JC, BUFFLER PA, GREENBERG SD: Environmental associations and histopathologic patterns of carcinoma of the lung: The challenge and dilemma in epidemiologic studies. Am Rev Resp Dis 128:195, 1983

16. JELINCK JS, REDMOND III J, PERRY JJ, ET AL: Small cell lung cancer: Staging with MR imaging. Radiology 177:837, 1990

17. KHOURI NF, STITIK FP, EROZAN YS, ET AL: Transthoracic needle aspiration biopsy of benign and malignant lung lesions. Am J Roentgenol 144:281, 1985

18. LILLINGTON EA: The solitary pulmonary nodule. Am Rev Resp Dis 110:699, 1974

19. MADEWELL JR, FEIGIN DS: Benign tumors of the lung. Semin Roentgenol 12:175, 1977

20. MAILE CW, MOORE AV, ULREICH S, ET AL: Chest radiographic–pathologic correlation in adult leukemia patients. Invest Radiol 18:495, 1983

21. MANIVEL JC, PRIEST JR, WATTERSON J, ET AL: Pleuropulmonary blastoma of childhood. Cancer 62:1516, 1988

22. MANUAL FOR STAGING OF CANCER, 1978 AMERICAN JOINT COMMITTEE FOR CANCER STAGING AND END RESULTS REPORTING, Chicago, Illinois

23. MATTHEWS MJ: Morphology of lung cancer. Semin Oncol 1:175, 1974

24. MCKENNA PJ JR, LIBSHITZ HI, MOUNTAIN CE, ET AL: Roentgenographic evaluation of mediastinal nodes for preoperative assessment in lung cancer. Chest 88:206, 1985

25. MITCHELL DM, SHAK SH, EDWARDS D, ET AL: Incidence of pulmonary nodules detected by computed tomography in patients with bronchial carcinoid. Clinic Radiol 37:151, 1986

26. MODAN B: Population distribution of histological types of lung cancer: Epidemiologic aspects in Israel and review of the literature. Isr J Med Sci 14:772, 1978

27. MOFFAT RE, CHANG CH, SLAVEN JE: Roentgen consideration in primary pulmonary artery sarcoma. Radiology 104:283, 1972

28. MUHM JR, BROWN LR, CROWE JK, ET AL: Comparison of whole lung tomography and computed tomography for detecting pulmonary nodules. Am J Roentgenol 131:981, 1978

29. MUHM JR, MILLER WE, FONTANA RS, ET AL: Lung cancer detected during a screening program using four-month chest radiographs. Radiology 148:609, 1983

30. MULLER NL: Differential diagnosis of chronic diffuse infiltrative lung disease in high resolution computed tomography. Semin Roentgenol XXVI(2):132, 1991

31. MULLER NL, MILLER RR: Computed tomography of chronic diffuse infiltrative lung disease: State of the art, Part I. Am Rev Resp Dis 142:1206, 1990

32. MURATA K, KHAN A, HERMAN PG: Pulmonary parenchymal disease: Evaluation with high resolution CT. Radiology 170:629, 1989

33. O'CONNELL RS, MCLOUD TC, WILKINS EW: Superior sulcus tumor: Radiographic diagnosis and workup. Am J Roentgenol 140:25, 1983

34. OHTOMO K, ARAKI T, YASHIRO N, ET AL: Pulmonary blastoma in children. Radiology 147:101, 1983

35. OLSSON HE, SPITZER RM, ERSTON WF: Primary and secondary pulmonary artery neoplasia mimicking acute pulmonary embolism. Radiology 118:49, 1976

36. OSBORNE DR, KOROBKIN M, RAVIN CE, ET AL: Comparison of plain radiography, conventional tomography and computed tomography in detecting intrathoracic lymph node metastases from lung carcinoma. Radiology 142:157, 1982

obstruction and no collapse may occur. In collateral air

Adhesive atelectasis refers to the nonobstructive ailessness found in patients with inactivation, decrease, or loss of surfactant. Hyaline membranes may then be formed within the alveoli, as in newborn respiratory distress syndrome, acute radiation pneumonitis, and uremia.

Cicatrization atelectasis refers to volume loss found in patients with local or general pulmonary fibrosis. Some prefer not to consider this a form of atelectasis, even though there is associated volume loss.

Chest radiographs are useful and reasonably accurate in patients with tumors causing bronchial obstruction and atelectasis, but when the cause of segmental or lobar atelectasis is not established with reasonable certainty on chest radiographs, CT should be performed.[96] MRI may have a place in determining the cause of atelectasis with associated infection, particularly in bone-marrow transplant patients.[42]

RADIOGRAPHIC CONSIDERATIONS

The fundamental alteration in the thorax produced by atelectasis is a decrease in volume of the segment, lobe, or lung involved. Therefore the interlobar fissure or fissures are displaced toward the airless lobe or segment. Crowding and displacement of vessels may be observed if they are surrounded by sufficient air-containing lung. Air bronchograms may be present, and bronchi may be displaced. There are other roentgen signs such as elevation of the diaphragm, shift of mediastinum to the side of involvement, hilar displacement, and narrowing of rib interspaces. Any of these signs may predominate in a given instance, depending on mediastinal and diaphragmatic fixation. In some patients the remaining lung on the involved side undergoes so much compensatory overinflation that there is no actual change in volume of the hemithorax and few of the signs mentioned are then present. The relative airlessness of the affected portion of lung may result in very little increased density unless enhanced by edema, blood, and/or retained secretions. So the amount of collapse doesn't necessarily correlate with the opacity of the involved lung. The classic ground-glass appearance is most likely caused by the opacity produced by collapsed lung which contains some fluid, plus air in a lobe or segment anterior or posterior to it. This appearance is noted most commonly in atelectasis of the left upper lobe. The opacity is uniform but has a grainy character that has been likened to the appearance of ground glass. It is usually relatively opaque medially and fades to a lesser opacity laterally. Wide variations in opacity are possible, however, depending on relative amounts of aerated, collapsed, and fluid-filled lung. Disease in the involved lobe may also add to its opacity. When atelectasis involves the entire lung, the opacity may be complete and homogeneous. The

bronchi as well as the lung may become airless in atelectasis caused by obstruction; then there is absence of an air bronchogram. If an air bronchogram is present, complete bronchial obstruction is unlikely. Absence of an air bronchogram does not necessarily mean obstruction, but suggests it. Associated with mediastinal shift there is often herniation of the opposite lung across the midline into the involved hemithorax; in chronic atelectasis this may become extensive. When there is right lower-lobe atelectasis the height of the right hemidiaphragm may not be ascertained. There is usually enough gas in the stomach or colon to outline the left hemidiaphragm, however. The cause of the atelectasis may be evident on the film and may add to the opacity (Fig. 30-1).

LOBAR ATELECTASIS

Lower-Lobe Atelectasis

Lower-lobe atelectasis is easily overlooked, particularly on the left side where the lobe may be hidden by the heart. The inferior pulmonary ligament attaches the medial aspect of the lower lobe to the mediastinum, so the lower lobe does not migrate upward toward the hilum. Also, the ligament keeps the base of a collapsed lower lobe in contact with the diaphragm. Occasionally, however, the inferior pulmonary ligament is incomplete, with no diaphragmatic attachment. In these cases, a paraspinal mass may be apparent on the PA projection, but the mass may not be visible on the lateral, and the hemidiaphragm is not obscured posteriorly by the adjacent density usually present in lower lobe atelectasis. This variation is usually present on the left side. When there are no pleural adhesions, the involved lobe moves medially to form ultimately a rather narrow triangle with the apex at the level of the hilum and the base at the diaphragm. In the lateral projection the earliest sign of decrease in volume of a lower lobe is downward and posterior displacement of the major interlobar fissure. Later, as the amount of atelectasis increases, the opacity of the atelectasic lobe may obliterate the shadow of the posterior aspect of the diaphragm on the affected side. If the collapsed lobe is sufficiently dense (e.g., retained secretions, fluid), the lower aortic silhouette and the paraspinal line may be effaced on the PA view, and on the lateral projection the density of the collapsed lobe adds to the density of the lower thoracic vertebrae, so they become as dense or slightly more dense than the upper thoracic vertebrae. The signs of mediastinal shift—downward displacement of the ipsilateral hilum which may be hidden by the collapse, diaphragmatic elevation, and decrease in size of the bony thorax—may be present to varying degrees or may be absent. If

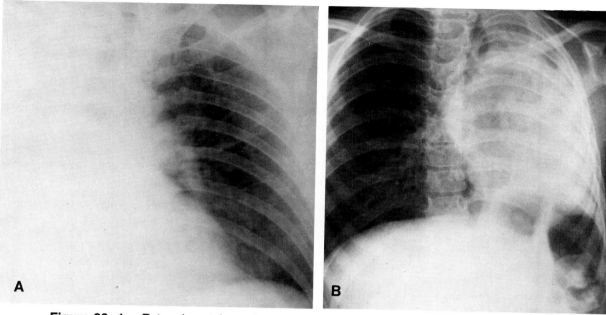

Figure 30–1. Extensive atelectasis. **(A)** There is a shift of the poorly outlined trachea to the right and almost complete density in the right lung. The heart is also shifted to the right. **(B)** Atelectasis of the left lung. In this patient, there is a marked shift of the mediastinal structures to the left, elevation of the left hemidiaphragm, and very little air in the atelectatic left lung.

they are absent, there is usually enough compensatory overinflation of the upper lobe on the left or of the upper and middle lobes on the right to alert the observer to the possibility of lobar collapse. When the roentgenogram is of sufficient penetration, the triangular shadow of the collapsed left lower lobe is usually outlined behind the heart on the frontal projection. Right lower-lobe collapse usually causes a similar shadow at the right medial base which may obliterate the cardiophrenic angle. On the lateral view, the inferior vena cava may be obliterated and the density of the lobe may simulate fluid in the major fissure.

Kattan has described upper mediastinal and aortic changes in lower-lobe atelectasis.[46] In right lower-lobe collapse, there may be an *upper triangle sign*. This is caused by a shift to the right of the anterior triangle consisting of the right and left anterior pleuromediastinal lines laterally and the clavicle above. The lines converge below as the anterior junction line. The triangle contains thymic, lymphoid, and areolar tissue and is not very dense. Although the triangle may shift to the left on left lower-lobe collapse, it is hidden by the aorta.

In severe left lower-lobe atelectasis, the heart shifts to the left and may rotate in a clockwise direction to such an extent that the appearance is that of a slight right anterior oblique rotation of the heart (flat waist sign).[46] Obliteration of the top of the aortic knob (top-of-the-knob sign) may also occur in left lower-lobe atelectasis. The lateral aspect of the left upper mediastinum is continuous with the left border of the pericardium below the aortic knob.

On the right side the vascular structures consisting of the right descending pulmonary artery, the superior pulmonary vein crossing it, the middle lobe artery, and arteries to the superior segment of the lower lobe form distinct converging points at the hilum. The right upper lobe arteries form a less distinct converging point above this level. In the presence of atelectasis of the right upper lobe, there is only one converging point. The same is true of right lower-lobe collapse. Therefore when one vascular converging point is present on the right, lobar collapse is suggested. The sign is not pertinent on the left, where there is only one converging point.[24]

Right Middle-Lobe Atelectasis

Right middle-lobe atelectasis may be complete or incomplete. When this lobe decreases in volume, the secondary interlobar fissure moves downward; it and the primary fissure can be outlined in contrast to the dense lung between them on the lateral projection. The middle lobe also tends to move medially so that in the PA view, a triangular shadow appears medially above the diaphragm. Its base is at the mediastinum and the apex points toward the lateral chest wall. As atelectasis becomes complete, the lobe may shrink to a very small size and may be difficult to see clearly in the PA projection. The opacity caused by the atelectatic lobe blurs the right cardiac margin. When this blurring is noted, the lateral view is confirmatory. In the lateral view, varying degrees of collapse are readily outlined. The appearance is that of a dense triangle, the apex of which is at or near the hilum and the base points downward and anteriorly. The upper and lower borders of this dense triangle may be slightly concave.

Collapse of the lateral segment only does not cause blurring of the right cardiac margin. Usually there is no discernible mediastinal shift, hilar displacement, alteration of the right hemidiaphragm, or detectable compensatory overinflation of upper and lower lobes because of the small volume of the middle as compared to the upper and lower lobes.

Upper-Lobe Atelectasis

In upper-lobe atelectasis the roentgen appearance depends on the presence or absence of adhesions between the visceral and parietal pleurae. When adhesions are present they may hold all or part of the lobe in its normal position; this peripheral upper lobe collapse can simulate local pleural disease or loculated pleural effusion, particularly in infants. The margins of the collapsed lobe are outlined by the overinflated lower lobe. When diagnosis becomes a problem, CT may be useful.[23] When there are no adhesions, the lobe tends to shrink uniformly and move toward the hilum. In *right upper-lobe atelectasis* the first sign is elevation of the interlobar fissure. If there are lateral adhesions the inferior aspect of the lobe becomes concave, with elevation of the minor fissure in its central aspect. There may be a slight increase in opacity of the lobe if fluid is present within it. With progressive collapse, the lobe shrinks and flattens against the apex and upper mediastinum. Partial adherence of the lobe in one area or another may alter the general contour, so a considerable variety of forms is possible. In the lateral view the major fissure tends to move anteriorly with increasing atelectasis and is usually visible; the upward displacement of the minor fissure may also be outlined in this projection. However, the atelectatic upper lobe may be difficult or impossible to identify in the lateral view. The middle lobe moves upward anteriorly and the lower lobe upward posteriorly. Its superior segment may actually occupy the apex and rotate forward to lie in a caplike manner over the collapsed upper lobe. This can sometimes be outlined in the lateral projection and can be predicted by the appearance of normally aerated or hyperaerated lung at the apex above the more dense atelectatic upper lobe in the frontal projection. The signs of mediastinal and tracheal displacement toward the involved side, elevation of the right hemidiaphragm and hilum, and decrease in size of the hemithorax, resulting in narrowing of the intercostal spaces, may also occur in varying degrees, but compensatory hyperinflation of the middle and lower lobes may be sufficient so that none of the other signs will be present. Mediastinal displacement may be a prominent feature when there are extensive adhesions holding the upper lobe to the lateral parietal pleura. The hilum may also be elevated and retracted to the ipsilateral side in such cases. When atelectasis is relatively complete and there are no adhesions, the shadow of the upper lobe tends to move toward the hilum and upper mediastinum. On the right side, it may then resemble slight mediastinal widening and occasionally may become so small that it is difficult to recognize.

Kattan and associates have described a local elevation of the diaphragm, the *juxtaphrenic peak*, which is seen on the PA roentgenogram as a small shadow projecting upward from the highest point on the dome of the diaphragm.[47] The shape varies from a narrow-based peak to a broad tent and is sometimes more round than angular. A similar peak may be caused by an inferior accessory fissure or by tangential projection of the medial aspect of the major fissure, so differentiation must be aided by other signs of atelectasis in some patients. The cause is uncertain, but it may be that a small amount of basal pleura with or without a wedge of lung tissue is pulled upward by negative intrathoracic pressure that increases when lobar collapse occurs. An unusual localized pneumothorax has been described in right upper-lobe obstructive atelectasis in children.[8]

Atelectasis of the left upper lobe is somewhat similar to that of the right upper lobe but the lobe moves superiorly, medially, and anteriorly rather than superiorly and anteriorly and early change is more difficult to recognize in the frontal projection because there is no minor interlobar fissure. A ground-glass opacity is helpful if there is enough fluid in the collapsed lobe to produce it. In the lateral view the major fissure tends to move forward and the opacity produced by the collapse is noted anteriorly with the lingula occupying a position similar to that of the middle lobe on the right. The partially collapsed lobe tends to be narrower inferiorly, owing to the smaller volume occupied by the lingula, and tends to extend upward and toward the periphery (Fig. 30-2). At times, the overinflated lower lobe may extend forward medially to a collapsed left lower lobe, where it produces a clearly defined area of lucency medial to the more opaque atelectatic upper

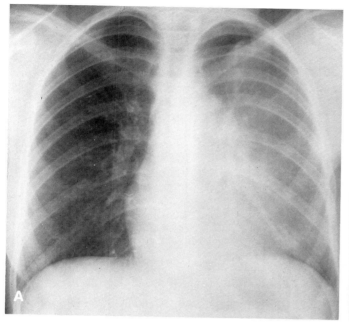
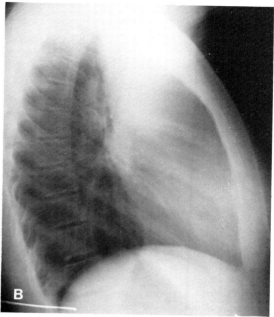

Figure 30–2. Left upper-lobe atelectasis. (**A**) Note the opacity on the left, which tends to fade toward the periphery. The border of the left side of the heart is blurred so the heart is not clearly defined. (**B**) A lateral view shows the opacity to be anterior. Note that the lower lobe extends to the apex above the partially atelectatic upper lobe. This is manifested on the frontal projection by the relatively normal aeration at the extreme left apex.

lobe. The secondary signs of mediastinal shift—hilar and diaphragmatic displacement as well as compensatory overinflation—may be somewhat greater than in right upper-lobe collapse because of the difference in volume. The juxtaphrenic peak may be present. Volume loss produces similar shift of the mediastinum to that noted in right upper-lobe disease, except that it is in the opposite direction. When collapse occurs in patients with chronic pulmonary inflammatory disease such as tuberculosis, there is often a considerable amount of associated pleural disease and contracting fibrosis of the lung. The lobe or segment involved is then difficult to evaluate on routine projections. In these instances, CT and rarely bronchography may be necessary for study of segmental anatomy.

Segmental Atelectasis

It is often possible to ascertain with a fair degree of accuracy the segment involved by segmental collapse, since the area of opacity produced by the atelectasis occupies the general area usually occupied by that segment in the absence of severely distorting associated pulmonary disease. By using frontal, lateral, and oblique projections as necessary, the site of the opacity

can be established and its relation to the interlobar fissures ascertained. The fissure tends to bow toward the site of the atelectasis; for example, in anterior segmental atelectasis of the right upper lobe, the secondary interlobar fissure elevates centrally to indicate that the volume of this lobe has decreased and in the lateral view the density will lie anteriorly. The same rules apply for lower-lobe segments, but the basal segments are very difficult to identify accurately (Fig. 30-3). In questionable cases, CT may be helpful.

Focal Atelectasis (Plate or Lobular)

When there is obstruction of a small subsegmental bronchus, a small area of atelectasis may result. This produces a thin horizontal or platelike line that is most often seen in the basal lung, where it occurs frequently. These small areas of atelectasis have been termed as "plate," "focal," or "lobular" atelectasis. They vary in size and sometimes cannot be distinguished from small areas of fibrosis. In some instances, these linear opacities are caused by a combination of subpleural collapse of lung plus an invagination of overlying pleura. They tend to occur in areas of pleural clefts, indentations, scars, and incomplete fissures—all sites

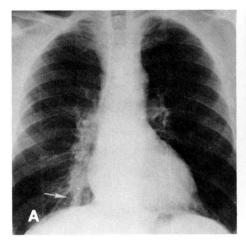
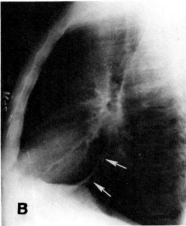

Figure 30–3. Segmental atelectasis. (**A**) There is partial atelectasis of the anterior segment of the right lower lobe, producing an irregular, poorly defined opacity at the right medial base (*arrow*). (**B**) In the lateral view, the opacity is immediately posterior to the major fissure, which is bowed backward (*arrows*). A bronchogram revealed obstruction of the anterior basal segmental bronchus in this patient.

of pre-existing pleural invagination. Pulmonary embolism is present in many patients with focal atelectasis, but the areas of atelectasis do not represent infarcts or occluded vessels. It is likely that focal atelectasis often indicates more widespread peripheral atelectasis than is radiographically evident. Therefore, it may indicate a greater disturbance in ventilation than is apparent.[89] Films exposed at frequent intervals will show disappearance or change in position of the linear areas of density, and when this is evident, the diagnosis of focal atelectasis is confirmed. The amount of involved lung is small, so the finding may be of little clinical significance, but as indicated above it does indicate poor ventilation in the area. When it is observed postoperatively, it implies that aeration is incomplete and that there probably is an accumulation of secretions causing obstruction of some of the basal subsegmental bronchi. Restriction of diaphragmatic movement and elevation of the diaphragm are additional factors in production of this type of atelectasis (Fig. 30-4).

It is fundamental to remember that atelectasis causes an area of increased opacity because of a combination of airlessness or relative airlessness and some fluid, in the involved segment, lobe, or lung and that the resultant decrease in volume must be compensated by a decrease in total volume of the involved hemithorax or by an increase in volume of the uninvolved lobe or segments.

Chronic isolated atelectasis of the middle lobe has been described and termed *middle-lobe syndrome*. Although it is usually thought to be caused by inflammatory disease, several studies have indicated a high incidence of malignancy. In one study of 135 patients, 43% were found to have malignant tumors, so persistent atelectasis of the middle lobe is potentially caused by malignancy and should be managed as such.[10]

Round Atelectasis (Folded Lung)

Round atelectasis was originally described in Europe and more recently in the American literature.[40] This lesion is formed in patients with pleural effusion, including those with asbestos-related pleural disease. A mass-like density is produced which must be differentiated from pleural and pulmonary tumors. The tumor-like mass is formed when a partially aerated portion of

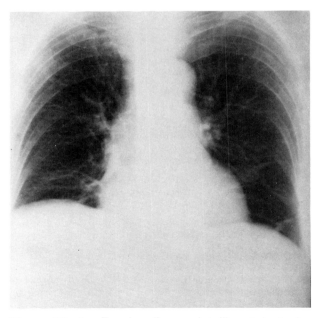

Figure 30–4. Focal or linear platelike atelectasis. Note the horizontal opacities in both lower lungs. These disappeared in 1 week. At times, linear fibrosis may occur in the lung and simulate focal atelectasis.

peripheral parenchyma floats on a pleural effusion and a collapsed section forms a groove, cleft, or fold on the lung surface. The floating lung tilts and if this portion is lifted by the fluid, adhesions form. As the fluid recedes, a round mass of atelectatic lung is left adherent to the pleura. The adhesions cause the tilted lung to remain atelectatic. The normal lung then expands around the mass as the pleural disease regresses. At times, the round atelectasis retracts centrally and is surrounded by aerated lung. Some lesions persist while others gradually regress.

On plain film, there is evidence of pleural disease as well as a pleural-based round or oval mass ranging from 2.5 to 5 cm in diameter. A convergence of vessels and bronchi resembling a comet tail may be observed entering the mass. Tomography or CT may be necessary to confirm the diagnosis.[59] Eight major and five minor CT signs have been described.[25] The major signs are:

1. Round mass 4 to 7 cm in diameter
2. Mass most dense at periphery, air bronchogram centrally
3. Mass forming an acute angle with the pleura
4. Pleural thickening present, usually greatest adjacent to the mass (fairly common with asbestos exposure)
5. Bronchi and vessels curving into the mass
6. At least two sharp margins present
7. Central margin blurred by entering vessels—the comet tail
8. Air bronchogram usually present centrally

The minor signs are:

1. Adjacent lung hyperinflated
2. When right-sided, posterior displacement of the right main bronchus
3. Interlobar fissure thickened and displaced owing to pleural scarring
4. Bilateral masses present
5. No change for a year or more; occasionally resolution

At times, the mass may be irregular, lobulated and poorly defined, so it must be suspected in a patient with a juxtapleural mass with evidence of pleural disease.[20]

COMPUTED TOMOGRAPHY IN LOBAR COLLAPSE

When plain film findings are atypical or equivocal, collapsed lung is associated with a pulmonary mass, fluid obscures the lung, and when it is necessary to follow patients with lung tumor and atelectasis, CT may be of value in patients with suspected atelectasis.[64, 65, 73] Lobar collapse causes compensatory overinflation, which usually can be identified on CT except

in middle-lobe atelectasis where volume loss is so small that there is little overinflation of the other lobes. Therefore this is a finding common to collapse of all but the middle lobe.

In *lower-lobe atelectasis*, the lateral border of the collapsed lobe is concave or straight in the upper portion and either convex or concave inferiorly, so a convexity superiorly indicates an associated mass. The lobe collapses posteromedially and usually maintains contact with the diaphragm when the pulmonary ligament is complete. If the inferior pulmonary ligament is incomplete, the lobe may collapse toward the hilum. The major fissure is displaced medially and the mediastinum is shifted toward the side of the lesion. Compensatory overinflation may be identified in contrast to the normal opposite lung. When pleural fluid is present, the collapsed lobe may be surrounded by the fluid, which may be less dense than the collapsed lobe.

When the *right middle lobe* is collapsed, the configuration is triangular, with the apex directed laterally. The triangle is small at the hilar level and its inferior aspect. If the lobe is high (rotated or tipped upward) the volume of the triangle of density is increased. The triangle is decreased when the lobe is low (rotated inferiorly); since it is more vertical in position, it is seen on more CT planes than in the more horizontal position (rotated upward). Many variations in position of this lobe are possible when it is atelectatic, particularly if there is distortion secondary to adhesions.

The *right upper lobe* collapses toward the mediastinum, and may move toward the anterior chest wall and the lung apex to a varying extent. It presents as a mass in the anteromedial aspect of the upper thorax on CT. If a tumor is present in the lobe, there is a convexity of the posterolateral aspect of the lobe; the size and location of the convexity are indicative of the size and location of the tumor. When the *left upper lobe* is collapsed, the lobe tends to move anteriorly and medially, and may move superiorly, so it presents as an anteromedial density on CT. Pleural adhesions may alter the position of any collapsed lobe, so an atypical appearance is produced. When the upper lobe is collapsed peripherally in an anterior position, the superior segment of the lower lobe may move anteriorly between the upper lobe and mediastinum to produce a radiolucent triangle medial to the posterior aspect of the upper lobe. This radiolucency may appear on the PA film as a stripe between the aortic arch and the collapsed lobe. As a result the aortic arch is very clearly defined. Lingular collapse alone is usually against the left heart border.

Endobronchial tumors can be identified within the lumen of a bronchus in most patients with *obstructive atelectasis*. The diagnosis of neoplasm is made more certain when a bolus of contrast material is used to aid in defining the tumor. Benign versus malignant tumors cannot be differentiated, however. Mucous plugs causing obstruction can usually be identified because of the branching pattern of the intrabronchial opacity, and the wall of the bronchus is visible distinct from the mucous plug.

In nonobstructive atelectasis, CT is useful in demonstrating patency of bronchi when the bronchi are identified by careful evaluation of the bronchial tree in the involved area. Collapse secondary to pleural effusion can be seen and any underlying pleural mass can be detected. In *cicatrization atelectasis*, the lung is often distorted; therefore, CT can provide valuable information regarding the location of the collapse, the absence of endobronchial mass, and the frequent association with bronchiectasis.

ATELECTASIS AND LUNG TORSION

Atelectasis is usually present when there is torsion of the lung, a rare complication found following traumatic pneumothorax and thoracic surgery. Occasionally it appears to occur spontaneously.[30, 61] The radiographic signs include: (1) a collapsed or consolidated lobe in an unusual position; (2) hilar displacement in an inappropriate direction for the involved lobe; (3) alteration in normal position and sweep of pulmonary vessels; (4) rapid opacification of the involved lobe following trauma or surgery; (5) marked change (usually opacification) of the involved lobe on sequential films. When the condition is suspected on the chest radiograph, CT is usually indicated if there is any question of the diagnosis because mortality is high if surgical fixation is delayed.

Pulmonary angiography may also be useful and may be diagnostic.[63] Findings include slow filling and decrease in caliber of the arteries to the involved lobe and little filling of the veins except for possible retrograde filling of a short segment of the venous stump near the heart. The contrast tends to clear very slowly from the involved lobe.

When the middle lobe collapses following right upper lobectomy, findings may be similar to those of other lobe torsion, so close clinical observation is necessary in these patients.[79]

RESPIRATORY DISTRESS SYNDROME OF THE NEWBORN (HYALINE MEMBRANE DISEASE)

Hyaline membrane disease of newborn infants is characterized by increasingly labored breathing, expiratory grunting, retraction of interspaces, cyanosis, and hypercapnia. Diffuse atelectasis of the adhesive type is present and the terminal bronchioles are dilated. The hyaline membrane lines the bronchioles, alveolar ducts, and alveoli. The disease may lead to death by asphyxiation in the first 48 to 72 hours of life. In 90% or more of cases it occurs in premature infants, in infants delivered by cesarean section, or in offspring of diabetic mothers.[7] It may also occur in full-term infants who have some condition that interferes with normal ventilation such as pneumothorax, diaphragmatic hernia, meconium aspiration, pneumonia, and birth trauma. The process is found in infants who breathe after birth, not in the stillborn. Respirations may be normal at or shortly following birth, but within a few hours dyspnea and cyanosis appear. In this disease a chest roentgenogram obtained very shortly after birth may be normal, but abnormalities are apparent within a few hours. The disease is usually the result of a deficiency of surfactant in an immature lung. Histopathologic examination reveals dilated bronchioles, thick interstitial septa, collapsed alveoli, and the presence of a hyaline material lining the alveoli, the bronchioles, and the alveolar ducts. The hyaline membrane causes atelectasis of alveoli, which is accompanied by dilatation of the alveolar ducts and terminal bronchioles. Therefore the volume of the lung is not necessarily decreased, even though there is peripheral atelectasis. The hyaline membranes are the residua of pulmonary edema and are secondary to the surfactant deficiency.

ROENTGEN FINDINGS

Four stages in the evolution of the disease have been described and identified radiographically.[66, 67] The first recognizable abnormality is an air-bronchogram pattern greater than normal. In the second stage, there is a fine miliary granularity associated with a slight increase in the reticular pattern of the lungs. This may be so minor as to be very difficult to ascertain; however, the air-bronchogram pattern stands out more clearly in this stage. The third stage consists of a gradual progression resulting in a confluent opacification or an unequivocal dense, reticular pattern. Infants who recover show gradual clearing, which is often irregular over a period of 3 to 10 days. The fourth stage is one of confluent opacity that may vary in extent. It is usually bilateral but it is not unusual to note some asymmetry. The roentgen pattern does not always follow the described stages in each instance, however. The most characteristic appearance is that of a granular pattern of marked increase in opacity, corresponding to stage three, with associated demonstrable bronchial air shadows that are sharply outlined and extend well out into the lungs (Fig. 30-5). There is no outward bulge of soft tissues in the intercostal spaces, as is noted in many other conditions that cause respiratory distress.[93]

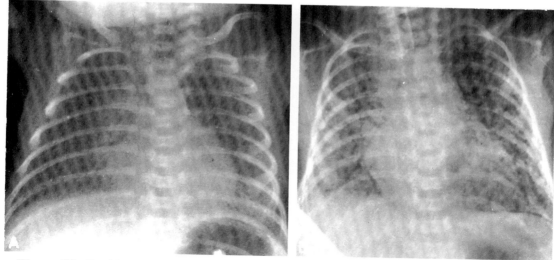

Figure 30–5. Hyaline membrane disease (RDS). **(A)** Premature infant at 2 days of age shows a rather diffuse granular reticular density, with streaks of air representing an air-bronchogram pattern noted particularly well at the bases. **(B)** Three days later, an endotracheal tube is in place. There is now a considerable amount of alveolar density interspersed with streaks of gas representing interstitial emphysema, which is also noted along the right cardiac margin and at the left base.

Pulmonary interstitial emphysema may appear, usually related to positive-pressure assisted ventilation. The air trapped in the interstitium does not change much on expiration. There are elongated (1 to 3 cm) lucent areas that tend to radiate outward from the hilum. They are often somewhat tortuous. Mediastinal emphysema and/or pneumothorax may also be present.

At times the changes of hyaline membrane disease may be localized to the lower lobes, and at other times the clearing occurs first in the upper lobes when there is improvement. This suggests that upper lobes mature earlier than the lower lobes, a pattern similar to that in lambs and rabbits. Sometimes the distribution of the disease may be very uneven and atypical.[2]

In other neonatal respiratory distress syndromes caused by pulmonary disease, usually pulmonary opacities are evident. However, these tend to be coarse and irregular, often bilateral but not necessarily symmetric. This pattern is usually associated with bronchopneumonia or aspiration pneumonitis.

TRANSIENT RESPIRATORY DISTRESS (WET-LUNG DISEASE) OF THE NEWBORN (TRDN)

The roentgen findings in another neonatal distress syndrome, transient respiratory distress of the newborn (TRDN), have been described by Swischuk.[83] This syndrome occurs in infants delivered of diabetic mothers, in premature infants, and in infants delivered by breech extraction or by cesarean section. The distress (tachypnea) is noted early in the neonatal period and clears in 1 to 4 days. The cause appears to be incomplete or delayed clearing of alveolar fluid after birth. As a result the lungs are "wet." This is manifested radiographically by findings resembling those of alveolar edema with an air-bronchogram pattern, or, in less severe cases, interstitial edema, often with what appear to be Kerley's A lines and small amounts of pleural fluid. Minimal to moderate overaeration is common. At times, the roentgen findings may be similar to those of hyaline membrane disease, but in wet-lung disease there is progressive and rapid improvement (Fig. 30-6).[83, 90]

Total opacity of the right lung or an opaque to semiopaque right upper lobe has been reported in eight neonates with very little respiratory distress. The opacity clears in 24 to 48 hours. Whether or not it is related to TRDN is not known, and the cause is not clear.

BRONCHOPULMONARY DYSPLASIA

Prolonged oxygen therapy can cause pulmonary damage, particularly in infants with hyaline membrane disease, causing recognizable pathologic and radiologic

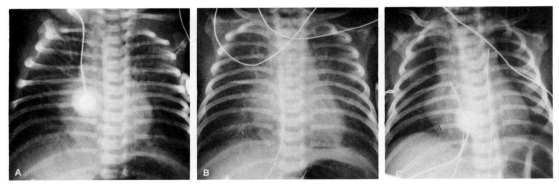

Figure 30–6.   Newborn infant with transient respiratory distress (wet lung). **(A)** Shortly after birth, some central alveolar density with some linear interstitial density extending well into the lung fields is manifest. **(B)** Ninety minutes later, some improvement has taken place peripherally. **(C)** Five hours later, the lungs are clear. Such rapid improvement is characteristic of this condition.

changes. This is often accompanied by damage caused by positive-pressure breathing apparatus (barotrauma). Northway and associates describe four stages in which the findings are somewhat characteristic.[66] In stage 1, occurring in the first 2 or 3 days, the findings are those of severe respiratory distress syndrome. In stage 2, occurring in 4 to 10 days, opacification of lungs is marked, with a clearly defined air-bronchogram pattern. Stage 3, occurring between 10 and 20 days, is a period of transition to chronic disease. The roentgen pattern is one of a spongy appearance produced by a combination of atelectasis and emphysema; plus interstitial pulmonary emphysema with multiple small bullae or air cysts throughout the lungs. In stage 4, a stage of chronic disease, the bullae enlarge and they may become large enough to resemble pneumatoceles. This occurs in patients who survive more than a month. Histologic studies have corresponded well with Northway's staging of bronchopulmonary dysplasia, especially in the later (third and fourth) stages. Stages 1 and 2 are similar to those of respiratory distress syndrome and usually cannot be differentiated from it. The incidence of bronchopulmonary dysplasia is high (35% or more) when mechanical ventilation is required for long periods in neonates with respiratory distress syndrome. These patients develop evidence of pulmonary interstitial air—interstitial emphysema. The emphysema and cysts usually disappear spontaneously. Wood and co-workers studied the lungs of 22 infants soon after death and found that the air was in the lymphatics of the interlobular septa and visceral pleura in all, and in the interstitial space in six.[95] It is likely, therefore, that much of the "interstitial" air observed in bronchopulmonary dysplasia is in the lymphatics rather than in the interstitium.

Although survivors seem to have increased susceptibility to respiratory infections and some have alterations in pulmonary function, little anatomic change is observed. Several studies of radiographic and morphologic changes in survivors of bronchopulmonary dysplasia show very little change.[27, 38] Linear shadows, predominantly basal, owing to fibrosis and deep pleural fissuring and slight thickening of interstitial tissues were observed radiographically, along with slight decrease in the AP diameter of the thorax. In one study, autopsy cases showed: (1) variably sized regions of interstitial fibrosis with distortion of air spaces in more than 50% of cases, and (2) normal conducting bronchi, uniform distal air space enlargement indicating failure of alveolar development and little interstitial fibrosis.[27]

In adults, prolonged exposure to oxygen presumably without evidence of barotrauma may also cause pulmonary disease. There is an exudative reaction that may progress to interstitial fibrosis. Initial roentgen changes consist of a diffuse alveolar opacity caused by edema. Later, linear and nodular opacities appear, commonly in the bases; these represent a proliferative phase. These changes occur in the adult respiratory distress syndrome, in which other pulmonary conditions may contribute to the roentgen findings.

ADULT RESPIRATORY DISTRESS SYNDROME (ARDS)

The term "adult respiratory distress syndrome" is used widely to describe a syndrome resulting from a number of conditions in which there is pulmonary injury leading to severe-permeability (non-cardiogenic) pulmonary edema. Mortality is 60% or more, usually as a result of pulmonary sepsis but also caused by respiratory failure and by the underlying disease or injury. The clinical signs include marked dyspnea, increased respiratory effort, hypoxemia which is often severe, and cyanosis.[3, 45, 69] The basic process is probably a combination of diffuse alveolar epithelial and capillary endothelial injury in the pulmonary microvasculature causing increased permeability and pulmonary edema with a high protein content. Neutrophils also play a role in many patients. Circulating neutrophils respond to certain toxic substances, which cause the neutrophils to migrate to extravascular structures where they are unable to function normally. This results in tissue injury in the lung. Neutrophils are not a factor in all patients, however. A number of other factors have been implicated, including alterations in the clotting system, unstable oxygen molecules, and a variety of enzymes. Alterations in production of surfactant are probably secondary in adults.

A variety of causes have been implicated including hemorrhagic or septic shock; massive trauma, either pulmonary or general; severe viral pneumonia; a number of other organisms causing extensive pneumonia; aspiration of gastric contents; drug overdose; cardiopulmonary bypass; inhalation of corrosive chemicals; smoke inhalation; hypoxemia associated with near drowning; thoracic irradiation[17]; and hemorrhagic pancreatitis. Hypovolemic shock appears to develop in most of the patients, but disseminated intravascular coagulation involving the pulmonary microcirculation is a major pathogenic factor in most, if not all, patients. Other factors include surfactant deficit and left ventricular failure; in some instances, oxygen toxicity and prolonged respiratory care may add to the injury. The disease progresses through three pathophysiologic phases:

1. Increased extravascular protein-rich fluid with an increase in lymph flow caused by damage to the alveolar endothelium and epithelium
2. An intermediate phase with hypoxemia, severe damage to alveolar epithelial cells, a marked amount of high-protein alveolar edema, hyaline membrane formation, and an infiltrate of mixed cells, predominantly neutrophils
3. A proliferative phase with deposition of connective tissue and formation of honeycomb-like cysts

There is a difference of opinion regarding the use of the term adult respiratory distress syndrome; many would apply the etiologic terms "acute pulmonary insufficiency associated with shock, drug overdose, near-drowning," and so forth. Other synonyms include shock lung, posttraumatic pulmonary insufficiency, hemorrhagic lung syndrome, stiff lung syndrome, solid lung syndrome, adult hyaline membrane disease, respirator lung, congestive atelectasis, progressive pulmonary consolidation, pump lung, posttransfusion lung, transplant lung, postperfusion lung, and respiratory insufficiency associated with oxygen toxicity, fat embolism, and disseminated intravascular coagulation. None of these terms describe the respiratory distress syndrome seen in premature infants.

Roentgenographic findings are variable, but, in most instances, no abnormalities are noted in the first 12 hours following initiation of the syndrome. The earliest changes are those of interstitial edema, which is not often observed. This may be associated with or followed by patchy alveolar edema causing local, ill-defined, acinar-type opacities. After 24 hours or so, this may progress to more typical and massive consolidation representing extensive alveolar edema with very dense lungs and clearly defined air bronchograms. The extent of edema is usually greater than that in cardiac failure. Usually the heart is not enlarged, and there is no pleural effusion. Complications such as gram-negative pneumonias may result in multiple cavitations. The massive edema regresses in 4 to 7 days, so there appears to be radiographic improvement. Proliferative changes in the lung, which may appear as early as 2 days after the onset, but usually take 5 to 7 days, are manifested as an increase in interstitial markings observed as the acute edema regresses. The pulmonary opacities are not as variable or rapidly reversible as in patients with pulmonary edema who do not have respiratory insufficiency. Finally, after a week or so there is a mixed pattern of interstitial and alveolar densities—usually bilateral but not always symmetric. Evidence of barotrauma is common in these patients when high pressures are used in administration of oxygen. Often a cystlike or bubbly pattern is observed in some areas or throughout the lung. This usually represents pulmonary interstitial emphysema resulting from barotrauma and is probably a part of bronchopulmonary dysplasia in those who have been treated for long periods with high pressures of positive end expiratory pressure (PEEP) and high concentrations of oxygen. More subtle findings include parenchymal stippling, which represents small, round opacities surrounded by lucent areas, which probably represent small vessels surrounded by air. Areas of lucent mottling also represent interstitial air. Subpleural cysts, parenchymal cysts, or bullae also indicate air leak into the pulmonary interstitium. Early recognition is important, since complications such as pneumothorax, secondary infection, and pulmonary fibrosis may be life-threatening.[85] If the patient recovers, the changes may clear completely.

There are no radiographic signs of elevation of pulmonary venous pressure in this syndrome in that there is no redistribution of blood flow. Left ventricular failure in these patients is nearly impossible to diagnose radiographically, so the Swan-Ganz catheter is used. This provides the most dependable method now available for detecting left ventricular failure. Duration of the clinical and roentgenographic findings is quite variable. In the advanced stage when respiratory insufficiency is refractory, there is usually a mixed pulmonary lesion consisting of alveolar and interstitial opacities that are bilateral, may not be symmetric, and may be associated with cavitation if the condition is complicated by anaerobic infection. The use of PEEP may be crucial in patient management in some instances. As indicated, it may cause barotrauma, resulting in interstitial emphysema, mediastinal emphysema, subpleural air cysts, pneumothorax, or tension pneumothorax. Because these patients are hypoxemic, tension pneumothorax is a grave complication. Its presence must be suspected in those patients whose dyspnea and hypoxemia increase suddenly.

HAMMAN-RICH SYNDROME

This condition, originally described by Hamman and Rich,[39] is characterized by an insidious onset of general malaise, fever, occasional dry cough, chest pain, and dyspnea, which soon becomes severe. The original patients died within 1 to 6 months of pulmonary insufficiency. Respiratory insufficiency and right-sided heart failure occur and recurrent infections are common in the late stage of the disease. Microscopic examination shows marked fibroblastic proliferation in the alveolar walls, often associated with edema and an infiltration of lymphocytes and plasma cells. The presence of eosinophils has been noted by several investigators. Later the fibroblastic proliferation results in extensive thickening of alveolar walls and interstitial tissues, causing severe respiratory dysfunction leading to death. Review of the original case material indicates that the disease is actually acute interstitial pneumonia, similar to the adult respiratory distress syndrome, but the cause is usually not apparent.[6, 68] The organized phase of diffuse alveolar damage is fibrosis. It does not represent the common chronic interstitial pneumonias or the usual chronic interstitial pulmonary fibrosis. Therefore, the term Hamman-Rich syndrome should probably be abandoned or used only to signify the acute, diffuse alveolar fibrosing disease that leads to death in less than a year. It is not a chronic interstitial pulmonary disease.

ROENTGEN FINDINGS

Early in the disease there is a slight increase in pulmonary interstitial markings and a slight decrease in diaphragmatic motion that can be noted fluoroscopically or on roentgenograms obtained in inspiration and expiration. As the fibrosis progresses, the interstitial markings become more prominent, resulting in thick linear shadows extending outward from the hila and a reticular pattern of increased density in the peripheral lung fields. The change is not necessarily symmetric but is usually bilateral. In far-advanced disease there is extensive strandlike thickening with considerable lucency surrounded by the thick strands resembling a coarse honeycomb or cystic pattern. The volume of the lung decreases progressively (see Fig. 30-18). Because the roentgen findings are not characteristic, the diagnosis must be based on clinical manifestations, with the history of rapidly progressing dyspnea with failure to find any definite cause. Lung biopsy is necessary to make the diagnosis.

PNEUMOTHORAX

The presence of air or gas in the pleural cavity is termed *pneumothorax*. Under normal conditions the pressure in the pleural space is less than atmospheric pressure. When there is communication with the atmosphere, either through a defect in the parietal pleura and chest wall, mediastinal pleura in patients with pneumomediastinum, or through a defect in the visceral pleura, air enters the pleural space. The amount of air that enters depends on a variety of factors, including the elasticity of the lung, the presence or absence of pleural adhesions, and the type of defect in the pleura. There are a number of conditions in which pneumothorax is sometimes observed. In the respiratory distress syndrome, pneumothorax may develop in addition to pneumomediastinum, particularly when positive-pressure respiratory assistance is used. It also occurs in patients with chronic obstructive pulmonary disease and with pulmonary histiocytosis X. It has been reported in women, related to the onset of menses; usually the right hemithorax is involved. Trauma is also a common cause. Bullous emphysema, severe asthma, sarcoidosis, and a number of pulmonary infections may also cause pneumothorax. Many cases are iatrogenic, caused by transthoracic needle biopsy, thoracentesis, misplaced catheters, thoracic surgery, and so forth.

SPONTANEOUS PNEUMOTHORAX

The term *spontaneous pneumothorax* is usually reserved to designate pneumothorax that occurs without apparent cause in healthy individuals, particularly in young males. The air enters the pleural cavity through an opening in the visceral pleura. In most instances the cause is obscure and the site of the defect not accurately localized. In some of these, pulmonary interstitial emphysema is probably the cause. In others, sub-pleural blebs are visible and it is presumed that rupture of one of these may introduce the pneumothorax. Once the pneumothorax is established (Fig. 30-7), the course depends on the defect in the pleura. If the defect closes promptly, the air in the pleural space is absorbed in a few days and the pneumothorax disappears. If the defect remains open in a manner that allows air to enter the pleural space, the size of the pneumothorax increases and some type of tube drainage is usually instituted.

TENSION PNEUMOTHORAX

Occasionally there is a check-valve or one-way-valve type of defect through which air can enter the pleural space but cannot leave it. This results in a much more serious condition, tension pneumothorax. When this occurs there is rapid or slow accumulation of air in the pleural space, resulting in collapse of the lung provided there are no adhesions to hold it out. This is followed by a shift of mediastinal structures away from the side of the pneumothorax as well as an increase in size of the involved hemithorax and depression of the hemidiaphragm on the side of the lesion (Fig. 30-8). This condition is particularly hazardous in the newborn and, if not treated promptly, can cause death.

TRAUMATIC PNEUMOTHORAX

Air may enter the pleural space through the parietal pleura as the result of penetrating wounds of the thorax. It may also be secondary to renal surgery, sympathectomy, and other upper abdominal surgical procedures, or it may be introduced through a needle at the time of thoracentesis or biopsy. Trauma to the lungs or bronchi may also result in defects in the visceral pleura, causing pneumothorax. When associated with rib fractures it is often caused by a rent in the pleura produced by sharp bony spicules. There is injury to the visceral and parietal pleurae in these instances, but the air usually enters through the defect in the visceral pleura. The pneumothorax commonly seen in the newborn is very likely traumatic in origin in most instances. Pneumothorax of this type may also follow bronchoscopy. In addition to the findings of pneumothorax, the cause may be apparent on the chest roentgenogram.

PNEUMOTHORAX SECONDARY TO BRONCHOPLEURAL FISTULA

Regardless of the cause, bronchopleural fistula results in pneumothorax that usually persists for a long time. Tuberculosis is a common cause and the fistula can be produced by rupture of a subpleural lesion into the pleural space or by rupture of a tuberculous empyema

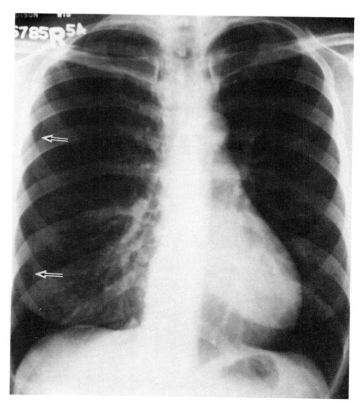

Figure 30–7. Spontaneous pneumothorax. Arrows indicate the visceral pleural line of the upper and lower lobes.

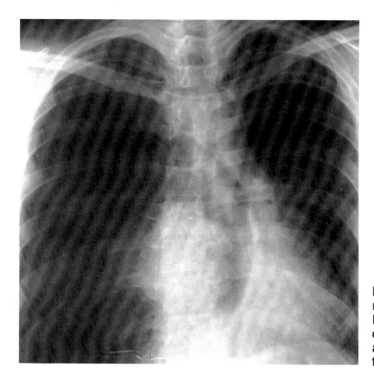

Figure 30–8. Tension pneumothorax. The right lung is collapsed and displaced to the left. Part of it is herniated across the midline. Note complete absence of lung markings on the right and the considerable shift of mediastinal structures to the left.

through the pleura into the lung with subsequent formation of a fistula. Other inflammatory diseases of the lung, both acute and chronic, may also cause bronchopleural fistula with resultant pneumothorax. Other infectious diseases of the pleura producing empyema may also result in bronchopleural fistula with rupture of the empyema through the visceral pleura leading to bronchial communication. CT is sometimes helpful in detecting the site of the fistula.

RADIOGRAPHIC CONSIDERATIONS

The presence of a large pneumothorax is identified readily on chest radiographic examination and in many instances, when it is secondary to disease or trauma, the cause can be established. The air in the pleural space is more radiolucent than the lung adjacent to it, particularly if the lung is decreased in volume, compressed, or is involved by disease that increases its density. When pleural adhesions are present, small amounts of loculated pneumothorax may be very difficult to see unless lateral or oblique projections are obtained. Such spaces often contain a small amount of fluid, and when a horizontal exam is used for radiography the presence of a horizontal fluid level indicates that gas as well as fluid is present. When the amount of pneumothorax is very small and is apical in position, its presence is indicated by a thin, smooth, curved, linear

opacity representing the visceral pleura. Above this line no pulmonary markings are visible. Occasionally the pneumothorax is so small that its presence at the apex can only be suspected on the usual roentgenogram obtained with the patient in deep inspiration. A roentgenogram obtained during maximum expiration will aid in confirming the diagnosis, because the lung then is relatively more dense than the pneumothorax. The lung decreases in volume during expiration but the pneumothorax space does not change. There is, therefore, relatively more pneumothorax in relation to lung in expiration than in inspiration and there is presumably a smaller visceral pleural surface in contact with the pneumothorax, which is easier to define. The lateral decubitus position (involved side up) with the film exposed when the patient is in expiration may be very helpful; a horizontal beam is used and the visceral pleura may be more clearly defined than at the apex where bone density (of ribs and clavicle) may make identification of pleura very difficult.[55]

When pneumothorax occurs in patients with lobar atelectasis, air collects in the pleural space adjacent to the collapsed lung. Therefore, abnormal distribution of air in these patients suggests lobar collapse. In *tension pneumothorax* the shift of mediastinal structures, compression of the lung, and depression of the diaphragm are readily seen. When fluid is present in addition to air or gas, horizontal-beam films showing an air–fluid level are diagnostic. At times, the intrapleural air is trapped in unusual positions by adhesions. Occasionally, pneumothorax may be seen in a subpulmonary position, particularly in patients with COPD and a decrease of lung compliance. It may also be observed along the medial surface of the lung in newborn infants who are often examined in the supine position.[62] In this situation, it must be differentiated from pneumomediastinum. When the anterior junction line is visible in neonates, it indicates bilateral pneumothorax, since this line is ordinarily not visible in these patients.[56] In young infants, pneumothorax may be best evaluated with anteroposterior and lateral films exposed at about the same time.

In critically ill adults who are examined in the supine or supine semirecumbent position, air in the pleural space may appear anteromedially along the mediastinum, in a subpulmonic position, in an apicolateral position or posteromedially in the paraspinal area.[84] Air may be observed in the interlobar fissures, particularly the minor fissure in right-sided pneumothorax.[81] The deep sulcus sign was described by Gordon in supine films of patients with pneumothorax.[36] This consists of relative radiolucency of the depth of the lateral costophrenic sulcus, indicating air in this area. Diagnosis may not be possible on plain films. Therefore, CT can be used if information regarding presence or absence of pneumothorax is vital, since pneumothorax is relatively easy to detect on axial CT.

Pneumothorax may be loculated between the lung and mediastinum, posterior to the inferior pulmonary ligament. This probably accounts for the air in what has been described as a pulmonary ligament pneumatocele.[33] Most authors believe that although air may dissect from the mediastinum into the pulmonary ligament in neonates, this rarely, if ever, occurs in adults. CT is useful in determining the location of air in these patients. On the PA view, the air is usually on the left side inferomedially, and is bounded anteriorly by the pulmonary ligament as seen on the lateral projection.

In summary, the diagnosis of pneumothorax may be difficult to make on radiographic examination of the chest, particularly in supine films. The lateral projection may serve to confirm the presence of pneumothorax when the frontal projection is equivocal. When the pneumothorax is small, a film in expiration is often of value; and, occasionally, when peripheral loculated pneumothorax is present, lateral and oblique views are needed for distinct visualization. A round opacity is occasionally observed, at or below the hilum in patients with a large pneumothorax. This has been shown to represent torsion in a partially atelectatic upper lobe. This may also happen to the middle lobe, but the pulmonary ligament prevents lower-lobe torsion.[9] In addition to the value of radiographs in making the diagnosis, progress films are used to follow its course.

DIFFERENTIAL DIAGNOSIS

Occasionally a peripheral emphysematous bleb or bulla may stimulate a localized pneumothorax, but in most instances the round or geometric form of its inner wall indicates the nature of the lesion and differentiates it from pneumothorax. When the diagnosis is particularly difficult, CT can usually but not always solve the problem. Occasionally these emphysematous bullae become very large (tension bullae) and may displace the lung and mediastinum in a manner simulating displacement by tension pneumothorax. In these instances, differentiation cannot be made with certainty on plain film radiographic examination alone. CT is very helpful in such situations. In patients with far-advanced tuberculosis, large peripheral cavitation, often involving the greater part of an upper lobe (usually the left), may be difficult to distinguish from pneumothorax secondary to bronchopleural fistula. If serial roentgenograms are available, the progress of the lesion indicates its nature in most instances, but there are some patients in whom the nature of the lesion remains uncertain, and even at autopsy or at surgery the disease may be so extensive that the visceral pleura cannot be identified. The same type of lesion may follow other pulmonary infections but is less common.

ALTERED IMMUNITY AND THE LUNG

The immune system is composed of lymphocytes: the B (bursa) and T (thymic-derived) cells. The B-cells secrete immunoglobulins and are responsible for humoral immunity. The immunoglobulins are: IgG, IgA, IgM, IgE, and IgD. The T-lymphocyte or T-cell is responsible for cellular immunity. The *immune responses* are classified into four types: *Type I*—IgE–dependent, in which the antibody is E. There is an immediate skin test; the clinical examples are extrinsic asthma and anaphylaxis. *Type II*—tissue-specific antibody. Antibodies are G and M. A clinical example is Goodpasture's syndrome. *Type III*—immune complexes. Antibodies are G and M. Clinical examples are extrinsic alveolitis produced by organic and inorganic dust and intrinsic alveolitis including collagen–vascular diseases and fibrosing alveolitis. The first three are examples of humoral immune responses. *Type IV*—cell-mediated (delayed hypersensitivity). Clinical examples are intracellular infections, graft rejection, and cancer suppression.[74] Some of the conditions mentioned here are described in greater detail in the sections that follow.

BRONCHIAL ASTHMA

Bronchial asthma is very common, occurs at all ages, and is characterized by wheezing, prolongation of the expiratory phase of respiration, dyspnea, and cough.[5] It tends to appear in recurrent attacks. Early in the course of the disease there are no radiographic findings in the chest between the acute episodes. During an acute asthmatic attack there is increased lucency of the lungs because of acute overdistention. Small areas of focal atelectasis often cause scattered patchy opacities parallel to the bronchovascular markings. They are often widespread throughout both lungs. The interstitial markings may also be thickened, particularly in the parahilar and central pulmonary zones. There is also depression of the diaphragm and decreased diaphragmatic motion that can be detected on fluoroscopic examination. During an acute asthma attack, pneumomediastinum or pneumothorax may occur. This is most commonly observed in children and young adults. In patients with severe and constant asthma, some roentgen changes may become permanent. These patients are subject to recurrent pulmonary infections leading to pulmonary fibrosis associated with emphysema. The roentgen findings then consist of prominence of interstitial markings in a chest that is otherwise more radiolucent than normal. The anteroposterior diameter of the chest is increased, the diaphragm is low and flat, and the ribs are often more horizontal than normal (Fig. 30-9). The emphysema may become severe, leading to formation of large emphysematous bullae peripherally. Parallel lines and tubular shadows representing thickened bronchial walls have been observed in patients with asthma, probably caused by bronchial infection. Mucous plug or impaction may also occur in asthma patients often associated with allergic aspergillosis (Fig. 30-10). The bronchial obstruction produced by the impaction may result in atelectasis, an accumulation of secretions in the obstructed segment, and infection. Eventually, bronchiectasis may result; this may produce plain-film findings similar to those of bronchiectasis in nonasthmatic patients. There appears to be some predilection for the upper lobes. Roentgen findings depend on the nature of the associated pulmonary disease and, when segmental atelectasis or an apparent pneumonitis is found in an asthmatic, mucous plug or impaction should be suspected. Occasionally, during an acute asthma attack, the central pulmonary arteries enlarge as compared to baseline film, probably indicating temporary arterial hypertension. Cavitary pulmonary infarction has been reported as a complication in steroid-dependent asthma.[37]

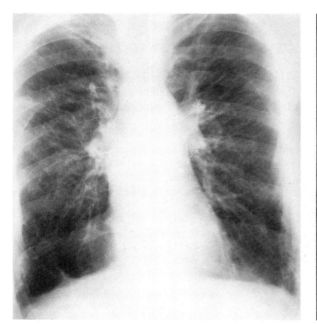
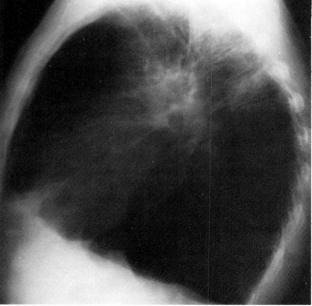

Figure 30–9. Pulmonary changes in a 44-year-old male with a long history of bronchial asthma. Note the lower, flat diaphragm, deep anteroposterior diameter of the chest, and an increase in interstitial markings throughout the lungs. The increase in central pulmonary arteries indicates arterial hypertension associated with COPD.

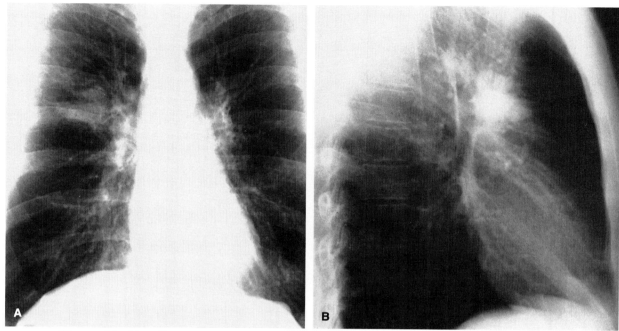

Figure 30–10. Severe asthma with bronchopulmonary aspergillosis and mucoceles. **(A)** Note fingerlike projections above and lateral to the right hilum, representing a mucous plug. The chest is overinflated and there is minimal bronchial wall thickening, probably secondary to chronic bronchial inflammation. **(B)** Lateral projection showing overinflation and large mucoceles overlying the anterior upper hilum.

IDIOPATHIC PULMONARY HEMOSIDEROSIS

Hemosiderosis is a term used to indicate the presence of macrophages filled with hemosiderin deposited in the alveoli and interstitial tissues of the lung. The etiology is unknown, but because some immunologic mechanism is a distinct possibility, the disease is discussed here. There is an injury at the level of the alveolocapillary membrane allowing the leakage of blood into the interstitium and ultimately into the alveolar space of the lung. This is manifested by recurrent episodes of acute illness in which dyspnea, cyanosis, and weakness along with cough, hemoptysis, and chest pain occur. The attack lasts a few days or weeks before subsiding. Recurrent episodes of bleeding ultimately produce marked roentgenographic changes. The prognosis is generally poor, although the disease may progress very slowly in some patients. It is somewhat more frequent in children than in adults. In children there is no sex predominance, but when it develops in adults, there is a preponderance of males of about 2 or 3 to 1.

The roentgen findings in the acute phase are those of alveolar hemorrhage which cause widespread, patchy alveolar opacities that clear gradually over a period of days. Residual deposition of hemosiderin in the interstitium produces thickening that appears roentgenographically as an increase in interstitial markings, producing a reticular or reticulonodular appearance (Fig. 30-11). The diagnosis is made by correlating the clinical history with the roentgenographic changes. MRI may be of value[76] in demonstrating the presence of widespread deposits of ferric iron throughout the lung. This may obviate biopsy or other invasive diagnostic methods, particularly in a critically ill patient. An association with celiac disease has been reported, but a pathogenetic link between the two diseases has not been established.[71] The disease must be differentiated from a number of other diseases that cause widespread interstitial change of this type and from other diseases that cause lung hemorrhage.

Pulmonary Changes Following Hemoptysis

When hemoptysis occurs and blood is aspirated, the roentgen findings vary with the amount and distribution of the blood. An opacity comparable to that of a

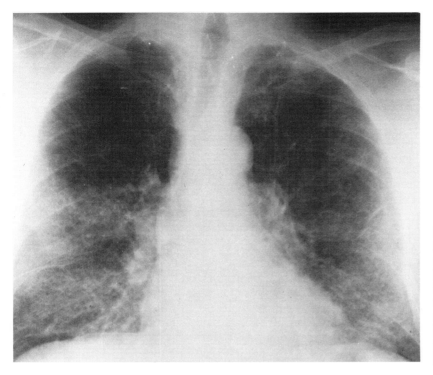

Figure 30–11. Idiopathic pulmonary hemisiderosis in a 42-year-old male with a long history of repeated hemoptysis. Note the extensive interstitial disease, which is somewhat linear in the upper lung and is reticulonodular in the central and basal lungs. There is pulmonary arterial hypertension manifested by large central pulmonary arteries.

patch of pneumonia of similar size is produced. It is usually hazy and poorly defined and may be local or widely scattered, depending on the site(s) and amount of the bleeding. The opacity usually clears within 2 or 3 days, which aids in differentiating hemorrhage from inflammatory disease. Evidence of the disease causing the hemoptysis may or may not be present. In patients with pulmonary contusion causing hemorrhage, a relatively clearly defined mass (hematoma) may appear which is unlike the more diffuse change usually observed in patients with hemoptysis. It changes more slowly.

GOODPASTURE'S SYNDROME

Goodpasture's syndrome is an autoimmune disease in which circulating antibodies have been demonstrated against the alveolar basement membrane and against glomerular basement membrane. In contrast to idiopathic pulmonary hemosiderosis, it occurs in young adults with a male predominance of 7 or 8 to 1.

The roentgen findings are related to extensive intra-alveolar hemorrhage, which produces diffuse opacity of an extent proportional to the amount of bleeding. It is usually bilateral and is often more prominent in the parahilar areas and in the central and lower lungs than in the apices. If the hemorrhage stops, the blood quickly clears leaving a reticular interstitial pattern

that increases with additional bleeding as the disease progresses. Often the clearing is partial, then another hemorrhage produces additional opacity. Septal lines are not ordinarily observed. Adenopathy sufficient to produce recognizable hilar enlargement may be present. Pleural effusion rarely occurs. The diagnosis should be suspected when a combination of hemoptysis and renal disease occurs in a young man. The prognosis in Goodpasture's syndrome is generally poor.

EOSINOPHILIC LUNG DISEASE— PULMONARY INFILTRATES WITH EOSINOPHILIA (PIE)

Eosinophilic disease includes a group of widely varied disorders. Several classifications have been used, none of them entirely satisfactory because of the number of etiologic factors, the diversity of clinical syndromes, and the fact that tissue eosinophilia occurs in some patients, blood eosinophilia in others and both tissue and blood eosinophilia in still others.[22] One of the classifications is termed the *PIE syndrome*, in which there are five major categories: (1) Löffler's syndrome; (2) chronic eosinophilic pneumonia or a chronic form of pulmonary opacities with eosinophilia; (3) chronic PIE with asthma; (4) tropical eosinophilia; (5) polyarteritis or vasculitis in association with pulmonary opacities,

LÖFFLER'S SYNDROME (TRANSIENT PULMONARY INFILTRATION WITH EOSINOPHILIA, ACUTE EOSINOPHILIC PNEUMONIA)

Löffler's syndrome consists of fleeting pulmonary opacities associated with eosinophilia. Usually the subjects are allergic individuals and it is believed to represent a pulmonary reaction to a variety of allergens. The symptoms are usually mild and consist of cough, malaise, low-grade fever, dyspnea with occasional wheezing, mild chest pain, and metallic taste in the mouth. It is associated with eosinophilia, that ranges from 10% to 70%, and usually also with leukocytosis. The amount of pathologic material available is small because this is a relatively benign condition, but the findings in patients who have died accidentally consist of eosinophilic pneumonia in which the involvement is interstitial as well as alveolar. There is also some associated pulmonary edema, probably secondary to increased permeability of capillaries. Acute eosinophilic pneumonia can cause non-infectious respiratory failure, however.

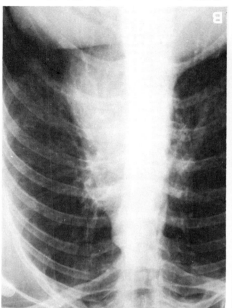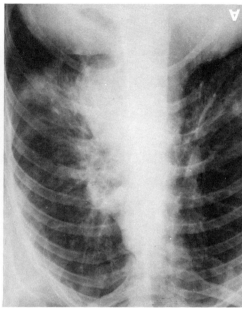

Figure 30–12. Eosinophilic pneumonia (Löffler's pneumonia). **(A)** Note the poorly defined, scattered disease in the left central and lower lung, with a lesser amount of disease superiorly. **(B)** Examination 15 days later shows the disease has cleared. The patient had eosinophilia, had eosinophils in the sputum, and was allergic.

which are the predominant part of the disease. There may be many manifestations in other organ systems in polyarteritis.[52]

Although the symptoms may be severe, the disease usually responds quickly to corticosteroids.[4]

Roentgen Findings

The disease produces poorly defined opacities that may be single or multiple, unilateral or bilateral. The volume of lung affected varies considerably and the individual areas of involvement are patchy in type and usually poorly outlined. They resemble pneumonia due to other causes but are unique in that the homogeneous densities are usually peripheral and rapid change is the rule. It is not unusual to observe clearing or partial clearing in one area and progression in another area of the same lung or of the opposite lung. In severe cases, pulmonary consolidation may be extensive and bilateral. Without therapy, change may be very slow. At times, the findings remain stable for several days. When such a changing opacity is observed and the patient is found to have eosinophilia, the diagnosis of Löffler's syndrome can be made (Fig. 30-12). A minor amount of pleural reaction resulting in small amounts of pleural effusion may occur, but the presence or absence of effusion is of no diagnostic significance.

Because similar eosinophilic pneumonias may be caused by a variety of parasitic infestations, by infections, and by drugs, the term "eosinophilic pneumonia" should be used to denote those of unknown cause. The others are better designated as eosinophilic pneumonia caused by a drug (name of drug), by infestation (name of parasite), and so on. The administration of cortisone usually produces rapid clearing of the pulmonary disease and a decrease in the circulating eosinophils.

CHRONIC EOSINOPHILIC PNEUMONIA

Chronic eosinophilic pneumonia is similar to Löffler's syndrome except that the symptoms are prolonged and the course more malignant. The disease usually occurs in women. Its onset may be sudden and its duration may extend from months to years. Episodes of weakness, weight loss, fever, cough, dyspnea, and hemoptysis may occur. Roentgen findings consists of a variety of patterns of opacity, some resembling confluent pneumonia, others consisting of coarse, strandlike densities which may be widespread. Although the disease tends to be peripheral in the upper lung zones, it may or may not appear so on plain films (Fig. 30-13).

CT is more likely to identify the peripheral location of the pulmonary consolidation when location is not certain in patients suspected of having chronic eosinophilic pneumonia. Mediastinal adenopathy has also been reported on CT studies.[38] Changes in the pulmonary disease are common, as in Löffler's syndrome. Eosinophils are found in the biopsy specimens which show interstitial pneumonia of varying degrees of severity, sometimes associated with fibrosis. There is also an elevated eosinophil count in the circulating blood. The lesions do not respond to antibiotics, but clear dramatically with steroid therapy.

COLLAGEN–VASCULAR (CONNECTIVE-TISSUE) DISEASES

The collagen–vascular diseases consist of a heterogeneous group of conditions in which involvement of connective tissue, particularly the intercellular amorphous ground substance, is the common morphologic feature. They appear to be related to hypersensitivity in some instances, but hypersensitivity is not the only

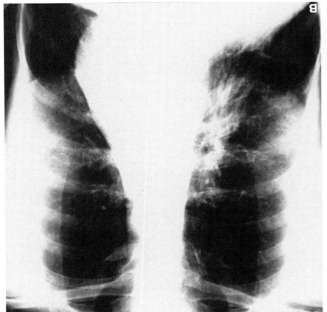
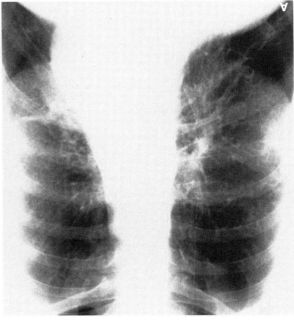

Figure 30-13. Chronic eosinophilic pneumonia in a patient with cough and slight fever. (**A**) Initial radiograph shows peripheral consolidation laterally on the right and some disease adjacent to the heart on the left. (**B**) Two months later the lateral disease adjacent to the heart has cleared, but the lateral alveolar disease persists on the right and some lateral disease has also developed on the left. The patient had eosinophilia and eosinophils in the sputum.

RHEUMATIC PNEUMONIA

Rheumatic fever is a disease in which cardiac lesions are common and may result in secondary pulmonary congestion and edema. The "pneumonia" seen in this disease is often caused by pulmonary edema and congestion and there is a considerable difference of opinion as to the incidence of actual pulmonary involvement in this disease. The roentgen findings of rheumatic pneumonia simulate those of pulmonary edema and congestion. They consist of hazy opacities, usually in the parahilar and midlung areas. They may be confluent or patchy and are often associated with basal changes indicating pulmonary congestion. At times there does appear to be involvement of lungs, so scattered opacities in the absence of cardiac failure in a patient with rheumatic fever is most likely indicative of rheumatic pneumonia.[28] Histopathologic study is often necessary to differentiate rheumatic pneumonia from pulmonary edema and congestion, but the clinical findings, along with radiographic findings, may permit the presumptive diagnosis.

SYSTEMIC LUPUS ERYTHEMATOSUS

Systemic lupus erythematosus is commonly found in young and middle-aged women, with a female-to-male ratio in the range of 10 to 1. It is a multisystem disease with autoantibodies and circulating immune complexes which cause inflammatory changes in connective tissue, vessels, and serosal surfaces. Pulmonary or pleural involvement of some type occurs in 50% to 70% of patients at some time in the course of the disease, and may be higher in patients with severe disease. In children, pulmonary hemorrhage is common and is associated with high mortality. The disease is chronic and often fatal, but may undergo repeated remissions and exacerbations. A number of drugs are capable of inducing systemic lupus erythematosus. Pleural and pulmonary involvement are not as common in drug-inducing systemic lupus erythematosus, and the symptoms are milder because there is no renal or CNS disease in drug-induced lupus. The disease subsides when the drugs are discontinued.

Roentgen Findings

Pleural effusion is the most common finding. The effusion is bilateral and usually small, but may be massive. Eventually, pleural fibrosis occurs following repeated episodes of effusion. The diaphragm may move poorly and basal lung volume may decrease. Pericardial effusion may also occur. The pulmonary parenchymal changes are varied as in polyarteritis and range from the soft, patchy opacity of pulmonary edema to strand-

cause since the tissue changes are known to be produced by a variety of dissimilar diseases. Polyarteritis (periarteritis) nodosa, rheumatic fever, rheumatoid arthritis, disseminated lupus erythematosus, Behçet's disease, mixed connective-tissue disease, and scleroderma (progressive systemic sclerosis) are all members of this group. Polymyositis, dermatomyositis, Sjögren's syndrome, and, possibly, ankylosing spondylitis are also included.[43] Wegener's granulomatosis, lymphomatoid granulomatosis, and immunoblastic lymphadenopathy are related and are included by many in this group of conditions. There is a considerable amount of overlap in the clinical findings, so lesions that are usually predominant in one entity may be seen in another. Individual cases have been reported in which four or five varieties of involvement have been present.

POLYARTERITIS (PERIARTERITIS) NODOSA

In polyarteritis nodosa there is a necrotizing vasculitis involving the medium-sized arteries; their small branches are also affected, so the lesions are often found throughout the body. Pulmonary involvement is rare but can cause a variety of radiographic changes. Massive pulmonary edema may occur in patients who are acutely ill, possibly related to renal disease in most, if not all of them. Other pulmonary changes consist of scattered patchy opacities, some of which are secondary to infarcts; these may excavate and cause small cavities. When present this cavitation is often multiple and it is characteristic that one cavity becomes smaller and closes while another is in the process of forming. Clearly defined or hazy nodules may appear. Some may resemble hematogenous metastases while others simulate inflammatory nodules and may raise the possibility of tuberculosis. At times the interstitial markings are increased. Basal congestion resulting in enlargement of vascular shadows and blurring of vessels is often noted and pleural effusion may occur. Enlargement of the cardiac silhouette is not uncommon. In some patients this is caused by pericardial effusion, while in others there is dilatation of the heart. These pulmonary and pleural changes may undergo rapid clearing or may progress rapidly. There is nothing characteristic about the roentgen findings, but, in a chronically ill patient with involvement of other systems, these pulmonary, pleural, and pericardial findings are suggestive of this disease. The pulmonary roentgen changes usually respond rapidly and clear following institution of steroid therapy.

As indicated, in classic polyarteritis nodosa, pulmonary involvement is rare. In the variants, systemic necrotizing vasculitis, allergic angiitis, and granulomatosis, pulmonary involvement is much more common.

like accentuation of bronchovascular markings, indicating diffuse interstitial disease, which is uncommon. Occasionally the lesions assume a nodular appearance and rarely may cavitate. Pulmonary opacities are usually transitory. The pulmonary alterations, including atelectasis, tend to be basal in position (Fig. 30-14). In addition to pericardial effusion, pancarditis may cause enlargement of the cardiac silhouette. When the pulmonary disease becomes chronic, resulting in basal fibrosis, there is often elevation of the diaphragm and its motion is restricted. The combination of bilateral pleural effusion, pericardial effusion causing enlargement of the cardiac silhouette, and a changing bilateral pulmonary disease suggests systemic lupus erythematosus. Pulmonary changes are less frequent than pleural and cardiac involvement, but may be bizarre, with cavitation in nodules, formation of pneumatoceles, and rapid alteration. Subpleural opacities are common; they are probably infarcts. Pulmonary infection may be superimposed on the lung changes produced by lupus; radiographic differentiation may be very difficult.

PROGRESSIVE SYSTEMIC SCLEROSIS (SCLERODERMA)

Progressive systemic sclerosis is characterized by atrophy and sclerosis of many organ systems including the skin, musculoskeletal system, and heart as well as the lungs. Raynaud's phenomenon with trophic changes in the fingers occurs in 80% to 90% of patients and may antedate other signs of the disease for years. Pulmonary manifestations occur in approximately 10% of the patients. As in the other collagen–vascular diseases, a variety of lesions may be observed, but the findings tend to be more stable in this disease than in the others. The basic lesion is interstitial fibrosis, which may take the form of accentuated interstitial markings, resulting in a fine reticular pattern that becomes more coarse and dense as the disease progresses, eventually producing a reticulonodular pattern. Although the lesion is usually basal with slow progression, rarely it ultimately may involve the entire lung. There is often some scattered nodulation in the parahilar areas and in the bases as well. Pleural effusion may occur late in the disease, but is not a prominent feature, and pleural fibrosis is also an unusual finding. In a few patients with long-standing disease, subpleural cysts have been described that are apparently caused by a loss of alveolar tissue. This results in small cystic spaces, surrounded by thick fibrous walls. CT is capable of detecting the linear basal opacities and small cystic spaces earlier in the disease than chest radiography (Fig. 30-15). Occasionally, pneumothorax is observed, presumably caused by rupture of one of the cysts into the pleural space. The

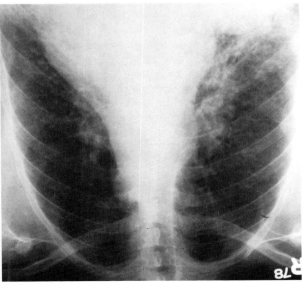

Figure 30-14. Disseminated lupus erythematosus. Note the basal interstitial disease with a small pleural effusion on the right. This patient was a male. This disease is more common in females, and pleural effusion is usually a more prominent feature of the disease in the thorax.

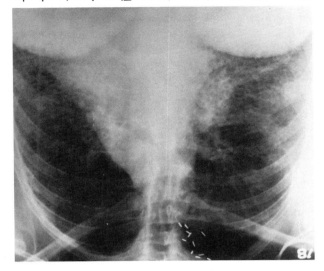

Figure 30-15. Scleroderma. There is extensive interstitial disease, chiefly in the bases and central lung. Apices are relatively spared. This interstitial disease is largely reticulonodular in type.

apices are spared in this manifestation of the disease (Fig. 30-16). Decreased volume of the lower lobes is characteristic of the disease. When the esophagus is involved, aspiration with the basal lung changes caused by aspiration pneumonia may occur in addition to the changes produced by pulmonary scleroderma. There is a fairly high incidence of bronchioloalveolar carcinoma in patients with long-term scleroderma.

MIXED CONNECTIVE-TISSUE DISEASE

Mixed connective-tissue disease is an overlap syndrome combining scleroderma, systemic lupus, polymyositis, dermatomyositis and a non-deforming arthritis to varying degrees. Pulmonary involvement is common, with a large percentage of patients having pulmonary dysfunction and abnormal chest roentgenograms. The chest findings include basal interstitial disease and pleural and pericardial fluid. Pulmonary hypertension is sometimes observed in conjunction with severe interstitial pulmonary involvement. Although peripheral adenopathy is common, mediastinal adenopathy is rare. Findings on the chest roentgenogram are similar to those of the overlap syndrome of scleroderma and systemic lupus, so the roentgen findings are not specifically diagnostic.

RHEUMATOID DISEASE OF THE LUNG

Rheumatoid arthritis is occasionally accompanied by pulmonary disease, which is a part of the generalized disease. Chest radiographic findings can be placed in the following categories: (1) Pleurisy with or without effusion is most frequent (50%); (2) necrobiotic nodules; (3) Caplan's syndrome; (4) Diffuse interstitial pattern; (5) Pulmonary arteritis and hypertension. The pulmonary lesions tend to occur in patients with high titers of rheumatoid factor and subcutaneous rheumatoid nodules.

As indicated, the most common finding in the thorax is pleuritis which is often accompanied by pleural effusion that is minimal to moderate in amount and usually bilateral. The fluid may remain for months or years with very little variation. Pleural thickening may eventually occur in these patients. The most common pulmonary change (30% to 40%) is that of an interstitial pneumonitis, which may produce a reticular pattern of interstitial opacity similar to that in idiopathic interstitial fibrosis. The distribution of the interstitial opacities may be diffuse, but at times tends to be parahilar and basal (Fig. 30-17). Sometimes, diffuse interstitial disease can be demonstrated on biopsy in patients with abnormal pulmonary function and normal chest roentgenograms. Occasionally the interstitial process may coalesce to form patchy areas resembling an alveolar

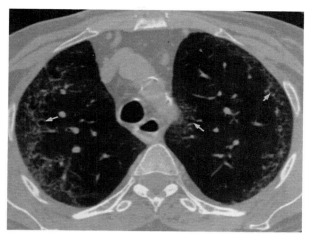

Figure 30–16. Scleroderma. There are bilateral peripheral sublobular areas of fibrosis. Multiple small cystic areas consistent with honeycombing are present peripherally and along the left mediastinal border (*arrows*). High-resolution CT scan, 1.5-mm collimation, bone algorithm. (Courtesy of Julie K. Mitby, MD)

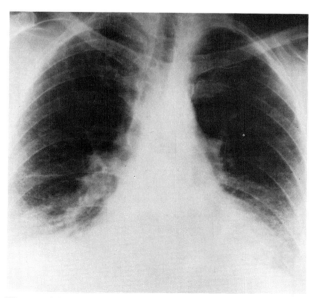

Figure 30–17. Rheumatoid disease of the lung. In this patient, there is basal interstitial disease that is quite similar to that often noted in scleroderma. Pleural effusion is a more common manifestation of rheumatoid disease of the lung.

type of pneumonia. Rarely, upper-lobe fibrosis and cystlike cavitation may be observed in rheumatoid arthritis. The incidence of diffuse interstitial disease is high in severe arthritis, which it may precede by years. It may rarely progress to end-stage pulmonary fibrosis, or "honeycomb lung." Males are affected twice as often as females.

Rheumatoid necrobiotic nodules of the lung are somewhat less common than the diffuse change. They may be multiple or solitary and vary from a few millimeters to several centimeters in size. It is common to observe them in a subpleural position, so occasionally pneumothorax may complicate this manifestation. Cavitation may occur, and is often associated with pleural effusion, bronchopleural fistula, or both. The nodules occur most frequently in males, often associated with subcutaneous rheumatoid nodules. They may disappear spontaneously, or may persist and sometimes grow over a period of years.

Caplan's syndrome has been described in patients with coal worker's pneumoconiosis who have rheumatoid arthritis. The patients have crops of pulmonary nodules varying from 0.5 to 5 cm in diameter, often peripheral on a background of pneumoconiosis and usually associated with exacerbation of rheumatoid arthritis and new subcutaneous rheumatoid nodules. At times, a single pulmonary nodule may be observed. This syndrome has been expanded to include asbestosis and silicosis acquired in industries other than coal mining. All pulmonary findings in rheumatoid arthritis are increased in cigarette smokers.

Pulmonary arteritis leading to pulmonary arterial hypertension may occur as the only pulmonary manifestation of rheumatoid arthritis. It causes enlargement of central pulmonary arteries and right ventricular enlargement. Other pulmonary manifestations of rheumatoid arthritis may be present, however.

ANKYLOSING SPONDYLITIS

Ankylosing spondylitis is accompanied by pulmonary disease in rare instances. The roentgenographic findings are those of bilateral upper-lobe fibrosis manifested by small nodular and linear shadows, which may coalesce to form linear and nodular opacities that may be very large. Obliterative bronchiolitis is present in some, if not all, of the patients with upper-lobe disease. In these patients, the coalescent lesions may be caused by obstructive pneumonitis. This may also occur in the rare similar upper-lobe disease observed in rheumatoid arthritis. Cavitation is frequent and in many instances is associated with aspergilloma. The disease may be stable for years or may progress steadily until extensive fibrosis results in upward retraction of one or both hila and upper-lobe bronchiectasis. In these instances, the roentgenographic appearance is quite similar to that of chronic pulmonary tuberculosis. In addition there may be apical pleural thickening that may become extensive. These changes usually occur in patients with long-standing and extensive involvement of the spine and often involvement of the large joints as well. There is restriction of the chest wall, caused by involvement of costovertebral joints which become ankylosed.

POLYMYOSITIS AND DERMATOMYOSITIS

Interstitial lung disease is known to be associated with polymyositis and dermatomyositis, but with less frequency than with other collagen–vascular diseases (5% or less). It may occur at any age, with a mean of 50 years. Female-to-male ratio is 2:1. The roentgen pattern is one of a diffuse reticulonodular interstitial process, usually localized to the lung bases. In the more acute disease, there may be a mixed alveolar and interstitial pattern. Pleural effusion seldom occurs. Rarely, fibrosing alveolitis may complicate dermatomyositis and may progress rapidly. It causes an interstitial pattern which also increases in severity rapidly as the disease progresses. If there is pharyngeal or esophageal involvement, aspiration pneumonia may develop. When the diaphragmatic muscle is involved, there is elevation of the diaphragm and loss of lung volume.

SJÖGREN'S SYNDROME

Sjögren's syndrome is a chronic inflammatory process characterized by atrophy of the lacrimal and salivary glands and leading to decreased production of tears and dryness of the mouth in the primary form. In the secondary form it is usually associated with rheumatoid arthritis (50%), but systemic lupus erythematosus, dermatomyositis, and scleroderma have also been reported to be associated with this syndrome. Pulmonary manifestations are frequent and consist of an interstitial process that is reticulonodular or nodular, similar to that found in rheumatoid arthritis (15%). Pleurisy and/ or pleural effusion may also occur. The pathologic change is that of a benign lymphocystic infiltration. There is an associated broad spectrum of lymphoproliferative disorders ranging from extraglandular lymphocytic infiltration or lymphoid interstitial pneumonitis to pseudolymphoma, which may progress to malignant neoplasm such as lymphoma and Hodgkin's disease in patients with Sjögren's syndrome.

BEHÇET'S SYNDROME

Behçet's syndrome is a vasculitis resulting in aphthous ulceration of oral and genital mucosa and relapsing iritis. It occurs in young adults, usually in the third decade of life. The incidence is greater in males than

females. Vascular involvement manifested by migratory thrombophlebitis may result in obstruction of the superior or inferior vena cava. Pulmonary involvement is rare, with vasculitis and thrombosis involving the pulmonary arteries appearing along with exacerbations of the disease elsewhere. The pulmonary radiographic findings include fleeting bilateral alveolar opacities produced by hemoptysis, which is likely a result of vasculitis. There may be round opacities, some of which represent aneurysms of lobular arteries; if they rupture, massive hemoptysis may occur. Central nervous system involvement appears to be the major cause of the high mortality (40%) observed in this disease, but massive exsanguinating hemoptysis may result from pulmonary involvement as indicated.

IMMUNOBLASTIC LYMPHADENOPATHY (ANGIOIMMUNOBLASTIC LYMPHADENOPATHY)

Immunoblastic lymphadenopathy is characterized by an acute or subacute onset of fever, generalized lymphadenopathy, and hepatosplenomegaly. In about one third of patients, a history of drug ingestion is obtained and a skin rash occurs at the onset of the disease. Histologically, this condition resembles Hodgkin's disease with an infiltration of histiocytes, plasma cells, eosinophils, and immunoblasts that replace lymphocytes and efface lymph-node architecture. There is also hyperproliferation of postcapillary venules and amorphous interstitial deposits consisting of cellular debris. In some patients the disease may evolve into a lymphoma. Although the cause is not certain, an abnormal immune state is likely, so this condition is included in this section. Radiographic findings consist of pulmonary opacities, evidence of hilar and mediastinal adenopathy in 50%, and bilateral pleural effusion. The pulmonary opacities are varied and range from the signs of diffuse interstitial linear or reticulonodular disease, usually basal, to an alveolar pattern which may resemble that secondary to pulmonary edema. It may be associated with an interstitial pattern in other parts of the lung. Superimposed infection may add to the pulmonary opacity and result in asymmetry. The response to steroids is dramatic in some of these patients.[97]

PULMONARY ANGIITIS AND GRANULOMATOSIS

Most of the diseases discussed in this section have a histopathologic similarity in that pulmonary vasculitis (angiitis) and granulomatosis, often with necrosis, are present in varying degrees. However, there are significant clinical differences, and there is some disagreement as to how they should be classified. The comprehensive review is given by Churg.[21] He includes a larger variety of condi-

tions, including bronchocentric granulomatosis, angiitis associated with various bacterial and mycotic infections, as well as rheumatoid nodules in this category. Weisbrod[88] has also reviewed these diseases, dividing them into two categories: *angiocentric*, which includes Wegener's granulomatosis, allergic angiitis, allergic granulomatosis (Churg-Strauss syndrome), lymphomatoid granulomatosis, and necrotizing sarcoid granulomatosis; and *bronchocentric*, which consists of bronchocentric granulomatosis, described in Chapter 27.

Wegener's Granulomatosis

Midline lethal granuloma is a destructive process of unknown cause, probably a hyperimmune reaction which some investigators believe is related to the collagen–vascular diseases. It is often a fatal condition in which there is extensive destruction of the bony structures of the nose and paranasal sinuses. When this condition is associated with necrotizing granulomatous vasculitis of the lungs and necrotizing glomerulonephritis, which may be focal or general, the syndrome is known as Wegener's syndrome or necrotizing granulomatosis. The three main pathologic features are: (1) necrotizing granulomatous lesions of the upper respiratory tract, (2) necrotizing angiitis of arteries and veins, and (3) glomerulitis. When the kidneys are not involved and the disease is confined to the respiratory system, the term "limited Wegener's" is used. The roentgen changes in the sinuses are those of soft-tissue opacity plus destruction of bone that cannot be differentiated from the destruction produced by malignant neoplasm. The granulomatous lesion of the lung, which is characteristic of the disease, is a nodule which may be solitary or multiple. Its size varies from 1 to 8 cm in diameter. The round nodules may cavitate (60% to 70% do). The cavity is usually small in relation to the size of the nodule, with an irregular inner wall, but the nodule may excavate completely leaving a thin wall, and then eventually may disappear. The outer margins of the nodules may be sharply defined or may be indistinct and have a shaggy appearance. When multiple, the nodules tend to be few in number, and may resemble pulmonary metastases (Fig. 30-18). Occasionally a solitary mass resembling a primary lung tumor may occur. Other findings include areas of poorly defined consolidation resembling pneumonia. When the vasculitis extensively involves alveolar capillaries, massive pulmonary hemorrhage may occur. This is a very rare complication in this disease. As in the other granulomatous diseases with angiitis there is nothing specific about the roentgen pulmonary changes. Pleural effusion rarely occurs late in the disease. On occasion, an endobronchial mass may cause atelectasis of a lobe or lung. This may be associated with pleural disease accompanied by effusion or pleural thickening. The effu-

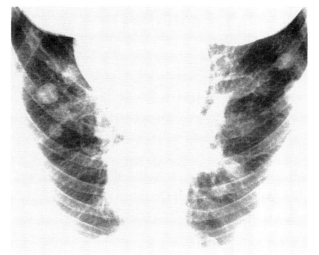

Figure 30-18. Wegener's granulomatosis in a middle-aged male with recent onset of arthralgia and mild cough. Note bilateral nodules, many of which are clearly defined and none of which are cavitary.

sion may be massive. Pneumothorax is a relatively rare complication.

Lymphomatoid Granulomatosis

Lymphomatoid granulomatosis is a type of granulomatous vasculitis that resembles malignant lymphoma histologically because of prominent lymphoreticular proliferation.[41] A necrotizing vasculitis differentiates it from lymphoma. Symptoms are cough, fever, malaise, dyspnea, weight loss, arthralgia, and occasionally hemoptysis. Skin lesions are found in nearly 50% of patients. It occurs in the 30- to 60-year age group, and there is slight male predominance. It generally involves the lungs, so the chest roentgenogram is usually abnormal. The most characteristic radiographic appearance is that of multiple, bilateral masses that are fairly well circumscribed and in more than 50% of cases resemble metastatic nodules. Some of the nodules may have a shaggy appearance, however. The lesions are usually confined to the mid and lower lungs. In those that do not resemble metastases, the most common appearance is that of large, poorly defined subpleural opacities, which may cavitate and resemble pneumonia. The cavities may have thick or thin walls and sometimes contain fluid levels. Hemoptysis—sometimes massive—may occur in patients with cavitation. At times the nodules are smaller, more numerous, and poorly defined. The presence of a single, large, unilateral mass has also been reported in patients with this disease. Occasionally mixed alveolar and interstitial disease may be observed, so that radiographic diagnosis cannot be made. Hilar adenopathy may be present but is unusual, and pleural effusion is occasionally observed.[54] In about 10% of patients, the disease progresses to lymphoma, usually of the plasmacytoid or immunoblastic type. Biopsy is necessary to make the diagnosis. If untreated, the disease often progresses rapidly, with death caused by pulmonary disease, CNS disease, or frank malignancy.

Necrotizing Sarcoidal Granulomatosis

Necrotizing sarcoidal granulomatosis is another rare type of granulomatous angiitis in which there is marked infiltration with sarcoidlike granulomas around blood vessels. Radiologic findings consist of bilateral nodules or poorly defined opacities with or without cavitation. A miliary type of disease has also been reported. Pleural effusion may occur, but hilar adenopathy is infrequent.[32] The etiology is not clear, but altered immunity is likely.

Allergic (Non-infectious) Granulomatosis and Angiitis (Churg-Strauss Syndrome)

Churg-Strauss syndrome is a rare disease characterized by pulmonary vasculitis, neuropathy, extravascular granulomas, tissue and blood eosinophilia, and frequently, asthma.[57] Small and medium arteries are involved; the granulomas are perivascular and contain giant cells and eosinophils. Pulmonary roentgen findings may closely resemble those of polyarteritis nodosa and in 25%, an eosinophilic pneumonia is present, with peripheral distribution similar to that of other eosinophilic pneumonias. Nodules are common. Diffuse interstitial disease, at times with a miliary pattern, hilar adenopathy, and pleural effusions, may also occur. High-resolution CT has been used in the study of patients with this disease and may be of value because thickened arterial walls caused by eosinophilic infiltration indicating vasculitis may be visible.[16]

Pulmonary Hyalinizing Granuloma

Pulmonary hyalinizing granuloma is probably caused by an exaggerated immune response and is therefore included in this section. The clinical course is benign with minimal signs or symptoms. Cough, malaise, fever, dyspnea, fatigue and/or pleuritic pain may occur, however. Histologic findings in the pulmonary nodules consist of concentric hyaline lamellae with perivascular collections of lymphocytes and plasma cells. Radiographic findings are those of multiple pulmonary nodules (occasionally solitary), usually bilateral, well cir-

circumscribed, and solid. Their size ranges from a few millimeters to 15 cm in diameter. At times the lesions are irregular and poorly defined. Cavitation is not common. Most of the lesions resemble nodular pulmonary metastases. Sclerosing mediastinitis may complicate this disease.[26]

IMMUNE-DEFICIENCY SYNDROMES

The immune deficiency diseases result in increased susceptibility to respiratory infections as well as infections elsewhere.[91] A number of types of deficiency states have been described: (1) decrease or absence of all immunoglobulins; (2) decrease or absence of a specific immunoglobulin; (3) lack of complement; (4) inability to handle various antigens; (5) defect in leukocyte function; and (6) the presence of inhibitors of essential components of the immune system. Because findings of repeated pulmonary infection are common to many of these diseases, a specific diagnosis cannot be made radiographically.

The syndromes are classified as *primary*, indicating a genetic abnormality, and *secondary*, indicating that some disease has interfered with normal function of the immune system.

AGAMMAGLOBULINEMIAS

The agammaglobulinemias are states in which antibodies cannot be formed because of an absence or deficiency of gammaglobulins. The congenital form is a sex-linked recessive genetic defect transmitted by females to male offspring (Bruton's disease).[14] Secondary agammaglobulinemia, or hypogammaglobulinemia, may be acquired, as in patients with multiple myeloma, leukemia, or lymphoma. However, there is also a group in whom, although the disease is of genetic origin, it is not manifested in infancy. Repeat infections are commonly observed in the lungs in patients with the agammaglobulinemias. Infections of the paranasal sinuses and mastoids are also very common, as are infections of the urinary tract and skin. The radiographic findings in the lungs are therefore those of recurrent bronchopneumonia, which may lead to postinflammatory fibrotic changes and to bronchiectasis. No hilar adenopathy is present, and the decrease or absence of lymphoid tissue in the pharynx results in a large pharyngeal airway that is characteristic of these conditions in young children. This is readily observed in a lateral radiograph of the nasopharynx. In older children, lymph nodes and lymphoid tissue may become evident when there is hyperplasia of reticulum cells. In the acquired type of agammaglobulinemia, there may be hyperplasia of lymphoid tissue and the mediastinal nodes may be enlarged.

DYSGAMMAGLOBULINEMIAS

The term "dysgammaglobulinemia" refers to conditions in which there is a deficiency in one or two of the immunoglobulins with normal or elevated levels of others. The patients may be susceptible to respiratory infections, which are observed as repeated pneumonias and are ultimately associated with bronchiectasis, atelectasis, and fibrosis.

COMBINED IMMUNODEFICIENCIES

The basic abnormality in this group of deficiencies is cellular, but there is impairment of humoral immunity also. In severe disease, both B- and T-lymphocyte functions may be markedly depressed or absent. Children having these deficiency diseases are susceptible to viral infections in addition to bacterial, fungal, and parasitic infections.

COMPLEMENT DEFICIENCY

Patients with complement deficiency have normal antibody production, leukocyte function, and cellular immunity, but lack certain components of complement and are therefore subject to frequent infections, usually with staphylococcal or gram-negative organisms.

HYPERIMMUNOGLOBULINEMIA E SYNDROME

The immunodeficiency syndrome known as hyperimmunoglobulinemia E syndrome was described in 1972.[60] It is characterized by susceptibility to staphylococcal infections of the skin and respiratory tract beginning in infancy. There is depressed cellular immunity and deficient antibody formation, as well as extreme elevation of serum IgE. Radiographic findings reflect the clinical syndrome of repeated pneumonias, with formation of cysts. Some of the cysts originate as pneumatoceles, others as abscesses with cavitation. The pneumonia is segmental or lobar and the cysts appeared from 2 to 8 years after the initial pneumonia in Merten's series of 11 patients (10 males, 1 female).[60] Single cysts were found in 7 and multiple cysts in 4 patients. The cysts resolved spontaneously with antibiotic treatment in 5 patients while in the others, the cysts persisted or recurred. The cyst walls vary in thickness and fluid levels may be present. Some cysts become chronically infected with fungi and saprophytic bacteria. Cysts may become very large and require resection. Nine patients had sinus infections and 4 had mastoiditis manifested on roentgenograms.

CHRONIC INTERSTITIAL PNEUMONIAS (DIFFUSE FIBROSING ALVEOLITIS)

The term "chronic interstitial pneumonia," as used by Liebow and Carrington, indicates a pneumonia in which the most significant or persistent component of the tissue response in the lung is in the interalveolar septa and more proximal supporting tissues.[53] Others, including Scadding and Hinson,[77,78] prefer the term "fibrosing alveolitis" to describe these diseases, many of which are of unknown cause. They believed that the categories described by Liebow and Carrington are not very clear, so the entire group of chronic interstitial pneumonias (fibrosing alveolitis) remains somewhat controversial. They then restrict the term "pneumonia" to denote inflammation of the lung characterized by consolidation produced by exudates filling the alveoli. Some believe the group of idiopathic interstitial pneumonias represent inflammatory responses of the alveolar walls to injuries of different types, durations, and intensities and are thus different aspects of a multifaceted "fibrosing alveolitis."

In view of the lack of knowledge regarding etiology, two partial classifications are necessary—one histopathologic, the other etiologic. They are not mutually exclusive, as the etiology is not often determined. The chest film findings in chronic interstitial lung disease progress at varying rates. The earliest manifestation is a fine nodularity followed or associated with a fine reticular or reticulonodular pattern. This may change to a coarse reticular or reticulonodular pattern with cystic areas. The most chronic form of the interstitial pneumonias is represented by interstitial fibrosis. In this end stage there is usually breakdown of alveolar walls in addition to fibrosis, which produces the so-called honeycomb pattern of pulmonary interstitial fibrosis. The honeycomb pattern usually implies far-advanced disease in that part of the lung, but not necessarily in all of the lung. Since the chest film findings are not a sensitive indicator of progression of interstitial lung disease, biopsy and/or examination of cells obtained by alveolar lavage as well as gallium scans are used for this purpose. About 30% of patients with biopsy-proved alveolitis have normal chest roentgenograms.

The radiologist does have a role in the study of the interstitial lung disease and should evaluate the following: (1) distribution of disease and lung volume; (2) progression of the opacities; (3) presence of hilar nodes; (4) pleural abnormalities; (5) presence of conglomerate masses; and (6) malignant change.[45] A high degree of radiographic diagnostic accuracy is not possible.

On the basis of histologic criteria and to some extent on radiographic and clinical criteria, Liebow and Carrington have described the following interstitial pneumonias: (1) *UIP*—the classic, undifferentiated, or

usual; (2) *BIP*—nonbacterial bronchiolitis obliterans superimposed on UIP; (3) *DIP*—desquamative; (4) *LIP*—lymphoid; and (5) *GIP*—giant cell.[53]

As will be noted in the following descriptions, the interstitial pneumonias exhibit a rather wide variety of roentgenographic patterns. The use of CT, including high-resolution, thin-section CT, in the study of patients with the various forms of chronic interstitial pneumonias including end-stage disease has been studied by many. Its ultimate role in patient management and diagnosis has yet to be determined. Because of this the differential diagnosis is based on lung biopsy with study of histologic sections. In most instances, the etiology is not clear. As indicated, many prefer the term "fibrosing alveolitis" for these conditions in which there is ultimately more or less interstitial fibrosis.

CLASSICAL OR UNDIFFERENTIATED INTERSTITIAL PNEUMONIA (UIP)

This disease is the result of diffuse alveolar damage from a large variety of agents, including a number of inhalants such as oxygen in high concentrations, particularly when administered by intermittent positive pressure breathing (IPPB) machines; viruses and mycoplasma; and conditions with altered immunity, such as scleroderma and rheumatoid arthritis. A number of drugs, bleomycin in particular, also can cause fibrosing alveolitis. In some cases a genetic factor may be involved. However, the cause of most chronic interstitial pneumonias is unknown. Whatever the cause, diffuse alveolar damage is produced, probably with some necrosis of alveolar epithelium and proteinacious exudates. The basement membrane is usually preserved. Hyaline membranes comprised of exudate and remnants of necrotic alveolar lining cells may be present. Interstitial infiltrations of lymphocytes and mononuclear cells are also noted in this stage. Interstitial proliferation and fibrosis eventually occur in some areas. During the acute phase, the exudates plus the swelling of alveolar cells and the interstitial infiltrate produce a roentgen picture simulating the hazy appearance of pulmonary edema. Roentgenographic findings vary considerably. In the early fibrotic phase, a fine reticular pattern may be observed, often predominantly basal, and in the more chronic forms of UIP the opacity produced is coarse and strandlike and tends to extend radially from the hilum. Small, round radiolucencies may appear and become more prominent with increasing fibrosis and destruction of the alveolar walls; this represents the honeycomb pattern of pulmonary fibrosis. There is often an associated loss of lung volume, which suggests either UIP or scleroderma. As mentioned, radiographic findings are not specific.

DIFFUSE ALVEOLAR DAMAGE AND BRONCHIOLITIS OBLITERANS (BIP)

When there is damage to bronchioles superimposed on the lesion of UIP, BIP is produced. Although the cause is not clear, this kind of damage can be the result of inhalation of corrosive fumes of strong acids. However, it appears to occur much more commonly as a result of a necrotizing bacterial bronchiolitis superimposed on viral pneumonia. The radiographic findings consist of streaks of flamelike opacity noted chiefly in the upper and central lung, although they may occur anywhere in the lungs. This may represent UIP with superimposed bacterial infection rather than a distinct entity and is very rare in our experience.

DESQUAMATIVE INTERSTITIAL PNEUMONIA (DIP)

DIP is an interstitial pneumonia characterized by extensive proliferation and desquamation of granular pneumocytes (type II alveolar-lining cells). It is associated with a mild interstitial cellular infiltration of plasma cells, lymphocytes, and eosinophils and with some septal and pleural edema. These desquamated cells and large aggregated macrophages may fill the bronchioles as well as alveoli. As in the other diseases affecting the alveolar walls, the cause is not certain, but in many an immunologic mechanism is a factor.

Roentgenographic findings consist of bilateral basal shadows which often are hazy and may have a ground-glass appearance. As the disease progresses, the basal density increases. The pattern is variable, however, with more density in upper than in lower lungs in some patients. In many of our patients, the disease has been widely scattered with pulmonary opacities of varying configuration, often with a mixed interstitial and alveolar pattern (Fig. 30-19). We have observed very few patients with "classical" medial basal "ground glass" disease originally described by Liebow.[53] There is usually a favorable response to steroids; occasionally, however, the disease may progress to a nonspecific, honeycomb pattern of fibrosis with loss of pulmonary volume—the end-stage lung.[29, 34]

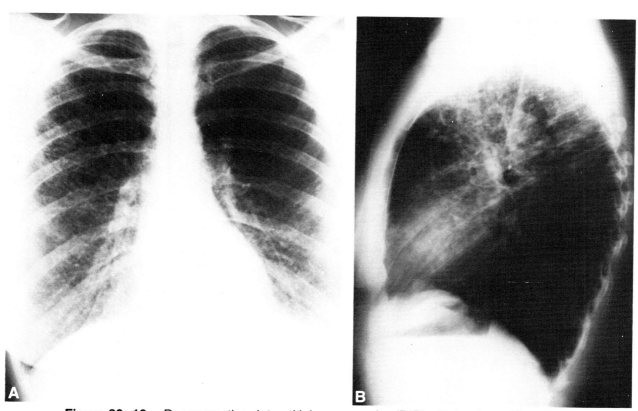

Figure 30–19. Desquamative interstitial pneumonia (DIP). Note the widespread, somewhat stringy, interstitial disease, which is noted best at the bases in (**A**) the frontal projection and (**B**) in the upper lung in the lateral projection. In our experience, there has been no characteristic roentgenographic pattern in this disease.

LYMPHOID INTERSTITIAL PNEUMONIA (LIP)

In lymphoid interstitial pneumonia there is massive and widespread infiltration of both lungs by lymphoid tissue, which resembles lymphoma very very closely histologically. The history is that of a very chronic interstitial pneumonia with cough, dyspnea, fever, and weight loss over a long period. The infiltration is interstitial in the interalveolar septa and in the peribronchiolar and perivenous spaces. Local lymph nodes and extrapulmonary tissues are not involved. The infiltrate is a mixture of small lymphocytes, plasma cells, and occasional large mononuclear cells, with the small lymphocytes predominating. Although the cause is not certain, some type of hypersensitivity appears to be a factor in most patients. Radiographic changes are variable and range from bilateral diffuse nodular opacities to peripheral opacities, which may be linear or branching, sometimes appearing rather poorly defined and conglomerate. Some of the peripheral linear opacities resemble Kerley's B lines. As the disease progresses, alveoli are compressed and obliterated by dense, linear opacities. The disease is usually bilateral but not necessarily symmetric. Ultimately, fibrosis may lead to honeycombing, and the end-stage lung. This disease does not respond to steroids and tends to progress slowly. At times it can be relatively local, producing a rather conglomerate-appearing, poorly defined, mass-like opacity.

GIANT-CELL INTERSTITIAL PNEUMONIA (GIP)

This unique interstitial pneumonia is characterized by the presence of intra-alveolar giant cells and an interstitial infiltrate that is predominately lymphocytic. The giant cells are very large and a single cell may nearly fill an alveolus. Clinically, the condition is manifested by cough and dyspnea; there may be some weight loss and fever. Roentgen findings are varied. A confluent nodular process may be present in one or both lungs and in either upper or lower lobes. Sometimes, mottled nodular densities and strandlike or streaklike densities extending from the hilum to the periphery of the lung may be noted. In our experience this condition is very rare.

DIFFUSE PULMONARY FIBROSIS OF UNKNOWN ETIOLOGY

Fibrosis of the lungs may result from a number of diseases. These include infections such as tuberculosis, the fungal diseases, bronchiectasis, sarcoidosis, the collagen–vascular and other diseases with altered immunity, the pneumoconioses, and others. The cause can sometimes be ascertained in this group if clinical history, physical findings, laboratory findings, and roentgen alterations are correlated. The roentgen manifestations of the diseases of known etiology are discussed in the appropriate sections. There is a large group of conditions in which fibrosis may be localized or scattered and in which there is no evidence of cause—nonspecific fibroses of obscure etiology. As more knowledge is gained regarding histopathology of the lung, however, it is likely that the number of patients placed in this idiopathic category will decrease. The roentgen findings are those of an increasing thickening of interstitial lung markings that is often more prominent in the bases than elsewhere. This produces a fine reticular pattern that gradually becomes more coarse. In end-stage disease a honeycomb pattern may be observed. In other instances, a more linear pattern is produced which at times may be associated with a fine nodular or granular pattern. Secondary pulmonary hypertension may develop, resulting in a gradual increase in the size of the pulmonary artery and its hilar branches, as well as evidence of right ventricular enlargement. The roentgen changes develop over a period of years or many months. The etiology may never be determined; even at autopsy the findings can only be described as nonspecific fibrosis of unknown cause (Fig. 30-20).

LUNG DISEASE IN NEUROFIBROMATOSIS

Interstitial pulmonary fibrosis occurs in about 10% of patients with neurofibromatosis who are over 30 years of age. The pulmonary disease does not become manifest until adult life. The cause is not known, but there probably is a genetic influence. Radiographic findings consist of linear interstitial opacity that is bilateral and tends to be basal. The interstitial changes may also be extensive, with a reticular and linear pattern involving most of the pulmonary parenchyma. Large upper-lobe bullae also are part of the disease, which produces relatively minor dyspnea.[87] Bullae may occasionally be predominantly basal. The presence of numerous cutaneous nodules is very helpful in making a radiologic diagnosis of this condition.

AMYLOIDOSIS

Amyloidosis is usually classified into the *primary* and *secondary types*. The secondary type is found in patients with chronic inflammatory disease, such as chronic osteomyelitis, bronchiectasis, and tuberculosis. It also develops in patients with rheumatoid arthritis and in those having malignant neoplasms; it is much more common than the primary type.[92] Amyloid

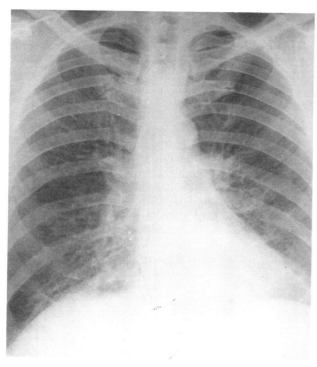

Figure 30–20.   Diffuse pulmonary fibrosis. The interstitial change is very extensive in this patient, whose history provided no clue to the cause of the disease. Lung biopsy revealed diffuse pulmonary fibrosis of unknown cause.

is deposited in the spleen, liver, adrenal glands, and kidneys secondary to the chronic inflammatory disease or malignancy. Radiographically detectable amyloid deposits in the lung are rare in this form of amyloidosis. In the rare primary form of the disease the amyloid is typically deposited in the heart, gastrointestinal tract, lungs, muscle, and skin. It develops in patients with no other disease and in those with plasma-cell abnormalities, such as multiple myeloma, or with abnormal immunoglobulins; however, the cause is unknown. There is pulmonary involvement in 30% to 70% of patients with primary amyloidosis. Amyloid is made up of a protein matrix consisting of fragments of immunoglobulin polypeptide chains. There are several chemical types of amyloid. In tissue, the deposits are polymers of a basic protein. Light-chain polymers are found in multiple myeloma and other plasma cell dyscrasias in which deposits may be found in the lungs. This material is deposited in the alveolar walls and around the interalveolar capillaries, as well as in the walls of the smaller blood vessels in the lung when pulmonary involvement is present. The myocardium is

affected in approximately 70% of patients with the primary form of the disease. Deposits may also occur in bronchial and tracheal walls.

The patterns of pulmonary amyloid deposition can be classified into three major types: (1) tracheobronchial in which amyloid deposition in the wall results in a diffuse thickening and distortion of the tracheobronchial tree; (2) nodular pulmonary in which single or multiple parenchymal nodules are produced by masses of amyloid that increase very slowly in size; and (3) diffuse alveolar septal in which amyloid is deposited in interstitial tissues, often perivascular, but also in alveolar walls and septa. Less commonly there may be diffuse tracheobronchial infiltration or, rarely, hilarnode involvement.

ROENTGEN FINDINGS

The roentgen findings in the tracheobronchial form of amyloidosis are related to obstruction causing atelectasis or overinflation and sometimes postobstructive pneumonia. Bronchial distortion, tracheal irregularity, and luminal narrowing can be observed on bronchoscopy and CT. The nodular form consists of single or multiple masses that can become calcified or may cavitate. The alveolar septal form may show a miliary nodular or reticulonodular pattern. There may also be a form resembling diffuse fibrosis with radiating strands extending outward from the hilum into the central lung. In the alveolar septal type there is often associated pleural effusion that may appear, regress, and then reappear. Pleural deposits may cause pleural thickening. As the disease progresses, the radiating strands increase and, in some instances, fine granular or more coarse nodular lesions develop. Calcification and bone formation may be observed in the pulmonary lesions and in the hilar and mediastinal nodes. The bone formation is peculiar and resembles spikelike pieces of broken glass. The roentgen progression is accompanied by increasing dyspnea. This generalized type of involvement must be distinguished from other chronic diseases that cause interstitial fibrosis. It may resemble sarcoidosis. The nodular form of the disease consists of one or more homogeneous masses that may be somewhat lobulated and resemble primary lung tumor closely; the local form is usually found in elderly men. When nodes are involved, there is deposition of amyloid in hilar and mediastinal nodes with a gradual increase in the hilar size and blurring of mediastinal borders. The prognosis is poor in the tracheobronchial and the alveolar septal forms of the disease. Decreasing pulmonary volume and respiratory insufficiency are observed in the alveolar septal form and obstruction is noted in the tracheobronchial form. All forms of pulmonary amyloidosis are relatively rare.

HISTIOCYTOSIS X

Eosinophilic granuloma is the most benign of a group of diseases of unknown cause which include Hand-Schüller-Christian disease and Letterer-Siwe disease and have been termed "histiocytosis X." Letterer-Siwe disease occurs in infants; it is acute and often rapidly fatal. Hand-Schüller-Christian disease occurs in older children and is more benign, while eosinophilic granuloma occurs in young adults and is often localized and benign when occurring in bone. Eosinophilic granuloma has been found as a lesion occurring only in the lung with increasing frequency. In some patients (about 20%) the typical bone lesion is associated with the pulmonary disease, but in others the lung appears to be the sole site of involvement. Now the term histi-

ocytosis X is used to indicate eosinophilic granuloma of the lung.

The roentgen manifestations of pulmonary histiocytosis X are reasonably characteristic. Generalized involvement is noted, manifested by a reticular pattern with small nodular lesions on the order of 1 to 3 mm in size. These nodules may be poorly defined, with hazy borders (Fig. 30-21A). They may be scattered generally throughout the lungs but tend to be somewhat more pronounced in the upper lungs (Fig. 30-21B). The disease may regress spontaneously in about one third of patients. In one third the disease persists, but does not progress. In one third it progresses, with increasing interstitial involvement. The appearance is then that of a reticulonodular pattern which gradually becomes more coarse and develops small foci of cyst-

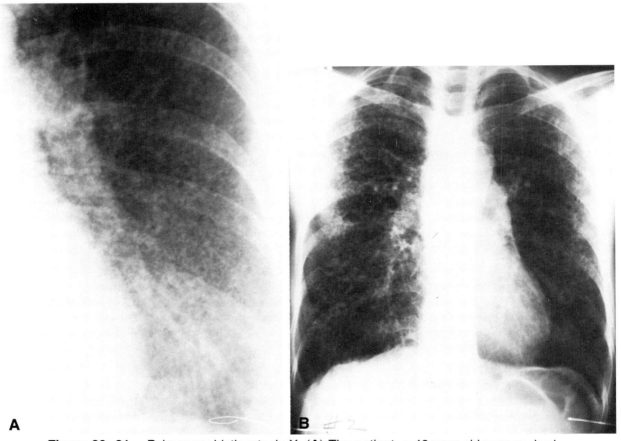

Figure 30–21. Pulmonary histiocytosis X. (**A**) The patient, a 40-year-old woman, had extensive pulmonary involvement consisting largely of tiny nodules and very few cystlike areas, as shown in this close-up view. (**B**) In another patient with chronic disease, a considerable amount of fibrosis has produced a "honeycomb" lung, noted best in the lateral aspect of the left central and upper lung. Elsewhere there are small granuloma-appearing nodules. There is a little emphysema with bullae at the left apex.

like rarefaction, resulting in a honeycomb lung (Fig. 30-22). There is usually no hilar adenopathy and usually no pleural involvement. However, with the advent of CT, enlarged paratracheal nodes and mediastinal nodes at other sites have been reported.[11] High-resolution CT reveals diffuse nodules, some of which may cavitate, cysts with either thin (more common) or thick walls, a reticular pattern, and occasionally "ground-glass" opacities (Fig. 30-22).[12] Spontaneous pneumothorax is fairly common and some of the patients have diabetes insipidus.

We have observed several patients in whom the radiographic findings were very unusual, consisting of scattered and patchy areas of what appeared to be alveolar-type disease, most likely representing an active phase. Others have also observed local alveolar disease, a few upper-lobe nodules, a large area of alveolar consolidation, and other unusual features.[72]

Because the roentgen findings are not characteristic and simulate those of other chronic interstitial pulmonary disease, the diagnosis must be based on clinical manifestations. The presence of the typical roentgen changes observed in bone is helpful when present. Lung biopsy is often necessary, but the diagnosis can be suspected in asymptomatic young patients with extensive pulmonary disease and little adenopathy or pleural involvement. There may be few symptoms, but some patients have chronic cough and later develop dyspnea. In the progressive form, the dyspnea increases and there is fibrosis resulting in cor pulmonale and end-stage lung disease.

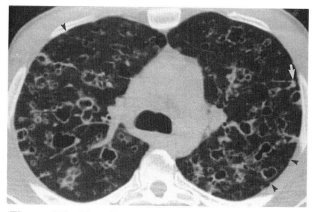

Figure 30–22. Eosinophilic granuloma (histiocytosis X). There are multiple thin- and thick-walled cysts throughout the lung parenchyma. A nodule (*white arrow*) and several subpleural micronodules (*black arrowheads*) are present. High-resolution CT scan, 2-mm collimation, bone algorithm. (Courtesy of Julie K. Mitby, MD)

GAUCHER'S DISEASE AND NIEMANN-PICK DISEASE

Gaucher's disease is caused by an inborn error of metabolism in which there is an accumulation of glucosylceramide in reticuloendothelial cells. The lung may be involved with roentgen findings of interstitial disease manifested by a diffuse reticulonodular or miliary pattern of pulmonary opacity.[94] Niemann-Pick disease is a related lipid storage disorder of phospholipid metabolism. Pulmonary involvement causes diffuse nodular disease with linear strands producing a honeycomb effect or a coarse reticulonodular pattern on the roentgenogram of the chest. Basal Kerley's B lines may also be present, and there may be some pulmonary calcifications.[50]

LYMPHANGIOMYOMATOSIS (LYMPHANGIOLEIOMYOMATOSIS, MUSCULAR HYPERPLASIA, MYOMATOSIS)

Tuberous sclerosis is a hereditary disease characterized by mental deficiency, seizures, adenoma sebaceum (acneform rash) on the face with butterfly distribution, and hamartomatous tumors that may affect various parts of the body, including the central nervous system, liver, spleen, kidneys, and bones. Mental deficiency is common. There is reasonably good evidence to show that lymphangioleiomyomatosis is a *forme fruste* of tuberous sclerosis. *Lymphangiomyomatosis* usually occurs in adults in whom there is no mental deficiency and no clinical evidence of central nervous system damage even though calcifications may be noted intracranially.[15]

In these patients without tuberous sclerosis, *lymphangiomyomatosis* is a rare disease, usually occurring in young women, in which there is an overgrowth of atypical smooth muscle along the lymphatics of the lung. There may also be involvement of the extrapulmonary thoracic lymphatics and abdominal lymphatics. The disease is sufficiently similar to tuberous sclerosis to warrant an assumption by some authorities that it is a *forme fruste* of tuberous sclerosis, as indicated earlier. Others believe there are enough differences to make the diseases separate entities. Radiographic findings that are often observed late in the course of lymphangiomyomatosis are similar to those in tuberous sclerosis. Recurrent spontaneous pneumothorax may occur before any pulmonary abnormalities are visible on the chest roentgenogram. The earliest pulmonary findings are those of a diffuse pattern of tiny opacities described as reticulonodular, granular, miliary, or interstitial. Later, a coarse reticular pattern is observed, often with septal lines. Eventually, a honeycomb pattern is seen, but its appearance is more delicate than the usual honeycomb pattern noted in end-stage interstitial disease. The lungs tend to increase rather than decrease in volume. Chylous effusions may occur similar to those in tuberous sclerosis.[19, 82, 86] The effusions are usually large and tend to recur. CT has been used to study these patients.[1] The findings on CT are largely those of many cysts or cystlike spaces ranging from 3 to 40 mm in diameter distributed throughout both lungs, with some sparing of the apices (Fig. 30-23). No nodularity was observed on CT, and no reticular pattern was present. Aberle and associates believe the reticular pattern on plain films is probably a summation of the walls of overlying cysts (Fig. 30-24).[1] CT findings appear earlier than changes observed on chest radiographs and tend to correlate well with pulmonary function studies. Although the diagnosis depends on lung biopsy, the disease may be suspected in young women having chylous pleural effusions and repeated spontaneous pneumothorax with or without a reticulonodular pulmonary interstitial pattern and progressive increase of lung volume. Some authors believe that in the absence of tuberous sclerosis, muscular hyperplasia represents the end stage of chronic interstitial pneumonia, primarily DIP or UIP.[70]

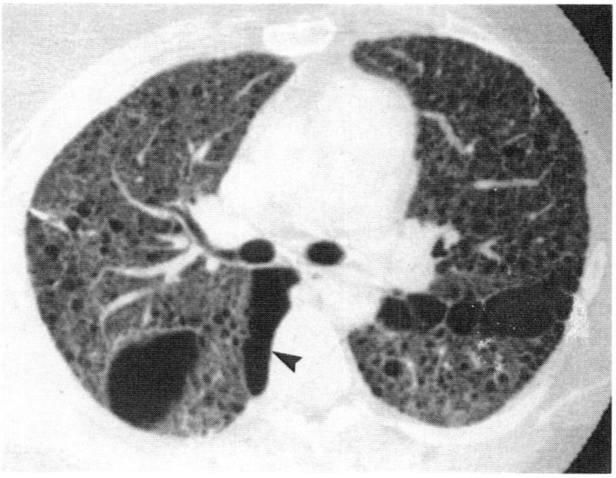

PULMONARY ALVEOLAR MICROLITHIASIS

Pulmonary alveolar microlithiasis is a rare disease characterized by the presence of small calcium-containing bodies in the alveoli of the lung. The cause is not known but there is a high familial incidence (50%) indicating that there may be a hereditary factor.[35, 80] The disease is asymptomatic for long periods but eventually dyspnea appears, followed by cough, cyanosis, and right-sided heart failure. Because of the late appearance of symptoms the disease is usually first discovered on routine chest roentgenography.

ROENTGEN FINDINGS

The appearance of the chest is characteristic. There is widespread uniform distribution of fine sandlike particles of calcific density, which are usually less than 1 mm in diameter. They are uniform in size and there is no tendency to conglomeration. When extensive, some of the tiny calcifications may overlap and be difficult to define as individual particles. Overexposed films using a grid are of value in visualizing them, particularly when the disease is far advanced. The opacity is often great enough to obscure the heart and mediastinal outlines as well as the diaphragm. In some patients, the pulmonary opacity is so great that the pleura ap-

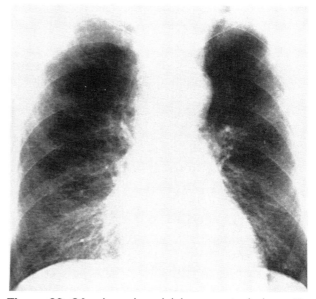

Figure 30–23. Pulmonary lymphangioleiomyomatosis. There are multiple large and small air cysts diffusely involving the lung parenchyma. A loculated medial pneumothorax is present on the right (*arrowhead*). High-resolution CT scan, 1.5-mm collimation, bone algorithm. (Courtesy of Donald Yandow, MD)

Figure 30–24. Lymphangioleiomyomatosis in a 43-year-old female. A reticulonodular pattern is observed in the central and lower lung bilaterally. There was some upper lobe change, but it is not seen well on this reproduction.

pears as a negative or black-line shadow instead of a white one, and even the heart may appear radiolucent in contrast to the extensive pulmonary calcification.[49] There is no other disease that resembles this condition, because the tiny particles are calcified and are more dense than particles of comparable size in any of the miliary diseases.

Pulmonary calcifications or ossifications can be caused by a number of other conditions, but there is no resemblance to alveolar microlithiasis. Infections such as histoplasmosis, chicken pox pneumonia in adults, chronic renal failure, renal transplantation, hypervitaminosis D, parathyroid neoplasms, altered calcium and phosphorus metabolism, chronic mitral stenosis, and metastatic tumors can cause pulmonary calcification or ossification. The appearance is quite variable. Rarely, pulmonary ossification may be idiopathic.

FAMILIAL DYSAUTONOMIA (RILEY-DAY SYNDROME)

Familial dysautonomia results from dysfunction of the autonomic nervous system. It is a familial congenital disorder transmitted as an autosomal recessive trait that occurs in infants and children, usually Jewish. It was originally described in five children in 1949. Clinical findings consist of defective (decreased) lacrimation, excessive perspiration, blotchy skin, drooling, emotional instability, motor incoordination, hyporeflexia, and indifference to pain. Death is usually caused by pulmonary disease. The pulmonary findings are related to bronchial hypersecretion and resultant obstruction that often leads to infection. Pulmonary manifestations sufficient to produce roentgen changes on the chest film occur in approximately 65% to 75% of the patients.[31] Early changes consist of diffuse accentuation of markings resulting from interstitial infiltration. Patchy bronchopneumonia is common and often persists for long periods. The repeated episodes of pneumonia accentuate the findings and may produce areas of homogeneous opacity scattered in the lungs; these areas appear and disappear. Atelectasis of a lobe or segment is common and tends to persist for several weeks. The right upper lobe is frequently involved. Bronchiectasis is not commonly found. The pulmonary disease is usually more focal and not as widespread as in cystic fibrosis of the pancreas, but there is some similarity in the roentgen findings of these two diseases.

POLYCYTHEMIA

Polycythemia may be secondary to anoxia in a variety of chronic pulmonary diseases and in congenital heart disease. In these instances it is a compensatory phenomenon and there are no pulmonary roentgen findings indicating its presence. Polycythemia vera or primary polycythemia is a hematologic disorder characterized by hyperplasia of the red bone marrow, resulting in an increase in circulating red blood cells and in leukocytosis. In these patients, vascular engorgement results in prominence of vascular shadows in the lungs. Basal fibrosis resulting in increased basal markings is sometimes noted, along with changes suggesting basal congestion. Discrete rounded densities in the midzones of the lungs that are believed to represent venous thromboses have also been reported; they vary in size and appear and disappear in a few weeks. Pulmonary thromboembolism is common. These findings are not diagnostic, but when pulmonary vascular distention is present without cardiac or pulmonary disease evident to account for it, the diagnosis can be suggested.

CHOLESTEROL PNEUMONITIS (ENDOGENOUS LIPID PNEUMONIA)

Cholesterol pneumonitis is a rare type of chronic interstitial inflammation of the lung in which the exudate consists of large mononuclear cells filled with cholesterol and cholesterol esters. These cells are noted to infiltrate the interstitial tissues and alveolar walls and to fill the alveoli. The etiology is not clear and the disease does not appear to be related to lipid pneumonia of the aspiration type. It is sometimes called endogenous lipid pneumonia and deposits are often found associated with chronic pulmonary diseases that produce bronchial obstruction. For example, it may occur in chronic bronchial obstruction by an endobronchial neoplasm or in bronchiolitis obliterans with diffuse alveolar damage (BIP). It may also occur in the absence of obstruction in slowly resolving pneumonias—the "inflammatory pseudotumor."

ROENTGEN FINDINGS

In the obstructive types, the signs of BIP or of an obstructive tumor may be observed. In the nonobstructive type, the disease is characterized by a single confluent homogeneous density that may be lobar or segmental in distribution. There is usually a decrease in the volume of the lobe affected by the disease. The process extends to the pleura. Hilar node enlargement may occur, and pleural fluid or pleural thickening is often present. The absence of endobronchial block and the fact that only a part of a segment is involved in the segmental type of disease are factors in favor of cholesterol pneumonitis over tumor. The disease is more compact and clearly defined than exogenous lipid pneumonia and its distribution, with the lesion extending to the pleura, is unlike that in exogenous lipid pneumonia. The diagnosis is usually made by biopsy.

PULMONARY ALVEOLAR PROTEINOSIS

Pulmonary alveolar proteinosis was described by Rosen and associates in 1958.[75] It is characterized by the presence in the alveoli of PAS-positive (periodic acid-Schiff stain) proteinaceous material rich in lipid. The exact nature of the material has not been determined; it appears to be produced by septal lining cells which slough into the lumen and become necrotic. Cellular infiltrate and reaction are absent or minimal. The cause is not known; inhalation of some of the newer chemical agents used in sprays and the like has been suggested, along with an infectious agent antigenically allied to *Pneumocystis carinii*. In some instances, the disease is associated with immunoglobulin deficiency and the incidence appears to be increased in patients with lymphoma or a hematologic malignant lesion.[18] The disease occurs in adults who are 20 to 50 years of age, but may occasionally be observed in children. It appears to be a new disease, since no examples of it were observed before 1955. It often runs an insidious course with no symptoms early in the disease or when pulmonary involvement is minimal. Later or in more severe disease symptoms may occur characterized by malaise, cough, dyspnea, and weight loss. Physical findings are minimal and gross radiographic abnormality may be observed in patients with few symptoms. The course of the disease may also be variable; in a few patients it is rapidly progressive, leading to pulmonary insufficiency with cyanosis, clubbing of the fingers, and death caused by the progressive loss of pulmonary function or intercurrent infection. It is particularly lethal in children, where the mortality approaches 100%, as opposed to less than 30% in adults. Secondary fungal infection is the cause of most deaths in this disease. *Nocardia* is the most common of these organisms, but *Candida*, *Mucor*, and *Cryptococcus* may also be the cause. In other patients the symptoms may regress, with partial clearing of pulmonary changes; occasionally the disease may clear completely. Tracheobronchial lavage of the involved lobes with saline solution has been used with definite improvement in some patients. Steroids are ineffective and their use is contraindicated.

The roentgen findings at the height of the disease are those of parahilar opacities simulating pulmonary edema. The opacity appears to radiate from the hila chiefly to the bases; it is indistinct or "soft" and may have a somewhat irregular pattern resembling nodularity. There are variations of this pattern; at times the disease appears to be unilateral and it need not be perihilar; it is predominantly basal and central, however. A number of cases have been reported in which distribution of the alveolar opacity was quite atypical, so the disease must be kept in mind when alveolar opacities persist in an afebrile, relatively asymptomatic patient (Figs. 30-25 and 30-26). Roentgen findings change slowly and when clearing occurs there may be some residual fibrosis represented by linear opacities and small nodules. The diagnosis can be suspected on the basis of clinical and roentgen findings. The presence of PAS-positive material in the sputum is diagnostic, but, if it is not obtained, lung biopsy may be necessary to establish the diagnosis.

NEAR-DROWNING

When a patient is recovered from the water in a state of apnea and subsequently revived, pulmonary changes occur which are evidently caused by hypoxia or a combination of aspiration of water and hypoxia. In "dry" near-drowning, there is enough laryngospasm to prevent inhalation of water and the pulmonary changes are secondary to hypoxia. Recovery rate is highest in this

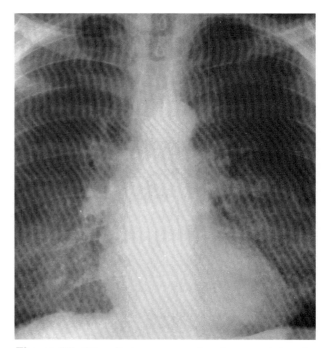

Figure 30–25. Pulmonary alveolar proteinosis. There is bilateral basal involvement medially. It is somewhat confluent on the right and indistinct on the left. The medial basal distribution of the disease is characteristic but is not always present.

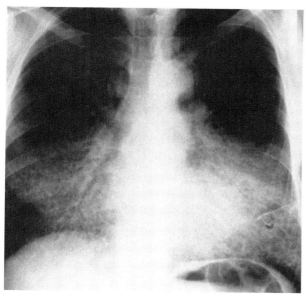

Figure 30–26. Pulmonary alveolar proteinosis in a 56-year-old male with some cough and dyspnea. There is a greater amount of alveolar filling than that noted in Figure 30-25.

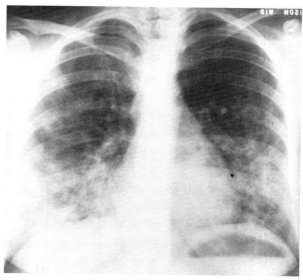

Figure 30–27. Near-drowning. Immediately following resuscitation, there were no abnormalities noted on the chest film. This film, exposed 3 hours later, shows bilateral opacity, with a central and basal distribution resembling alveolar edema.

group. In "wet" near-drowning, water is aspirated in varying amounts and may contribute to the clinical and roentgen findings. In experimental animals, sea water, being hypertonic, increases pulmonary alveolar fluid and leads to hypovolemia; while hypotonic fresh water is absorbed quickly leading to hemodilution and hemolysis of red cells. Clinically and radiographically, no clearly defined differences have been reported in humans who have aspirated water.[44] Pulmonary edema and hemorrhage have been observed histopathologically in drowning victims, and the roentgen findings in the near-drowning patient resemble those of pulmonary edema of varying degrees of severity. There may be a delay in appearance of roentgen changes for several hours. The findings consist of bilateral, poorly defined, alveolar opacities which may be very extensive and confluent, sparing the periphery (Fig. 30-27). In other patients the involvement is less marked and tends to be reticulonodular and poorly defined. Clearing is usually rapid and is complete in 2 to 6 days. As the process resolves, the appearance changes from that of alveolar edema to a pattern resembling interstitial edema. Aspiration of foreign material may complicate the picture by causing atelectasis and pulmonary infection. When recovery is delayed, pulmonary infection is usually found as a complication. Pneumothorax and pneumomediastinum are complications of resuscitation efforts.

THE POSTSURGICAL CHEST

The roentgenographic appearance of the chest following *pulmonary resection* varies with the type of surgery. There is also considerable variation in the ability of the remaining lung to expand and fill the hemithorax. Immediately following lobar or segmental resection, the roentgenogram often outlines pneumothorax that varies in amount and position, depending on the volume of pulmonary tissue removed and the presence or absence of pleural adhesions. The hemidiaphragm on the operated side is usually elevated, and there is often a mediastinal shift to that side. A drainage tube is left in place, and this is visible along with some emphysema in the lateral chest wall that often extends up into the neck. This emphysema is manifested by streaks of radiolucency within the soft tissues (Fig. 30-28). There may be some fluid in the soft tissues, along with air. This produces fluid levels that may overlie the lung parenchyma. These accumulations in the wound space can usually be differentiated from loculated pockets of air and fluid in the pleural space by their position in relation to the chest wall. A segment of rib is sometimes resected, and surgical section or fracture of a rib above or below the missing rib is often observed. It is not unusual to note some diffuse opacity at the surgical site, even on roentgenograms obtained very shortly following completion of

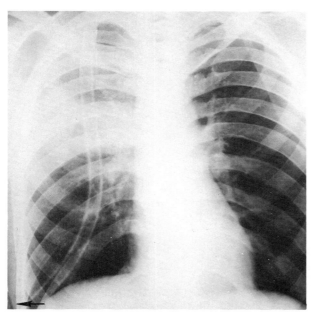

Figure 30–28. Postoperative chest. Portable film exposed 1 day following segmental resection of the apical and posterior segments of the right upper lobe. The hazy opacity in the right midlung most likely represents edema and some hemorrhage at the surgical site. The remaining lung is well expanded. The large drainage tube is easily identified. The arrow at the right base indicates a small amount of postoperative subcutaneous emphysema.

the procedure. This is caused by a combination of edema and possibly hemorrhage at the surgical site, along with some fluid in the adjacent pleural space. The opacity varies considerably with the type of resection, being most commonly observed when a segmental resection is performed. Within 24 hours, there usually is fluid in the pleural space at the base and surrounding the remaining lung. The amount of pneumothorax is often decreased in that period of time.

It is not unusual to observe some atelectasis in the remaining lobe. It often clears within 24 hours, resulting in an increase in lung volume and a decrease in the size of the pneumothorax. Subsequent roentgenograms show a gradual decrease in the size of the residual pneumothorax and an increase in expansion of the remaining lung. The subcutaneous emphysema usually disappears in 7 to 10 days. Severe subcutaneous emphysema is occasionally seen to extend into the neck on both sides and into the soft tissues of the opposite hemithorax, as well as into the mediastinum. This requires a longer time to clear. Eventually the pneumothorax and fluid disappear, leaving a relatively small

amount of residual pleural thickening or perhaps some irregular adhesive tenting of the diaphragm manifested by local elevation of it. When segmental resection is performed and no rib is removed, it is often difficult or impossible to detect recognizable residues on the side of resection after a period of 6 months.

Pneumonectomy is occasionally necessary in the treatment of tumor or tuberculosis, and following this operation a large amount of pneumothorax is usually noted in the immediate postoperative film, along with subcutaneous emphysema, as in segmental and lobar resections. Rib removal and surgical section can also be recognized. As times passes, fluid accumulates in the hemithorax; this gradually replaces the air (Fig. 30-29). Elevation of the diaphragm and shift of the mediastinal structures to the surgical side vary considerably but are almost always present, along with herniation of the normal lung across the midline (Fig. 30-30).

Complications may occur and can be recognized on the roentgenograms. Bronchopleural fistula is manifested by continuing pneumothorax for an unusually long period of time or by sudden increase in the

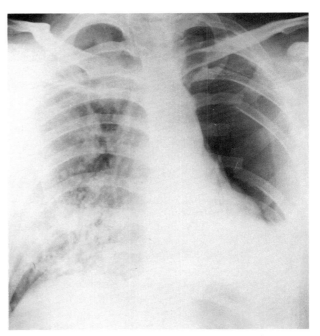

Figure 30–29. Postoperative chest. A left pneumonectomy was performed 2 days before this examination was made with portable equipment. Fluid and air fill the left pleural space. Much of the opacity at the right base is secondary to iodized oil residual from previous bronchography. There has been resection of the posterior arc of the sixth rib and surgical section of the fifth and seventh ribs.

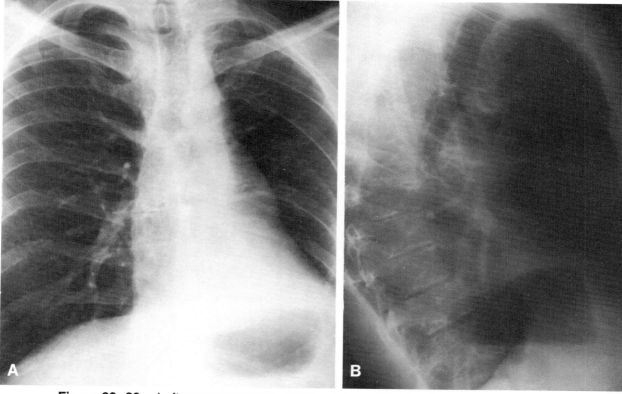

Figure 30–30. Left pneumonectomy. (**A**) Frontal and (**B**) lateral roentgenograms show remarkable shift of the right lung into the left hemithorax through the anterior mediastinum. The heart is displaced posteriorly. The mediastinal shift and elevation of the left hemidiaphragm are rather minimal. Radiolucency of the remaining lung is indicative of compensatory overexpansion.

amount of pneumothorax, along with decrease in fluid without aspiration. When lobar or segmental resections are performed, the remaining segments or lobes may collapse or undergo torsion and then collapse (see under Lobar Atelectasis). These atelectatic areas are recognized as areas of increased opacity.

REFERENCES AND SELECTED READINGS

1. ABERLE DR, HANSELL DM, BROWN K, ET AL: Lymphangiomyomatosis: CT, chest radiographic and functional correlations. Radiology 176:381, 1990

2. ABLOW RC, ORZALESI MM: Localized roentgenographic pattern of hyaline membrane disease. Am J Roentgenol 112:23, 1971

3. ADAMS FG, LEDINGHAM IMCA: The pulmonary manifestations of septic shock. Clin Radiol 28:315, 1977

4. ALLEN JN, PACHT ER, GADEK JE, ET AL: Acute eosinophilic pneumonia as a reversible cause of noninfectious respiratory failure. N Engl J Med 321:569, 1989

5. AMERICAN THORACIC SOCIETY: Definitions and classification of chronic bronchitis, asthma and pulmonary emphysema. Am Rev Resp Dis 85:762, 1962

6. ASKIN FB: Back to the future: The Hamman-Rich syndrome and acute interstitial pneumonia. Mayo Clin Proc 65:1624, 1990

7. BAGHDASSARIAN OM, AVERY ME, NEUHAUSER EBD: A form of pulmonary insufficiency in premature infants: Pulmonary dysmaturity? Am J Roentgenol 89:1020, 1963

8. BERDON WE, DEE GJ, ABRAMSON SJ, ET AL: Localized pneumothorax adjacent to a collapsed lobe: A sign of bronchial obstruction. Radiol 150:691, 1984

9. BERKMEN YM, YANKELEVITZ D, DAVIS S, ET AL: Torsion of the upper lobe in pneumothorax. Radiol 173:447, 1989

10. BERTELSON S, STRUVE-CHRISTENSEN E, AASTED A: Isolated middle lobe atelectasis: Aetiology, pathogenesis and treatment of the so-called middle lobe syndrome. Thorax 35:449, 1980

11. BRAMBILLA E, FONTAINE E, PISON CM, ET AL: Pulmonary histiocytosis X with mediastinal node involvement. Am Rev Resp Dis 142:1216, 1990

12. BRAUNER MW, GRENIER P, MONELHI MM, ET AL: Pulmonary histiocytosis X: Evaluation with high-resolution CT. Radiol 172:255, 1989

13. BRETTNER A, HEITZMAN ER, WOODIN WG: Pulmonary complications of drug therapy. Radiology 96:31, 1970

14. BRUTON OC: Agammaglobulinemia. Pediatrics 9:722, 1952

15. BRUWER AJ, KIERLAND RR, SCHMIDT HW: Pulmonary tuberous sclerosis. Am J Roentgenol 85:748, 1956

16. BUSCHMAN DL, WALDRON JA JR, KING TE JR: Churg-Strauss pulmonary vasculitis. High resolution computed tomography scanning and pathologic findings. Am Rev Resp Dis 142:458, 1990

17. BYHARDT RW, ABRAMS R, ALMAGRO U: The association of adult respiratory distress syndrome (ARDS) with thoracic irradiation (RT). Int J Radiation Oncol Biol Phys 15:1441, 1988

18. CARNOVALE R, ZORNOZA J, GOLDMAN AM, ET AL: Pulmonary alveolar proteinosis: Its association with hematologic malignancy and lymphoma. Radiology 122:303, 1977

19. CARRINGTON CB, CUGELL DW, GAENSLER EA, ET AL: Lymphangioleiomyomatosis. Physiologic–pathologic–radiologic correlations. Am Rev Resp Dis 116:977, 1977

20. CARVALHO PM, CARR DH: Computed tomography of folded lung. Clin Radiol 41:86, 1990

21. CHURG A: Pulmonary angiitis and granulomatosis revisited. Human Pathology 14:868, 1983

22. CITRO LA, GORDON ME, MILLER WT: Eosinophilic lung disease (or how to slice P.I.E.). Am J Roentgenol 117:787, 1973

23. DON C, DESMARAIS R: Peripheral upper lobe collapse in adults. Radiol 170:657, 1989

24. DON C, HAMMOND DI: The vascular converging points of the right pulmonary hilus and their diagnostic significance. Radiol 155:295, 1985

25. DOYLE TC, LAWLER GA: CT features of rounded atelectasis of the lung. Am J Roentgenol 143:225, 1984

26. ENGLEMAN P, LIEBOW AA, GMELICH J, ET AL: Pulmonary hyalinizing granuloma. Am Rev Resp Dis 115:997, 1977

27. ERICKSON AM, DE LA MONTE SM, MOORE GW, ET AL: The progression of morphologic changes in bronchopulmonary dysplasia. Am J Pathol 127:474, 1987

28. ESPOSITO MJ: Focal pulmonary hemosiderosis in rheumatic heart disease. Am J Roentgenol 73:351, 1955

29. FEIGIN DS, FRIEDMAN PJ: Chest radiography in desquamative interstitial pneumonitis: A review of 37 patients. Am J Roentgenol 134:91, 1980

30. FELSON B: Lung torsion: Radiographic findings in nine cases. Radiol 162:631, 1987

31. FISHBEIN D, GROSSMAN RF: Pulmonary manifestations of familial dysautonomia in an adult. Am J Med 80:709, 1986

32. FISHER MR, CHRIST ML, BERNSTEIN JR: Necrotizing sarcoid-like granulomatosis: Radiologic–pathologic correlation. J Can Assoc Radiol 35:313, 1984

33. FRIEDMAN PJ: Adult pulmonary ligament pneumatocele: A loculated pneumothorax. Radiology 155:575, 1985

34. GAENSLER EA, GOFF AM, PROWSE CM: Desquamative interstitial pneumonia. N Engl J Med 274:113, 1966

35. GOMEZ GE, LICHTEMBERGER E, SANTAMARIA A, ET AL: Familial pulmonary alveolar microlithiasis. Radiology 72:550, 1953

36. GORDON R: The deep sulcus sign. Radiol 136:25, 1980

37. GRAY AW JR, MARTINEZ FJ, STREITZ JM JR, ET AL: Upper lobe cavitary mass in a steroid-dependent asthmatic patient. Chest 99:1261, 1991

38. GRISCOM NT, WHEELER WB, SWEEZEY NB, ET AL: Bronchopulmonary dysplasia: Radiographic appearance in middle childhood. Radiol 171:811, 1989

39. HAMMAN L, RICH AR: Acute diffuse interstitial fibrosis of the lungs. Johns Hopkins Med J 74:177, 1944

40. HANKE R, KRETZSCHMAR R: Round atelectasis. Semin Roentgenol 15:174, 1980

41. HEITZMAN ER, MARKARIAN B, DELISE CT: Lymphoproliferative disorders of the thorax. Semin Roentgenol 10:73, 1975

42. HEROLD CJ, KUHLMAN JE, ZERHOUNI EA: Pulmonary atelectasis: Signal patterns with MR imaging. Radiol 178:715, 1991

43. HUNNINGHAKE GW, FAUCI AS: Pulmonary involvement in the collagen vascular diseases: State of the art. Am Rev Resp Dis 119:471, 1979

44. HUNTER TB, WHITEHOUSE WM: Fresh-water, near-drowning: Radiological aspects. Radiology 112:51, 1974

45. JOFFE N: Roentgenologic findings in post-shock and postoperative pulmonary insufficiency. Radiol 94:369, 1970

46. KATTAN KR: Upper mediastinal changes in lower lobe collapse. Semin Roentgenol 15:183, 1980

47. KATTAN KR, EYLER WR, FELSON B: The juxtaphrenic peak in upper lobe collapse. Semin Roentgenol 15:187, 1980

48. KERR IH: Interstitial lung disease: The role of the radiologist. Clin Radiol 35:1, 1984

49. KINO T, KOHARA Y, TSUJI S: Pulmonary alveolar microlithiasis. Am Rev Resp Dis 105:105, 1972

50. LACHMAN R, CROCKER A, SCHULMAN J, ET AL: Radiological findings in Niemann-Pick disease. Radiology 108:659, 1973

51. LI YW, SNOW J, SMITH WL, ET AL: Localized pulmonary lymphangiectasis. Am J Roentgenol 145:269, 1985

52. LIEBOW AA, CARRINGTON CB: The eosinophilic pneumonias. Medicine (Baltimore) 48:251, 1969

53. LIEBOW AA, CARRINGTON CB: The interstitial pneumonias. In Simon M, Potchen EJ, LeMay M (eds): Frontiers of Pulmonary Radiology. New York, Grune & Stratton, 1969

54. LIEBOW AA, CARRINGTON CRB, FRIEDMAN PJ: Lymphomatoid granulomatosis. Human Path 3:457, 1972

55. MACEWAN DW, DUNBAR JS, SMITH RD, ET AL: Pneumothorax in young infants: Recognition and evaluation. J Can Assoc Radiol 22:264, 1971

56. MARKOWITZ RL: The anterior junction line: A radiographic sign of bilateral pneumothorax in neonates. Radiol 167:717, 1988

57. MASI HT, HUNDER GG, LIE JT, ET AL: The American College of Rheumatology 1990 criteria for the classification of Churg-Strauss syndrome (allergic granulomatosis and angiitis). Arthritis Rheum 33:1094, 1990

58. MAYO JR, MÜLLER N, ROAD J, ET AL: Chronic eosinophilic pneumonia: CT findings in six cases. Am J Roentgenol 153:727, 1989

59. MCHUGH K, BLAQUIERE RM: CT features of rounded atelectasis. Am J Roentgenol 153:257, 1989

60. MERTEN DF, BUCKLEY RH, PRATT PC, ET AL: Hyperimmunoglobulinemia E syndrome: Radiographic observations. Radiol 132:17, 1979

61. MOSER ES JR, PROTO AV: Lung torsion: Case report and literature review. Radiol 162:639, 1987

62. MOSKOWITZ PS, GRISCOM NT: The medial pneumothorax. Radiol 120:143, 1976

63. MUNK PL, VELLET AD, ZWIREWICK C: Torsion of the upper lobe of the lung after surgery: Finding on pulmonary angiography. Am J Roentgenol 157:471, 1991

64. NAIDICH DP, MCCAULEY DI, KHOURI NF, ET AL: Computed tomography of lobar collapse: 1. Endobronchial obstruction. J Comput Assist Tomogr 7:745, 1983

65. NAIDICH DP, MCCAULEY DI, KHOURI NF, ET AL: Computed tomography of lobar collapse: 2. Collapse in the absence of endobronchial obstruction. J Comput Assist Tomogr 7:758, 1983

66. NORTHWAY WH JR: Bronchopulmonary dysplasia and research in diagnostic radiology. Am J Roentgenol 156:681, 1991

67. NORTHWAY WH JR, ROSAN RC, PORTER DY: Pulmonary disease following respirator therapy of hyaline-membrane disease: Bronchopulmonary dysplasia. N Engl J Med 276:357, 1967

68. OLSON J, COLBY TV, ELLIOTT CG: Hamman-Rich syndrome revisited. Mayo Clin Proc 65:1538, 1990

69. OSTENDORF P, BIRZLE H, VOGEL W, ET AL: Pulmonary radiographic abnormalities in shock: Roentgen–clinical–pathological correlation. Radiol 115:257, 1975

70. OVENFORS C-O, DAHLGREN SE, RIPE E, ET AL: Muscular hyperplasia of the lung: A clinical, radiographic and histopathologic study. Am J Roentgenol 135:703, 1980

71. PACHECO A, CASANOVA C, FOGUE L, ET AL: Long-term clinical follow up of adult idiopathic pulmonary hemosiderosis and celiac disease. Chest 99:1525, 1991

72. POMERANZ SJ, PROTO AV: Histiocytosis X: Unusual confusing features of eosinophilic granuloma. Chest 89:88, 1986

73. RAASCH BN, HEITZMAN ER, CORSKY EW, ET AL: A computed tomographic study of bronchopulmonary collapse. Radiographics 4:195, 1984

74. ROBERTS SR JR: Immunology and the lung: An overview. Semin Roentgenol 10:7, 1975

75. ROSEN SH, CASTLEMAN B, LIEBOW AA (with collaboration of ENZINGER FM, HUNT RTN): Pulmonary alveolar proteinosis. N Engl J Med 258:1123, 1958

76. RUBIN GD, EDWARDS DK III, REICHER MA, ET AL: Diagnosis of pulmonary hemosiderosis by MR imaging. Am J Roentgenol 152:573, 1989

77. SCADDING JG: Diffuse pulmonary alveolar fibrosis. Thorax 29:271, 1974

78. SCADDING JG, HINSON KFW: Diffuse fibrosing alveolitis (diffuse interstitial fibrosis of the lungs). Thorax 22:291, 1967

79. SHIPLEY RT, MAHONEY MC: Right middle lobe collapse following right upper lobectomy. Radiology 166:725, 1988

80. SOSMAN MC, DODD GD, JONES WD, ET AL: Pulmonary alveolar microlithiasis. Am J Roentgenol 77:947, 1957

81. SPIZARNY DL, GOODMAN LR: Air in the minor fissure: A sign of right-sided pneumothorax. Radiol 160:329, 1986

82. STOVIN PGI, LUM LC, FLOWER CDR, ET AL: The lungs in lymphangiomyomatosis and in tuberous sclerosis. Thorax 30:497, 1975

83. SWISCHUK LE: Transient respiratory distress of the newborn (TRDN): A temporary disturbance of a normal phenomenon. Am J Roentgenol 108:557, 1970

84. TOCINO IM, MILLER MH, FAIRFAX WR: Distribution of pneumothorax in the supine and semirecumbent critically ill adult. Am J Roentgenol 144:901, 1985

85. UNGER JM, ENGLAND DM, BOGUST GA: Interstitial emphysema in adults: Recognition and prognostic implications. J Thorac Imag 4:86, 1989

86. VALENSI QH: Pulmonary lymphangiomyoma, a probable forme frust of tuberous sclerosis. Am Rev Resp Dis 108:1411, 1973

87. WEBB WR, GOODMAN PC: Fibrosing alveolitis in patients with neurofibromatosis. Radiology 122:289, 1977

88. WEISBROD GL: Pulmonary angiitis and granulomatosis: A review. J Can Assoc Radiol 40:127, 1989

89. WESTCOTT JL, COLE S: Plate atelectasis. Radiology 155:1, 1985

90. WESENBERG RL, GRAVEN SN, MCCABE EB: Radiological findings in wet-lung disease. Radiology 98:69, 1971

91. WILLIAMS JL, MARKOWITZ RI, CAPITANIO MA, ET AL: Immune deficiency syndromes. Semin Roentgenol 10:83, 1975

92. WILSON SR, SANDERS DE, DELARUE NC: Intrathoracic manifestations of amyloid disease. Radiology 120:283, 1976

93. WOLFSON SL, FRECH R, HEWITT C, ET AL: Radiographic diagnosis of hyaline membrane disease. Radiology 93:339, 1969

94. WOLSON AH: Pulmonary findings in Gaucher's disease. Am J Roentgenol 123:712, 1975

95. WOOD BP, ANDERSON VM, MAUK JE, ET AL: Pulmonary interstitial air: Locating "pulmonary interstitial emphysema" of the premature infant. Am J Roentgenol 138: 809, 1982

96. WOODRING JH: Determining the cause of pulmonary atelectasis: A comparison of plain radiography and CT. Am J Roentgenol 150:757, 1988

97. ZYLAK CJ, BANERJEE R, GALBRAITH PA, ET AL: Lung involvement in angioimmunoblastic lymphadenopathy (AIL). Radiology 121:513, 1976

*Paul and Juhl's Essentials of Radiologic Imaging,
Sixth Edition,* edited by John H. Juhl and
Andrew B. Crummy. J.B. Lippincott Company,
Philadelphia, © 1993.

CHAPTER **31**

Diseases of the Pleura, Mediastinum, and Diaphragm

John H. Juhl

THE PLEURA

Pleural disease is common and its detection and evaluation are an important part of imaging of the chest. Pleural and chest-wall disease is evaluated by chest radiography, including oblique, lateral decubitus, and highly penetrated films if necessary. When the chest radiograph is equivocal, computerized tomography is indicated and is usually helpful. CT is also useful when the extent of disease is uncertain. Ultrasound is employed in detecting and localizing pleural fluid, often for guided thoracentesis, and in differentiating between solid masses and fluid in or adjacent to the pleural space.

PLEURAL EFFUSION

General Considerations

The pleural space is lined by a smooth serous membrane that is lubricated by a small amount (5 to 15 ml) of serous fluid. Except for this thin layer of lubricating fluid, the pleural surfaces are in contact; therefore the pleural space is a potential one in the normal person. The formation of excess fluid is caused by many conditions, a number of which are significant diseases either involving the lungs primarily or as a secondary manifestation of systemic disease. The causes include infections by many types of bacteria. Infections caused by viruses, rickettsia, parasites, or fungi may also cause effusion. Massive pleural effusion has been reported in children with coccidioidomycosis; when present, this suggests a severe form of the disease.[55] Renal failure is a frequent cause of pleural effusion, which may be large in some cases. Many patients with collagen–vascular disease develop pleural effusion during the course of the disease. This is particularly true in systemic lupus erythematosus, but also occurs in rheumatoid arthritis and Wegener's granulomatosis. Effusion is common in asbestos-related pleural disease. Subcapsular splenic hematoma may be associated with pleural effusion on the left. Small amounts of effusion occur very frequently in the post partum period. Rarely it occurs in myxedema; pleural endometriosis is also a rare cause of fluid, usually bloody. Malignant tumors of the lung, mediastinum, and chest wall and metastatic tumors may also cause pleural effusion that is often bloody or blood-tinged. In lymphoma, pleural effusion, which may be chylous, is not common but indicates a poor prognosis when it occurs. Diseases that cause lymphatic obstruction, produce hypoproteinemia, cardiac failure, and pulmonary infarction are also accompanied by pleural effusion in many instances. Accidental and surgical trauma produce effusions that are often bloody or blood-tinged. Massive pleural effusion, usually on the left side but sometimes bilateral, may complicate pancreatitis. The fluid contains high levels of amylase and of protein and tends to recur following thoracentesis.

Small pleural effusions are common following upper-abdominal surgery.[38] They tend to disappear spontaneously and do not represent a significant complication, even though a number are exudates. Spontaneous esophageal rupture (Boerhaave's syndrome) is rare but may be followed by pleural effusion. In some patients the cause cannot be found.[66]

Chylous effusion or chylothorax is usually the result of thoracic-duct obstruction or injury (traumatic or surgical) but may be idiopathic.

There is some difference of opinion as to the amount of pleural fluid necessary to produce enough opacity to be visible on a posteroanterior roentgenogram of the chest. Experimentally, in human cadavers as little as 5 ml of fluid was visible in the pleural space in properly exposed lateral decubitus films.[10] If a lateral view can be obtained, small amounts of fluid can be detected by the characteristic appearance of obliteration of the sharp, posterior costophrenic angle by homogeneous opacity that is slightly concave. This concavity can be simulated by thickened pleura and adhesions. Therefore, if detection of a small amount of fluid is necessary, the lateral decubitus view should be obtained with the affected side down. If there is fluid in the posterior sulcus, a vertical beam will then outline a normal acute posterior angle, since the free fluid will move to the dependent lateral thorax. When the posterior costophrenic angle appears normal, the best method for detection of small amounts of fluid is to have the patient lie with the affected side down, following which a horizontal-beam PA or AP film is exposed with the patient in inspiration. Small amounts of fluid will then be visible along the lateral chest wall, because the fluid produces homogeneous density that lies between the inner rib margin and the visceral pleura of the lung. If there is a question as to the presence of fluid producing obliteration of a lateral costophrenic sulcus in the frontal projection, the patient is placed in the lateral decubitus position on the side opposite the affected one and a horizontal beam is directed to obtain an AP or PA roentgenogram. In this instance, if fluid is present it will gravitate to the mediastinum, leaving the costophrenic sulcus sharply angulated. In the critically ill patient, roentgen examination may be limited to the supine projection; it is estimated that 175 to 500 ml of fluid are needed for accurate detection. Signs of fluid in the supine position include (1) homogeneous opacity in the affected hemithorax; (2) obliteration or partial obliteration of the diaphragmatic silhouette; (3) meniscus sign, particularly if the upper thorax can be elevated somewhat; (4) apical capping by fluid, if a large amount is present; and (5) widening of a minor fissure and/or visible lateral aspect of a major fissure.

If a semisupine position can be obtained, oblique films may be very helpful in detecting pleural fluid, which collects posteromedially in the lower thorax in this view. When hydropneumothorax is present in such a patient, one or more of the following signs may lead to its detection: (1) air in the lateral costophrenic angle—the deep sulcus sign; (2) air in the anterior costophrenic angle—the anterior sulcus sign; (3) air in the subpulmonic pleural space; (4) a lucency lateral to pleural line usually indicates pneumothorax, but if the zone between the chest wall and pleural line is dense and the pleural line obscured, fluid is present; (5) a visible pleural line plus increased opacity of the pleural space. If an erect film can be obtained, a fluid level indicates the presence of hydropneumothorax.[51] When findings are equivocal, ultrasound and/or CT can be very useful in detecting fluid.

Large amounts of fluid in the free pleural space gravitate with change in position and these decubitus positions can be used to demonstrate the parts of the pulmonary parenchyma that are obscured by the fluid in the routine upright frontal and lateral chest roentgenograms. For example, the prone position can be used for better visualization of the posterior lung bases. Posteroanterior and horizontal-beam lateral views are obtained.[64] The earliest roentgen sign of fluid on the routine upright chest film is obliteration of the sharp angle produced by the normal costophrenic sulcus. As the amount of fluid increases, more of the diaphragm and the basal lung become obscured by it. The superior border of the fluid is concave and often blurred, because some of the fluid extends upward into the pleural space surrounding the lung. As a rule, the fluid extends higher laterally than medially because of differences in elastic recoil of the lung. When fluid occupies a sizable portion of the volume of the affected hemithorax there is increasing compression of the lung, depression of the diaphragm, and often a shift of the mediastinum to the opposite side. When the effusion is massive and fills one hemithorax, the pulmonary compression and mediastinal shift may become marked.

When films are exposed with the patient in the supine or prone position, free fluid shifts to the most dependent part of the thorax. Therefore it causes a homogeneous hazy opacity that is uniformly distributed throughout the involved hemithorax unless there is loculation. The degree of opacity then varies with the amount of fluid. CT studies have shown that there may be general volume loss without local atelectasis in some patients with large effusions.[52] In others, local atelectasis (segmental or subsegmental) may occur. Total or subtotal lobar atelectasis is present in some patients with large effusions (Fig. 31-1). The lower lobe is usually involved and tends to be elevated, with attenuation of the pulmonary ligament.

Atypical arrangements of pleural fluid may occur as a

Loculated Pleural Effusion

Pleural fluid in varying amounts may become loculated or encapsulated adjacent to any pleural surface, including the interlobar fissures. This occurs commonly in patients with empyema, or hemothorax and in those with pleural adhesions. It is also seen in some patients with cardiac failure. Small amounts of fluid in the interlobar fissures are identified best in lateral and oblique views. The one exception is the minor interlobar fissure on the right, which is usually visible on the PA projection (Fig. 31-2). As the amount of fluid increases, the opacity increases until it may become round or oval and simulate tumor. The differentiation between tumor and loculated fluid can usually be made without difficulty when oblique and lateral views are obtained, because the characteristic elongated or elliptic shape, often with tapering ends in the plane of the fissure, tends to be more prominent in these projections than in the frontal view (Fig. 31-3). The clearly defined borders of these loculated effusions are also of differential diagnostic significance. Fluid in the major interlobar fissures often produces a poorly defined increase in opacity when viewed in the frontal projection; lateral views are usually needed to identify clearly the nature of the process. When fluid is loculated adjacent to the mediastinum, it produces a local or general mediastinal widening that may simulate a mediastinal or pleural tumor. When the fluid adjacent to the mediastinum simulates tumor, decubitus views to show alteration in the shape of the "mass" are helpful in the differential diagnosis and the presence of fluid elsewhere or in the opposite hemithorax is a useful sign whenever loculated fluid simulates mass. The pulmonary ligament anchors the lower lobe to the mediastinum and fluid may be loculated posterior (usually) or anterior to it. Posterior loculation of fluid may simulate retrocardiac atelectasis or mass on the left and an inferomedial mediastinal mass on the right. Decubitus projections usually make the differential diagnosis, but at times, ultrasound or CT must be used to solve the problem. When the fluid is located along the costal surface, it does not ordinarily present a diagnostic problem, but when there is doubt as to the nature of the process or the type of transudate or exudate present, the lesion may be localized and thoracentesis performed.

Infrapulmonary Pleural Effusion

At times, a large pleural effusion may be present in a basal hemithorax, elevating the lung base without distorting it and simulating elevation of the diaphragm.[29] This is observed in upright films, particularly on the right side where the fluid opacity blends with that of the liver and diaphragm below it. On the left, there is

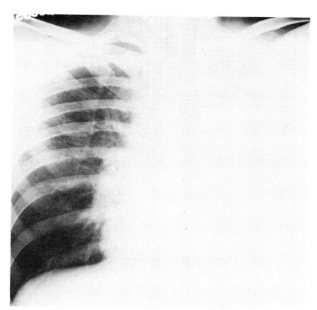

Figure 31–1. Massive pleural effusion, in this case on the left. Note the shift of the mediastinal structures to the right and the complete opacity of the left hemithorax. Massive atelectasis causing complete opacity results in a shift toward the involved side, a helpful differential point.

result of disease in the underlying lung. The differential collapse of diseased pulmonary tissue observed in tuberculosis was the basis for the use of therapeutic pneumothorax. The elasticity of the lung also plays an important part in distribution of fluid. When a change caused by disease modifies the uniform recoiling tendency of the lung, atypical distribution of fluid occurs in the absence of loculation. The presence of fluid without true loculation in these instances can be confirmed by decubitus and other views as needed.

Although the cause of pleural effusion may be obvious in many instances, in many others it is obscure. Fluid can be obtained by thoracentesis and appropriate bacteriological, chemical and cytologic studies obtained, depending on the clinical situation. If fluid is loculated, ultrasound guidance for thoracentesis may be helpful. Sonography is also useful to differentiate pleural fluid from a pleural mass in patients with local pleural opacity.[43] It is of particular value when a bedside examination is needed in a patient who is critically ill. When pleural biopsy is necessary, sonography may also be helpful. Occasionally, CT guidance is necessary to obtain fluid and to characterize and localize pleural masses that may be associated with effusion.

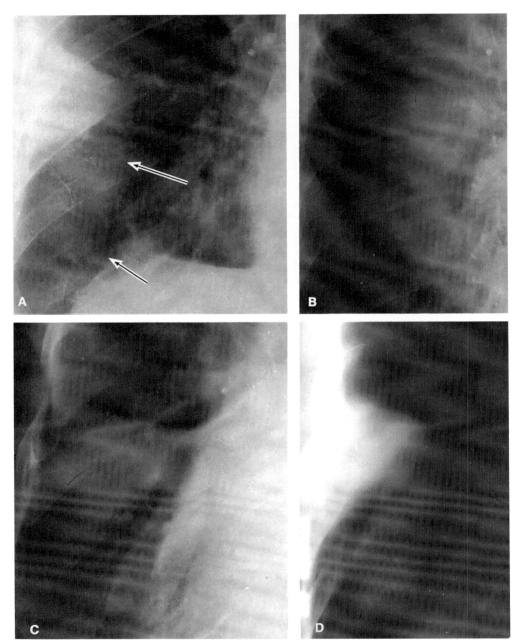

Figure 31–2. Loculated pleural effusion. Some fluid is loculated in the lateral aspect of the minor fissure, and there is an elongated loculation in the major fissure. (**A**) Frontal projection. Arrows outline the lower loculation, which is faintly visualized since it does not cause much density in this projection. (**B**) Left anterior oblique view. (**C**) Right anterior oblique view. (**D**) Tomogram, which outlines the fluid in the major and minor fissures.

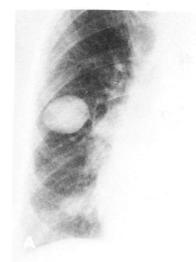
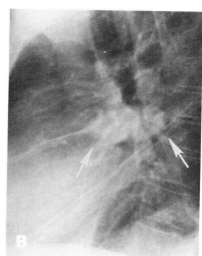

Figure 31–3. Loculated pleural effusion simulating tumor (pseudotumor). The mass in the right central lung is noted to be round in (**A**) the frontal view and elongated in (**B**) the lateral view (*arrows*). In the lateral projection, it can be clearly recognized as fluid in the interlobar fissure.

usually enough air in the stomach or colon to localize the diaphragm. In some instances the costophrenic angle appears to be preserved while in others there is slight blunting or concavity of the normally acute angle. In the latter instance, infrapulmonary effusion can be suspected, but when the lateral inferior lung margin is maintained so that a costophrenic sulcus is simulated, a high index of suspicion is necessary to make the diagnosis. At times, a very small amount of fluid in an interlobar fissure will be the only sign of effusion. In most instances the costophrenic sulcus appears to be displaced a few millimeters away from the inner chest wall; oblique projections may be needed to demonstrate this sign. Another sign is absence of visible intrapulmonary vessels below the level of the dome of the diaphragm. Normally these vessels can be observed well below this level. Alterations in the superior surface of the subpulmonary opacity produced by fluid also aid in the diagnosis in some instances. The dome of the diaphragm tends to be more lateral than in the normal person, with a rather sharp downward inclination laterally. This tends to be accentuated on expiration and may be demonstrated only on a film exposed with the patient in expiration. This is probably caused by central fixation of the lower lobe to the mediastinum by the pulmonary ligament.

When an infrapulmonary effusion is present on the left, the diagnosis is made more readily because the presence of air in the stomach usually outlines its fundus and identifies the position of the diaphragm in the routine frontal and lateral chest roentgenograms. Fluoroscopy or roentgenograms with the patient in the lateral decubitus position are used to confirm the presence of infrapulmonary effusion. The fluid is then distributed in the dependent hemithorax and causes an opacity along the chest wall. In addition, the diaphragm can be identified. Its position is noted to be lower than the opacity simulating diaphragm in the upright view (Fig. 31-4). If the effusion is loculated, ultrasound or CT may be needed to differentiate it from other conditions.

Large pleural effusions may invert the left hemidiaphragm so a pseudomass is produced in the left upper quadrant of the abdomen.[67] When the effusion is massive and there is significant inversion, paradoxical diaphragmatic motion may be observed on the ipsilateral side. When inversion is present, the diagnosis can be confirmed by supine or decubitus projections; also the "mass" disappears after thoracentesis. Rarely the right hemidiaphragm may be inverted by massive effusion, usually in patients with some pleural adhesions. In these patients, a pseudomass of the liver is produced which may be difficult to assess, even with CT.[28] Occasionally, fluid below the diaphragm will simulate subpulmonary effusion. We have observed one patient with a left subphrenic abscess which displaced the stomach downward, simulating infrapulmonary effusion with some diaphragmatic inversion. Ascites can occasionally widen the distance between the diaphragm and stomach, simulating subpulmonary effusion. Also on CT a band of basal atelectasis can simulate a hemidiaphragm in the presence of infrapulmonary effusion.[18] Usually, however, the band is tapered or thickened and is often interrupted rather than continuous, so careful observation will usually make the correct diagnosis possible. Several signs have been described on CT studies which, when taken together, differentiate pleural fluid from ascites or demonstrate

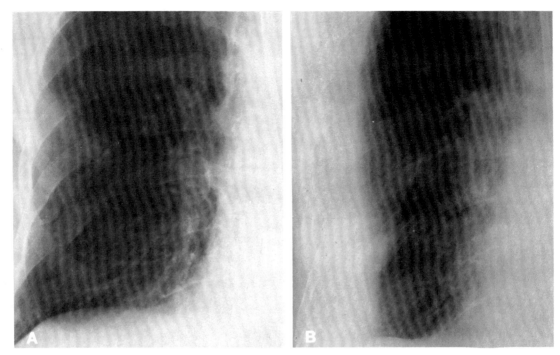

Figure 31–4.   Infrapulmonary pleural effusion. **(A)** Upright frontal projection. The right lower lung and dome of the diaphragm are included. The costophrenic angle is clear, but the cardiohepatic angle is slightly blurred. In comparison to the left side, the right hemidiaphragm was high, therefore effusion was suspected. **(B)** This right lateral decubitus projection shows a large amount of fluid along the right lateral thoracic wall, confirming the presence of infrapulmonary fluid, which was suspected in the initial examination.

that both are present.[25] The signs are: (1) The diaphragm sign—pleural fluid is outside the diaphragm, ascites is inside the diaphragm. (2) Displaced crus—the crus of the diaphragm is displaced anteriorly and laterally away from the spine by pleural effusion. (3) Interface sign—the interface between fluid and liver is indistinct with pleural effusion and distinct with ascites. (4) Bare area sign—there is lack of fluid opacity in the hepatic bare area in ascites.

Summary

Pleural fluid causes a homogeneous opacity that does not vary significantly with the type of fluid. In the upright chest roentgenogram obtained in the frontal projection, several hundred cubic centimeters of fluid may be present without producing any roentgen change, but much smaller amounts, ranging from 25 (or less) to 100 ml, can be detected when lateral decubitus views are obtained. Small amounts can also be detected using CT. As the amount of fluid increases, it gradually obscures the diaphragm and lower lung and,

when large, tends to depress the diaphragm and displace the mediastinum to the opposite side. Free fluid is often concave superiorly, unless air or gas is present, in which case a straight, horizontal gas–fluid level is present. Loculated fluid may simulate tumor but recumbent, lateral, and decubitus views plus progress roentgenograms to show the rapid changes that often occur are usually sufficient to make the proper diagnosis. If not, ultrasound or CT may be used. Pulmonary disease may alter pulmonary elasticity and lead to atypical accumulations of free pleural fluid. Fluid within pre-existing peripheral cysts or bullae may simulate loculated pleural effusion. Usually sonography or CT is of value, but occasionally loculated pleural fluid cannot be differentiated from parenchymal disease or intracystic intrapulmonary fluid.[71]

Ultrasound is a relatively inexpensive, rapid method that can be used to differentiate loculated pleural fluid from pleural masses when conventional studies cannot make this determination (Fig. 31-5). It also can be used to direct aspiration of fluid or needle biopsy of a mass. Real-time scanning is particularly useful. The dia-

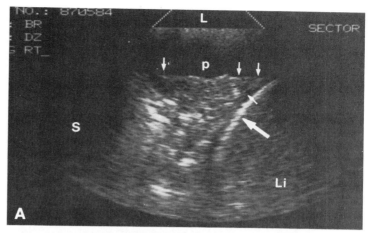

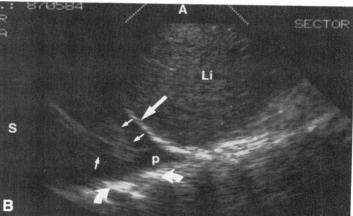

Figure 31–5. Ultrasonogram of lower thorax showing pleural effusion. (**A**) Coronal plane from right side, upper abdomen between ribs. Superior (*S*) and lateral (*L*); liver (*Li*) in an inferior position; pleural effusion (*p*); atelectatic lung (*small arrows*); diaphragm (*large arrow*). (**B**) Longitudinal plane shows anechoic fluid (*p*); surrounding nonaerated (echogenic) lung (*small arrows*); and ribs with acoustic shadowing (*curved arrows*). Anterior (*A*), superior (*S*), and liver (*Li*). (Courtesy of Robert Rosenberg, MD)

phragm can usually be identified and inversion, if present, can therefore be detected. When ultrasound fails to resolve the problem, CT can be used to identify and localized fluid and to guide aspiration (Fig. 31-6).

INFLAMMATORY DISEASES

Acute Pleuritis

Acute infection of the pleura results in a serofibrinous inflammatory reaction that causes some pleural thickening and edema. This produces opacity that can sometimes be recognized radiographically, provided the area of involvement is situated in a region in which the thickness of the pleura can be determined. This condition is often associated with considerable pain, resulting in some fixation of the thorax and decrease in diaphragmatic motion as well as elevation of the diaphragm; in some instances these diaphragmatic changes may be the only roentgen signs. A correlation of history, clinical findings, and roentgen findings usu-

ally makes the diagnosis but may not determine etiology. A small amount of pleural effusion may result and, if it is large enough in amount, it can be recognized. The diagnosis of acute fibrinous or serofibrinous pleurisy is not ordinarily difficult to make on clinical examination, but chest roentgenography is of value in excluding the possibility of other disease even though the small area of pleural thickening or fluid associated with it may not be visible.

Chronic Pleural Thickening (Fibrosis)

Chronic, nonsuppurative pleural disease may be caused by a variety of bacteria; tuberculosis is among the common causes. Pleuritis of tuberculous origin is often localized to the apex of the lung. The apical pleural thickening or cap may not indicate previous tuberculosis, however. In some instances, the pleural cap consists of thickening of the visceral pleural plus nonspecific fibrosis of the subpleural lung.[58] Its inci-

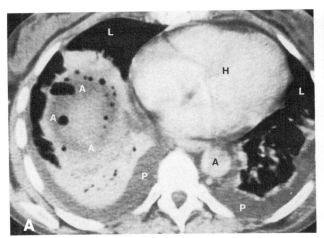
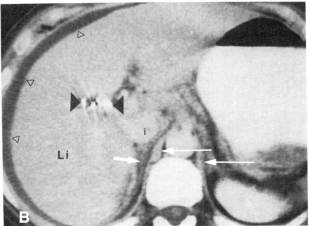

Figure 31–6. CT showing bilateral pleural effusion in a patient with right subphrenic abscess. (**A**) Lower chest section. Pleural fluid bilaterally (*p*) above diaphragm; abscess containing bubbles of gas (*white A's*) separated from the pleural effusion by the diaphragm, which is obscured by the inflammatory disease; heart (*H*); descending aorta (*black A*); lung (*L*). (**B**) This section is 10 cm lower than **A**. Subphrenic fluid or abscess (*open arrowheads*); liver (*Li*); crus of diaphragm (*long arrows*); right adrenal (*short arrow*); inferior vena cava in liver (*i*); surgical clips in gallbladder bed (*black arrowheads*). (Courtesy of Richard Logan, MD)

dence increases with age, so nonspecific infection of the subpleural lung associated with some ischemia may be the cause in some cases. Chronic pleuritis results in pleural thickening manifested by soft-tissue opacity between the inner aspect of the ribs and the adjacent lung. The inner surface is often irregular. The amount varies from a very thin linear band to a large amount of homogeneous density, representing grossly thickened fibrotic pleura. In other instances, pleural thickening may extend along the lateral chest wall to the base and occasionally may surround the entire lung, resulting in gradual fibrotic contraction leading to decrease in size of the involved hemithorax, along with the homogeneous opacity produced by the thickened fibrotic pleura. It is not uncommon to find large, thick, calcium plaques in the pleura in these patients. Occasionally a shell of pleural calcification may encase large portions of the lung and may also extend into the interlobar fissures. It is manifested by irregular linear plaques of opacity that are more opaque than the soft-tissue density produced by thick pleura alone. Any organism that produces chronic granulomatous inflammatory disease may cause these changes. Such pleural fibrosis may result in marked decrease in volume of the hemithorax and consequent loss of pulmonary function may require decortication to free the lung and allow functional improvement.

When extensive bilateral pleural thickening is pres-

ent, particularly if linear calcific plaques are visible in the diaphragmatic pleura, asbestos exposure is nearly always the cause. Noncalcified local pleural thickening is somewhat more frequent in asbestos workers than are the linear calcifications just described. These pleural plaques may be quite thin and inconspicuous. Apical involvement is rare in asbestos exposure, and costophrenic angle obliteration is also rare. Calcification is usually a late finding and is most frequently observed in the parietal pleura of the diaphragm (Fig. 31-7). Calcific plaques may also occur along the mediastinal pleura and along the lower lateral chest wall (parietal pleura) bilaterally. They are usually seen as linear or irregular plaques which are not very thick, in contrast to the heavy, irregular plaques that may occur in chronic inflammatory disease. Parenchymal pulmonary involvement need not be roentgenographically visible in asbestos-related pleural disease.

CT is of particular value in determining the presence of pleural plaques in asbestos workers. They may be difficult or impossible to detect on plain chest radiographs. Extrapleural fat is common and can be differentiated from fibrous pleural plaques by differences in attenuation.

In many instances, small amounts of pleural thickening are noted along one or both thoracic walls in patients with no history of antecedent disease, so that the cause cannot be established. Often this may be caused

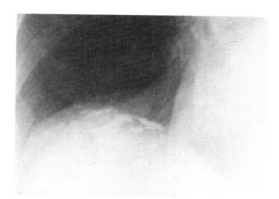

Figure 31–7. Asbestos-related pleural calcification. Note the dense linear masses of calcium in the diaphragmatic pleura. No basal pulmonary disease is present.

by asbestos in patients who may not have a history of working in an industry in which known exposure has occurred.

Unilateral pleural thickening with calcification is nearly always secondary to inflammatory disease or to trauma with calcification in a hematoma. It is not infrequent to observe obliteration of a costophrenic sulcus in patients who previously have had pneumonia with associated pleuritis. Pleural infection results in more or less obliteration of the pleural space as a result of fibrous adhesions between the visceral and parietal layers. These adhesions are recognized roentgenographically by their effect on adjacent structures as well as by visualization of the bandlike density representing them. Adhesions over the diaphragm may produce small, local tentlike elevations of the diaphragm. Similar distortion may be caused by contraction of local pulmonary lesions, however. Adhesions between the pleura and pericardium can sometimes be recognized roentgenographically by small spikelike irregularities of the outline of the pericardium. When sizable pneumothorax is present, the presence of adhesions can be readily detected because the lung pulls away from the parietal pleura if there are no adhesions.

Empyema

Thoracic empyema, or pyothorax, is an inflammatory disease of the pleura with suppuration that results in an accumulation of pus in the pleural space. A number of organisms may cause this disease, including *Mycobacterium tuberculosis*. Staphylococcal pneumonia is frequently complicated by empyema. It is likely that any organism capable of causing pulmonary infection may also produce empyema, the latter is usually, but not

always, a complication of the former. Roentgenograms outline the empyema as a mass that may vary in size from a large lesion that obscures most of the lung to a relatively small loculated mass along the chest wall or in an interlobar fissure. Postpneumonic empyemas usually occur along the posterior pleural space or within an interlobar fissure. Anterior empyema from this cause is very rare. There need not be evidence of associated pulmonary disease. If present, the type of alteration in the lungs resulting from the disease may aid in determining the cause of the empyema. In the acute stage there is usually some inflammation in the lung adjacent to the empyema and this results in fuzzy irregularity of the margin. The fluid may not be loculated early in the disease. In the more chronic empyema the pulmonary inflammatory reaction may subside so the mass is more clearly defined and sharply demarcated from the adjacent aerated lung (Fig. 31-8). Air or gas within the empyema causes a fluid level and indicates communication with a bronchus, the skin surface, or an infection by gas-forming organisms. The pleural infection is usually peripheral, with one part of the empyema adjacent to the costal pleura. It can be localized roentgenographically or fluoroscopically but may be difficult to differentiate from peripheral lung abscess in some cases. Ultrasound is helpful in differ-

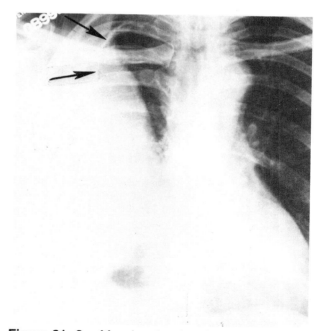

Figure 31–8. Massive loculated pleural density. Arrows indicate some linear calcification in the pleura. This large loculation was found to represent a chronic empyema.

entiating empyema from a solid pleural mass. If this examination doesn't yield sufficient information, CT can be used. The CT signs of empyema are: (1) The wall is oval or lenticular, in contrast to the round appearance of a lung abscess. (2) Empyema wall is smooth and relatively uniform in thickness, in contrast to the variable thickness and irregular outline of the exterior wall of the lung abscess. (3) Bronchi and vessels are compressed, displaced, or distorted and do not end abruptly as in abscess. (4) Pleural separation, the "split pleural sign" caused by a fibrin peel surrounding the pus in the empyema, is present in about two thirds or more. (5) Compression of the lung occurs in empyema, but not with an abscess. Empyema may be loculated in the subpulmonic space and simulate subpulmonic effusion or subphrenic abscess; CT is valuable in making the differential diagnosis. However, a loculated intrapleural hematoma may simulate empyema and differentiation from lung abscess may be difficult at times, particularly in empyema involving an interlobar fissure, so CT must be interpreted very carefully to minimize errors. When contrast is used, CT usually demonstrates enhancement of the parietal pleura, thickening of the parietal pleura, and thickening of extrapleural subcostal tissues; sometimes there is also some enhancement (increased attenuation) of extrapleural fat.[70] When empyema develops in a postpneumonectomy space, the concavity produced by the herniated normal lung may become a convexity extending to the contralateral side if the empyema attains sufficient size.[27]

TUMORS OF THE PLEURA

Benign Tumors

Pleural-based tumors include lipoma, fibroma, fibromyxoma, hemangioma, chondroma, and neurofibroma; these tumors actually originate in the chest wall and project into the thorax. Lipoma is the most common of this group and can be differentiated from the others on CT because of its low attenuation. Thin-needle biopsy can then be done if necessary to avoid thoracotomy. The other tumors usually cannot be distinguished from one another unless typical calcifications are visible in a hemangioma or chondroma. The one possible exception is liposarcoma, where areas of low attenuation are interspersed with areas of higher opacity, often poorly defined, representing the malignancy (malignant cells) within the lipomatous mass. Recognition of this pattern on CT should lead to the inclusion of this tumor in the differential diagnosis.[47] Most pleural-based tumors have obtuse angles with the thoracic wall, in contrast to the acute angle observed with intrapulmonary masses, however, this is not a reliable sign, with pedunculated mesothelioma a notable exception. The fibrous pleural mesothelioma is the only benign tumor that originates in the pleura. It is localized and may be pedunculated and move in relationship to other thoracic structures. It may be lobulated, usually arises from the visceral pleura (75%), and its pleural origin may not be obvious because there may be an acute angle between it and the chest wall. When pedunculated, the appearance may change markedly; this can be observed particularly well at fluoroscopy or on decubitus films. The pleural-based or chest-wall tumors may become very large and produce large, smoothly rounded or lobulated densities, the internal aspects of which are clearly outlined by the air-filled lung. The outer aspects blend into the chest wall and may produce some widening of the intercostal space and rib erosion or deformity to indicate that they are primary chest-wall tumors. At times it is necessary to differentiate them from tumors arising in the lung. CT is useful in defining the extent of these masses. It also outlines the relationship of the lung and chest wall to the mass. When the tumor occurs in the fissures, it simulates a pulmonary mass. However, if it can be localized to a fissure on radiographs obtained in several projections or on CT, the possibility of fibrous mesothelioma should be considered.[65] However, there are no pathognomonic CT signs.[14]

Primary Malignant Tumors

Diffuse pleural mesothelioma is usually malignant; its relationship to asbestos exposure has been well documented. These tumors are usually unilateral but may spread to the pericardium or opposite pleural surface late in the course of the disease. They arise in the pleura, often in the interlobar fissures, and extend rapidly to involve a large part of the pleural space. The roentgen findings consists of a somewhat scalloped-appearing mass involving the pleura. It is often extensive when first observed, and may surround the entire lung (Fig. 31-9). Earlier, an irregular nodular or scalloped pleural mass may be observed. Pleural effusion is common and may obscure the tumor.

Effusion may be the first sign of the tumor and may be massive in the presence of a relatively small mass arising in the pleura. When massive effusion is present, mediastinal shift toward the contralateral side may not occur because of fixation of the mediastinum by tumor. Fluid tends to reaccumulate rapidly following thoracentesis. When extensive, these tumors may block the lymphatics sufficiently to result in accumulation of interstitial fluid in the lungs, so that severe interstitial edema is observed. The major differential problem is metastatic malignancy with extensive pleural involvement. If the fluid is drained the tumor may be visible. Even then, the appearance simulates that of pleural thickening and loculated fluid associated

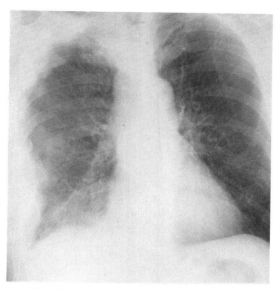

Figure 31–9. Malignant mesothelioma of the pleura on the right. Note the irregular lobulated pleural density, surrounding the lung, representing the tumor. There is very little pleural effusion.

with the pleural disease, so diagnosis usually depends on biopsy.[1] Local mesothelioma occasionally may be malignant, although it is usually considered benign. Radiographically, the only sign suggesting malignancy is rib erosion caused by the invasion of the chest wall.

CT is used extensively in the study of patients suspected of having malignant mesothelioma. Three patterns have been described: (1) focal round tumor nodules with intervening areas of normal pleura (29%); (2) focal round tumor nodules superimposed on diffuse pleural thickening (43%); and (3) focal plaque like areas of tumor (29%).[61] Pleural effusion is present in 80%, pleural calcification in 55%, lung invasion in about 80%, and hilar or mediastinal adenopathy in 19%. Although the extent of the mass can be determined by CT, invasion of the chest wall and/or lung may be very difficult to assess. Final diagnosis must be made by biopsy, because the tumor type cannot be determined by CT. MRI has also been used in the study of these tumors; its major value seems to be in the assessment of mediastinal involvement.[1, 40]

Metastatic Tumors

Metastatic pleural tumors occur much more frequently than the malignant primary neoplasms. Of these, bronchogenic carcinoma is the most common, either by direct invasion or by tumor emboli to the visceral pleura as the result of pulmonary artery invasion. The metastatic pleural tumor arising from a distant primary source in many instances is very small and forms tiny nodules in the visceral or parietal pleura that are not visible roentgenographically. Bloody pleural effusion is common, so the major roentgen finding is often that of pleural effusion. There may be direct extension into the pleura from a chest-wall metastasis in which rib is also involved. Then a soft-tissue chest-wall mass and irregular rib destruction indicate there is a malignant neoplasm present to account for the pleural effusion and mass projecting into the pleural space. The history of primary tumor elsewhere is of great importance in making the roentgen diagnosis. Aside from lung, breast carcinoma is the most common cause of pleural metastases, but the primary tumor may be in the pancreas, ovary, colon, or other sites of adenocarcinoma. Lymphoma may also invade the pleura, usually in far advanced disease in conjunction with recurrent mediastinal or pulmonary involvement.[63] Plasma-cell myeloma involving ribs often results in a chest-wall mass, displacing and sometimes invading the pleura. Roentgen signs of pleural metastases may be indirect (e.g., a pleural effusion containing blood and malignant cells) or direct (e.g., a pleural mass visible on chest roentgenogram). When a malignant pleural effusion is present, CT is useful in detecting small pleural nodules that may not be visible on conventional studies.

NON-NEOPLASTIC PLEURAL MASSES
Thoracic Splenosis

Thoracic splenosis is a rare condition that occurs when there is simultaneous splenic and diaphragmatic rupture.[45] Splenic implants on the pleura grow into small masses of splenic tissue. There may also be implants on the pericardium and peritoneum. The splenic implants are functional and need not be removed if they are asymptomatic. Single or multiple small (usually less than 3 cm) pleural nodules may be observed on the roentgenogram. The nodules are usually discovered months to years after the inciting trauma on incidental chest radiographs. When such a nodule is seen and the diagnosis suspected, a radionuclide spleen scan (using 99mTechnetium sulfur colloid) can be done. If uptake is high, indicating the likelihood of splenosis, it can be confirmed using 99mTc-labelled heat-damaged erythrocytes, which are sequestered by splenic tissue.

Pleural Endometriosis

In the rare instances when pleural endometriosis is present, symptoms are cyclical. Pleural endometriosis may occur in patients with diaphragmatic defects. Multiple small pleural nodules, pleural fluid, and defects in the diaphragm may be observed. CT and sonography may be needed to make the diagnosis.[30]

Fibrin Bodies

Fibrin bodies—or fibrin "balls"—are made up of masses of fibrin that resemble tumor within the pleural space. They form in patients with fibrinous pleuritis with effusion and are usually obscured by the fluid during formation. When the fluid is removed by means of thoracentesis or is absorbed, the fibrin bodies become apparent. The roentgen findings are those of round or oval, single or multiple masses, usually appearing at the base, which become visible after an effusion has been drained or absorbed. Alteration of the patient's position may result in displacement of these bodies. When this is observed, the diagnosis is almost certain. However, occasionally a pedunculated tumor such as a fibrous pleural mesothelioma may change position in a similar manner. A fibrin body may disappear spontaneously, or may persist for years. Fluoroscopy may be of value if the masses move freely. CT may also be helpful.

THE MEDIASTINUM

Because a number of structures lie within the mediastinum and tumors metastasize there, several diagnostic possibilities arise when abnormality is seen. CT has proved to be the most productive study when a mediastinal abnormality is observed on plain films. CT used to study 71 patients with mediastinal widening correctly identified masses, anatomic variants, and vascular abnormalities in 92%.[3] CT findings were indeterminate in 4% and incorrect in 4%. A correct specific diagnosis was made in 58%, which obviated further diagnostic evaluation.

There have been a number of studies comparing CT with MRI in lung cancer staging. As a rule these modalities are complementary, although CT is the first study done when mediastinal disease is observed or suspected on chest radiography.

MRI has also been used experimentally and clinically in mediastinal disease.[2] Because several imaging sequences are usually required, MRI is more time-consuming and expensive; therefore, it is often necessary to limit the clinical use of MRI in mediastinal disease. Invasion of vascular structures is often demonstrated better on MRI than on CT; the same is true of subtle invasion of other mediastinal structures. The ability to produce coronal and sagittal images is an advantage of MRI which is of definite value in some situations, such as superior pulmonary sulcus (Pancoast) tumor where vascular and CNS invasion is more clearly defined. The ultimate place of these two modalities in relation to various abnormalities in the mediastinum and thorax has yet to be determined.

INFLAMMATORY DISEASES

Acute Mediastinitis

Acute inflammations of the mediastinum, although rare, usually arise following injury of the esophagus caused by ingestion of sharp foreign bodies or instrumentation of the esophagus. When esophageal rupture is suspected, it can be confirmed quickly by the demonstration of extravasation of ingested contrast material into the mediastinum or pleural space. Occasionally inflammation extends into the mediastinum from infections involving the sternum, spine, anterior chest wall, and mediastinal lymph nodes, and rarely from infections originating in the anterior neck or the subdiaphragmatic area. These mediastinal infections may result in the formation of abscesses, which may rupture into the esophagus, tracheobronchial tree, or pleural space. These ruptures may cause a rapid change in the mediastinal contour as well as a sudden clinical change. When antibiotics are given early following an esophageal injury, abscess formation is uncommon, so the incidence of mediastinal abscess is now relatively low. The chest radiographic findings include a diffuse increase in opacity and widening of the mediastinum to both sides of the midline in the region of involvement. If the process extends downward from a retropharyngeal abscess, roentgenograms of the neck obtained in lateral projection often show the soft-tissue mass displacing the pharynx and trachea anteriorly. When the infection has resulted from esophageal injury it is not uncommon to observe a small amount of mediastinal emphysema manifested by streaks of radiolucency. If an abscess becomes chronic, it may be large and clearly defined so its appearance may simulate that of mediastinal tumor. It is not unusual to have enough pleural reaction to produce effusion. The suspicion of acute mediastinitis arises on the basis of correlation of roentgen findings with the clinical history. CT can then be used to define more clearly the mediastinal abnormalities. The findings are varied. In some, there is diffuse involvement leading to loss of tissue planes and mediastinal widening, local or diffuse (Fig. 31-10). In others, a local mediastinal abscess is present. There may also be gas in the soft tissues if the esophagus is ruptured or if the infection is caused by gas-forming organisms. In patients who have had surgery with sternotomy, soft-tissue planes are effaced so benign postoperative changes may not be differentiated from acute mediastinitis.[6, 8] In more subacute or chronic situations, osteomyelitis of the sternum may be present, usually after sternotomy. A rapid accumulation of blood, chyle, or edema fluid may also cause acute mediastinal widening. The history and clinical findings are usually helpful in differentiating these conditions.

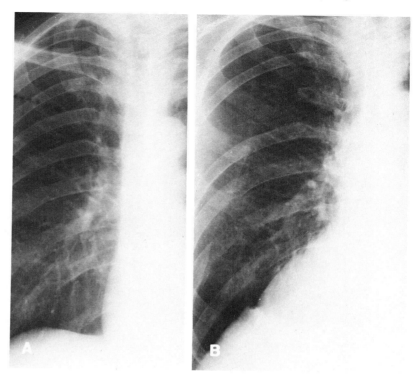

Figure 31–10. Acute mediastinitis. **(A)** No mediastinal abnormalities are noted in this preliminary examination. **(B)** Examination performed 2 weeks following resection of an esophageal neoplasm. The patient had developed an acute febrile illness. Now the mediastinal border on the right is indistinct superiorly. There is some widening, and the infection resulted in mediastinal pleuritis, with loculated pleural fluid producing the mass at the right medial base.

Chronic Mediastinitis

Granulomatous Mediastinitis

Tuberculosis, histoplasmosis, and rarely actinomycosis may produce a chronic granulomatous infection in the mediastinum. Other organisms are less commonly the cause. The involvement is usually in the upper mediastinum at and above the level of the hila and usually anterior to the trachea. Slight mediastinal widening is often the only finding. The radiographic findings are not characteristic and may be very minor, consisting of slight mediastinal widening, which is usually more evident on the right. There may or may not be calcified nodes associated with the chronic disease, which often is asymptomatic. Occasionally diffuse mediastinal inflammation caused by histoplasmosis results in enough fibrosis to obstruct the superior vena cava, and in these patients roentgen findings may be minimal. There may be associated pulmonary involvement. Enlargement of mediastinal nodes is common early in the disease. These nodes may decrease in size and disappear in the chronic phase, however. In other patients they may calcify and may gradually increase in size. If they are adjacent to the superior vena cava, they may produce caval obstruction many years after the initial infection.

Chronic Fibrous (Sclerosing) Mediastinitis

Occasionally, signs of superior caval obstruction will appear in a patient with no history of pulmonary, esophageal, tracheal, or pharyngeal disease. These signs evidently may be caused by a number of conditions, most commonly histoplasmosis, but there may be other infectious causes as well as an idiopathic process similar to that noted in retroperitoneal fibrosis.[26, 42] Nocardia may occasionally cause mediastinitis with caval obstruction, and rarely sarcoidosis is responsible. The location of the disease is the same as in chronic granulomatous mediastinitis—namely, the upper anterior half of the mediastinum. Roentgen findings consist of slight mediastinal widening, often slightly more in the right paratracheal area than elsewhere. Hilar enlargement may or may not be present, sometimes with evidence of calcified nodes. Some tracheal narrowing may also be present. Venography can be used to demonstrate venous obstruction, but CT with intravenous contrast can also be used. MRI is better at assessing vascular patency without the use of contrast agents. As indicated above, CT or MRI are sometimes of value, particularly when a well-defined granulomatous mass is observed, which may be amenable to surgery.[39, 59] When the fibrosis is diffuse and CT shows obliteration of fat planes, narrowing or obstruction of vessels or proximal airways, or narrowing of the esophagus, surgery may have little to offer. When the mediastinal fibrosis is a part of systematic fibrosis, which often begins in the retroperitoneum, the process is often predominantly posterior.[35] Granulomatous histoplasmosis may also be posterior.[36] Calcifications are present in some patients. The clinical findings must be correlated with radiographic findings to determine diagnosis. If tissue diagnosis is needed, mediastinoscopy or surgical exploration may be necessary.

Inflammatory Diseases of the Mediastinal Lymph Nodes

In nearly all infectious diseases of the lungs and bronchi there is histopathologic involvement of the mediastinal nodes, but most of these diseases do not usually cause enough enlargement to be of roentgen importance. There are chronic pulmonary inflammatory diseases, however, in which there is sufficient enlargement of hilar and mediastinal nodes to produce recognizable opacity on chest radiographs.

Acute Nonspecific Lymphadenopathy
Some enlargement of the hilum shadow is often present in pneumonia, but is so minimal it usually escapes detection or is obscured by the pulmonary infection. Lung abscess is frequently accompanied by hilar and/or mediastinal adenopathy. Rarely, infectious mononucleosis is associated with mediastinal adenopathy. Occasionally an infected node may undergo suppuration, leading to acute mediastinitis or mediastinal abscess.

Chronic Inflammations
Occasionally, lymph nodes are enlarged in patients with chronic suppurative disease of the bronchi and in some patients with mucoviscidosis, leading to recognizable hilar enlargement which is often poorly defined and is associated with the accentuation of basal markings and patchy pneumonia often found in bronchiectasis. A number of fungi are capable of producing pulmonary disease and they also involve the hilar nodes, resulting in enlargement. Adenopathy is most commonly found in the acute phase of coccidiodomycosis and histoplasmosis and may be present in other infectious diseases, such as actinomycosis and blastomycosis. In these diseases the pulmonary infection produces changes that have been described in the previous chapters relating to these infections. This involvement of hilar and mediastinal nodes often leads to calcification in the nodes, which requires 1 or 2 years to develop. It is most commonly observed in histoplasmosis.

Primary tuberculosis is almost always associated with mediastinal lymphadenopathy, particularly in children. The enlargement of hilar or paratracheal nodes may or may not be associated with a visible parenchymal lesion. Characteristically, in primary tuberculosis a single group of nodes is involved. If more than one group is affected, one group is usually considerably larger than the other. The roentgen findings are those of a somewhat lobulated node enlargement; the outline of the hilum may be moderately fuzzy and indistinct. A visible parenchymal lesion may be present. When the acute phase is over, the borders of the hilum become more distinct and nodes gradually decrease in size. Calcification is often noted after a year or more.

All of these chronic inflammatory diseases that involve the lungs, as well as the mediastinal nodes, must be differentiated from one another by appropriate skin tests and bacteriologic studies, as indicated in Chapters 25 and 26. Node enlargement is noted in a variety of noninfectious diseases of the lungs, including some of the pneumoconioses. In these patients the pulmonary lesions are usually predominant. Massive mediastinal lymph-node enlargement has been reported occasionally in patients without other disease. The large nodes simulate mediastinal tumors or malignant lymphomas. Biopsy reveals a nonspecific chronic lymphadenitis. Sarcoidosis is usually associated with lymphadenopathy sufficient to produce recognizable enlargement of hilar and mediastinal lymph nodes at some time during the course of the disease.

Other Causes of Mediastinal Node Enlargement
Giant mediastinal lymph node hyperplasia (Castleman's disease) is an asymptomatic, idiopathic, massive adenopathy usually appearing as a solitary mass—most commonly in the middle or posterior mediastinum.[31] The mass becomes extremely large but does not calcify. *Benign lymphoid hyperplasia* may be associated with abnormalities of the immune system such as hypergammaglobulinemia. *Angioimmunoblastic (immunoblastic) lymphadenopathy* is a hyperimmune disorder that may resemble Hodgkin's disease. It causes enlargement of mediastinal nodes similar to that noted in Hodgkin's disease. It occurs in men more often than in women, usually in those older than 50 years of age. Roentgenographic findings are similar to those in Hodgkin's disease. The three disorders just described must be differentiated from disseminated malignant disease by laboratory methods and by biopsy.

MEDIASTINAL TUMORS AND ALLIED LESIONS

There are a number of structures within and extending through the mediastinum. Tumors, cysts, and other masses may arise from any of them. There is a correlation between location within the mediastinum and the type of mass. Table 31-1 lists the causes of mass lesions

located in each mediastinal compartment. When large, any of the masses may occupy portions of two or even three compartments. The conditions causing lymph node enlargement, although predominantly in the middle mediastinum, may also involve the anterior mediastinum. Hematoma may occur in any of the com-partments.

In addition to routine roentgenograms in frontal and lateral projections, it may be useful to obtain oblique projections. Esophagrams or vascular studies may be needed in some cases. CT is very useful to determine the location, site, extent, and relative density of medi-astinal masses and is indicated unless some obvious cause such as esophageal hiatus hernia is present. Its utility in locating obscure lesions and in determining relative tissue density and extent of mediastinal tumors as well as in the investigation of abnormal plain-film findings has been demonstrated, as previously indi-cated. When the mass is localized in relation to other mediastinal structures and its characteristics are deter-mined, it is often possible to be reasonably certain of the diagnosis. In other instances, biopsy is necessary to make the histologic diagnosis. MRI has also been used in the study of mediastinal masses, as mentioned earlier.

TUMORS OF THE MEDIASTINAL LYMPH NODES

The Lymphomas

Hodgkin's Disease

Four histologic types of Hodgkin's disease are classified by the Committee on Nomenclature of the American Cancer Society:[41]

Cell Type	Frequency[7]
1. Lymphocytic	5% to 7%
2. Nodular sclerosis	60% to 65%
3. Mixed cellularity	25%
4. Lymphocyte depletion	5%

The same report on staging lists the following:

Stage I—disease limited to one anatomic region or two contiguous anatomic regions on the same side of the diaphragm

Stage II—disease in more than two anatomic regions or in two noncontiguous regions on the same side of the diaphragm

Stage III—disease on both sides of the diaphragm, but not extending beyond the involvement of lymph nodes, spleen, and/or Waldeyer's ring

Stage IV—Involvement of the bone marrow, lung parenchyma, pleura, liver, bone, skin, kidney, gastrointestinal tract, or any tissue or organ in addition to lymph nodes, spleen or Waldeyer's ring

The stages are subclassified as A, absence of, or B, presence of systemic symptoms of weight loss, fever, night sweats, or pruritus not explained by other dis-ease. A classification of non-Hodgkin's lymphomas, published in 1982, is presented in Table 31-2.[48] Several other classifications are included in that paper for those interested.

Of 164 patients with untreated Hodgkin's disease studied by Filly and co-workers, 67% had radiographic evidence of intrathoracic disease.[20] They compared these with a group of 136 patients with non-Hodgkin's

Table 31-1. Location of Mediastinal Masses

ANTERIOR	MIDDLE	POSTERIOR
Thymic cysts and tumors	Hodgkin's disease	Neurogenic tumors
Dermoid cyst	Non-Hodgkin's lymphoma	Meningocele
Teratoma	Lymph-node metastases	Neurenteric cyst
Choriocarcinoma	Sarcoidosis	Gastroenteric cyst (also middle)
Seminoma	Infectious mononucleosis	
Thyroid mass	Bronchogenic cyst	Spindle cell tumors
Parathyroid adenoma	Pericardial cyst	Esophageal hernias
Lipoma	Tracheal tumors	Esophageal cyst
Fibroma	Thyroid masses	Esophageal tumor
Hemangioma	Aortic aneurysm	Esophageal diverticula
Lymphangioma	Pulmonary artery aneurysm	Extramedullary hema-topoiesis
Foramen of Morgagni hernia	Amyloidosis*	Thoracic spine masses
	Castleman's disease*	
	Immunoblastic lymphadenopathy*	

* Rare lesions
† With permission of Waverly Press, Inc., 428 E. Preston Street, Baltimore, MD 21202.

Superior mediastinal nodes—involved in 46% of patients with intrathoracic non-Hodgkin's lymphoma

Single-node involvement—15% of Hodgkin's and 40% of non-Hodgkin's lymphomas

Posterior mediastinal and paracardiac lymphadenopathy as sole site of thoracic disease—found only in non-Hodgkin's lymphoma

Tracheobronchial nodes—Hodgkin's, 45%; non-Hodgkin's, 14%

Paratracheal nodes—Hodgkin's, 40%; non-Hodgkin's, 14%

Bronchopulmonary nodes—Hodgkin's, 21%; non-Hodgkin's, 8%

Subcarinal nodes—Hodgkin's, 12%; non-Hodgkin's, 4%

Internal mammary nodes—Hodgkin's, 7%; non-Hodgkin's, 1%

Posterior mediastinal nodes—Hodgkin's, 5%; non-Hodgkin's, 1%

Paracardiac nodes—Hodgkin's, 2%; non-Hodgkin's, 4%. (Note: The nodes in the anterior cardiophrenic area can usually be detected on CT, not on chest radiography).

Radiographic Considerations in Lymphoma

As indicated, the lymphomas commonly involve the hilar and mediastinal lymph nodes and often cause massive enlargement of them. The involvement is characteristically bilateral and the nodes affected produce mass shadows corresponding to their location. The roentgen findings vary widely with the amount and distribution of the enlargement (Figs. 31-11 and 31-12). Often there is a single large mass projecting to both sides of the superior mediastinum with bilateral hilar enlargement. In other patients, individual nodes are outlined, resulting in a more lobulated appearance. The latter is somewhat more common in Hodgkin's disease, while the single massive enlargement is often found in non-Hodgkin's lymphoma. In non-Hodgkin's lymphoma, intrathoracic disease is present in 40% to 50% at the time of diagnosis, compared to 85% in Hodgkin's disease. Non-Hodgkin's lymphoma occurs on pleural and pericardial surfaces, in contrast to node enlargement in Hodgkin's disease. In the lateral view the masses usually appear in the anterior and middle mediastinum. When unilateral, the trachea may be displaced but this is not commonly noted in lymphoma. Tracheal compression may be observed, particularly in children, when adjacent masses are large. Occasionally there are stringy opacities extending outward into the pulmonary parenchyma, indicating involvement of the lungs by direct extension. This results in some blurring of the hilar or mediastinal mass along its outer borders. Pulmonary parenchymal involve-

lymphoma, of whom 43% had intrathoracic disease. They found the following node involvement:

Internal mammary nodes—10 times more frequent in Hodgkin's disease

Anterior mediastinal, tracheobronchial, and/or paratracheal nodes—3 to 4 times more common in Hodgkin's disease

Superior mediastinal nodes—involved in 90% of patients with intrathoracic Hodgkin's disease

Table 31-2. The International Working Formulation of Non-Hodgkin's Lymphoma

I. Low Grade
A. Malignant lymphoma
  1. Small lymphocytic consistent with chronic lymphocytic leukemia
  2. Plasmacytoid
B. Malignant lymphoma, follicular—predominantly small cleaved-cell
  1. Diffuse areas
  2. Sclerosis
C. Malignant lymphoma, follicular—mixed, small cleaved- and large-cell
  1. Diffuse areas
  2. Sclerosis
II. Intermediate Grade
D. Malignant lymphoma, follicular—predominantly large-cell
  1. Diffuse areas
  2. Sclerosis
E. Malignant lymphoma, diffuse—small cleaved-cell
  1. Sclerosis
F. Malignant lymphoma, diffuse—mixed, small- and large-cell
  1. Sclerosis
  2. Epithelioid cell component
G. Malignant lymphoma, diffuse—large-cell
  1. Cleaved cell
  2. Noncleaved cell
  3. Sclerosis
III. High Grade
H. Malignant lymphoma—large-cell, immunoblastic
  1. Plasmacytoid
  2. Clear cell
  3. Polymorphous
  4. Epithelioid cell component
I. Malignant lymphoma—lymphoblastic
  1. Convoluted cell
  2. Nonconvoluted cell
J. Malignant lymphoma—small noncleaved-cell
  1. Burkitt's
  2. Follicular
K. Miscellaneous
  1. Composite
  2. Mycosis fungoides
  3. Histiocyte
  4. Extramedullary plasmacytoma
L. Unclassifiable
M. Other

National Cancer Institute sponsored study of classifications of non-Hodgkin's lymphoma. Cancer 49: 2121, 1982. With permission.

ment is more frequent in Hodgkin's disease (11.6%) than in non-Hodgkin's lymphoma (3.7%)[20]. In addition to direct extension, pulmonary involvement takes the form of pulmonary nodules, which may be unilateral or bilateral, may cavitate, and may be clearly outlined or poorly defined.

When the chest radiographs (PA and lateral) are negative, in many instances no further chest studies may be indicated. When mediastinal adenopathy is noted, CT with contrast and in some instances MRI may be necessary, particularly when intravenous contrast is contraindicated.[7]

Metastases

Lymph-node metastases are often a part of generalized lymphangitic spread to the lungs, resulting in enlargement of mediastinal nodes plus strands of density radiating outward from the hilum into the lung (Figs. 31-13 and 31-14). Pleural involvement resulting in pleural effusion is commonly associated with this type of disease. Enlarged mediastinal nodes may also be associated with the multiple nodular hematogenous type of metastases. Occasionally, enlarged nodes may be the only roentgen manifestation of metastatic disease in the chest. Small-cell tumor of the lung may appear as a mediastinal mass, whereas the primary lesion in the lung may not be visible. In the latter instance, differentiation between metastasis and lymphoma cannot be made solely on the basis of roentgen findings. When enlarged mediastinal nodes are observed and suspect-

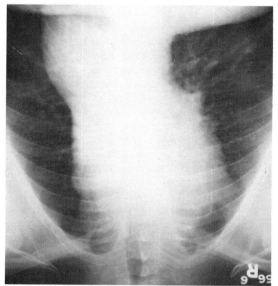

Figure 31-11. CT using bolus contrast and mediastinal windows to show anterior mediastinal nodes (*N*) in a patient with Hodgkin's disease. Superior vena cava (*v*), aortic arch (*A*), trachea (*T*). (Courtesy of Robert Rosenberg, MD)

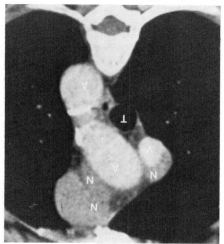

Figure 31-12. Mediastinal Hodgkin's disease. The large mass is bilateral and lobulated. It appears to involve left hilar as well as mediastinal nodes. The trachea is deviated to the left but is not well visualized in its intrathoracic portion because of the density of the tumor. There is very little evidence of pulmonary involvement.

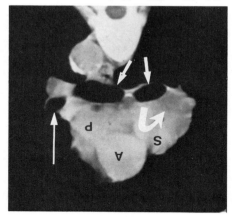

Figure 31-13. CT with intravenous contrast and mediastinal windows showing mediastinal adenopathy (*curved arrow*) in a patient with lung cancer; ascending aorta (*A*); superior vena cava (*S*); pulmonary artery (*P*); right and left main bronchi (*short arrows*); and left upper-lobe bronchus (*long arrow*). (Courtesy of Richard Logan, MD)

-ed to represent malignancy, a definite diagnosis must be made. A history of primary tumor elsewhere favors metastasis, while the presence of lymph-node enlargement elsewhere favors lymphoma. If nodes are not available elsewhere for biopsy, it is necessary to biopsy the mass of nodes, using percutaneous or transbronchial thin-needle aspiration, mediastinoscopy, mediastinotomy, or thoracotomy as the situation warrants.

Neurogenic Tumors

Ganglioneuroma and *neurofibroma* (*neurilemoma*) are the two most common tumors of neurogenic origin found in the mediastinum. The neurofibromas arise from intercostal nerves and occur most commonly in the posterior mediastinum, where they produce a round density that may reach a large size (Figs. 31-15 and 31-16). Some neurofibromas arise in the region of a spinal foramen and extend into the spinal canal, producing the so-called dumbbell type of tumor. These neurofibromas often cause pressure erosion of the adjacent pedicles and vertebral body. Oblique views are usually necessary to determine the presence or absence of bony involvement, and when bony involvement is manifest the diagnosis of neurogenic tumor can be made with great accuracy. Ganglioneuroma arises in the sympathetic ganglia of the thoracic region and also produces a posterior mediastinal tumor that may be-

come very large. Occasionally the thoracic neurofibroma may be a manifestation of multiple neurofibromatosis and is then associated with numerous subcutaneous neurofibromas. There are some slight differences that aid in the differentiation of the neurogenic tumors. The neurofibroma tends to have a narrow mediastinal base, as seen in the frontal projection, whereas the ganglioneuroma tends to have a broad mediastinal base. The angle between the tumor and the mediastinum tends to be acute in the neurofibroma and obtuse in the ganglioneuroma. As a general rule the neurofibroma or neurilemoma tends to be a round mass, while the ganglioneuroma is more elongated, (i.e., its vertical diameter is greater than the transverse or sagittal diameter) (Fig. 31-17).

The neurogenic tumors are usually fairly smooth and clearly defined, but occasionally they may be lobulated. They are usually benign, but occasionally a neurofibrosarcoma is found in the same location in the mediastinum as that in which a benign neurogenic tumor may arise. Rarely a neurogenic tumor may arise from the vagus nerve and present as a middle mediastinal mass. Bilateral neurofibroma of the vagus has been reported in patients with neurofibromatosis. Rarely, neuroblastoma may involve the mediastinum. This tumor, which occurs during childhood, tends to metastasize widely and grow rapidly. When primary in the mediastinum, it often contains some punctate calcifica-

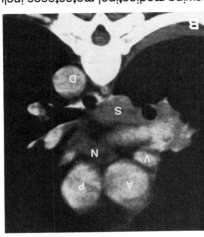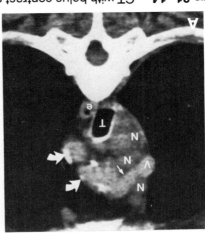

Figure 31-14. CT with bolus contrast showing mediastinal metastases including subcarinal nodes in a patient with esophageal carcinoma. (A) CT at the level of calcified aortic arch (*curved arrows*), showing metastatic nodes (N); trachea (T); esophagus (e). The superior vena cava (V) and left brachiocephalic vein (*small arrow*) are indicated. (B) At 1 cm inferior to the carina showing subcarinal (S) and retroaortic (N) adenopathy. Ascending (A) and descending aorta (D) as well as the pulmonary artery (P) are somewhat opacified, along with the superior vena cava (V). (Courtesy of Robert Rosenberg, MD)

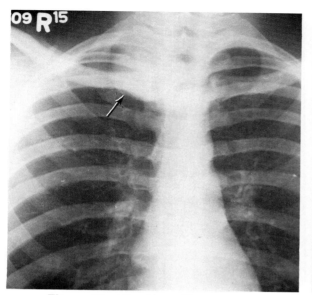

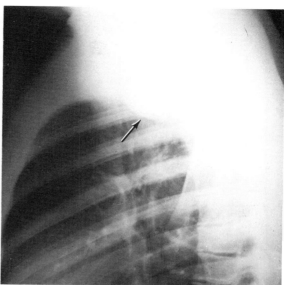

Figure 31–15. Neurofibroma. (**A**) Note the smooth outline of the tumor and its posterior location (*arrow*), also evident on (**B**) the lateral view (*arrow*). Since the tumor extends to the apex of the right thoracic cavity, it must lie posteriorly.

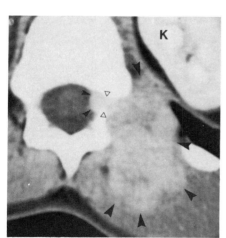

Figure 31–16. Aggressive neurilemoma in a patient with a low left paraspinal mass noted on a chest film. CT with contrast and soft-tissue window at the level of the upper pole of the left kidney. Large extrapleural mass displacing medial basal lung laterally (*large arrowheads*), encroaching on the spinal canal (*small arrowheads*), and causing bone erosion of the pedicle (*open arrowheads*). (Courtesy of Richard Logan, MD)

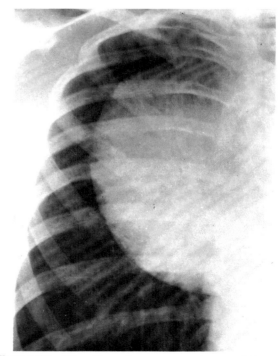

Figure 31–17. Ganglioneuroma. Large right posterior mediastinal mass with a vertical diameter greater than transverse diameter, a characteristic of this tumor.

tion, and there may be rib or vertebral erosion. In contrast, metastatic neuroblastoma does not contain calcium, does not erode bone, and often appears as multiple mediastinal masses. Pheochromocytoma also may occasionally originate in the posterior mediastinum. It has no distinguishing roentgen features. Paraganglioma (chemodectoma) is another rare tumor of neurogenic origin; it may arise anywhere in the mediastinum.

Pleural fluid is occasionally present in patients with neurogenic tumors and does not necessarily indicate malignancy. Calcification is rarely seen in these tumors, except in primary neuroblastoma of the mediastinum.

Teratoid Tumors

Benign Lesions

Mediastinal teratoma is an anterior mediastinal lesion that grows very slowly and may reach great size before producing symptoms. When it contains only ectodermal derivatives it may be called a "dermoid cyst."

Because histologic examination usually reveals derivatives of the other germ layers, the term "teratoma" or "teratoid cyst" is more accurate. The tumor is usually found in young adults. When benign, it is usually a well-encapsulated cystic tumor that is multilocular and smooth but may be somewhat lobulated. Calcification is often present in the wall, but it is uncommon to find bone and poorly formed teeth within the mass.

The roentgen findings are those of an anterior mediastinal mass, the bulk of which extends to one side. Calcification in the wall and within it can be more clearly demonstrated on well-penetrated roentgenograms (Fig. 31-18) or CT. It may be round, oval, or lobulated and is usually clearly defined laterally while the medial wall blends with mediastinal structures. Very often there is fat in the teratoid tumor or cyst which may be detected on CT scan. When poorly formed teeth or fat or both are detected on CT, the diagnosis is virtually certain. The tumor elements must be present at birth, but because the mass often grows slowly it is usually found in young adults. Rarely, massive benign teratoma is present at birth.

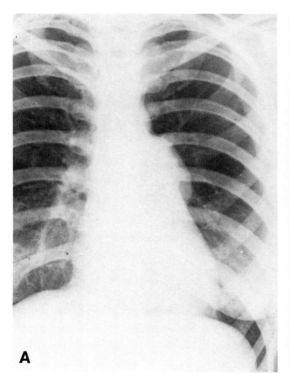
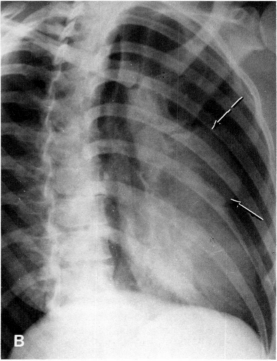

Figure 31–18.   Mediastinal dermoid cyst. **(A)** Frontal view showing a mass projecting to the left just below the transverse aortic arch. The mass obscures the left pulmonary artery and the left hilum. **(B)** In the right anterior oblique view, the mass is seen to lie anteriorly (*arrows*). There is no calcification within the mass or its walls.

Malignant Lesions

A *malignant teratoma* may also occupy the anterior mediastinum, but this lesion grows rapidly and usually causes death within a year of discovery. It produces symptoms and is discovered because of them, unlike the benign teratoma that is often discovered on routine roentgen study of the chest. The chest radiographic and CT findings are those of an anterior mediastinal mass that is often less clearly defined and more lobulated than benign teratoma. Extension into the lung as well as into mediastinal structures blurs the margins. Pleural extension may result in effusion. The prognosis is poor in such a malignant teratoma.

Seminoma is another malignant tumor that may arise in the mediastinum from aberrant germ cells. This rare tumor is found in young men in the third and fourth decades. The radiographic study reveals a lobulated anterior mediastinal mass, often extending to both sides of the midline. This tumor may or may not cause symptoms of dyspnea, cough, and substernal pain. The prognosis is generally good with proper treatment.

Endodermal sinus (yolk sac) tumor is a rare cause of an anterior mediastinal mass.[21] It occurs in young males who are usually symptomatic when the mass is discovered. The prognosis is poor. There are no distinctive radiographic signs, except that the patient with a large, often lobulated, anterior mediastinal mass has symptoms of fever, chest pain, and sometimes cough and dyspnea.

Mediastinal Cysts

The mediastinal cysts usually appear as rounded or oval mass lesions that are smooth and clearly defined. They tend to change slightly in shape with alteration in position and with respiration. CT or ultrasound are helpful in delineating the cystic nature of these masses. In addition to the congenital cysts in which low attenuation contents are usually present, it must be remembered that areas of low attenuation may be present in areas of hemorrhage or necrosis in bronchogenic neoplasms, enlarged neoplastic nodes, in areas of cystic degeneration in neurogenic tumors, and in lymphangiomas and meningoceles.[24]

Bronchogenic Cyst

Cysts of bronchogenic origin are lined with ciliated columnar epithelium and are usually asymptomatic. They commonly occur in the middle mediastinum near the trachea and in the region of the carina but may be found anywhere in the mediastinum (Fig. 31-19). They range considerably in size, are clearly defined, and are not lobulated. They may compress or displace the bronchi and/or trachea in children, resulting in symp-

toms. In adults they do not usually compress or displace these structures and are ordinarily asymptomatic. Rarely, "milk of calcium" is observed within the cyst. CT is useful in outlining the cyst. Ordinarily the contents are near water density, so the diagnosis can be made. Occasionally there is greater density, so tumor cannot be excluded on CT. As in other benign mediastinal cysts, the contour may change with positional changes. A somewhat pointed appearance has been reported on CT and may be helpful in the diagnosis when high attenuation cysts are present.[16]

Gastroenteric Cyst (Duplication)

Gastroenteric cysts probably represent small local duplications of the intestinal tract. They contain secretory cells and may grow to a large size early in life. They produce symptoms because of pressure on mediastinal structures and are often discovered during infancy, usually before the child is 2 years old. They appear as large rounded or oval opacities in the posterior mediastinum near the esophagus and usually extend to one side of the midline (Fig. 31-20). Sonography may establish the cystic nature of the mass, but CT may be necessary. They are related to neurenteric cysts but have no connection to the neural canal. Many are associated with vertebral anomalies and other abnormalities such as meningocele, intestinal malrotation, and esophageal atresia; congenital heart disease may also be present. They are also related to bronchopulmonary foregut malformations but usually have no connection with the gastrointestinal tract. Partial pericardial defect may accompany the type that is more closely related to bronchopulmonary foregut malformation.

Neurenteric Cyst

A neurenteric cyst is a rare mediastinal cyst that appears to be formed from a remnant of the neurenteric canal that forms an evanescent communication from the gut through the dorsal midline structures to the dorsal surface of the embryo—the neural canal.[49] The lesion consists of a mediastinal cystic mass that may be continuous with a duplication or giant diverticulum of the intestinal tract, and may be associated with a diaphragmatic hernia. There is also a defect in the anterior aspect of the spine and faulty vertebral development such as a butterfly vertebra. A fibrous stalk connects the cyst to the meninges in the spinal canal. These cysts may connect with the gut by way of a tubular structure. Therefore, various combinations of closed cysts or communicating cysts with the gut and/or neural canal may be found, at times with associated congenital anomalies. They do not appear to be related to bronchial or pericardial cysts. CT is very useful, be-

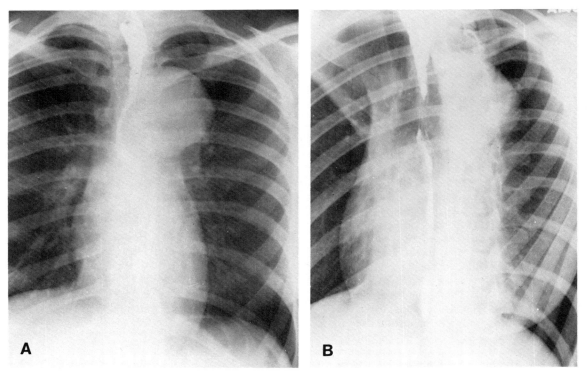

Figure 31–19. Bronchogenic cyst. (**A**) A clearly defined mediastinal mass is noted on the left, overlying the aortic arch. (**B**) The left anterior oblique view shows the mass to lie at about the level of the posterior aortic arch and upper descending aorta. No expansile pulsation was noted at fluoroscopy.

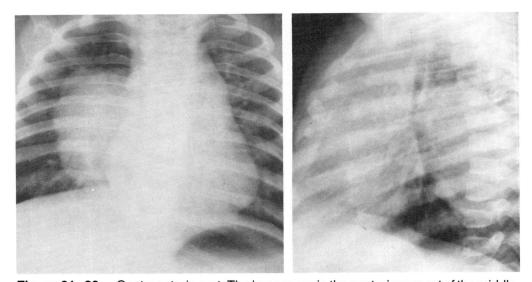

Figure 31–20. Gastroenteric cyst. The large mass in the posterior aspect of the middle mediastinum produced some esophageal compression and resulted in a feeding problem in this infant. The symptoms had been present since birth but had progressed. This examination, performed when the infant was 3 months old, was followed by excision, with relief of symptoms.

cause defects in the vertebra can be readily detected. MRI is useful when the spinal canal is separated by the anomaly. Occasionally a communication with the intraabdominal gastrointestinal tract is demonstrated during an upper GI study.

Pericardial Cyst

Pericardial cysts usually arise near and are attached to the parietal pericardium.[19] They are lined by flat cells that may be endothelial or mesothelial in origin. They contain clear fluid and are sometimes termed "clearwater" or "simple" cysts. When a small cyst of this type is found in the region of the cardiohepatic angle, it may extend into the primary interlobar fissure. The interlobar portion is then tear-drop– or pear-shaped (Fig. 31-21). The usual location of the oval mass adjacent to the heart and attached to the pericardium is helpful in making the diagnosis. The pericardial cyst is often basal and may simulate a diaphragmatic tumor or a foramen of Morgagni hernia (Fig. 31-22). CT can usually define the mass as a cyst. However, these cysts may contain thick viscous material and have high CT numbers. Ultrasonography may then be of value in demonstrating that the mass is cystic. If so, cyst puncture and aspiration may be performed for confirmation. In some instances, sonography followed by cyst puncture is sufficient.

Mediastinal Pancreatic Pseudocyst

Rarely a pancreatic pseudocyst will migrate or extend into the posterior mediastinum through the aortic or esophageal hiatus. Usually thoracic and abdominal pain and dyspnea along with a mass in the lower posterior mediastinum are present. There are a few reports of very large pseudocysts extending into the superior aspect of the mediastinum. The esophagus and stomach may be displaced by the mass.

Cystic Hygroma (Lymphangioma)

Lymphangioma or cystic hygroma may extend into the superior mediastinum from the neck and produce a mass that can be visualized radiographically. The presence of the spongy mass in the neck plus apparent continuation of it into the superior mediastinum usually permits the diagnosis. This lesion is soft and pliable, and alteration in contour may be visible in different phases of respiration on films or at fluoroscopy. Anterior mediastinal lymphangioma may also occur in the absence of a cervical mass. The mass is soft and spongy, so it does not ordinarily displace or compress the trachea. It molds to the mediastinal contours and surrounds vessels but does not invade or displace them. They are not calcified. These characteristics should lead to the diagnosis on CT when such a low attenuation mass is present.

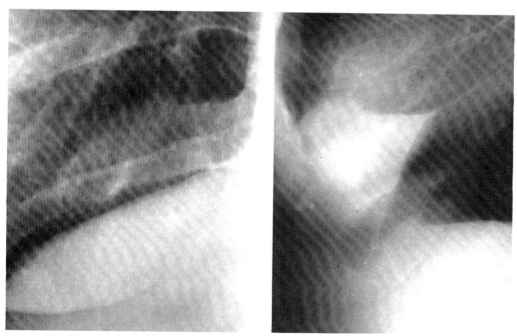

Figure 31–21. Pericardial cyst at the cardiohepatic angle. Note the typical teardrop appearance in the lateral view.

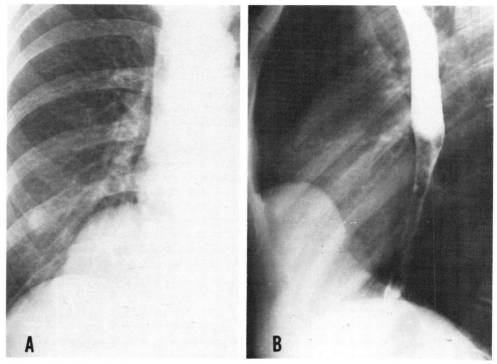

Figure 31–22.   Pericardial cyst. (**A**) Mass of water density is noted at the cardio-hepatic angle. (**B**) The anterior location of the mass is confirmed. Hernia of Morgagni's foramen usually occurs in the same position.

Intrathoracic Thyroid

Intrathoracic thyroid is a relatively common tumor, noted in the anterior mediastinum, which is usually connected by an isthmus of tissue to the thyroid gland in the neck. Rarely there is no connection. This isthmus is often wide enough to be recognized roentgenographically so that the connection between the intrathoracic mass and the thyroid is demonstrated. Even if the tumor is bilateral, it is usually eccentric enough to produce tracheal deviation and often compression; this becomes a significant finding for the diagnosis of intrathoracic goiter. The lateral view often shows posterior displacement of the trachea as well (Fig. 31-23). It is not uncommon to observe calcification within the mass (Fig. 31-24). The intrathoracic thyroid often moves on swallowing but may be fixed. It may be posterior in position and produce a mass in the posterior mediastinum behind the trachea, almost always on the right side. The mass of thyroid tissue may also extend far downward into the inferior aspect of the anterior mediastinum. We have observed one patient in whom the goiter encircled the esophagus in a manner that simulated esophageal leiomyoma. The mass may reach great size without producing symptoms. When the

mediastinal thyroid is posterior in position, there is usually some displacement of the esophagus as well as the trachea. This is helpful in making the diagnosis. Brachiocephalic vessels may be displaced or compressed. Rarely esophageal compression produces dysphagia and occasionally tracheal compression results in respiratory distress. If calcification is minimal, it may be observed only on CT. When the reaction is positive, scans using radioactive iodine (^{131}I) are diagnostic; but there may be no function, so a negative scan does not exclude the possibility of intrathoracic thyroid.

Parathyroid Adenoma

Parathyroid adenoma is usually found in the anterior aspect of the superior mediastinum or in the anterior mediastinum. It is usually relatively small, eccentric, and presents on either side. There is rarely any calcification in the tumor. There is nothing diagnostic about the appearance of the mass as visualized on the roentgenogram. When renal lithiasis or bone lesions of hyperparathyroidism are present in association with an anterior mediastinal mass, the diagnosis of parathyroid adenoma causing hyperparathyroidism can be made. CT scanning plays a major role in the examination of

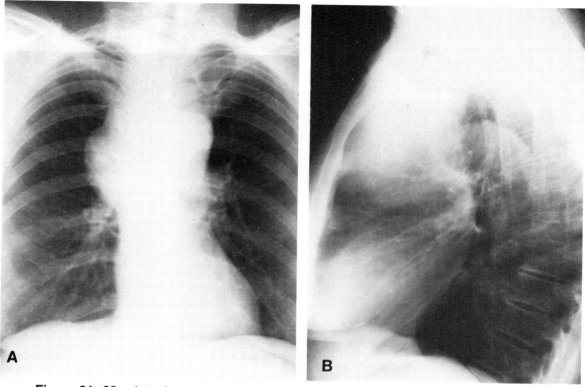

Figure 31–23. Intrathoracic thyroid. (**A**) Note the mediastinal mass above the right hilum, with widening of the superior mediastinum, which extends up into the neck. The trachea is displaced somewhat to the left. (**B**) The lateral view shows the anterior position of the mass and posterior displacement of the upper trachea. The patient was asymptomatic.

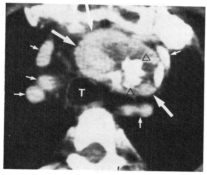

Figure 31–24. Anterosuperior mediastinal mass containing calcification. This CT above the aortic arch using mediastinal windows, and bolus intravenous contrast shows the inhomogeneous intrathoracic goiter (*large arrows*), containing calcium (*small arrowhead*). The trachea (*T*) and the five upper mediastinal vessels (*small arrows*) are indicated. Note displacement of the vessels on the left by the large mass. (Courtesy of Robert Rosenberg, MD)

these patients with hypercalcemia, even though no mass is visible on the chest radiograph. Small tumors can be detected and localized to reduce surgical time in exploring for parathyroids, particularly in the posterior mediastinum. CT is also indicated in patients who have had surgery without change in their hyperparathyroidism. In these patients, the parathyroid is often ectopic and may lie in the posterior superior mediastinum near the groove between the trachea and esophagus. Parathyroid adenoma may also occur in the neck. High-resolution ultrasound may be very useful in detecting and localizing cervical tumors (Fig. 31-25).

Lesions of the Thymus

The normal thymus, a bilobed pyramidal structure, lies in a retrosternal position largely behind the manubrium, but in children, in whom it is often large, it may extend well down into the retrosternal space anterior to the heart. The retrosternal line formed by the anterior mediastinal pleural reflections is seen above the heart on the lateral view of the thorax. There is usually

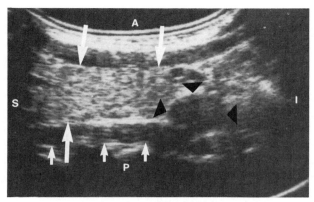

Figure 31–25. Longitudinal ultrasonogram on the right shows a hypoechoic parathyroid adenoma (*black arrowheads*), which measured 11 mm in length. Anterior (*A*), posterior (*P*), superior (*S*), inferior (*I*), thyroid gland (*large arrows*), and jugular vein (*small arrows*). (Courtesy of Richard Logan, MD)

some soft tissue between the sternum and this line, which ranges from 2 or 3 mm to a maximum of 8 mm in length. The thymic shadow in infants and children tends to obliterate the line. If there is more than 8 mm between the line and the sternum, the possibility of abnormalities such as tumor, internal mammary artery, vein or node enlargement, and hematoma must be considered in adults and older children. However, a large normal thymus may persist into the middle teens and cannot be differentiated from other anterior mediastinal masses. Rarely the thymus may be in an aberrant position, such as behind the trachea or adjacent to the base of the heart, or it may extend upward above the left brachiocephalic vein to the level of the inferior aspect of the thyroid. Occasionally it may be in the posterior mediastinum.[13] In these situations, CT may make the diagnosis and occasionally MRI may be necessary to confirm it, because it appears to be better than CT in distinguishing between mediastinal fat and thymus replaced by fat.[11, 15] The only plain-film finding that might suggest the diagnosis is a change in size and shape of the mass on inspiration and expiration.

Benign Thymic Lesions. Benign thymomas are located in the anterior mediastinum at the level of the junction of the heart and great vessels. They grow slowly and may become very large. They account for about 15% of mediastinal tumors. They occur in adults with an average age of 50 years. At times the tumor is in the midline and may be difficult or impossible to visualize in the frontal projection, but is readily visible in oblique or lateral views. Mottled calcification is occasionally noted within it.

Myasthenia gravis is found in about 30% of patients with thymoma. Of patients with myasthenia gravis, 10% to 15% have thymic tumors, some of which are malignant and invasive. Patients with myasthenia gravis should be examined for thymic tumor. In addition to PA and lateral views, a shallow (20%) oblique projection may be helpful in patients younger than 21 years. CT is indicated only when there is a questionable lesion on chest radiography or when clinical symptoms and signs suggest thymic abnormality.[17] CT should remain the procedure of choice when no obvious abnormality is found on chest radiography.[4] However, it cannot differentiate the various causes of thymic enlargement in many instances. There is no way to be certain on roentgen examination that a thymic mass is benign or malignant.

Thymic Cyst. Thymomas may be cystic and contain calcium which outlines the wall and suggests the cystic nature of the tumor. Thymic cyst location is similar to that of the solid type of thymoma (Fig. 31-26), but it is much less common. The cystic elements should be readily apparent on CT. Rarely they may extend into the neck.

Thymolipoma. A thymolipoma is an uncommon benign fatty tumor that originates in the atrophic thymus. It usually becomes very large and is asymptomatic. The presence of this tumor may be suggested when a large, fatty, anterior mediastinal mass is observed in an asymptomatic adult. There is no association with myasthenia gravis. The fatty nature of the mass is readily detected on CT.

Malignant Thymic Lesions. Early in its development, the malignant thymic tumor resembles a benign thymoma in appearance and location. It grows rapidly, however, and is invasive, so the margins become blurred. It often becomes very large, extends to both sides of the midline, and then resembles lymphoma. It spreads by direct invasion, and sometimes there may be implantation of tumor on the adjacent pleura or pericardium. The tumor may be carcinomatous or sarcomatous. CT is useful in defining the extent of tumor, and sometimes can detect invasion of adjacent structures.[33] MRI may be necessary when findings of invasion are equivocal on CT.

Intrathoracic Meningocele

Intrathoracic meningocele is a herniation of the meninges laterally to cause a posterior mediastinal mass.[62] It is rare and is usually mistaken for the more common posterior mediastinal neurofibroma. Kyphoscoliosis frequently accompanies this abnormality, and its presence may aid in suggesting the diagnosis. An intrathoracic

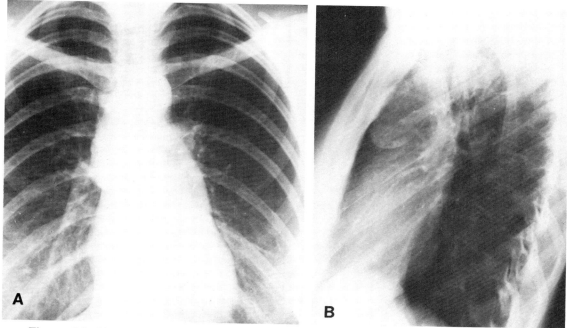

Figure 31–26. Thymic cyst. **(A)** In the frontal projection, a mass is seen in the right upper mediastinum. This extends downward below the level of the inferior branch of the right pulmonary artery. Its upper extent is not clearly defined. **(B)** In the lateral view, the mass is noted to lie anteriorly and, again, its upper extent is not clearly defined. There is a little calcification inferiorly, causing a slightly mottled appearance of the smooth lower margin.

meningocele is often associated with neurofibromatosis (von Recklinghausen's disease). There may be erosion about the intervertebral foramen through which the meninges protrude, and skeletal defects are commonly associated with it. These meningoceles may be single or multiple, unilateral or bilateral. When the presence of this lesion is suspected, it can be confirmed by myelography. CT with or without intrathecal contrast can identify the lesion and determine the presence of any associated bone abnormality.

Mediastinal Lipomatosis Caused by Steroids
In patients with morbid obesity or with the use of long-term, large-dose steroid therapy in organ transplantation and in treatment of various chronic diseases, there may be deposition of large amounts of fat in the mediastinum.[57] The patients on steroids usually manifest Cushing's syndrome, often with fat deposition in supraclavicular and epicardial areas, as well as in the mediastinum. The condition is important only in that it must be differentiated from other conditions that may cause mediastinal widening. Roentgen findings consist of mediastinal widening, which is relatively radiolucent

and poorly defined when compared to other mediastinal masses (Fig. 31-27). The trachea is not compressed or displaced, and excess epicardial fat may also be present. The diagnosis is usually made readily on chest radiography, but if there is any question CT is very useful in making the diagnosis and in determining whether or not fat is the cause of the mediastinal abnormality.

Miscellaneous Masses
Benign tumors such as lipoma, fibroma, chondroma, and hemangioma occur rarely within the mediastinum. There is nothing characteristic about the chest radiographic appearance of a *lipoma* or *fibroma*, but lipoma can usually be recognized on CT. If necessary, thin-needle aspiration biopsy can be used to confirm the diagnosis if the tumor is accessible. Other fat-containing masses that must be differentiated include liposarcoma, benign teratoma, thymolipoma, steroid-induced fat, and benign lipomatosis. The *chondroma* may contain a considerable amount of irregular calcification that helps to identify it. *Hemangiomas* are often poorly defined, widespread masses that may con-

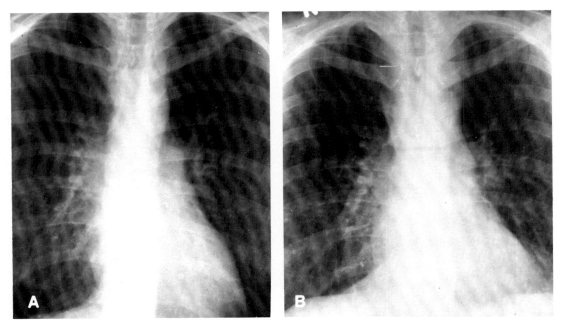

Figure 31–27. Mediastinal lipomatosis. The patient, an 18-year-old female, had a renal transplant and was on long-term steroid therapy. (**A**) Initial chest film. (**B**) Film obtained 1 year later shows mediastinal widening superiorly, which is very poorly defined. There is more epicardial fat at the apex and the cardiohepatic angle than was present earlier.

tain small rounded calcifications that represent phleboliths. When the latter are present, the diagnosis can be made with a reasonable degree of certainty. Most hemangiomas occur in the anterior mediastinum. They tend to be defined clearly in the anteroposterior projection but are often difficult to outline in the lateral projection.[32]

Varices or venous aneurysms involving mediastinal veins may cause asymptomatic mediastinal widening. *Desmoid tumors* arising in the chest wall may project into the mediastinum but more commonly are pleural-based and tend to resemble fibrous pleural mesotheliomas. Rarely, *pheochromocytoma* may occur in the thorax; as indicated earlier, its posterior location is similar to that of neurogenic tumor. Otherwise unexplained hypertension plus the mass should lead to the suspicion of this tumor. *Fibrosarcoma* and other sarcomas arising in the mediastinal soft tissues are extremely rare. Soft-tissue sarcoma may arise posteriorly and can present as a paravertebral mass; however, there is nothing characteristic about the radiographic appearance.

Extramedullary hematopoiesis may occur in a number of diseases in which there is chronic anemia. It has also been reported in Paget's disease of bone. Occasionally, the heterotopic bone marrow may develop in the paravertebral region of the thorax, presenting as a posterior mediastinal mass that may be very large. It may be unilateral or bilateral and may extend for some distance along the thoracic spine in a lobulated manner. It is believed to represent extruded bone marrow that results from progressive lysis of the cortex of ribs or vertebrae by the hyperactive marrow cells. Continuity with the marrow space may be lost, and longitudinal growth occurs in the extrapleural paraspinal space producing the elongated, lobulated paraspinal masses. The diagnosis can be suspected if the patient has a long history of anemia. CT readily identifies fat in the extramedullary hematopoiesis in the paraspinal area.

Occasionally, *esophageal diverticula* may attain large size and appear as mediastinal masses. There is usually enough air within them that a gas–fluid level is demonstrated, indicating the type of lesion. An esophagram readily outlines and defines this type of lesion. In *achalasia* (cardiospasm), the esophagus becomes grossly dilated and may simulate mediastinal tumor. On occasion, a fluid level may be present and allow the diagnosis to be made. If large, the fluid-filled mass extends the length of the mediastinum and the diagnosis is then apparent.

Paraspinal abscess secondary to tuberculosis or

other chronic infection of the thoracic spine often produces a shadow that may simulate tumor. The abscesses are usually somewhat spindleshaped and the opacity produced merges with the normal paraspinal shadow above and below the mass. Lateral and oblique projections that outline the vertebral bodies and intervertebral discs usually indicate the cause for the lesion, since varying amounts of destruction of one or more vertebral bodies, along with narrowing of the intervening intervertebral disc space, are common findings. There is also calcification within the chronic abscess in many instances. CT is very useful in defining the soft-tissue mass and the extent of bone destruction. Conventional tomography can also be used for this purpose. *Tumors of the thoracic spine* may produce masses but their location is usually clearly defined in lateral views so that there is no difficulty in differentiation between these lesions and mediastinal tumor.

Mediastinal hematoma may also produce a mediastinal mass. Usually there is a history of trauma or of a recent surgical procedure, so a presumptive diagnosis can be made. Rapid changes in the size of the mass are characteristic when they occur. Rarely in patients with a mediastinal hematoma caused by an aortic rupture, the blood may dissect along bronchovascular sheaths to resemble pulmonary edema (Fig. 31-28).[54] This is a very unlikely complication, however.

Cardiac disease and lesions of the great vessels within the mediastinum are discussed in Chapter 32.

THE DIAPHRAGM

The diaphragm is the muscle of respiration that separates the thorax from the abdominal cavity. The anatomy and variations are described by Panicek and asso-

ciates.[53] The muscle fibers of the diaphragm originate from the xiphoid process and from the eighth to twelfth ribs and insert into the central tendon. Posteriorly, the diaphragmatic crura arise from the upper lumbar vertebral bodies, originating as low as the third lumbar body. The central tendon lies somewhat anterior to the middle thorax and roughly parallels the anterior chest wall. The muscle fibers anteriorly are relatively short and posteriorlaterally are two to three times longer, so the major muscle mass is in the posterior aspect of the diaphragm. The position of the diaphragm is described in Chapter 22. There are a number of openings in it through which structures such as the esophagus and aorta pass to enter the abdomen (Fig. 31-29). The superior surface of the diaphragm is readily seen in the roentgenogram of the normal chest because it is clearly outlined by the radiolucent lung above it. Its lower margin is often visible on the left, at least in part, because there is usually some gas in the fundus of the stomach and gas or fecal material in the splenic flexure of the colon that define a portion of its undersurface. On the right side, the liver is of comparable density, so the undersurface of the diaphragm cannot be seen unless pneumoperitoneum is present. The right hemidiaphragm is usually one interspace higher than the left. In full inspiration the dome of the right leaf of the diaphragm is at the approximate level of the tenth rib posteriorly, while the left is at the level of the eleventh rib posteriorly. Using the anterior ribs as landmarks, the dome of the right hemidiaphragm lies between the level of the fifth rib and the level of the sixth interspace measured on the standard 6-foot roentgenogram obtained with the patient in moderately deep inspiration. The dome tends to be higher in hypersthenic and obese patients and may be lower in asthenic subjects. The height of the diaphragm appears to be related to

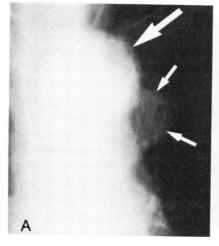
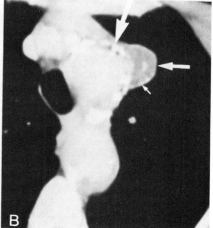

Figure 31–28. (**A**) Chest film shows mass (*small arrows*) in the region of the aortopulmonary window below the aortic arch (*large arrow*). (**B**) CT with contrast bolus at the level of the inferior aspect of the aortic arch shows the extensive calcification in the aorta (*large arrow*), the mass (*medium arrow*) with some calcification in its wall (*small arrow*). It proved to be a focal dissecting hematoma. (Courtesy of Richard Logan, MD)

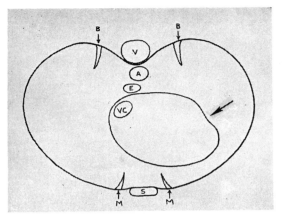

Figure 31–29.   Diagram to show the normal openings and areas of potential weakness in the diaphragm. The sketch is drawn viewing the diaphragm from above. The vertebral body (*V*) and the sternum (*S*) are labeled for orientation purposes. Foramen of Bochdalek (*B*); aorta (*A*); esophageal hiatus (*E*); opening for the inferior vena cava (*VC*); Morgagni's foramen (potential opening) (*M*); attachment of the pericardium to the diaphragm (*arrow*).

the position of the apex of the heart rather than to the position of the liver (i.e., the low hemidiaphragm is on the side of the cardiac apex); this is observed in patients with dextrocardia and normal abdominal situs.

CHANGES IN THE DIAPHRAGM WITH AGE

The esophageal hiatus gradually enlarges with advancing age.[9] Diaphragmatic defects (areas of thinning) increase from zero in the third decade to 56% in patients in the seventh and eighth decades. The most severe defects consist of an area of discontinuity of the diaphragm associated with herniation of omental fat into the thorax. Defects are found largely posteromedially. Emphysema is a factor in the development of the defects, which have been found in 84% of patients with emphysema. The defects are more common in females, if the presence of emphysema is excluded. The status of skeletal muscle and obesity do not appear to be factors. Diaphragmatic muscle generally does not change in thickness with aging.

MOTION OF THE DIAPHRAGM

Asynchronous motion is common, and there is often more excursion on the left than on the right. Average range of motion is 3 to 6 cm, but it can be increased by training. In patients with emphysema, the motion range is often less than 3 cm. On rapid inspiration that

is induced by a rapid inspiratory "sniff," there is often a minimal temporary paradoxical motion, usually on the right. Then the hemidiaphragm moves downward normally. The momentary paradoxical motion is normal. With the patient in a lateral decubitus position, the dependent hemidiaphragm is high, and excursion is greatly enhanced. This position is helpful in assessing diaphragmatic weakness and significant paradoxical motion.

FUNCTIONAL DISTURBANCES OF THE DIAPHRAGM

The most common disturbance of the diaphragm is hiccough (singultus). This consists of sudden diaphragmatic contraction associated with closure of the glottis. It is either local in origin, caused by irritation of the diaphragm, or central, in which case it may be produced by encephalitis, uremia, or brain tumor. Occasionally it is hysterical in origin. Attacks are usually very short, but occasionally paroxysms may last for months or years. Radiography is of value only if it may serve to identify an irritating lesion producing the contraction. Fluoroscopy can be used to determine the severity of the contraction and to determine whether one or both hemidiaphragms are involved.

Tonic contraction or splinting of the diaphragm often results when basal pleuritis, subphrenic abscess, or trauma has produced diaphragmatic injury. In any of these instances there is elevation of the diaphragm, which may be bilateral but is usually unilateral, and may be confined to one portion of a hemidiaphragm. Chest roentgenography outlines the height of the diaphragm and fluoroscopy will reveal the amount and location of the limitation of motion.

PARALYSIS AND PARESIS OF THE DIAPHRAGM

When the diaphragm is paralyzed, it is elevated, because intra-abdominal pressure is greater than intrathoracic pressure. The amount of elevation varies considerably and paresis or paralysis may be unilateral or bilateral. When paralysis is complete on one side, paradoxical motion is usually visible at fluoroscopy. This means that during inspiration the paralyzed hemidiaphragm rises while the normal hemidiaphragm descends; during expiration the normal hemidiaphragm rises and the paralyzed one descends. This paradoxical motion can be accentuated by having the patient sniff. This causes a rapid but shallow inspiration. In paresis of the diaphragm there may or may not be elevation visible on chest roentgenograms, but a lag in contraction of the involved hemidiaphragm is readily visible fluoroscopically and this is also accentuated by having the patient sniff. Normally there may be a slight difference in motion on the two sides. In our experience, the left hemidiaphragm moves slightly more rapidly than the right on deep, rapid inspiration. When there is much difficulty in determining relative diaphragmatic motion on the two sides, fluoroscopy with the patient in the lateral decubitus position is helpful, because motion on the dependent side is augmented and comparison is easier with greater excursion.

EVENTRATION OF THE DIAPHRAGM

Eventration of the diaphragm is the term used to describe an abnormal elevation of the diaphragm. It is thought to result from a deficiency of muscular development that may be general or local. The local form is occasionally bilateral, but bilateral general eventration is very rare. Local eventration is nearly always on the right side anteromedially. There is some difference of opinion as to the cause of eventration. Some observers believe there is a deficiency of nervous as well as of muscular tissue. The diagnosis is based on observation of the elevated diaphragm on a chest roentgenogram. There is no disease or tumor visible to produce the elevation, and at fluoroscopy the involved hemidiaphragm is usually observed to move. The movement may be normal or diminished and paradoxical motion can be observed on rapid inspiration in some instances. It is often difficult to differentiate from hernia and may be impossible to differentiate from phrenic

paralysis or paresis. Congenital eventration (Fig. 31-30), manifested in childhood, is usually on the right, in contrast to eventration developing in adults, which is usually on the left and in males.[37] When eventration is left-sided, there is often a long fluid level in the gastric fundus when the patient is in the upright position. The afferent and efferent limbs of the stomach or colon are widely separated in eventration, but are together or nearly so in congenital or acquired hernia, being constricted at the hernial opening. Ultrasound can be used to identify the intact diaphragm in these patients with eventration.

Localized Eventration

Local weakness of the diaphragm with upward protrusion of the liver is the most common manifestation of localized eventration. It usually occurs on the anteromedial aspect of the right hemidiaphragm, through which a portion of the right lobe of the liver bulges. This has been termed the "anteromedial hump" of the liver. The smoothly rounded appearance of the bulge is usually characteristic, but, if the bulge simulates tumor, liver scan or CT will make differentiation possible. In our experience, primary or metastatic hepatic tumor does not cause this type of local elevation. Local eventrations may occur elsewhere, particularly posteriorly, where upward displacement of the kidney may produce a rounded mass density simulating tumor.

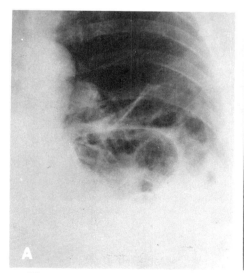 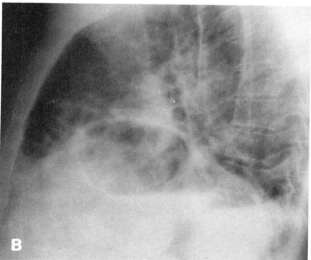

Figure 31–30. Eventration of the diaphragm. The dome of the diaphragm is difficult to visualize in (**A**) the frontal projection because of changes in the basal lung on the left. (**B**) The dome is more clearly defined in the lateral view and is noted to be elevated. Since the patient experienced respiratory symptoms secondary to poor diaphragmatic function, surgical repair was carried out, and the diagnosis of congenital eventration confirmed.

This probability should be considered when the mass is comparable in size to the upper pole of the kidney. When suspected, intravenous urography can be used to outline the kidney and determine its relationship to the diaphragm. However, ultrasound of the kidney is diagnostic in most instances.

DIAPHRAGMATIC DISPLACEMENTS

In addition to the elevation of the diaphragm noted in eventration, paralysis, and paresis, a number of intrathoracic and intra-abdominal conditions may result in elevation of the diaphragm. On the right side, tumors and cysts of the liver, subphrenic abscess, and right renal tumors may elevate the diaphragm generally or locally. On the left side the causes include enlargement of the spleen, left renal tumors, and dilatation or tumors of the stomach and of the splenic flexure of the colon. Ascites, obesity, large intra-abdominal tumors, and pregnancy may result in bilateral elevation. Intrathoracic diseases that decrease pulmonary volume cause elevation on the involved side. These include pulmonary fibrosis, chronic pleural disease, and atelectasis. The elevation may be relatively uniform or rather irregular. The amount depends on the severity of the lesion producing it. If the disease causing it is bilateral, elevation is bilateral.

Irregularity of the diaphragm superiorly is often secondary to previous pulmonary inflammatory disease. This is termed "tenting" or "adhesive tenting" and is often associated with basal pulmonary fibrosis and obliteration of the costophrenic sulcus.

The diaphragm is displaced downward by lesions that produce an increase in thoracic volume, such as large intrathoracic neoplasms, massive pleural effusion, pulmonary emphysema, and tension pneumothorax. Massive pleural effusion may cause inversion of the left hemidiaphragm, displacing the kidney, spleen, and stomach downward. This inversion may produce a pseudomass in the left upper abdominal quadrant which disappears when thoracentesis and removal of pleural fluid are accomplished (Fig. 31-31).[67] Less commonly, the right hemidiaphragm is inverted by massive pleural effusion.[28] Ultrasound can usually identify the diaphragm in this condition, since it cannot be detected on chest radiography.

DIAPHRAGMATIC TUMORS

Primary diaphragmatic tumors are rare and may be benign or malignant.[34] The most common benign tumor is lipoma, but numerous other benign tumors have been reported; they include fibroma, chondroma, neurofibroma, angiofibroma, and angioma as well as congenital cysts such as cystic teratoma. Benign cystic teratoma is extremely rare, but can be diagnosed on CT because it contains fat, calcium and/or teeth, and soft tissue quite similar to ovarian cystic teratomas. Because malignancy cannot be excluded by any imaging method, these cystic masses should be removed surgically.[46] The malignant tumors are all sarcomas; fibrosarcoma is the most common but others such as fibromyxosarcoma, fibroangioendothelioma, undifferentiated sarcoma, myosarcoma, hemangioendothelioma, heman-

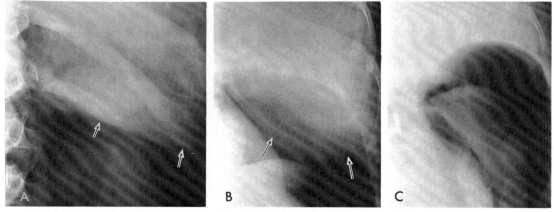

Figure 31–31.   Inversion of the diaphragm caused by massive left pleural effusion. (**A**) This film shows the mass in the left upper quadrant, which was continuous with massive left pleural effusion (*arrows*). (**B**) Pneumoperitoneum shows the inverted diaphragm projecting downward into the abdominal cavity (*arrows*.) (**C**) Pneumoperitoneum following thoracentesis shows the diaphragm to have assumed its normal upward convexity. There is still a moderately large left pleural effusion that obscures the lower lung on the left.

giopericytoma, leiomyosarcoma, or mesenchymoma may occur. Malignant tumors predominate in a ratio of three to two over benign tumors arising in the diaphragm. These tumors produce basal masses that usually project above the normal rounded opacity produced by the diaphragm. They may be smooth or lobulated and vary considerably in size. When the tumor is on the left, it may project downward to encroach on the gastric air bubble. The limits of the tumor may then be outlined inferiorly as the tumor projects into the stomach and superiorly as it projects above the diaphragm. Conventional roentgen studies serve only to identify a mass. CT is used to determine the site and extent of the mass, and if a lipoma is present, the diagnosis can be made. Because the other cell types produce no characteristic findings, biopsy or surgical exploration is usually indicated when a tumor is found in the diaphragm.

DIAPHRAGMATIC HERNIAS

Esophageal Hiatal Hernia

Herniation of all or part of the stomach through the esophageal hiatus into the thorax produces a mass shadow at the left medial base that is often visible on the frontal roentgenogram. Not infrequently, gas and fluid within the thoracic portion of the stomach make the diagnosis apparent on plain-film roentgenograms; if not, the lesion can be readily identified by means of a barium swallow. This examination also serves to identify the occasional diverticulum of the esophagus in this region and to differentiate the esophageal lesions from pulmonary cyst or abscess as well as from diaphragmatic tumor.

Morgagni Hernia

Foramen of Morgagni hernia is a rare diaphragmatic hernia that may result in a basal mass shadow, usually in the region of the cardiohepatic angle because it occurs mainly on the right (Fig. 31-32). It is most often observed in obese adults. This type of hernia through the retrosternal foramen of Morgagni (space of Larrey) on either side of the midline is usually small and often contains omentum. Theoretically a hernial sac should be present, but is not always demonstrated at surgery. Occasionally a portion of bowel may lie within the hernial sac. In the latter instance, it may be possible to make the diagnosis on routine roentgenographic study of the chest, but a CT or sonographic study is usually required. If omentum is herniated, the fat can be identified. Other studies include barium enema, which may show upward angulation of the mid-transverse colon when the hernial sac contains omen-

tum. The pyloric end of the stomach and proximal duodenum may also be displaced upward toward the diaphragm.

Rarely, the liver may herniate through the foramen of Morgagni into the thorax in infants and young children. This is usually accompanied by partial obstruction of the inferior vena cava.[60] Inferior vena cavography demonstrates the kinking and partial obstruction of the vena cava. When Morgagni hernia presents in infancy, it is usually accompanied by one or more anomalies. In one study, 13 of 17 patients had significant congenital defects including cardiac defects such as dextrocardia, ventricular septal defect; anomalous pulmonary venous return, trisomy 21, and large omphaloceles.[56] Liver, colon, and small bowel are often found in the hernia in infants, in contrast to the adult presentation where omental fat is often the only structure in the hernia and there are no associated congenital anomalies.

Bochdalek Hernia

Normally the pleuroperitoneal hiatus or foramen is posterolateral in position, but in congenital hernias arising in this area, the foramen may be very large, with absence of much of the involved hemidiaphragm. In such instances, most of the abdominal viscera may be in the thorax, leading to severe ipsilateral pulmonary hypoplasia. The presenting complaint may then be neonatal respiratory distress. These hernias occur predominantly on the left side (two to one). In contrast to the foramen of Morgagni hernias, true pleuroperitoneal hiatal hernias do not have a hernial sac. This is because the abdominal contents enter the thorax before the space between the septum transversum and the pleuroperitoneal membrane is closed.

Herniation through the pleuroperitoneal foramen of Bochdalek is often large and loops of bowel can be visualized and identified, so differential diagnosis is not difficult. When the hernia is smaller and does not contain gas-filled bowel, the diagnosis is more difficult to make. The use of CT to examine the thorax and upper abdomen has revealed a higher incidence of Bochdalek hernias than was previously reported (Fig. 31-33). An incidence of 6% was reported in a CT study of 940 patients.[22] The size of the diaphragmatic defect did not correlate with the size of the hernia. Most hernias contained fat and were frequently incidental findings on abdominal or chest scans of adults. Large Bochdalek hernias usually present at birth and produce respiratory distress and unilateral pulmonary hypoplasia. In some patients, however, no symptoms may appear for several months. In newborns with respiratory distress in the first 12 hours of life, mortality rate is about 50%. High risk factors include: right-sided her-

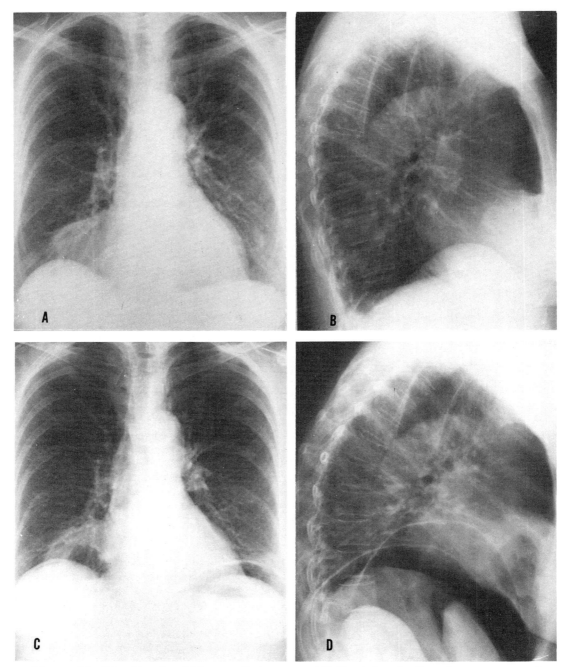

Figure 31–32. Hernia of Morgagni's foramen. (**A**) Frontal projection shows a mass at the cardiohepatic angle. (**B**) The anterior location of the mass is noted. (**C**) Following diagnostic pneumoperitoneum, air is seen to extend up into the thorax through a defect in the diaphragm. (**D**) Air extends upward anteriorly.

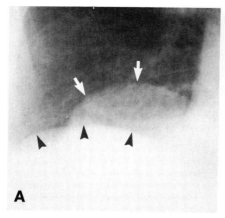

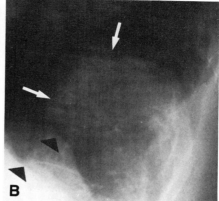

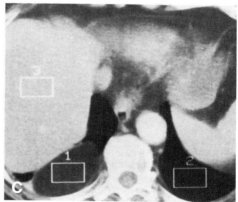

Figure 31–33. Hernia of the foramen of Bochdalek. (**A**) Frontal and (**B**) lateral films showing a posteromedial mass (*white arrows*) in an asymptomatic male; diaphragm (*black arrowheads*). (**C**) This CT with contrast at the level of the mass (box 1: −80 HU) shows the left lung (box 2: −700 HU) and the liver (box 3: +60 HU). The mass projects upward into the thorax in a retrohepatic position. (Courtesy of Richard Logan, MD)

nia; stomach in thorax; pneumothorax; non-aeration of the ipsilateral lung; and less than 50% aeration of the contralateral lung.[69] The roentgen findings vary with the amount of herniation. Gas-filled bowel is recognized within the thorax when the defect is on the left. The liver may also extend into the thorax when the defect is on the right. The remaining diaphragm is often visible. CT can be used to identify the diaphragm and its relation to the intrathoracic mass. Ultrasound also is sometimes useful in identifying the diaphragm in these patients, and real-time sonography may be particularly valuable as a bedside technique in critically ill patients.

Traumatic Hernia of the Diaphragm

Although gunshot wounds and knife wounds may lacerate the diaphragm, immediate surgery is usually necessary, so the defect is identified, at times before any radiographic studies are done. Traumatic rupture of the diaphragm usually results from severe blunt injury to the abdomen and less commonly to the thorax.[68] In severely traumatized patients, the combination of rib fractures and pelvic or vertebral fractures should raise

the possibility of diaphragmatic rupture—especially in patients wearing seatbelts.[5] About one third of diaphragmatic ruptures present immediately after the injury and are diagnosed then. The diaphragm may be ruptured completely with defects in the parietal pleura and peritoneum so there is no hernial sac. In other instances, either the pleura or peritoneum may form a sac. The left hemidiaphragm is involved in about 90% of patients who survive their injury. The rupture usually involves the posterior central portion of the diaphragm, but there may be avulsion of the diaphragm from the ribs. The stomach is the organ most often herniated, but colon, small bowel, spleen, liver, or gallbladder may also herniate. The radiographic signs in this condition vary with the extent of the rupture and depend on upward displacement of abdominal content. At times, no abnormality is observed. There may be elevation of the hemidiaphragm or apparent elevation, since herniated viscera may parallel the diaphragm on both frontal and lateral projections. This pseudoelevation may change in shape with change in position, however. In these instances it is strongly suggestive of rupture with hernia. Apparent normal diaphragmatic motion does not exclude the possibility of hernia. Recognizable bowel shadows may be visible in the thorax and sometimes in the pericardial sac. Administration of barium by mouth and by rectum to identify the relationship of the gastrointestinal tract to the diaphragm usually confirms the diagnosis. Both loops of gut are kept close together by the diaphragm surrounding the rupture—an hourglass appearance—so ordinarily there is no problem in differentiation from eventration. Because there may not be immediate herniation of abdominal viscera into the thorax following trauma, serial films are sometimes useful in the posttraumatic period and should be obtained if there is any suspicion of diphragmatic rupture. Other signs which suggest rupture include ipsilateral pleural effusion, mediastinal shift to the opposite side, and poor definition of the involved hemidiaphragm.

Because the defects do not heal spontaneously, traumatic rupture of the diaphragm may be followed by a traumatic hernia—sometimes years after the traumatic event. The roentgen findings are similar to those in the immediate type of posttraumatic herniation. Oblique and lateral views often permit localization of the defect. There may be partial or complete obstruction of the involved gut, either with or without vascular compromise in both immediate and delayed herniation. Hemothorax or hydrothorax may also be present and raises the possibility of strangulation. The combination of a high left hemidiaphragm and splenic flexure obstruction in a patient with history of trauma is very suggestive. Right-sided rupture, which may be more common than reported figures would indicate, also may cause diaphragmatic elevation with partial or total herniation of the liver. A high index of suspicion when diaphragmatic abnormality is observed in a patient who has suffered thoracoabdominal trauma is necessary to suggest, then confirm, the diagnosis. Immediate surgery is necessary in many instances.

In patients with suspected diaphragmatic rupture, chest x-ray is more useful than is generally reported, particularly if a follow-up film is obtained 6 to 12 hours after the initial radiograph.[23] CT has been disappointing. MRI may be of more value because coronal and sagittal images can be obtained.[44] Sonography is of great value in outlining diaphragmatic defects, but its use may be limited in some instances by interstitial emphysema of the overlying soft tissues and in others by severe pain in the area.[50]

Epicardial Fat Pads

Localized fat deposits are often present at the cardiac apex and in the cardiohepatic angle. Those at the apex are usually readily identified. When the amount of fat is unusually great it can produce a mass in the cardiohepatic angle that simulates foramen of Morgagni her-
nia or diaphragmatic tumor. Deposits of fat are usually of less density than are the adjacent heart and diaphragm, but this difference is small and not entirely reliable because the omentum, frequently present in foramen of Morgagni hernia, is of similar opacity. It is probable that a small foramen of Morgagni hernia is sometimes the cause of the shadow, but this is usually asymptomatic and the differentiation is then of no clinical importance. The fat pads tend to occur in obese patients, and when a fat pad is present in the cardiohepatic angle, there is usually a fat pad at the cardiac apex. The association of these opacities is of some diagnostic importance. CT can be used to identify the fat in these masses, if necessary.

ACCESSORY DIAPHRAGM

Accessory diaphragm (venolobar syndrome, duplication of the diaphragm), is very rare and occurs on the right side.[12] It consists of a sheet of fibrous and muscular tissue, which represents a partial duplication, extending from the anterior aspect of the normal diaphragm upward and posteriorly to insert along the fifth to seventh ribs. It parallels the major fissure and may extend into it to separate the lower lobe from the upper and middle lobes. It is usually attached to the pericardium medially and has a medial hiatus. Pulmonary anomalies associated with accessory diaphragm include partial fissure anomalies, aplasia or hypoplasia of a lobe, partial diversion of the lower lobe by the anomalous diaphragm, and anomalous pulmonary vascular supply including lower lobe venous drainage into the inferior vena cava, the scimitar syndrome, and anomalous arterial supply to the lower lobe from the aorta. This is the reason this complex of anomalies is sometimes called the "venolobar syndrome."

Roentgen findings include a shift of the mediastinum to the involved side because of hypoplasia and lack of clarity of the mediastinum on the same side with hazy opacity of the central lung. On the lateral view the accessory diaphragm may be visible; it resembles the major fissure but extends to the diaphragm and is more anterior in position than the normal fissure (Fig. 31-34). Bronchography may show the lobar hypoplasia and angiography may demonstrate the anomalous arterial supply and venous drainage that often accompany this anomaly.

CYSTS OF THE DIAPHRAGM

Intradiaphragmatic cysts usually represent extralobar sequestration in which aberrant lung tissue is enclosed within the diaphragm. The left hemidiaphragm is involved in about 90% of cases. Occasionally, a coelomic cyst may be found in the diaphragm. Roentgen find-

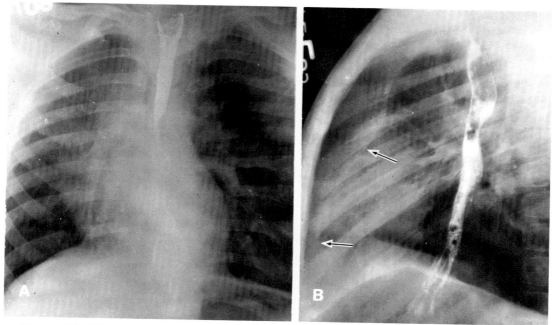

Figure 31–34. Accessory diaphragm on the right. (**A**) Note the mediastinal shift to the right, with poor definition of mediastinal structures on the involved side. There is also hazy density in the medial aspect of the upper half of the right hemithorax. (**B**) The lateral projection shows a somewhat curved line resembling an anteriorly displaced major fissure, except that it extends down to the diaphragm anteriorly (*arrows*). An aortogram showed an anomalous artery originating below the diaphragm, supplying a portion of the right lower lobe.

ings of a diaphragmatic mass are similar to those produced by benign diaphragmatic tumors. Sonography and CT are useful to demonstrate the cystic nature of the diaphragmatic mass.

REFERENCES AND SELECTED READINGS

1. ADAMS VI, UNNI KK, MUHM JR, ET AL: Diffuse malignant mesothelioma of pleura: Diagnosis and survival in 92 cases. Cancer 58:1540, 1986

2. ARONBERG DJ, GLAZER HS, SAGEL SS: MRI and CT of the mediastinum: Comparison, controversies, and pitfalls. Radiol Clin North Am 23:439, 1985

3. BARON RL, LEVITT RG, SAGEL SS, ET AL: Computed tomography in the evaluation of mediastinal widening. Radiology 138:107, 1981

4. BATRA P, HERRMANN C JR, MULDER D: Mediastinal imaging in myasthenia gravis: Correlation of chest radiography, CT, MRI and surgical findings. Am J Roentgenol 148:515, 1987

5. BERGQVIST D, DAHLGREN S, HEDELIN H: Rupture of the diaphragm in patients wearing seatbelts. J Trauma 18:781, 1978

6. BREATNACH E, NATH PH, DELANEY DJ: The role of computed tomography in acute and subacute mediastinitis. Clinic Radiol 37:139, 1986

7. CABANILLAS F, FULLER LM: The radiologic assessment of the lymphoma patient from the standpoint of the clinician. Radiol Clin North Am 28:683, 1990

8. CARROL CL, JEFFREY RB JR, FEDERLE MP, ET AL: CT evaluation of mediastinal infection. J Comput Assist Tomogr 11:449, 1987

9. CASKEY CI, ZERHOUNI EA, FISLMAN EK, ET AL: Aging of the diaphragm: A CT study. Radiology 171:385, 1989

10. COLLINS JD, BURWELL D, FURMANSKI S, ET AL: Minimal detectable pleural effusions. Radiology 105:51, 1972

11. CORY DA, COHEN MD, SMOTH JA: Thymus in the superior mediastinum simulating adenopathy: Appearance on CT. Radiology 162:457, 1987

12. DAVIS WS, ALLEN RP: Accessory diaphragm: Duplication of the diaphragm. Radiol Clin North Am 6:253, 1968

13. DAY DL, GEDGAUDAS E: The thymus. Radiol Clin North Am 22:519, 1984

14. DEDRICK CG, MCLOUD TC, SHEPARD JAO, ET AL: Com-

puted tomography of localized pleural mesothelioma. Am J Roentgenol 144:275, 1985

15. DeGeer G, Webb WR, Gamsu G: Normal thymus: Assessment with MR and CT. Radiology 158:313, 1986

16. Demos TC, Budorick NE, Posniak HV: Benign mediastinal cysts: Pointed appearance on CT. J Comput Assist Tomogr 13:132, 1989

17. Ellis K, Auston JHM, Jaretzki A III: Radiologic detection of thymoma in patients with myasthenia gravis. Am J Roentgenol 151:873, 1988

18. Federly MP, Mark AS, Guillaumin ES: CT of subpulmonic pleural effusion and atlectasis: Criteria for differentiation from subphrenic fluid. Am J Roentgenol 146:685, 1986

19. Feigin DS, Fenoglio JJ, McAllister HA, et al: Pericardial cysts. Radiology 125:15, 1977

20. Filly R, Blank N, Castellino RA: Radiographic distribution of intrathoracic disease in previously untreated patients with Hodgkin's disease and non-Hodgkin's lymphoma. Radiology 120:277, 1976

21. Fox MA, Vix VA: Endodermal sinus (yolk sac) tumors of the anterior mediastinum. Am J Roentgenol 135:291, 1980

22. Gale ME: Bochdalek hernia: Prevalence and CT characteristics. Radiology 156:449, 1985

23. Gelman R, Mirvis SE, Geus D: Diaphragmatic rupture due to blunt trauma: Sensitivity of plain chest radiographs. Am J Roentgenol 156:51, 1991

24. Glazer HS, Siegel MJ, Sagel SS: Low attenuation mediastinal masses on CT. Am J Roentgenol 152:1173, 1989

25. Halvorsen RA, Fedyshin PJ, Korobkin M, et al: CT differentiation of pleural effusion from ascites: An evaluation of four signs using blinded analysis of 52 cases. Invest Radiol 21:391, 1986

26. Hansen KF: Idiopathic fibrosis of the mediastinum as a cause of superior vena caval syndrome. Radiology 85:433, 1965

27. Heater K, Revzani L, Rubin JM: CT evaluation of empyema in post-pneumonectomy space. Am J Roentgenol 145:39, 1985

28. Hertzmann Y, Solomon A: Inversion of the right diaphragm: A thoracoabdominal CT pitfall. Gastrointest Radiol 11:200, 1986

29. Hessen I: Roentgen examination of pleural fluid. Acta Radiol [Suppl] (Stockholm) 86, 1951

30. Im JG, Kang HS, Choi BJ, et al: Pleural endometriosis: CT and sonographic findings. Am J Roentgenol 148:523, 1987

31. Inada K, Kawai K, Katsumura T, et al: Giant lymph node hyperplasia of the mediastinum. Am Rev Tuberc 79:232, 1959

32. Keegan JM: Hemangioma of the mediastinum. Am J Roentgenol 69:66, 1953

33. Keen SJ, Libshitz HI: Thymic lesions: Experience with computed tomography in 24 patients. Cancer 59:1520, 1987

34. Keirns MM: Tumors of the diaphragm. Radiology 58:542, 1952

35. Kountz PD, Molina PL, Sagel SI: Fibrosing mediastinitis in the posterior thorax. Am J Roentgenol 153:489, 1989

36. Landay MJ, Rollins NK: Mediastinal histoplasmosis granuloma: Evaluation with CT. Radiology 172:657, 1989

37. Laxdal OE, McDougall H, Mellen GW: Congenital eventration of the diaphragm. N Engl J Med 250:401, 1954

38. Light RW, George RB: Incidence and insignificance of pleural effusion after abdominal surgery. Chest 69:621, 1976

39. Loyd JE, Tillman BF, Atkinson JB, et al: Mediastinal fibrosis complicating histoplasmosis. Medicine 67:295, 1988

40. Lonigan JG, Libshitz HI: MR imaging of malignant pleural mesothelioma. J Comput Assist Tomogr 13:617, 1989

41. Lukes RJ, Craver LF, Hall TC, et al: Report of the Nomenclature Committee. Cancer Research 26:1311, 1966

42. Lull GF Jr, Winn DF Jr: Chronic fibrous mediastinitis due to histoplasma capsulatum. Radiology 73:378, 1959

43. McLoud TC, Flower CDR: Imaging the pleura: Sonography, CT and MR imaging. Am J Roentgenol 156:1145, 1991

44. Nirvis SE, Keramati B, Buckman R, et al: MR imaging of traumatic diaphragmatic rupture. J Comput Assist Tomogr 12:147, 1988

45. Moncada R, Williams V, Fareed J, et al: Thoracic splenosis. Am J Roentgenol 144:705, 1985

46. Miller NL: CT features of cystic teratoma of diaphragm. J Comput Assist Tomogr 10:325, 1986

47. Munk PL, Muller NL: Pleural liposarcoma: CT diagnosis. J Comput Assist Tomogr 12:709, 1988

48. National Cancer Institute sponsored study of classifications of non-Hodgkin's lymphomas: summary and description of a working formulation for clinical usage. Cancer 49:2112, 1982

49. Neuhauser EBD, Harris GBC, Berrett A: Roentgenographic features of neurenteric cysts. Am J Roentgenol 79:235, 1958

50. Nilsson PE, Aspelin P, Ekberg O, et al: Radiologic diagnosis in traumatic rupture of the right diaphragm: Report of a case. Acta Radiol 29:653, 1988

51. Onik G, Goodman PC, Webb WR, et al: Hydropneumothorax: Detection on supine radiographs. Radiology 152:31, 1984

52. Paling MR, Griffin GK: Lower lobe collapse due to pleural effusion: A CT analysis. J Comput Assist Tomogr 9:1079, 1985

53. Panicek DM, Benson CB, Gottlieb RH, et al: The diaphragm: Anatomic, pathologic and radiologic considerations. Radiographics 8:385, 1988

54. PANICEK DM, EWING DK, MARKARIAN B, ET AL: Interstitial pulmonary hemorrhage from mediastinal hematoma secondary to aortic rupture. Radiology 162:165, 1987

55. PINCKNEY L, PARKER BR: Primary coccidioidomycosis in children presenting with massive pleural effusion. Am J Roentgenol 130:247, 1978

56. POKORNY CW, McGILL, HARBERG FJ: Presentation of Morgagni hernias during infancy: Presentation and associated anomalies. J Pediatr Surg 19:394, 1984

57. PRICE JE JR, RIGLER LG: Widening of the mediastinum resulting from fat accumulation. Radiology 96:497, 1970

58. RENNER RR, MARKARIAN B, PERNICE NJ, ET AL: The apical cap. Radiology 110:569, 1974

59. RHOLL KS, LEVITT RG, GLAZER HS: Magnetic resonance imaging of fibrosing mediastinitis. Am J Roentgenol 146:255, 1985

60. ROSENBLUM D, NUSSBAUM A, SCHWARTZ S: Partial obstruction of the inferior vena cava by herniation of the liver through the foramen of Morgagni. Radiology 68:399, 1957

61. SELTZER GC, ANTMON K, FINBERG H, ET AL: Computed tomography of malignant pleural mesothelioma. J Comput Assist Tomogr 7:626, 1983

62. SENGPIEL GW, RUZICKA FF, LODMELL EA: Lateral intrathoracic meningocele. Radiology 50:515, 1948

63. SHUMAN LS, LIBSHITZ HI: Solid pleural manifestations of lymphoma. Am J Roentgenol 142:269, 1984

64. SIMONDS B, FRIEDMAN PJ, SOKOLOFF J: The prone chest film. Radiology 116:11, 1975

65. SPIZARNY DL, GROSS BH, SHEPARD JAO: CT findings in localized fibrous mesothelioma. J Comput Assist Tomogr 10:942, 1986

66. STOREY DD, DINES DE, COLES DT: Pleural effusion: A diagnostic dilemma. JAMA 236:2183, 1976

67. SWINGLE JD, LOGAN R, JUHL JH: Inversion of the left hemidiaphragm. JAMA 208:863, 1969

68. TARVER RD, GODWIN JD, PUTMAN CE: The diaphragm. Radiol Clin North Am 22:615, 1984

69. TOULOUKIAN RJ, MARKOWITZ RI: A preoperative x-ray scoring system for risk assessment of newborns with congenital diaphragmatic hernia. J Pediatr Surg 19:252, 1984

70. WAITE RJ, CARBONNEAU RJ, BALIKIAN JP, ET AL: Parietal pleural changes in empyema Appearances at CT: 35 cases of patients with empyema. Radiology 175:145, 1990

71. ZINN WL, NAIDICH DP, WHELAN CA, ET AL: Fluid within pre-existing pulmonary air spaces: A potential pitfall in the CT differentiation of pleural from parenchymal disease. J Comput Assist Tomogr 11:441, 1987

*Paul and Juhl's Essentials of Radiologic Imaging,
Sixth Edition*, edited by John H. Juhl and
Andrew B. Crummy. J.B. Lippincott Company,
Philadelphia, © 1993.

CHAPTER **32A**

The Cardiovascular System

Andrew B. Crummy

METHODS OF EXAMINATION

The importance of plain film examination of the heart has decreased in recent years because of the advent of newer noninvasive examinations such as ultrasound, including Doppler evaluation, computed tomography (CT), and, most recently, magnetic resonance imaging (MRI). Nevertheless, plain films can provide a plethora of anatomic and physiologic information about the cardiovascular system in a well-accepted, safe, and inexpensive manner. The recognition of cardiovascular abnormalities on chest films taken for other reasons is very important, also. In some conditions, the cardiovascular diagnosis can be made by roentgenographic methods alone, but it must be recognized that these studies usually form only a part of the complete evaluation, and that the x-ray findings must be correlated with other findings including clinical history, physical, electrocardiographic data as well as more complex examinations such as echocardiography and MRI.

On roentgen examination, the size and shape of the heart can be determined in various projections and indications of diseases of the pulmonary artery and aorta as well as shunts and anomalous vessels may be seen. In addition, the roentgenogram furnishes a permanent record of the cardiac size and shape.

ROENTGENOGRAPHY

A complete roentgen study of the heart usually requires a minimum of four projections: posteroanterior, left anterior oblique at approximately 60°, right anterior oblique at approximately 45°, and lateral. The films are exposed at a 6-foot distance, with the patient in the upright position and in moderately deep inspiration. Magnification resulting from divergent distortion is minimized by obtaining posteroanterior and anterior oblique views to place the heart closer to the film (the anterior chest is adjacent to film). A left lateral view (with the left side adjacent to film) also tends to minimize magnification. To outline the esophagus, we use a barium suspension as an aid in determining position and size of the aortic arch. In addition, alteration in esophageal contour may reflect changes in the left-sided chambers. The use of ultrasound in determining cardiac chamber size has decreased the use of the oblique projections, so that frequently the cardiac examination is restricted to PA and lateral projections, usually without barium in the esophagus.

FLUOROSCOPY

Cardiovascular fluoroscopy no longer has widespread use and in our institution is largely limited to the evaluation of specific questions: i.e., the presence of large pericardial effusions and the evaluation of aortic arch anomalies. Generally, calcium is better seen on fluoroscopy then on plain films and these observations may be made at the time of cardiac catheterization. Minor amounts of calcification are best seen on CT.[71] In our department, the use of fluoroscopy has virtually disappeared in the study of congenital heart disease because in general the patients require more definitive studies such as cardiac catheterization, angiocardiography, ultrasonography, and MRI.

There are several disadvantages in cardiac fluoroscopy, one of the most important of which is the amount of radiation to which the patient is exposed.

This can be kept to a minimum by observing the rules described in Chapter 22. The second disadvantage is distortion. Because the distance between the target of the x-ray tube and the patient is short, there is considerable enlargement of the cardiac silhouette and distortion of other thoracic structures. This can be decreased by using longer distances between target and the patient, and by using a small shutter opening, producing the central-beam effect. The third disadvantage is lack of permanent record. This is obviated to a certain extent by the use of cine or videotape recording and by roentgenograms obtained before the procedure.

ANGIOCARDIOGRAPHY

This method of contrast cardiac visualization has been used widely for examination of patients with all types of cardiac and pulmonary diseases (Fig. 32-1). The technique and indications are discussed briefly in Chapter 22. The method is used in the diagnosis of congenital and acquired cardiac disease. Selective angiocardiography in which a small amount of opaque medium (an organic iodide) is injected into a specific chamber or vessel during cardiac catheterization is used almost exclusively.

CORONARY ARTERIOGRAPHY

Selective catheterization of the coronary arteries followed by injection of a contrast medium (one of the organic iodides) is used in combination with cineradiography rapid serial filming or videotaping to study the coronary arteries. Details of technique are beyond the scope of this discussion.

AORTOGRAPHY

This examination consists of the injection of one of the organic iodides into the aorta through a catheter introduced into one of its major branches and placed into a desired position in the aorta. The examination has a place in the investigation of patients with congenital and acquired problems of the aortic arch. It is used in infants with congestive heart failure in whom there is evidence of a left-to-right shunt and in whom patent ductus arteriosus is suspected. Coarctation of the aorta in infants may also cause congestive heart failure. The lesion can be defined by aortography. In adults, aortography is used to define anomalies of the aortic arch and its branches as well as in the study of the aortic valve and the coronary arteries. It is also useful in patients with masses adjacent to the aorta in whom

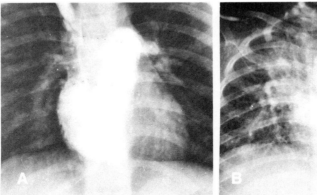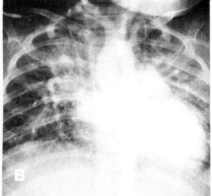

Figure 32–1. Angiocardiogram—normal findings. (**A**) Filling of the right side of the heart. Some medium is in the superior vena cava and can be seen entering the right atrium. The right ventricle is partially obscured by the atrium. Note relative radiolucency of the left side of the heart. The pulmonary outflow tract and artery are well visualized, but there is no opacification of the branches of the pulmonary artery as yet. (**B**) This is a later phase in a younger child to show filling of the left side of the heart. The left ventricle is clearly defined, making up the left lower cardiac border. The aorta and its brachiocephalic branches are outlined. The left atrium is well filled and is noted to overlie the root of the aorta, with the appendage projecting to the left above the ventricle. A considerable amount of the medium remains in the pulmonary vascular system.

aneurysm is a possibility and in patients suspected of having dissecting hematoma, and traumatic or other aneurysms.

ULTRASONIC INVESTIGATION OF THE HEART

The use of ultrasound in examination of the heart has increased greatly in the past 20 years, and it is now well established and a widely used diagnostic tool. Ultrasonic investigation is a noninvasive, safe, and comfortable study that will demonstrate valve and chamber motion wall thickness and size. Doppler examination allows determination of the cross-sectional area of a valve as well as quantification of gradients that may be present. It is of value in the study of the hypertrophic cardiomyopathies both with and without associated subaortic stenosis and in the study of the congestive type in which there is chamber dilatation. With ultrasound, left ventricular diameter and outflow configuration can be determined; qualitative assessment of right and left ventricular size is possible, also. The size of the left atrium can be measured accurately and left atrial myxomas or other intraatrial tumors can be detected. Ultrasound is also useful in the investigation of congenital heart disease, particularly in patients with hypoplastic left-heart syndrome, double-outlet right ventricle, and right ventricular volume overload. In addition, it is the most sensitive method for determining the presence of pericardial effusion.

DETERMINATION OF CARDIAC SIZE

The size of the heart is related to body weight and height as well as to surface area, sex, and age. A number of methods of correlation of these factors with cardiac size, as measured on the roentgenogram, have been described. It is unfortunate that in the borderline cases in which determination of possible cardiac enlargement is most needed, the mathematic formulas are most faulty since there is a normal variation of approximately plus or minus 10%. Numerous factors such as depth of respiration, thoracic deformity, and pulmonary and abdominal diseases that elevate or depress the diaphragm affect the size of the cardiac silhouette. Because normal and the abnormal size cannot be determined specifically in an individual patient, most of the methods of measurement are chiefly of statistical value. These methods are usually based on direct measurement on teleoroentgenograms. The most commonly used are (1) measurement of transverse diameters; (2) measurement of surface area; and (3) cardiothoracic ratio. The transverse diameter of the heart is the sum of the maximum projections of the heart to the right and to the left of the midline; the measurement

should be made so as not to include epicardial fat or other noncardiac structures (Fig. 32-2). The diameter can then be compared with the theoretic transverse diameter of the heart for various heights and weights as described by Ungerleider and Clark.[84] Surface area estimations based on artificial construction of the base of the heart and of the diaphragmatic contour of the heart have been described by Ungerleider and Gubner.[85] A nomogram used for measuring children's hearts has been reported by Meyer.[56] The cardiothoracic ratio is the ratio between the transverse cardiac diameter and the greatest internal diameter of the thorax, measured on the frontal teleoroentgenogram. This is the easiest and quickest method of measurement of cardiac size; an adult heart that measures more than one half of the internal diameter of the chest is considered enlarged. The method is gross, because the cardiothoracic ratio varies widely with variations in body habitus. It can be useful, however, as a rough estimate of cardiac size. The cardiothoracic ratio is most useful in assessing changes in heart size or monitoring progression of disease, or as a response to therapy.

These are a few of the many methods described and there are a number of objections to each of them. In borderline cases, the numeric exactness of the various measurements is not matched by the reliability of the method. Most of the measurements are relatively simple and easy to apply and do serve as a basis for discrimination between hearts that are obviously normal and those obviously enlarged. They are accurate enough for most statistical studies.

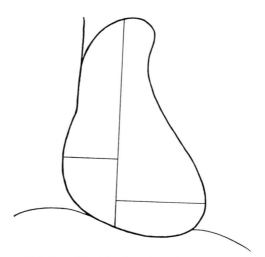

Figure 32–2. Sketch showing the method of measuring the transverse diameter of the heart. The sum of the horizontal projections from the vertical line is the transverse diameter.

Ultrasonography is now used widely in determination of cardiac size including individual chambers and wall thickness. Cardiac chamber size and ventricular wall thickness can be determined with considerable accuracy by ultrasonic methods and increases or decreases can be assessed by serial examination.

THE NORMAL HEART

THE ADULT HEART

The heart and its major vessels occupy the middle mediastinum and normally produce a uniform density that is readily recognized on the roentgenogram. The density of the great vessels and the heart is comparable, so that the contours of the silhouette are visible in contrast to the adjacent radiolucent lungs. The inferior cardiac border has a density comparable to that of the diaphragm and often is not clearly defined. On the right side the shadow of the liver below the diaphragm blends into that of the heart, but on the left side there is frequently enough air in the stomach immediately below the dome of the diaphragm to outline the inferior left border of the heart. Marked individual variations are noted in the relationships inferiorly, resulting in an inferior border that is difficult or impossible to define in some patients, while in others it is clearly outlined. The heart lies approximately two thirds to the left of the midline and one third to the right of the midline in the average person.

The Posteroanterior Projection

In the posteroanterior projection, the right side of the cardiovascular silhouette is divided into two segments. The lower segment is usually convex and represents the lateral border of the right atrium. This segment is often separated from the upper border by an indentation. The upper segment is nearly vertical in the young adult and is usually formed by the superior vena cava.

In older adults, the aorta tends to dilate and elongate so that the right upper border becomes more convex. The convexity represents the right lateral aspect of the ascending aortic arch. In asthenic persons with a vertical heart, it is sometimes possible to outline the reflection of the pericardium down to the inferior vena cava. It appears as a small, straight, or slightly concave downward continuation of the convex shadow of the right atrium. On the left side there are usually three visible segments. The uppermost is rounded and convex laterally. It represents the aortic knob, or transverse aortic arch. The descending aorta may also form a portion of the left border, particularly in the persons with vertical hearts. The left lateral wall of the aorta can often be followed downward behind the heart, in the left paraspinal area almost to the diaphragm, especially on over-penetrated films. Immediately below the aortic knob is another short segment, the contour of which varies considerably. It represents the pulmonary artery and occasionally its left main branch. In most normal adults it is straight or slightly convex.

Considerable prominence of the pulmonary artery is a common finding in normal young women and should not be considered abnormal. The left pulmonary artery passes over the lower portion of the left main bronchus and the proximal left upper lobe bronchus. The main pulmonary artery arises just below the level of the left main bronchus. There is some variability, but the left auricular appendage usually forms the short segment of the left border of the heart just below the pulmonary artery.

In some persons, a portion of the distal right ventricular outflow tract may form the border in this area. The left ventricle forms the remainder of the left cardiac margin, including the apex, and is by far the largest segment. The contour of this border is usually dependent upon the habitus of the person. It tends to be relatively straight and descends sharply in the asthenic individual, while in the hypersthenic person it is convex and angles outward considerably. There is thus a considerable range between the extremes of vertical and transverse cardiac configuration. There has been some difference of opinion, but the wide use of angiocardiography has demonstrated rather clearly that the left auricular appendage normally does not project beyond the left ventricle along the left border of the heart. In patients with disease resulting in enlargement of the left atrium, the appendage may project to the left of the ventricle and produce a convexity immediately below the level of the pulmonary artery. The amount of this change varies with the amount and type of left atrial enlargement.

These various segments can usually be identified on the roentgenogram, and alterations aid in the diagnosis of various cardiovascular abnormalities. The cardiac apex usually forms the lower left border of the heart and is usually at or near the level of the dome of the diaphragm; it is somewhat angular, with the apex of the angle rounded (Fig. 32-3). A shadow that is less than the density of the heart often extends lateral to the cardiac apex. This is the apical fat pad.

The Right Anterior Oblique (RAO) Projection

In the RAO projection, the person being examined is rotated to the left 45° so that the right anterior chest wall is nearest the cassette and the left posterior chest wall is nearest the tube. In the RAO projection, the left or most anterior cardiac border consists from above downward of the ascending aortic arch, the pulmonary

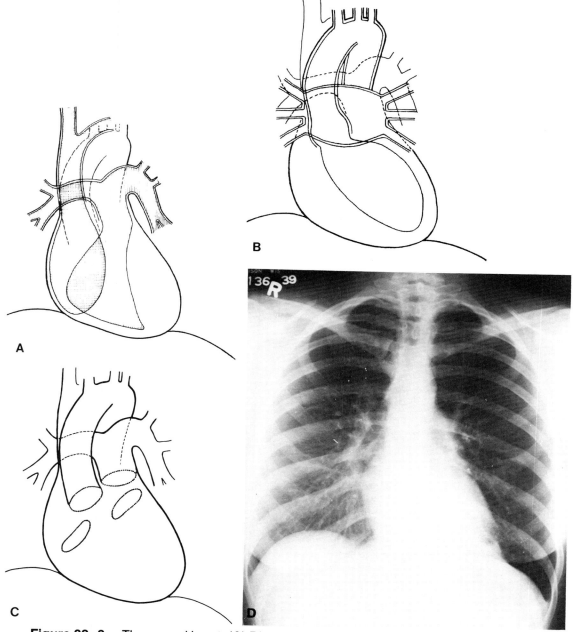

Figure 32–3. The normal heart. (**A**) Diagram to show the relative position of the chambers of the right side of the heart in the AP projection. Horizontal lines outline the vena cava and right atrium. The position of the aorta is also indicated. (**B**) The left side of the heart in frontal projection. Note that the left ventricle forms most of the left border of the heart. The position of the left atrium in the diagram is slightly above its usual position. (**C**) Sketch to show approximate position of valves in the frontal projection. The mitral valve is above to the left of the tricuspid. Aortic and pulmonic rings are noted at the root of their respective arteries. (**D**) Roentgenogram showing the normal cardiovascular silhouette. There are many variations, as indicated in the test. (From Dotter CT, Steinberg I: Angiocardiography. Annals of Roentgenology, vol 20, 1951)

artery, pulmonary conus (conus infundibularis) or out-flow tract of the right ventricle, and a portion of the left ventricle. If the subject is rotated more than 45°, an increasing amount of the left border is made up of right ventricle accompanied by a decrease in the left ventricular contribution to this border. The posterior (right) contour in this projection is formed cranial to caudad by the left atrium, right atrium, and a short segment of the inferior vena cava. These contours are outlined in Figure 32-4. This projection is useful in detecting enlargement of the left atrium and in determining the prominence of the pulmonary outflow tract and artery.

The Left Anterior Oblique (LAO) Projection

In the LAO projection, the patient is turned to his or her right about 60° so that the left anterior chest is nearest the cassette, while the right posterior aspect is nearest the tube. The anterior (right) contour in the LAO is formed by the ascending aorta, the right atrial appendage, right atrium, and occasionally the right ventricle from above downward. In most instances, the right atrium forms the lower anterior border in this projection, although the posterior (left) contour is formed by the left atrium above and the left ventricle below. Occasionally the shallow indentation representing the atrioventricular groove can be discerned along the posterior border. The contours are indicated in Figure 32-5. The left anterior oblique view is also useful in examining the aorta because the arch is "opened," with very little overlapping.

The Lateral Projection

In the lateral projection, the anterior aspect of the cardiovascular silhouette is formed superiorly by the ascending aorta, then by the pulmonary artery, the right ventricular outflow tract, and the right ventricle. Slight rotation in the lateral position will project the right ventricle to be formed by the border anteriorly. The posterior silhouette is formed by the left atrium above and left ventricle below. The contours are indicated in Figure 32-6.

THE HEART IN INFANCY AND CHILDHOOD

At birth the right ventricle is relatively large and is approximately the same size as the left ventricle. During early life the left ventricle grows more rapidly than the right and its wall becomes thicker. The globular heart of the newborn extends to the right almost as far as it does to the left, in contrast to the adult heart, two thirds of which lies to the left of the midline. In addition to the globular heart shape noted on the frontal projection in infants, the chambers and great vessels are not defined as clearly. There is great variability in the size and shape of the heart in the newborn and during the first few weeks of life. Therefore, the diagnosis of cardiac enlargement should be made with caution. There is often more prominence in the region of the pulmonary artery and right ventricular outflow tract than in the adult, and the aortic knob is not readily visible in the newborn and in the young infant.

In infants and young children, there is frequently enough thymic tissue to obscure the cardiac base and great vessels. Slight local displacement of the trachea away from the side of the aortic arch may provide a clue about its position.

The heart generally maintains its globular shape for the first six months of life. It then begins to descend in the thorax and, as it does, the long axis shifts from horizontal to a more oblique and then to an obliquely vertical position. This is a gradual process, so that when the child is 5 to 7 years of age the silhouette approaches that of the adult heart, although the ascending aortic arch and knob are not as prominent as they will be later. As in the adult, the general contour of the heart is related to body habitus. This becomes apparent in the 5- to 10-year-old child.

Measurements of cardiac size in children show that the size of the heart in relation to the thoracic size is somewhat greater than in adults. The long axis of a child's heart tends to be more horizontal than in adults so the cardiothoracic index ranges from an upper limit of 0.65 in the first year to 0.50 in the fifth year and from then on the ratio is in the range of 0.50. Measurements of the heart in children are subject to the same errors as indicated in the discussion on heart size in the adult,

Figure 32–4.   The normal heart in the right anterior oblique projection. (**A**) The right side of the heart. The vena cava, right chambers, and pulmonary arteries are outlined. (**B**) Left side of the heart. Note that the left atrium forms the left upper posterior contour, and the apex of the left ventricle forms the lower anterior contour. (**C**) Sketch to show the approximate position of the valves in the right anterior oblique position. The mitral valve is posterior to the tricuspid. Aortic and pulmonic rings are noted at the roots of their respective arteries. (**D**) Roentgenogram in this position showing the normal cardiac configuration. Barium in the esophagus tends to outline the posterior cardiac border below the carina. (From Dotter CT, Steinberg I: Angiocardiography. Annals of Roentgenology, vol 20, 1951)

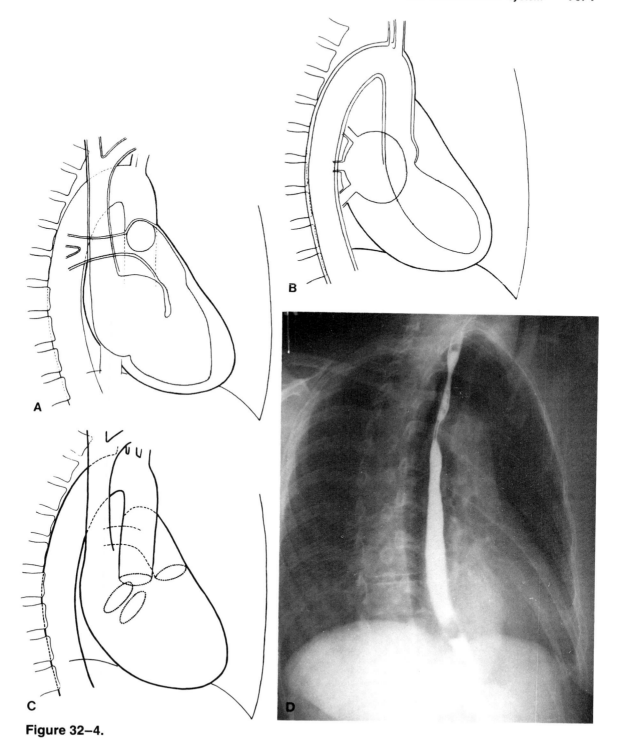

Figure 32–4.

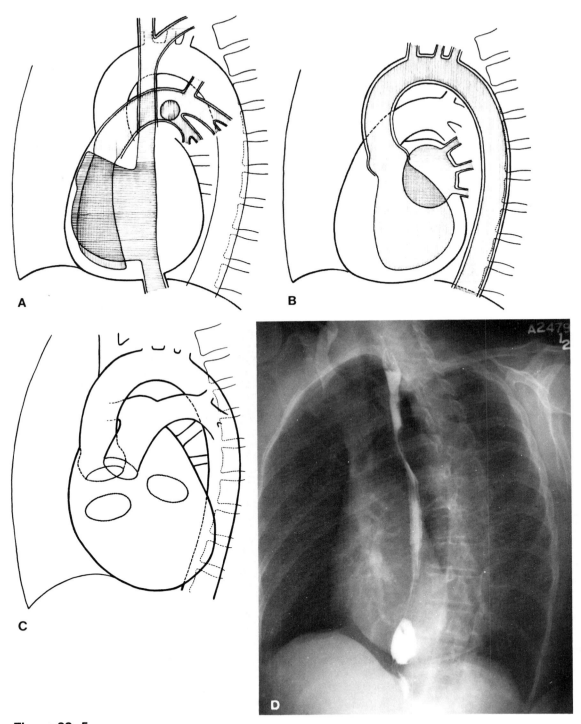

Figure 32–5.

and there is the additional factor of inability to control the depth of respiration in infants and young children.

THE NORMAL AORTA

The border-forming contours of the aorta have been mentioned previously and are outlined in Figures 32-3 though 32-5. The right lateral contour of the ascending aorta is partially border-forming in adults with aortic dilatation or elongation. The medial border of the ascending aorta is not visible in the frontal projection, but the superior and lateral borders of the aortic knob are visualized as the upper left margin of the cardiovascular shadow, and, in older adults, a portion of the descending aorta may be border forming just below the aortic knob. It is often possible to outline the descending aorta although it is not border forming. It appears as a slightly convex, linear shadow extending downward, overlying the left upper cardiac silhouette. In the right anterior oblique view, the upper anterior portion of the cardiovascular silhouette is formed by the ascending aorta.

In the RAO, the descending arch and part of the thoracic aorta can often be outlined posterior to the cardiac silhouette. The aortic arch is defined more clearly in the left anterior oblique view. Again, the ascending arch forms the upper anterior portion of the cardiovascular silhouette; the transverse and descending portions of the arch, as well as the remaining thoracic aorta, are often visible in this projection. The aorta is often defined clearly in older adults in whom arteriosclerotic changes have resulted in deposition of calcium in the aortic walls. With advancing age the aorta becomes elongated so that the ascending arch and knob become more prominent and its silhouette of the ascending portion more convex. The aortic knob is larger in diameter and there is often considerable tortuosity of the aorta.

Numerous methods of aortic measurement have been described. They are subject to the same errors as the various mathematic formulas used in determining cardiac size. The measurements are most faulty in the borderline group in which accurate determination is most necessary. There is a gradual decrease in diameter of the aorta as it is more distant from the heart so that the ascending portion of the arch is the widest, followed by the transverse, the descending, and the lower thoracic aorta. Dotter and Steinberg measured the inner diameter of the aorta by means of angiocardiography and observed a wide range. In 100 patients the diameter of the ascending aorta ranged from 16 to 38 mm with an average of 28.6 mm. Measurements elsewhere showed comparable wide ranges.

Detailed studies of the aorta can be performed with water-soluble iodine containing contrast agents. The contrast can be injected on the venous side of the circulation and propelled forward by cardiac action and deposited directly into the aorta. The latter method provides better opacification. Indications for these studies are the evaluation of vascular disease such as aneurysm, atherosclerosis, trauma, dissecting hematoma, or nonvascular disease such as juxtaaortic masses. Recently CT and MRI have assumed important roles in vascular studies. The details of the examination are beyond the scope of this book.

THE PERICARDIUM

The pericardium is a closed, endothelium-lined sac that envelops the heart. It consists of a visceral layer covering the heart and a parietal layer reflected to form a continuous sac. It normally contains 15 to 25 mL of clear fluid. The parietal pericardium fuses with the diaphragm below and the mediastinal pleura laterally and anteriorly, except in the sternal area, where there is no pleura. The reflection of the parietal pericardium occurs in a line that begins at the superior vena cava above its junction with the right atrium on the right side, and continues to the left over the anterior aspect of the ascending aorta to the pulmonary artery, which is

◀ **Figure 32–5.**   The normal heart in the left anterior oblique projection. (**A**) The right side of the heart. The vena cava and right atrium are outlined by horizontal lines. The right ventricle and outflow tract along with the pulmonary artery are outlined. The aortic arch is also indicated. This is a somewhat exaggerated left oblique projection, and it differs very little from the lateral. Note that the anterior contour is made up of the right atrium and ventricle. (**B**) The left side of the heart. The left atrium is outlined by horizontal lines. The left ventricle, aorta, and the pulmonary artery are also indicated. (**C**) Sketch to show approximate position of the valves in the left anterior oblique position. The mitral valve is posterior to the tricuspid, and the aortic and pulmonary rings are noted at the roots of these arteries. (**D**) The left anterior oblique roentgenogram shows the normal cardiac contour in this projection. The esophagus, outlined by barium, is normal. (From Dotter CT, Steinberg I: Angiocardiography. Annals of Roentgenology, vol 20, 1951)

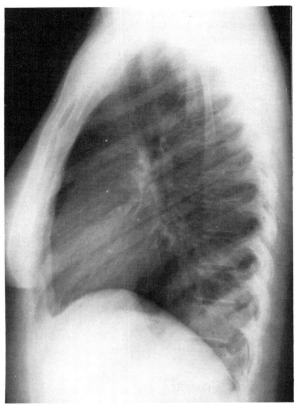

Figure 32–6. The normal heart, shown in the lateral roentgenogram. The contours are described in the text and are similar to those seen in Figure 32–5.

covered by pericardium nearly to the level of the ligamentum arteriosus. Posteriorly the pericardium extends up as far as the proximal superior vena cava and down to the inferior vena cava. The pericardium cannot be visualized on a film in the normal person. However, it is well demonstrated by CT and ultrasound examination. The apical fat pad frequently seen at the left cardiodiaphragmatic angle lies between the parietal pericardium and a reflection of the parietal pleura as it extends downward and laterally to cover the diaphragm in this region. A similar situation exists on the right, and a fat pad is occasionally noted in the cardiohepatic angle.

ENLARGEMENT OF THE HEART

GENERAL CARDIAC ENLARGEMENT

General cardiac enlargement may be caused by disease that produces a toxic effect on the myocardium and weakens it, and by conditions that cause an increase in the workload on the heart. This load is usually initially on a single chamber, and when that chamber fails a second one becomes enlarged; eventually all chambers may be involved. Therefore, in the latter type of disease, single- or double-chamber enlargement may predominate while in myocardiopathies there is more likely to be uniform and generalized cardiac enlargement.

The roentgen appearance of the heart in myocardiopathies varies considerably, but the lateral contours on both sides often become more convex inferiorly and the normal slight alterations in the contour indicating the various segments are frequently effaced. The transverse diameter is usually increased more than the vertical diameter. Evidence of pulmonary congestion manifested by prominent and poor definition of pulmonary basal vascular markings may also be present. At fluoroscopy or ultrasound examination, pulsations are diminished, and, in extreme cases, are so poor as to be difficult to define. When single- or multiple-chamber enlargement is present, the cardiac contour often shows characteristic changes that can be recognized roentgenographically.

LEFT VENTRICULAR ENLARGEMENT

When there is an increased workload on a cardiac chamber, the muscle fibers elongate in response to the added work and dilatation results. When this load is maintained over a period of time, the dilatation is followed by hypertrophy, which is represented by actual increase in the size of the individual muscle fibers. The initial dilatation that precedes hypertrophy is the means by which heart muscle increases its ability to work. When the workload becomes great there is secondary dilatation that results from failure of the heart muscle to do its work adequately. This type of dilatation indicates cardiac decompensation and failure.

Hypertrophy of the heart muscle is a clearly defined pathologic finding, but the roentgen changes are often minimal or absent, making it difficult to determine in many instances. However, hypertrophy may cause alteration in cardiac shape, usually manifested by rounding of the contour of the ventricle involved. Little if any change in size results when hypertrophy is present without dilatation. Conversely, dilatation causes an increase in size and may also alter the shape of the cardiac silhouette. The ventricles may be divided into two functional components, the inflow tract and the outflow tract. The blood flows into the left ventricle from the left atrium through the mitral valve that lies posterior and somewhat caudad to the aortic valve. The inflow tract extends from the valve along the posterior wall of the left ventricle and posterior half of the septum to the apex. The outflow tract is anterior and extends from the apex along the anterior half of the septum and anterior portion of the lateral ventricular wall and anterior leaflet of the mitral valve.

Any disease that causes an increased workload on the left ventricle may cause enlargement of this chamber. This is manifested first by elongation of the outflow tract. This produces an increase in the length of the left ventricular segment making up the left lateral cardiac contour as visualized roentgenographically. The second sign of enlargement of this tract is rounding of the contour of the left ventricle. As a result of this downward and leftward enlargement, the cardiac apex may extend below the dome of the diaphragm. This may be seen in the air-filled gastric fundus. Enlargement of the inflow tract of the left ventricle, which follows that of the outflow tract, produces posterior enlargement best outlined on the roentgenogram obtained in the left anterior oblique projection. This posterior enlargement has led to the use of the angle of clearance between the left ventricle and spine in the left anterior oblique position as a criterion for left ventricular enlargement. The angle of clearance of the left ventricle is the angle through which the patient must be rotated to his right from the posteroanterior position into the left anterior (or right posterior) oblique position to clear the posterior silhouette of the left ventricle from the thoracic spine. The angle is measured at a point where these structures do not quite overlap. Normal variation is so high, however, that the specific angle of 55°, which is often quoted, is most likely too high in some individuals and too low in others. In addition to the enlargement downward and to the left as well as posteriorly, disease resulting in increased left ventricular work may result in concentric hypertrophy of this chamber. This indicates that the ventricle is hypertrophied without significant dilatation so that there is very little actual enlargement. The hypertrophy is manifested roentgenographically by rounding of the left ventricular contour and apex as visualized in the frontal projection. Enlargement of the left ventricle is demonstrated in the posteroanterior, lateral, and left anterior oblique projections.

The most marked enlargement of the left ventricle is caused by hypertension, aortic insufficiency, and myocardiopathy. Other lesions that produce enlargement of this chamber are aortic stenosis, mitral insufficiency, coarctation of the aorta, arteriovenous shunts that may be intracardiac or extracardiac, arteriosclerotic cardiovascular disease, and hyperthyroidism.

RIGHT VENTRICULAR ENLARGEMENT

The right ventricle is enlarged in persons having diseases that increase the work of this chamber. These diseases include a number of pulmonary diseases as well as primary vascular disease in the pulmonary arteries that results in pulmonary hypertension. Stenosis of the pulmonary valve or infundibulum and other congenital cardiac lesions, such as truncus arteriosus and septal defects, may also result in enlargement of this ventricle. Mitral valvular disease is also a common cause. When enlargement occurs, the outflow tract is the site of the earliest dilatation. Enlargement of the outflow tract extends from the apex of the right ventricle to the pulmonic valve and includes the anterior wall along with the upper half of the interventricular septum. The inflow tract that extends from the tricuspid valve to the apex includes the lower half of the interventricular septum inferiorly, and the lower part of its outer wall anteriorly. Enlargement of the outflow tract of the right ventricle results in lengthening of the anterior ventricular wall, which is manifested radiographically by prominence of the distal right ventricle or pulmonary conus. The result is an anterior bulge in the upper anterior cardiac contour just below the pulmonary artery noted in the right anterior oblique projection. There is often associated enlargement of the pulmonary artery, which adds to the anterior prominence of the upper border of the heart in this projection. When this occurs, there is more prominence and convexity of the pulmonary artery segment in the frontal projection than is normal. This results in straightening or convexity of the left upper cardiac contour below the aortic knob. When the enlargement of the right ventricle becomes greater, the heart tends to be rotated to the left (counterclockwise as viewed from the front) so that the conus of the right ventricle may become border forming. In the RAO projection, the anterolateral bulge in the region of the outflow tract of the right ventricle reduces the size of the retrosternal space between the upper cardiac border and the sternum. The pulmonary artery also contributes to this narrowing. There is also a fullness superiorly in the retrosternal space in the lateral projection.

When the inflow tract of the right ventricle enlarges, the diaphragmatic portion of this ventricle is increased in length, resulting in an anterior rounding or bulge in the right ventricular area as visualized in the left anterior oblique projection. This enlargement may also displace the left ventricle posteriorly and elevate the cardiac apex. The latter is a common finding in infants and children with congenital cardiac disease resulting in right ventricular enlargement. When right ventricular dilatation is associated with enlargement of the left ventricle, the differentiation and evaluation of the relative size of each chamber are often very difficult to make.

LEFT ATRIAL ENLARGEMENT

Rheumatic mitral valvular disease had been the most common cause of the left atrial enlargement until the antibiotic era. Now, other diseases such as right-to-left shunts and myocardiopathies are more common causes. Left atrial enlargement also occurs in other diseases such as congenital cardiac lesions resulting in intracardiac shunts, and in left ventricular failure. The left atrium lies posteriorly and does not form any part of the cardiac contour in the frontal projection in the normal subject. Small amounts of enlargement are often entirely posterior. The earliest radiologic sign is displacement of the esophagus posteriorly and slightly to the right, which can be demonstrated on a chest film exposed following the oral administration of barium to outline the esophagus. In the normal person, the esophagus is relatively straight as visualized in the right anterior oblique projection and a small amount of atrial enlargement produces a localized posterior bulge in the region of the atrium that lies just below the level of the carina. As this chamber becomes larger, it enlarges to the right and left as well as posteriorly. The left auricular appendage may then project beyond the left ventricle to produce a straightening of the left or localized convexity of the cardiac border just below the pulmonary artery segment. The atrial appendage is usually relatively larger in patients with rheumatic heart disease than in those with comparable left atrial enlargement secondary to other disease. This enlargement causes the contour change often termed the "mitral silhouette" in which the appendage produces a considerable convexity of the left upper cardiac margin just below the level of the pulmonary artery. The enlargement to the right may be sufficient to make the right border of this chamber extend beyond the upper aspect of the right atrium and the superior vena cava. This results in a double contour on the right as visualized in the frontal projection. There may also be a visible double contour on the right when the left atrium does not project beyond the right atrial border. This is caused by the increased density of the large left atrium. Elevation of the left main bronchus may also be visible; when the enlargement reaches this stage, the mass of this chamber is often large enough to produce an oval localized density that can be seen through the heart in the frontal projection. When enlargement is massive, the left atrium may form most of the right cardiac contour and part of the left upper cardiac contour in the frontal projection. Rarely, the left atrium projects only to the left when it enlarges. In the left anterior oblique projection, enlargement of the left atrium produces a posterior bulge just below the left main bronchus. This is a relatively constant and sensitive indicator of enlargement of this chamber provided that the proper obliquity of approximately 45° is obtained.

Westcott and Ferguson have described a method for measuring left atrial size on lateral films.[87] This method depends on clear visualization of the right pulmonary artery because it relies upon a line drawn downward from the anterior wall of the right pulmonary artery parallel to the barium-filled esophagus. The anteroposterior diameter is measured from this line to the anterior esophageal wall. The anterior wall of the right pulmonary artery indicates the level of the anterior wall of the left atrium and the anterior esophageal wall outlines the posterior atrial margin. They found the normal diameter of the left atrium to range from 25 to 42 mm for men 25 years of age, and 17 to 38 mm for women of the same age. The male mean is 30.04 ± 3.9 mm and the female mean is 28 ± 3.9 mm. This correlated well with echocardiographic measurements in the study.

A method for measuring the left atrial diameter on the frontal film has been described by Higgins and associates.[34] In this method, measurement is made from the midpoint of the curvilinear margin of the double density produced by the left atrium on the right side to the midpoint of the inferior wall of the left bronchus. By this method the diameter of the left atrium was found to be less than 7 cm in 96% of normal persons and greater than 7 cm in 90% of patients with left atrial enlargement as determined by echocardiography. The method is not very reliable in children. It is simple to obtain and permits comparison of left atrial size in patients with mitral valvular disease. Measurements were not corrected for magnification. Generally, these most accurate and reliable measurements of left atrial size are obtained with ultrasound examination.

RIGHT ATRIAL ENLARGEMENT

The right atrium is enlarged in atrial septal defect, tricuspid stenosis and insufficiency, and in right ventricular failure. The right auricular appendage enlarges first and enlargement of the right atrium can be suspected when there is a bulge or prominence in the right atrial segment in the left anterior oblique projection. This bulge represents the auricular appendage; occasionally, this enlargement produces actual angulation between the appendage and the right ventricle in the left oblique projection. When the body of the atrium enlarges, it produces enlargement of the lower right cardiac contour to the right with increased convexity of this contour. Marked increase of this chamber produces great enlargement to the right in the frontal projection and a local prominence to the right and posteriorly as visualized in the right anterior oblique projection. In this view, the local enlargement lies just above the diaphragm and below the area in which the left atrium is visible when it is increased in size. Slight enlargement of the right atrium is very difficult to detect radiographically, particularly when other chambers are enlarged as in severe rheumatic valvular disease with chronic congestive failure.

CONGENITAL HEART DISEASE

Accurate diagnosis of the nature of congenital cardiac malformations is now imperative because surgical techniques are available for the cure of a number of lesions and palliation of others. The radiographic methods are a very important part of the examination of patients with congenital defects, but accurate diagnosis depends upon correlation of all clinical and laboratory findings, including echocardiography and cardiac catheterization with angiocardiography. In acyanotic patients, the presence of a cardiac defect such as an atrial septal defect with the shunt may be recognized on a chest film taken for an unrelated reason.

There are wide variations in the roentgen findings in any single defect because of the extended range of severity of single or multiple defects. For example, septal defects may be small and produce little shunting of blood and very little alteration in the appearance of the cardiovascular silhouette; they may be very large and accompanied by a large shunt and marked changes in the cardiovascular silhouette. The same is true of the defects that produce cyanosis. A broad spectrum of physiologic and anatomic alteration is possible for each defect.

The differential diagnosis of many of these lesions is difficult to make and it is helpful to classify the defects into those that produce cyanosis and those that do not. These can then be subdivided according to the radiographic appearance of the pulmonary vessels and to the presence or absence of cardiac enlargement. By using this approach, each defect can be placed in a relatively small group and special studies can differentiate the members of that group. Comprehensive review of all congenital defects is not within the scope of this volume. Echocardiography is the most useful noninvasive technique, while selective angiocardiography is the most useful invasive imaging method for the diagnosis of the congenital cardiac diseases. MRI is assuming a rapidly increasing and important role in the evaluation of congenital heart disease (infra vide).

CYANOTIC DEFECTS

Tetralogy of Fallot

The tetralogy of Fallot consists of two fundamental defects: (1) pulmonic stenosis and (2) high interventricular septal defect. The third and fourth alterations described in this tetralogy are secondary and consist of the aorta overriding the ventricular septum with dextroposition, and hypertrophy of the right ventricle. The pulmonic stenosis causes an elevation of pressure in the right ventricle; the septal defect and overriding of the aorta allow blood from the right ventricle (venous blood) to be shunted directly into the general circula-

tion. This right-to-left shunt from the right ventricle into the aorta results in cyanosis resulting from unsaturation of the arterial blood. In addition to the abnormalities originally described, other anomalies often occur in combination. The most common is a patent foramen ovale. True atrial septal defect is less common; when this defect is present, the term "pentalogy of Fallot" is sometimes used. A right-sided aortic arch is present in about 25% of patients with tetralogy. Extracardiac anomalies consisting of malformations of the aortic arch system are also common. Rarely, abnormalities such as stenosis of peripheral pulmonary arteries, partial anomalous venous return, absence or hypoplasia of the pulmonary valve, persistent common atrioventricular canal, and tricuspid insufficiency may be associated with tetralogy of Fallot. The pulmonic stenosis is usually infundibular in type. The infundibulum generally is constricted into a long, narrow channel and there may be an associated valvular stenosis. Valvular stenosis alone, however, is unusual in tetralogy. When this occurs there may be some poststenotic dilatation of the pulmonary artery that alters the configuration of the left cardiovascular border. Occasionally, the stenosis is localized to the proximal infundibulum, the ostium infundibula. When this occurs the infundibulum dilates to a greater or lesser extent, forming a "third" ventricle. The degree of stenosis varies from a very slight narrowing to pulmonary atresia. In the latter instance, which is very rare, the bronchial arteries or a patent ductus arteriosus and pulmonary arteries provide the pulmonary blood supply. The roentgenographic findings vary with the degree of pulmonic stenosis and the amount of shunt. This lesion has been called a pseudotruncus.

Roentgen Findings

Heart Size. The heart is usually within the normal limits of size and may appear to be somewhat smaller than normal. Appreciable cardiac enlargement in this condition is unusual unless the patient survives into adult life. The right ventricle hypertrophies, but usually does not dilate.

Pulmonary Artery. The pulmonary artery segment, as visualized in the frontal projection, is small, resulting in concavity of the upper left cardiac margin in the region of this segment. The degree of concavity depends on the degree of stenosis, and varies from marked concavity to a pulmonary artery segment that cannot be distinguished from the normal. In the occasional patient with stenosis of the ostium infundibula, the dilated infundibulum may produce a convexity in the left side of the heart border at and just below the level of the left main bronchus, which represents the distal right ventricle. When poststenotic dilatation of the pulmonary artery is present in patients with valvular stenosis, there is slight convexity rather than concavity in the region of this artery.

Pulmonary Vascularity. Pulmonary vascularity decreases, resulting in a decrease in the size of the vessels making up the hilum on both sides, and relative avascularity of the lung fields. This is an indication of decreased pulmonary blood flow. In severe stenosis and in patients with pseudotruncus, the branching of the dilated bronchial arteries may produce a brushlike appearance, with small vessels of uniform caliber in contrast to the decreasing caliber of pulmonary arteries usually noted. In patients with minimal defects resulting in the so-called "acyanotic" tetralogy, the vascularity is usually normal.

Heart Shape. The enlargement of the right ventricle results in elevation of the apex and a rounded configuration of the lower left cardiac margin. In the LAO projection, the right ventricular enlargement produces rounding of the anterior cardiac contour and, when the enlargement is significant, the left ventricle is elevated and displaced posteriorly so that the left or posterior cardiac border has a convex prominence in its central portion well above the diaphragm. This represents the left ventricle in an abnormal position, sometimes termed the "left ventricular cap." There is also noted unusual radiolucency in the region of the pulmonary artery that lies below and within the arch of the aorta. This is sometimes termed the "aortic window." In the RAO projection there may be rounding of the anterior cardiac contour in the region of the right ventricle, with decrease in the region of the distal pulmonary outflow tract and pulmonary artery segment. In the lateral view there is anterior and upward bulging of the heart, tending to fill the retrosternal space superiorly.

The Aorta. The findings in the right aortic arch that occur in approximately 25% of patients consist of absence of aortic shadow on the left and presence of a vascular shadow on the right at the aortic level. This is readily detected in adults and in older children, but in infants the aortic arch may not be visible. The superior vena cava is displaced laterally, however, and the resulting convex density in the right upper mediastinum may suggest the aortic position. Sometimes barium in the esophagus is helpful along with visualization of the trachea, where an indentation on the right may identify the site of the aortic arch. The aorta is enlarged in rough proportion to the amount of right-to-left shunt.

Other Findings. When poststenotic dilatation of the main pulmonary artery occurs, as has been indicated, the pulmonary artery is normal or slightly larger than normal. The presence of a "third" ventricle also may alter the silhouette as noted previously. It is apparent that the appearance of the heart in tetralogy varies from one in which there is very little deviation from the normal to one in which there is marked alteration (Figs. 32-7 through 32-9).

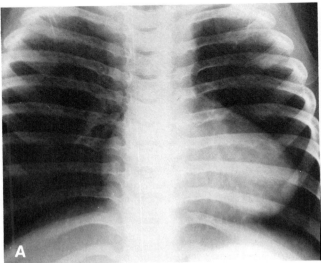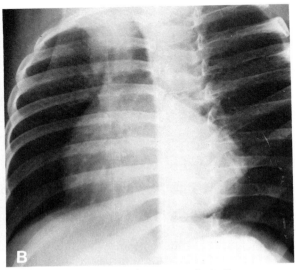

Figure 32–7. Severe tetralogy of Fallot in a 6-month-old child. Note the concavity in the left upper cardiac border, the elevation of the apex, and the relative avascularity of the hila and lungs (**A**). The left anterior oblique projection (**B**) shows the prominence of the chambers of the right side of the heart as well as the elevation of the apex and the avascularity.

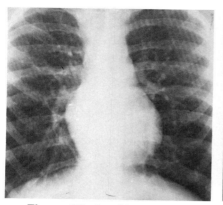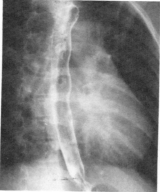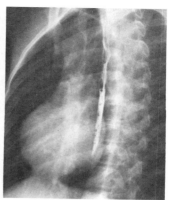

Figure 32–8. Moderately severe tetralogy of Fallot in an 11-year-old child. Note the round apex and the prominence of the right border of the heart in the left anterior oblique projection. The diminution of vascularity is minimal.

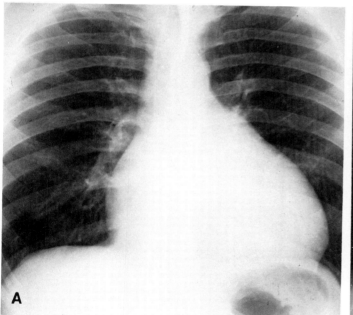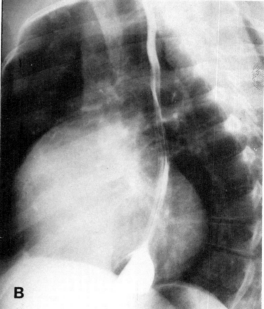

Figure 32–9. Tetralogy of Fallot in a man, age 35, with moderate cyanosis. (**A**) Note that the heart is enlarged but the hilar vessels are small, and there is scanty vascularity in the lungs. There is no concavity in the region of the main pulmonary artery. (**B**) In this left anterior oblique projection, the marked prominence of the cardiac silhouette anteriorly indicates the massive enlargement of the right side of the heart.

Angiocardiography. Angiocardiography outlines the right ventricle and shows immediate filling of the aorta from the right ventricle, often with little if any shunt into the left ventricle. The site of stenosis is usually outlined, particularly in the right anterior oblique or lateral view. Pulmonary artery size is also defined.

Pulmonary Stenosis With Intact Ventricular Septum and Atrial Right-to-Left Shunt. In this entity, sometimes referred to as trilogy of Fallot, the atrial defect is usually a patent foramen ovale. Cyanosis appears when right atrial pressure has increased enough to cause a right-to-left shunt through the patent foramen ovale or atrial septal defect. This often occurs early in life but may be delayed.

Roentgen Findings

Heart Size. The heart is moderately to markedly enlarged, with elevation of the apex indicating right ventricular enlargement. The aorta is usually normal in size and the arch is on the left side.

Pulmonary Artery. Poststenotic dilatation of the main and left pulmonary artery results in prominence of the pulmonary artery segment in the frontal and oblique projections but is not always present. Poststenotic dilatation occurs with valvular stenosis, which usually occurs in this condition. Infundibular stenosis may result as a secondary change when muscular hypertrophy occurs in the infundibulum, or it may be primarily responsible for the high right ventricular pressure that occurs in an estimated 10% of patients. A small pulmonary artery distal to the narrowing occurs in infundibular stenosis (Fig. 32-10).

Pulmonary Vascularity. Pulmonary vascularity tends to be decreased but may appear normal when shunting is not marked.

Heart Shape. The silhouette is that of right atrial and right ventricular enlargement; poststenotic dilatation results in prominence of the pulmonary artery. The left atrium may be enlarged. The apex is elevated and the right ventricle is prominent in the left anterior oblique and frontal projections.

Angiocardiography. Angiocardiography is a valuable examination in this condition. The films are exposed in rapid succession, or cine or videotape recording is performed after caval or right atrial injection. These recordings show the defect at the atrial level, with a jet of opaque material propelled through the defect rapidly filling the left atrium, left ventricle, and then the aorta. This results in rapid opacification of the right chamber and simultaneous, or nearly simultaneous, opacification of the pulmonary artery and aorta. The pulmonary stenosis may be directly visible in some cases. The poststenotic dilatation frequently present is also recognized easily on the angiocardiogram. Selective right ventricular injection is the most effective in showing the enlarged right ventricle associated with muscular hypertrophy. The pulmonary valve is usually thickened and often dome shaped, with a jet of opaque medium crossing the valve into a moderately dilated pulmonary artery. The infundibulum is long

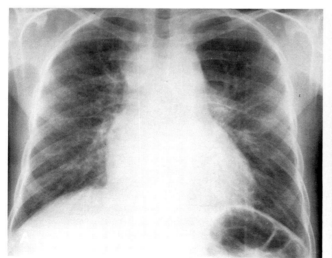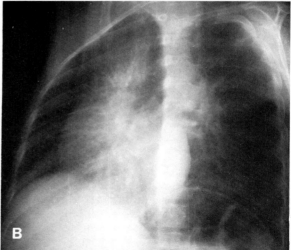

Figure 32–10. Pulmonary stenosis with interatrial septal defect. The stenosis was severe, and the lungs were supplied by bronchial arteries to a great extent. This accounts for the absence of normal hilar vessels, noted particularly on the right. The brushlike arteries that are present represent bronchial arteries that supplied the lungs. Frontal (**A**) and the left anterior oblique (**B**) projections.

and smooth and shows rather marked change in diameter from systole to diastole, in contrast to the findings in tetralogy of Fallot.

Complete Transposition of the Great Vessels

The relative positions of the pulmonary artery and the aorta are reversed in complete transposition. This results in two closed circulations because the blood from the lungs enters the left atrium by way of the pulmonary veins, then enters the left ventricle and passes through the pulmonary artery back to the lungs. The systemic venous return enters the right atrium, goes into the right ventricle, and exits through the aorta back into the systemic circulation. Because this situation is not life sustaining, complete transposition must be accompanied by other anomalies that will allow intra- or extracardiac shunts or both. These consist of patent ductus arteriosus, and interatrial and interventricular septal defects. Ventricular septal defects occur in less than one half of patients, while an interatrial defect that may be a small atrial septal defect or a patent foramen ovale is usually present. The ductus arteriosus may be patent. Rarely, anomalous pulmonary venous return shunts blood from the lungs to the right side of the heart.

This anomaly is more frequent in males than females in a ratio of two or four to one. Prognosis is poor, but is improving with advances in cardiac surgery.

Roentgen Findings

Heart Size. The heart is usually normal or nearly normal in size at birth and for the first two weeks of life. Increasing size leads to definite enlargement in most patients in a few weeks. Nearly all of these infants have enlargements by the age of 2 months.

Heart Shape. Both ventricles are enlarged and the general contour of the heart is oval or egg shaped. The right ventricle is usually enlarged to a greater extent than the left. The shape of the heart in the lateral and LAO positions tends to be round. As the obliquity is increased, the vascular pedicle tends to become larger in its transverse diameter. In the frontal projection, however, the base usually produced by the great vessels is narrow. Furthermore, the absence of normal thymic tissue accentuates this finding. The thymus may also be small or absent in other severe congenital heart conditions and in infants with severe, stressful, noncardiac disease.

Pulmonary Artery and Aorta. There is narrowing of the shadow of the great vessels in the frontal projection, the result of a more anteroposterior course of the aorta that arises anteriorly and tends to course directly backward. This produces a widening of the shadows of the great vessels in the oblique projections, because the vessels that are superimposed in the frontal projection are separated by obliquity. Because the pulmonary infundibulum is not formed normally and the pulmonary artery lies closer to the midline than normal, the convexity usually formed by the infundibulum and pulmonary artery is not present. In some instances, a distinct concavity is noted in the left upper cardiac border. The outline of the aortic arch is absent (Fig. 32-11).

Pulmonary Vascularity. Pulmonary vessels are enlarged and prominent. Occasionally, when there is pulmonic stenosis or the shunts are small, the pulmonary vascularity associated with transposition will be decreased in size. Because the heart is not as large and the contour is not abnormal, the diagnosis of transposition with pulmonic stenosis may be very difficult to make.

Angiocardiography. Venous angiocardiographic findings consist of a sequential filling of the right atrium, the right ventricle, and of an anteriorly placed aorta from the right ventricle. There is usually very poor opacification of the pulmonary artery and the shunt that makes this condition compatible with life may be visualized. If an atrial septal defect is present it is usually apparent, with rapid opacification of the left atrium. A patent ductus may be demonstrated but an interventricular septal defect is very difficult to define. The enlargement of the right-sided heart chambers can also be noted on the angiocardiogram. There tends to be some difference in relationship of the great vessels, ranging from a pulmonary artery that lies posterior and slightly to the left of the aorta to one that lies directly posterior or rarely directly to the left of the aorta.

Selective, right-ventricular angiocardiography is somewhat more satisfactory than a venous injection, particularly in outlining ventricular septal defect and the pulmonary artery.

Tricuspid Atresia

Tricuspid atresia with hypoplasia or aplasia of the right ventricle is associated with several other malformations in order that circulation may be sustained. The tricuspid valve is atretic and there is hypoplasia or absence of the right ventricle. Edwards and associates classify these anomalies based on the relationship of great vessels and the presence or absence of pulmonary

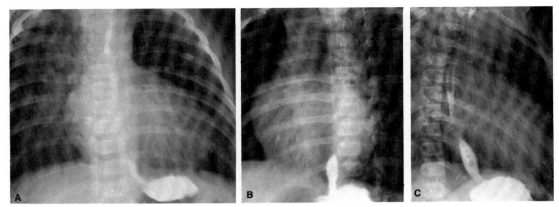

Figure 32–11. Transposition of the great vessels. **(A)** Frontal projection. **(B)** Left anterior oblique projection. **(C)** Right anterior oblique projection. There is cardiac enlargement. The large pulmonary vessels are best seen in the right hilum and central lung. The apex is elevated, indicating right ventricular enlargement. The vascular pedicle is narrow in the frontal projection and broad in both oblique views. This is characteristic of transposition.

stenosis.[16] In type I the great vessels are normally related and there are (1) coexistent tricuspid and pulmonary atresia; (2) a narrow septal defect between the left ventricle and the infundibular portion of the right ventricle, a small vestigial right ventricle, and a small pulmonary artery (this is the most common form); or (3) a large interventricular septal defect with valvular stenosis and normal pulmonary artery. Rarely, transposition of the great vessels occurs in this form. In type II, transposition of the great vessels without pulmonic stenosis occurs, and there is essentially a common ventricle. Rarely, this anomaly is found without transposition. As indicated, in type I there is some type of right ventricular or pulmonary artery obstruction. In these patients, an atrial septal defect is present so that the blood flows into the right atrium, is shunted across the septal defect to the left atrium, and to the left ventricle. The blood is then distributed to the lungs by way of an interventricular septal defect and hypoplastic right ventricle through the pulmonary artery to the lungs. If the right ventricle or pulmonary artery is atretic, the blood must get to the lungs by way of a patent ductus.

TRICUSPID ATRESIA WITH PULMONARY STENOSIS

Roentgen Findings

Heart Size. The heart is usually enlarged, but there is considerable variation; at times the enlargement is slight, but in others it is marked.

Heart Shape. The heart is often boot shaped and may resemble the silhouette of tetralogy of Fallot. The right heart border is relatively straight or flat and may not extend to the right of the spine. The pulmonary artery segment is concave. The left atrium may be enlarged; this is a helpful diagnostic sign. The right atrium is usually enlarged, sometimes significantly. Evidence of left ventricular preponderance on the electrocardiogram is helpful in determining the presence of left ventricle enlargement, because right ventricular enlargement can rotate the heart and produce a similar silhouette. The left side of the heart border is rounded with apparent elevation of the apex, simulating the elevation associated with right ventricular enlargement. The change in the contour of the heart commonly described to indicate absence hypoplasia of the right ventricle is not often found in this condition. This change consists of diminished convexity or actual concavity of the right lower heart border in the frontal projection and of the anterior inferior border in the left anterior oblique view. The reason for the absence of this sign is that the right atrium enlarges to the extent that it fills the deficit resulting from right ventricular absence or hypoplasia.

Pulmonary Artery. There is concavity in the region of the main pulmonary artery in the frontal projection. It may be extreme, resulting in an angular junction between the aorta and the upper left ventricular silhouette.

Pulmonary Vascularity. Pulmonary vascularity is usually decreased, unless there is complete transposition of the great vessels. When this is present, vascularity is normal or increased.

The Aorta. The aorta is generally enlarged.

Angiocardiography. This examination is useful in establishing the anatomic diagnosis in tricuspid atresia. The finding indicates a large right atrium, below which is a triangular radiolucent notch, representing the defect caused by absence of filling of the right ventricle. A shunt from the right to the left atrium is observed, resulting in rapid opacification of the left side of the heart. The size of the pulmonary vessels is demonstrated, but the root of the pulmonary artery, the site of stenosis, and the right ventricular chamber may be difficult to outline.

Tricuspid Atresia Without Pulmonary Stenosis

As has been indicated, this form of the anomaly is usually associated with transposition of the great vessels and a common ventricle.

Roentgen findings consist of gross cardiac enlargement, narrowing of the great vessels at the base, indicating transposition, and some left atrial enlargement. The pulmonary vascularity is greatly increased. Correlation with electrocardiographic findings of left ventricular preponderance in a cyanotic child with hypervascularity is highly suggestive of the diagnosis.

In patients with transposition and tricuspid atresia, the right atrial appendage may lie to the left of the aorta and the pulmonary artery, and behind the great vessels. It projects above the left atrial appendage. The term "juxtaposition of the atrial appendages" is used to describe this anomaly, which produces a characteristic large bulge high on the left cardiac border that suggests the diagnosis.

Tricuspid Stenosis

Congenital tricuspid stenosis is very rare and is usually combined with other congenital cardiac defects. The only consistent roentgen finding is hypovascularity of the lungs. The enlargement of the right atrium present in these patients may not be recognized readily. In some cases, the appearance simulates that of tetralogy of Fallot. No consistent roentgen appearance has been described.

Persistent Truncus Arteriosus

There are four types of this rare anomaly in which there is only one large arterial trunk that overrides the ventricular septum. The pulmonary artery may arise (Type I) as a branch of the common trunk. This is the most common type (48%) and carries the worst prognosis. A second form consists of separate origin of pulmonary arteries from the dorsal wall of the truncus (29%). In a third form, one or both pulmonary arteries arise independently from either side of the truncus (11%). In

these anomalies, the pulmonary vascularity is usually increased. Type IV consists of absence of the pulmonary artery with a truncus arteriosus that supplies the lungs by way of the bronchial arteries or other collateral vessels (12%). There is marked decrease in pulmonary vascularity in this type.

Roentgen Findings. The truncus is usually large and produces a convexity in the region of the ascending arch. There is often prominence of the peripheral pulmonary vessels, despite a concavity in the region of the main pulmonary artery. The heart is usually enlarged. Right ventricular enlargement predominates, resulting in elevation of the cardiac apex that may be striking, so that the silhouette resembles that of severe tetralogy of Fallot, although it tends to be larger in truncus. In the fourth type and in pseudotruncus (see the section about tetralogy of Fallot) the ascending aortic arch is prominent and the pulmonary artery segment is concave. The pulmonary vascularity is markedly diminished. The bronchial arteries that supply the lungs are visualized as small vessels extending outward in a fine brushlike pattern from the hila on both sides. The comma-shaped pattern of the pulmonary arteries is absent in these patients. The shape of the heart is often distinctive in the frontal position. There is a sharp right-angled junction between the vascular pedicle on the left and the upper left ventricular border, or an acute angle may be present. Right aortic arch is present in about 25% of these patients. Angiocardiography demonstrates opacification of the large truncus from the large right ventricle and shows the pulmonary artery filling after the truncus has filled. In the fourth type and in pseudotruncus the appearance is similar to that in severe tetralogy on the angiocardiogram.

Ebstein's Anomaly

This malformation consists of downward displacement of the tricuspid valve far into the right ventricle. The upper portion of the right ventricle is incorporated into the right atrium. As a result, the ventricle is small and the atrium is large. The myocardium proximal to the abnormally placed valve is thin and the large right atrium is unable to empty itself properly. Cyanosis is often present in this disease because venous blood is shunted from the right to the left atrium through an interatrial septal defect that is usually present. If there is no intracardiac shunt, cyanosis is not produced.

Roentgen Findings. The heart is usually greatly enlarged and the lungs are hypovascular. The right atrium and ventricle are the chambers involved. Enlargement to the right with a shoulder-like prominence of the right upper cardiac enlargement is characteristic. The left upper cardiac contour often enlarges in a more sloping manner, caused by enlargement of the outflow tract of the right ventricle. This gives the heart a square or boxlike shape with a narrow vascular pedicle and a small aortic arch (Fig. 32-12). When this is found, along with hypovascularity of the lung and a small aorta, the roentgen diagnosis can be made with reasonable certainty, particularly when correlated with electrocardiographic findings. Angiocardiography, therefore, may not be needed. On venous angiocardiography, the large right atrium fills and empties slowly through the foramen ovale or atrial septal defect into the left atrium and through the tricuspid valve into the right ventricle. The right side of the heart remains opacified for an unusually long period of time. Selective injection of contrast medium into the right ventricle identifies the level of the tricuspid valve and shows tricuspid insufficiency when present. Occasionally, there is an associated pulmonic valvular stenosis that may be defined by this examination. In these patients, there may be a considerable right-to-left shunt manifested by marked hypovascularity. In those patients without a shunt, the pulmonary vascularity is normal.

Total Anomalous Pulmonary Venous Return

In this anomaly the pulmonary veins empty into the right atrium by one of several pathways. The most common is by the left innominate vein. Others empty (1) directly into the coronary sinus; (2) directly into the right atrium; (3) through a large vein into the right superior vena cava; (4) into a persistent left superior vena cava; (5) into the portal vein, ductus venosus, or inferior vena cava below the diaphragm; or, (6) occasionally into the azygous or a hepatic vein. The latter type occurs predominantly in males. In patients with a persistent left superior vena cava or vertical vein, the blood flows upward in this vein for a short distance to the left of the superior aspect of the aortic arch and then flows centrally, in the left innominate vein, which empties into the superior vena cava on the right. When all the pulmonary venous blood is returned to the right side of the heart, a right-to-left shunt is needed to be compatible with life. The most common anomaly is an atrial septal defect or patent foramen ovale. As a result of this combination of defects, the right heart is overloaded and becomes enlarged while the left heart and aorta are relatively small. Desaturation is present but frank cyanosis is uncommon.

When the anomalous venous return is above the diaphragm, the pulmonary venous pressure is moderately increased, and minimal pulmonary edema is often present. In total anomalous venous return below the diaphragm, there is usually a greater increase in venous pressure and severe pulmonary edema is common in the newborn.

Roentgen Findings. In total anomalous pulmonary venous return above the diaphragm, the heart is enlarged. The enlargement is on the right side, although this may not be readily apparent. Pulmonary vessels are prominent because of the increased blood flow in the lesser circulation. When there is a persistent left vena cava, or left vertical vein with total anomalous pulmonary venous connection to the left innominate vein, there is a characteristic figure-of-eight deformity of the cardiovascular silhouette. This is best appreciated in older children. The upper limbs of the "eight" are formed by the vena cava on the right and the vertical vein on the left. They are dilated and form convexities on either side above the heart (Fig. 32-13A). The blood flows upward in the vertical vein, across to the right, and into the superior vena cava. In the occasional patient in whom the veins drain into the right superior or inferior vena cava, these veins may be visualized on the plain-film roentgenogram. CT will often outline the abnormal vessel to good advantage. The aorta is small and hypoplastic and the pulmonary artery is often enlarged to the extent that its upper border forms a horizontal shelf immediately below the hypoplastic aortic arch.

Angiocardiography can be used to establish the diagnosis, but when the figure-of-eight is present, along with the evidence of enlargement of pulmonary vessels, the diagnosis can be made with reasonable certainty on plain films alone. The thymic shadow may produce a figure-of-eight sign and must be differentiated. This "snowman" or "figure-of-eight" is often not apparent in the first few weeks of life. The lateral view may then be helpful, since the shadow of the anomalous vertical vein or left superior vena cava is denser and has a sharper anterior border than the shadow of the thymus. Most of the other sites of return show no characteristic vascular pattern, but, because there is a bidirectional shunt, pulmonary hypervascularity is present despite the patient's desaturation. There is right-sided cardiac enlargement with no evidence of left atrial enlargement. Anomalous venous return into the coronary sinus dilates this structure and may cause a local indentation on the anterior aspect of the barium-filled esophagus.

Total anomalous pulmonary venous return below the diaphragm presents a different roentgen picture. The heart is usually normal in size and shape, but the lungs are abnormal. The findings are of pulmonary vascular congestion and edema. The vascular changes resemble those seen in adults with venous hypertension secondary to mitral valvular disease, except that the hilar vessels are not prominent in these infants (this observation requires an upright film). This association of normal-sized heart and roentgen and clinical evidence of congestive failure in a cyanotic male infant with no heart murmurs is highly suggestive of the diagnosis.

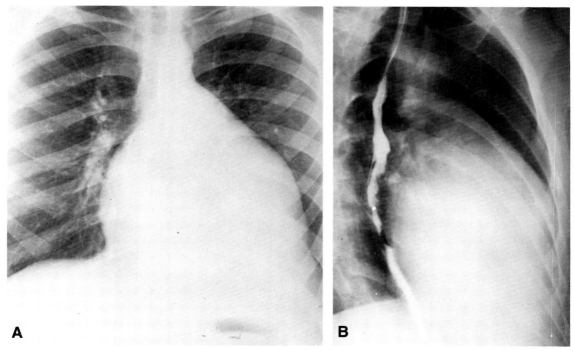

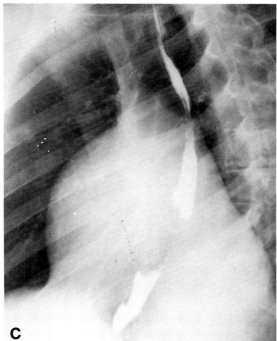

Figure 32–12. Ebstein's anomaly. The heart is greatly enlarged. Massive enlargement of the right atrium in the oblique projections is noted. Frontal (**A**), right anterior oblique (**B**), and left anterior oblique (**C**) positions.

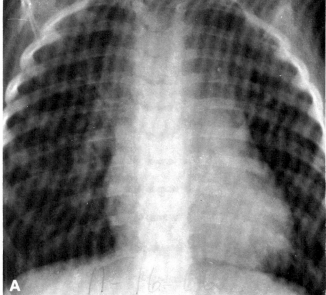

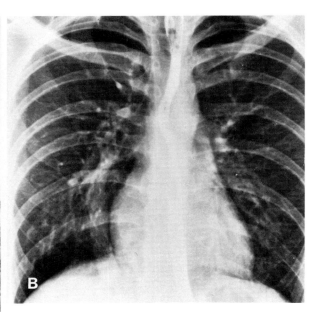

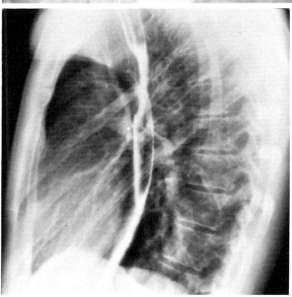

Figure 32–13. (**A**) Total anomalous pulmonary venous return. This is a reasonably typical example of a figure-of-eight deformity, with the large veins forming a convexity on either side in the upper mediastinum. The pulmonary vascularity is not very well seen in this illustration but was distinctly increased. (**B**) Partial anomalous pulmonary venous return (scimitar syndrome). Note the hypervascularity and the large vessel paralleling the border of the right side of the heart and extending below the level of the diaphragm. (**C**) This vessel is seen posteriorly. It somewhat overlies the vertebral bodies in the lower thorax. This vein emptied into the inferior vena cava. There is also an azygous fissure in this patient.

The lungs may have a "ground-glass" appearance. Angiocardiography can then be used to demonstrate the draining vein that extends below the diaphragm.

Partial Anomalous Venous Return

The most common partial anomalous venous connection is to the right atrium. This results in a left-to-right shunt of modest proportions which usually does not cause symptoms and is often found upon study of patients with atrial septal defect. Roentgen findings are

similar to those of atrial septal defect and include pulmonary arterial enlargement and hypervascularity related to the size of the shunt. A rare combination of hypoplasia of the right lung and anomalous right pulmonary venous return into the inferior vena cava is termed the "scimitar syndrome" because the anomalous vein is visible as a curved shadow in the lower right lung (Figs. 32-13A and B). There may also be other associated anomalies such as accessory hemidiaphragm, sequestration, and hepatic herniations. An anomalous systemic artery that may arise below the diaphragm frequently supplies a portion of the lung at the base. The term "congenital pulmonary venolobar syndrome" has been used to describe this combination of anomalies, some of which may be absent in a given patient.[60]

Partial anomalous drainage of the left upper lobe may be by way of an anomalous vertical vein that produces a left paramediastinal density lateral to the aortic knob with a smooth, curvilinear border outlined against the lung. This appearance is similar to that of the left side of the "snowman" sign observed in total anomalous pulmonary venous return, but the anomaly causes no symptoms and the finding is often incidental. Linear or CT may be used for better definition of the density.

OTHER CYANOTIC DEFECTS

Transposition of the Taussig-Bing Type

This is a variant of transposition in which the aorta arises from the right ventricle while the pulmonary artery overrides the ventricular septum. A high ventricular septal defect is present. When this defect is above the crista supraventricularis and is closely applied to the origin on the pulmonary trunk, it represents the Taussig-Bing type of transposition. Another type is one in which the ventricular septal defect is below the crista supraventricularis, remote from the pulmonary valve. In the latter, the left ventricular bloodstream is directed to the pulmonary artery. This results in enlargement of the right ventricle and atrium. The pulmonary artery is dilated but its branches are often diminished in size as compared with the large main vessels. This is the result of vascular changes that cause pulmonary hypertension.

Roentgen Findings. Cardiac enlargement occurs primarily because of the enlarged right ventricle. This is associated with enlargement of the pulmonary artery segment and hilar vessels. The midzone pulmonary vascular channels may be full but become small when pulmonary hypertension develops. There may be left atrial and left ventricular enlargement as well. On plain films the two types cannot be differentiated. In the Taussig-Bing type, angiocardiography shows immediate filling of the aorta from the right ventricle with relatively poor filling of the pulmonary artery and its branches from this chamber. The pulmonary trunk is wider than the aorta. The aortic and pulmonary valves are at the same horizontal level and are superimposed in the lateral view.

When the septal defect is below the crista supraventricularis, there is better filling of the pulmonary artery from the right ventricle. The valves are on the same horizontal plane or the pulmonary valve may be slightly higher than the aortic valve. Similar lateral superimposition is noted.

Congenital Heart Disease in the Neonatal Period

According to Gyepes and Vincent,[28] nine congenital heart lesions commonly produce cyanosis or distress in the first two weeks of life that may be life-threatening and require emergency diagnostic studies. They are (1) pulmonary atresia or severe pulmonic stenosis with intact ventricular septum; (2) pulmonary atresia or severe pulmonic stenosis with ventricular septal defect; (3) Ebstein's malformation; (4) tricuspid atresia; (5) transposition of the great arteries; (6) syndrome of coarctation of the aorta; (7) total anomalous pulmonary venous return with obstruction; (8) hypoplastic left heart syndrome; and (9) severe coarctation of the aorta. These lesions are grouped into three categories related to cardiovascular pathophysiology (see Table 32-1). Group I is characterized by decreased pulmonary blood flow; pulmonary atresia, tricuspid atresia, Ebstein's malformation, and pulmonary atresia with ventricular septal defect are included in this group. Intense cyanosis occurs early, and, usually, in this group of patients, there is a severely hypoplastic right ventricle incapable of dilatation. About 10% have a normal right ventricle that, however, is dilated; and when the right ventricle is dilated the right atrium may also be dilated. Group II consists of lesions with increased blood flow; transposition of the great arteries and the syndrome of coarctation of the aorta are included in this group. Group III consists of lesions with severe pulmonary venous congestion; this group includes total anomalous venous return, hypoplastic left heart, and severe coarctation with intact ventricular septum. In the coarctation syndrome in which there is a ventricular septal defect associated with severe coarctation, the ventricular shunt volume becomes greater than in patients with isolated ventricular septal defect, and failure typically occurs when the patient is 2 weeks of age.

The chest roentgenogram in the posteroanterior projection may be very helpful, particularly in differentiating the groups. In group I, in which decreased pulmonary blood flow results in decreased vascularity, it is likely that the patient has pulmonary atresia, severe pulmonic stenosis, or Ebstein's anomaly. If gross enlargement of the right atrium can be detected, Ebstein's anomaly is likely. If the heart is only moderately enlarged or normal, the combination of pulmonary atresia or stenosis plus ventricular septal defect, or pulmonary atresia or stenosis with intact ventricular septum and a hypoplastic right ventricle, is likely. In tricuspid atresia, the heart may be normal or slightly enlarged. In some instances, there is discrete enlargement of the right atrium in these patients.

In the second group in which there is normal or moderately increased pulmonary arterial pattern, transposition of the great arteries or coarctation syndrome are the most likely. If the heart is oval or egg shaped, transposition is likely, while infants with coarctation syndrome have a combination of a large heart, increased pulmonary blood flow, plus some degree of pulmonary venous congestion. Identification of the site of the coarctation is usually not possible in this age group.

In the third group in which there is cardiomegaly and pulmonary venous congestion, it is likely that the infant has either severe coarctation of the aorta or some form of the hypoplastic left-heart syndrome. When the heart is normal or slightly enlarged in these infants with pulmonary venous congestion, it is likely that total anomalous pulmonary venous return with obstruction is present. Although these diagnoses or differentials can be suggested, the severity of the problem indicates that emergency echocardiography or MRI imaging, or cardiac catheterization and angiocardiography are usually necessary. The procedures are usually abbreviated, and only crucial diagnostic information is sought.

Hypoplastic Left Heart Syndrome

This syndrome consists of hypoplasia of the left ventricle associated with a number of anomalies including aortic valvular stenosis or atresia, an atretic aortic arch, and/or mitral stenosis or atresia. As has been noted, the hypoplastic left heart syndrome is one of the causes of congestive failure in the first week of life, usually within two or three days after birth. Roentgen findings consist of progressive cardiomegaly, increased pulmonary vascularity caused by venous congestion, and a somewhat globular-appearing heart. Failure is often impossible to control, with death occurring in the first week of life.

Other Anomalies

A number of other rare anomalies may be associated with cyanosis. They include the bilocular and trilocular heart, atrioventricularis communis, and a number of others often associated with obstruction to pulmonary flow. The roentgen findings are not characteristic in these conditions, but the heart is usually enlarged.

NONCYANOTIC DEFECTS

The cardiovascular anomalies to be discussed in this section consist of defects that cause left-to-right shunts under ordinary circumstances and of other anomalies, chiefly involving the valves. The shunting of blood from left to right is dependent upon the pressure gradient across the defect. The pressure is usually higher on the left side so that the shunt is maintained from left to right; if pulmonary hypertension results, the pressure in the right-sided heart chambers and pulmonary artery may exceed that on the left. The shunt is reversed and cyanosis or arterial unsaturation develops. The roentgen diagnosis of this group of congenital anomalies often rests in part upon differentiation between right and left ventricular enlargement. The criteria for enlargement of these chambers described in the sections on "left ventricular and right ventricular enlargement" may be useless in these patients because enlargement of one chamber may simulate that of another. Therefore differentiation cannot be made on plain-film study alone, and radiographic findings must be correlated with clinical, electrocardiographic, echocardiographic, angiocardiographic magnetic resonance, and catheterization data. In patients with left-to-right intracardiac shunts, pulmonary inflammatory disease is common. Obstruction with lobular, segmental, and even lobar atelectasis may be found. These findings may be significant when the cardiac silhouette does not suggest the type of congenital anomaly. The large pulmonary artery associated with left-to-right shunts plus a large left atrium may cause complete atelectasis of the left lung. The bronchus is evidently compressed between the artery and the atrium in these cases. The result is a small, opaque, left hemithorax.

Patent Ductus Arteriosus

The ductus arteriosus serves to shunt blood into the systemic circulation from the pulmonary artery in intrauterine life and is patent at birth. Functionally, the ductus closes very early in life. Anatomic closure is usually completed in two months, but is sometimes delayed up to six months and, rarely, for a year. The ductus arises near the origin of the left pulmonary artery and empties into the aorta just distal to the left subclavian artery. Occasionally, a right-sided ductus is found.

Roentgen Findings. The findings on the routine frontal, oblique, and lateral roentgenograms are not always diagnostic, particularly in infants and young children, and must be correlated with clinical data. The left atrium and left ventricle are enlarged and there is enlargement of the aorta proximal to the ductus. The pulmonary artery and peripheral pulmonary vessels are enlarged. The findings roughly parallel the amount of left-to-right shunt. In patients with small shunts, no detectable cardiovascular abnormalities may be noted radiographically. In left-to-right shunts, the pulmonary-to-systemic flow ratio must be at least 2:1 to be recognized as increased flow in the lungs.

Heart Size. Slight cardiac enlargement is present in about half the patients; in large shunts, a considerable amount of enlargement may be present.

Heart Shape. There may be enough left atrial enlargement to produce recognizable displacement of the esophagus in the right anterior oblique projection. Left ventricular enlargement is also present, causing elongation of the left border of the heart in the frontal view and rounding of the left ventricular silhouette in the left anterior oblique projection. Continued increase in pulmonary blood flow may result in some degree of pulmonary hypertension, which in turn causes right ventricular enlargement.

Pulmonary Artery. The most consistent finding in patent ductus arteriosus is enlargement of the pulmonary artery segment. This produces convex prominence in the region of the segment in the frontal projection (Fig. 32-14).

Pulmonary Vascularity. The vascularity in the hila and peripheral lungs is increased. Measurement of pulmonary arteries is ordinarily not very useful in the detection of enlargement because there is a wide range of normal. However, the diameter of the right descending pulmonary artery has been found to be nearly that of the trachea in children over 2 years of age.[12] When a left-to-right shunt was present, the artery diameter was never less than that of the trachea in a study of 102 children with left-to-right shunts. In 90% of a group of 112 normal children, these structures measured the same or varied within 2 mm. Measurement of pulmonary arteries may be used to corroborate the subjective impression of arterial enlargement. A shunt is unlikely if the diameter of the descending artery is smaller than that of the trachea.

The Aorta. The aorta is often enlarged (Fig. 32-15). There may be a slight bulge of the descending aortic wall below the prominent knob indicating minor enlargement in this region. This represents the infundibulum of the patent ductus. It is not a frequent sign in children and is not diagnostic, because similar slight convexity can occur in patients without patent ductus. Rarely there is calcification at the aortic end of the ductus in adults. This has not been reported in children. Occasionally, the ductus itself is visible as a small convexity between the aortic knob or transverse arch and the pulmonary artery.

Angiocardiography. This examination is often disappointing but may show reopacification of the pulmonary artery from the aorta and slight enlargement of the left heart chambers. The demonstration of the local aortic enlargement at the site of the ductus or of a

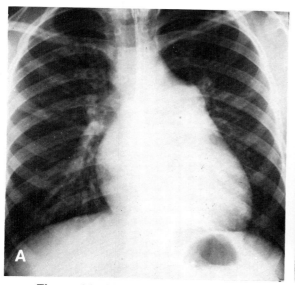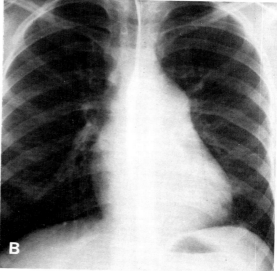

Figure 32–14. Patent ductus arteriosus. (**A**) Moderate cardiac enlargement, considerable prominence of the pulmonary artery resulting in convexity of the left upper cardiac border below the aortic arch, and hypervascularity noted best in and adjacent to the right hilum. (**B**) This film obtained one year after ligation of the ductus shows diminution in heart size and pulmonary vascularity without much change in the size of the main pulmonary artery.

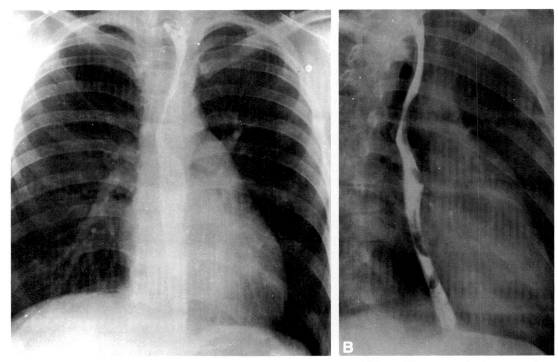

Figure 32–15.   Patent ductus arteriosus in a 12-year-old boy. The aorta is large and indents the esophagus in both frontal (**A**) and right anterior oblique (**B**) views. The main pulmonary artery is enlarged, and there is moderate hypervascularity. The slight indentation of the esophagus below the carina noted in the oblique view indicates left atrial enlargement, and there is probably a little left ventricular enlargement as well.

ductus diverticulum is helpful but not conclusive. A transient local defect in the opacification of the pulmonary artery at the site of the ductus, caused by a jet of nonopacified blood shunted through the ductus, is diagnostic when visualized.

Retrograde Aortography.   This examination is much more useful than angiocardiography. The opaque material is injected directly into the aorta and the opacified blood traverses the ductus and outlines the pulmonary artery and its branches.

Patent Ductus With Right-to-Left Shunt

In this condition, flow is reversed because the pulmonary arterial pressure exceeds that in the aorta. The pulmonary arterial systolic pressure is normally much lower than systemic arterial pressure. In large patent ductus arteriosus the pulmonary and systemic arterial pressures are equal. Equalization depends on a large-volume, left-to-right shunt, increased pulmonary resistance, or a combination of the two. Pulmonary arte-

rial disease may eventually develop to the point where pulmonary arterial resistance is greater than systemic resistance. When this degree of pulmonary hypertension is reached, the ductus acts as a safety valve for the lesser circulation. A right-to-left shunt results and the patient becomes desaturated. Cyanosis may be apparent in the lower extremities but absent in the upper extremities because the desaturated blood enters the descending aorta.

As a result of the pulmonary hypertension, the right ventricle becomes enlarged and the main pulmonary artery is often increased further in size along with the vessels in the hila, while the vessels in the central and peripheral lung are relatively small. This difference in size of proximal and peripheral pulmonary vessels is reliable, however, only when it is unequivocal. There may be calcification in the pulmonary artery and aorta adjacent to the ductus as well as in the ductus in these patients. Isolated calcification in the pulmonary artery may occur in association with pulmonary valvular stenosis, pulmonary artery aneurysm, or pulmonary hypertension from any cause. However, when calcifica-

tion occurs in the pulmonary artery and the adjacent aortic arch, the combination is suggestive of patent ductus with or without reversal of flow.[62] The left atrium tends to decrease in size when the shunt is reversed in patients with patent ductus arteriosus.

Interatrial Septal Defect

Atrial septal defects are among the most frequent congenital heart lesions. Several types exist. The most common is a patent foramen ovale that is large enough to result in a shunt. When there is a defect at the fossa ovalis, it is termed an "ostium secundum defect." A persistent ostium primum is a defect at the base of the atrial septum and is part of a spectrum of lesions that are associated with anomalies of the endocardial cushion. There also is a high atrial septal defect, sinus venosus type, which is usually associated with anomalous pulmonary venous return from the right lung. As a result of these defects there is free communication between the two atria, permitting a shunt. The anatomic location of the defect is not as important in determining the volume of the shunt as is its size and the difference in atrial pressures. Because left atrial pressure is usually higher than the pressure in the right atrium, the shunt is from left to right. As a result, the pulmonary blood flow is increased and this increases the amount of right ventricular work.

Roentgen Findings

Heart Size. The heart is usually slightly enlarged, but may be normal in size.

Heart Shape. Enlargement of the right ventricle and atrium occurs and may be typical enough to be recognized, but differentiation between right and left ventricular enlargement is not always possible. The left atrium is not enlarged.

The Pulmonary Artery. The pulmonary artery is enlarged and this may be quite marked, causing a large convexity that may partially obscure the smaller aortic knob. The size of the pulmonary artery segment in this anomaly is usually larger than in the other two common anomalies that produce left-to-right shunts, patent ductus arteriosus, and ventricular septal defect (Fig. 32-16).

Pulmonary Vascularity. The hilar and pulmonary vascularity is also increased.

The Aorta. The shunting of blood away from the left side of the heart into the lesser circulation results in decreased flow through the aorta. The aorta tends to be smaller than normal in size. This may be visualized easily, particularly in adults, but in infants and small children aortic size is often difficult to determine.

Angiocardiography. Angiocardiography is used occasionally to visualize the shunt and indicate its size and location.

Atrial Septal Defect With Right-to-Left Shunt

Pulmonary hypertension may occur, causing a reversal of the shunt when the right atrial pressure exceeds that in the left atrium. It is caused by organic changes in pulmonary arteries resulting in increasing vascular resistance. Arterial unsaturation occurs and cyanosis may then be observed. The right-sided heart chambers become more enlarged, particularly the right ventricle. The pulmonary artery also increases in size and there may be a marked decrease in size of peripheral pulmonary arteries, a sign of pulmonary hypertension. This may result in a considerable difference in diameter of central and peripheral pulmonary arteries.

Atrial Septal Defect With Mitral Stenosis (Lutembacher's Syndrome)

This rare condition consists of atrial septal defect combined with either congenital or acquired mitral stenosis. It results in a greater increase in right ventricular workload than does an uncomplicated atrial septal defect of similar size, because the increased left atrial pressure results in an increased left-to-right shunt. An enlarged pulmonary artery is the characteristic feature noted on the roentgenogram. The heart is generally enlarged and pulmonary vascularity is increased. The right ventricle and atrium are considerably increased in size and there may be some enlargement of the left atrium as well.

Angiocardiographic findings in this condition are similar to those in atrial septal defect. A jet of opaque medium crossing the plane of the septum from the left atrium to the right atrium is diagnostic of atrial septal defect. The mitral stenosis may also be demonstrated. There are other indirect angiocardiographic signs that may aid in the diagnosis. They consist of (1) enlargement of the right atrium and ventricle along with the pulmonary artery, (2) reopacification of the right side of the heart following left-sided opacification, and (3) dilution in the right atrium when a large shunt is present.

Ventricular Septal Defect

This is the most common of the congenital cardiac lesions. The defects may occur low in the septal wall but more commonly the defect is high. When the opening occurs high and adjacent to the mitral and

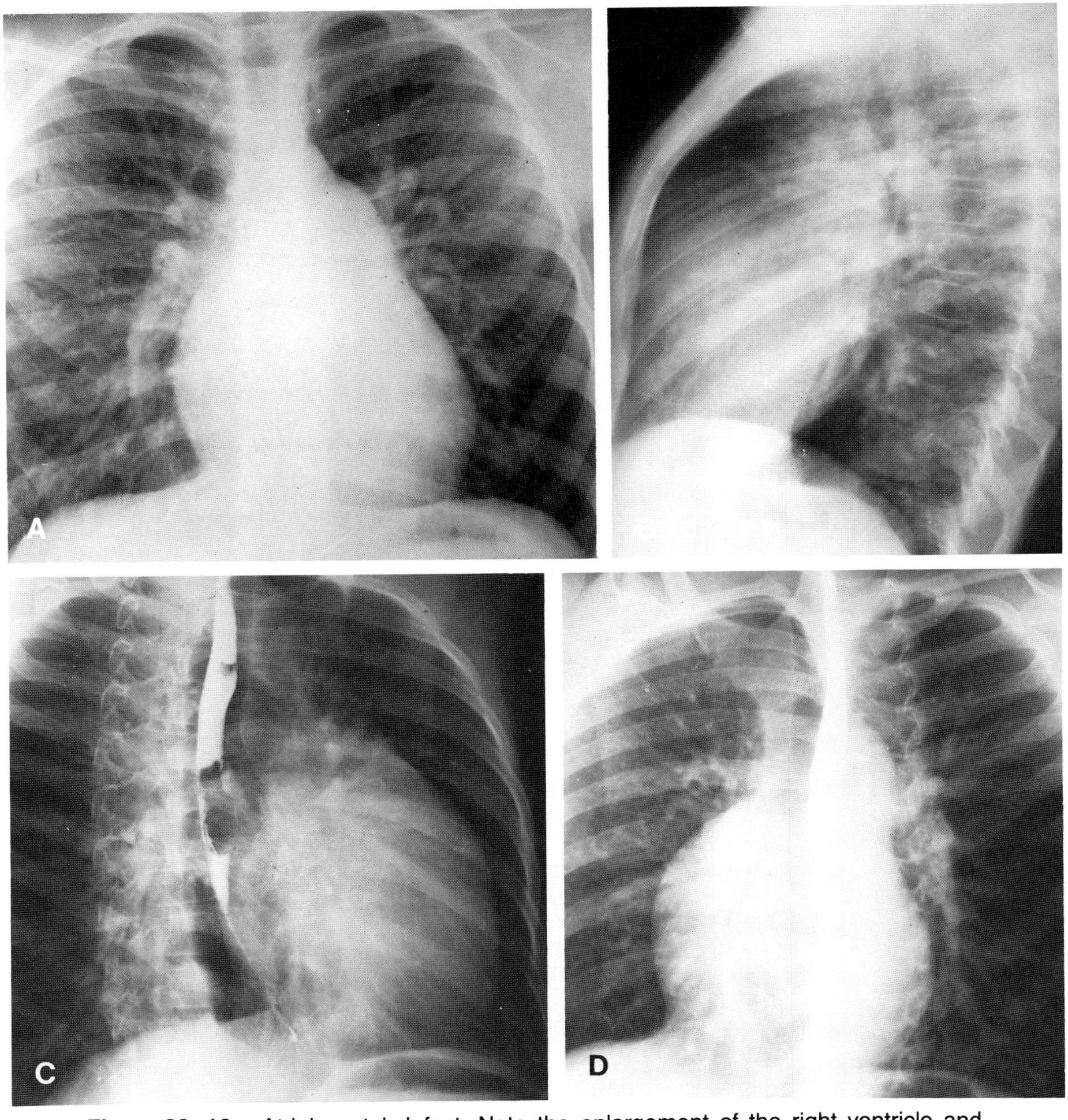

Figure 32–16. Atrial septal defect. Note the enlargement of the right ventricle and pulmonary artery; the lungs are hypervascular. Frontal (**A**), lateral (**B**), right anterior oblique (**C**), and left anterior oblique (**D**) projections.

tricuspid valves, it may involve the atrial septum and result in an anomaly known as atrioventricularis communis. Ventricular septal defect results in a left-to-right shunt because the left ventricular pressure is usually higher than the pressure in the right ventricle. As in the atrial septal defects, the size of the shunt is determined by the relationship of pressures on the two sides of the shunt and the size of the defect. There may be very little change in the size and shape of the heart when the defect is small and there is not much shunt. If a sizeable shunt is present, there will be alterations that can be visualized on the chest roentgenogram.

Roentgen Findings. The left ventricle and left atrium are enlarged, along with the right ventricle. The right ventricle increases in size as pulmonary arterial pressure rises. It is often difficult to determine which ventricle predominates. The aorta is normal in size.

Heart Size. The heart may be normal in size but is often enlarged.

Heart Shape. Ventricular work is increased on both sides so that both ventricles may enlarge. The left ventricle often enlarges first. There may be left atrial enlargement resulting in recognizable displacement of the esophagus by this chamber in the right oblique and lateral projection (Fig. 32-17).

The Pulmonary Artery. This vessel is enlarged and prominent.

Pulmonary Vascularity. Hilar and peripheral pulmonary vascularity is increased when the shunt is large.

The Aorta. The aorta is normal in size.

Angiocardiography. Angiocardiography shows a shunt of opaque material across the defect from the left into the right ventricle. Cardiac catheterization is a reliable diagnostic method in the study of this anomaly. Selective angiocardiography can be used to localize the site of the defect. The shunt may also be seen with echocardiography.

Ventricular Septal Defect With Right-to-Left Shunt

Occlusive pulmonary vascular changes develop in patients with ventricular septal defect, leading to reversal of the shunt when the pulmonary arterial pressure exceeds the systemic pressure. The term "Eisenmenger's complex" has been used to indicate this complication of shunt reversal with cyanosis developing in adolescence or in adult life.

Roentgen findings indicate cardiac enlargement, usually biventricular and moderate in amount. The pulmonary artery segment and central hilar vessels are very large, with disproportionate decrease in midzone and peripheral arteries indicating pulmonary hypertension (Fig. 32-18). When there has been a small left-to-right shunt or a right-to-left shunt from early childhood, the heart is not as large and the arterial disproportion is minimal. In the latter type, plain-film study may reveal very minor changes or changes resembling those of isolated pulmonic stenosis. As the

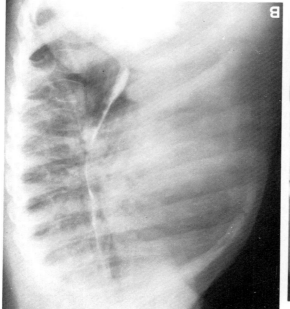
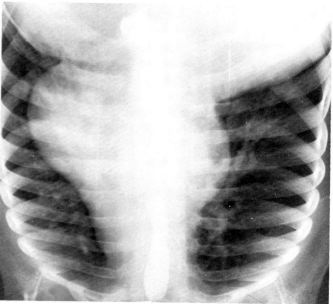

Figure 32-17. Ventricular septal defect in a 16-month-old child. (A) The heart is enlarged, and there is some hypervascularity in the lungs. The posterior displacement of the mid esophagus noted in the lateral projection (B) indicates some left atrial enlargement. The size of the aorta is very difficult to assess in a child of this age.

shunt reverses, the heart may decrease in size and become normal until cardiac failure occurs.

Persistent Common Atrioventricular Canal (A–V Communis)

This defect may vary from the complete form in which there is a low atrial septal defect, a high ventricular septal defect, and clefts in mitral and tricuspid valves to a lesser form in which the tricuspid valve is normal, or one in which the tricuspid valve is abnormal, or one in which the ventricular septum is intact and the tricuspid valve is normal.

As in other left-to-right shunts, the roentgen findings depend upon the magnitude of the shunt and the presence or absence of pulmonary hypertension. Cardiac enlargement, usually biventricular, is present along with hilar prominence and peripheral hypervascularity. The heart is generally larger than in patients with atrial or ventricular septal defect (Fig. 32-19). There may be left atrial enlargement. The aorta tends to be small. If pulmonary hypertension develops, the changes are similar to those noted in ventricular septal defect with right-to-left shunt.

Pulmonic Stenosis

The term "pulmonic stenosis" is used to refer to the two types of right ventricular outflow obstruction, namely, valvular and infundibular stenosis. Valvular pulmo-nary stenosis is much more frequent as an isolated lesion. Occasionally supravalvular stenosis may occur.

Roentgen Findings. In a number of patients no recognizable abnormality is noted. The characteristic findings in valvular stenosis are right ventricular enlargement and prominence of the main and left pulmonary arteries in a patient with normal peripheral pulmonary vascularity. The right atrium is sometimes enlarged. Isolated infundibular stenosis is rare.

Heart Size. The heart may be normal in size but is enlarged in about half of these patients.

Heart Shape. The enlargement is right sided and results in a rounded, right lower cardiac contour in the frontal projection and rounding of the right upper cardiac border in the LAO projection. The apex may be elevated and blunted. The outflow tract of the right ventricle is often prominent in the RAO projection.

Pulmonary Artery. The most characteristic finding is enlargement of the main pulmonary artery, resulting in convexity of the left upper cardiac margin below the aortic knob. This enlargement of the main pulmonary artery is due to poststenotic dilatation. The dilatation involves the main pulmonary artery and the left pulmonary artery, which result in prominence of the arterial silhouette of the left hilum. The change in the left pulmonary artery may be best seen in lateral projec-

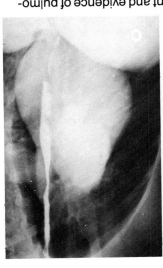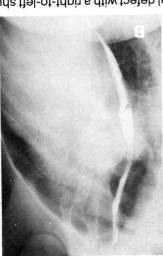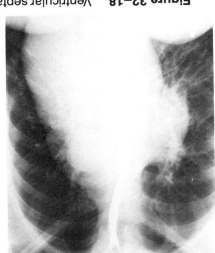

Figure 32-18. Ventricular septal defect with a right-to-left shunt and evidence of pulmonary hypertension. (A) The heart is generally enlarged, and there is great enlargement of the pulmonary artery and central hilar vessels in contrast to peripheral hypovascularity. Right ventricular enlargement is manifested by prominence of the distal right ventricle in the right anterior oblique projection (B) and of the right side of the heart in the left anterior oblique projection (C).

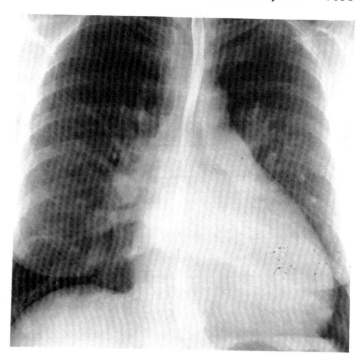

Figure 32–19. Persistent common atrioventricular canal. Note the gross cardiac enlargement and hypervascularity, particularly marked in the central lungs. The enlargement appears to be biventricular.

tion as it arches over the left bronchus. The right pulmonary artery may be dilated, but this vessel is hidden by mediastinal density. Therefore, the size of hilar vessels tend to be asymmetric in contrast to the symmetry often observed in pulmonary hypertension. This is a helpful differential diagnostic sign. Poststenotic dilatation occurs in valvular stenosis (Fig. 32-20), while in infundibular and supravalvular stenosis, the pulmonary artery is not prominent, and there may be no roentgen findings to indicate a cardiovascular disease.

Pulmonary Vascularity. The large main artery change is associated with normal size of the vessels in the lungs and in the right hilum.

Angiocardiography. Angiocardiography may show enlargement of the right atrium and ventricle, but generally provides a superb demonstration of the actual site and degree of pulmonic stenosis, along with the poststenotic dilatation of the pulmonary artery.

Aortic Stenosis

Congenital aortic stenosis may be subvalvular, valvular, or supravalvular. The valvular type of stenosis is more common than subaortic stenosis of the ventricular outflow tract, and supravalvular stenosis is quite rare. The valve may be bicuspid, but, more commonly, there is one cusp with a single commissure. Usually the bicuspid valve is not stenotic ad primam, but there is a

tendency to acquire deposits of fibrin and platelets that organize and become calcified. As this process continues, stenosis develops and the patients become symptomatic in the fifth or sixth decade of life.

Roentgen Findings. Poststenotic dilation of the aorta usually occurs in valvular stenosis. The dilatation is characteristically located in the ascending aorta and results in increased convexity of the right lateral aspect of the ascending aorta. It may be more clearly defined in the left anterior oblique than in the frontal projection. The transverse arch or aortic knob is not enlarged. Left ventricular hypertrophy and dilatation also occur in this condition and result in increased prominence of the left oblique projection and enlargement of the heart downward and to the left. The heart is usually not greatly enlarged unless it has begun to decompensate. In nearly half of our patients (in whom the stenosis was minimal to moderate) no detectable roentgen abnormalities were found except for the slight prominence of the ascending aorta. When present, the findings are characteristic.

Calcification of the aortic valve is diagnostic of aortic stenosis. It is best detected by fluoroscopy or CT. If seen on a plain film, most readily detected in the lateral view, and the patient is not in cardiac failure, the gradient is usually 50 mm of Hg or greater. Generally, because this type of a gradient is considered an indication for surgery, this observation is significant.

Subaortic stenosis is particularly difficult to diagnose

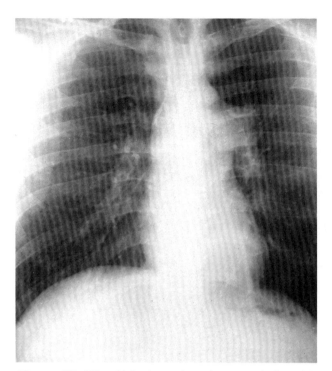

Figure 32–20. Valvular pulmonic stenosis in a 23-year-old man. Note the great enlargement of the pulmonary artery and the proximal aspect of the left pulmonary artery, resulting in large hilar vessels on the left in contrast to the small hilar vessels on the right.

roentgenographically because, in idiopathic hypertrophic subaortic stenosis, there is little if any poststenotic dilation; in the membranous type of stenosis, there is often no poststenotic dilatation, and the left ventricular hypertrophy is often minimal. The pulmonary artery, right side of the heart, and pulmonary vascularity are normal. In membranous, subaortic stenosis, there is a discrete, fibrous membrane below the aortic valve. This anomaly results in poststenotic dilatation in about 50% of patients. It is associated with other abnormalities in descending order of frequency: thick aortic valves, aortic insufficiency, ventricular septal defect, dilated sinuses of Valsalva, coarctation of the aorta, and mitral insufficiency.[2]

Corrected Transposition of the Great Vessels

Two major components in this anomaly are (1) transposition of the origins of the aorta and pulmonary artery, so that the aortic root is anterior and to the left of the pulmonary artery; and (2) inversion of the ventri-

cles with their accompanying atrioventricular valves. There is also inversion of the coronary arteries. Venous blood then enters the right atrium and flows through a bicuspid (mitral) valve into the anatomic left ventricle and to the lungs through the posteriorly placed pulmonary artery. Arterial blood returns from the lungs into the left atrium, and flows through a tricuspid valve into the anatomic right ventricle and to the general circulation through an anteriorly placed left-sided aorta.

When this lesion occurs alone, no functional circulatory abnormality is present and no symptoms occur. In the majority of these patients, however, there is an associated cardiovascular anomaly. Septal defects, especially ventricular, are the usual ones, and mitral valve anomalies are common. Pulmonic stenosis is also frequent.

The roentgen appearances depend on the associated defects. Signs caused by the anomalous position of the great vessels, however, may be quite characteristic. The ascending aorta often forms the upper left border of the heart and may produce a slight convexity, a long straight line, or a very slight concavity of this border (Fig. 32-21). The pulmonary artery does not form a part of the left border, but may indent the esophagus below the normal position of the aortic indentation. In some of these patients, the outflow tract of the right ventricle is directed to the right, resulting in greater perfusion of the right lung and enlargement of the right pulmonary artery and its major branches. The right

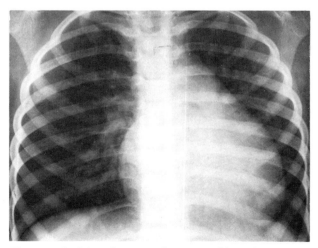

Figure 32–21. Corrected transposition of the great vessels. Note the slight convexity of the left upper cardiovascular border produced by the ascending aorta. No aortic shadow is noted on the right. There was an associated atrial septal defect with a very small left-to-right shunt.

hilar vessels may then be much more prominent than the left. Angiocardiography can be used to confirm the diagnosis as the anomalous position of the great vessels is readily determined.

Endocardial Fibroelastosis

Endocardial sclerosis, congenital subendothelial myofibrosis, congenital idiopathic hypertrophy of the heart, prenatal fibroelastosis, fetal endocarditis, endocardial dysplasia, and elastic-tissue hyperplasia are all synonyms for endocardial fibroelastosis. The disease is probably congenital or developmental in origin, although the cause is not definitely known. It is manifested by marked endocardial thickening that involves the left ventricle. The endocardium is involved by fibrous and elastic tissue without evidence of inflammation. The myocardium is usually markedly hypertrophied, and the left ventricle is dilated but is occasionally small in the contracted form of fibroelastosis, which is usually associated with aortic stenosis. Valves are often involved by contracture, thickening, and sometimes adhesions of the leaflets. The mitral valve is the most commonly and the most severely affected and mitral regurgitation is common. The patients usually show no evidence of heart disease at birth and may develop normally for a variable period of time. Symptoms progress rapidly and consist of dyspnea and evidence of congestive failure that may lead to death in a very short time. In some, the process appears to de-

velop more slowly and the patient survives for some length of time.

Roentgen Findings. The heart is usually enlarged, sometimes significantly. It tends to be globular in shape and there is often evidence of pulmonary congestion indicative of failure. The involvement of the mitral valve produces left atrial and ventricular enlargement. This can be recognized by the characteristic posterior displacement of the esophagus, bulging of the left upper cardiac border, double contour on the right, and enlargement of the left ventricle downward and to the left. Pulmonary venous congestion may be present as well as pulmonary edema. When the history is reasonably typical and these radiographic findings are noted, the diagnosis is fairly certain. In many instances, the diagnosis is made largely by the exclusion of the possibility of other diseases (Fig. 32-22).

Coarctation of the Aorta

This congenital malformation consists of an area of constriction in the aorta. It varies in degree from slight stenosis to atresia. The most commonly associated abnormality is bicuspid aorta valve, which is found in about 85% of patients with coarctation. Two general types, or groups, are recognized. The most common is the type in which the site of constriction is at or distal to the ductus arteriosus. The constriction develops early in intrauterine life, resulting in stimulus to the forma-

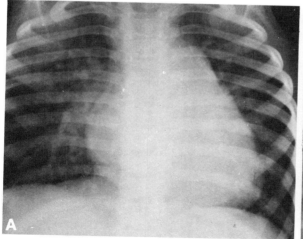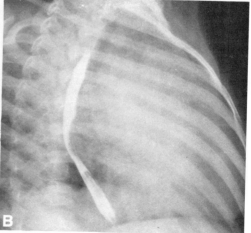

Figure 32–22. Endocardial fibroelastosis. **(A)** There is general cardiac enlargement and some evidence of pulmonary congestion. **(B)** In addition to the generalized backward displacement of the esophagus by the large heart, there is local displacement caused by enlargement of the left atrium. The patient was found to have mitral valvular involvement producing stenosis.

tion of collateral circulation to the lower body. As a result the infant is born with some collaterals and there is no change in the circulation when the ductus closes. The other general group, termed the "preductal type," consists of constriction proximal to the ductus. The coarctate segment is usually longer than in the other form and this lesion is often associated with other congenital cardiovascular anomalies. In this type there is no stimulus to the development of collateral circulation for the lower extremities during intrauterine life because blood from the pulmonary circulation is shunted into the descending aorta through the ductus. The preductal type, usually associated with other defects, is termed the "coarctation syndrome."

After birth, the ductus closes and the pulmonary blood flow to the descending aorta is shut off, causing a sudden increase in left ventricular work. This often results in decompensation before collaterals are developed. If the patent ductus persists in coarctation of the preductal type, cyanosis of the lower extremities with normal oxygenation of the head and upper extremities may occur. Associated cardiac anomalies may result in intracardiac right-to-left shunt. Desaturation is then generalized. In the infant, the roentgen findings are not characteristic. The heart is often grossly enlarged and there is evidence of pulmonary congestion. When coarctation results in congestive cardiac failure in infants, the roentgen and clinical findings are usually not

diagnostic. Retrograde aortography may be used to make the diagnosis. The use of MRI looks promising in this situation.

Roentgen Findings. The signs in the postductal type are usually characteristic enough to permit the diagnosis of coarctation on routine roentgen studies.

Rib Notching. Rib notching, an important radiologic sign, is caused by dilatation and tortuosity of the intercostal arteries that serve as collaterals between the proximal aorta, the internal mammary, and the aorta distal to the coarctation. It is almost universally present in adults but may not be demonstrated in children in the first five or six years of life. The sign consists of an irregular, scalloped sclerotic appearance of the inferior margins of the ribs laterally. It is usually most common and discernible in the fourth through the eighth ribs. The third rib is sometimes involved but the first and second are rarely notched because they are not involved in the collateral pathway. The irregularity is usually bilateral, but is not necessarily symmetric (Fig. 32-23). A number of other causes for rib notching are described elsewhere. They include subclavian artery obstruction, arteriovenous fistula of the intercostal vessels, tetralogy of Fallot, and superior caval obstruction with longstanding venous engorgement. In this group

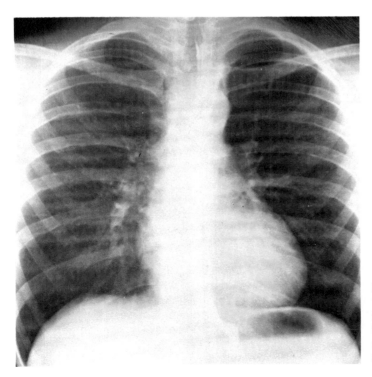

Figure 32–23. Coarctation of the aorta in a 10-year-old girl. There is clearly defined rib notching, which is very helpful in determining the diagnosis, since the site of the coarctation is not demonstrated, nor is there a very clearly defined area of poststenotic dilatation.

of diseases, the rib notching is often local and almost invariably unilateral.[48, 54]

The Aorta. The appearance of the aorta may be characteristic. The ascending arch is wide, producing convexity on the right side while the aortic knob or transverse aortic arch is small. Normally the left contour of the descending aorta can be visualized as a straight or gently convex line extending downward from the knob until it is obscured by the shadow of the heart below the hilum. In coarctation, a small indentation may be visible just below the knob that represents the actual site of coarctation. This is often associated with convexity below the coarctation site representing poststenotic dilatation. The appearance is that of two convexities that represent the aortic knob and the dilated aorta distal to the coarctation. In other patients the actual indentation is not visible; the normal, clearly visualized, left aortic border, however, is discontinuous. In the frontal projection, when the esophagus is filled with barium, there may be two clearly defined indentations on its left border, one above and one below the coarctation, which is sometimes termed the "reverse-3 sign." There is frequently enough dilatation of the left subclavian artery to result in convexity or prominence of the left superior mediastinal contour; this is often noted to be continuous with the shadow of the aortic knob. In the LAO projection, the notch and dilatation below it may be visible and the esophagus is often displaced by the dilated aorta immediately below the coarctation, as noted previously. This displacement is to the right, slightly anterior, and is definitely below the transverse aortic arch (Fig. 32-24). Congenital nonstenotic "kinking" of the aorta has also been described that may cause roentgen changes in this artery resembling those of coarctation. The other roentgen findings are absent, however, and there is no clinical evidence of coarctation.

Heart Size and Shape. The heart may be normal in size and shape, but the left ventricular workload is increased; eventually, left ventricular hypertrophy and dilatation result in enlargement of this chamber. The left atrium may also be enlarged. In infants with the coarctation syndrome and cardiac failure, the heart is relatively larger and there is evidence of pulmonary venous congestion as well as arterial hypervascularity, because the associated anomaly such as patent ductus arteriosus and interventricular septal defect result in a left-to-right shunt. It is difficult to ascertain how much

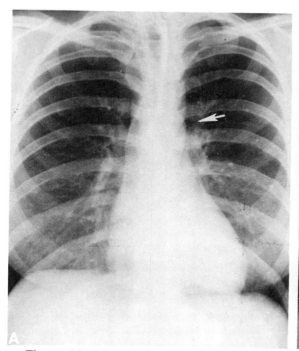
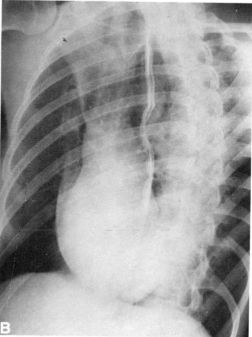

Figure 32–24. Coarctation of the aorta. (**A**) In this patient, the rib notching is relatively minor. The aortic knob is small, but there is a dilatation below it representing poststenotic dilatation of the aorta (retouched) (*arrow*). In the left anterior oblique projection (**B**), the esophagus is seen to be displaced slightly by the dilated aorta below the coarctation.

of the change is secondary to shunting and how much to congestive failure in these infants who often go into failure one or two weeks after birth.

Angiocardiography. This method is not ordinarily employed for the diagnosis of coarctation.

Retrograde Aortography. This examination is more useful than angiocardiography and clearly defines the coarctate segment as well as the aorta and its branches above and below it.

Kinking of the Aortic Arch (Pseudocoarctation)

Kinking or buckling of the aortic arch is sometimes termed "pseudocoarctation" because it simulates coarctation roentgenographically. No aortic constriction or gradient is present, however. The abnormality is presumably caused by a short, taut ligamentum arteriosum; because this does not account for the elongation of the arch that may be observed in this condition, a more likely cause is variation in normal differential growth rate of the aortic arch segments in early development.

Roentgen findings are variable, depending on the amount of elongation. The high aortic arch casts a round or crescentic shadow projecting to the left in the superior mediastinum, which may simulate a mediastinal tumor. Below this a second convexity projects to the left. The latter represents the arch at and distal to the kink, and may be more dense than the upper shadow. In other patients, the appearance is that of an unusually large aortic knob with an abrupt indentation at its inferior margin and a second convexity immediately below it, caused by actual dilatation of the aorta distal to the kink. Either or both of the shadows may indent the esophagus. The LAO and lateral views are usually diagnostic, since the indentation at the site of buckling can usually be identified (Fig. 32-25). CT in these projections may aid in the diagnosis. There is no left ventricular enlargement or rib notching. Aortography is diagnostic but usually not necessary.

Aneurysm of the Sinus of Valsalva

The aortic sinuses are three dilatations in the root of the aorta just above the aortic valves. They are named according to their corresponding aortic valve cusps: the right, left, and posterior. The right and left coronary arteries originate in or above the corresponding sinus of Valsalva and the posterior sinus is sometimes termed

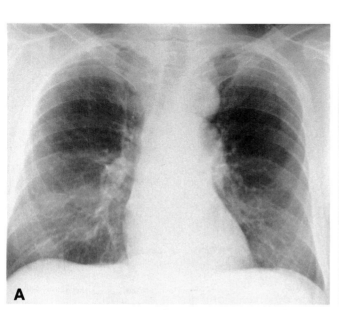
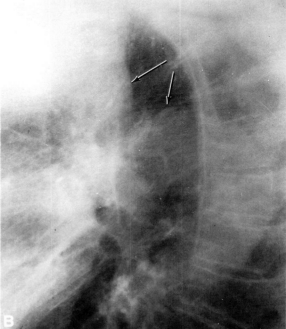

Figure 32–25. Pseudocoarctation of the aorta. (**A**) The transverse aortic arch is high, and there is a very large, broad convexity of the aorta to the left below the arch. (**B**) The severe kinking is demonstrated in the lateral view (*arrows*).

the "noncoronary sinus." Aneurysm is a rare congenital anomaly, usually involving the right aortic sinus. This sinus lies adjacent to the ventricular septum; occasionally, a fistulous tract develops into the right ventricle.

Rupture into the right atrium has been reported also. When this occurs, a left-to-right shunt is created and an increase in size of the right ventricle and the pulmonary artery and its branches occurs. When the aneurysm remains confined to the sinus, there is usually no alteration of the cardiovascular silhouette, but the aneurysm may be recognized by the calcification in the aneurysm wall. In the acquired type of aneurysm caused by cystic medial necrosis with or without Marfan's syndrome, however, there is usually aortic regurgitation leading to left ventricular enlargement and general dilatation of the ascending aorta. Aortic dissection is a frequent complication. The most common roentgen finding in any acquired type of aneurysm of the sinus of Valsalva is a local bulge of the right anterolateral cardiac contour. Aortography is useful to define the site and size of the aneurysm. Rarely, aneurysmal dilatation of all the sinuses of Valsalva may be associated with coarctation of the aorta.

Anomalous Left Coronary Artery

In this anomaly the blood supply to the myocardium is affected because the left coronary artery arises from the pulmonary artery. As a result, the left ventricle dilates early in life, leading to marked cardiac enlargement. The roentgen findings are not characteristic, but the large heart is visualized and there is often evidence of pulmonary congestion. Although the left ventricle is enlarged, the signs commonly associated with enlargement of this chamber are not necessarily present. When large collateral vessels form, the blood flows into the

Table 32–1. Definitions

Right and left ventricles and atria	Denotes morphology only; no functional or positional connotation
Inversion	Relationship between ventricles and feeding atria Noninverted: RV fed by RA, and LV fed by LA Inverted: RV fed by LA, and LV fed by RA
Transposition	Aorta arises from RV anterior to pulmonary artery, which arises from the LV

RV, right ventricle; LV, left ventricle; RA, right atrium; LA, left atrium. (Rosenbaum HD: The roentgen classification and diagnosis of cardiac alignments. Radiology 89:466, 1967)

pulmonary artery through the anomalous coronary. The patient has a left-to-right shunt. Pulmonary and coronary arteriography are necessary to make the diagnosis.

Rotation Anomalies of the Heart

The literature on classification and descriptions of various rotation and alignment anomalies is voluminous and somewhat confusing. Rosenbaum's classification of cardiac alignments based on patterns of blood flow is presented because of its consistency with current embryologic thought, as well as its relative simplicity and precision.[68] His definitions are indicated in Table 32-1. The possible courses of blood flow are given in Figure 32-26.

Using these definitions and combining them with the positional designations, a description of cardiac alignment includes designation of the ventriculotruncal alignment (eg, isolated ventricular inversion, inverted transposition, etc.), and a secondary indication of (1) the presence of situs solitus or situs inversus, and

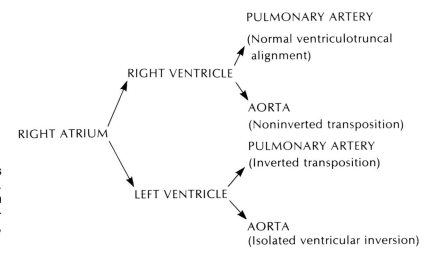

Figure 32–26. Possible courses of blood flow from the right atrium. (Rosenbaum HD: The roentgen classification and diagnosis of cardiac alignments. Radiology 89:466, 1967)

(2) a left-sided or right-sided heart. The abdominal visceral situs (situs solitus indicates the stomach is on the left; situs inversus indicates the stomach is on the right) indicates the position of the atria according to Rosenbaum, except in rare instances of isolated gastric inversion.[68] Elliott, Jue, and Amplatz believe that atrial position is more consistent with the side of the aortic arch.[17] If the right atrium is on the side opposite the stomach and on the same side as the liver, nearly all of the possible alignments can be determined with good biplane angiocardiograms. A few exceptions include the abnormalities associated with asplenia and polysplenia as well as some causes of common atrium. Although Rosenbaum's classification is not commonly used, it is valuable in defining the four fundamental ventriculotruncal alignments (Fig. 32-27). Figure 32-28 outlines the possible variations in abdominal situs and cardiac position and their relation to ventriculotruncal alignments.

Dextrocardia with situs solitus is nearly always associated with severe congenital cardiac malformation. Dextrocardia that is a part of complete situs inversus, a mirror image of the normal, almost always has a nor-mal ventriculotruncal alignment. A right-sided heart that result from pulmonary, diaphragmatic, or spinal abnormalities usually has no associated cardiac malformations.

ANOMALIES OF THE AORTIC ARCH AND ITS LARGE BRANCHES

The embryologic development of the aortic arch and its branches is complex. Six pairs of aortic arches develop in the embryo of man but not all are present at the same time. They originate anteriorly in the aortic sac, which represents the proximal portion of the developing aortic arch. They course backward on both sides to join the dorsal aorta, which is bilateral. The arches develop in the fifth week, and their transformation occupies the sixth and seventh weeks of fetal development. The first and second arches disappear early. The dorsal aorta at these levels persists as part of the internal carotid and the third arch persists as the proximal part of the common carotid artery on either side. The external carotid arteries arise as separate buds from the aortic sac and later transfer their origins onto the third ar-

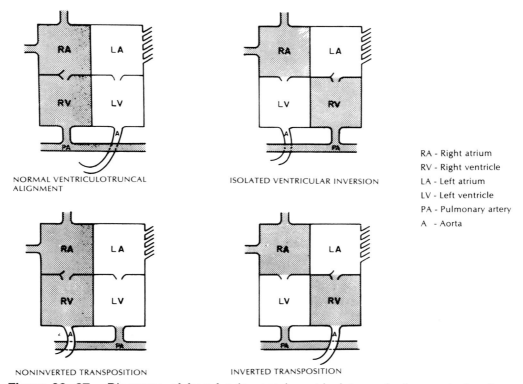

NORMAL VENTRICULOTRUNCAL ALIGNMENT

ISOLATED VENTRICULAR INVERSION

NONINVERTED TRANSPOSITION

INVERTED TRANSPOSITION

RA - Right atrium
RV - Right ventricle
LA - Left atrium
LV - Left ventricle
PA - Pulmonary artery
A - Aorta

Figure 32–27. Diagrams of four fundamental ventriculotruncal alignments in situs solitus. Relationships are reversed in situs inversus. (Rosenbaum HD: The roentgen classification and diagnosis of cardiac alignments. Radiology 89:466, 1967)

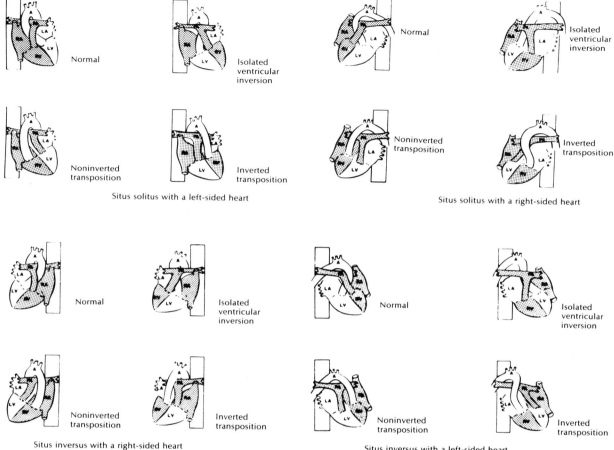

Figure 32–28. The four fundamental ventriculotruncal alignments in situs solitus and situs inversus, with both a right-sided heart and with a left-sided heart. Note that the alignments of situs solitus with the right-sided heart are identical to those seen with situs solitus and the left-sided heart. The only difference is the location of the cardiac apex. Similarly, the alignments for situs inversus and a left-sided heart are identical to those seen in situs inversus with a right-sided heart. (Rosenbaum HD: The roentgen classification and diagnosis of cardiac alignments. Radiology 89:466, 1967)

ches. The fourth arch persists on both sides. The left forms the permanent or left-sided aortic arch, while the right side forms the innominate artery. The fifth arches are transitory and disappear without a trace. The sixth arches arise from each dorsal aorta and extend across to the primitive pulmonary artery on either side to form the ductus arteriosus. The connection is lost on the right but persists on the left until after birth, when it closes to form the ligamentum arteriosum. Early in development the dorsal aorta fuses below the arch to form a single descending aorta.

Left Aortic Arch With Right Descending Aorta

In this rare anomaly, the left aortic arch arises normally and passes backward to the left of the trachea and esophagus and crosses to the right side of the mediastinum behind the esophagus where it continues as the right descending aorta. There is a left-sided aortic knob with absence of the aortic shadow below it on the left. An indentation on the posterior aspect of the esophagus courses from left to right in a cranial caudal direction. Often the descending aorta is visualized to the right of the midline.

Right Aortic Arch

The five types of right aortic arch are classified according to arrangement of arch vessels.[72] Type I right aortic arch, or mirror-image branching, is the more common of the mirror-image types. The first branch is the left innominate artery, followed by the right common carotid and the right subclavian. The aortic arch is to the right of the trachea and esophagus and descends on the right. This is the type usually associated with tetralogy of Fallot or truncus arteriosus and rarely with tricuspid atresia. The aortic knob can usually be identified on the right. It displaces the superior vena cava to the right and often produces a slight local deviation of the trachea to the left. When the esophagus is opacified, slight displacement to the left is often observed.

The second type is a rare type of mirror-image branching in which the left innominate artery is the first major branch, the right common carotid is the second, and the right subclavian is the third. The left ductus arteriosus extends from the upper descending aorta to the left pulmonary artery, forming a vascular ring. An aortic diverticulum may be present at the aortic origin of the left ductus. The arch descends on the right. This is a rare cause of a vascular ring, formed by the right arch on the right side and the ligamentum

or ductus on the left, which extends from the pulmonary artery posteriorly and to the right behind the esophagus where it joins the proximal descending aorta. Radiographic findings include the evidence of right aortic arch; barium study of the esophagus will show a posterior indentation produced by the ligamentum or ductus arteriosus.

Type III right aortic arch is one in which four vessels originate from the arch in the following order: left common carotid artery, right common carotid artery, right subclavian artery, and an aberrant left subclavian artery, which arises from the upper descending aorta. In this anomaly, the aorta may descend either to the right or to the left of the spine. There are two variations. In one, the aorta ascends to the right of the trachea and esophagus, and the arch passes to the left behind the esophagus and usually descends on the left side (Fig. 32-29). The left subclavian originates from the left posterior diverticulum of the distal aortic arch. In this variation, there is a large retroesophageal arch. A left ductus arteriosus may extend from the aortic diverticulum to the left pulmonary artery completing the vascular ring (Fig. 32-30). In the other variation, the aorta ascends and descends to the right of the spine. The left subclavian artery arises from a diverticulum of the descending aorta and courses obliquely behind the esophagus on which it causes extrinsic compression posteriorly. This rarely causes dysphagia. This type with the aberrant left subclavian artery is the most

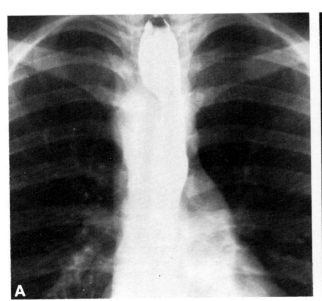
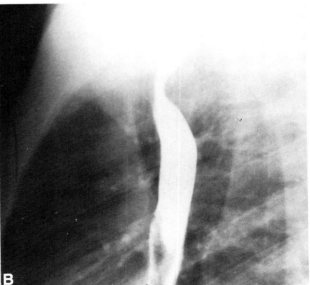

Figure 32–29.   Right aortic arch. (**A**) In the frontal view, no arch is noted on the left, and a vascular shadow on the right resembles the transverse aortic arch, which indents the esophagus. (**B**) In the lateral view, there is posterior indentation of the esophagus, indicating that the arch turns to the left and, in this patient, descends on the left.

Figure 32–30. Right aortic arch with a left patent ductus forming a vascular ring that resulted in moderate dysphagia. (**A**) In the frontal projection, the aortic knob is absent on the left and the aorta is noted on the right, where it indents the right lateral aspect of the esophagus. It also descends on the right. Some indentation is noted on the left lateral aspect of the esophagus slightly below the level of the aorta. (**B**) Spot film exposed during fluoroscopy, showing the esophageal narrowing clearly outlined. The ductus arteriosus crossed behind the esophagus from below upward, producing the well-marked posterior indentation noted. The ductus was ligated and sectioned, relieving the patient's symptoms.

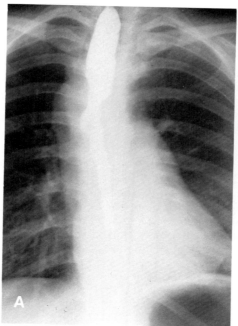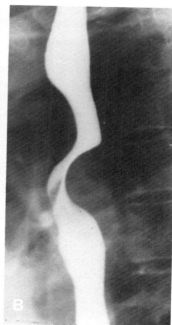

common of all types of right aortic arch and is often encountered as an incidental finding on routine chest film.

The incidence of associated congenital heart disease is very low, approximately 5% in these patients. Chest-film findings are those of the aortic mass to the right side of the trachea, often indenting it. The arch is often higher in position than the normal left arch. On the lateral film the retroesophageal aorta may be visible as a round mass displacing the trachea anteriorly; it will be noted to displace the esophagus anteriorly if the esophagus is filled with barium. The descending aorta may be seen coursing inferiorly on the left side.

In type IV right aortic arch, the left innominate artery is aberrant, arising as the third branch from the distal right arch and passing behind the esophagus, then dividing to form the left common carotid and subclavian arteries. The vascular ring is formed by the right arch, the retroesophageal innominate artery, and the left ductus arteriosus. In this anomaly, which is very rare, the right common carotid is the first branch, and the right subclavian is the second. Chest-film findings include evidence of right aortic arch with posterior compression of the esophagus produced by the aberrant left innominate artery.

In type V right aortic arch, the left common carotid, the right common carotid, and the right subclavian arteries arise from the arch in that order. The left subclavian is connected to the left pulmonary artery by

the left ductus arteriosus and has no connection to the aorta (isolation of the left subclavian artery). This anomaly is also uncommon. The chest-film findings include a right aortic knob and descending aorta. There may also be signs of cyanotic congenital heart disease, which is frequently associated with this malformation, the most common of which is tetralogy of Fallot. There is no vascular ring. In some patients, there is a subclavian steal syndrome in which this artery is supplied by the left vertebral artery.

Cervical Aortic Arch

Cervical aortic arch is a rare congenital anomaly in which the ascending aorta extends higher than usual so that the aortic arch is in the neck.[59] The incidence of right and left arches is approximately equal and the branching of the great vessels may vary from one patient to another. The plain-film findings consist of absence of the normal aortic arch in the thorax, an apparent cutoff of the tracheal air column in the superior mediastinum, a mass on either side caused by the arch that displaces the trachea, and superior mediastinal widening on the side of the descending aorta. The origin of the anomaly is uncertain because it may represent failure of descent of an otherwise normal fourth arch or persistence of one of the higher arches as the aortic arch.

Other Anomalies of the Aortic Arch and Its Large Branches

The innominate artery may arise more distally than normal and cross anterior to the trachea from left to right. It produces slight indentation on the trachea and occasionally may cause respiratory distress in infants. Similar anterior indentation and compression may be caused by the left carotid artery when it arises more proximally than normal, and must cross from right to left anterior to the trachea.

Anomalies Forming Vascular Rings

Double Aortic Arch. The double aortic arch comprises a large group of anomalies in which there are many variants. The fundamental defect results from persistence of both the right and the left aortic arches that encircle the trachea and esophagus and often produce partial obstruction of these structures. Either or both of the arches may function and may be comparable in size or one may be larger than the other. A portion of the smaller arch may be fibrous and nonfunc-

tioning but may nevertheless form the ring. The aorta may descend on either the right or the left side and anomalous origins of one or more of the great vessels often accompany this anomaly. The roentgen and fluoroscopic findings consist of evidence of compression of the trachea and esophagus by an encircling vascular ring (Fig. 32-31). The double arch produces densities on either side of the midline that may be symmetric. If necessary, aortography or MRI may be used to define in more detail the vascular ring.

Aberrant Right Subclavian Artery. This is the most common of the anomalies of the great vessels. The right subclavian originates as the most distal of the branches of the arch and reaches the right side by coursing obliquely upward and to the right, usually behind the esophagus. This defect is most often asymptomatic but may be associated with other cardiovascular anomalies. The major roentgen finding is an oblique indentation of the posterior aspect of the esophagus above the aortic arch, which extends upward and to the right. It is usually outlined best in the lateral and LAO projec-

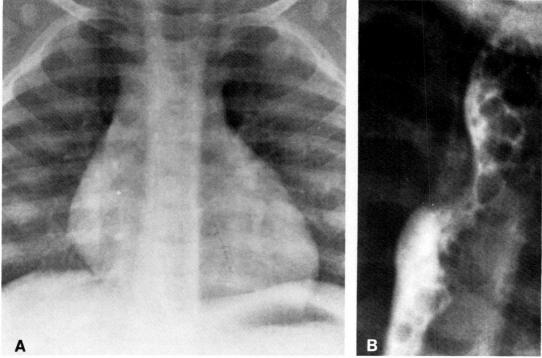

Figure 32–31.   Double aortic arch. (**A**) Note the very slight deviation of the trachea to the left in this 6-month-old infant with feeding problems. The vascular shadow on the right at the level of the aortic arch is somewhat larger than on the left. (**B**) Spot film with barium in the esophagus shows the indentation on the right to be higher and larger than the one on the left, which is smaller and lower, lying just above the left bronchus.

tions. Fluoroscopic examination with barium swallow will outline this defect and its effect on the esophagus (Fig. 32-32).

CONGENITAL ANOMALIES OF THE PULMONARY ARTERY AND ITS BRANCHES

Agenesis of the Pulmonary Artery

This is an uncommon anomaly in which there is absence of one pulmonary artery. It is associated with an anomalous systemic arterial blood supply to the lung that arises either from the aorta or from one of its major branches. The anomaly is often associated with other congenital anomalies of the cardiovascular system. Occasionally the systemic artery supplying the involved lung is very large; this results in a large arteriovenous shunt that may eventually cause cardiac failure. The high pressure in this anomalous system is believed to be the cause of hemoptysis, the most common symptom of the condition.

Roentgen Findings. The roentgen findings are characteristic enough in most instances to make the diagnosis or strongly suspect it. The involved hemithorax is smaller in size than normal. In addition to the difference in size of the bony thorax, the hemidiaphragm is often elevated and mediastinal structures are shifted to the affected side. There is often some herniation of the normal lung across the midline anterior to the aorta. The normal shadows of the pulmonary arterial branches in the hilum and in the lung are absent and the vessels that are visible form a relatively fine reticular vascular pattern caused by the branching bronchial arteries. The result is an absence of the hilum shadow or an inconspicuous one. Plain tomography or CT may be very useful to define clearly the difference in the hilar vessels on the two sides. Bronchography outlines the normally branching bronchial tree and excludes the possibility of atelectasis, while angiocardiography can be used to define the main pulmonary artery and its remaining branch and to show the lack of filling on the opposite side (Fig. 32-33). Agenesis of a lobe, or lobes, may occur in conjunction with agenesis of the pulmonary artery. Hypoplasia of one pulmonary artery may result in similar but somewhat less marked roentgen findings. Unless the hypoplasia is relatively severe, however, it is unlikely that the diagnosis can be made without the use of angiocardiography.

Congenital Absence of the Pulmonary Valve

Congenital absence of the pulmonary valve is a rare malformation. It is usually associated with tetralogy of Fallot and occasionally with ventricular septal defect, but it may occur as an isolated anomaly. Roentgen findings in patients with associated anomalies include

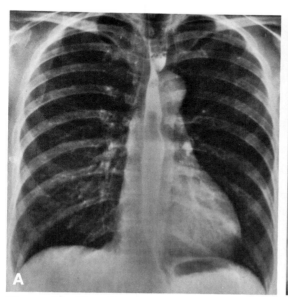
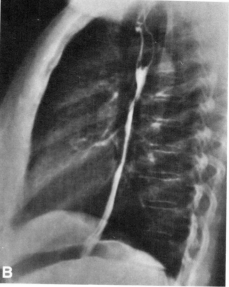

Figure 32–32. Aberrant right subclavian artery. Posteroanterior (**A**) and left lateral (**B**) projections show an oblique indentation of the left posterior aspect of the esophagus above the aortic arch. In the lateral view, note calcium in the aortic valve. The patient presented with symptoms related to aortic stenosis.

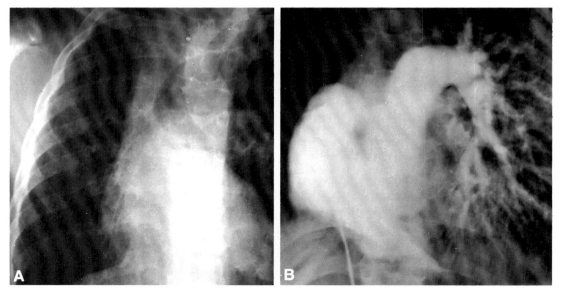

Figure 32–33.   Agenesis of the right pulmonary artery. (**A**) Frontal chest film shows a marked shift of the heart and mediastinal structures to the right. The branches of the right pulmonary artery are absent so that no hilar vessels are visible, and the entire right lung shows very little vascularity. (**B**) The angiocardiogram shows the main pulmonary artery and its left branch. Note that the right pulmonary artery is absent.

dilatation of one or both pulmonary arteries. The dilatation may be of such magnitude that wheezing due to obstructive emphysema on one or both sides is usually present. To-and-fro murmurs along the left sternal border and absent or diminished pulmonary second sounds are common. Absence of the pulmonary valve without associated anomalies produces much less dilatation of the pulmonary arteries centrally, so that respiratory distress is not produced. Varying amounts of right ventricular dilatation and hypertrophy alter the shape of the cardiac silhouette. CT will demonstrate the bronchial compression caused by the large artery.

Aberrant Left Pulmonary Artery

This anomaly, termed "pulmonary sling," consists of a distal origin of the left pulmonary artery. The origin may be from the right pulmonary artery or from the distal main pulmonary artery.[31] The aberrant artery passes over the right main bronchus, then passes backward and to the left between the trachea and esophagus to the left hilum. If it compresses the right main bronchus, obstructive symptoms result in respiratory distress. Roentgen findings include evidence of obstructive emphysema on the right, a low, small, left hilum, and, on the lateral view, a round mass indenting the barium-filled esophagus anteriorly, the key finding

in this condition. Dysphagia is not usually present. The anomalous artery may also produce a right-sided mediastinal mass, particularly if it causes no symptoms and is observed in the older child or in an adult. There is sometimes decreased vascularity of the left lung. Pulmonary arteriography will confirm the diagnosis.

Aberrant Vascular Connection Between Right Pulmonary Artery and the Left Atrium

This is a very rare anomaly. It causes cyanosis and clubbing of fingers and toes.[44] The distinctive roentgen finding indicates a small rounded mass that, on frontal projection, is seen overlying the midright atrium and protruding to the right beyond it; the lateral and inferior border is clearly defined. On the LAO projection, the density overlies the lower anterior aspect of the left atrium; again, its inferior border is clearly defined. The diagnosis can be confirmed by right-sided angiocardiography.

Pulmonary Arteriovenous Malformations

A pulmonary arteriovenous malformation (AVM) is a congenital vascular anomaly, sometimes termed a fistula or aneurysm (we prefer the term "arteriovenous malformation") through which a relatively large amount of nonoxygenated blood flows; therefore, the lesion represents a right-to-left shunt and is associated with varying degrees of unsaturation of the arterial blood. This malformation is usually multiple and occurs more frequently in the lower lobes than elsewhere. Because the caliber of the vessels within the mass varies, there is no quantitative correlation between the size of the anomaly and the amount of shunt. The pulmonary lesions may be accompanied by telangiectases elsewhere and are then a part of a generalized angiomatous process. Because these are right-to-left shunts that may be quite large, the filtering effect of the pulmonary capillary circulation is lost and any embolic process arising in the systemic venous system may result in systemic embolization. For example, brain abscess is a common complication.

Roentgen Findings. The malformation is represented by a round, oval, or lobulated mass or several masses, usually in the lower lobes. The lesion is clearly defined and it is often possible to see a large pulmonary artery extending from the hilum to the lesion: another vessel, the pulmonary vein, extends from the lesion to the region of the left atrium. If large vessels enter and drain the lesion, the diagnosis should be strongly suspected. CT is useful in outlining the blood supply and in clearly defining the lesions. When one is visualized, it is wise to look carefully for others because often they are multiple. The malformations may appear as nodules (single or multiple) in patients in whom no such lesions have been seen in the area previously. This may present a very difficult diagnostic problem, because primary or metastatic tumor is then a consideration. Pulmonary arteriography is diagnostic. These AVMs may be occluded with detachable balloons, or coils inserted transvascularly, which avoids resection of normal lung (Fig. 32-34). Because the fistulae increase in size with age, repeat treatment may be necessary.

Diffuse Pulmonary Hemangiomatosis

Diffuse pulmonary hemangiomatosis is a rare condition in which the lungs are the major sites of multiple hemangiomas that occur primarily along the bronchi, arteries, veins, and within the septa as well as in the pleura.[69] Hemangiomas may also occur in other sites such as the spleen and the thymus. Radiographic findings are those of diffuse, interstitial disease simulating fibrosis in children who have a history of repeated, often bloody, pleural effusions, as well as pulmonary infections, usually with hemoptysis. Thrombocytopenia and anemia develop, and eventually dyspnea and cyanosis appear associated with increasing interstitial disease and bloody pleural effusion. The prognosis is poor.

Pulmonary Varices

Pulmonary varix is another rare anomaly in which the arteries are normal and there is no capillary shunting.[5] In the venous phase, the veins feeding the varix (or varices) become filled at the same time as normal veins are filling, but there is delay in emptying of the varix, which drains directly into the left atrium. This anomaly should not be confused with pulmonary arteriovenous malformations that cause right-to-left shunting of blood. Plain-film findings are those of densities resembling dilated, tortuous vessels, usually in the parahilar area. Pulmonary angiography confirms the diagnosis.

Pulmonary Artery Coarctations

A wide variety of pulmonary coarctations have been reported. The stenosis may involve the pulmonary artery above the valve and either or both of its main branches. Multiple peripheral stenoses involving many segmental arterial branches may also occur. The stenosis may be sharply localized or involve a relatively long segment of the affected artery. The coarctation may be unilateral or bilateral and is associated with valvular pulmonic stenosis in 60% of patients. Supravalvular aortic stenosis also may be associated with pulmonary artery coarctations.

Roentgen findings are varied and depend upon the location of the stenotic lesion, its length, and the presence or absence of poststenotic dilatation. In the central types, poststenotic dilatation may result in an increase of the hilar vascular shadow. When the stenosis involves a long segment of either the right or left pulmonary artery or both, the hilar vascular shadow may be decreased, often with distinct increase in vessel size a short distance from the central hilum. In patients with multiple peripheral stenoses, the poststenotic dilatations may produce a nodular vascular pattern in the parahilar region unilaterally or bilaterally. These findings strongly indicate a diagnosis of pulmonary coarctation. Pulmonary arteriography is needed for definitive diagnosis and, in many instances, the lesions are discovered on arteriographic study performed for identification of other lesions or conditions.

Idiopathic Enlargement of the Pulmonary Artery

Dilatation of the pulmonary artery in diseases of the heart and lungs has been described. Occasionally, marked dilatation of the pulmonary artery occurs as an isolated finding. The dilatation may extend into the left main branch for a short distance and occasionally into the right branch. When all clinical and laboratory studies, including cardiac catheterization, fail to dem-

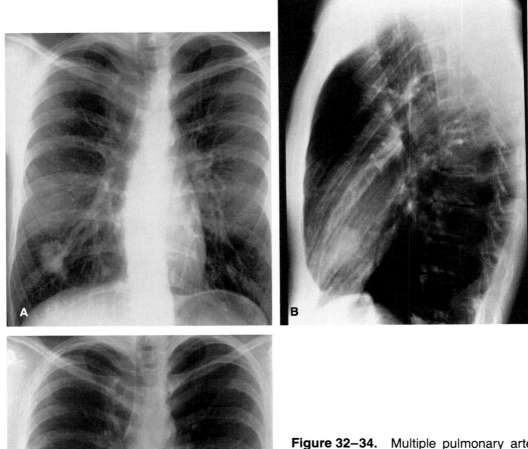

Figure 32–34. Multiple pulmonary arteriovenous malformations. (**A**) In the frontal chest film, several nodular densities are present. The largest is at the right base. Two large vessels are noted to extend from the mass to the hilum. (**B**) The large right basilar mass is located anteriorly in the middle lobe. (**C**) Film in the frontal projection taken postembolization shows the presence of some radiopaque Gianturco coils that were used to occlude the major fistula. The artery to the fistula was thrombosed and both it and the malformation itself are no longer as apparent.

onstrate a cause, this enlargement probably represents a true congenital aneurysm. The diagnosis is made by exclusion, however, because there are many known cardiac and pulmonary diseases that can result in considerable dilatation of the pulmonary artery. The only roentgenographic finding is prominence in the region of the artery, resulting in convexity and enlargement of the artery segment as seen in the frontal projection. The enlargement can also be observed in oblique and lateral views. The diagnosis is made with caution because it is one of exclusion and cannot be made on the basis of roentgenographic findings alone.

The pulmonary artery is often prominent in childhood and early adult life. The convexity produced by the pulmonary artery is moderately enlarged, with no sign of cardiac or pulmonary disease on roentgenographic examination. Examination reveals no cause for it and the vessel evidently decreases in size because the finding is uncommon in older adults.

ACQUIRED VALVULAR CARDIAC DISEASE

Mitral Stenosis

Acquired mitral valvular disease usually results from rheumatic heart disease. Mitral stenosis is most common but there is often some degree of mitral insufficiency. The left atrium must empty itself against increased resistance caused by the mitral stenosis and the chamber enlarges. The increased pressure is reflected back through the lesser circulation to the right ventricle. This results in changes in the pulmonary vessels and in the right side of the heart.

Roentgen Findings. The appearance of the cardiovascular silhouette in mitral valvular disease is often characteristic (Fig. 32-35). Left atrial enlargement causes alterations. This may be the only change in the cardiac silhouette for some time. Often, enough stenosis is great enough to ultimately cause right ventricular

enlargement and enough insufficiency to cause some left ventricular enlargement. There are also pulmonary vascular alterations. The signs of left atrial enlargement appear in frontal projection: (1) Convexity of the left upper cardiac margin occurs below the level of the left main bronchus. This represents enlargement of the auricular appendage (Fig. 32-36). In patients with a transverse heart the only alteration may be a straightening of the left upper cardiac margin in contrast to its usual slight concavity below the pulmonary artery. (2) A double contour or double convexity occurs on the right. The atrium may be large enough to be border forming on the right side, in which case a double convexity is visible. When it is not border forming, the atrium is often sufficiently dense to be identified within the right atrial border, forming a more dense convexity within the longer, right atrial convexity. (3) Sufficient posterior enlargement of the atrium enables it to be seen as an area of increased density within the cardiac margins on either side below the level of the carina. (4) Elevation of the left main bronchus is apparent. (5) In the lateral and right anterior oblique projections, a posterior and sometimes slightly rightward bulge will cause displacement of the esophagus, which is best seen when it is filled with barium. This results in a posterior convexity of the esophagus in this region. (6)

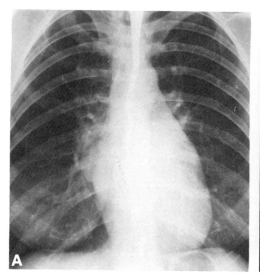
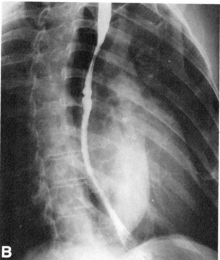

Figure 32–35. Mitral stenosis. **(A)** There is a double convexity on the right and a prominence of the left upper cardiac border. These signs indicate left atrial enlargement. The overall cardiac size is normal. Note the scarcity of pulmonary vessels at the bases despite sizable hilar arteries. **(B)** The right anterior oblique view shows posterior displacement of the esophagus by the enlarged left atrium. Also noted is some prominence of the outflow tract of the right ventricle, manifested by some convexity of the upper cardiac border on the left. The vascular redistribution indicates pulmonary venous hypertension.

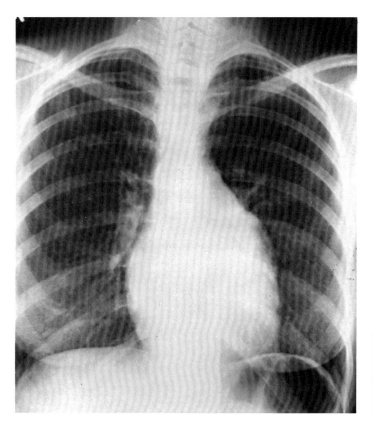

Figure 32–36.   Mitral stenosis. In this patient, the left atrium is very large and the appendage produces a marked local bulge below the left pulmonary artery in the upper left cardiac margin. Vascularity is approximately equal in the upper and lower lungs.

In the LAO projection, visualization of the enlarged atrium just below the left bronchus.

Calcium is often deposited in the mitral valve and its annulus. This may be difficult to demonstrate on roentgenograms of the chest but is usually easily seen fluoroscopically. The valvular calcification generally indicates mitral stenosis, while calcium in the mitral annulus may not necessarily be associated with valvular abnormality. The latter has a somewhat elliptical shape; the ellipse is usually open medially in a "u" or horseshoe shape.

Calcification in the left atrium is observed occasionally in patients with mitral stenosis. The calcium may be in the atrial wall or within a thrombus attached to the wall. When calcification in the atrium is suspected but not positively identified on the chest film, fluoroscopy can be used to confirm the diagnosis. When the calcification is in the atrial appendage, it is usually associated with mitral stenosis. Calcification in the wall of the atrium as well as in the appendage often indicates severe stenosis. This is an unfavorable prognostic sign.

If the disease results in pulmonary arterial hypertension, eventually the right ventricle enlarges and the signs of an increase in size of this chamber are ob-

served. Enlargement of the central pulmonary arteries is helpful in indicating right ventricular enlargement.

As has been noted, alterations in pulmonary vascular pressure tend to cause progressive pulmonary changes. Initially there is venous hypertension. The first sign is slight general venous distention or engorgement that is difficult to assess. It is most readily identified when earlier films are available for comparison. As the hypertension becomes more marked, constriction of the lower-lobe arteries and veins and distention of the upper-lobe vessels results in a reversal of the usual pattern in which the lower-lobe vessels are more prominent (Fig. 32-37). Most of the blood flow is then maintained through the upper lobes.

This alteration in the vascular pattern is usually readily identified early, but in longstanding chronic venous hypertension there may be enough interstitial change to obscure the vascular findings. As the venous pressure increases, more fluid escapes into the perivascular tissues and the lymphatis become dilated.

The edematous interlobular septa can be identified as dense lines of varying length, depending on their location. These lines were first described by Kerley in 1930. He described three lines, which he designated

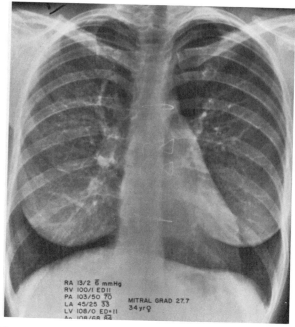

RA 13/2 6 mmHg
RV 100/I ED11
PA 103/50 70
LA 45/25 33   MITRAL GRAD 27.7
LV 108/0 ED=11   34 yr ♀
Ao 108/68 84

Figure 32–37. Pulmonary vessels in mitral steno-sis. The lower lung vessels are constricted and ap-pear to be smaller than the vessels in the upper lung.

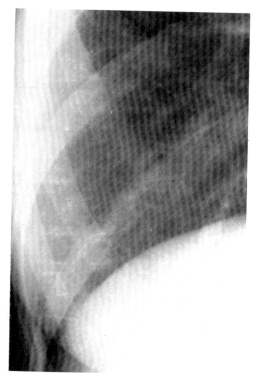

Figure 32–38. Kerley's B lines. This close-up view of the right lateral lung base of a patient with mitral stenosis shows short, horizontal, dense lines repre-senting interstitial edema.

A, B and C. The A lines are 5 to 10 cm long, nonbranch-ing, and extend obliquely upward and outward from pulmonary hilum in a fanlike manner. The B lines are best seen in the lower zones of the lung, perpendicular to the pleural surface, and generally are less than 2 cm in length. They are often best seen in oblique projec-tion. The combination of A and B lines will form a reticular pattern, designated as C lines. They all repre-sent edematous interlobular septa. The difference in size and orientation of the B lines is a reflection on the size and orientation of the interlobular septa. The pul-monary lobules tend to be large and oriented obliquely to the pleura in the upper lobes, while in the lower lobes they are shorter and are lateral to the pleural surface. This causes the appearance of Kerley's B lines, which are short, dense lines representing interlobular septa extending to the pleural surface.[42] They are ob-served in the lower lung and are at right angles to the pleural surface (Fig. 32-38). They do not bifurcate and are often observed best on oblique films. Interstitial edema fluid causes the density. The deep septal lines, Kerley's A lines, may also become visible. They are about 2 to 5 inches long, normally straight, and extend outward and upward in a somewhat fanlike manner from the upper hilar area into the periphery of the upper lung. Kerley's C lines also represent interstitial structures or lymphatics within the interstitial struc-

tures. They tend to be transient and difficult to visual-ize but cause a fine spider web or reticular pattern throughout the lung. In chronic venous hypertension associated with chronic passive congestion, deposits of hemosiderin are added to the other causes for promi-nence of the septal lines.

Eventually pulmonary arterial hypertension may oc-cur. This results in dilatation of the main pulmonary artery and its branches centrally, which is associated with a constriction of arteries in the midlung and pe-ripheral lung zones. These findings are then superim-posed on those of chronic venous hypertension and right ventricular hypertrophy.

Pulmonary hemosiderosis (deposition of blood pig-ments in the interstitial tissues) secondary to mitral disease is a frequent pathologic finding but is not com-monly recognized as such on chest films. Sufficient amounts of the deposits are visible roentgenographi-cally as fine granular or miliary shadows throughout the lungs (Fig. 32–39). They may become large enough to produce nodular densities ranging from 2 to 5 mm in diameter. The appearance of the lungs may resemble

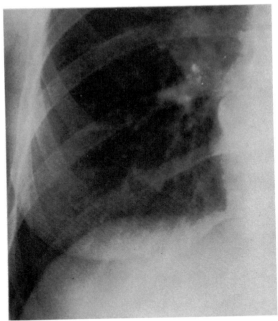

Figure 32–39. Hemosiderosis in a patient with mitral stenosis. Close-up view of the right lower lung shows numerous small, granular-appearing nodules that developed over several years of observation.

that noted in miliary tuberculosis or early nodular silicosis. The associated findings of mitral disease are usually obvious, however, so that there is no difficulty in making the differential diagnosis.

Pulmonary ossification or calcification is an uncommon finding in mitral stenosis. It is usually found in the lower lobes and produces multiple opacities resembling the calcified lesions of histoplasmosis scattered widely in the lung bases.

Mitral Insufficiency

Mitral insufficiency is often associated with mitral stenosis. This valvular defect increases the left ventricular workload and leads to dilatation of this chamber. It is manifested by enlargement of the heart downward and to the left with lengthening and rounding of the left lower cardiac contour. The left atrium is also enlarged and causes the signs described previously for enlargement of this chamber. Pulmonary congestion develops as in mitral stenosis. Often it is difficult to differentiate mitral stenosis and insufficiency. Relative mitral insufficiency commonly occurs in diseases that produce left ventricular dilatation. Its presence, although suspected, often may be difficult to detect radiographically. Acute mitral insufficiency caused by ruptured chordae ten-

dinea may occur as a result of bacterial endocarditis, rheumatic endocarditis, blunt trauma, or myocardial infarction. Idiopathic or spontaneous rupture may also occur. Usually there is an abrupt onset or sudden increase in dyspnea in a patient with existing cardiopulmonary disease. The chest film reveals pulmonary edema, moderate to no enlargement of the left atrium, and little if any cardiac enlargement.

Combined Mitral Stenosis and Insufficiency Disease

In many instances gross changes indicate a double lesion, while in others the findings are sufficiently characteristic to warrant the diagnosis of mitral stenosis without significant regurgitation. There is a third group in which differential diagnosis is difficult to make on roentgen study. As a rule, the left atrium is larger in combined stenosis and insufficiency than in stenosis alone. Left ventricular enlargement usually accompanies insufficiency, but this may be very difficult to detect. The posterior curve of the enlarged left atrium in the RAO projection tends to be longer in insufficiency than in isolated stenosis. Rheumatic heart disease also causes aortic stenosis and insufficiency that result in left ventricular enlargement.

These lesions must be kept in mind in addition to mitral insufficiency when left ventricular enlargement is present (Fig. 32–40). When surgery is contemplated in patients with mitral valve disease, cardiac catheterization is used to assess pulmonary arterial and venous pressures, as well as to define the amount of stenosis or insufficiency, or both, if present. Selective angiocardiography may be used in conjunction with catheterization to assess the amount of regurgitation, the severity of the stenosis, and the pliability of the valve.

Aortic Stenosis

Rheumatic heart disease had been the most common cause of acquired aortic stenosis. It may develop, however, as a degenerative process in patients with bicuspid aortic valves, leading to a calcified valve. This is now the primary etiology of aortic stenosis. Calcific aortic stenosis may also occur in patients without anomalous valves and with no history of rheumatic heart disease. This lesion causes increased workload on the left ventricle and results in hypertrophy. As a result, there is rounding of the left lower cardiac border. Hypertrophy is usually present without dilatation (concentric hypertrophy), the heart is within normal limits of size, and the only finding is rounding of the apex. When dilatation occurs, the left border elongates, moving the apex downward and to the left. The

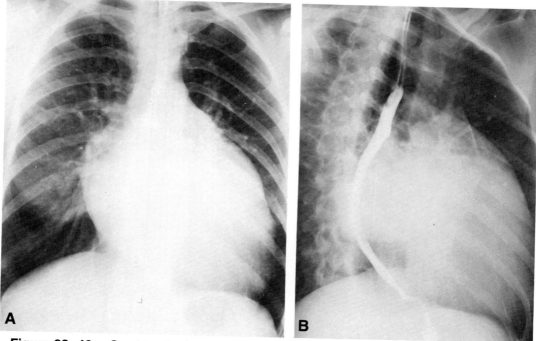

Figure 32–40. Combined mitral stenosis and insufficiency. Marked cardiac enlargement with massive enlargement of the left atrium noted on the frontal (**A**) and right anterior oblique (**B**) projections. There is also marked prominence of the pulmonary outflow tract. Note the paucity of basal vessels.

aortic knob is normal in size and the ascending aortic arch is enlarged, resulting in convexity of the right upper cardiac margin. This may be observed best in the LAO projection. This enlargement represents post stenotic dilatation. There may be a considerable amount of calcification in the aortic valve. This is usually readily visible fluoroscopically, but is difficult to see in the frontal roentgenogram because the valve is projected over the shadow of the spine. It is often visible in the right and left oblique projections, however, it is best seen in lateral projection. Value calcification is specific for aortic valve disease (Fig. 32–41).

Aortic valve calcification is also a reliable indication that the stenosis is severe, particularly when present in young patients. If the patient is not decompensated, visible calcification on the plain chest film usually indicates a gradient of 50 mm Hg or more across the valve. The roentgen findings in aortic stenosis may be diagnostic, but in some cases must be supported by clinical findings to make the diagnosis. As a general rule, left ventricular enlargement is found late in the course of the disease as a result of dilatation, which may result in left ventricular failure.

Aortic Insufficiency

Aortic insufficiency may be caused by rheumatic fever (rheumatic valvulitis), bacterial endocarditis, and less often by syphilis and arteriosclerosis. Incompetence of the aortic valve results in dilatation of the left ventricle along with hypertrophy. The outflow tract of this chamber is the first to enlarge, resulting in an increase in length of the left lower cardiac contour that represents the ventricular segment. The apex then extends below the dome of the diaphragm. The lower left ventricular contour is also rounded. As enlargement progresses with involvement of the inflow tract, the left ventricular segment increases further and the upper left contour tends to become more rounded. Posterior enlargement with rounding of the lower posterior cardiac margin as visualized in the LAO projection becomes evident (Fig. 32–42). The aorta may dilate, resulting in convexity of the aortic segment that makes up the upper right cardiovascular margin, and the aortic knob is often prominent. Enlargement of the heart may be extreme in aortic regurgitation and when massive left ventricular enlargement occurs, sometimes described

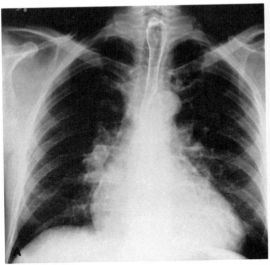

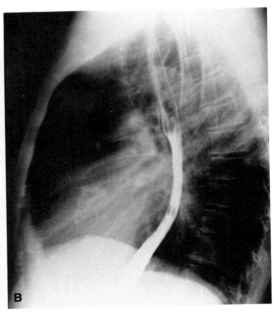

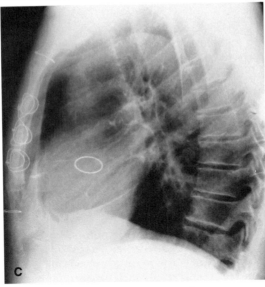

Figure 32–41. Calcific aortic stenosis. (**A**) The heart is moderately enlarged secondary to left ventricular dilatation and hypertrophy. There is slight prominence of the ascending aorta. (**B**) In the lateral projection dense calcification is present in the aortic valve. (**C**) A lateral projection postoperatively shows metal sutures in the sternum. These were used to close the median sternotomy. In addition, there is a radiopaque ring that is part of a Hancock aortic valve prosthesis. Note the absence of the calcium, which was present in the diseased valve.

by the term "cor bovinum." Combined stenosis and regurgitation may be present, but there is no way to ascertain the predominant lesion on roentgen study. When aortic valvular disease results in cardiac failure, the signs of pulmonary congestion develop along with the appearance of relative mitral insufficiency resulting in left atrial enlargement.

In rheumatic valvular disease, both the aortic and mitral valves are often involved and there may be massive generalized cardiac enlargement along with enlargement of the chambers in which work is increased. At times it is possible to determine the pre-

dominant defect, but this is not always the case. When a proximal valve (such as the mitral) is involved by stenosis and insufficiency, it becomes difficult to assess change in the distal (aortic) valve by roentgen means short of angiocardiography and aortography.

PULMONARY VALVULAR DISEASE

Pulmonary stenosis is usually a congenital anomaly; the roentgen findings produced by this lesion have been described in the section on pulmonic stenosis.

Pulmonary insufficiency is rare, but is usually ac-

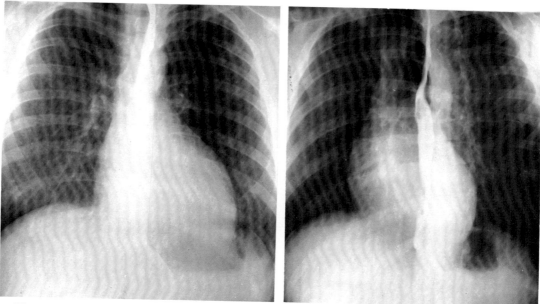

Figure 32–42. Aortic insufficiency. The left ventricle is considerably enlarged, and there is very little dilatation of the aorta.

quired. It usually results from endocarditis of the valve that is septic in character. This may cause repeated pulmonary emboli. Right ventricular enlargement accompanied by enlargement of the pulmonary artery may be recognized. The findings in congenital absence of the pulmonary valve were described previously.

TRICUSPID VALVULAR DISEASE

Acquired tricuspid valvular disease is uncommon, but this valve may be involved by rheumatic disease. Relative tricuspid insufficiency is also caused by excessive dilatation of the right ventricle. Disease involving the tricuspid valve is manifested by enlargement of the right atrium, which may be extreme. The enlargement causes widening of the heart to the right and increased convexity of the right lower cardiac margin. In the LAO and frontal views there may be a shoulder-like projection of the right auricular appendage, producing a sharp angulation between it and the ascending aorta; this indicates marked right atrial enlargement and suggests tricuspid disease. The superior and inferior venae cavae tend to be enlarged and, in tricuspid insufficiency, pulsation of the great veins may be recognized. Because tricuspid disease tends to decrease the load on the lesser circulation, unusual clarity of the lung fields has been described but is not a very helpful sign. Mitral defects result in dilatation of the right atrium because of increased venous pressure, the result of stasis. In the presence of mitral disease the roentgen

diagnosis of tricuspid insufficiency is difficult to make. Thus, the roentgen signs of tricuspid valvular disease may only be suggestive and not diagnostic.

MISCELLANEOUS CARDIAC CONDITIONS

Hypertensive Cardiovascular Disease

Persistent systemic arterial hypertension results in an increased workload on the left ventricle. Because the disease varies from a relatively mild form that causes little or no alteration in the cardiac silhouette to severe longstanding disease that produces marked changes, it is evident that the degree of roentgen change varies greatly. The heart may remain normal in size and shape for some time, but, in patients with persistent high pressures, left ventricular hypertrophy develops. The earliest change is rounding of the left lower cardiac border caused by concentric hypertrophy. The heart then enlarges downward and to the left with lengthening of the left ventricular contour and rounding of the apex, often resulting in displacement of the apex below the dome of the diaphragm. This enlargement also causes posterior convexity noted in the lateral and LAO projections. These latter changes indicate dilatation in addition to the hypertrophy that preceded it. The cardiac silhouette is similar to that seen in aortic insufficiency. It is important to remember that in transient or early hypertension no roentgen abnormalities are recognized. In addition to the alteration in the size and shape of the heart, aortic changes are a result of this disease. There is dilatation of the aorta that may be sufficient to produce convexity of the aortic segment of the right upper cardiovascular silhouette and enlargement of the aortic knob (Fig. 32–43).

When hypertension is relieved the heart may decrease in size. This represents primarily a decrease in the amount of dilatation. In many instances, irreversible changes have occurred, precluding the heart from regaining its normal contour following surgical or medical correction of the underlying disease. When decompensation occurs, there is often relative mitral insufficiency resulting in left atrial enlargement, pulmonary congestion, edema, and pleural effusion.

ARTERIOSCLEROTIC CARDIOVASCULAR DISEASE

General Arteriosclerotic (Ischemic Disease)

Arteriosclerotic disease is probably the cause of cardiac failure in the elderly patient with normotensive, non-valvular heart disease. Most of these patients will be found to have moderate-to-severe coronary sclerosis, which presumably causes myocardial changes leading to eventual failure. Because ischemia is the likely cause, "ischemic heart disease" is probably a better term.

Arteriosclerotic changes in the aortic valve may pro-duce stenosis or insufficiency, resulting in some enlargement of the left ventricle. The changes in the heart are accompanied by changes in the aorta that result from arteriosclerosis. They consist of dilatation and elongation of the aorta, resulting in enlargement and tortuosity. Calcific plaques are often present, particularly in the transverse arch.

The roentgen findings of ischemic cardiovascular disease vary considerably with the severity and duration. They consist of left ventricular cardiac enlargement, which is usually moderate in degree. Because dilatation is more prominent than hypertrophy, there is less rounding of the ventricle than in hypertensive disease. The two diseases are often combined, however. Calcification may be noted in the annulus fibrosus. The aortic knob is prominent and may contain calcium. It is often dilated. In the left oblique and lateral views, the aorta is noted to curve forward more than normal and extends farther upward, resulting in elongation of the vertical diameter of the silhouette. When decompensation occurs, generalized cardiac enlargement follows along with pulmonary congestive changes described previously (Fig. 32–44).

Coronary Artery Disease

Roentgen examination in sclerotic disease of the coronary arteries is usually not helpful because marked clinical and electrocardiographic signs of coronary insufficiency may be present without any alteration noted

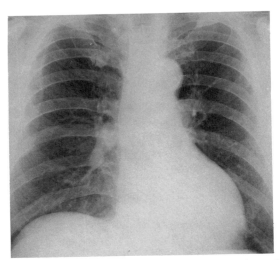

Figure 32–43. Hypertensive cardiovascular disease. There is moderate cardiac enlargement and rounding of the apex, indicating hypertrophy of the left ventricle. The transverse aortic arch is prominent, and there is a little calcification in it. The patient had a history of hypertension of long duration. The calcification indicates arteriosclerosis as well as hypertension.

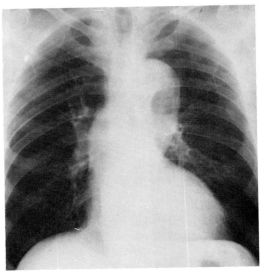

Figure 32–44. Arteriosclerotic (ischemic) cardiovascular disease. There is moderate cardiac enlargement, mainly in the left ventricle. The aorta is dilated, elongated, and tortuous.

on the roentgenogram. Occasionally there is enough calcification in the coronary arteries to be visualized on roentgenograms of good quality. Fluoroscopy or cine-angiography with an image intensifier may also permit visualization of calcified vessels. CT is the most sensitive method for detecting coronary artery calcifications. The circumflex and anterior descending branches of the left coronary artery are most often visible and appear as linear streaks of calcification, usually along the left margin of the heart below the pulmonary artery segment. Right coronary artery calcification may also be seen in oblique or lateral cineangiographies; the calcification can be seen to move horizontally with a wind-shield-wiper-like motion especially in the lateral projection. Whether this observation is of clinical use is debatable.[71] Selective coronary arteriography demonstrates stenosis and occlusion of major vessels and outlines the collateral circulation. Further discussion of the various findings of this important and widely used examination is beyond the scope of this book.

Coronary Artery Occlusion

Coronary occlusion that results in myocardial infarction may produce cardiac failure and lead to generalized cardiac enlargement. Marked cardiomegaly is usually a grave prognostic sign, particularly when it persists. Not infrequently, however, a chest roentgenogram obtained within a few hours of a coronary occlusion will not show significant enlargement but it is common to see some degree of pulmonary edema. Alveolar edema that persists indicates a poor prognosis, while persistent interstitial edema is slightly less ominous. When the infarct heals, the scar may be large enough to produce changes that can be recognized fluoroscopically. The area of scar does not contract and therefore does not pulsate normally. This lack of pulsation is local. Occasionally there is some slight paradoxical pulsation that can be recognized fluoroscopically and recorded on cine, videocine, or videotape. Later, following a myocardial infarct, there may be calcification in the myocardial scar or in the adjacent pericardium.

Ventricular Aneurysm

The most common cause of ventricular aneurysm is coronary occlusion. Rarely, trauma or inflammation may produce a cardiac aneurysm.[7] As a result of weakening of the myocardial wall at the site of infarct, a local bulge develops. It is most often noted at the left cardiac margin in the distribution of the left anterior descending coronary artery. The roentgen findings are those of localized or somewhat diffuse bulge along the left heart border that results in a bizarre silhouette (Fig. 32-45).

Fluoroscopically a paradoxical pulsation can sometimes be recognized and, occasionally, calcification is visible in the wall of the aneurysm. Many "aneurysms" in which there is no bulge or significant alteration in cardiac shape are observed on left ventriculography. There may be alteration in function because of the lack of contraction or paradoxical motion results in a decreased ejection fraction, which identifies the aneurysm in these patients. These changes may be seen with echo or isotope cardiography studies but are best evaluated with contrast left ventriculography. Occasionally, coronary artery aneurysms may develop and produce masses simulating ventricular aneurysms.

False aneurysms of the left ventricle result from local rupture of an infarcted area of the wall, thus no muscle fibers are present. Pericardium and organized clot then form the wall at the site of the pseudoaneurysm. Most of these false aneurysms extend posteriorly in contrast to the usual anterior or anterolateral presentation of true aneurysms. Often a narrow ostium connects the false aneurysm to the ventricular chamber, the sac of which is usually large. Rupture is frequent, while later rupture of true aneurysms is rare.

Left ventricular diverticulum is a congenital anomaly often associated with an anterior midline defect, such as a sternal, upper abdominal wall, anterior diaphragmatic, diaphragmatic pericardial, or intracardiac defect.[3] The lesion is important because of the danger of rupture. Some are so small that there are no roentgen findings; in others, an anterior cardiac soft-tissue bulge is present, often associated with one or more of the defects just listed. Rarely, a similar type of diverticulum may be found in the right ventricle, usually associated with another defect such as atrial septal defect, tetralogy of Fallot, or ventricular septal defect.

THE HEART AND LUNGS IN CONGESTIVE FAILURE

In cardiac failure there is nearly always dilatation of one or more cardiac chambers, resulting in cardiac enlargement. The generalized enlargement may obscure the single-chamber enlargement that had been present earlier. The transverse diameter of the heart usually increases, while the vertical diameter may actually decrease with the patient in the upright position, because the cardiac muscle may be weakened to the extent that it does not maintain the normal cardiac contour against the pull of gravity. There is one general exception to the rule that the heart in failure is considerably enlarged and that it is in acute left ventricular failure secondary to coronary thrombosis. In these patients there may be marked pulmonary congestion and edema with very little cardiac enlargement. In ischemic cardiovascular disease in which there is a consid-

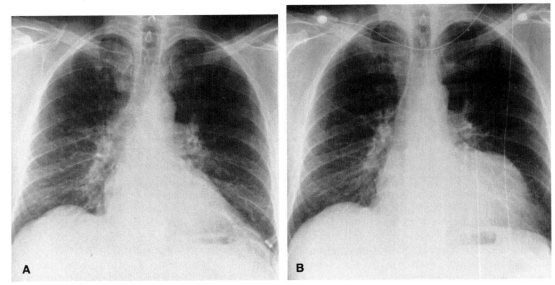

Figure 32–45.   Left ventricular aneurysm. **(A)** Frontal projection of the chest shows a slightly enlarged heart due to left ventricular dilatation. In addition, the pulmonary vascular pattern is congested and there are some Kerley B-lines present at the right base, indicating interstitial edema. A diagnosis of congestive heart failure secondary to myocardial infarction was made. **(B)** Repeat frontal film taken approximately three weeks later shows that the congestive heart failure has resolved. However, the heart has increased in size, and there is a bulge along the left ventricular border indicating a presence of a left ventricular aneurysm secondary to occlusion of the left anterior descending coronary artery.

erable amount of coronary involvement, failure may also occur with less enlargement than in other diseases.

When the left ventricle fails to expel blood at the same rate as the right side of the heart, left ventricular failure is said to occur. In this situation, left atrial pressure increases, resulting in an increase in pulmonary venous pressure and, finally, pulmonary congestion and edema result. The roentgen findings consist of dilatation of the pulmonary veins, causing accentuation of vascular markings. The vessels, both arteries and veins, in the upper zones are noted to be more prominent than at the bases. The individual vessels often appear blurred and less distinct than is normal, indicating perivascular edema. Interstitial markings throughout the lungs also become increasingly prominent as fluid accumulates there. Kerley's A and B lines may become visible. Small amounts of pleural effusion produce basal densities that obliterate the costophrenic sulci and often extend into the interlobar fissures. In acute left ventricular failure, alveolar edema is common. This produces bilateral parahilar and basal density that may be diffuse or patchy but is poorly defined in either instance. Effusion and edema may become

marked depending upon the severity of the failure (Fig. 32–46).

In right ventricular failure the blood accumulates on the venous side of the major circulation, and dependent edema as well as congestion of the abdominal viscera occurs. The lungs may be relatively clear. Right ventricular failure is normally secondary to left ventricular failure, so the findings mentioned previously may predominate.

COR PULMONALE

"Chronic cor pulmonale" is the term used to indicate the right ventricular hypertrophy that may lead to right-sided heart failure, produced by any disease or abnormality (exclusive of primary cardiac disease) that results in increased pressure in the lesser circulation. Numerous pulmonary diseases can cause cor pulmonale. These include congenital and acquired alterations in the thorax such as kyphoscoliosis and thoracoplasty; pulmonary artery disease such as chronic recurrent pulmonary emboli; and chronic pulmonary inflammatory disease, e.g., pulmonary tuberculosis,

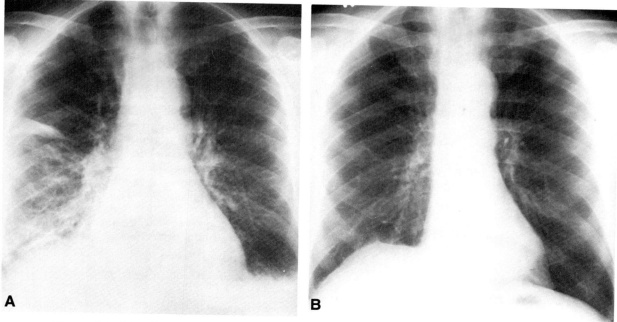

A   **B**

Figure 32–46. Congestive heart failure. (**A**) The heart is enlarged. There is some pleural effusion bilaterally, producing hazy density at the bases, obscuring the diaphragm, and blunting the costophrenic angles. There is also some fluid in the minor fissure on the right. The basal vessels are poorly defined, and on the right side there is considerable basal density, some of which is interstitial, and some appears to be alveolar, indicating edema. (**B**) Follow-up film taken 2 weeks later. There is no longer evidence of edema or pleural effusion, and the heart has decreased in size.

the pneumoconioses, and suppurative diseases such as chronic bronchiectasis. Pulmonary emphysema is the most common cause. Usually the diseases cause changes in peripheral arteries and arterioles or there is a primary disease of these vessels that leads to pulmonary hypertension. There is some controversy regarding pathogenesis in some of the conditions. In addition to the findings described in the following paragraphs, pulmonary changes caused by the underlying disease may be present.

Roentgen Findings. The heart is not necessarily enlarged and in the frontal projection is often vertical in type and appears small and round. There is prominence of the pulmonary artery segment in the left upper silhouette along with increase in the size of the hilar arteries bilaterally. The pulmonary infundibulum is enlarged along with the pulmonary artery. This is manifested by convex prominence of the pulmonary outflow tract and infundibular segment in the RAO projection. There is a discrepancy between the caliber of pulmonary arteries; the hilar arteries are enlarged

and the midzone and peripheral arteries are either normal or smaller than normal in diameter.

In some instances, there is a rapid and striking diminution in caliber of arteries in the parahilar areas. Not infrequently, the vascular changes must be used to suggest the diagnosis because the cardiac silhouette may not be typical. When right ventricular hypertrophy is marked, there may be some increased convexity of the lower right anterior cardiac silhouette noted in the LAO projection and the apex may be elevated and rounded. There is no enlargement of the left atrium or left ventricle in this condition. Pulmonary emphysema is often present and may be severe. When the ventricular enlargement becomes great there may be sufficient anterior protrusion and convexity to result in decrease in the retrosternal space anterior to the base of the heart as viewed in the lateral or extreme LAO projection. Additionally, marked enlargement of the pulmonary outflow tract may produce a longer convexity in the region of the pulmonary artery segment than is normally outlined.

In patients with severe thoracic deformities or

marked pulmonary disease, the disease causing the increase in pulmonary artery pressure may distort the heart to the point where chamber enlargement cannot be ascertained but the enlargement of the pulmonary artery is usually visible. In order to determine the diagnosis, correlation with clinical history, physical findings, and electrocardiographic findings should be made; when they are typical, the roentgen findings are reasonably reliable.

Acute cor pulmonale is found in the other conditions that cause acute hypoxia or anoxia, including massive pulmonary embolism, pulmonary edema, and tension pneumothorax. The various conditions are discussed under the pulmonary disease in question.

THE HEART IN THORACIC DEFORMITIES
Kyphoscoliosis

The heart is usually displaced to the side opposite the convexity of the dorsal spine. When the convexity is to the right, the right side of the heart border is often obscured by the shadow of the lower thoracic vertebrae. When the thoracic deformity is marked there is often rotation and torsion sufficient to interfere with cardiac function. In these patients there is so much deformity of the heart produced by the thoracic change that normal landmarks are altered and evaluation of chamber size and identification of chambers is very difficult.

Funnel Chest (Pectus Excavatum)

This deformity consists of depression of the sternum, which may be severe, and results in backward displacement of the heart to the left. On the lateral view the position of the sternum is easily recognized so that the diagnosis is made without difficulty in this projection. In the frontal view several radiographic signs are diagnostic. They consist of the following: (1) sharp downward angulation of the anterior arcs of the ribs with the degree of slant roughly proportional to the amount of depression; (2) displacement of the cardiac shadow to the left with some convexity in the left upper border so that the silhouette suggests mitral disease with enlargement and prominence of the left atrial appendage; (3) indistinct border of the right side of the heart, often obscured by the thoracic spine; (4) decreased density of the heart with more severe deformity, due to the decrease in its anteroposterior diameter; in these patients the lower thoracic spine is more readily visible than in the normal person; (5) increased density and cloudiness of the medial aspect of the right lung base, caused by some compression of the underlying lung, and accentuated by the visibility of pulmonary vessels that are often hidden by the right lower cardiac border; (6) some straightening of the normal rounded curve of the

thoracic spine or, in some instances, actual reversal of the curve; and (7) occasional backward displacement and compression of the heart between the sternum and thoracic spine resulting in actual widening with an increase in the transverse diameter to the right as well as to the left. If most of these signs are present, diagnosis of this deformity in the frontal projection is not difficult to make. The differentiation from mitral valvular disease in the frontal projection is important (Fig. 32-47). Fixation of the sternum to the central tendon of the diaphragm may result in paradoxical cardiac enlargement during inspiration in children with pectus excavatum. The diaphragm pulls the lower sternum posteriorly as it moves downward in inspiration, reducing the space between the spine and sternum and flattening the heart so that it appears wider and thus larger in the frontal projection.

DISEASES OF THE MYOCARDIUM (CARDIOMYOPATHY)

The cardiomyopathies have been divided pathophysiologically into three main groups: (1) *Congestive myopathy*. This group includes idiopathic myopathies, the majority of which occur with a known systemic disease such as infectious, postpartum, or connective tissue disease, or with a neuromuscular myopathy. (2) *Constrictive myopathy*. This includes conditions that simulate constrictive pericarditis, including infiltrative lesions of the myocardium and endocardium, e.g., endomyocardial fibrosis and endocardial fibroelastosis, either of which may also present as a congestive myopathy. (3) *Obstructive myopathy*. The clinical manifestations suggest an obstructive valve lesion. Included in this category are idiopathic, hypertrophic, and subaortic stenoses (hypertrophic obstructive cardiomyopathy), and malignant infiltration of the myocardium by tumors.[76]

The roentgen manifestations of these diseases are not specific, but there is usually cardiac enlargement that may be massive. The enlargement is generally caused by dilatation of all the chambers. The contractility of the heart is decreased, and fluoroscopy indicates marked diminution of pulsation. The transverse diameter often increases more than the longitudinal diameter. The heart appears broad, and normal contours are effaced. Although the heart may be markedly enlarged, there may be no signs of failure. In these patients, the differentiation from pericardial effusion is often difficult.

Infectious Myocarditis (Cardiomyopathy)

In infectious myocarditis, the degree of cardiac dilatation is proportional to the severity of muscle damage, and there may be rapid progression to gross generalized

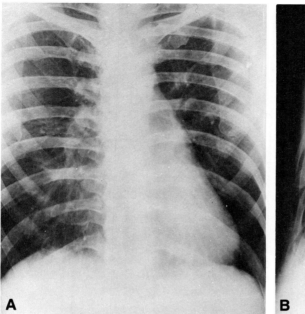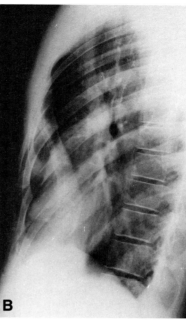

A   **B**

Figure 32–47. Funnel-chest deformity. **(A)** Most of the signs described in the text are present, including prominence of the left upper cardiac border, shift of the heart to the left, slight increase in density below the right hilum, failure to visualize the border of the right side of the heart, and accentuation of the downward angulation of the ribs. **(B)** The lateral view shows the marked posterior displacement of the lower sternum.

enlargement of the heart augmented by some pericardial effusion that is often present. The amount of effusion is often small. The roentgen findings of generalized enlargement of the cardiac silhouette are similar regardless of the infectious agent. However, in parasitic disease, such as hydatid myocarditis, calcification may occur.

Anemia

In severe anemias there may be considerable cardiac enlargement. Correction leads to regression to normal unless there has been a great deal of muscle damage. Radiographically, the enlargement tends to be general with some pulmonary artery prominence.

Postpartum Cardiomyopathy

Postpartum cardiomyopathy is rare, but when heart failure develops for the first time in the postpartum period, cardiomyopathy is a likely diagnosis.

Connective-Tissue Diseases

In systemic lupus erythematosus, polyarteritis, or scleroderma, a cardiomyopathy often associated with pericardial effusion may be present. In rheumatoid ar-

thritis, there is a greater tendency of involvement of the endocardium and the aortic and mitral valves than in any of the other three conditions.

Alcoholic Cardiomyopathy

Alcoholism may result in cardiomyopathy with severe myocardial damage and gross enlargement of the heart in some patients. In others with less severe myocardial damage, the findings are not as great and recovery may be complete, unlike the prospects for the more severe group in whom the prognosis is poor. Roentgen findings of cardiac enlargement vary with the severity of the disease. Thiamine deficiency may be a factor; it is possible that there is a combination of causes in some patients.

THE CONSTRICTIVE MYOPATHIES

The constrictive myopathies include infiltrative lesions of the endocardium and myocardium, such as endocardial fibroelastosis and myocardial fibrosis. The findings in endocardial fibroelastosis were described previously. Endomyocardial fibrosis is found most often in the tropics and may be right or left sided; in some patients, both ventricles are involved. Roentgen findings are those of cardiac enlargement with evidence of right atrial dilatation. Often, pericardial effusion is present making chamber identification difficult. The right ventricle is small, but the outflow tract and pulmonary arteries are large. When the left ventricle is involved, pulmonary venous hypertension and mitral incompetence result in an appearance simulating that of mitral valvular disease. In the biventricular form, the right-sided features tend to dominate, but there is usually evidence of enlarged upper-lobe pulmonary veins in contrast to pulmonary oligemia observed in isolated right-sided disease.

OBSTRUCTIVE CARDIOMYOPATHY

Obstructive cardiomyopathy includes hypertrophic obstructive cardiomyopathy or idiopathic hypertrophic subaortic stenosis. The muscle hypertrophy may be patchy, preventing outflow tract obstruction. Therefore, alteration in the cardiac configuration will not result. When there is outflow tract obstruction producing increased left ventricular workload, the heart may enlarge, and secondary mitral insufficiency may develop, producing a mitral configuration. There is usually no significant poststenotic dilatation of the aorta. Unless the mitral valve is involved, the only finding is that of left ventricular enlargement. Therefore, the diagnosis is usually made by left ventriculography.

The Heart in Beriberi

Vitamin B1 (thiamine) deficiency resulting in beriberi is uncommon in the United States, but is occasionally encountered. The roentgen findings are those of cardiac dilatation that may be diffuse and symmetric, producing generalized enlargement of the cardiac silhouette. The right ventricle is occasionally damaged more than the rest of the myocardium. This results in dilatation of the pulmonary artery and of the right ventricle and atrium. Pericardial effusion may be present and contribute to the enlargement of the cardiac shadow. Successful treatment results in prompt regression of the enlargement and reabsorption of pericardial fluid.

The Heart in Diseases of the Thyroid

Hypothyroidism. Hypofunction of the thyroid gland resulting in myxedema causes general dilatation of the cardiovascular silhouette. Pericardial effusion is common in myxedema and may contribute to part, if not all, of the increase in cardiac size. Some patients with "myxedema heart" have been shown to have massive pericardial effusions that have contributed to most of the enlargement. In treated patients with myxedema,

the heart returns to normal quickly, but, in chronic myxedema heart disease, return to normal may require many months of treatment.

Hyperthyroidism. The heart of a patient with hyperthyroidism is hyperactive and the pulse pressure is usually high. The cardiac configuration is not characteristic, but cardiac enlargement is frequently present. The enlargement may be left ventricular with rounding and elongation of the left ventricular border, but often the right ventricle is mainly affected and the pulmonary artery and right ventricular outflow tract are enlarged. Some investigators believe that right ventricular enlargement is more characteristic of this disease than is left ventricular enlargement. It is generally agreed that there is cardiac enlargement in severe hyperthyroidism and that the size of the heart decreases when the disease is controlled, but may not return to normal because of extensive myocardial damage.

CARDIAC INJURIES

Blunt cardiac injury may be suggested when chest films reveal fracture of the sternum or evidence of soft-tissue injury in the precordial area. Contusion of the myocardium often occurs with no external evidence of chest injury, and may simulate myocardial infarction, including the formation of posttraumatic ventricular aneurysm. Trauma may cause rupture of the papillary muscles or chordae tendinea, which may result in acute mitral insufficiency manifested by acute pulmonary edema with a normal-size heart.

Penetrating injuries may cause death before the patient can be treated, but occasionally a wound may cause hemopericardium without enough tamponade to cause immediate death. The roentgen signs are similar to those of pericardial effusion described in the section on diseases of the pericardium. In addition, the injury that produces the hemopericardium may cause hemothorax or pneumothorax. Occasionally, metallic foreign bodies such as bullets can penetrate the heart wall and even enter one of the cardiac chambers without causing death. They are readily visualized and may be localized by fluoroscopy. The motion of the opaque foreign body can be used as an aid in identifying its position. When the projectile is within a cardiac chamber, a considerable amount of movement is usually visualized in a somewhat irregularly circular or pendulous type of motion, while a projectile imbedded in the myocardium moves in a more uniform manner. Study of the heart shortly before surgery is important when foreign bodies are found within the heart or in its wall; since the foreign body may move out through the aorta into the systemic circulation when on the left side or into the lesser circulation when on the right. Occasionally, small, opaque, foreign bodies such as lead shot have been observed to move through the venous system to the heart.

TUMORS OF THE HEART

Benign or malignant primary cardiac tumors are rare. The more common tumors are fibroma, myxoma, rhabdomyoma, and rhabdosarcoma along with primary tumors of vascular origin. The most common benign tumor is the myxoma. It is found in the left atrium in about 75% of cases, and usually arises from the septum near the foramen ovale. Most of the remainder arises in the right atrium. Ventricular myxoma is rare. The tumor is usually pedunculated and may cause intermittent obstruction of an adjacent valve. Roentgen findings in myxoma may then resemble those of mitral or tricuspid stenosis, depending upon the site of origin. Left atrial myxoma can be suspected when there is roentgen evidence of mitral stenosis with no previous history of rheumatic fever, an inconstant and changing murmur, and embolic phenomena occurring without atrial fibrillation (Fig. 32–48). Right atrial myxoma results in roentgen findings, suggesting tricuspid stenosis or Ebstein's anomaly. Again, the murmur is inconstant, and embolic (pulmonary) phenomena occur. About 10% of atrial myxomas calcify enough to be visible at fluoroscopy. Right atrial myxoma does not interfere with valvular function as often as myxoma of the left atrium. Therefore, the right atrial tumor tends to be larger than the left before causing symptoms. Echocardiography and angiocardiography are useful in delineating intracardiac tumors. The other benign tumors tend to be intramural and include fibroma, hamartoma, rhabdomyoma, and lipoma. Most involve the left ventricular wall. They tend to produce cardiac enlargement, to calcify (20%), and are most frequent in children.

Rarely, intraventricular thrombi may calcify and resemble intracardiac tumors. Symptoms depend on the size and mobility of the hematoma. Its location, usually in the right ventricle, can be observed readily at fluoroscopy. Echocardiography is very useful in the study of intracardiac tumors.

Malignant tumors such as rhabdomyosarcoma or fibrosarcoma are rare and usually arise in the ventricular walls, while angiosarcoma apparently occurs most commonly in the right atrial wall. Echo and angiocardiography may be required to make the diagnosis. Masses projecting from the outer cardiac surface may produce bizarre cardiac shapes; the diagnosis, however, may be suspected on roentgen examination. CT is of great value for the demonstration of the site and extent of a bizarre mass, which appears to be intimately associated with the heart.

Metastatic myocardial tumors are much more common than the primary tumors. Cardiac involvement by lymphoma and various carcinomas often results in pericardial effusion. The roentgen findings, therefore, may be caused by hemopericardium. An irregular cardiac mass occurring alone (or associated with hemopericardium) in a patient with known Hodgkin's disease, lymphoma, or carcinoma virtually indicates myocardial metastasis.

Pericardial tumors, like those of the heart muscle, are rare. Of the primary tumors, the benign and malignant forms occur equally, but metastatic pericardial tumors are much more common than the primary ones. Fibroma, fibrosarcoma, benign and malignant mesothelioma, vascular tumors such as hemangioma and lymphangioma, teratoma, thymoma, leiomyoma, hamartoma, and intrapericardial bronchial cyst may arise in the pericardium. All are rare and cannot be differentiated radiographically. They may cause pericardial or pleural effusion. The major radiographic feature of the tumor itself is alteration of the cardiac contour, which varies with the size and shape of the mass.

ACQUIRED DISEASES OF THE AORTA

Arteriosclerosis of the Aorta

A certain amount of alteration in the appearance of the aorta with advancing age is secondary to loss of elasticity. The change consists of elongation and dilatation; it eventually occurs in all persons who live long enough. As a result of these anatomic changes, the configuration of the aortic arch changes roentgenographically. The ascending arch becomes more enlarged and thus results in more convexity of the right upper cardiac margin. The aortic knob on the left side becomes more prominent and somewhat enlarged. The descending aorta curves to the left in the posteroanterior view and back to midline or even to the right side before passing through the diaphragm. In the left oblique view and in the lateral projection, the arch of the aorta swings in a wider arc so that it often angles forward and upward, and finally, backward. The result is widening of the area between the limbs of the arch. The descending aorta may curve far backward to overlie the thoracic spine in the lateral view.

In arteriosclerotic disease of the aorta, the manifestations of elongation and dilatation occur earlier in life and plaques of calcium are often visualized in the transverse aortic arch. The amount of calcification varies considerably. The plaques are noted as dense linear shadows and are most commonly seen in the aortic knob but may be extensive throughout the aorta distal to the transverse arch, so that the entire wall of this structure may be outlined by calcium in extreme instances (Fig. 32-49). Aortic arteriosclerotic disease may not be significant unless complicated by dissection

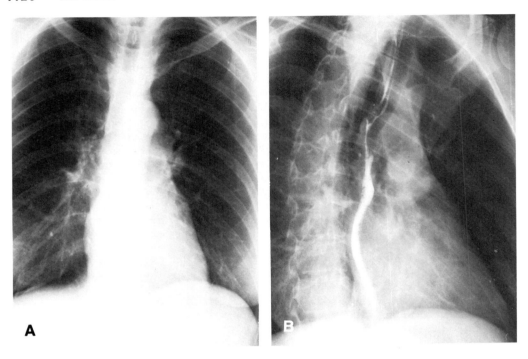

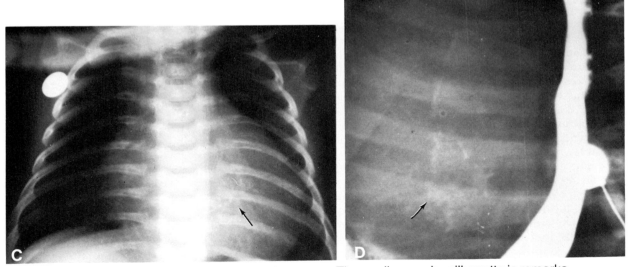

Figure 32–48. (**A** and **B**) Left atrial myxoma. The cardiovascular silhouette is remarkably similar to that of mitral stenosis, including slight constriction of basal vessels in the lungs. Note the definite posterior displacement of the esophagus by the enlarged atrium in the right anterior oblique view (**B**). (**C** and **D**) Calcified left ventricular tumor in a 7-week-old infant. In the frontal projection (**C**), the arrow points to the site of the tumor. Spot film with barium in the esophagus (**D**) shows mottled calcification in the intraventricular tumor (*arrow*).

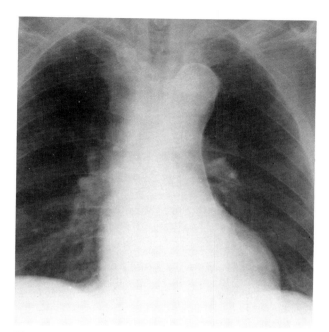

Figure 32–49. Arteriosclerotic disease of the aorta. Note the extensive calcification in the thoracic aorta. The aorta is slightly dilated, elongated, and tortuous. The patient also had extensive generalized arteriosclerosis.

or aneurysm, but it is often associated with arteriosclerotic disease elsewhere, e.g., in the carotid, renal, and coronary arteries, which may cause morbidity and mortality. Atheromatous fibrous plaques consist principally of an accumulation of intimal, smooth muscle cells loaded with lipid, chiefly cholesterol. The cells are also surrounded by lipid and by collagen elastic fibers. These cells are extracellular material which cover a large, deeper deposit of free extracellular lipid intermixed with cell debris. The plaque may become altered as a result of hemorrhage, calcification, cell necrosis, and/or mural thrombosis. The most distinct characteristic of this complicated lesion is the presence of calcification. This is the type of lesion that often is associated with occlusive disease. The latter usually occurs at a site of bifurcation or arterial fixation. Arteriography is used to outline these lesions. This technique and findings are discussed elsewhere.

Takayasu's Arteritis

Takayasu's arteritis was initially called "pulseless disease." It involves the aorta and its branches as well as the pulmonary arteries in an extensive manner.[6] Peripheral arteries are not usually involved. Most of the patients are under 30 years of age. The female to male

ratio is about 8:1. Although its etiology is not definitely known, it probably represents an autoimmune disease in which granulation tissue destroys the media of the large vessels and inflammatory cells are also present. As the inflammatory reaction subsides, scar tissue in the arterial walls causes marked thickening, resulting in luminal narrowing and occlusion. Plain films show widening of the aorta with irregularity of aortic contour and aortic calcifications that are linear, and may involve short or long segments of the aortic arch or the descending or the abdominal aorta. Aortic insufficiency that results from dilatation of the aortic root is present in 10% to 20% of the patients. The aortic valve is normal. Rarely, aortic dissection may occur in this disease. When the pulmonary arteries are involved, the roentgen findings may be those of pulmonary hypertension with prominence of the central pulmonary arteries. Partial occlusions of the branches may result in hypovascularity in the involved areas, which may be difficult to define roentgenographically. The possibility should be considered, however, in young women with a dilated, irregular aorta containing calcium. Arteriography is useful in demonstrating the type and extent of involvement.

SYPHILITIC AORTITIS

Luetic aortitis produces alterations that can often be recognized radiographically before clinical signs of specific aortic involvement are present. Circumscribed dilatation of the ascending aortic arch may occur and be recognized as enlargement of this portion of the aorta before the signs of aneurysm appear, but, because similar dilatation may occur in arteriosclerosis and in aortic stenosis (poststenotic dilatation), this finding cannot be considered as pathognomonic. The dilatation in arteriosclerotic disease is usually more diffuse than in luetic aortitis. Calcification in the wall of the ascending aortic arch is a more reliable sign of luetic aortitis. It is manifested by a thin, curvilinear shadow of calcific density in the outer wall of the ascending aorta, which may be visible in the frontal projection but is often more readily visualized in the LAO and lateral projections. This is in contrast to the calcification in arteriosclerotic disease that is most marked in the transverse aortic arch. Calcification may occur in the ascending aortic arch in arteriosclerosis, but this is usually found in elderly patients in whom the disease is severe. Furthermore, the plaques are thicker and more irregular than the somewhat thin linear shadows noted in syphilis. On pathologic examination of the aorta in arteriosclerosis, calcification is often found in the ascending aorta but is most prominent in the inner wall of the arch and may not be roentgenographically visible. Late syphilis is now so rare that it can be assumed that most patients with calcification in the ascending aorta have advanced arteriosclerotic disease. Aneurysms of the ascending aorta are frequently found in association with vascular syphilis.

AORTIC ANEURYSM

An aneurysm is a circumscribed axial or lateral area of localized widening in the wall of a blood vessel. Some dilatation of the aorta occurs in arteriosclerosis, and there is no sharply defined differentiation between simple dilatation and an aneurysm. The latter term is generally reserved to designate a clearly defined local area of cylindrical or saccular enlargement. Aneurysms involving the ascending aortic arch in the past were often of syphilitic origin, particularly when saccular in type, but connective-tissue disorders with medial necrosis such as in Marfan's syndrome may also be associated with aneurysm. Aneurysms of the descending aorta may be arteriosclerotic in origin; less frequently their origin is mycotic, traumatic, or congenital. Roentgen studies frequently are sufficient to make the diagnosis.

Local aneurysms of the descending thoracic aorta often produce no symptoms and are detected as incidental findings on chest roentgenograms. They usually project from the posterolateral aspect of the mid- or lower-descending thoracic aorta and appear as left-sided masses. They are usually of arteriosclerotic origin, although chronic traumatic and mycotic aneurysms are not rare.

Roentgen Findings. An aneurysm results in a mass shadow continuous with the aortic silhouette that varies considerably in size and shape among patients. It is not unusual to note widening of the superior mediastinum above the arch on the right when the aneurysm involves the ascending aorta and extends into the innominate artery. The mass of the aneurysm in the ascending aortic arch usually projects to the right while that of the descending arch projects to the left in the frontal plane (Fig. 32–50).

Occasionally the communication between the aorta and the aneurysm is very narrow (pedunculated aneurysm). The aneurysm may project in a direction not usually observed with the more common saccular lesions. The relationships can be studied in the lateral and in the oblique projections. Barium in the esophagus is used to show the relationship of the aortic mass to the esophagus in fluoroscopic and roentgen examinations. Generally, the lesion is defined most clearly in the LAO projection. Usually these studies are omitted and a CT examination provides the essential information. Occasionally, there may be more than one saccular aneurysm with an area of fusiform dilatation

between them. It is often possible to make the diagnosis of aneurysm on roentgenographic evidence alone. When the differentiation between aortic aneurysm and mediastinal mass due to other causes cannot be made roentgenographically, CT with a contrast bolus is valuable in demonstrating the nature of the mass, as well as the relationship of the mass to the heart and aorta. Aortography is the most definitive method of assessing the nature and relationship of the aorta and juxta-aorta masses. It is usually reserved for detailed study before surgery. Arteriosclerotic aneurysms usually occur in the abdominal aorta but may occur in the arch and descending portion of the thoracic aorta. They are generally smaller than those of luetic origin and often show calcification. Rarely, there may be erosion of bone secondary to aortic aneurysm. When the ascending arch is involved, the erosion occurs along the posterior aspect of the sternum; erosion through this bone was described previously. Aneurysms of the distal arch may erode one or more of the dorsal vertebral bodies. This bone erosion is more commonly seen in syphilitic aneurysms, although it is currently rare. The vertebrae involved have a scalloped appearance because the discs resist the erosion. The vertebral bodies are then concave anteriorly. Aortography clarifies the nature and extent of any aneurysm.

TRAUMATIC ANEURYSM

Rupture of all layers of the aorta caused by trauma usually leads to exsanguination and sudden death. When the adventitia is spared and rupture is incomplete, the patient may survive. Survival in others is evidently dependent upon mediastinal hematoma, which may temporarily prevent exsanguination. Temporary tamponade is afforded by the mediastinal tissues. Organization of the clot will result in formation of a false aneurysm. The disruption is often circumferential and the ruptured layers may retract. The usual site of this rupture is in the aortic arch, immediately distal to the left subclavian artery at the site of the ligamentum arteriosum. The roentgen findings in the acute phase consist of evidence of hematoma in the vicinity of the aortic arch. The hematoma may obscure the aortic outline in the region as well as widen the mediastinum. This is an important finding. Slight deviation of the trachea to the right also appears to be a significant finding.[23] This may be present in the absence of mediastinal widening. The esophagus may be displaced similarly by the mediastinal hematoma. This is evident because of displacement of a nasogastric tube. Extrapleural hemorrhage may cause an apparent apical pleural thickening or mass, another significant plain-film finding. Hemorrhage into the pleural space and lung is common and there may be evidence of rib or sternal

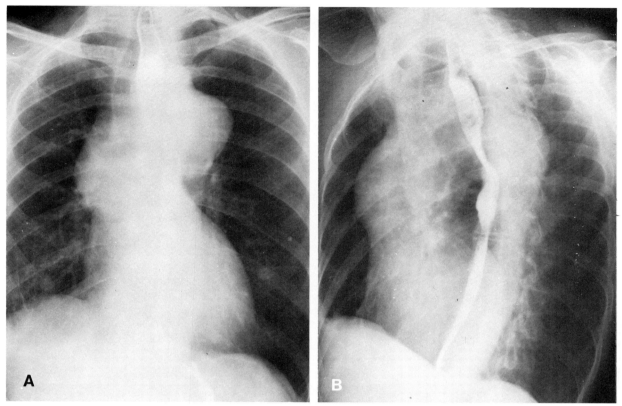

Figure 32–50. Aortic aneurysms. Note the fusiform dilatations of the ascending and transverse portions of the aortic arch in both frontal (**A**) and left anterior oblique (**B**) projections.

fracture. Pneumomediastinum and pneumothorax may occur but are not of particular diagnostic significance. When these signs are present in a patient who has suffered severe thoracic trauma, traumatic aortic fracture should be suspected. In our experience, there is an increased likelihood of aortic fractures when the pelvis, femurs, or mandible are fractured. Frequently, multiple fractures may be present, but these only attest to the severity of the injury.

A chest film should be obtained to detect aortic injury in all patients having severe deceleration accidents. Because the traumatic aneurysms are unstable and may rupture, prompt diagnostic and surgical measures are necessary. If multiple arterial injuries involving major arch branches are present, the innominate, carotid, and subclavian arteries should be examined at the same time. Percutaneous transfemoral arteriography is usually used to confirm the diagnosis (Fig. 32–51). However, if CT is used to assess other injuries, one should evaluate the aorta concurrently.

When a patient survives with an undetected traumatic aneurysm of the aorta or one of its major brachycephalic branches, the diffuse mediastinal density eventually clears, leaving fairly defined mass that represents the false aneurysm. Calcification develops in the wall in most of the lesions as they become chronic. Expansile pulsation is not necessarily present because of the organized thrombus in the wall. The diagnosis can usually be made on the basis of the roentgen findings in a patient who has a history of previous thoracic trauma. Aortography is then used to confirm the diagnosis and localize the site of origin (Fig. 32–52). When discovered, these aneurysms should be repaired.[22]

DISSECTING ANEURYSM

Dissecting Hematoma (Aneurysm)

A dissecting hematoma results from accumulation of blood in the aortic media. This accumulation may be the result of a primary bleed from the vasavasorum or through a tear in the intima. The overwhelming num-

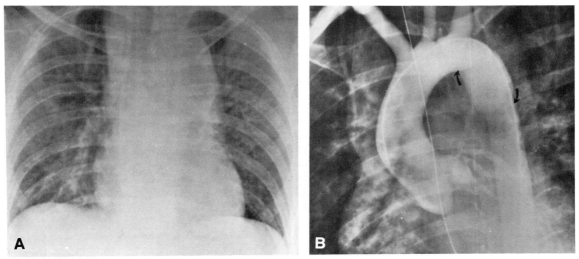

Figure 32–51. (**A**) An AP recumbent chest film shows widening of the mediastinum, displacement of the trachea to the right side, and an apical pleural cap. These findings suggest the presence of an extrapleural hematoma that has its epicenter to the left of the trachea. (**B**) Retrograde transfemoral aortogram shows a traumatic aneurysm (*curved arrows*). The appearance is typical of that of a traumatic aneurysm secondary to a deceleration injury.

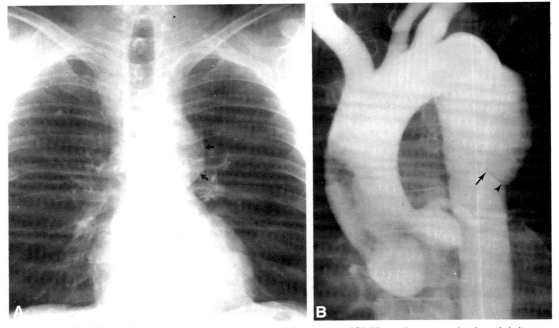

Figure 32–52. Chronic traumatic fracture of the aorta. (**A**) Note the mass in the vicinity of the transverse and upper-descending aorta (*arrows*). Note the thin curvilinear calcification in the wall of the mass (**B**). Aortogram shows the false aneurysm. A thin infolding of the aortic wall is also observed (*arrows*).

ber of dissecting hematomas occur in the face of an abnormal media, apparent in atherosclerosis or medial cystic necrosis. The exact cause of the medial bleed or the intimal disruption is not clear in most patients; however, there is a very high association with hypertension. A dissection produces a false channel, which may be so narrow that there is virtually no dilatation. In this instance, the term "aneurysm" is a misnomer.

The DeBakey classification is widely accepted because it is useful in the angiographic diagnosis and management of the dissecting hematomas as well as in providing some prognostic information. In this classification, dissecting hematomas are divided into three types. Type I: The dissection begins in the ascending aorta and extends through and beyond the aortic arch, often through the common iliac arteries. Type II: Dissection is limited to the ascending aorta. This is most commonly observed in Marfan's syndrome. Type III: Dissection begins in the thoracic or distal subclavian artery and extends distally, usually into the abdominal or pelvic vessels. Another simpler classification has been advocated. Type A includes those dissections in which the ascending aorta is involved; Type B includes dissections in which the ascending aorta is not involved. This classification has the advantage of reflecting the prognosis, which is much worse when the ascending aorta is the site of the section. Therapy differs, also. It is usually surgical if the ascending aorta is dissected.

Common sites of intimal defects are in or adjacent to a sinus of Valsalva and in the descending aorta near the ligamentum arteriosum. Dissections may also start at the site of an atheromatous plaque, and, in these instances, the abdominal aorta is the most common site.

The condition ends fatally in a few hours or days in a majority of patients. This is particularly true if the patient's hypertension cannot be controlled or aortic insufficiency results from involvement of the aortic valve ring. In about 10% of patients, there is reentry into the lumen, frequently in the abdominal aorta near its bifurcation. This permits the dissection to decompress and, in these instances, the patient may live for months or years. The weakened aorta may dilate eventually, and true aneurysm formation will occur.

The roentgen diagnosis is often difficult, and the findings must be correlated with the clinical history, which generally includes that of severe pain, frequently intrascapular, along with pallor and hemodynamic instability and shock. There may be widening of the aorta extending from the site of the dissection distally and occasionally proximally. This can be more readily apparent when a chest roentgenogram obtained before dissection is available for comparison.

Roentgenograms obtained on successive days may show extension of the area of widening. When this is observed in a patient with a typical clinical history and findings, the diagnosis of dissecting aneurysm is almost certain. When the false channel is very thin, there may be little, if any, increase in the apparent width of the aorta. When the false channel is wide, there may be some displacement of the trachea to the right, and displacement of the esophagus by the dissection may be visible on an esophagram or by displacement of a nasogastric tube. In the patients with extensive arteriosclerosis in whom calcification in atheromatous plaques is visible, it is sometimes possible to identify the inner wall of the aorta by means of this calcification. One can then judge the increased wall thickness caused by the dissecting hematoma because the outer wall is readily visible against the radiolucency of the lung. This is not an absolute sign, however, because circumferential neoplasm and periaortic fat may cause an apparent thickening of the wall.

Pleural effusion, usually left sided, is a common additional finding. Occasionally, recognizable enlargement of the branches of the aorta can be demonstrated, because dissection often extends into the walls of these vessels. When this enlargement is present, it is of considerable diagnostic significance. Because patients are often critically ill, roentgen examination is difficult. The use of this method of study is usually limited. In patients in whom the diagnosis is suspected early in the course of the disease, surgical measures may be warranted. In these instances, CT with a contrast bolus may be used to confirm the diagnosis. Angiography is essential to determine the extent of the dissection (false channel), the amount of deformity or narrowing of the true channel, and involvement of aortic branches if surgery is contemplated.

DISEASES OF THE PERICARDIUM

Pericardial Effusion

The pericardium is a thin membrane that is not ordinarily recognized as a separate structure because it is of the same density as the adjacent heart. It is relatively inelastic. Conditions that produce rapid accumulation of fluid within the pericardium may compress the heart enough to produce severe alteration of cardiac function, which may lead to death. This occurs most commonly as the result of hemorrhage secondary to trauma. Roentgenograms are not usually obtained because of the acuteness of the situation.

In chronic or subacute pericardial effusion, roentgen changes are produced when the amount of fluid reaches 400 or 500 mL. Smaller effusions up to 300 mL are not ordinarily diagnosed because they produce no significant alteration in the contour of the cardiovascular silhouette. This slow accumulation of fluid may reach massive proportions without producing tamponade.

Roentgen Findings. An increase in size of the cardiac silhouette depends upon the amount of fluid present. The shape of the cardiovascular silhouette is also altered. With moderate amounts of fluid, the enlargement is generalized and the cardiohepatic angle appears more acute than is normal. As the amount of fluid increases, there tends to be disproportionate enlargement of the heart inferiorly in the transverse diameter as compared with the increase in the vertical diameter. Demonstration of rapid progression, or regression, of these findings is a valuable sign in roentgen diagnosis (Fig. 32–53). At fluoroscopy, the pulsations are dampened or obliterated and there is some alteration in contour of the heart noted between the upright and the recumbent positions. This finding is often equivocal, however. Large effusions also tend to obliterate the normal segments noted on either side, and the cardiac enlargement extends to the right as well as to the left. Dilatation of the heart in myocardial failure can produce a silhouette that simulates that of pericardial effusion. Furthermore, in these patients the amplitude of pulsation is also small because of the myocardial weakness making differentiation very difficult. Mellins, Kottmeier, and Kiely found that fluid accumulated in dogs anteriorly, laterally, and superiorly, but not posteriorly in the pericardial space.[55] As a result, pericardial fluid dampened the cardiac pulsations anteriorly but not posteriorly. This sign was noted on a few patients and may be of value. Fluoroscopy in the lateral projection may show dampened or absent anterior pulsations and normal pulsations manifested by motion of the barium-filled esophagus posteriorly.

A layer of epicardial fat beneath the visceral pericardium may be identified on image intensification fluoroscopy and may allow one to demonstrate the epicardium, ie, the outer border of the heart. If this layer is separated from the pericardium, some material must be interposed between the epicardium and the visceral pericardium. In most circumstances, this represents fluid. In our experience, this fat is best demonstrated over the lower two thirds of the left cardiac margin in the frontal and lateral projections (Fig. 32–54). Because the heart in ordinary circumstances is closely apposed to the sternum, separation of the epicardial fat from the sternal border has the same significance as the separation of the epicardial fat from the lateral border of the cardiovascular silhouette. The use of supine cross-table lateral chest x-ray to demonstrate the separation of epicardial fat has been advocated (Fig. 32–55). If it can be demonstrated, this finding is of definite value; if it cannot be demonstrated, it is of no assistance. Therefore, in very young patients or pa-

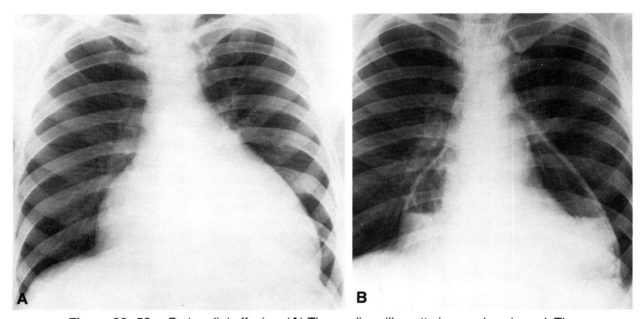

Figure 32–53.   Pericardial effusion. (**A**) The cardiac silhouette is grossly enlarged. The lungs are quite clear, and there is no evidence of pleural effusion. Two months earlier, the heart size had been normal. (**B**) This film was exposed following pericardial tap. Some fluid was removed, and air was injected to determine the thickness of the pericardial wall because there were leukocytes in the fluid. Note that the wall is several millimeters thick.

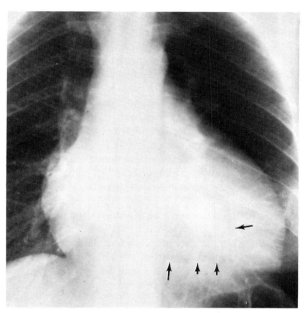

Figure 32–54. Large pericardial effusion. The epicardial fat line was easily observed on cineradiography and at fluoroscopy. It was faintly observed on this roentgenogram (*arrows*). It lies well within the silhouette and is indicative of the presence of a large pericardial effusion.

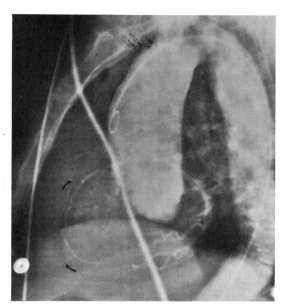

Figure 32–55. Hemopericardium. Thoracic aortogram outlines the dilated ascending aorta, with an anterior irregularity just above the aortic valve, indicating the presence of a leak. The arrows point to the epicardial fat, in which the coronary arteries can be seen. The epicardial fat is separated from the sternum, indicating the presence of a large amount of fluid—in this instance, blood.

tients with cachexia who will not have a sufficient amount of pericardial fat, one would not anticipate this examination to be useful.

The most sensitive method of demonstrating pericardial effusion is echocardiography. The cost of echocardiography is generally five times that of a fluoroscopic examination of the heart. Therefore, in patients suspected of having large effusions, the use of fluoroscopic examination can be cost effective. CT is also very sensitive to the presence of pericardial fluid.

Recently, milk of calcium pericardial fluid secondary to previous mediastinal irradiation was reported. The calcium was readily seen on plain films, fluoroscopy, and CT. Its liquid nature was recognizable by the distortion of the fluid by the beating heart.[70]

ADHESIVE AND CONSTRICTIVE PERICARDITIS

Adhesive pericarditis without constriction is usually of little clinical significance. Adhesions between the pleura and pericardium may result in some irregularity of the cardiac silhouette in the neighborhood of the adhesions. The cause of constrictive pericarditis is often obscure, although a number of possibilities exist, including infection and trauma. Whatever the cause,

the amount of pericardial fibrous-tissue reaction may reach the point at which constriction occurs. The visceral and parietal pericardium are adherent and also contracted. The basic abnormality is the inability of the ventricles to fill normally, resulting in diminution of stroke volume. Venous pressure is elevated. When this occurs, there may be severe clinical symptoms but the radiographic changes are minimal. The heart is often normal or small, and engorgement of the great veins may be evident. At fluoroscopy, diminished pulsations may be apparent. Calcific plaques often occur in the thickened pericardium and may be visible on plain film, especially in lateral projection. These are more readily seen with fluoroscopy, although CT best evaluates the presence and extent. At times the heart is nearly encased in a calcific shell. Occasionally, actual ossification occurs. When calcification is present, in a patient with clinical signs of constrictive pericarditis, the diagnosis is not difficult. When no calcification is present, roentgen findings are often equivocal. Calcification on plain films is present in about 50% of patients with constrictive pericarditis, but the number is much higher when CT is employed. The presence of pericardial calcification, however, does not necessarily indicate significant constriction. The classic finding is that of a quiet heart with clinical signs of failure, although the heart may be enlarged. Hepatic enlargement and ascites may be evident on abdominal examination. The symptoms of severe cardiac amyloidosis with noncompliant myocardium are similar to those of constrictive pericarditis, but there is usually more cardiac enlargement in amyloidosis than in constrictive pericarditis.

PERICARDIAL TUMORS

The most common mass lesion of the pericardium is the pericardial or clear-water cyst that has been described in Chapter 31 under "Pericardial Cyst." Primary pericardial tumors are rare and produce localized enlargements of various sizes and shapes that cannot be differentiated from cardiac tumors unless pneumopericardium or CT are used. Occasionally, sarcoma or mesothelioma arising in the pericardium can surround and enlarge the cardiac shadow. The pericardium is much more frequently involved by metastatic tumor, and the presence of pericardial and pleural effusion may obscure the actual lesion. Hodgkin's disease often involves the pericardium and malignant melanoma, occasionally metastasizing to the heart and pericardium. CT scanning and ultrasonography are widely used to evaluate patients with pericardial masses. The presence of masses elsewhere in the thorax suggests the diagnosis of metastatic disease. In the presence of a solitary pericardial or cardiac mass, thoracotomy or percutaneous transthoracic biopsy may be necessary for definitive diagnosis.

"SPONTANEOUS" PNEUMOPERICARDIUM

This is a rare condition for which there are a number of causes. Left subphrenic abscess may penetrate the pericardial portion of the diaphragm, with resultant purulent infection pus and, often, gas within the pericardial sac. Direct extension of esophageal carcinoma may produce a similar situation. Occasionally, congenital diaphragmatic hernia may occur through a defect in the pericardial portion of the diaphragm. In this situation, gas-filled loops of bowel may be noted within the pericardial sac. Similarly, gas-filled loops of intestine may also be visible within the pericardium following traumatic herniations.

CONGENITAL PERICARDIAL DEFECTS

The majority of congenital pericardial defects are on the left side. They vary from small defects overlying the pulmonary artery to absence of the entire left pericardium on the left, or, more rarely, absence of the entire pericardium. The parietal pleura is also involved, preventing a barrier between the heart and the lung. The defects occur predominantly in males with the ratio of 3:1. Left-sided defects are more common. Associated anomalies include patent ductus arteriosus, atrial septal defect, bicuspid aortic valve, pulmonary sequestration, bronchogenic cyst, diaphragmatic hernia, and tetralogy of Fallot. One or more of these are found in about 30% of patients with partial defects. The roentgen findings in complete absence of the left pericardium are characteristic enough to make the diagnosis or strongly suggest it. The heart is shifted to the left. The left border of the heart is flattened as the heart extends to the left over the dome of the diaphragm. The pulmonary artery segment is long and more sharply defined than usual and there is a radiolucent portion of lung between the aorta and pulmonary artery that provides the contrast necessary for the clear definition. The left ventricular segment is also distinct and clearly defined (Fig. 32-56). In the lateral view the pulmonary artery may be more distinct than usual. CT scanning is diagnostic. Partial defects may permit her-

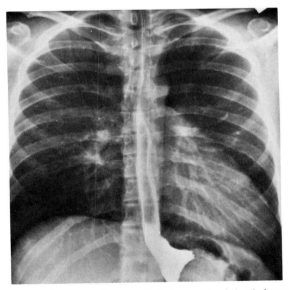

Figure 32–56.   Congenital absence of the left pericardium. This patient was asymptomatic but had a murmur detected on physical examination. The heart is shifted to the left, and the left border is flattened. The pulmonary artery segment is long and more sharply delineated than usual, and the lung extends between the aorta and pulmonary artery. Although this appearance is characteristic, confirmation, if desired, is best obtained with a CT scan.

niation of the left auricular appendage to produce a bizarre appearance of the left upper cardiac silhouette. Right-sided defects permit unusually clear visualization of the great vessels including the aortic root; lung tissue may herniate medial the superior vena cava to clearly outline this vessel. Protrusions of the heart, usually the atria, through surgical defects in the pericardium are not uncommon. This possibility must be considered when an unusual bulge or protrusion is noted in the postoperative period. Acute cardiac herniation with incarceration that causes obstruction of the superior vena cava may occur following surgery or major chest injury. Roentgen findings are usually diagnostic.

CARDIAC PACEMAKERS

Use of permanent cardiac pacemakers has increased in recent years.[73] Walter has described the roentgenographic appearance and characteristics of pacemakers used commonly.[86] The power source and generator are assembled together and are buried in the subcutaneous tissues of the chest wall; a soft-tissue tunnel is created to provide for their passage to the external surface of the myocardium or, more commonly, to the venous system for entry of transvenous pacemakers. Epicardial electrodes are sutured in place while the transvenous electrodes are placed at the apex of the right ventricle. Because the power source, the leads, and the electrodes are observed well radiographically, their position can be determined, and, in case of malfunction, follow-up studies may be useful. When the leads are not long enough, the electrodes may be displaced from the right ventricular apex into the high right ventricle or right ventricular outflow tract, or even into the right atrium or inferior vena cava. Initial malpositioning can also be detected.

Occasionally, the right ventricle is perforated by the electrodes projecting anteriorly to the cardiac wall. Fracture of the leads may be detected, usually at the fixation point in the myocardium when epicardial leads are employed, and at points of flexion over the margins of the clavicle or ribs when the transvenous type of leads are used (Fig. 32-57). Some fractures are subtle and can be demonstrated only with oblique views or with the patient in multiple positions during inspiration and expiration. Fluoroscopy is useful for these evaluations. The pacemaker generator may rotate and thereby pull the electrodes out of position. Misplacement in the coronary sinus occurs occasionally, and, in this case, the electrodes lie posteriorly instead of in their normal anterior position in the right ventricular apex. Battery failure can sometimes be detected by the presence of free mercury, which is radiopaque, in the radiolucent electrolyte areas that become indistinct and somewhat opaque.

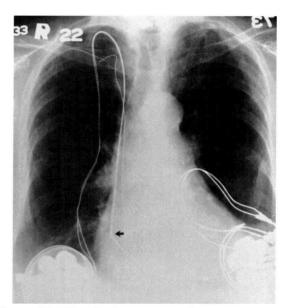

Figure 32–57. Broken pacemaker wire. Abrupt angulation of the pacemaker wire in the right atrium (*arrow*) indicates that the wire has been fractured.

CHANGES SEEN AS THE RESULT OF PREVIOUS CARDIOVASCULAR SURGERY

Changes seen on films of patients who have had previous cardiovascular surgery allow one to infer a great deal of information. Alterations in the bony thorax with the presence of radioopaque devices provide clues as to what has previously transpired. Most surgery on the descending aorta is performed through a left thoracotomy. Residuals of previous thoracotomy include resection or irregularity of the ribs where the rib retraction devices were placed. Alterations of the pleura such as thickening and blunting of the costal phrenic sulci are common. The presence of rib notching in a patient with changes secondary to a left thoracotomy suggest the diagnosis of a previous coarctation repair. The older a patient with a coarctation the more likely that rib notching will be present. Conversely, the younger the patient is at the time of repair the more likely that the rib notching will involute or even resolve completely.

Cardiac operations and surgery on the ascending aorta are usually performed through a median sternotomy. Continuity of the sternum is re-established with metal sutures that are easily recognizable (see Fig. 32-41C).

Many of the devices used for cardiovascular repair have radioopaque elements, and their configuration

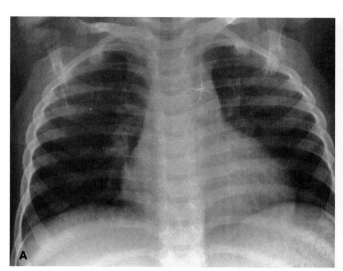
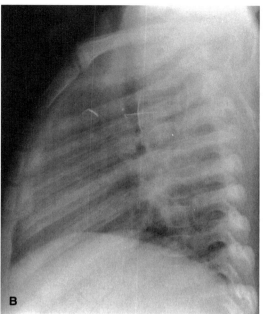

Figure 32–58. **(A)** Frontal and **(B)** lateral projections of a child show the metallic components of a Sideris occlusion device. The position indicates that it was placed in a patent ductus arteriosis.

and position will suggest their nature. Ring-like devices in the region of a valve herald a prosthetic valve or a support ring placed at the time of valvuloplasty (see Fig. 32-41C). Multiple vascular clips along the course of the internal mammary artery indicate its use as a bypass conduit that may be either uni- or bilateral.

Intravenous or epicardial pacemaker leads have a characteristic appearance. Fractures of the leads can be detected. Many surgeons place metallic markers at the site of the aortic ostium of saphenous vein bypass grafts to facilitate postoperative coronary arteriography if it becomes necessary. In the face of radioopaque sternal sutures and metallic markers on the ascending aorta, one can diagnose previous coronary artery bypass surgery.

Metallic components of a percutaneously placed device to close an atrial septal defect or patent dectus arteriosis can be recognized by their appearance and position (Figs 32-58A and B). Vascular occlusion coils also have a typical appearance and once seen are identified readily (see Fig. 32-34C).

Changes in the size and contour of the heart may offer important clues. During mitral valve surgery, the left atrial appendage is often resected. This will result in a concavity along the left heart border just below the pulmonary artery. Likewise, striking decrease in car-

diac size in very short period of time suggests the possibility of a cardiac transplant or a pericardiocentesis.

REFERENCES AND SELECTED READINGS

1. AMPLATZ K, LESTER RG, SCHIEBLER GL, ET AL: The roentgenologic features of Ebstein's anomaly of the tricuspid valve. Am J Roentgenol 81:788, 1959
2. BALTAXE HA, MOLLER JH, AMPLATZ K: Membranous subaortic stenosis and its associated malformations. Radiology 95:287, 1970
3. BANDOW GT, ROWE GG, CRUMMY AB: Congenital diverticulum of the right and left ventricles. Radiology 117:19, 1975
4. BANK ER, HERNANDEZ RJ: CT and MR of congenital heart disease. Radiol Clin N Amer 26(2):241–262, 1988
5. BARTRAM C, STRICKLAND B: Pulmonary varices. Br J Radiol 44:927, 1971
6. BERKMEN YM, LANDE A: Chest roentgenography as a window to the diagnosis of Takayasu's arteritis. Am J Roentgenol 125:842, 1975
7. BERKOFF HA, ROWE GG, CRUMMY AB, ET AL: Asymptomatic left ventricular aneurysm. A sequela of blunt chest trauma. Circulation 55:545, 1977

8. BRUWER AJ: Posteroanterior chest roentgenogram in two types of anomalous pulmonary venous connection. J Thorac Surg 32:119, 1956

9. CAPUTO GR, HIGGINS CB: Advances in cardiac imaging modalities: Fast computed tomography, magnetic resonance imaging, and position emission tomography. Invest Radiol 25:838–854, 1990

10. CAREY LS, EDWARDS JE: Roentgenographic features in cases with origin of both great vessels from the right ventricle without pulmonary stenosis. Am J Roentgenol 93:269, 1965

11. CASTILLO M, OLDHAM S: Cardiac volvulus: Plain film recognition of an often fatal condition. Am J Roentgenol 145:271–272, 1985

12. COUSSEMENT AM, GOODING CA: Objective radiographic assessment of pulmonary vascularity in children. Radiology 109:649, 1973

13. CRUMMY AB, HIPONA FA: The radiographic aspects of right ventricular myxoma. Brit J Radiol 37: 468, 1964

14. DAVES ML: Cardiac Roentgenology: Shadows of the Heart. Chicago, Year Book Medical Publishers, Inc., 1981

15. DAVIS GD, KINCAID OW, HALLERMANN FJ: Roentgen aspects of cardiac tumors. Semin Roentgenol 4:384, 1969

16. EDWARDS JE, CAREY LS, NEUFELD HN, ET AL: Congenital heart disease. Philadelphia, W. B. Saunders, 1965

17. ELLIOTT LP, JUE KL, AMPLATZ K: A roentgen classification of cardiac malpositions. Invest Radiol 1:17, 1966

18. ELLIS K, LEED NE, HIMMELSTEIN A: Congenital deficiencies in the parietal pericardium. Am J Roentgenol 82:125, 1959

19. EPSTEIN BS: Calcification of the ascending aorta. Am J Roentgenol 77:281, 1957

20. EYLER WR, ZIEGLER RF, SHEA JJ, ET AL: Endocardial fibroelastosis: Roentgen appearance. Radiology 64:797, 1955

21. FIGLEY MM: Accessory roentgen signs of coarctation of the aorta. Radiology 62: 671, 1954

22. FINKELMEIER BA, MENTZER RM, KAISER DL, ET AL: Chronic traumatic thoracic aneurysm. J Thorac Cardiovasc Surg 84: 257–266, 1982

23. FLAHERTY TT, WEGNER GP, CRUMMY AB, ET AL: Nonpenetrating injuries to the thoracic aorta. Radiology 92: 541, 1969

24. GAY BB JR, FRANCH RH, SHUFORD WH, ET AL: The roentgenologic features of single and multiple coarctations of the pulmonary artery and branches. Am J Roentgenol 90:599, 1963

25. GEDGAUDAS E, MOLLER JH, CASTANEDA-ZUNIGA WR, ET AL: Cardiovascular Radiology. Philadelphia, W. B. Saunders, 1985

26. GOETZ AA, GRAHAM WH: Aneurysm of the sinus of Valsalva. Radiology 67:416, 1956

27. GOTT VL, LESTER RG, LILLEHEI CW,, ET AL: Total anomalous pulmonary return. An analysis of thirty cases. Circulation 13:543, 1956

28. GYEPES MT, VINCENT WR: Severe congenital heart disease in the neonatal period. Am J Roentgenol 116:490, 1972

29. HARRIS EJ: Aneurysms of the sinus of Valsalva. Am J Roentgenol 76:767, 1956

30. HARRIS GBC, NEUHAUSER EBD, GIEDION A: Total anomalous pulmonary venous return below the diaphragm. Am J Roentgenol 84:436, 1960

31. HATTEN HP JR, LORMAN JG, ROSENBAUM HD: Pulmonary sling in the adult. Am J Roentgenol 128:919, 1977

32. HAYASHI K, MEANEY TF, ZELCH JV, ET AL: Aortographic analysis of aortic dissection. Am J Roentgenol 122:769, 1974

33. HEINSIMER JA, COLLINS GJ, BURKMAN MH, ROBERTS L, CHEN JTT: Supine cross-table lateral chest roentgenogram for the detection of pericardial effusion. JAMA 257(23):3266–3268, 1987

34. HIGGINS CB, REINKE RT, JONES NE, ET AL: Left atrial dimension on the frontal thoracic radiograph: A method for assessing left atrial enlargement. Am J Roentgenol 130:251, 1978

35. HIPONA FA, CRUMMY AB: Congenital pericardial defect associated with tetralogy of Fallot. Circulation 29:132, 1964

36. HODGES PC, EYSTER JAE: Estimate of transverse cardiac diameter in man. Arch Intern Med 37:707, 1926

37. HORIMOTO M, IGARASHI K, AOI K, OKAMOTO K, TAKENAKA T: Unlateral diffuse pulmonary artery involvement in Takayasu's arteritis associated with coronary–pulmonary artery fistula and bronchial–pulmonary artery fistula: A case report. Angiology (1):73–80, 1991

38. JONSSON G, SALTZMAN GF: Infundibulum of patent ductus arteriosus—diagnostic sign in conventional roentgenograms. Acta Radiol [Suppl] (Stock) 38:8, 1952

39. KEATS TE, KREIS VA, SIMPSON E: The roentgen manifestations of pulmonary hypertension in congenital heart disease. Radiology 66:693, 1956

40. KEATS TE, STEINBACH HL: Patent ductus arteriosus. A critical evaluation of its roentgen signs. Radiology 64: 528, 1955

41. KELLEY MJ, JAFFE CC, KLEINMAN CS: Cardiac Imaging in Infants and Children. Philadelphia, W. B. Saunders, 1982

42. KERLEY P: Lung changes in acquired heart disease. Am J Roentgenol 80:256, 1958

43. KLATTE EC, CAMPBELL JA, LURIE PR: Aortic configuration in congenital heart disease. Radiology 74:555, 1960

44. KRAUSE DW, KUEHN HJ, SELLERS RD, ET AL: Roentgen sign associated with an aberrant vessel connecting the right main pulmonary artery to the left atrium. Radiology 111:177, 1974

45. KUMAR S, MANDALAM KR, UNNI M, ROY S, GUPTA AK, RAO VRK: Left cervical arch and associated abnormalities. Cardiovasc & Intervent Radiol 12:88–91, 1989

46. LESTER RG, ANDERSON RC, AMPLATZ K, ET AL: Roentgenologic diagnosis of congenitally corrected transposition of the great vessels. Am J Roentgenol 83:985, 1960

47. LEVIN B, BORDEN CW: Anomalous pulmonary venous drainage into the left vertical vein. Radiology 63:317, 1954

48. LEVIN B, RIGLER LG: Rib notching following subclavian artery obstruction. Radiology 62: 660, 1954

49. LEVIN B, WHITE H: Total anomalous pulmonary venous drainage into the portal system. Radiology 76:894, 1961

50. LODWICK GE: Dissecting aneurysms of the thoracic and abdominal aorta. Am J Roentgenol 69:907, 1955

51. LODWICK GS, GLADSTONE WS: Correlation of anatomic and roentgen changes in arteriosclerosis and syphilis of the ascending aorta. Radiology 69:70, 1957

52. LOWE GM, DONALDSON JS, BACKER CL: Vascular rings: 10-year review of imaging. Radiographics 11:637–646, 1991

53. LUETMER PH, MILLER GM: Right aortic arch with isolation of the left subclavian artery: Case report and review of the literature. Mayo Clin Proc 65:407–413, 1990

54. MCCORD MC, BAVENDAM FA: Unusual causes of rib notching. Am J Roentgenol 67:405, 1952

55. MELLINS HZ, KOTTMEIER P, KIELY B: Radiologic signs of pericardial effusion. Radiology 73:9, 1959

56. MEYER RR: A method for measuring children's hearts. Radiology 53:363, 1949

57. MILLER SW: Cardiac Angiography. Boston, Little, Brown and Company, Boston, 1984

58. MONCADA R, BAKER M, SALINAS M, ET AL: Diagnostic role of computed tomography in pericardial heart disease: Congenital defects, thickening, neoplasms, and effusions. Am Heart J 103:263–282, 1982

59. MONCADA R, SHANNON M, MILLER R, ET AL: The cervical aortic arch. Am J Roentgenol 125:591, 1975

60. PARTRIDGE JB, OSBORNE JM, SLAUGHTER RE: Scimitar etcetera—the dysmorphic right lung. Clin Radiol 39: 11–19, 1988

61. PAUL LW, RICHTER MR: Funnel chest deformity and its recognition in posteroanterior roentgenograms of the thorax. Am J Roentgenol 46:619, 1941

62. POCHASZEVSKY R, DUNST ME: Coexistent pulmonary artery and aortic arch calcification. Am J Roentgenol 116:141, 1972

63. RAO PS, SIDERIS EB, CHOPRA PS: Catheter closure of atrial septal defect: Successful use in 3.6 kg infant. Am Heart J 121(6):1826–1829, 1991

64. RAO PS, WILSON AD, SIDERIS EB, CHOPRA PS: Transcatheter closure of patent ductus arteriosus with buttoned device: First successful clinical application in a child. Am Heart J 121(6):1799–1802, 1991

65. REICH NE, WITTER M: Roentgenographic visualization of the coronary arteries. Am J Roentgenol 77:274, 1951

66. ROEHM TU JR, JUE KL, AMPLATZ K: Radiographic features of the scimitar syndrome. Radiology 86:856, 1966

67. RONDEROS A: Endocardial fibroelastosis. Am J Roentgenol 84:442, 1960

68. ROSENBAUM HD: The roentgen classification and diagnosis of cardiac alignments. Radiology 89:466, 1967

69. ROWEN M, THOMPSON JR, WILLIAMSON RA, ET AL: Diffuse pulmonary hemangiomatosis. Radiology 127:445, 1978

70. SAROSI MG, CRUMMY AB, MCDERMOTT JC, KRONCKE GM: Case Report: Milk of calcium pericardial effusion. Cardiovasc Intervent Radiol 14(5):314–315, 1991

71. SCHULTZ KW, THORSEN MK, GURNEY JW, ET AL: Comparison of fluoroscopy, angiography and CT in coronary artery calcification. Appl Radiol (June):38–42, 1989

72. SHUFORD WH, SYBERS RG: The aortic arch and its malformations. Springfield, IL, Thomas, 1974

73. SORKIN RP, SCHUURMANN BJ, SIMON AB: Radiographic aspects of permanent cardiac pacemakers. Radiology 119: 281, 1976

74. STEINBERG I: Anomalies (pseudocoarctation) of the arch of the aorta. Am J Roentgenol 88:73, 1962

75. STEINBERG I, FINBY N: Roentgen manifestations of unperforated aortic sinus aneurysms. Am J Roentgenol 77: 263, 1957

76. STEINER RE: The roentgen features of the cardiomyopathies. Semin Roentgenol 4:311, 1969

77. STEVENS GM: Buckling of the aortic arch (pseudocoarctation, kinking): A roentgenographic entity. Radiology 70: 67, 1958

78. STRIFE JL, MATSUMOTO J, BISSETT GS, MARTIN R: The position of the trachea in infants and children with right aortic arch. Pediatr Radiol 19:226–229, 1989

79. STURM JT, BILLIAR TR, DORSEY JS, ET AL: Risk factors for survival following surgical treatment of traumatic aortic rupture. Ann Thor Surg 39:418–421, 1985

80. SUSSMAN ML, JACOBSON G: Critical evaluation of roentgen criteria of right ventricular enlargement. Circulation 11:391, 1955

81. SWISCHUK LE: Plain film interpretation in congenital heart disease. Philadelphia, Lea & Febiger, 1979

82. TEGTMEYER CJ: Roentgenographic assessment of causes of cardiac pacemaker failure and complications. CRC Crit Rev in Diag Imag, 9:1–50, 1977

83. TORRANCE DJ: Demonstration of subepicardial fat as an aid in the diagnosis of pericardial fluid or thickening. Am J Roentgenol 74:850, 1955

84. UNGERLEIDER HE, CLARK CP: Study of transverse diameter of heart silhouette, with prediction table based on teleroentgenogram. Am Heart J 17:92, 1939

85. UNGERLEIDER HE, GUBNER R: Evaluation of heart size measurements. Am Heart J 24:494, 1942

86. WALTER WH III: Radiographic identification of commonly used pulse generators—1970. JAMA 215:971, 1974

87. WESCOTT JL, FERGUSON D: The right pulmonary artery—left atrial axis line. Method for measuring left atrial size on lateral radiographs. Radiology 118:265, 1976

88. WHITE RI JR, MITCHELL SE, BARTH KH, ET AL: Angioarchitecture of pulmonary arteriovenous malforma-

tions: An important consideration before embolotherapy. Am J Roentgenol 140:681–686, 1983

89. WYMAN SM: Congenital absence of a pulmonary artery. Radiology 62:321, 1954

90. WYMAN SM: Dissecting aneurysm of the thoracic aorta: Its roentgen recognition. Am J Roentgenol 78:247, 1957

CHAPTER 32B MAGNETIC RESONANCE IMAGING OF THE HEART

Murray G. Baron

Clinical evaluation of cardiac disease requires an accurate delineation of the anatomy of the heart as well as determination of its global and regional function. Much of this data can be acquired with magnetic resonance imaging (MRI), noninvasively and without the use of ionizing radiation.[4]

Because of the difference in the signal strengths of flowing blood, and that of myocardium and other soft tissues, the internal structure of the cardiac chambers is seen as well as the chamber walls and the pericardium. In contrast to angiocardiography, intravascular contrast agents are not required. MR images can be obtained in any plane, unlike echocardiography, which is limited by the available acoustic windows. Images acquired in rapid succession show the chambers at multiple points in the cardiac cycle so that chamber volumes and segmental ventricular wall motion and thickening can be measured accurately. Review of the images in cine mode provides a detailed study of the mechanics of ventricular wall motion.

TECHNICAL CONSIDERATIONS

CARDIAC GATING

Each MR image is constructed from data acquired from multiple radio frequency (RF) excitations during the course of a scan. Because the heart is a dynamic structure, acquisitions that occur at random in relation to the cardiac cycle would represent the heart in a different state of contraction and different position, so that the final image would simply be a blur. By triggering the acquisition from the R wave of the EKG, the heart is always imaged at the same point in the cardiac cycle, thus producing a sharply delineated image.

PULSE SEQUENCES

Spin-echo imaging provides maximum contrast between the heart and the blood within it. The technique involves exposing the tissues to two separate radiofrequency pulses for each data acquisition. Rapidly flowing blood does not remain in the imaging plane long enough to receive both pulses and, therefore, does not generate any signal, appearing as a black void against the grayish tones of the stationary tissues. If flow is sufficiently slow, some of the blood may receive both pulses and generate a signal, mimicking the appearance of clotted blood. This slow flow often occurs adjacent to an akinetic segment of ventricular wall but it can also be seen in the normal heart or aorta, toward the end of diastole.

Only a single RF pulse is needed for gradient echo imaging, and the entire sequence is short; a scan can be completed in less than half the time required for a spin-echo image. Smoothly flowing blood gives off a strong signal and appears whiter than the surrounding tissues. When flow is not coherent, there is a rapid loss of signal so that areas of turbulence appear as black voids. Because the intensity of the emitted signal is roughly proportional to the speed of flow, this technique can be used to quantify the velocity of blood flow.

IMAGING PLANES

MRI is a tomographic technique that allows visualization of only those structures that lie within the imaging plane. Although this increases their visibility by excluding overlying shadows, it also creates problems in picturing structures that extend over more than one section. Even with multiple sections that are adjacent to each other, it may be difficult to follow a structure from one slice to the next. This problem can be minimized by the proper choice of imaging planes. By necessity, this is an interactive process requiring the presence of the physician, so that subsequent sections can be chosen on the basis of what has already been seen.

Most scans begin with images made in one or more of the standard orthogonal projections. The coronal (Fig. 32-59) and sagittal (Fig. 32-60) views are comparable to the frontal and lateral views of an angiocardiogram, while the transverse image (32-61) shows the heart in cross section. If oblique or compound oblique sections are needed, they can be planned from one or more of the basic views.

Two commonly used oblique sections correspond to views used in echocardiography. The four-chamber view is a tilted transverse section that provides maximum visibility of all four cardiac chambers, the mitral

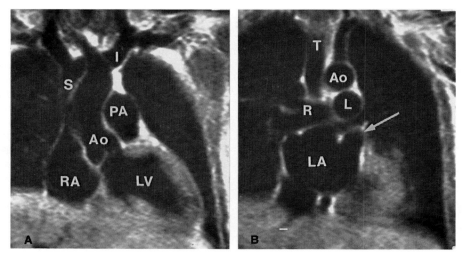

Figure 32–59. Normal. Spin-echo image, coronal plane. **(A)** Level of the aortic valve. The aortic valve is seen as a thin line of soft-tissue density between the left ventricle (LV) and the ascending aorta (Ao). The main pulmonary artery (PA) is sectioned obliquely as it courses upward and posteriorly. RA—right atrium; S—superior vena cava; I—left innominate vein. **(B)** Several centimeters posteriorly, the section cuts through the body of the left atrium (LA) and its appendage (*arrow*), immediately posterior to the division of the main pulmonary artery and just in front of the tracheal bifurcation. The right pulmonary artery (R) courses to the right and slightly posteriorly, while the left pulmonary artery (L) heads straight backward. The distal portion of the aortic arch (Ao) is seen in cross section just before it turns down to become the descending aorta. This is the part of the arch that forms the aortic knob on plain films. T—trachea.

and tricuspid valves, and the interventricular, inter-atrial, and atrioventricular septa (Fig. 32-62*A*). A section 1 to 2 cm toward the head demonstrates the outflow tract of the left ventricle leading to the aortic valve (Fig. 32-62*B*). Sections in the short-axis view (Fig. 32-63) are oriented perpendicular to the long axis of the left ventricle. The left ventricle is seen in true cross section with a minimum of distortion. The muscular interventricular septum is seen on end and the outflow tract of the right ventricle is also visualized clearly.

FUNCTIONAL PARAMETERS

The ventricular stroke volume and ejection fraction are calculated from the systolic and diastolic volumes of the ventricle. These volumes are measured directly from the MR images without the need for compensatory mathematical formulas. The short-axis view is the most accurate for calculation of left ventricular volume. Contiguous slices through the entire ventricle are acquired

in both systole and diastole. The cavity area is determined on each slice and multiplied by the thickness of the section. The total of the values gives the ventricular volume for that phase of the cardiac cycle. The inaccuracies of the method stem from difficulties in identifying the exact level of the mitral valve marking the base of the ventricle, and in accurately measuring the chamber on slices near the ventricular apex because of distortion due to the sharp slope of its walls.

Normally, the thickness of the left ventricular wall is roughly the same in all areas. Localized thinning of the wall is a sign of previous myocardial infarction (see Fig. 32-61*A*). Thickening of the wall, with a width greater than 1.5 cm and a ratio of the thickness of the septum to the posterior wall of greater than 1.5:1, is diagnostic of hypertrophic cardiomyopathy. These measurements are best made in the short-axis view.

As the normal myocardium contracts, it thickens evenly around the circumference of the ventricle. A decrease in the degree of thickening of the myocardium between diastole and systole is a more sensitive

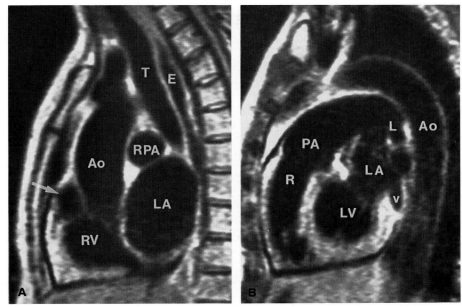

Figure 32–60. Normal heart. Spin-echo image, sagittal plane. (**A**) Midline section. The ascending aorta (Ao) is tilted slightly to the right as it courses upward so that it lies in the same sagittal plane as the inflow portion of the right ventricle (RV). The anterior extent of the right atrial appendage (*arrow*) is seen above the ventricle. The right pulmonary artery (RPA) is cut in cross section as it courses horizontally through the mediastinum to the right lung. LA—left atrium; T—trachea; E—esophagus. (**B**) Several centimeters to the left of (**A**), the section passes through the midportion of the outflow tract of the right ventricle (R) and the root of the pulmonary artery (PA). The muscular portion of the interventricular septum is seen on end between the right ventricle and the left ventricle (LV). L—left pulmonary artery; v—left inferior pulmonary vein.

sign of ischemic myocardial damage than is an absolute thinning of the wall (see Fig. 32-63).

ACQUIRED HEART DISEASE[6]

CORONARY ARTERY DISEASE[7]

Because of their irregularly curving course, none of the coronary arteries can be included completely in a single tomographic section of reasonable thickness. Furthermore, because they are often sectioned at oblique angles, a factitious appearance of stenosis or occlusion can be created as the coronary arteries pass out of a slice. For these reasons, MRI is of little use in evaluating patency of the coronary arteries.

It is of value, however, in detecting the effects of coronary disease, as well as the presence, severity, and the results of myocardial ischemia. An acute myocardial infarct usually appears as an area of increased signal intensity on spin-echo images because of the increased water content of the edematous, ischemic tissue. These changes can be detected in the experimental animal within three to four hours of coronary occlusion, and persist for about three weeks. The findings are not specific, however, for infarction, because similar areas of increased signal intensity can occur in the normal heart and they are not seen with all infarcts. A localized decrease in the systolic thickening of the ventricular wall is a better and more sensitive sign of myocardial ischemia.

Two complications of myocardial infarction that can produce confusing clinical signs are mitral insufficiency due to rupture of an infarcted papillary muscle and a ventricular septal defect following infarction and necrosis of the septum. These are detected easily and

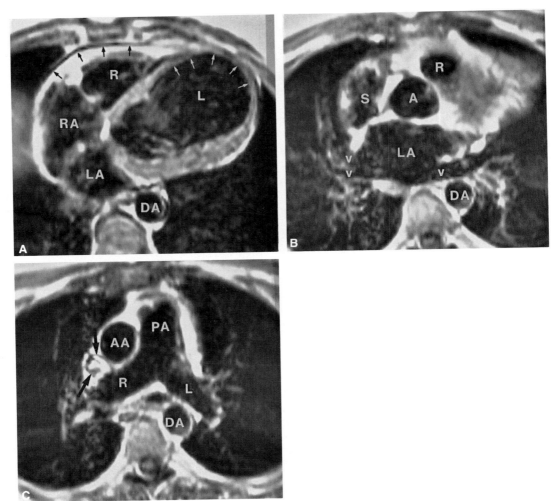

Figure 32–61.   Left ventricular aneurysm, postmyocardial infarction. Spin-echo images, transverse plane. (**A**) Level of the midleft ventricle. The apical portion of the interventricular septum and the anterior free wall of the left ventricle are thinned. The myocardium in this region has been replaced by fibrous scar tissue and bulges outward to form an aneurysm (*white arrows*). The dark curvilinear shadow anterior to the right ventricle (*black arrows*) represents the pericardium and pericardial space. R—right ventricle; RA—right atrium; LA—left atrium; DA—descending aorta. (**B**) Level of the midleft atrium. R—right ventricular outflow tract; A—aortic valve; S—junction of superior cava and right atrium; v—pulmonary veins; LA—left atrium; DA—descending aorta. (**C**) Level of pulmonary artery bifurcation. Signal within the superior cava (*arrows*) is due to slow bloodflow and not clot. AA—ascending aorta; PA—main pulmonary artery; R—right pulmonary artery; L—left pulmonary artery; DA—descending aorta.

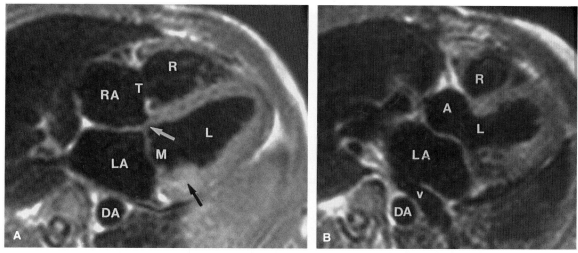

Figure 32–62. Loffler's endocarditis. Four-chamber view, spin-echo images. (**A**) Mid-ventricular level. The tricuspid valve (T) lies anterior to the mitral valve (M). The atrioventricular septum (*white arrow*) lies between the insertion of the two valves and separates the left ventricle (L) from the right atrium (RA). An endocardial plaque (*black arrows*), typical of this disease, is seen in the inflow tract of the left ventricle (L) just in front of the mitral valve. R—right ventricle; LA—left atrium; DA—descending aorta. (**B**) Level of the left atrium. The outflow tact of the left ventricle (L) leads into the aortic valve (A). v—pulmonary vein.

Figure 32–63. Short axis view, spin-echo images. Previous septal infarction. The left ventricle (L) is seen in cross section, separated from the right ventricle (R) by the interventricular septum. The septum is abnormally thin during diastole (**A**) and shows no evidence of thickening during systole (**B**). (Courtesy of Dr. R. I. Pettigrew).

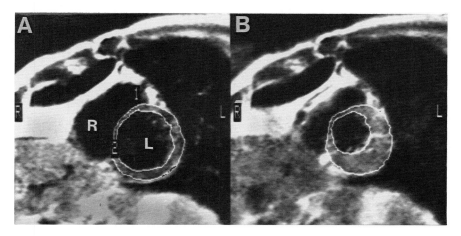

distinguished from one another by the intracardiac cardiac flow patterns seen on gradient-echo movies.

Older infarcts usually appear thinner than the normal myocardium during diastole, and show little or no thickening during systole (see Fig. 32-63). A localized outward bulging of the wall indicates a ventricular aneurysm (see Fig. 32-61A).

The MR evaluation of a decrease in myocardial per-

fusion secondary to narrowing of a coronary vessel can be enhanced by the intravenous injection of a paramagnetic "contrast" material such as gadolinium-DTPA.[8] This substance increases the relaxation times of tissue so that its MR signal increases in intensity. When the Gd-DTPA is combined with a large molecule such as albumin, its distribution is limited to the intravascular space so that it can be used as a valid indicator of myocardial perfusion. Muscle with a normal blood supply, which is well perfused by the gadolinium-laden blood, will appear brighter on the MR image than will ischemic myocardium.

A common problem following acute infarction is the differentiation of dead muscle from "stunned" myocardium. This is important, because stunned muscle can recover with adequate reperfusion. Following the intravenous injection of Gd-DTPA, both the stunned and the dead myocardium in the experimental animal emit weak signals shortly after the acute vascular insult. With reperfusion, signal from the stunned myocardium rapidly increases in intensity to reach equilibrium with the normal myocardium. An irreversibly infarcted segment shows an even greater increase in signal following restoration of blood flow, its signal intensity exceeding that of normal myocardium, presumably because of loss of vascular integrity in the infarcted region and leakage of the contrast material into the extravascular space.[9]

VALVULAR DISEASE

A transient signal void on gradient-echo movies, extending retrograde from the tricuspid or mitral valve during ventricular systole, or from the aortic or pulmonic valve during diastole, indicates incompetence of that valve (Fig. 32-64). Because the regurgitation does not continue through an entire cardiac cycle, the signal void becomes progressively more diffuse until it disappears, only to recur with the next cycle. A similar signal void can be caused by a tumor such as a myxoma that prolapses through the atrioventricular valve, but it will persist throughout the cardiac cycle.

The severity of the valvular insufficiency can be estimated by comparing the size of the signal void to that of the recipient chamber. This can also be quantified by comparing the stroke volumes of the two ventricles.[3] Normally, these are just about equal. With an insufficient valve, the increase in the stroke volume of the involved ventricle will represent the regurgitant volume.

Because of the force with which blood is ejected from the ventricles, a broad area of signal loss is normally seen in the pulmonary artery and aorta during systole. When either semilunar valve is stenotic, the "lucent" jet spurting through it becomes narrowed. The pressure gradient across the stenotic valve cannot be determined accurately with current MRI techniques.

PERICARDIAL DISEASE[1]

The pericardium appears on spin-echo images as a dark (low-signal intensity), curvilinear stripe, representing the combined images of the pericardium, the epicardium, and the pericardial fluid. It is best seen over the

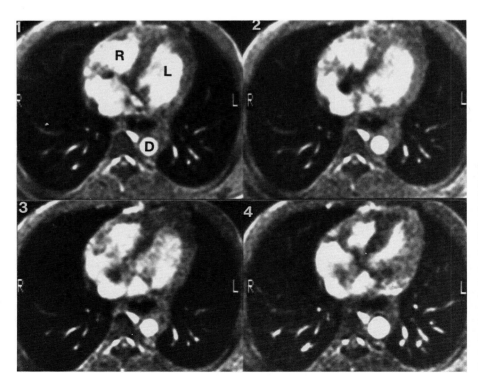

Figure 32–64. Tricuspid insufficiency. Selected frames from gradient echo movie, transverse plane. Start of systole (**1**) through end systole (**4**). As the right ventricle (R) contracts, the insufficient stream causes a signal void (*arrow*) in the right atrium. This becomes more diffuse with time, as the regurgitant jet ceases and normal flow is restored. L—left ventricle; D—descending aorta.

anterolateral margins of the heart where it is set off between the brighter signals of the extrapericardial fat and the subepicardial fat (Figs. 32-61 and 32-65*B*). As the amount of fluid between the two layers increases, the pericardial stripe widens. A thickness of more than 4 mm is abnormal (see Fig. 32-65).

Regardless of whether the pericardial fluid is a transudate or an exudate, it will have a low-signal intensity because the irregular motion of the fluid caused by the beating heart results in a rapid dephasing of its nuclear spins. When a pericardial effusion is loculated, the fluid cannot move and its signal is of similar intensity to that of myocardium (Fig. 32-65*B*).

Involvement of the pericardium is not uncommon in patients with metastatic malignancy. The most frequent finding is a pericardial effusion; a thickened rind of infiltrated pericardium often can be seen enclosing the fluid. In more advanced cases, the pericardial space may be completely obliterated by the tumor involving the pericardium.

CARDIAC TUMORS[1]

About 75% of cardiac tumors are benign and most of these are atrial myxomas. This tumor can be recognized equally well by echocardiography and MRI, although MRI more accurately demonstrates the point of attachment of the tumor to the atrial wall or septum. The MR diagnosis of a myxoma depends on the location and mobility of the tumor. MRI cannot distinguish between benign and malignant lesions from the intrinsic characteristics of the mass itself, nor can it accurately determine the extent of the lesion.

CONGENITAL HEART DISEASE[2, 5]

A detailed delineation of the cardiac anatomy is essential for the diagnosis of congenital heart disease. The presence, size, and position of the cardiac chambers and great vessels, their relationship to each other, the integrity of the cardiac septae, and the status of the

cardiac valves must all be determined. Most of this data can be obtained by MR scanning, and, in some cases (e.g., coarctation of the aorta), this is all that is needed in addition to the clinical findings before surgery.

IDENTIFICATION OF CARDIAC STRUCTURES

In patients with acquired cardiac disease, the heart is assumed to be normally formed so that the chambers and great vessels can be identified from their position and their connections to each other. In many instances of congenital heart disease, these relationships are distorted or grossly abnormal and the identification of the chambers must depend on their intrinsic anatomic characteristics.

The most constant, potentially visible, anatomic feature that differentiates the two atria is the configuration of their appendages. The right atrial appendage is trapezoidal in shape and communicates with the atrium through a broad opening, while the left atrial appendage is more finger-like and has a narrow communication with its atrium. Because the appendages lie on an oblique plane however, they are not always well seen on MR scans, and these criteria may be of little practical value. The atria can be identified reliably on scans because their side-to-side relationship is almost always coherent with the thoracic situs. In situs solitus, the right atrium lies to the right of the left atrium. The thoracic situs can be identified from a coronal section through the tracheal bifurcation. In normal situs, the right lung has an eparterial bronchus that courses over the right pulmonary artery, while the left lung shows a hyparterial bronchial pattern with both the upper and lower lobar bronchi coursing under the pulmonary artery. Another valid identifier is a complete inferior vena cava emptying into the right atrium.

Except in rare instances, the right ventricle can be identified because it has a muscular outflow tract, the infundibulum, that separates its inflow and outflow valves. In the left ventricle, the two valves insert on the same fibrous tendon and touch each other. The infundibulum is best visualized in the coronal or sagittal

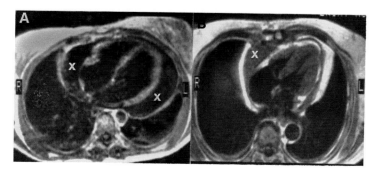

Figure 32–65. Pericardial effusion. (**A**) Free effusion. Because of the motion of the fluid causing the rapid dephasing of the nuclear spins, the large effusion (x) presents as a signal void. (**B**) Loculated effusion. The loculated fluid (x) has a signal density similar to that of myocardium.

views (see Fig. 32-60*B*). The greater thickness of the right ventricular wall and its accentuated trabeculation (Fig. 32-66A) are less reliable signs. The right ventricle can also be identified if the moderator band is seen. This is a prominent muscular trabeculum that arises from the lateral wall of the ventricle and courses anteriorly, toward the septum. It often can be seen on transverse sections, crossing the right ventricular cavity near its apex.

The great vessels are identified by their branches and the organs they supply.

ROTATIONAL ANOMALIES

These tend to be complex abnormalities. Although MRI is usually adequate for defining the underlying anomaly and some of the associated lesions (Fig.

32-66), it cannot replace cardiac catheterization and angiocardiography. Conversely, MRI is valuable because the orientation of the chambers and vessels may be so abnormal that the limited choice of views available from other diagnostic techniques may not be adequate to demonstrate the cardiac anatomy.

SEPTAL DEFECTS

The atrial septum is best examined in the four-chamber view. A discontinuity in the septum usually represents an atrial sepral defect (ASD), but in some cases it is simply an artefact due to signal dropout.

Because of its size and curved shape, the ventricular septum is projected on end in several views. Although it is clearly seen in the transverse, four-chamber, and sagittal views, it is perhaps best studied, in the LAO

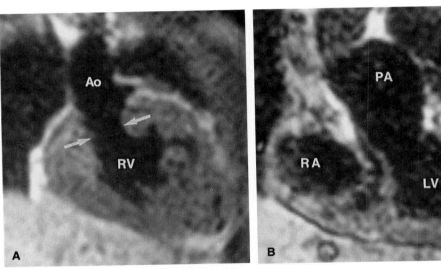

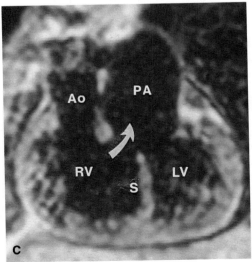

Figure 32–66. Transposition of the great arteries. (**A**) Coronal section through the right ventricle (RV). The aorta (Ao) arises from the infundibulum (*arrows*). In this case, the ventricular wall is characteristically thick and heavily trabeculated. (**B**) Coronal section through the left ventricle (LV), which gives rise to a markedly dilated pulmonary artery (PA). The cause for the dilatation is not apparent. RA—right atrium. (**C**) Section corresponding to a left anterior oblique view. The aorta (Ao) arises anteriorly to the pulmonary artery (PA). The interventricular septum (S) is incomplete, and the pulmonary artery arises across the septal defect (*arrow*) and receives blood from both ventricles.

projection, as it is in angiocardiography. In this view, the muscular septum is seen as a soft-tissue wall, separating the bodies of the right and left ventricles. Because of the thickness of the septum, visualization of a gap is a reliable sign of a septal defect (Fig. 32-66C). Although the resolution of the technique is inadequate to demonstrate small septal defects, the turbulence caused by the transeptal shunt is usually obvious on gradient-echo movies. The same is true with a patent ductus arteriosus.

ABNORMALITIES OF THE VALVES

The MR appearances of congenital valvular stenosis and insufficiency are essentially the same as in the acquired form of the disease. Valvular atresia is considerably more serious and usually affects the development of one or more of the cardiac chambers.

When the tricuspid valve is atretic, there is no direct communication between the right atrium and the right ventricle, and the inflow portion of the right ventricle is underdeveloped. The two chambers are separated by a fibrofatty septum extending inward from the atrioventricular sulcus, best visualized in transverse sections through the right atrium and ventricle. A diminutive right ventricular (RV) chamber is also associated with isolated pulmonic valve atresia. The tricuspid valve is usually small but patent. Atresia of the mitral and/or aortic valves results in hypoplasia of the left side of the heart and the aorta.

An endocardial cushion defect is recognized most effectively on the four-chamber view. The atrioventricular septum is absent so that the mitral and tricuspid valves insert at the same anteroposterior level on the crest of the muscular ventricular septum. A single atrioventricular valve spanning both atrioventricular (A-V) orifices is indicative of a complete atrioventricular canal (Fig. 32-67). Anterior displacement of the tricuspid valve into the right ventricle is characteristic of Ebstein's anomaly.

VENTRICULAR ABNORMALITIES

In tetralogy of Fallot, a tilted coronal view is usually best in evaluating the degree of infundibular stenosis. The angle of the imaging plane is determined from the sagittal section and is set to the angle of the long axis of the infundibulum. The ventricular septal defect (VSD) in tetralogy is usually large and involves the base of the interventricular septum. It can be seen well in the oblique sagittal or transverse views.

Differentiation of a double outlet right ventricle from a tetralogy requires demonstration of a separation of the aortic and mitral valves by a ridge of myocardium in a heart where the aorta arises from the right ventri-

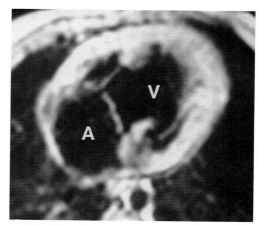

Figure 32–67. Two-chambered heart. Note single ventricle (V) and a common atrium (A). The linear soft tissue density between the two is the common atrioventricular valve.

cle. The left ventricle communicates with the aorta through a defect at the base of the ventricular septum.

In a persistent truncus arteriosus, the pulmonary arteries arise directly from the aorta and there always is a VSD immediately beneath the truncus valve. Both lesions can be demonstrated in the coronal view.

PRECATHETERIZATION AND POSTOPERATIVE STUDIES

With the more complex lesions, especially in the infant, cardiac catheterization is extremely difficult because little can be predicted about the position of the chambers within the heart. Often, one or two angiocardiographic runs are needed simply for orientation. Because only a limited amount of contrast material can be injected safely at one examination, a second catheterization is often needed to complete the study. Time can be saved by performing the scout work with MRI and then planning the catheterization (Fig. 32-67).

Postoperative patients frequently require repeated follow-up studies to monitor the results of surgery, to evaluate the patency of created shunts, and postsurgical areas of stenosis. Frequently, the entire examination can be performed by MRI, saving the patient significant radiation exposure as well as the considerable cost of multiple catheterizations.

The value of an MR examination of the heart depends largely on the design of the study. The maximum value will not be realized if standard "recipes" that prescribe a set of views in advance are employed. As with angiocardiography, cardiac MRI is a physician-intense, interactive procedure that requires interpretation of each scan in order to determine the optimal orientation of subsequent sections.

In most instances, the informational content of the MR study is greater than that of two-dimensional, or Doppler echocardiography. However, use of MRI is limited because of problems of logistics and availability; MRI remains an adjunct to echocardiography for the study of the cardiac patient.

REFERENCES AND SELECTED READINGS

1. BARON MG. MRI of pericardium, cardiomyopathy and cardiac masses. Cardiovascular Imaging. Categorical course syllabus. Casarella WJ, ed. ARRS, 1990
2. FLETCHER BD, JOCABSTEIN MD. Magnetic Resonance Imaging of Congenital Heart Disease. Anatomic, Angiographic and Echocardiographic Correlations. St. Louis, C. V. Mosby, Co., 1988
3. GLOGAR D, GLOBITS S, NEUHOLD A, MAYR H. Assessment of mitral regurgitation by magnetic resonance imaging. Magnetic Resonance Imaging. 7:611, 1989
4. HIGGINS CB. MR of the heart: Anatomy, physiology & metabolism. Am J Roentgenol 151:239, 1988
5. HIGGINS CB, SILVERMAN NH, KERSTING-SOMMERHOFF BA, SCHMIDT K. Congenital Heart Disease. Echocardiography and Magnetic Resonance Imaging. New York, Raven Press, 1990
6. PETTIGREW RI. Dynamic magnetic resonance imaging in acquired heart disease. Seminars in Ultrasound, CT, and MR. 12:61, 1991
7. VAN DER WALL EE, DE ROOS A, VAN VOORTHUISEN AE, BRUSCHKE, AVG. Magnetic resonance imaging: A new approach for evaluating coronary artery disease? Am Heart J 121:1203, 1991
8. WOLFE CL. Role of magnetic resonance contrast agents in cardiac imaging. Am J Cardiol 66:59 F, 1990
9. WOLFE CL, MOSELEY ME, WIKSTROM MG, SIEVERS RE, ET AL. Assessment of myocardial salvage after ischemia and reperfusion using magnetic resonance imaging and spectroscopy. Circulation 80:969, 1989

The Face, Mouth, and Jaws

*Paul and Juhl's Essentials of Radiologic Imaging,
Sixth Edition,* edited by John H. Juhl and
Andrew B. Crummy. J.B. Lippincott Company,
Philadelphia, © 1993.

CHAPTER **33**

The Paranasal Sinuses

June M. Unger

Considerable progress in paranasal sinus imaging during the past decade is primarily a result of refinements in CT and MRI. Although its inherent value has been overshadowed by the potential of the more advanced imaging methods, the conventional films continue to provide definitive diagnostic information in certain clinical situations, and serve as a relatively cost-effective screening tool in others. In this chapter we will, therefore, attempt to incorporate all appropriate current imaging methods, emphasizing those that provide optimal information in a particular diagnostic problem.

CONVENTIONAL RADIOGRAPHY

Conventional (plain film) radiography of the paranasal sinuses should provide optimal anatomic detail with maximum contrast. This is accomplished with x-ray beam collimation, the use of a suitable grid to eliminate scatter, and an appropriate film–screen combination. Ideally, the area of interest should be closest to the film in order to reduce unsharpness due to magnification, and all views should be taken with the patient erect in order to demonstrate fluid levels. In the critically ill patient some compromises in positioning may be necessary, including the use of the supine cross-table lateral view for fluid level detection.

The conventional paranasal sinus examination should consist of a minimum of three views: the Caldwell (PA), Waters (occipitomental), and lateral (Figs. 33-1 through 33-3). The primary purpose of the Caldwell view is to visualize the frontal and ethmoid sinuses, while the maxillary sinuses are best demonstrated in the Waters view. In the lateral view the

anterior and posterior walls of the frontal and maxillary sinuses are demonstrated, and there is a moderately unobstructed view of the sphenoid sinus.

If CT is not available, additional information may be gained in problem cases with additional views, such as the base or submentovertical view (Fig. 33-4), and Rheese or optic foramen view (Fig. 35-5). The submentovertical view visualizes the bones of the skull base, as well as providing and axial view of the maxillary sinuses, and portions of the ethmoid and sphenoid sinuses. The Rheese view is the only conventional projection in which the posterior ethmoid cells may be seen without the superimposition of extraneous osseous structures.

EMBRYOLOGY AND ANATOMY

The paranasal sinuses are derived from ectoderm and originate as outpouchings from the nasal cavity. All are normally paired, with the exception of the ethmoid air cells that are multiple.

The maxillary antra or sinuses are the first to appear embryologically, with recognizable development evident during the fourth month of gestation. They are located inframedially with respect to the orbits in the newborn, but extend laterally as they pneumatize the maxillary bone (Fig. 33-6A) until the usual adult configuration has been achieved, at approximately 12 years of age. The mature maxillary sinus consists of a roof, floor, and three walls: the medial, facial, and infratemporal. The roof and medial walls are shared with the orbit and nasal cavity, respectively, forming the orbital floor and lateral wall of the nose. The normal antrum may be

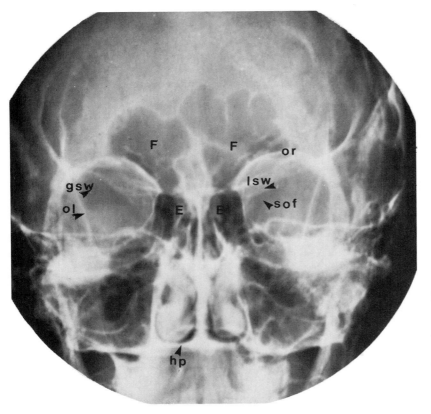

Figure 33–1. Caldwell (PA) view. Frontal sinuses (F), ethmoid sinuses (E). Some of the additional structures visualized include the oblique line of the orbit (ol), superior orbital fissure (sof), orbital rim (or), hard palate (hp), lesser (lsw), and greater sphenoidal wings (gsw).

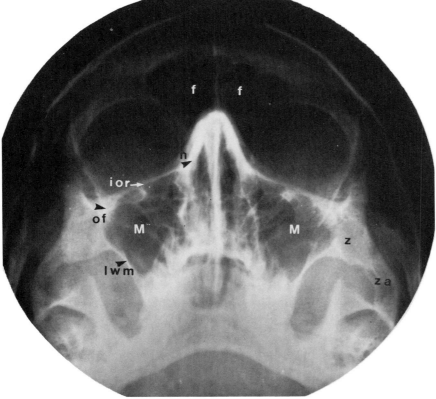

Figure 33–2. Waters view. Maxillary sinus (M). Other structures seen include the lateral wall of the maxillary sinus (lwm), inferior orbital rim (ior), orbital floor (of), zygoma (z), zygomatic arch (za), frontal sinus (f), and nasal bones (n).

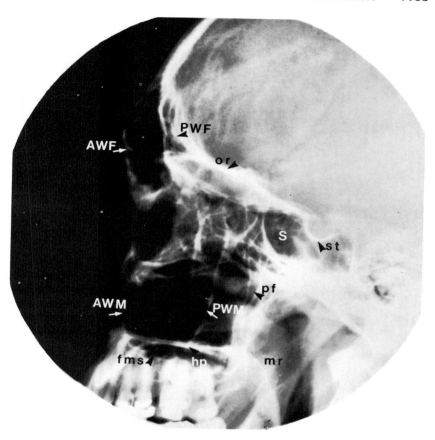

Figure 33–3. Lateral view. Anterior and posterior walls of the frontal sinuses (AWF, PWF), anterior and posterior walls of the maxillary sinuses (AWM, PWM), sphenoid sinus (S). Other structures include the floor of the maxillary sinus (fms), roof of the orbit (or), sella turcica (st), pterygomaxillary fossa (pf), hard palate (hp), and mandibular ramus (mr).

compartmentalized occasionally by membranous or bony septations.

The ethmoid sinuses do not begin to form until the fifth month of gestation, are extremely small at birth, and do not approach adult size until puberty. The number of paired cells, which may range from a few to 18 or more, are anatomically divided into anterior, middle, and posterior groups according to the location of the draining ostia. The ethmoid air cells may remain confined to the ethmoid bone, or invade the adjacent bones of the cranial vault or face.

The frontal sinuses originate as extensions of the anterior ethmoid cells and are usually not recognizable at birth. Development accelerates after infancy but may not be complete until adulthood. Septation, hypoplasia and aplasia are common.

The sphenoid sinuses begin to develop during the fourth intrauterine month but usually do not exceed 2 mm in diameter at birth. Pneumatization is slow until puberty (Fig. 33-6*B*), but is generally completed in the young adult. Pneumatization of other portions of the sphenoid bone, especially the pterygoid processes, is common. Failure of pneumatization resulting in a permanent infantile appearance occurs occasionally.

All of the paranasal sinuses drain into the superior or lateral aspect of the nose. The ostia of the frontal, maxillary, and anterior and middle ethmoid cells drain into a depression, the *hiatus semilunaris*, which is located in the lateral nasal wall at the level of the anterior aspect of the middle meatus. The sphenoid sinuses drain into the sphenoethmoidal recess, which lies above the superior nasal concha, and the posterior ethmoid cells drain into the superior meatus. Some anatomic variability exists (e.g., the frontal sinuses may occasionally drain into the anterior ethmoid air cells). Certain ostia, notably the maxillary and sphenoid, appear to be poorly located physiologically and, in the absence of normal mucociliary clearance, may complicate drainage of accumulated secretions, particularly with the head in the erect or supine position.

INFLAMMATORY DISEASE

Acute inflammation of the paranasal sinuses is usually caused by a rhinovirus and commonly occurs as an accompaniment of upper respiratory tract infection. Bacterial superinfection is most often a result of *Hemo-*

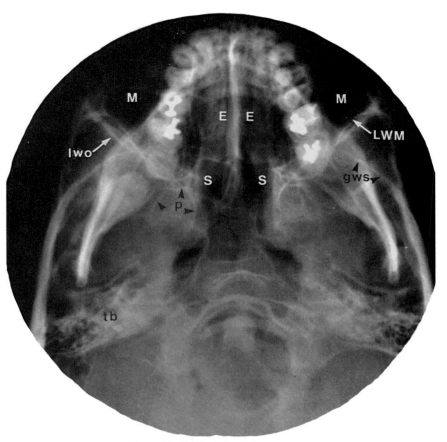

Figure 33–4. Submentovertical (base) view. Maxillary sinuses (M), lateral walls maxillary sinuses (LWM), sphenoid sinus (S), and ethmoid sinuses (E) superimposed on nasal turbinates. Other structures visualized include the lateral wall of the orbit (lwo), greater wing of sphenoid (gsw), pterygoid processes including medial and lateral wings (p), and temporal bone (tb).

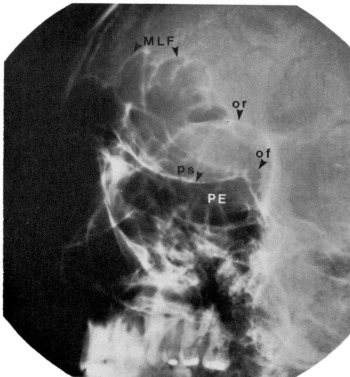

Figure 33–5. Rheese and (optic foramen) view. Posterior ethmoid cells (PE) and mucoperiosteal line of frontal sinuses (MLF). Other structures seen include the optic foramen (of), planum sphenoidale (ps), and orbital rim (or).

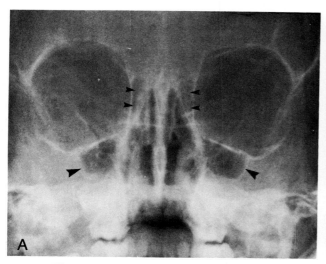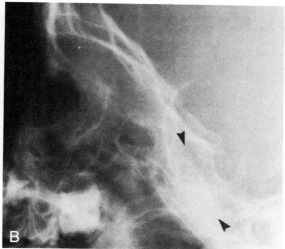

Figure 33–6. Paranasal sinuses in a 3-year-old child. **(A)** PA view. The maxillary antra have begun to extend laterally (*large arrowheads*). The ethmoid air cells are small (*small arrowheads*) and there are no frontal sinuses. **(B)** Lateral view. The body of the sphenoid is not pneumatized (*arrowheads*).

philus or *Streptococcus*. Chronic sinusitis is presumed to develop as an aftermath of acute or recurrent sinusitis that has proved refractory to treatment; cultures most frequently yield anaerobic organisms.

Sinusitis also occurs as an accompaniment of allergic rhinitis, as a complication of dental root infections and extractions, and, uncommonly, as the result of fungus infection. A variety of pathogenic fungi have been incriminated but the more frequent offenders include aspergillus and *Candida*. Sinusitis as a result of aspergillus may be produced by a form of the fungus that occurs in otherwise healthy individuals; *Candida* infections are generally opportunistic, occurring in patients either on long-term antibiotics or who are chronically ill or debilitated. The most devastating fungus infections, however, are those produced by the phycomycetes group, which causes rhinocerebral mucormycosis.

Conventional films usually confirm a diagnosis of sinusitis. Fluid levels, mucosal thickening, and opacification of the normally aerated sinus lumen establish the diagnosis. Air–fluid levels are most often the result of accumulated secretions in patients with sinusitis. They usually occur as a result of bleeding after acute trauma, and may also be found after antral lavage. Erect or cross-table lateral films are required for detection (Fig. 33-7).

Mucosal thickening produces a soft-tissue opacity of variable width that follows the inner contours of the sinus walls (Fig. 33-8). An opaque sinus is an airless

sinus that is filled with fluid, thickened mucosa, or a combination of both (Fig. 33-9).

Decrease in density of the bony sinus walls may accompany sinusitis. This is generally most apparent in the frontal sinuses when the sharp white boundary of the mucoperiosteal line is diminished (Fig. 33-10). The thin bony walls of the ethmoid air cells are indis-

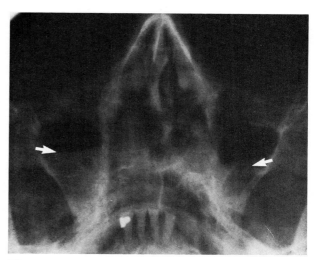

Figure 33–7. Erect Waters view. Note the bilateral fluid levels (*arrows*), consistent with acute sinusitis.

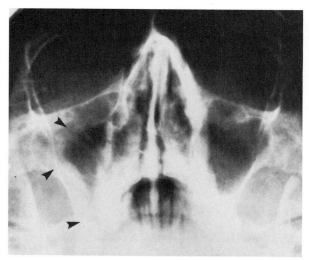

Figure 33–8. Waters view. The mucosa of the roof and lateral wall of the right maxillary antrum is thickened (*arrowheads*).

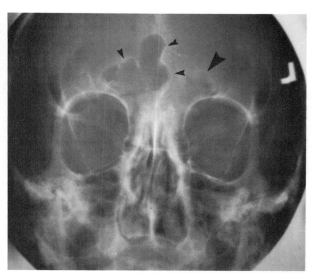

Figure 33–10. Caldwell view. The thin white mucoperiosteal line of the normal right frontal sinus is indicated by the small arrowheads. The left frontal sinus is diseased, and the mucoperiosteal line is indistinct (*large arrowhead*).

tinguishable in the presence of ethmoid opacification, and the density of the osseous walls of the remaining sinuses may more closely approximate that of the soft-tissue contents when there is mucosal thickening, fluid, or opacification present. Although these changes may indicate demineralization, they may also be artifactually produced as a result of the loss of the normal air–bone interface.

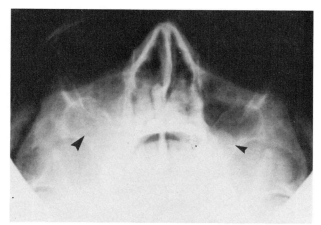

Figure 33–9. Waters view. Opacification of the right maxillary antrum (*large arrowhead*). A small mucous retention cyst or serous cyst is present at the base of the left maxillary antrum (*small arrowhead*).

In the presence of chronic infection, the early osseous changes of demineralization may be followed by sclerosis with an apparent increase in density and actual increase in thickness of the sinus walls, presumably as a result of stimulation of the periosteum by the irritant effect of the sinus contents. This is best seen in the maxillary sinuses (Fig. 33-11), but may also be apparent in the frontal sinuses.

It is often impossible to differentiate acute from chronic sinusitis by imaging methods because mucosal thickening and opacification are common to both. The single distinguishing feature of acute sinusitis is the air–fluid level, whereas the only characteristic finding in chronic sinusitis is the sclerotic, thickened bone of the sinus wall.

The maxillary sinuses are the most commonly involved of the paranasal sinuses in both acute and chronic sinusitis, followed by the ethmoid and frontal sinuses. Although sphenoid sinusitis is reputedly least frequent, it may also be underdiagnosed by conventional techniques. The common occurrence of sphenoid sinusitis on CT scans of the head suggests a higher incidence than usually assumed. Pansinusitis is prevalent in acute upper respiratory viral infections and in allergic states. Isolated sinus involvement is more frequently a result of acute or chronic bacterial superinfection.

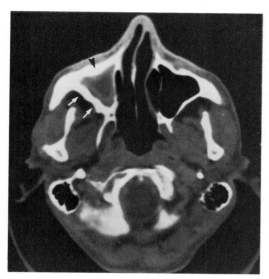

Figure 33–11. Axial CT, midplane of maxillary sinuses. There is appreciable thickening of the bone of the anterior and lateral walls of the right maxillary sinus (*black arrowhead* and *white arrows*). Thickened mucosa surrounds a central area of lower density that may represent fluid.

COMPLICATIONS OF INFLAMMATORY DISEASE

The complications of sinusitis include mucous retention cysts, serous cysts, mucoceles, osteomyelitis, and intraorbital and intracranial infections.

The mucous retention cyst is a true cyst with an epithelial lining. It is formed by the accumulation of secretions within an occluded mucous gland. The serous cyst is produced by submucosal fluid accumulation, has no epithelial lining, and is therefore not a true cyst. Either cyst may present as a smoothly marginated mass, usually in the inferior portion of a maxillary sinus. They are clinically asymptomatic, radiographically indistinguishable from each other, and may persist for months.

Mucoceles form secondary to accumulation of secretions as a result of occlusion of a sinus ostium by mucosal edema or inspissated mucus, often in patients with a history of previous facial trauma. They are characterized by total sinus opacification with thinning and expansion of the sinus walls. The mucocele contents occasionally appear relatively radiolucent, a phenomenon that was originally thought to be the result of the nature of the mucocele contents, but more recently has been attributed to the coexistent thinning of bone (Fig. 33-12).[2] Most mucoceles involve the frontal sinuses; approximately 25% occur in the ethmoids (Fig. 33-13).

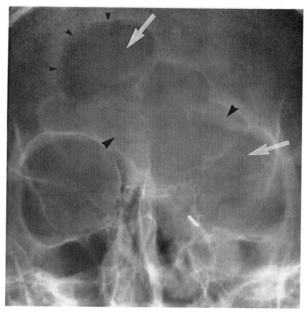

Figure 33–12. Caldwell view. Bilateral frontal mucoceles. Note the relative radiolucency of the mucoceles (*white arrows*) compared with the adjacent mucosal thickening (*black medium-sized arrowheads*). Expansion and thinning of the mucocele wall is better seen on the right (*small black arrowheads*). The expanded left superior orbital rim is no longer identifiable. Wire indicates previous surgery in the area of the frontonasal ducts.

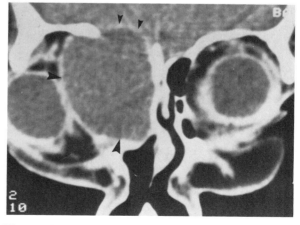

Figure 33–13. Coronal CT. A large mucocele replaces the right ethmoid air cells. The thickened lamina papyracea (*large arrowheads*) bulges into the right orbit and displaces the globe laterally. Marked thinning of the medial portion of the orbital rim has occurred (*small arrowheads*). (Case courtesy of F. Quiroz, MD).

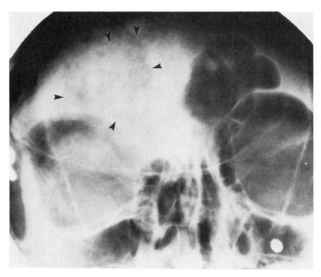

Figure 33–14. Caldwell view. Chronic osteomyelitis of the frontal bone. There is dense sclerosis with areas of relative radiolucency that probably represent involucra (*arrowheads*).

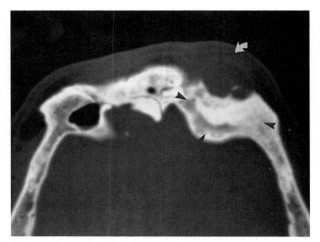

Figure 33–15. Axial CT, bone window. Pott's puffy tumor. There is soft-tissue swelling over the left frontal area (*white arrow*) and changes consistent with osteomyelitis in the walls of the opacified left frontal sinus (*black arrowheads*).

Maxillary mucoceles are uncommon, and sphenoid mucoceles are rare. An infected mucocele is called a pyocele.

Osteomyelitis usually develops as a complication of frontal sinusitis, but is occasionally found, following dental infection, in the maxillary sinuses of children. In the frontal sinuses there is loss of the normal mucoperiosteal line, followed by subsequent patchy osseous rarefaction that may progress to irregular areas of bone thickening, sclerosis, and sequestrum formation (Fig. 33-14). When there is associated anterior pericranial (subperiosteal) abscess, the overlying swelling of the forehead is known as Pott's puffy tumor (Fig. 33-15).[5]

Intracranial infection develops from sinusitis by direct spread through bone, along perineural soft tissues, or by a venous route. The frontal sinusitis is the usual source of infection, but it may also originate in the ethmoid and sphenoid sinuses. Intracranial abscess, meningitis, or cavernous sinus thrombosis may result. The formerly high incidence of these life-threatening situations has been reduced to approximately 3% through the use of antibiotics.

Infection of the orbits in paranasal sinus disease is most often a result of direct spread from the ethmoids or, rarely, the sphenoid sinuses, through sinus walls or by venous channels. It is more common in children than adults, possibly reflecting a higher incidence of upper respiratory tract infection. The usual complications include orbital cellulitis, retrobulbar neuritis, and orbital abscess. CT or MRI are the best imaging methods for establishing the diagnosis (Fig. 33-16).

POLYPOID RHINOSINUSITIS

Polypoid degeneration of the paranasal sinus mucosa has been considered by some to represent a complication of sinusitis, although the precise etiology has never been determined. Allergy, tobacco, and certain drugs have all been incriminated. Although principally a disease of adults occurring in approximately 4% of the

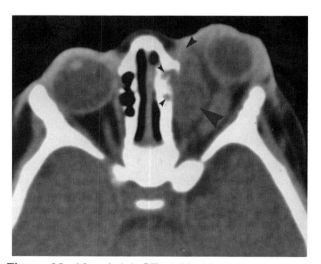

Figure 33–16. Axial CT, midorbital plane. Four-month-old child with left ethmoid sinusitis. A few opacified ethmoid air cells are visible (*small arrowheads*). The inflammatory process has produced both preseptal cellulitis (*medium arrowhead*) and intraorbital abscess (*large arrowhead*).

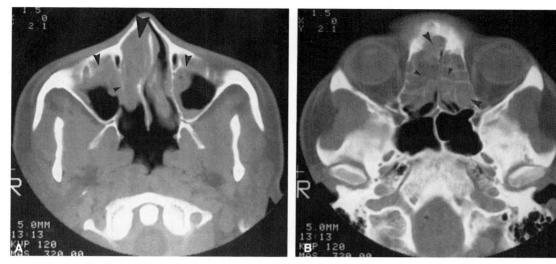

Figure 33–17. (**A**) Axial CT, maxillary sinuses. Polypoid rhinosinusitis. Polypoid mucosal hypertrophy involves the anteromedial wall of both maxillary sinuses (*medium arrowheads*), and fills the anterior portion of the right nasal cavity (*large arrowhead*), causing deviation of the nasal septum. Note the marked thinning and apparent destructive change in the medial wall of the right maxillary sinus (*small arrowhead*). A small fluid level is present in the left maxillary sinus. (**B**) Axial CT, ethmoid sinuses. The ethmoid air cells are opacified by a combination of polypoid mucosal hypertrophy (*large arrowheads*) and retained secretions (*small arrowheads*). The ethmoid expansion had produced hypertelorism.

population, it is also common in children who have cystic fibrosis.

The mucosal hypertrophy ultimately results in hypervascular polypoid masses that contain inflammatory cells and eosinophils. Although these masses generally present clinically in the nasal cavity, they almost always involve multiple sinuses simultaneously, and there is usually coexistent sinusitis. CT is useful in delineating their polypoid character and in differentiating them from simple mucosal thickening. Continuous proliferation of the polyps may result in expansile and destructive changes in the sinus walls, mimicking those produced by malignant disease (Fig. 33-17).

GRANULOMATOUS DISEASE

The nose and paranasal sinuses may be affected by a number of granulomatous diseases including tuberculosis, syphilis, Wegener granulomatosis, midline granuloma, and sarcoid. All of these originate in the nose and secondarily involve the sinuses, especially the maxillary antra. Initial mucosal thickening indistinguishable from sinusitis may result in varying degrees of destructive change that can involve the nasal septum, palate, and sinus walls, producing changes that simulate malignancy (Fig. 33-18).

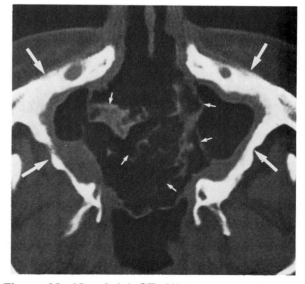

Figure 33–18. Axial CT. Wegener granulomatosis. The nasal cavity and medial maxillary sinus walls have been destroyed. Strands of abnormal tissue are present (*small arrows*). There is irregular thickening of the lateral antral walls (*large arrows*). (Case courtesy of K. Shaffer, MD).

BENIGN TUMORS

Only about one third of the neoplasms that occur in the paranasal sinuses are benign. With the exception of osteomas, these tumors usually arise in the maxillary sinuses, and are similar in appearance, presenting as well-circumscribed soft-tissue masses that may expand or thin sinus walls, but are not characteristically destructive. Osteomas, epithelial papillomas, antrochoanal polyps, and plasmacytomas are among the more typical lesions. A variety of relatively rare benign tumors may originate from any of the neurogenic, vascular, or osseous cellular elements. The sinuses may also be secondarily involved by extension of benign tumors from the pituitary gland, nasopharynx, orbit, and maxillary dental area.

The most common benign paranasal sinus tumor is the osteoma, which usually originates in the frontal sinuses near the frontoethmoid suture. Osteomas are also found in the ethmoids but are rare in the maxillary and sphenoid sinuses. Most osteomas are of the hard or ivory type and consist of compact bone. They present radiographically as dense, well-marginated intrasinus structures (Fig. 33-19). A variant, the soft or cancellous osteoma, occasionally may be sufficiently lacking in density to be confused with a soft-tissue mass. Most osteomas are characteristic radiographically and normally slow growing; unless there is obstruction of a sinus ostium or cosmetic deformity, they are usually not removed surgically.

The epithelial papilloma is a true polyp, as opposed to the pseudopolyps found in polypoid rhinosinusitis. Two types, squamous or inverting, depend on the histologic disposition of the surface epithelium. The squamous papilloma is a simple polypoid growth. The inverting papilloma, however, tends to exhibit certain aggressive growth characteristics, which include bone involvement, and may be difficult to differentiate radiologically from a malignant lesion (Fig. 33-20). Moreover, although malignant transformation is virtually unknown in the squamous papilloma, it has been reported in as many as 10% of inverting papillomas.

Extramedullary plasmacytomas are rare. Eighty percent occur in the head and neck, principally in the nose and paranasal sinuses, and most more often in middle-aged men. They generally present as solitary soft-tissue masses that may be polypoid or invasive; the prognosis is better with the polypoid type. Although these lesions are radiosensitive, the primary treatment consists of surgical removal. Radiotherapy is reserved for recurrence, which is common.

The antrochoanal polyp is an adenomatous polyp that, while similar histologically to the pseudopolyps found in polypoid rhinosinusitis, differs in behavior. It originates in a maxillary sinus and is extruded through the sinus ostium into the nose, subsequently presenting as a smooth, rounded mass in the nasopharynx (Fig. 33-21). Ipsilateral nasal and maxillary sinus opacification are usually present.

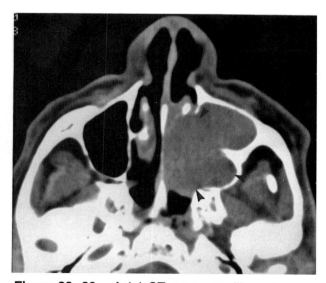

Figure 33–20. Axial CT scan, maxillary sinuses. Inverting papilloma. A large soft-tissue mass fills the left maxillary sinus and the major portion of the left nasal cavity. The medial antral wall has been destroyed and the posterolateral wall of the sinus is displaced (*arrowheads*). The papilloma also extended into the left orbit (Fig. 33–21).

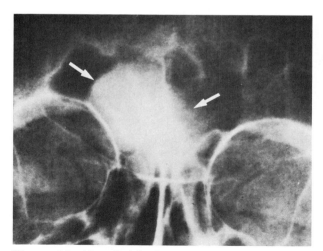

Figure 33–19. Caldwell view. Ivory osteoma. The large bony mass fills most of the right frontal sinus and extends into the left (*arrows*).

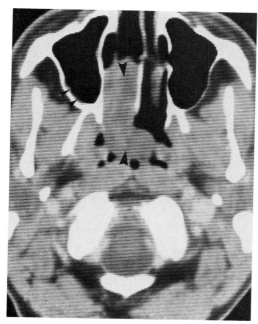

Figure 33–21. Axial CT. Antrochoanal polyp. A large soft-tissue mass fills the posterior aspect of the right nasal cavity and extends into the nasopharynx (*large arrowheads*). Minimal mucosal thickening is present in the right maxillary sinus (*small arrowheads*). This is exceptional; ipsilateral sinus opacification is usually present.

MALIGNANT TUMORS

Malignant neoplasms of the nose and paranasal sinuses constitute approximately 3% of cancers of the upper aerodigestive tract.[1] Most are squamous-cell carcinomas; the remaining neoplasms are large adenocarcinomas, adenoid cystic carcinomas, melanomas, and lymphomas. All other primary malignant sinus tumors are extremely rare and consist essentially of different types of sarcomas. The majority of these tumors arise in the maxillary sinuses, with the exception of melanomas, which more commonly originate in the nasal cavity. Because most of the neoplasms are advanced at the time of diagnosis, local invasion is prevalent. Five-year survival rates generally are poor, ranging from 10% to 25%, depending on cell type. In general, the best prognosis is found in squamous-cell carcinomas and lymphomas.

These cancers characteristically appear as aggressive soft-tissue masses that occlude sinus ostia, exhibit local soft-tissue invasion, and cause bone destruction (Fig. 33-22).[4] In advanced tumors the origin may be imposs-

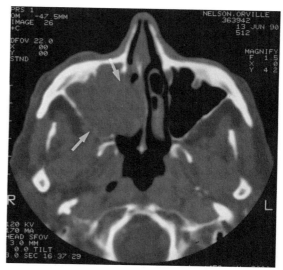

Figure 33–22. Axial CT, maxillary sinuses, bone window. Squamous-cell carcinoma. The right maxillary sinus and nasal cavity are opacified and there is destruction of both the medial and posterolateral sinus walls (*arrows*).

ible to determine, but statistically the epicenter is usually in the maxillary sinus. Any or all of the osseous sinus walls may be destroyed, as well as the adjacent bone of the face and skull (Fig. 33-23). Involvement of the pterygomaxillary and infratemporal fossae is a generally accepted contraindication to surgery (Fig. 33-24). CT is the best imaging method for evaluating bone destruction, while MRI is the method of choice for visualizing the soft tissues for extent of tumor, and separating tumor from retained secretions (Figs. 33-25A and B).

Approximately one third of patients will eventually develop metastasis to the cervical lymph nodes. Distant metastases to lung and bone are more frequently caused by adenoid cystic carcinomas than by the other cell types.

METASTATIC AND INVASIVE TUMORS

The paranasal sinuses may be invaded directly by malignant intracranial neoplasms, and tumors of the orbit, nasopharynx, oral cavity, and facial skin (Figs. 33-26 and 33-27). Metastasis to the paranasal sinuses from distant sites is uncommon and generally occurs through hematogenous spread. The kidney, lung, and breast are the most frequent sources.

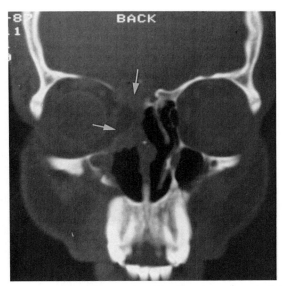

Figure 33–23. Coronal CT. Carcinoma of right maxillary sinus. There has been a partial right maxillectomy with resection of the inferior turbinate. Recurrent tumor has extended into the right ethmoid sinus and destroyed portions of the medial orbital wall and cribiform plate (*arrows*).

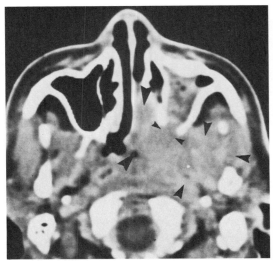

Figure 33–24. Axial CT. Mucoepidermoid carcinoma, left maxillary sinus. The tumor has extended into the left nasal cavity and nasopharynx (*large arrowheads*). There is destruction of the pterygoid process (*small arrowheads*) and extension of tumor into the infratemporal fossa (*medium arrowheads*).

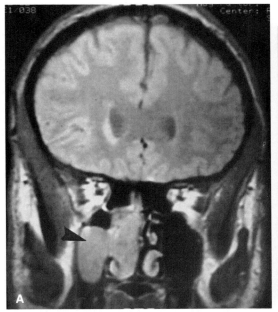
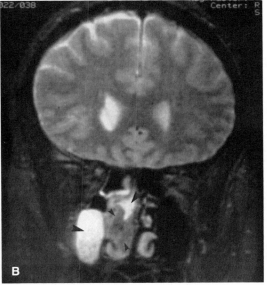

Figure 33–25. (**A**) Coronal MRI, T1-weighted. Squamous-cell carcinoma originating in the ethmoid sinus. A mass of intermediate echogenicity is seen filling the right nasal cavity and ethmoidomaxillary sinus complex (*arrowhead*). (**B**) The corresponding T2-weighted image clearly shows the demarcation between the intermediate signal of the tumor (*small arrowheads*), and the high signal of the retained secretions (*large arrowheads*).

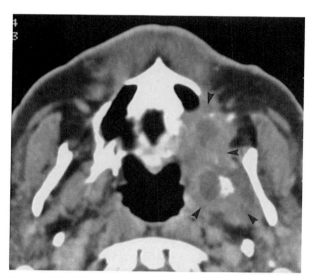

Figure 33–26. Axial CT. Carcinoma of the left alveolar ridge. Necrotizing tumor has invaded the left maxillary sinus, pterygomaxillary fossa, and parapharyngeal space (*arrowheads*). There is destruction of the hard palate, ipsilateral maxillary sinus walls, and pterygoid plates.

NONNEOPLASTIC LESIONS

Fibrous dysplasia, a bone disorder of unknown etiology, is characterized by fibroosseous proliferation with replacement of medullary cavities. Although it may involve one or more bones, the monostotic type is more common. The polyostotic form tends to produce asymmetric deformities and is associated with Albright's syndrome. The lesions may appear cystic, sclerotic or exhibit a ground-glass appearance, depending on the amount of fibrous tissue present. Facial involvement is asymmetric, and expansile, frequently obliterating one or more of the paranasal sinuses (Fig. 33-28). The radiographic appearance is usually sufficiently typical to establish the diagnosis without biopsy.

Craniometaphyseal dysplasia is a rare hereditary disorder that, unlike fibrous dysplasia, always produces densely sclerotic expansile changes in the bones of the face and skull. Involvement tends to be symmetric and produces appreciable deformity, often creating a leonine appearance. Splaying of the metaphysis of tubular bones is an associated finding.

Meningoceles and encephaloceles consist of herniated meninges or brain, respectively. They can be congenital or may be acquired as the result of trauma. Protrusion of intracranial contents into the nose or paranasal sinuses occurs through osseous defects and may resemble a polyp or other soft-tissue mass. The defect in the bone is usually well circumscribed and may have a sclerotic border.

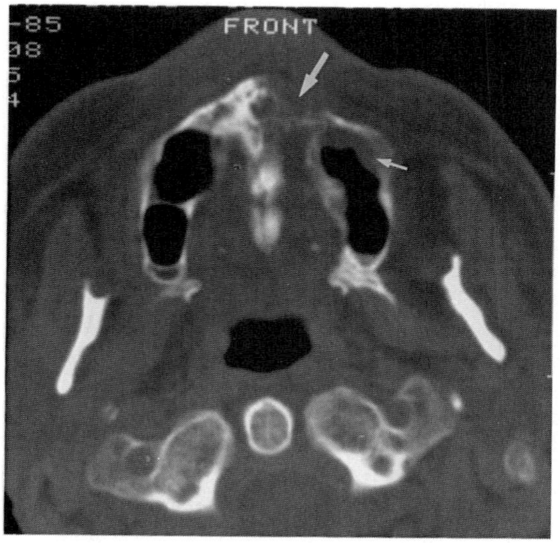

Figure 33–27. Axial CT. Basal cell carcinoma of the face invading the left maxillary sinus. Bone destruction is present anteriorly (*large arrow*). There is focal thickening of the antral mucosa (*small arrow*).

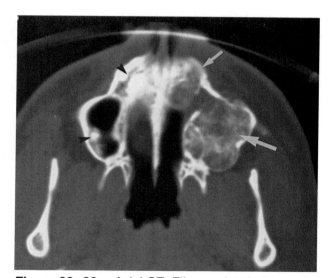

Figure 33–28. Axial CT. Fibrous dysplasia involving the maxillary sinuses. There is an expansile ground-glasslike mass enlarging the left sinus (*white arrows*), and early bone changes on the right (*black arrowheads*).

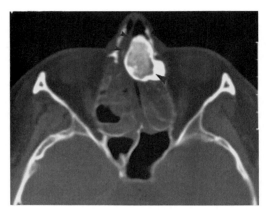

Figure 33–29. Axial CT, bone window. Rhinolith. A large calcified mass is in the anterior portion of the left nasal cavity (*large arrowhead*). Note the deviation of the nasal septum (*small arrowheads*).

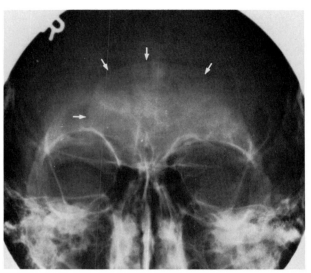

Figure 33–30. Caldwell view. Osteoplastic frontal flap. The margins are still distinct (*arrows*).

Rhinoliths are sclerotic masses that develop as a result of calcium deposition around a foreign body. While characteristically found in the nose (Fig. 33-29), they may occasionally occur in the maxillary sinus.

Other unusual, nonneoplastic masses include dermoids, nasal gliomas, hemangiomas, and globulomaxillary and odontogenic cysts.

THE POSTOPERATIVE SINUS

The postoperative appearance of a paranasal sinus will, obviously, vary with the type of surgery performed. Although similarities exist between related procedures, differences in surgical technique may produce considerable variability in the radiographic appearance. The following discussion will be limited to a few of the more common operations.

The osteoplastic frontal flap was devised as a cosmetically acceptable treatment for the complications of frontal sinusitis. Using a radiographic template cut from an unmagnified Caldwell view, the frontal bone overlying the sinuses is exposed and separated at the periphery of the frontal sinuses with a saw. The diseased mucosa is removed, the sinuses packed with muscle and fat, and the bone replaced. Postoperatively the sinuses will appear opacified, with changes that may occasionally be confused with those associated with a mucocele (Fig. 33-30).

The Caldwell-Luc approach is used principally for the treatment of chronic maxillary sinusitis, the removal of intrasinus masses and biopsy. Sinus exposure is created through a maxillary antrostomy, which is made by a sublabial incision in the anterolateral gingival buccal mucosa. A defect is then made in the lateral nasal wall, producing a nasoantral window for improvement of sinus drainage. After healing has occurred, the sinus may appear radiographically normal or reflect changes due to surgery. These include decrease in volume due to antral contraction, fibro-osseous proliferation causing thickening of sinus walls (Fig. 33-31), and compartmentalization of the sinus lumen by bony septa.[3]

Ethmoidectomy may be performed endoscopically, by the external approach (the Lynch procedure), the intranasal route or the transmaxillary route. The endoscopic route has become popular as a means of restoration of the ostiomeatal complex in patients with impaired mucociliary clearance due to localized disease.[6] Intranasal ethmoidectomy is generally performed as a means of eradicating chronic ethmoid sinusitis. The middle turbinate may be fractured or removed for purposes of exposure. An attempt is then made to remove all ethmoid cells and mucosa. Postoperative radiographs usually show loss of the middle turbinate and a monolocular space, which replaces the ethmoid air cells and communicates with the upper portion of the nasal cavity (Fig. 33-32). If a Caldwell-Luc procedure is performed at the time of ethmoidectomy in order to eradicate maxillary sinus disease, postoperative changes from this procedure may also be evident radiographically.

Partial or total maxillectomy is generally reserved for

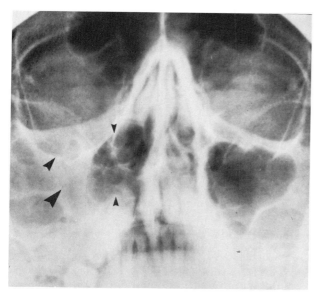

Figure 33–31. Waters view. Post right Caldwell-Luc procedure. There is marked fibroosseous proliferation (*large arrowhead*), which encroaches on the sinus lumen. The orbital floor is depressed (*medium arrowhead*), contributing to the reduction in sinus size. The large nasoantral window is indicated by the small arrowheads.

the treatment of rhinocerebral mucormycosis and malignant neoplasms. Because any of the adjacent bone or soft tissue may be sacrificed, the postoperative roentgenographic appearance can exhibit marked variability. Any reliable assessment of recurrence necessitates baseline postoperative CT or MRI for subsequent comparisons (Fig. 33-33).

Sphenoid surgery is usually performed for benign masses such as polyps or mucoceles, although the sphenoid sinus is also involved when pituitary tumors are removed by the transphenoidal route. CT is essential to identify surgical changes in the sphenoid wall. Some degree of pneumatization is almost always retained (Fig. 33-34).

RADIATION

Radiation therapy for malignant neoplasms can produce changes in both soft tissues and bone, the degree of which will depend on the initial tumor size, radiation dosage, and prior surgery. The usual reaction in bone consists of a sterile osteomyelitis or osteoradionecrosis, which appear as areas of rarefaction radiographically. It

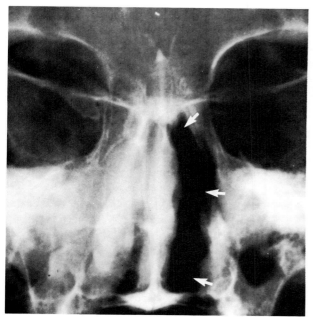

Figure 33–32. Caldwell view. Postintranasal ethmoidectomy for polypoid rhinosinusitis. The contents of the left nasal fossa and adjacent ethmoids have been removed (*arrows*). There is persistent disease in the remaining sinuses.

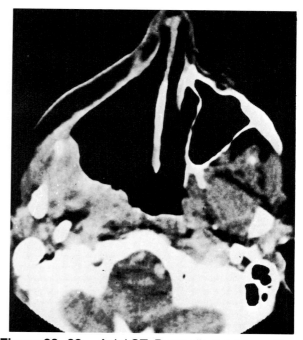

Figure 33–33. Axial CT. Postradical right maxillectomy. The right maxillary sinus, pterygoid process, and structures contained within the right nasal cavity have been removed. (Case courtesy of K. Shaffer, MD).

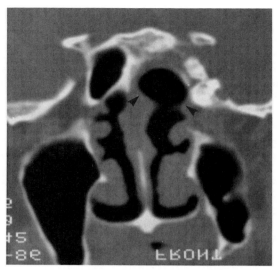

Figure 33–34. Coronal CT. Transphenoidal hypophysectomy. There is absence of bone in the anterior aspect of the floor of the left sphenoid sinus (*arrowheads*).

may be difficult to differentiate these changes from invasive or recurrent tumor.

REFERENCES AND SELECTED READINGS

1. BATSAKIS JG. Tumors of the Head and Neck, 2nd ed. Baltimore, Williams & Wilkins, 1979
2. SOM PM. Sinonasal cavity. In Som PM, Bergeron RT (Eds.). Head and Neck Imaging, 2nd ed. St. Louis, CV Mosby, 1991
3. UNGER JM. Head and Neck Imaging. New York, Churchill–Livingstone, 1987
4. WEBER AL, STANTON AD: Malignant tumors of the paranasal sinuses: Radiologic, clinical, and histopathologic evaluation of 200 cases. Head Neck Surg 6:761, 1984
5. WELLS RG, STY JR, LANDERS AD. Radiological evaluation of Pott puffy tumor. JAMA 255:1331, 1986
6. ZINREICH SJ, KENNEDY DW, ROSENBAUM AE, ET AL. Paranasal sinuses: CT imaging requirements for endoscopic surgery. Radiology 163:769–775, 1987

Paul and Juhl's Essentials of Radiologic Imaging, Sixth Edition, edited by John H. Juhl and Andrew B. Crummy. J.B. Lippincott Company, Philadelphia, © 1993.

CHAPTER **34**

Facial Trauma

June M. Unger

The facial skeleton is conveniently divided into upper, middle, and lower thirds for purposes of fracture description. The upper third consists primarily of the frontal bone and orbits; the middle third largely comprises the maxillae, nasal bones and zygomatic arches; and the lower third is principally made up of the mandible. Fractures involving any one of these areas have distinctive features that merit separate consideration.

Conventional radiography and CT are the imaging methods of choice. MRI is currently reserved for visualization of the complications of trauma, such as intraorbital hematoma, and may even be contraindicated in certain acute injuries, particularly those in which there may be ferromagnetic foreign bodies present.[6]

FRONTAL SINUS FRACTURES

Frontal sinus fractures can be caused by direct trauma, represent an extension of cranial vault or base of skull fractures, or accompany other facial fractures. They may be linear, comminuted, or complex. Linear fractures usually involve only the anterior sinus wall, whereas complex fractures, which are commonly associated with other facial trauma, consist of fractures of both the anterior and posterior walls (Fig. 34-1). A fluid level or sinus opacification as a result of hemorrhage or mucosal edema is typical, and depending on the fracture location, there may be orbital emphysema or pneumocephaly. These fractures are ordinarily demonstrated on conventional Caldwell and lateral views, but fragment displacement is better identified with CT.

ORBITAL FRACTURES

Fractures of the orbit occur as isolated injuries or in combination with other facial or cranial fractures. They may be simple or complex.

SIMPLE FRACTURES

Simple fractures are of two kinds: those that involve only the orbital rim, and those of the blowout type, which involve the orbital walls. Because the orbital rim is the strongest part of the orbit, isolated rim fractures are uncommon.

Blowout fractures are produced by a sudden increase in intraorbital pressure caused by violent impact from an external force, such as a fist or ball. The weaker portions of the orbit are fractured, usually the orbital floor and frequently the medial wall. A blowout fracture is considered pure if only the orbital floor or medial wall is involved, and impure if there is a coexistent fracture of the orbital rim.

Radiographic findings in blowout fractures include floor disruption, ipsilateral sinus opacification because of hemorrhage, and orbital emphysema resulting from interruption of the roof of the adjacent maxillary sinus or *lamina papyracea* of the ethmoid sinuses.[3] These abnormalities are usually visible on conventional Waters, Caldwell, and lateral views; CT may be required for more precise fracture detail (Fig. 34-2) and is essential for the diagnosis of most medial wall fractures (Fig. 34-3).

The major complication of blowout fractures is mus-

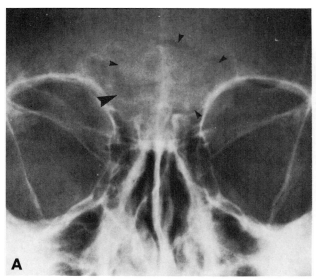
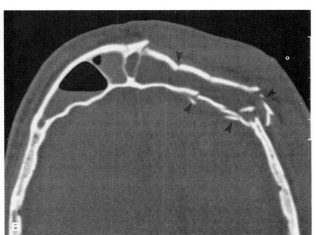

Figure 34–1.   Complex frontal sinus fracture. **(A)** Caldwell view. There is opacification of the frontal sinus (*large arrowhead*). Multiple comminuted fracture fragments are present (*small arrowheads*). **(B)** Axial CT scan in a different patient. There is comminution of both the anterior and posterior walls of the left frontal sinus (*arrowheads*), accompanied by sinus opacification and an air–fluid level in the right frontal sinus.

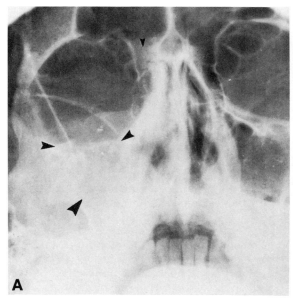
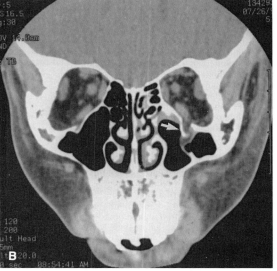

Figure 34–2.   Blowout fractures. **(A)** Waters view. The right orbital floor is depressed (*medium arrowheads*) and there is opacification of the right maxillary sinus (*large arrowhead*). The right ethmoid air cells are also opacified (*small arrowhead*) suggesting the presence of a medial wall blowout fracture, which was subsequently confirmed by tomography. **(B)** Coronal CT in a different patient. A trapdoor fragment (*arrow*) consisting of a portion of the left orbital floor is within the left maxillary sinus. A small amount of herniated orbital fat accompanies the fragment.

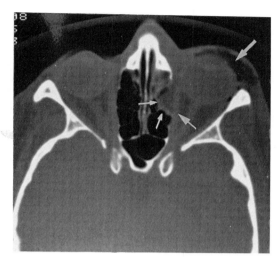

Figure 34–3. Axial CT. Isolated medial wall blowout fracture. There is depression of fracture fragments into the adjacent ethmoid air cells, which are opacified (*small arrows*). There is no evidence of entrapment of the medial rectus muscle (*medium arrow*). Orbital emphysema is present (*large arrow*).

cle entrapment. Both the inferior rectus and inferior oblique muscles can be trapped in floor fractures, whereas medial rectus entrapment may occur in medial wall fractures. Fractures that involve the infraorbital foramen may produce anesthesia over the distribution of the infraorbital nerve.

COMPLEX FRACTURES

Complex fractures of the orbit are produced in tripod fractures, Le Fort II and III injuries, and may be an accompaniment of trauma to the cranial vault or base. The inferior and lateral orbital rim and floor are fractured in the usual tripod fracture (see Fig. 34-16). Complications are related to the injury sites and similar to those described in impure blowout fractures. The sites of orbital involvement in Le Fort II and III injuries differ (see Fig. 34-9). In the Le Fort II fracture complex, the medial portion of the orbit is damaged, whereas both the medial and lateral aspect of the orbit are included in Le Fort III fractures (Fig. 34-4).

Severe cranial trauma may produce fractures limited to a particular site, such as the orbital roof, or, by extension of fracture lines, involve the orbital apex, which contains both the optic foramen and the superior orbital fissure. Orbital apex fractures may be linear and undisplaced, comminuted (Fig. 34-5), or consist of complete avulsion of the apex, with the apical fragment containing an intact optic foramen.[5] Complications include optic nerve damage; the superior orbital fissure syndrome because of injury to cranial nerves III, IV, and VI; and the orbital apex syndrome, which is due to a combination of optic nerve damage and the superior orbital fissure syndrome. All suspected complex fractures, with the possible exception of the uncomplicated tripod fracture, should be imaged with CT; small fracture fragments and damage to intraorbital contents cannot be demonstrated adequately by conventional techniques.

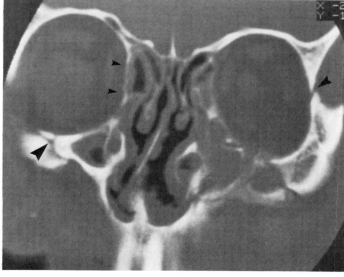

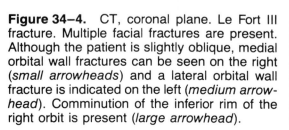

Figure 34–4. CT, coronal plane. Le Fort III fracture. Multiple facial fractures are present. Although the patient is slightly oblique, medial orbital wall fractures can be seen on the right (*small arrowheads*) and a lateral orbital wall fracture is indicated on the left (*medium arrowhead*). Comminution of the inferior rim of the right orbit is present (*large arrowhead*).

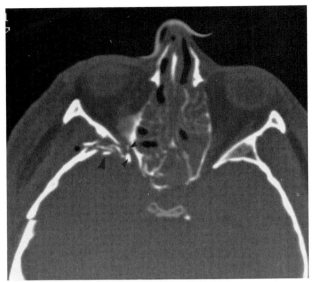

Figure 34–5. Axial CT. Comminuted right orbital apex fracture. The right sphenoid wing is fractured (*large arrowhead*) and there is displacement of fragments into the superior orbital fissure (*small arrowheads*).

MIDFACE FRACTURES

Fractures of the midfacial skeleton may be isolated to a single bone or may present as a complex group of associated fractures, such as those originally described by Le Fort, or as the more laterally situated tripod fracture. Although fractures of the nasal bones and zygomatic arches are actually midface fractures, they are usually considered separately by virtue of their genesis and management.

ISOLATED MEDIAL AND LATERAL MIDFACE FRACTURES

Isolated medial and lateral midface fractures are usually the result of a direct blow to a small area. If nasal bone fractures are excluded, midface fractures can be considered to principally involve the maxilla and zygoma. The anterolateral wall of the maxillary sinus and alveolar process of the maxilla are frequent sites of predilection. Either fracture may be difficult to diagnose with conventional views of the facial bones, and are more adequately visualized with CT (Figs. 34-6 and 34-7).

The zygoma is frequently fractured in complex midface fractures (*vide infra*), but isolated fractures of the zygomatic arch are relatively uncommon. The arch

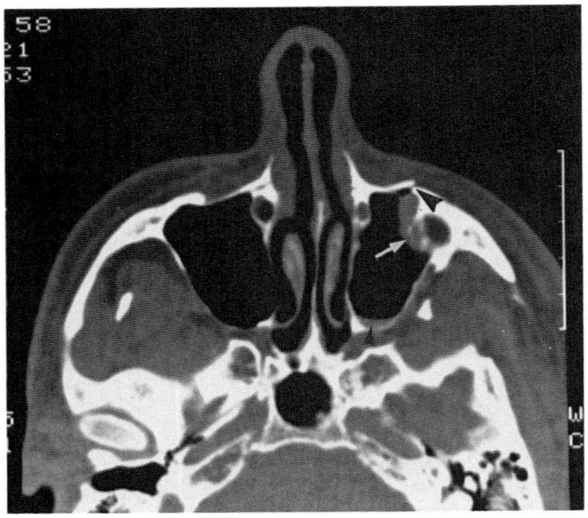

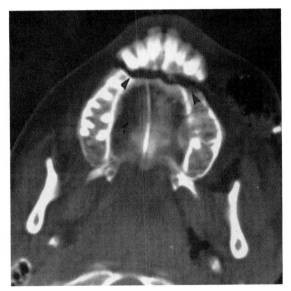

Figure 34–6. Axial CT. Fracture of anterior wall of the left maxillary sinus. There is minimal anterior displacement of the fragment (*large arrowhead*). Adherent blood clot (*white arrow*) and a small fluid level are present in the sinus (*small arrowhead*).

Figure 34–7. Axial CT. Fracture through the alveolar process of the maxilla. The diastatic fracture line crosses the anterior aspect of the hard palate (*arrowheads*).

tends to fracture anteriorly, in the midportion or posteriorly, and fractures may be single, multiple, displaced, or undisplaced. Treatment is not required for the undisplaced single fracture. Multiple fractures, which are more common, are often displaced and require reduction to prevent permanent facial deformity (Fig. 34-8).[4]

Conventional radiography of the zygomatic arch is generally sufficient for detection of zygomatic arch fractures. The submentovertical projection, or an oblique variation of it, known as the "jug-handle" view is ordinarily used. CT may be necessary to confirm suspected

coronoid process impingement due to arch fragment displacement.

LE FORT FRACTURES

Le Fort fractures involve the midfacial skeleton in a predictable manner (Fig. 34-9). They are bilateral and, as originally described, symmetric. The Le Fort I, or Guerin fracture is a transverse fracture that transects the inferior aspect of the maxilla above the line of

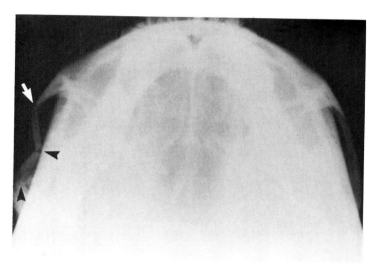

Figure 34–8. Submentovertical projection. Comminuted, depressed fracture of the right zygomatic arch. Fractures can be identified anteriorly, posteriorly, and in the midportion of the arch (*arrowheads* and *arrow*). Elevation of fragments is necessary to prevent facial deformity.

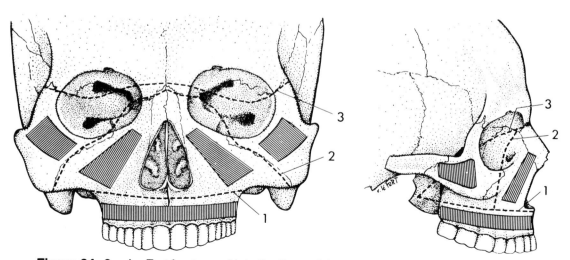

Figure 34–9. Le Fort fractures. Note the lines of the Le Fort I (1), II (2), and III (3). (Dodd GD, Jing B: Radiology of the Nose, Paranasal Sinuses, and Nasopharynx. Baltimore, Williams & Wilkins, 1977, with permission.)

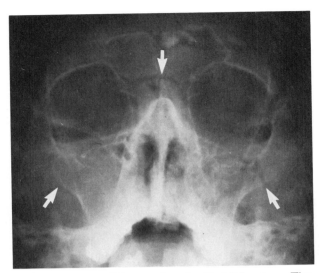

Figure 34–10. Waters view. Le Fort II fracture. The pyramidal configuration of the major fragment is denoted by the arrows. There are accompanying bilateral fractures of the inferior portions of the orbits and comminution of the left maxillary bone is present. The frontal and maxillary sinuses are opacified with hemorrhage.

dentition, the nasal septum, and the most inferior portions of the pterygoid plates. It effectively results in a mobile or "floating palate." The Le Fort II fracture produces a major fragment that is pyramidal in shape (Fig. 34-10). The apex is at or near the root of the nasal bones, and the oblique lateral walls extend from the medial portions of the orbits to the lateral walls of the maxillae. The posterior continuation of the fracture lines terminates in the midportions of the pterygoid plates. Le Fort III fractures result in craniofacial separation. The fracture line is essentially a horizontally oriented zigzag that transects the nasal frontal suture, orbital walls (including the sphenoid portion), and zygomatic arches, ending in the pterygoid bases.[4]

The pterygoid processes are almost invariably fractured in any of the Le Fort injuries (Fig. 34-11). Other associated fractures include central or paramedian splitting of the hard palate (Fig. 34-12), and fracture of the anterior nasal spine of the maxilla (Fig. 34-13). When the midface injury is so severe that it defies categorization, it is commonly referred to as a panfacial fracture, or "facial smash."

The advantage of the Le Fort classification is that it allows the radiologist to categorize an aggregate of complex fracture lines in a meaningful manner to the clinician. The disadvantage is that Le Fort injuries seldom precisely fit the classical description, and the types tend to overlap or be asymmetric (Fig. 34-14). In

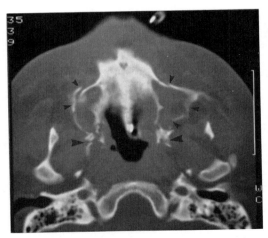

Figure 34–11. Axial CT scan. Le Fort II fracture. There are bilateral comminuted fractures of the maxillary sinuses (*small arrowheads*), and pterygoid processes of the sphenoid bones (*large arrowheads*).

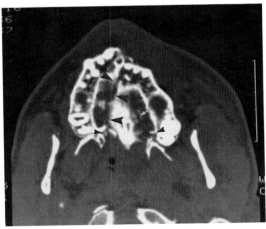

Figure 34–12. Axial CT. Comminuted midpalatal split, Le Fort II. The main fracture line is diagonal (*large arrowheads*), and the left half of the hard palate is displaced posterior to the right. Small fracture fragments are also seen adjacent to the pterygoid processes (*small arrowheads*). A mildly diastatic fracture is present on the left (*white arrow*).

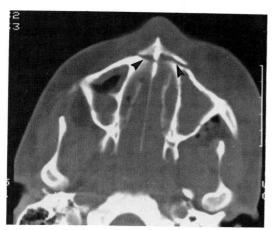

Figure 34–13. Axial CT. Le Fort I. Fracture through anterior nasal spine of the maxilla (*arrowheads*).

order to obviate this problem, other methods of describing facial trauma have been devised; one of the more notable relates the significance of fracture type to the inherent facial struts.[2]

Plain films are of limited value in the delineation of midface fractures, and should be considered, at best, a screening method; CT is the diagnostic procedure of choice. Reconstruction in orthogonal planes is frequently helpful, and many clinicians consider three-dimensional reconstruction valuable in planning and assessing the effects of treatment.

TRIPOD FRACTURES

Although the zygoma is considered to be the second most commonly fractured bone of the midface, the fracture actually occurs more often at the articulations of the zygoma or in the adjacent bones rather than in the zygoma. (Fig. 34-15). The four major articulations are formed with the maxilla, temporal bone, frontal bone, and greater wing of the sphenoid. The tripod fracture is either the result of separation at three of these suture lines, fracture of the adjacent bones, or, most commonly, a combination of sutural separation and fracture. Although considerable variability may be exhibited, the orbital floor, zygomaticofrontal suture, posterior portion of the zygomatic arch, and lateral wall of the maxilla are usually involved. Displacement is common. The tripod fracture can usually be diagnosed on the conventional Waters views (Fig. 34-16)[1] but coexistent orbital soft-tissue damage is better evaluated with CT.

FRACTURES OF THE NASAL BONES

Fractures of the nasal bones are the most common fractures of the midfacial skeleton. Approximately half are isolated to the nasal bones; the remainder occur as part of a complex facial fracture, such as a Le Fort injury.

Most of the isolated fractures are linear and trans-

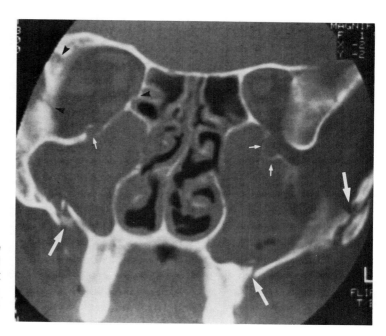

Figure 34–14. Coronal CT. Facial fracture that has features of both Le Fort II and III fractures. The black arrowheads on the right indicate fractures found in Le Fort III injuries, whereas the white arrows denote fractures consistent with a Le Fort II injury.

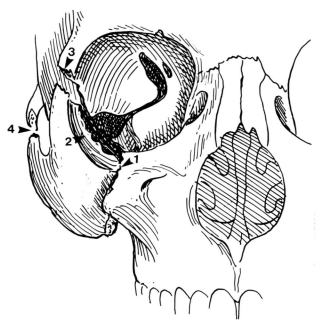

Figure 34–15. Tripod fracture. Common sites of zygomatic suture separation; zygomaticomaxillary, (2) zygomaticosphenoidal, (3) zygomaticofrontal, zygomaticotemporal. (Zizmor J, Noyek A: Orbital trauma. In Newton TH, Potts Radiology of the Skull and Brain. The Skull, Vol I. St. Louis, CV Mosby, with permission.)

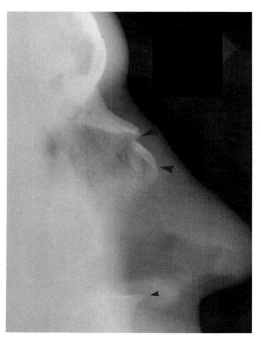

Figure 34–17. Nasal bones, lateral view. There is a transverse fracture (*top arrowhead*) through the anterior portion of the nasal bones with depression of the distal fragment (*middle arrowhead*). The anterior nasal spine of the maxilla is intact (*bottom arrowhead*).

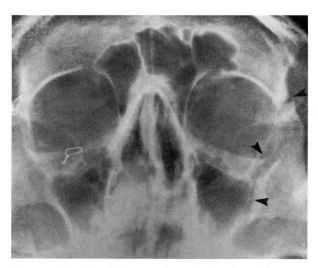

Figure 34–16. Waters view. Left tripod fracture. The upper arrowhead designates the zygomaticofrontal suture separation; the middle arrowhead points to a fracture in the area of the zygomaticosphenoid suture, and the inferior arrowhead indicates a fracture in the lateral wall of the maxilla. The wire sutures on the right are related to an old tripod fracture.

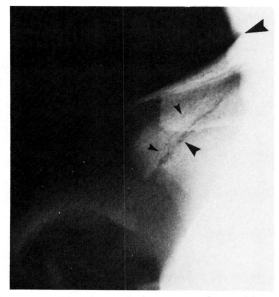

Figure 34–18. Lateral view, normal nasal bones. The large arrowhead indicates the site of the nasofrontal suture, the small arrowheads point to nasociliary grooves, and the medium arrowhead indicates the nasomaxillary suture.

verse, with the fracture usually occurring through the thinner lower third of the nasal bones. Depression of the distal fragment is common (Fig. 34-17). Longitudinal fractures, which parallel the long axis of the nose, may occasionally be more difficult to diagnose because of confusion with the groove for the nasociliary nerve or supernumerary suture lines (Fig. 34-18).

Fragment displacement is almost always present in comminuted fractures, and does not follow any particular pattern (Fig. 34-19). There may be an accompanying fracture of the anterior nasal spine of the maxilla, or separation of the nasal bones at the nasofrontal suture.

Conventional techniques are generally sufficient for imaging nasal bone fractures. The lateral view is the most useful in determining the amount of distal fragment depression in transverse fractures, and assessing the general orientation of fragments in longitudinal fractures. In addition to the Waters view, an axial view using occlusal film is often a valuable method of assessing the degree of medial and lateral displacement of nasal bone fragments.

FRACTURES OF THE MANDIBLE

The mandible is the second most commonly fractured facial bone. Although the mandible contains major areas of strength that serve to withstand the pressures of mastication, there are also sites of inherent structural weakness predisposed to fracture. These include the mental foramen and the thinner bone of the angle and condylar neck. Any area containing a dental socket or unerupted or impacted tooth is also a weaker area.

Various types of fractures occur in the mandible and vary from the simple break with relatively little soft-tissue injury, to the compound fracture, in which there is cutaneous or mucous membrane disruption (Fig. 34-20). Either type may be comminuted. Greenstick fractures, which involve only one surface of the bone, are more common in children but are important to recognize and treat, because significant displacement may develop subsequently as the result of muscle traction.

Fracture location and type are related to the site of contact and velocity of the initiating force. The most common fracture is a result of a blow to the body of the mandible, and consists of a fracture through the parasymphyseal area or mental foramen on the side of the blow, and an angle or subcondylar fracture on the opposite side (Fig. 34-21). A blow that is directed to the symphysis can produce parasymphyseal or bilateral condylar fractures, or both (Fig. 34-22). Low-velocity blows tend to produce undisplaced fractures with a contralateral component, whereas high-velocity blows more often produce comminution limited to the point

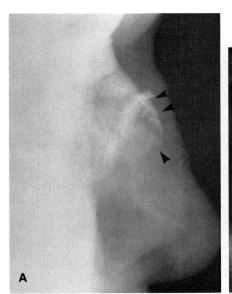 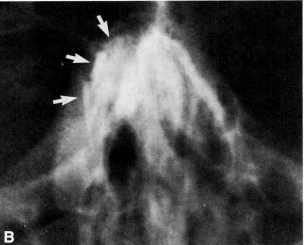

Figure 34–19. Comminuted nasal bone fractures. (**A**) Lateral view. There are multiple displaced fragments (*arrowheads*). (**B**) Waters view in a different patient. The lateral displacement of the right nasal bone fragments (*arrows*) is considerably greater than was suspected from the lateral view.

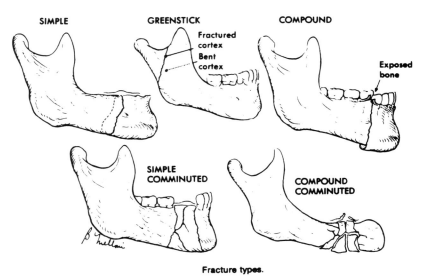

Figure 34–20. Types of mandibular fractures. (Kruger GO: Textbook of Oral and Maxillofacial Surgery, 6th ed. St. Louis, CV Mosby, 1984, with permission.)

of impact. The majority of mandibular fractures are, however, multiple and bilateral.

Displacement of mandibular fractures is dependent on the fracture site, direction of the fracture line, and muscle traction. Fracture stability also is determined largely by the direction of the fracture line and is dependent on muscle attachments or slings. The mas-

seter muscle is particularly influential in the determination of the disposition of fractures involving the area of the mandibular angle (Fig. 34-23). In subcondylar fractures, contraction of the lateral pterygoid muscles produces medial displacement of the proximal condylar fragment (Fig. 34-24). The anterior mandibular fragment, which is the result of parasymphyseal frac-

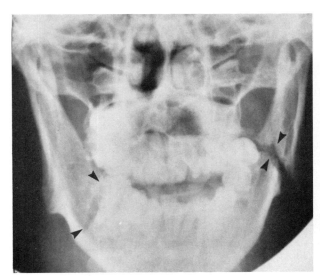

Figure 34–21. PA view. Mandible fractures resulting from a blow to the body of the right mandible. Fracture lines are present adjacent to the right mental foramen and at the left mandibular angle (*arrowheads*).

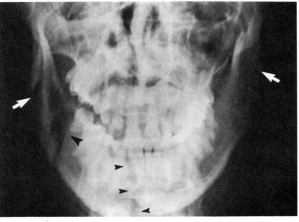

Figure 34–22. PA view. Mandible fractures produced by a blow to the mandibular symphysis. There is a mildly displaced right parasymphyseal fracture (*small black arrowheads*). Bilateral condyle fractures are present (*white arrows*), and there is a comminuted fracture of the right mandibular angle (*large black arrowhead*).

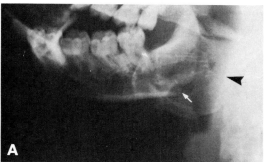
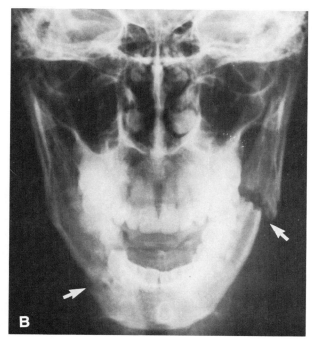

Figure 34–23. Unstable fracture, left mandibular angle. (**A**) Oblique view, left mandible. There is displacement and rotation of the proximal fragment (*black arrowhead*) due to the pull of the masseter muscle. The anteriorly oblique orientation of the fracture line, which is indicated by the white arrow, predisposes to this type of displacement. (**B**) PA view. The orientation of the left mandibular fragments is less well identified; a contralateral fracture through the right mental foramen, however, is now apparent (*arrows*).

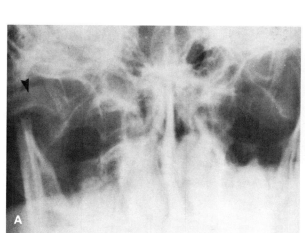
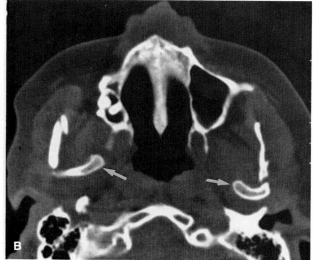

Figure 34–24. (**A**) AP view of the mandible. Left subcondylar fracture. There is characteristic medial displacement of the proximal condylar fragment (*arrowhead*) due to contraction of the lateral pterygoid muscle. (**B**) Axial CT scan in a different patient. Bilateral mandible fractures. Note the medial displacement of the proximal condylar fragments (*arrows*).

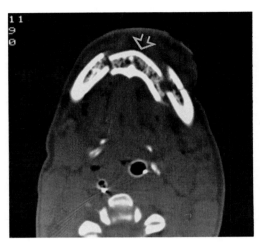

Figure 34–25. Axial CT scan. Parasymphyseal fracture. There is posterior displacement of the central fragment (*arrow*) due to contraction of the muscles of the floor of the mouth and anterior neck.

tures, may undergo posterior displacement as a result of the combined contraction of the genioglossus and suprahyoid muscles (Fig. 34-25).

The treatment of mandibular fractures varies with the fracture type and location. In general, it consists of splinting and fixation through wiring of fragments, or intermaxillary fixation with arch bars or wire loops. Because the mandible is essentially a membranous bone, bone union is primarily fibrous; the time interval between the achievement of clinical stability and radio-graphic evidence of healing may be considerable. Complications related to healing included infection, malunion, malocclusion, and facial deformity.

Conventional techniques are commonly used for imaging of the mandible. The preferred views are the PA, Towne, and oblique projections of the mandible. Panoramic tomography provides an additional means of fracture definition. CT, although not considered the primary means of imaging in this situation, occasionally proves more efficacious than the conventional methods for establishing both the number and position of fragments.

REFERENCES AND SELECTED READINGS

1. DOLAN KD, JACOBY CG, SMOKER WRK: Radiology of Facial Injury, 2nd ed. New York, Macmillan, 1988
2. GENTRY LR, MANOR, TURSKI PA, STROTHER CM: High-resolution CT analysis of facial struts in trauma: Osseous and soft tissue complications. Am J Roentgenol 140:533, 1983
3. LLOYD GA: Radiology of the Orbit. Philadelphia, WB Saunders, 1985
4. ROWE NL, WILLIAMS JLI: Maxillofacial Injuries, Vols 1 and 2. New York, Churchill–Livingstone, 1985
5. UNGER JM: Orbital apex fractures: The contribution of computed tomography. Radiology 150:713, 1984
6. WEISS RA, HAIK BG, SAINT–LOUIS A, ELLSWORTH RM: Advanced diagnostic imaging techniques in ophthalmology. Adv Opthalmic Plast Reconstr Surg 6:207, 1987

*Paul and Juhl's Essentials of Radiologic Imaging,
Sixth Edition*, edited by John H. Juhl and
Andrew B. Crummy. J.B. Lippincott Company,
Philadelphia, © 1993.

CHAPTER **35**

The Temporal Bone

June M. Unger

METHODS OF EXAMINATION

During the first half of the twentieth century, the radiographic examination of the temporal bone was accomplished using conventional filming techniques, some of which remain applicable under certain circumstances. Greatly improved anatomic detail was made possible in the 1950s, when equipment capable of providing complex motion tomography became commercially available. Since 1980, however, thin-section, high-resolution CT has effectively supplanted other techniques by virtue of its inherent superior resolution. More recently, MRI has become the procedure of choice in the diagnosis of tumors involving the internal auditory canal and adjacent cerebellopontine angle.

CONVENTIONAL RADIOGRAPHY

When conventional radiography was the only method available for imaging of the temporal bone, many projections were devised to minimize the interference produced by the adjacent bones of the skull. Lateral, oblique, AP, and semiaxial views, and modifications of these views produced by angulation of the x-ray beam or patient's head, were all employed. Currently, the

lateral mastoid view (Fig. 35-1) is the only projection still used in most imaging centers, largely to confirm a diagnosis of acute mastoiditis, or substantiate previous mastoid disease.

COMPUTED TOMOGRAPHY

CT of the temporal bone is the method of choice for evaluation of bone detail and soft-tissue changes produced by inflammation and both nonneoplastic and peripheral neoplastic masses. Specialized techniques of image reconstruction that can provide high resolution and a section thickness of 2 mm or less are essential.[3] Whether images should be obtained in the coronal as well as the standard axial plane depends on the particular disease process and potential sites of involvement. Pertinent anatomic details of the significant axial and coronal planes are illustrated in Figures 35-2 and 35-3.

MAGNETIC RESONANCE IMAGING

The contrast resolution, soft-tissue discrimination, and potential tumor enhancement following administration of a paramagnetic contrast agent such as gadolinium have made MRI the method of choice in the diagnosis

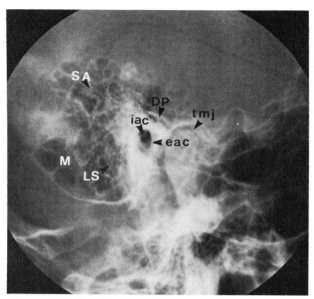

Figure 35–1. Temporal bone. Lateral (Law) projection. Mastoid air cells (M); dural plate (DP); area of the anterior wall of the lateral venous sinus (LS); sinodural angle, or angel of Citelli (merging of DP and LS) (SA); temporomandibular joint (tmj); external auditory canal (eac); and internal auditory canal (iac).

of central neoplastic lesions that involve either the cerebellopontine angle or internal auditory canal. With continuing refinements in MR angiography, additional detail of vascular abnormalities related to tumors and anomalies such as vascular loops is becoming possible without the potential hazards of invasive techniques.

ANATOMIC CONSIDERATIONS

The temporal bone consists of five parts: the squamous, mastoid, petrous, and tympanic portions, and the styloid process. The squamous portion contributes to the lateral aspect of the cranial vault; the petrous portion creates the division of the skull base into middle and posterior cranial fossae and contains the structures of the inner ear. The tympanic portion contributes primarily to the external ear, and the mastoid consists chiefly of air cells that communicate with the middle ear. The styloid process serves as a point of origin for muscles and ligaments.

CONGENITAL ABNORMALITIES OF THE TEMPORAL BONE

Although congenital abnormalities of the temporal bone are relatively uncommon, some are correctable, and precise definition of the abnormality and related anatomic changes becomes important before surgery is considered. CT is ordinarily the imaging procedure of choice.

These malformations basically consist of two groups, divided on the basis of embryologic derivation. The first group comprises developmental defects of the external and middle ear, both of which are derived from the first branchial arches and clefts, and includes those conduction defects most amenable to surgical correction. The second group, which consists of structures that originate from the auditory vesicle, includes all of the inner ear anomalies. These lesions are associated with sensorineural deafness and, although not

Figure 35–2. Temporal bone, coronal CT images, high-resolution, bone algorithm. (**A**) ▶ (Most anterior) Plane of head of malleus and geniculate ganglion. First cochlear turn (c), geniculate ganglion fossa (gg), head of malleus (m), mastoid air cells (mc), occipital bone (o), tympanic cavity (tc), tendon of tensor tympani muscle (tt). (**B**) Plane of ossicular mass and midcochlea. Cochlea (c), carotid canal (cc), first and second portions of facial nerve canal (f), lateral wall of the attic (lwa), neck of malleus (n), ossicular mass (malleus and incus) (om), bony spur or scutum (s). (**C**) Plane of incus. Basal turn of cochlea (c), external auditory canal (eac), body of incus (i), head of malleus (black m), manubrium of malleus (white m), cochlear promontory (p). (**D**) Plane of oval window. Body of incus (i), internal auditory canal (iac), incudostapedial articulation (is), oval window (ow), superior semicircular canal (ssc). (**E**) Plane of round window. Vertical portion of facial nerve canal (f), horizontal semicircular canal (hsc), jugular fossa (jf), round window (rw), superior semicircular canal (ssc), sinus tympani (st), tegmen tympani (t). (**F**) (Most posterior) Plane of cochlear aqueduct. Mastoid antrum (a), ampulla of posterior semicircular canal (ap), cochlear aqueduct (ca), area of stylomastoid foramen (f), superior semicircular canal (ssc).

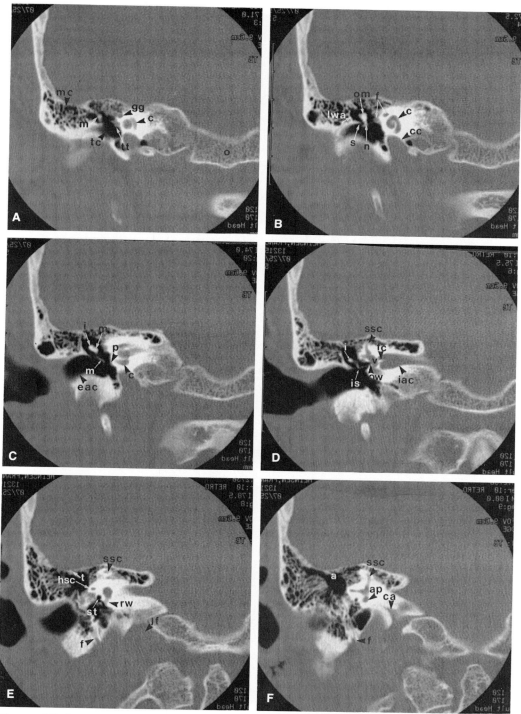

Figure 35–2.

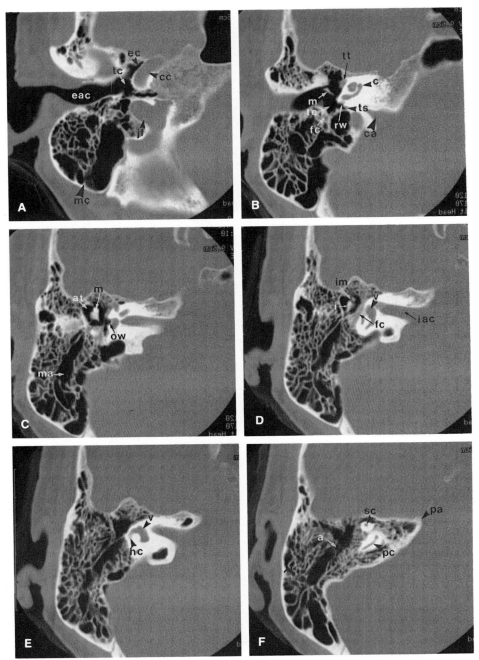

Figure 35–3.

◄ **Figure 35–3.** Temporal bone, axial CT images, high-resolution, bone algorithm. (**A**) (Most inferior) Plane of the hypotympanum. Carotid canal (cc), external auditory canal (eac), eustachian canal (ec), jugular fossa (jf), mastoid air cells (mc), tympanic cavity (hypotympanum) (tc). (**B**) Midcochlear plane. Basal turn of cochlea (intermediate and apical turns are adjacent) (c), cochlear aqueduct (ca), vertical portion of facial nerve canal (fc), handle of malleus (m), tympanic cavity (tc), tympanic sinus (ts), tensor tympani muscle (tt). (**C**) Plane of the oval window. Attic (epitympanic recess) (at), head of malleus (m), mastoid antrum (ma), oval window (ow). (**D**) Plane of incudomalleolar articulation. Facial canal (fc), body of incus (i), internal auditory canal (iac), incudomalleolar articulation (im), vestibule (v). (**E**) Plane of horizontal semicircular canal. Horizontal canal (hc), vestibule (v). (**F**) Plane of additus ad antrum. Additus ad antrum (a), petrous apex (pa), posterior semicircular canal (pc), superior semicircular canal (sc).

surgically correctable, may be helped by devices such as cochlear implants.

Defects related to branchial arch development include deformity of the auricle, partial or complete atresia of the external auditory canal, and abnormalities of the ossicles (Fig. 35-4). Any of these may be accompanied by peculiarities in the position of the facial nerve canal that must be identified before corrective surgery.

Inner ear anomalies vary from those solely involving the semicircular canals to complete aplasia of the otic capsule. A rare but well-known abnormality, the Mundini defect, is caused by partial or total absence of the cochlear turns (Fig. 35-5).

INFLAMMATORY DISEASE

Most of the inflammatory changes that occur in the temporal bone are the result of uncontrolled external or middle-ear infections. The most common etiologic organism is either the B-hemolytic streptococcus or pneumococcus, except in children under 5 years of age, who may be infected by *Hemophilus influenzae.* Acute mastoiditis, a frequent complication of otitis media before administration of antibiotics, has become uncommon and rarely is seen radiographically (Figs. 35-6 A and B). Acute petrositis, which may develop from extension of mastoid infection into petrosal air cells, has also become a rarity.

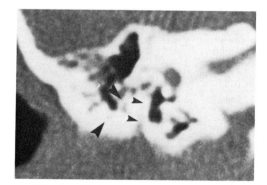

Figure 35–4. Temporal bone, CT, coronal plane. Aplasia of the external auditory canal. Thick bone replaces the external auditory canal and extends into the posterior aspect of the tympanic cavity (*large arrowheads*). The vertical portion of the facial nerve canal is anterior to the normal location (*small arrowheads*).

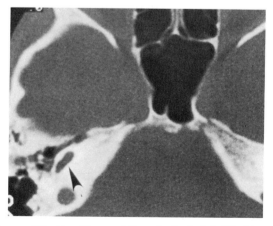

Figure 35–5. Base of the skull. Axial CT. Mundini defect. The right cochlear turns are absent (*arrowhead*). The left cochlea appeared normal. (Courtesy of D. Johnson, MD).

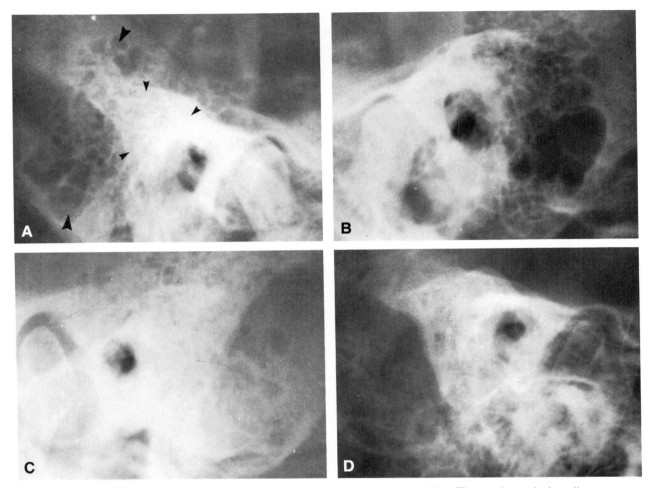

Figure 35–6.   Mastoiditis. Lateral views. (**A**) Acute mastoiditis. The periantral air cells are hazy (*small arrowheads*). The peripheral mastoid cells appear uninvolved (*large arrowheads*). (**B**) Normal side for comparison. (**C**) Subacute mastoiditis. There is considerable opacification and coalescence of air cells, consistent with early septal breakdown. (**D**) Chronic mastoiditis. The entire mastoid appears sclerotic and there are no recognizable air cells.

Subacute and chronic mastoiditis, which are usually the consequence of recurrent otitis media, result in breakdown of mastoid septa, thickening of mucous membranes, and eventual bony sclerosis (Figs. 35-6 C and D). Secondary or acquired cholesteatomas are common complications of chronic mastoiditis and are the result of invasion of the middle ear or contiguous areas by keratinizing squamous epithelium. The route usually runs from the external canal through a tympanic membrane perforation into the epitympanic recess. As epithelial debris accumulate, bone is eroded either by pressure necrosis or from collagenase activity from the the cholesteatoma matrix. Initial destruction of the lateral attic wall, particularly in the area of the bony spur, may be followed by ossicular damage with the production of a conduction defect (Fig. 35-7). Erosion of the bony covering of the lateral aspect of the horizontal semicircular canal may create a labyrinthine fistula and cause vestibular symptoms. Destruction of the bony covering of the facial nerve canal or roof of the tympanic cavity (the tegmen tympani) may result in neurologic complications.

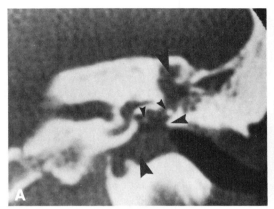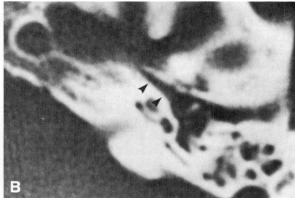

Figure 35–7. Cholesteatoma. (**A**) Coronal CT, plane of oval window. A soft-tissue mass fills the middle ear and epitympanic recess (*large arrowheads*). The bony spur is blunted (*medium arrowhead*), and there is partial destruction of the ossicles (*small arrowheads*). (**B**) Axial CT, plane of cochlea. The cholesteatoma extends into the eustachian tube (*arrowheads*).

CT is the imaging procedure of choice for the identification of early cholesteatomas. Although relatively large cholesteatomas that have produced bone erosion may be identifiable by conventional views, at this stage, surgical restoration of hearing may no longer be possible. Recurrent cholesteatoma may be found occasionally in the postoperative ear and will need to be differentiated from granulation tissue. This is not always possible with imaging techniques.

Other causes of inflammatory changes in the temporal bone include fungus infections, and, rarely, tuberculosis and syphilis. An uncommon, but potentially lethal inflammation may be produced by *Pseudomonas aeruginosa* under appropriate circumstances, typically in the elderly diabetic. The advanced osseous destruction of the temporal bone that occurs has led to the designation of this entity as malignant external otitis (Fig. 35-8).

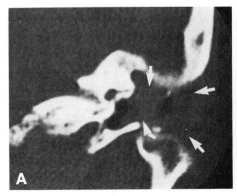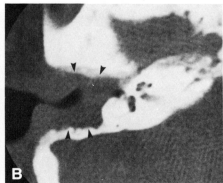

Figure 35–8. Malignant external otitis. (**A**) Coronal CT, left temporal bone. The inflammatory mass (*arrows*) has destroyed the ossicles and walls of the external canal. (**B**) Axial CT, right temporal bone. The extent of destruction of the anterior and posterior canal walls is demonstrated (*arrowheads*).

OSTEODYSTROPHIES

The osteodystrophies that occur in the temporal bone may be isolated to the temporal bone, such as otosclerosis, or may represent an additional manifestation of a primarily extratemporal skeletal disorder such as Paget's disease, histiocytosis X, fibrous dysplasia, or craniometaphyseal dysplasia.

Otosclerosis is a disease of the labyrinthine capsule. It is somewhat more common in women than in men and usually does not become clinically evident before 20 years of age. Early or active otosclerosis consists of osseous rarefaction or otospongiosis. There is eventual maturation into sclerotic or inactive foci, constituting the end or stable stage of the disease.

The earliest pathologic change occurs in the bone just anterior to the oval window. Involvement of the oval window and stapedial foot plate commonly results in ankylosis of the foot plate in the oval window. The hearing loss is conductive, and surgical procedures are directed toward restoration of the ossicular chain. Progression of disease with involvement of the round window, basal turn of the cochlea, or other portions of the labyrinthine capsule may result in a noncorrectible sensorineural hearing loss. (Fig. 35-9).

The purpose of imaging in otosclerosis, therefore, is to assess the type and degree of labyrinthine capsule involvement and to establish a diagnosis in questionable cases. CT is essential; conventional radiographic methods are of no value in the detection of minute changes that may be present.

The other osteodystrophies, although less common than otosclerosis, occasionally have distinguishing features that may be diagnostic. The changes of Paget's disease, for example, are fairly characteristic. Expansion of the base of the skull by thickened, abnormal bone produces an appearance of increased density on conventional film that is, in reality, artifactual; although the amount of bone is increased, it is actually decalcified. The changes of fibrous dysplasia are also expansile but more often sclerotic (Fig. 35-10). In other diseases in which hyperostosis is a prominent feature, such as craniometaphyseal dysplasia (Fig. 35-11), the dense, expanded sclerotic bone may eventually encroach on the otic capsular structures, producing luminal narrowing.

TRAUMA

Fractures of the temporal bone are the second most common fractures of the base of the skull, superseded only by sphenoid fractures.[5] They are classified according to the predominant plane of the fracture line as longitudinal or transverse. Longitudinal fractures follow the long axis of the petrous bone, whereas transverse fractures cross it. Comminution can occur with

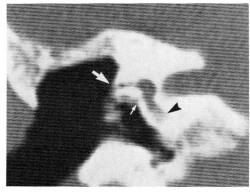

Figure 35–9.   Mature otosclerosis. Coronal CT. There is sclerosis in the basal turn of the cochlea (*black arrowhead*) and marked thickening of the bone adjacent to the oval window (*small white arrow*). The patient had multiple surgical procedures for restoration of hearing; a fenestration defect is indicated by the large white arrow.

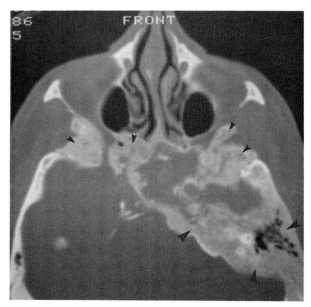

Figure 35–10.   Fibrous dysplasia. Axial CT scan. There is expansion and sclerosis of the left temporal bone (*large arrowheads*) and sphenoid bone (*small arrowheads*).

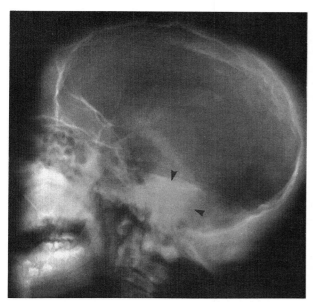

Figure 35–11. Craniometaphyseal dysplasia. Lateral skull. There is marked sclerosis and thickening of the facial bones, temporal bones (*arrowheads*) and remaining skull base as well as portions of the cranial vault.

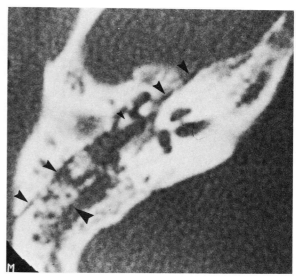

Figure 35–12. Axial CT. Longitudinal fracture, right temporal bone. The fracture line follows the long axis of the temporal bone (*medium arrowheads*). The incus is subluxed laterally (*small arrowhead*). The mastoid air cells are opacified with blood (*large arrowhead*).

either type of fracture and may obscure the basic fracture type. Fractures can also be classified according to their relationship to the bony labyrinth as extralabyrinthine, tympanolabyrinthine, or labyrinthine.

Approximately 80% of temporal bone fractures are of the longitudinal type and are usually caused either by a direct blow to the temporal area or an indirect blow in which force has been transmitted to a mandibular condyle. Clinical features include bleeding from the ear and conductive hearing loss secondary to ossicular dislocation. The incus, because of relatively loose ligamentous attachments, is the most frequently dislocated ossicle (Fig. 35-12). Although the facial nerve is damaged in 20% of longitudinal fractures, the damage is transient in 75%. Dural tears may occur when the fracture involves the roof of the tympanic cavity or tegmen tympani.

The less common transverse fracture is usually the result of a blow to the occiput. These fractures may involve the labyrinthine capsule, effectively destroying the cochlear and vestibular system (Fig. 35-13). Signs and symptoms of labyrinthine fracture include hemotympanum behind an intact tympanic membrane, vertigo with spontaneous nystagmus, sensorineural hearing loss, and permanent facial paralysis in 50% of

patients. Conventional films may show gross fracture lines and bleeding into the mastoid air cells (Fig. 35-14); however, CT is essential for demonstrating fracture line detail, small bone fragments and ossicular damage. Coexistent damage to intracranial contents may be evaluated at the same time.

TUMORS

Most discussions of temporal bone tumors include not only tumors that originate in the osseous or soft-tissue structures of the temporal bone, but also those that occur in the immediately adjacent cerebellopontine angle. Either group may be subdivided into benign or malignant, and primary or secondary neoplasms.

Glomus tumors, which originate from paraganglion cells, are the most common primary tumors of the temporal bone. These benign neoplasms most frequently arise on or adjacent to the promontory of the middle ear where they are referred to as glomus tympanicum tumors (Fig. 35-15). In this location, their CT appearance may mimic inflammatory disease and be difficult to differentiate from granulation tissue or secondary cholesteatomas. Glomus jugulare tumors, which occur

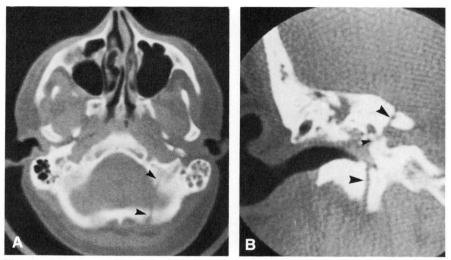

Figure 35–13. (**A**) Axial CT, base of skull. A fracture line crosses the left occiptal bone and extends to the petrous portion of the left temporal bone (*small arrowheads*). (**B**) Coronal CT, right temporal bone. A fracture line (*large arrowhead*) crosses the otic capsule between the vestibule and basal turn of the cochlea (*small arrowhead*).

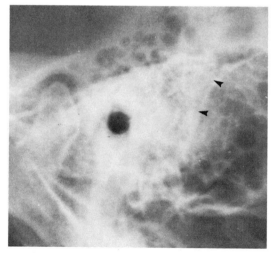

Figure 35–14. Longitudinal fracture. Conventional lateral view. There is air cell opacification, resembling that seen in acute mastoiditis, adjacent to the barely perceptible fracture line (*arrowheads*).

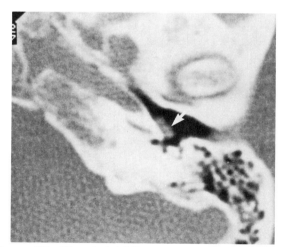

Figure 35–15. Axial CT, plane of basal turn of cochlea. A soft-tissue mass (*arrow*) is adherent to the inferior aspect of the promontory. Pathologic diagnosis: glomus tympanicum.

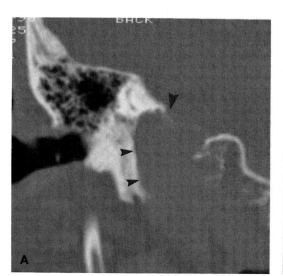

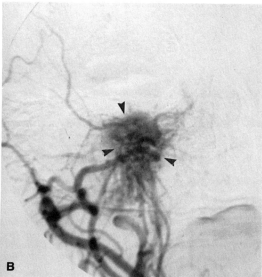

Figure 35–16. Glomus jugular tumor. (**A**) Coronal CT. There is expansion of the jugular fossa (*small arrowheads* indicate lateral wall) and destruction of the petrous apex (*large arrowhead*). (**B**) Digital subtraction angiogram, AP projection, external carotid artery injection. There is pronounced tumor vascularity (*arrowheads*). The arterial supply of the tumor is from the external carotid circulation, usually from the ascending pharyngeal branch of the external carotid artery.

in the area of the jugular foramen, are less common but potentially more locally invasive and destructive (Fig. 35-16).

Other benign tumors of the middle and external ear include tumors originating in the tympanic portion of the facial nerve, and a variety of external auditory canal tumors and tumor like lesions such as ceruminomas, osteomas, and exostose.

The malignant tumors that affect the temporal bone are usually secondary, and the result of local invasion from adnexal structures such as the salivary glands; primary malignant tumors are relatively uncommon. Metastasis from distant sites, most frequently breast, kidney, and lung, also occurs. Primary rhabdomyosarcoma of the middle ear occurs more often in children than in adults (Fig. 35-17), whereas squamous cell carcinoma originating in the external auditory canal is a neoplasm more commonly found in adults (Fig. 35-18).

Almost all of the tumors and tumor-like masses that occur in the cerebellopontine angle are benign. Eighty percent of these are acoustic schwannomas; the remainder include meningiomas, primary cholesteatomas or epidermoid tumors, neuromas of cranial nerves

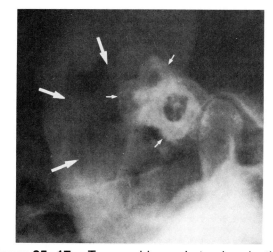

Figure 35–17. Temporal bone. Lateral projection. There has been marked osteolytic destruction of the mastoid portion of the temporal bone (*large arrows*). The enchondral bone of the otic capsule is preserved (*small arrows*). Pathologic diagnosis: rhabdomyosarcoma.

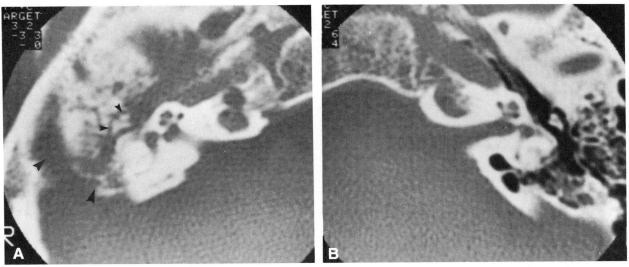

Figure 35–18.   Squamous cell carcinoma. (**A**) Axial CT, right temporal bone, plane of cochlea, and horizontal semicircular canal. Marked osteolytic destruction of the mastoid (*large arrowheads*) is apparent. A soft-tissue mass fills the tympanic cavity and surrounds the ossicles (*small arrowheads*). (**B**) Normal side for comparison.

V and VII, aneurysms and other vascular lesions, and arachnoid cysts.

Before MRI, CT was considered the appropriate imaging method for establishing the diagnosis of cerebellopontine angle tumors (Fig. 35-19), particularly acoustic schwannomas (Fig. 35-20). Diagnosis was based on widening of the medial aspect of the internal auditory canal, enhancement of an intracanalicular or cerebellopontine mass following injection of intravenous iodinated contrast (Fig. 35-20), or demonstration of a

mass related to the internal auditory canal following subarachnoid instillation of air. Although CT remains a viable alternative for the detection of eighth-nerve tumors, the current imaging method of choice is magnetic resonance, using a paramagnetic contrast agent such as gadolinium. With MRI it is possible to diagnose

Figure 35–19.   Axial CT. A large, enhancing mass on the right extends into the posterior fossa. It previously had been shown to contain calcium on a noncontrast scan. Pathologic diagnosis: meningioma.

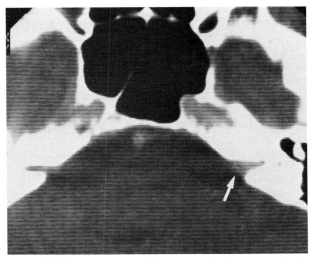

Figure 35–20.   Axial CT. A small, almost entirely intracanalicular, left acoustic schwannoma is present (*arrow*). Note the funnel-like enlargement of the involved internal auditory canal in comparison with the normal side.

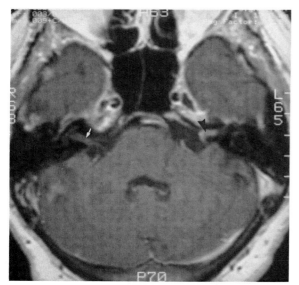

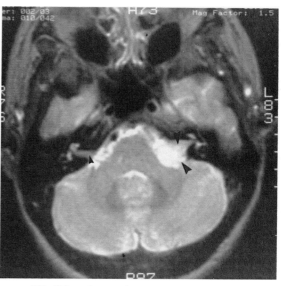

Figure 35–21. Acoustic schwannoma. Axial MRI, T1-weighted, postintravenous gadolinium. Marked enhancement of the small tumor involves the medial aspect of the intracanalicular portion of the left eighth nerve (*large arrowhead*). The normal right eighth nerve is indicated (*small arrow*).

Figure 35–22. Acoustic schwannoma. Axial MRI, T2-weighted. The large, high-signal mass has enlarged the intracanalicular portion of the left eighth nerve, and fills the cerebellopontine angle (*large arrowheads*). The nerves in the right internal auditory canal are normal (*small arrowhead*).

extremely small tumors, as well as confirm larger masses in the cerebellopontine angle (Figs. 35-21 and 35-22).

The other tumor and tumor like lesions of the petrous apex are also generally preferentially diagnosed

with MRI (Figs. 35-23 and 35-24). Neurogenic tumors elsewhere in the temporal bone may be preferentially imaged by CT if bone erosion is a diagnostic consideration (Fig. 35-25).

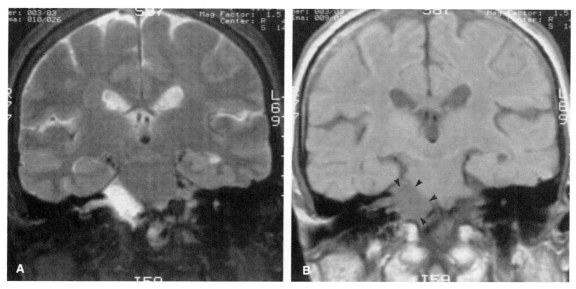

Figure 35–23. Epidermoid. (**A**) Coronal MRI, T1-weighted. A large homogeneous mass, which is slightly higher in signal than CSF, fills the right cerebellopontine angle (*arrowheads*). (**B**) On a T2-weighted image, the lesion is again noted to be hyperintense to CSF.

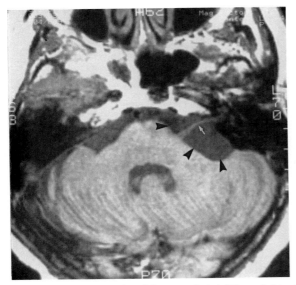

Figure 35–24. Arachnoid cyst. Axial T1-weighted MRI. The large fluid-filled structure expands the left cerebellopontine angle cistern (*arrowheads*). Note the elongation and thinning of cranial nerves VII and VIII (*white arrow*).

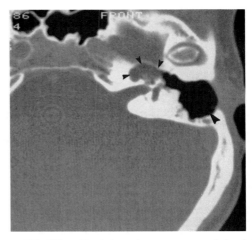

Figure 35–25. Facial schwannoma, labyrinthine segment. Axial CT scan. A large circumscribed osteolytic area is seen anterior to the cochlear capsule (*small arrowheads*). The bone changes appear more expansile than destructive. An adjacent old surgical defect is present (*large arrowhead*).

REFERENCES AND SELECTED READINGS

1. CHAKERES DW, KAPIL A: Computed tomography of the temporal bone. Med Radiogr Photogr 60:3, 1984
2. SHAFFER KA. Temporal bone imaging. In Unger JM: Handbook of Head and Neck Imaging. New York, Churchill–Livingstone, 1987
3. SHAFFER KA, HAUGHTON VM, WILSON CR: High resolution computed tomography of the temporal bone. Radiology 134:409, 1980
4. SOM PM, BERGERON RT, CURTIN HD, REEDE DL (EDS): Head and Neck Imaging. St. Louis, CV Mosby, 1991
5. UNGER JM, GENTRY LR, GROSSMAN JE: Sphenoid fractures: prevalence, sites and significance. Radiology 175: 175, 1990

Paul and Juhl's Essentials of Radiologic Imaging,
Sixth Edition, edited by John H. Juhl and
Andrew B. Crummy. J.B. Lippincott Company,
Philadelphia, © 1993.

CHAPTER **36**

The Teeth, Jaws and Salivary Glands

John H. Juhl

The roentgen examination of the teeth is used by the medical profession largely to determine the presence or absence of infection involving the teeth and jaws. Certain changes in the alveolus result from generalized disease, and examination of the teeth is also helpful in these conditions. Tumors arising on the alveolar ridge, tongue, or other intraoral sites may involve the bony alveolus. Roentgen examination is used to detect, plan therapy, and follow the progress of these tumors.

Specific techniques for dental radiography include intraoral dental radiographic study and the panoramic type of extraoral examinations. Three general intraoral methods of examination used are the intraoral dental, bitewing, and occlusal. The standard intraoral films are placed in position and held there by the patient while the exposure is being made. A total of 14 of these small films are exposed for a complete dental survey. These exposures should include the crowns and roots of all teeth. Bitewing films are used to examine the crowns of the teeth. These films have a central flap that is held between the teeth with the mouth closed. Each film then includes upper and lower dental crowns. A total of seven exposures is used in examination of all the teeth in this manner. The occlusal film is larger and is also employed as an intraoral film. It is used most widely in patients who are edentulous in a search for retained root fragments or local infection of the alveolus. It is also useful in the examination of small cysts or tumors of the alveolar ridge and jaw.

Panoramic devices save time and radiation exposure. They are used as a dental screening device and as a method of examining the alveolar ridges and adjacent portions of the maxilla as well as the mandible. A number of panoramic devices are available with a variety of special features to suit the needs of physicians interested in the teeth and jaws as well as those of the oral surgeon and dentist (see Fig. 36-11). These devices rotate around a fixed head position during filming. A single exposure may be used to survey all of the teeth as well as the jaws. In our experience, because dental detail is not as good as in dental films, we use these devices for the examination of the mandible and maxilla and as a screening examination of the teeth. The panoramic methods reduce radiation exposure considerably, from a dose of about 15 rad for a full-mouth dental survey with two bitewing exposures to about 3 rad for a panoramic exposure, plus bite wings. Lead-lined cones are effective in reducing skin exposure in dental radiography. The mandible is examined by means of special views in frontal and lateral oblique projection. The temporomandibular joints also require special techniques and are examined with the mouth opened and closed. Films of the normal as well as the abnormal joint are usually obtained for comparison purposes. Tomography, CT, and MRI are of considerable value in the examination of the temporomandibular joints. There is also a place for arthrography of these joints using contrast.

THE NORMAL TEETH

The discussion of dental and jaw problems is necessarily limited in this text. Those interested in more detailed information should refer to *Stafne's Oral Radiographic Diagnosis* by Gibilisco.[7]

The teeth appear in two sets. The first are termed deciduous or temporary teeth. There are 20 deciduous teeth, 10 in each jaw, 5 in each quadrant. They are named from the midline as follows: central incisor, lateral incisor, cuspid, first molar (premolar), and second molar (premolar). In the adult jaw there are normally 32 teeth; 8 in each quadrant named as follows from the midline: central incisor, lateral incisor, cuspid (canine), first bicuspid, second bicuspid, and first, second, and third molar. Examples of these teeth are shown in Figures 36-1 through 36-3.

Each tooth consists of a crown and a root. The junction between them is called the neck or cervix. The roots lie in sockets in the alveolar process of the jaw and are attached by alveolar periosteum. Many variations in opacity are noted on dental radiographs, listed in decreasing order: (1) metal crowns and fillings; (2) enamel of the teeth; (3) dentine; (4) cementum; (5) cortical bone; (6) cancellous bone; and (7) medullary spaces, canals, foramina, and soft tissues. The crown of the tooth is therefore slightly more dense than the root and within each tooth is a narrow radiolucency termed the root canal. Immediately surrounding each tooth is a radiolucent space representing the alveolar periosteum (periodontal membrane). Adjacent to this is a thin, dense structure composed of compact bone called the lamina dura (Fig. 36-4).

The mandible or lower jaw is composed of two equal halves united at the symphysis anteriorly. Each half consists of a body extending from the midline backward in a roughly horizontal direction and a ramus at somewhat less than a right angle so that the ramus is nearly vertical. It articulates with the base of the skull by means of a condylar process that projects upward from the posterior aspect of the ramus. The other upward projection anteriorly is termed the coronoid process. The lower teeth are set in the alveolar process. The upper teeth are set in the alveolar process of the maxilla. The lower aspect of the maxillary antrum is visible on dental films of the upper teeth. The mental foramen appears as a radiolucency below and between the lower bicuspids. The mandibular canal extends forward, parallel to the alveolar ridge, and is a radiolucency that should not be mistaken for disease (Fig. 36-5).

There are a few structures in the maxilla that should also be mentioned. The intermaxillary suture is ob-

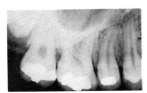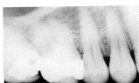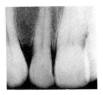

Figure 36–1. Examples of teeth in the upper jaw. From left to right: partially outlined unerupted third molar, second molar, first molar, second bicuspid, first bicuspid, partially visualized second molar, first molar, second bicuspid, first bicuspid, partially visualized cuspid, remainder of the cuspid, lateral incisor, central incisor. Note the radiolucency representing the floor of the maxillary antrum. There are metallic restorations (fillings) in the molar teeth.

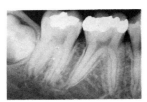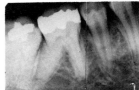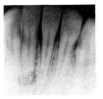

Figure 36–2. Examples of teeth in the lower jaw. From left to right: partially visualized and unerupted third molar, second molar, first molar, partially visualized second bicuspid, partially visualized second molar, first molar, second bicuspid, first bicuspid, lateral incisor, central incisor, lateral incisor, cuspid. Note metallic fillings in the molar teeth.

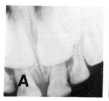
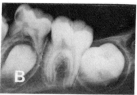

Figure 36–3. Examples of developing teeth. The unerupted permanent teeth are noted in the alveolus, with some resorption of the roots of the deciduous teeth. **(A)** Upper incisors. **(B)** Lower bicuspid and molars.

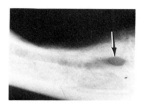

Figure 36–5. Mental foramen. The arrow indicates the foramen. The mandibular canal extends posteriorly from the foramen in this edentulous mandibular alveolus.

served in children and often in young adults. It appears as a midline radiolucent suture extending from the alveolar crest between the upper central incisors back to the posterior aspect of the palate. It may be interrupted in some areas. It has cortical margins that are smooth or slightly irregular. Usually there is no difficulty in differentiating it from a fracture. The incisive foramen (anterior palatine foramen) varies in size from a slit near the sagittal plane of the maxilla near the level of the apices of the central incisors to a rather large round or oval foramen, usually clearly marginated and occasionally appearing somewhat bilobed. The radicular cyst, from which it must be differentiated, maintains its relation to the dental root in contrast to the foramen (see "Chronic Rarefying Osteitis with Cyst Formation" under the section entitled "Periapical Infections" in this chapter).

DENTAL INFECTIONS

DENTAL CARIES

The presence of a cavity may escape detection by clinical methods of examination and yet be readily visible on a radiograph. Regardless of their cause, dental caries

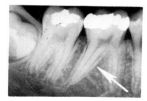

Figure 36–4. Lower molar teeth. Lamina dura surrounds the dental root (*arrow*). The bony alevolus extends to the neck of the tooth. The crown is above it, and the roots are embedded in the bone. The dental root canal is represented by the thin radiolucent line extending into the dental root. The alveolodental periosteum (periodontal membrane) forms a radiolucent line between the lamina dura and the dental root.

may lead to foci of infection involving the periapical tissues of the jaw and are, therefore, important lesions. On the roentgenogram a carious area is radiolucent and appears as an area of decreased opacity that is usually slightly irregular and may occur anywhere on the crown of a tooth or in its neck (Fig. 36-6).

PULP CHANGES

The dental pulp contains the blood and nerve supply of the tooth. The cellular elements include odontoblasts and mesenchymal cells capable of differentiating into odontoclasts. Therefore, irritation caused by a number of external stimuli including occlusal wear, dental caries, and minor trauma may lead to formation of calcifications (pulp stones) or thickening of the walls of the pulp chamber. There may be resorption with pulp chamber enlargement when infection is severe; this is caused by metaplasia with formation of osteoclasts.

PERIAPICAL (PERIRADICULAR) INFECTIONS

All of the periapical inflammatory lesions represent chronic disease when they are advanced enough to produce roentgen changes. Chronic infection around the apex of a dental root is manifested by several changes that can be recognized and classified. At times

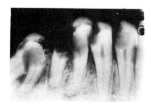

Figure 36–6. Dental caries. Note the multiple radiolucent defects in the crowns of the teeth, particularly the first and second molars, and to a lesser extent in the bicuspids.

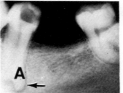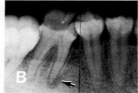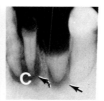

Figure 36–7. Periapical infections. **(A)** Chronic periapical periostitis. The arrow indicates an increase in radiolucency between the dental apex and the lamina dura. This tooth is also carious. **(B)** Periapical granuloma. The arrow indicates destruction of bone adjacent to the apex of the root of the first molar. Note that the crown is carious. **(C)** Periapical abscess. An abscess results in considerable destruction of bone around the apices of the involved teeth (*arrows*).

the division into the various types by means of radiographic pattern is difficult. The lesions may occur in the absence of clinical signs, which makes radiographic examination doubly important. Usually the infection follows the death of the pulp, and bacteria pass through the root canal into the periapical tissues.

Chronic Periapical Periostitis. This condition may be caused by occlusal trauma as well as by infection. It results in some thickening of the periosteum (periodontal membrane) at the apex of the root and is manifested on the roentgenogram by increased width of the radiolucent space between the lamina dura and the dental apex. The lamina dura is usually intact but may be thinned and partially resorbed (Fig. 36-7A) or may be thickened and sclerotic.

Periapical Granuloma. This represents the chronic stage of periapical infection in which there is destruction of bone adjacent to the apex of the tooth. The resultant space is filled with granulation tissue. Roentgenographically there is a radiolucent zone, usually with clearly defined margins, which is located at the dental root apex. The lamina dura is usually destroyed but the bony margin of the radiolucent zone is clearly outlined (Fig. 36-7B). It should be realized that a granuloma, radicular cyst, and abscess may be similar roentgenographically and, in many instances, cannot be differentiated. Usually the granuloma is no more than 1 cm in diameter, much smaller than the usual radicular cyst.

Periapical Abscess. This is the stage of the disease in which there is actual suppuration. A radiolucent zone is noted around the apex of the tooth in this condition and the margin is somewhat irregular and poorly defined, but may be sclerotic in disease of long

duration. The lamina dura is destroyed in the area of the disease (Fig. 36-7C).

Radicular or Root Cyst. Proliferation of squamous cells frequently found in granulation tissue around a dental root apex is stimulated by chronic inflammation. This mass of epithelial cells breaks down to form a cystlike cavity that gradually enlarges because of slow, constant pressure produced by the cellular proliferation. Eventually, a cyst wall is formed by dense fibrous tissue. Roentgen findings are those of a radiolucent area around the apex of one or more teeth, which may be rather large. The margins are clearly defined, often with a thin layer of compact bone clearly outlining the cyst. A large cyst may expand the bone and displace contiguous teeth (Fig. 36-8).

At times the various manifestations of periapical infection are difficult to classify into one of the groups

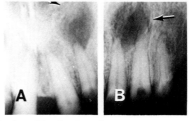

Figure 36–8. Radicular (root) cyst. **(a)** Note the large rarefied area extending into the alveolus from the root of the lateral incisor. The cyst is moderately well circumscribed, with a clearly defined margin. **(B)** Slightly different view in which the cyst overlaps the apex of the adjacent cuspid (*arrow*). Note the small abscess or granuloma involving the first bicuspid. All of the crowns are carious.

named in the foregoing discussion, but should be recognized as lesions caused by infection; that is, they represent a focus of infection that must be managed by dental surgery.

ALVEOLAR (PERIODONTAL) INFECTIONS

The earliest clinical manifestation of infection involving the alveolar tissues surrounding the teeth is that of gingivitis. The process begins with an accumulation of bacterial plaques on dental surfaces, which cause loss of the supporting structures because there is bacterial invasion of the gingival margins from the plaques. The accumulation of calculus above and below the gingival margin may play a role, but its relation to gingivitis is not clear. The infection progresses to the alveolodental periosteum, where chronic periostitis is produced. This results in absorption and destruction of bone surrounding the teeth representing periodontitis (alveolar recession). When the process involves a single tooth and extends downward toward or to the apex it may be termed the vertical type of alveolar periostitis. If it is more generalized and results in destruction of the alveolar septum between several teeth, it is termed the horizontal type of periodontitis (alveolar recession).[54]

Radiographic Findings. The radiographic changes parallel the destructive process. At first there is some widening of the radiolucency between the root and the lamina dura at the neck associated with some loss of the alveolar process. In the vertical type, the radiolucency around a single tooth increases. This indicates thickening of the periodontal ligament (membrane) and early bone involvement leading to loss of bony support and loss of the lamina dura. In the horizontal type, the alveolar ridge gradually disappears between the teeth until there is loss of bony support for several teeth. Roentgenographically, the presence of pus in these pockets of infection cannot be ascertained, but when the alveolar destruction is marked there usually is a considerable amount of local sepsis. Dense projections often appear at the neck of the affected teeth, which represent calculus. Occasionally, root resorption occurs, resulting in loss of the root in one or more areas. This is manifested on the radiograph by an area of irregular radiolucency indenting the normally smooth surface of the involved root (Fig. 36-9A, B, and C).

Hypercementosis (Exostosis of the Dental Root).
Cementum that is somewhat denser than cortical bone is produced and accumulates around the root of an affected tooth, usually a permanent one, to cause this abnormality. The premolars (bicuspids) are most commonly affected, with the first and second molars next in frequency. Radiographic findings reveal an enlarged,

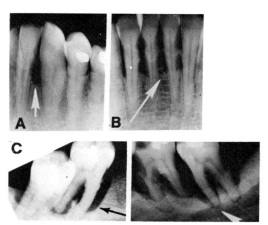

Figure 36–9. (**A**) Vertical periodontitis. Note loss of bone extending between the roots of the lateral incisor and cuspid in the lower jaw (*arrow*). The process is localized in this patient. (**B**) Horizontal periodontitis. The alveolus has been destroyed to a comparable extent throughout the incisor area (*arrow*). The density surrounding the necks of the teeth represents calculus. (**C**) Examples of severe periodontitis, with pockets extending nearly to the apices of the involved teeth (*arrows*).

bulbous, dense root that may be unusual in shape. The relationship of the lamina dura to the root does not change; it covers the abnormal root as in the normal state. The cause is not clear, and it may represent a dental anomaly.

DENTAL TRAUMA

Minimal trauma is a frequent occurrence, and there are no roentgen findings. If the pulp is damaged, it may be stimulated to lay down calcified scar tissue which may fill the pulp chamber. Root resorption may also result from minor trauma. These changes can be observed roentgenographically. Trauma to a deciduous tooth may injure and thus impair the developing permanent tooth.[38] The enamel may be hypoplastic in some; in others, there is failure of narrowing of the pulp chamber, caused by degeneration of the pulp that cannot form dentin. A wide pulp chamber in an adult, therefore, may be the result of childhood trauma. The opposite may also occur, eg, self-obliteration of the pulp by excess dentin deposition.

Various types of trauma that are important in children have been described. Complicated crown fracture or crown–root fractures expose the pulp. This makes prognosis poor for saving the tooth. In uncomplicated crown or crown–root fracture, the dentin is not exposed and prognosis is better. The root fracture that is usually missed clinically can be detected radiographically, but tomography may be required. Other complications of dental injury in children are failure of union, traumatic bone cyst, and apical cyst.

DENTAL MANIFESTATIONS OF GENERALIZED DISORDERS

In addition to outlining the teeth, intraoral dental films also include the alveolar process of the mandible, which may reflect changes in certain systemic diseases.

ENDOCRINE AND METABOLIC DISORDERS

Hypopituitarism. Delayed dentition along with delay in osseous development is characteristic of hypopituitarism and dental films will show the delay in development as well as the small underdeveloped jaw. There is a delay in general skeletal development, as well. There is also a delay in loss of primary teeth and development of permanent teeth. The teeth are normal in size.

Hyperpituitarism. In acromegaly and giantism there is an overgrowth of the mandible, so that the teeth are more widely separated than normal. The tongue is large and may protrude past the anterior teeth or past both teeth and lips. It also narrows the pharyngeal airway and may obliterate the valleculae. The greatest mandibular growth is in the incisor area. Rami may be normal or short. Radiographic study is helpful in differentiating this type of overgrowth from that associated with other conditions that produce abnormal enlargement of the jaw. Hypercementosis of the posterior teeth is common.

Hypothyroidism (Cretinism). Delayed development of the teeth that occurs in this condition is associated with underdevelopment of the jaw. Primary teeth remain for several years beyond the normal time for exfoliation, and there is a comparable delay in appearance of permanent teeth. In myxedema (adult onset), no definite dental alteration is present.

Hypoparathyroidism. Hypoplasia of the enamel occurs when the onset of the disease is early in life, before the enamel is completely formed. Hypoplasia of the dentine may also occur if the hypoparathyroidism occurs before the dental roots are developed. This is manifested by short, underdeveloped roots. In pseudohypoparathyroidism, dental changes are similar to those in hypoparathyroidism: hypoplasia of the enamel, short underdeveloped roots, and delayed or noneruption of affected teeth.

Hyperparathyroidism. There is thinning or loss of the lamina dura noted on dental roentgenograms along with marked decalcification of the alveolus. Dental films of the upper jaw also demonstrate a loss of the clearly defined outline of the bony floor of the maxillary antrum that is also a result of decalcification (Fig. 36-10). In severe disease, cystlike rarefactions may appear in the mandible. Following successful removal of the tumor causing the parathyroid hyperfunction, the alveolus tends to return to normal and the lamina dura reappears. This disease is now discovered at a relatively early stage in most instances, so no radiologic changes may be observed in the alveolus.

Cushing's Syndrome. Moderate decalcification of the alveolus is noted on the dental radiograph in this condition along with partial loss of the lamina dura. As a result, this structure is sometimes difficult to outline, but there are usually some areas in which it can be observed.

Diabetes Mellitus. In severe diabetes, particularly in children, dental infection is a problem so that periapical as well as periodontal disease is commonly present and may be severe. These changes are readily outlined on dental radiographs but are not present in all patients and are nonspecific.

Hypophosphatasia. There is loss of alveolar bone, enlargement of pulp chambers of root canals, and a decrease in thickness of the enamel and dentine. The roots, therefore, are thin with wide pulp cavities. Deciduous teeth are lost early because of absence of cementum without early eruption of permanent teeth (Fig. 36-11). Mild forms of the disease may have no dental findings.

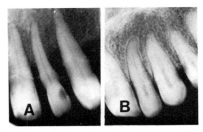

Figure 36–10. Hyperparathyroidism. (**A**) Note the absence of the lamina dura of the teeth. There is also loss of bone density in the alveolus and some alveolar periostitis. (**B**) Normal teeth with normal lamina dura and alveolar density.

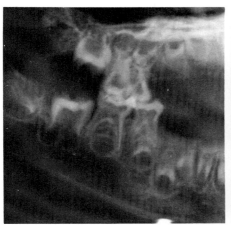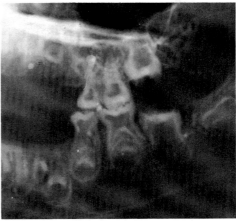

Figure 36–11. Hypophosphatasia in a 2-year-old child. Panorex film of the teeth and jaws. All deciduous teeth have been lost except the premolars. The roots are small, and the pulp cavities are very large.

DEVELOPMENTAL DISORDERS

Midline Facial Clefts. In cleft lip and cleft palate, there are dental anomalies ranging from deformity and malposition of some upper central teeth, to the presence of supernumerary teeth, to absence of a number of teeth. The films outline the osseous deformity as well as the dental alterations. A number of other isolated anomalies of the jaws and teeth are clearly defined on occlusal films or on panoramic films of mandible and maxilla. They include congenital hypoplasia and hyperplasia of the mandible, and unilateral hypoplasia of the face.

Osteogenesis Imperfecta. The characteristic dental alteration in this condition is replacement of the pulp canals by dentine, resulting in teeth that are uniformly dense. The finding of absent root canals is first observed in the incisor and the first molar teeth, which are the earliest to develop completely.

Dentinogenesis Imperfecta. This an autosomal dominant trait that is unrelated to osteogenesis imperfecta. The deciduous and permanent teeth are brown and wear away rapidly. Dental roots are small and conical; small molars have single roots. The root canal may be very small, partially obstructed, and pulp is diminished or absent.

Osteopetrosis. The dense, ivory-like bone characteristic of this disease is noted in the alveolus; the roots of the teeth are often incompletely developed.

Achondroplasia. There is delay in dental development in this condition that is readily observed on roentgenograms of the teeth. Many of the teeth remain unerupted into adult life.

Ectodermal Dysplasia. This disease is characterized by partial or complete absence of hair, sweat glands, and teeth. The degree of dental abnormality ranges from complete dental aplasia to congenital absence of a few of the teeth.

Oculodento-osseous Dysplasia. Hypoplasia of the enamel is associated with microphthalmia, skeletal dysplasia and sclerosis, digital malformations and in some patients, calcification in the basal ganglia.

Trichodento-osseous Syndrome. Dental abnormalities consist of delayed or partial dental eruption with wide and long pulp chambers. Dental caries with multiple periapical abscesses and associated condensing osteitis are frequent. In infancy there is dark curly hair that may become straight by the second decade.

Taurodontism. This condition is characterized by short dental roots, enlarged pulp chambers and elongated dental bodies. It is observed in about 20% of patients with Klinefelter's syndrome.

Chondroectodermal Dysplasia (Ellis-van Creveld). This disorder is characterized by dysplasia of fingernails, short stature caused by shortening of the tubular bones, polydactyly, carpal fusion, and dental abnormalities. Congenital cardiac abnormality may also be present. There is usually a decreased number of teeth that are widely spaced and peg shaped. Malocclusion is frequent; the mandible is always hypoplastic and the undersurface often markedly concave (antegonial notching).

Cleidocranial Dysostosis. Abnormal dentition and abnormality of the jaws are very frequent in this condition. There is often a delay in appearance of the teeth, with numerous supernumerary teeth. Permanent teeth are frequently malposed and fail to erupt. There is absence or hypoplasia of the clavicles and anomalies of the cranial bones; numerous wormian bones are common.

Unilateral Hyperplasia of the Face. The teeth develop prematurely on the hyperplastic side of the face; films of the jaws showing the difference in development of the teeth may permit early diagnosis of this rare condition. The jaw is deviated to the normal side, and malocclusion is common.

Unilateral Hyperplasia of the Coronoid Process. This is a rare anomaly of the mandible. Bilateral hyperplasia of the coronoid process may also occur.[25, 29] The elongated coronoid process impinges on the zygomatic arch. This causes restricted mandibular motion, so the elongated process must be resected. There is marked elongation of the coronoid process noted radiographically.

Mandibulofacial Dysostosis (Treacher-Collins Syndrome).[33] The teeth may be malposed, widely separated, hypoplastic and displaced; malocclusion is common in this syndrome in which there is hypoplasia of the facial bones, particularly the zygoma and mandible. Cleft palate, absence of the palatine bones or high palate, and underdevelopment of paranasal sinuses and mastoids may also be observed on roentgenograms of the facial bones.

Other Anomalies. There are a number of other developmental disorders in which abnormality occurs, but most are very rare. They include *Rutherfurd's syndrome*, in which deciduous teeth are unerupted and absorb with permanent teeth visible below them.[18] This is evidently caused by gingival hyperplasia to an extent that eruption of the teeth is prevented. *Oculomandibulodyscephaly* (Hallermann-Streiff syndrome) is another rare condition in which teeth are malformed, erupt early and irregularly, and may be erupted at birth. The palate is high and narrow, and there is hypoplasia of the mandible.

Dental and jaw abnormalities may also occur in *dysosteosclerosis* in which there is dental hypoplasia and the permanent teeth fail to erupt. Sclerosis of bone is noted in the base of the skull, ribs, and vertebral bodies. *Micrognathia* may be congenital and is associated with a number of syndromes; it is sometimes acquired secondary to trauma or infection. In juvenile

rheumatoid arthritis, the mandible is often underdeveloped and a rather deep local notch may be observed on the undersurface of the mandibular body, just anterior to the angle (gonion). There is also a congenital form of notching (antegonial), which is a uniform concavity of the entire undersurface of the body of the mandible. *Melnick-Needles syndrome* reveals radiographic alterations in the mandibular rami, in which appear thin medial cortex, and absence of the outer cortex produces cystlike lesions. Coronoid processes are hypoplastic and molar teeth are absent or impacted. *Radiotherapy* of the jaw in childhood may cause dental anomalies and hypoplasia, depending on age of the child and radiation dose.

Other causes of dental and jaw abnormalities include achondroplasia, the mucopolysaccharidoses, chondrodystrophia calcificans congenita, hypotelorism, hypertelorism, Marchesani's syndrome, Marfan's syndrome, and mental deficiencies of various types including mongolism. It is beyond the scope of this book to include all of these abnormalities.

MISCELLANEOUS DISORDERS

Eosinophilic Granuloma (Histiocytosis X) of Bone. This lesion often involves the jaw, resulting in destruction of the area of bone affected, with no visible reaction. It is not unusual to observe the bone destroyed so completely that teeth are left with no visible bony supporting structure, the so-called "floating" teeth. The bony lesions may be solitary or multiple within the mandible and may involve other bones. Several other diseases may destroy the mandible in a similar way; they include several of the non-Hodgkin's lymphomas, metastatic neuroblastoma, and Ewing's tumor. The teeth may appear to "float," but there are often soft-tissue changes and other signs that tend to make the diagnosis. MRI using surface coils is helpful in defining extent of bone and soft-tissue disease in these patients.

Acrosclerosis and Scleroderma. An increase in the thickness of the periodontal membrane results in uniform widening of the radiolucent space between the dental roots and the lamina dura. The uniform widening of this space in all of the teeth differentiates acrosclerosis and scleroderma from inflammatory disease of the alveolus in which the widening is rarely uniform.

Osteomalacia. The decalcification caused by this disease is noted in the alveolus. The lamina dura is also involved, and is absent in some areas but usually can be visualized in others.

Rickets. A deficiency of vitamin D may cause dental disturbances as well as the classic skeletal abnormalities. Hypoplasia of the enamel is frequently observed because the disease usually occurs in young children and infants. When the onset is late as in rachitis tarda, the development of the dental roots may be retarded. This is caused by defective dentine and cementum that may result in poor attachment of the teeth and lead to periodontal infection. The pulp chambers are abnormally large.

Renal Osteodystrophy. The dental findings are similar to those of hyperparathyroidism, with demineralization of the alveolus and loss of the lamina dura. In the child, delayed dental development is also observed.

Congenital Lead Poisoning. This condition may cause a delay in development of the deciduous teeth as well as typical lead lines in the long bones and increased density of the cranial vault.

Infantile Cortical Hyperostosis. This disease frequently involves the mandible, causing soft-tissue swelling, pain, and varying amounts of periosteal new-bone formation. This is now very rare.

CYSTS AND TUMORS OF THE JAW

Many lesions in the mandible may cause a local radiolucent defect. Some of these are defined clearly by a sclerotic rim of bone, while others may have indistinct borders. There is so much similarity between benign cysts and tumors and low-grade malignancies in the jaw that roentgen findings are often equivocal. In these instances, biopsy must be performed. It is worthwhile to describe these lesions, however, because many can be clearly differentiated radiographically.

DENTAL CYSTS

Periodontal (Radicular or Dental Root Cysts).
These cysts are the result of chronic periapical infection and have been described in the section "Periapical Infections." The cystic cavity is clearly defined and usually unilocular. The relationship of the radiolucent cystic structure to the dental root is important in the differential diagnosis. This is the most common "cyst" of the jaw; all others are relatively rare.

Follicular Cysts. This type of cyst arises in relation to a tooth follicle. Three forms may occur, depending upon the cyst content. These are the (1) dentigerous, (2) simple follicular (primordial), and (3) cystic odontoma.

The most common type of follicular cyst is the *dentigerous cyst* formed about the crown of a tooth. It develops around an unerupted, malposed tooth. Char-

acteristically, it produces a sharply marginated, expansile, rarefied area with a formed or incompletely formed tooth projecting into the cavity along one side.

Roentgen examination shows the large rarefaction, usually in the molar area, which causes expansion of the mandible. Its edges are clearly defined and there is a tooth or a part of a tooth projecting into the radiolucent cyst (Fig. 36-12). These cysts may occur in the maxilla as well as in the mandible.

The *simple follicular (primordial) cyst* is rare; it arises from the epithelium of the enamel before development of the tooth, so that it is radiographically similar to the dentigerous cyst, except that there is no tooth associated with it. Because these follicular cysts are related to the developing teeth, they are usually found in patients under the age of 15 years. Occasionally, this type of cyst may originate in a supernumerary tooth bud, in which instance it can occur in a patient with a full complement of teeth.[43] Simple follicular cysts tend to occur in the third molar region of the mandible.

Cystic Odontoma. This is a follicular cyst that contains a mass of rudimentary teeth or a mass of very dense material that may be amorphous.

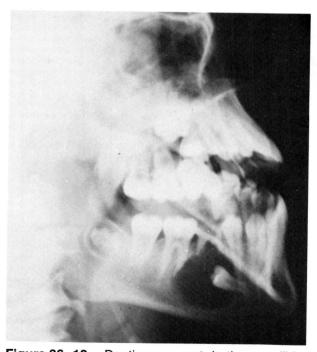

Figure 36–12. Dentigerous cyst. In the mandible, note the clearly defined radiolucent cyst that has resulted in erosion of the root of the second bicuspid and first molar. The small tooth projecting into it is typical and, when this is present, a positive diagnosis can be made.

Odontogenic Keratocyst. This cyst may occur as a solitary lesion but may be associated with the basal-cell nevus syndrome. Because the cyst resembles a primordial cyst radiographically, the diagnosis must be made histologically. These cysts are usually found associated with unerupted teeth. They are lined by squamous cells. The radiographic findings consist of a cystlike radiolucency of variable size, ranging from 1 to 9 cm. The cyst is clearly defined, but there is little or no sclerosis of the wall. It may be unilocular or loculated. Resorption of adjacent dental roots is rare. Occasionally some calcification is present within the cyst. The recurrence rate is high, up to 50%; therefore, it should be differentiated from a primordial and a dentigerous cyst. Symptoms consist of pain, tenderness, swelling, and persistent drainage after dental extraction.

Calcifying Epithelial Odontogenic Cyst. According to Gorlin, who first described it, this cyst occupies an anomalous position between cyst and neoplasm.[10] Most of them occur in the mandible and are situated either centrally (75%) or on the gingiva causing superficial erosion of bone. Radiographic findings are those of a central lucent lesion with scattered, irregular foci of calcification. The margins are defined clearly, but there is no limiting area of sclerosis. The cyst is apparently benign but is locally aggressive and, therefore, may recur.

Basal-Cell Nevus Syndrome. This is a hereditary disorder manifested by multiple, basal-cell epitheliomas of the skin, cysts of the jaws, and skeletal anomalies that include short fourth metacarpal, rib anomalies, vertebral anomalies, and ectopic calcifications in soft tissues.[2] The cysts in the jaw are usually symptomatic before the skin changes are noted, and appear to be either an odontogenic keratocyst or a simple follicular or dentigerous cyst.

ODONTOGENIC TUMORS

Ameloblastoma (Adamantinoma). The adamantinoma is a slowly growing tumor that is malignant; local recurrence with eventual widespread local involvement may occur. It arises from the anlage of the enamel organ. It is usually found in children and adults of ages varying from 7 to 82 years, with an average of 37 years. It may occur in either jaw but is more common in the mandible than the maxilla. The tumor may be divided into numerous compartments by bony septa, particularly in the mandible. The roentgen findings are those of a central tumor that produces destruction of bone and the dental roots, as well as expansion of the cortex through which numerous complete or incomplete trabeculations pass, giving the appearance of a multicystic mass (Fig. 36-13). Occasionally the tumor is unilocular with no trabeculation. This type is found in the maxilla more frequently than in the mandible. There is no attempt at new bone formation but the mass is clearly defined by a smooth-appearing bony wall. The recurrent or more malignant form is more invasive and its limits are not defined clearly. The unilocular adamantinoma may resemble a radicular cyst or simple follicular cyst. The polycystic type may resemble a central giant cell tumor and radiographic differentiation is not absolute. Rarely, this tumor secretes pseudoparathormone resulting in hypercalcemia. Removal of the tumor results in a return of calcium levels to normal. CT or MRI are helpful in defining the limits of the tumor.

Adenomatoid Odontogenic Tumor (Adenoameloblastoma). This tumor is benign. It is twice as frequent in females as in males, and usually occurs before the age of 30 and often before 20 years of age. It occurs commonly in the anterior maxilla, related to an unerupted tooth. Roentgen findings are those of a small (< 2 cm) radiolucent area, usually clearly defined. It contains foci of calcification that rarely is extensive.

Calcifying Epithelial Odontogenic Tumor (Pindborg Tumor). This tumor arises from odontogenic cells but is unlike the ameloblastoma.[34] Amyloid, which subsequently calcifies, is deposited in this tumor,

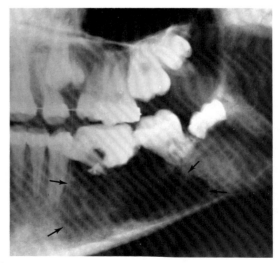

Figure 36–13. Ameloblastoma. This tumor in the body of the mandible is reasonably well defined (*arrows*). It has destroyed the bone and dental roots in the premolar and molar areas and appears to be somewhat multicystic anteriorly.

which usually occurs in the premolar–molar area of the mandible in association with an impacted or unerupted tooth. About one third of these tumors involved the maxilla, and rarely the maxillary antrum, where an ectopic tooth is observed surrounded by a cystlike cavity. As the tumor develops around the crown of an unerupted tooth, it resembles a dentigerous cyst, but often contains numerous calcifications. However, as it increases in size, the periphery becomes poorly defined and calcifies in an irregular pattern that eventually may resemble an osteosarcoma.

Complex (Complex Composite) Odontoma. This is a single mass made up of two or more of the solid dental tissues, including enamel, dentin, pulp, and cementum. Radiographically it is a densely opaque mass of malformed dental elements in either jaw, surrounded by a thin radiolucent line similar to the periodontal membrane. There is condensation of bone surrounding the mass resulting in an encapsulated appearance. The most common sites are the upper central incisor and the lower molar areas. Complex odontomas are usually found in the second and third decades of life. They are asymptomatic except that a mass is produced that may become very large.

Compound (Compound Composite) Odontoma. This is similar to the complex odontoma except that the dense mass is composed of a bundle of dwarfed misshapen teeth, which are recognizable as teeth. There is a radiolucent line surrounding the mass of teeth representing the pericoronal space usually observed around the crown of an unerupted tooth. It is found most often in the cuspid (canine) area with equal frequency in maxilla and mandible.

Odontogenic Fibroma (Fibromyxoma). This evidently arises from dental tissue and may be associated with an unerupted tooth. Radiographically it may be a multicompartmented, cystlike rarefaction; the fine trabeculations may be angular, forming the multilocular appearance. Some of them are unilocular, and have no trabeculation. The tumors may be expansile with well-defined margins in some and poorly defined margins in others. Although usually benign, some may become locally invasive, probably accounting for the poorly defined margins in some lesions. Thinning of the cortex is present in large lesions. At times the lesion is unilocular and associated with an unerupted tooth. It, therefore, cannot be differentiated from dentigerous cyst because roentgen appearances are identical. When the posterior maxilla is involved, the tumor may extend into and fill the antrum. MRI appears to be better than CT in evaluating the extent of the invasive-type lesions.[6]

Cementoma (Cementifying Fibroma). Cementoma is of mesenchymal origin and usually occurs in the mandible and is often multiple. It begins in the periapical region with proliferation of connective tissue at its site of origin, the periodontal membrane of a developed, erupted tooth. In this stage it resembles a periapical granuloma or root cyst because the mesenchymal mass is radiolucent. The second stage is one in which the fibrous tissue is converted into a calcified cementumlike substance. This dense mass then develops within the cystlike space. There may be some associated hypercementosis of the adjacent dental root. Most of these lesions occur in females. They are usually small, asymptomatic, and require no treatment.

Gigantiform Cementoma.[7] This lesion, originating in the periodontal membrane, consists of a lobulated mass of dense, slightly mottled calcified cementum. It appears to be familial. Usually there are simultaneous masses in the mandible and maxilla. It may become such a large dysplastic mass (masses) that differentiation from other lesions such as Paget's disease and fibrous dysplasia may be difficult. The lesion may be expansile. Some appear densely and uniformly calcified, while in others there are scattered areas of lucency.

Medial Mandibular Bone Concavity (Stafne's Defect or Cyst). This is an asymptomatic cystlike lesion of the posterior mandible anterior to the angle.[51] It is a medial concavity of the mandible that may be related to salivary gland hypertrophy. Ectopic salivary gland tissue may be present in the concavity. Radiographically it appears as a small (usually less than 3 cm), ovoid, cystlike lucency that is clearly defined by a narrow border of sclerotic bone. Unlike most other cysts or cystlike lesions, it lies below the mandibular canal. It may be bilateral.

NONODONTOGENIC CYSTS AND TUMORS

Incisive Canal Cyst (Anterior Palatine Foramen Cyst). As indicated earlier, the normal incisive foramen may vary considerably in size. The roentgen diagnosis of a cyst in this canal must be made on the basis of the clinical history of a slowly enlarging mass, either in the anterior palate or protruding into the nose, associated with a midline cyst that usually has clearly defined borders of condensed bone. Because incisive canal cysts are benign, their course can be followed if there is any doubt as to the diagnosis. Rarely, a median mandibular cyst may occur; its appearance is similar to that of the incisive canal cyst except for location.

Aneurysmal Bone Cyst. An aneurysmal bone cyst occurs very rarely in the mandible. As in aneurysmal bone cyst elsewhere, it tends to be a cortical lesion that expands the bone locally. It has the appearance of a trabeculated lytic cavity projecting from the bone in a manner that resembles a soap bubble. There may be marked expansion and thinning of the cortex. Its relation to trauma is not entirely clear, nor is its relationship to reparative giant-cell granuloma. CT may show a thin rim of newly formed bone surrounding the lesion that may not be detected on the radiographs of the jaw.[8]

Benign Giant-Cell Reparative Granuloma (Benign Giant-Cell Tumor). There is controversy as to how this lesion should be classified, but it is probably a nontumorous reparative process. The origin may be central or peripheral; a peripheral tumor originates in the alveolar soft tissue and may produce a smooth, pressure defect of the bone on the alveolar crest, but does not invade bone. The central tumor may be unilocular and expansile, and may resemble a large cyst, except that there is no condensation of bone forming the wall of the defect. Internal calcification occurs occasionally. Adjacent teeth may be displaced by the expanding mass, but there is rarely any dental resorption. However, the lamina dura may be eroded and lost. There may also be cortical thinning if the mass enlarges sufficiently.[17] The other form is multilocular. It may also expand the cortex and deform and displace adjacent teeth. The borders are not defined clearly by condensation of bone. This type cannot be differentiated from ameloblastoma on radiographic examination.

Osteoblastoma. Osteoblastoma is another rare benign tumor that may involve the mandible. It is a tumor of young adults (under 30 years of age). When a similar lesion is less than 1 cm in diameter, it is termed *osteoid osteoma*. When it occurs in the mandible, its roentgen appearance is that of a spherical ossified tumor surrounded by a clear radiolucent halo, which, in turn, is surrounded by smooth, dense bone. Osteoblastoma occurs adjacent to and may engulf a dental root. It has the potential to become moderately large, while osteoid osteoma is a small lesion, less than 1 cm in diameter. Osteoblastoma is usually relatively painless, while osteoid osteoma is frequently very painful.

Fibrous Dysplasia of the Jaw. The alveolar areas of one or both jaws may be involved by fibrous dysplasia locally or as part of general disease. This is not a true tumor but does cause expansion of the cortex in the area involved. It characteristically involves a considerable extent of bone and may occur in both the mandible and maxilla in the same patient. The roentgenographic findings consist of the appearance of an expanding bone lesion that may be extensive. At times, the lesion may be uniformly dense with a ground-glass appearance in which normal trabeculations are not seen. This sclerotic, expansile appearance is most frequently seen in the maxilla. These lesions may also be radiolucent with irregular trabeculations giving them a multicystic appearance. This appearance usually is found in the mandible. At times the disease may be localized, with a reasonably well-circumscribed area of mandibular expansion in which there are mottled areas of density and rarefaction. In some cases, a mixture of increased and decreased density is present. The teeth are not usually resorbed, but occasionally may be displaced. Cranial bones may be involved in the same patient.

OTHER BENIGN TUMORS

Cherubism. This is a familial disease characterized by symmetrical swelling of the mandible caused by a rather massive, fibrous tissue proliferation that expands the cortex. The tissue proliferation is centered in the region of the angle and extends to the ramus and body. The maxilla may also be involved occasionally. The swelling appears in early childhood (at about the age of 3 years, but may appear as early as 1 year of age) and is more common in males than females. Radiographic findings consist of expansive areas in the mandible that are bilaterally symmetrical. The cortex may be very thin and there are no teeth in the involved areas. These radiolucent expansile lesions are usually multiloculated and bilaterally symmetrical. Abnormal dentition with wide separation, poor development, or absence of teeth is common in the mandible, but there is more variability in the maxilla and the upper teeth may be normal.

Torus Palatinus and Torus Mandibularis. *Torus palatinus* is an exostosis arising at the margins of the palatal processes at the median palatal suture, usually bilaterally. The radiographic signs are those of a moderately flat mass of cortical bone projecting downward from the palate, often somewhat lobular with a midline groove (Fig. 36-14). *Torus mandibularis* is a similar dense exostosis projecting from the medial aspect of the anterior mandible. It is usually bilateral and may be accompanied by multiple masses that appear to be lobulated. The torus is significant only if it becomes large enough to interfere with speech or dental function.

Miscellaneous Benign Tumors. *Osteoma* of the jaw may occur and resemble osteoma elsewhere. Multiple osteomas are not uncommon. As in other bones, they may be flat and broad based, or somewhat pedunculated. They are more common in the mandible than in the maxilla. Osteomas of the jaws and other bones associated with multiple polyposis of the colon, multiple epidermoid cysts, and desmoid tumors occur in

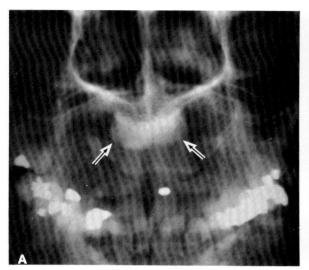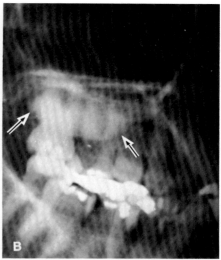

Figure 36–14. Torus palatinus. **(A)** Frontal projection showing the dense bone forming the torus extending downward from the palate (*arrows*). There is a poorly defined midline groove. **(B)** Note the somewhat elongated bony mass in the hard palate in this lateral projection (*arrows*).

Gardner's syndrome, a rare familial condition. Occasionally, *ossifying fibroma* may occur in the mandible or in the maxilla in the region of the maxillary antrum. The radiographic findings are those of a large radiolucent expanding lesion, which is usually found in young patients ranging from 10 to 30 years of age. At first the lesions are usually entirely destructive and therefore radiolucent. The wall is clearly defined. Later some calcification is noted within the tumor. *Hemangioma* of the jaw also presents an appearance typical of this lesion in other flat bones.

MALIGNANT TUMORS

Osteosarcoma. Osteosarcoma and *chondrosarcoma* rarely occur in the jaw and their appearance is similar to the appearance of these tumors elsewhere. As a rule, osteosarcoma of the jaw occurs 10 to 15 years later than peripheral osteosarcoma; therefore, it involves an older age group. The body of the mandible and the alveolar ridge of the maxilla are the most frequent sites. As a rule, the mandibular tumors are lytic and those in the maxilla are sclerotic, but lytic, sclerotic, or mixed patterns may occur at either site. A "sunburst" appearance also may occur.[5] *Ewing's tumor* is also found occasionally. The appearance of this tumor is similar to its appearance elsewhere. Solitary *plasma cell myeloma* (plasmacytoma) may occasionally arise in the jaw, producing a lytic expansile mass that is sometimes well margined. *Multiple myeloma* develops eventually in most of

these patients with solitary lesions. *Non-Hodgkin's lymphoma* is rare in the jaw but occurs occasionally.

Carcinoma of the alveolar ridge or carcinoma arising in the maxillary antrum may involve the alveolus by direct extension. This results in destruction of bone in an irregular manner, with no clearly defined wall and often with evidence of an associated soft-tissue mass (Fig. 36-15). In patients with carcinoma that involves the alveolar ridge, there is often ulceration, and infection may involve the bone. Infection is characterized by sequestrum formation (Fig. 36-16). Fragments of devitalized bone separating or separated from the area of disease are always highly suggestive of osteomyelitis. Differentiation between infection and carcinomatous destruction of bone is sometimes difficult; biopsy is then required to make the diagnosis. The most common malignant lesion of the jaw is a metastatic malignant tumor. Tumors of the lung, breast, and kidney are the most common primary source. In widespread multiple myeloma, lesions caused by this tumor may be visible. The manifestations are those of multiple areas of destruction without reaction in the osteolytic metastases, which are far more common in the jaw than the blastic metastases.

INFECTIONS OF THE JAWS

Osteomyelitis may be of hematogenous origin, but is more often secondary to dental infection and to carcinoma of the alveolus. Infection of bone may also follow

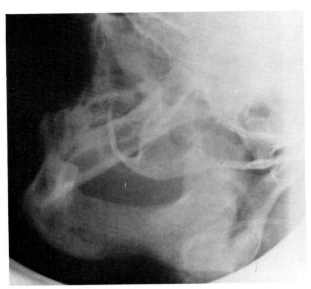

Figure 36–15.   Carcinoma eroding the mandible. Note the irregular destructive lesion on the inferior aspect of the body of the mandible just anterior to the angle. This was caused by direct extension of a squamous-cell carcinoma in the submandibular region. There is no bone reaction, and the outline is irregular.

jaw trauma and infection of the maxillary sinus. The roentgen findings of irregular bone destruction, sequestrum formation, periosteal reaction, and late sclerosis are similar to those of osteomyelitis elsewhere. Cellulitis adjacent to the mandible may cause periosteal new-bone formation without osteomyelitis. Chronic inflammations such as *tuberculosis* and *actinomycosis* may also involve the jaw, causing bone destruction. Soft-tissue involvement is common, especially in actinomycosis. Syphilis is rare but may cause a mixed lytic–sclerotic lesion of the jaw.

THE TEMPOROMANDIBULAR ARTICULATION

The temporomandibular (TM) articulation is examined using plain films with the patient's mouth open and closed, and by means of tomography. Hypocycloidal tomography appears to be used only occasionally now that CT is generally available. It is particularly valuable when there are bone changes or suspected bone changes. MRI is being used more frequently and, if available, is the method of choice, when there is dysfunction of the TM

joints. TM joint arthrography would then be reserved for those in whom the question of disc perforation is important and when the study of joint dynamics is important.[14, 19] CT remains the examination of choice in patients with acute trauma of the TM joints. Both joints are often examined, so that one can be compared with the other. Normally the articular surfaces are smooth and the mandibular condyle moves forward out of the glenoid fossa when the mouth is opened. The range of motion in the normal state is similar on the two sides and the appearances are similar but not necessarily identical (Fig. 36-17). Formation of the glenoid fossa ranges from a flat appearance to a deeply concave fossa. Pain upon motion of the jaw, along with crepitation and limitation of motion are often secondary to dental disease and malocclusion that may not be evident on radiographic study. Effusion in the joint is manifested by widening of the joint space. Degenerative changes are similar to those noted in other joints, with some eburnation of joint surfaces and narrowing of the radiographic joint space.

Rheumatoid arthritis may involve these articulations. In a study of 36 TM joints in 28 patients with rheumatoid arthritis, Larheim found that CT was not as useful as MRI in outlining the extent of bone abnormalities and the presence of associated soft-tissue abnormalities.[24] In another study, he found MRI to be superior to hypocycloidal tomography.[23] Loss of joint space, irregularity, poor definition of joint surfaces, and erosions of subchondral bone, subcortical cysts, subcortical sclerosis, and osteophyte formation are found in the mandibular condyle in these patients with rheumatoid arthritis. Ankylosing spondylitis is often accompanied by involvement of the TM joints with changes similar to those of rheumatoid arthritis, including narrowing of the joint space, erosions of bone, decreased motion, secondary changes of demineralization, extensive sclerosis, and, at times, joint-space widening. These diseases may also lead to fibrous and, occasionally, to bony ankylosis. Fibrous ankylosis may also result from trauma and may be incomplete so that the range of motion is markedly diminished. Various injuries of the TM joints may result in derangement of the meniscus, joint effusion, swelling of soft tissues in and around the joint, fracture of the condyle or condylar neck, and ischemic necrosis of the condyle. Patients with injuries leading to internal joint derangements who have had no previous fracture and intact dentition may develop secondary osteoarthritis and facial changes (remodeling) of the condyle and temporal bone.[39, 40] Occasionally, bony ankylosis occurs following septic arthritis. Roentgenograms show the continuity of bone between the condyle and glenoid fossa in this condition.

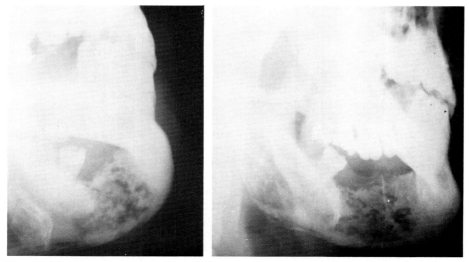

Figure 36–16. Osteomyelitis of the mandible. Two projections showing irregular moth-eaten destruction of bone. There are a number of moderately dense sequestra forming a mosaic pattern in the area of disease.

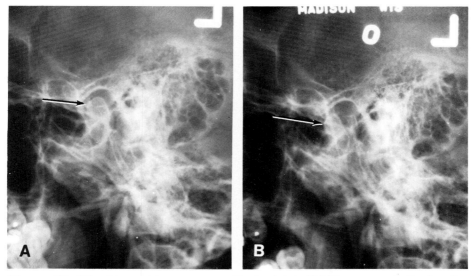

Figure 36–17. Normal temporomandibular joint. (**A**) The arrow indicates the mandibular condyle in normal relationship to the fossa and with a normal joint space. (**B**) Film exposed with patient's mouth open. Note the condyle, which has moved forward (*arrow*), and the difference in its relationship to the fossa.

UNCOMMON TEMPOROMANDIBULAR JOINT CONDITIONS

Joint Laxity

Patients with systemic joint laxity may have associated laxity of the TM joints, which often leads to joint dysfunction. This is found in patients with Ehlers-Danlos syndrome and in others with no definite detectable etiology.[12]

Osteochondritis Dissecans and Avascular Necrosis

The mandibular condyle may be involved by either of these lesions, presumably secondary to ischemia, which may be of unknown etiology. In a study of 40 patients with either of these conditions, it was found that there was internal TM joint derangement in 31 of 34 without previous surgery. There were alterations in condylar morphology found on MRI, as well.[41]

Synovial Osteochondromatosis

This is another rare condition involving the TM joints. It is characterized by synovial metaplasia with formation of foci of hyaline cartilage, which often contains calcification. Conventional radiography may show joint erosions, displacement of the condyles, swelling, and scattered intracapsular calcifications. CT is better at outlining these abnormalities, particularly in defining extensive erosions of bony structures.[30] MRI was advantageous in outlining the expansion of joint capsule, delineation of the boundaries of the capsule, bone erosions, and joint fluid. Both of these methods outline the typical loose bodies.[16]

Chondrosarcoma of the Joint

This is a very rare malignancy of the TM joint. The tumor presents as a soft-tissue mass, usually containing calcifications within the joint, which often breaks through the capsule and may destroy bone.[56]

Pigmented villonodular synovitis causes a smooth erosion of bone adjacent to the joint but is very rare. Clinically there is a soft-tissue mass in or in the vicinity of the joint, and this, in combination with smooth erosion, should suggest the lesion.[22] Findings are similar to those in other joints with this condition.

ARTHROGRAPHY OF THE TEMPOROMANDIBULAR JOINTS

Arthrography is helpful in demonstrating meniscal abnormalities of the TM joints in patients with joint dysfunction who may have minimal or no bone abnor-

mality.[14, 19, 26, 27] The examination may be performed with or without the use of local anesthesia. Under fluoroscopic guidance, a small (22 gauge) needle is inserted into the inferior joint space by placing the tip on the posterior surface of the condyle with the mouth slightly open. The needle hub moves with the condyle if it is in the proper position. A water-soluble iodinated contrast material is injected into the inferior space and should flow around the head of the condyle. About 0.5 to 0.8 mL of contrast is used. Many add 0.5 mL of 1:1000 adrenalin to 10 mL of the contrast agent to delay absorption. Double-contrast arthrography has also been described but its advantages have yet to be proved.[57] Although some examiners fill only the inferior space, many believe that complete demonstration of the configuration of the meniscus requires two-compartment filling.[31] The superior compartment is filled by reinserting and advancing the needle to contact the head of the condyle, then redirecting it into the space between the condyle and the temporal fossa. When both compartments are filled, the joint is examined fluoroscopically with opening and closing of the mouth. Spot films may be used to record any observed abnormality. Videotaping may then be used to study dynamic function. Finally, lateral roentgenograms and films in other projections as needed are obtained to complete the examination (Fig. 36-18). Some authors use polytomography as a part of the study, which is now used mainly when there is a question of disk perforation and/or when study of joint dynamics is important.[1]

CT is also used in the examination of the TM joints (Fig. 36-19).[15] It is likely that it may be replaced to a great extent by MRI in the future, as MRI becomes available in more institutions.

MRI is now being done using a surface coil.[37] Normal anatomy and pathology within the joint are demonstrated extremely well. Therefore, it is likely that this method will also replace arthrography in many instances. It is noninvasive, uses no ionizing radiation, and coronal and sagittal imaging can be performed. This is important in some cases because rotational and medial or lateral disk displacements apparently occur in about 25% of patients with internal derangements.[20, 42] This emphasizes the advantage of multiplanar capabilities of MRI. For these reasons, many authors recommend that MRI be the first imaging method to be used in these patients with suspected internal derangement of the TM joint (Figs. 36-20 and 36-21).[13, 32, 36]

Anatomic and Pathologic Considerations. Dysfunction of the TM joints occurs for a number of reasons. They include forced and prolonged opening of the jaw associated with anesthesia and dental pro-

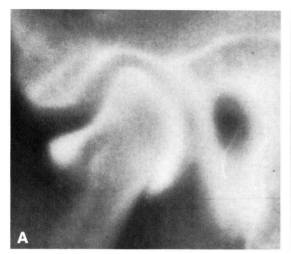
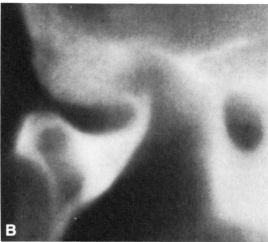

Figure 36–18.   Meniscus displacement with reduction. Arthrogram. **(A)** With the jaw in the closed position and with contrast in the lower joint compartment of the temporomandibular joint, the meniscus is noted to be displaced anterior to the condylar head. **(B)** With the jaw in the open position, the meniscus is now in a normal anatomic relationship to the condylar head and articular eminence. The contrast is now in the posterior recess of the lower joint compartment. (Courtesy of Richard W. Katzberg, MD)

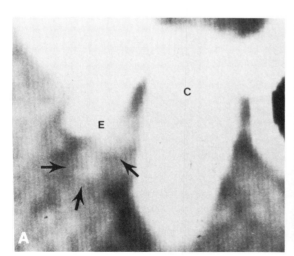
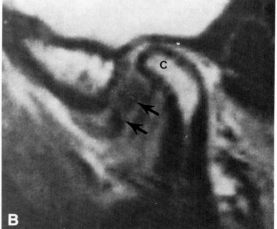

Figure 36–19.   Abnormal temporomandibular joint. **(A)** Direct sagittal CT of the temporomandibular joint with soft-tissue setting shows the meniscus to be displaced anteriorly (*arrows*) and with marked increase in density (131 HU), suggesting calcifications within the meniscus tissue itself. Condyle (C), articular eminence (E). **(B)** MRI with surface coil using the sagittal imaging plane shows the meniscus (*arrows*) to be displaced completely anteriorly, with good correlation with the CT shown in *A*. This is with the jaw in the open position. (Courtesy of Richard W. Katzberg, MD)

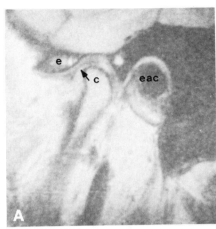
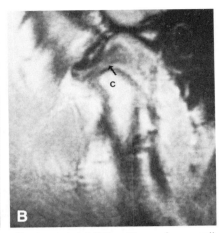

Figure 36–20.   Normal temporomandibular joint MRI with surface coil. **(A)** Closed jaw position. The normal meniscus has a biconcave lenslike configuration, and the posterior band is located at the 12 o'clock position relative to the condylar head (c). The thin zone of the meniscus is identified by the arrow. Articular eminence (e), external auditory canal (eac). **(B)** Normal temporomandibular joint with the jaw in the open position. Arrow demonstrates the thin zone of the meniscus that articulates with the convex surface of the condylar head (c). (Courtesy of Richard W. Katzberg, MD)

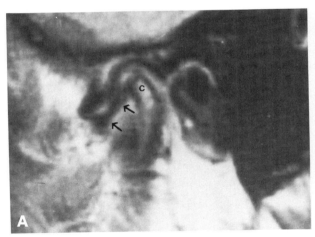
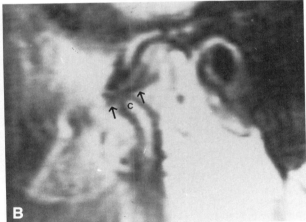

Figure 36–21.   Abnormal temporomandibular joint. MRI demonstrating anterior meniscal displacement with reduction. **(A)** The meniscus (*arrows*) is a low-signal intensity and is displaced completely anterior to the condylar head (c) with the jaw in the closed position. **(B)** Jaw in the open position and beyond the opening click. It shows the meniscus (*arrows*) to be recaptured relative to the condylar head (c) with anterior condylar translation. (Courtesy of Richard W. Katzberg, MD)

cedures, as well as trauma. In some instances, an inciting factor cannot be determined.

A thin fibrocartilaginous meniscus separates the joint into superior and inferior spaces. The meniscus measures about 1 mm in thickness centrally and 3 mm peripherally, and can be seen between the superior and inferior joint spaces. Anterior displacement of the meniscus is the most frequent abnormality; it may be persistent or may reduce spontaneously when the mouth is opened, often accompanied by a click or an irregularity of motion when the condyle slides over the thickened meniscus. The meniscus may reduce in some patients during mandibular movement, but does not reduce in others. History of locking of the jaw may be present in both situations. Perforation of the meniscus may be present, demonstrated by filling of superior space when the inferior space is filled. Care must be taken when doing arthrography that the needle has not traversed the meniscus, however. The site of the perforation is usually not determined at arthrography. Usually the perforation is at the posterior attachment of the meniscus.

In some instances, the meniscus may detach posteriorly or may become fragmented, followed by degenerative arthritic changes in the articular surfaces of the joint, which are accelerated by perforation, fragmentation, or detachment.

THE SALIVARY GLANDS

Roentgen methods are used to study the salivary glands in patients suspected of having calculi, strictures, inflammatory disease, tumors, autoimmune diseases, and sarcoidosis. The calculi are usually very dense and visualization is largely a matter of proper technique. Submandibular glands and ducts are examined by placing an occlusal film in the mouth and using a submentovertex type of projection. Parotid calculi may be in the gland or duct. Intraoral, lateral extraoral, and anteroposterior or tangential extraoral films are needed. Sialography can be used for localization if required. The discussion of the salivary glands including sialography is necessarily limited by space requirements. For those interested, the books by Rabinov and coworkers, Som and Bergeron, and articles by Som and colleagues are recommended.[35, 44, 47–49, 50, 53]

Sialography. This examination consists of filling the salivary ducts of the parotid or submandibular glands with an appropriate radiopaque medium. A preliminary film is taken to check for calcification. The duct is entered with a fine, thin-walled Teflon tube with a tapered end. A number of needles and cannulas have been used for this examination, including a butterfly infusion needle with the tip filed flat and smooth.[46] This can be held in place by using the butterfly for the patient to retain between teeth and buccal mucosa and taping the catheter to the face. Some prefer a blunt-tipped cannula that also can be taped in place. A dilator usually is not needed. The catheter is introduced for a distance of 1 to 3 cm, and can be kept in place during the exposure. Local anesthesia (Xylocaine [astra] or Lidocaine [Abbott]) may be used if necessary. When the parotid is to be examined, Stensen's duct can be catheterized for a short distance without much difficulty in most patients. Approximately 1 to 2 ml of the desired radiopaque medium is injected under very low pressure or hydrostatic pressure and films of the parotid gland and duct area are obtained in lateral and frontal projections with the catheter left in place (Fig. 36-22). The examination is best completed under fluoroscopic control because spot films can be exposed in suitable projections. We examine the submandibular gland much less frequently, and the injection of Wharton's duct is more difficult (Fig. 36-23). A fine dilator and a thin polyethylene catheter with guidewire are used; the catheter may be introduced for a distance of 2 to 5 cm, and 1 to 2 ml of an opaque medium is injected under fluoroscopic control. Following this, the films are checked. The patient is then given a few drops of lemon extract to stimulate salivary secretion and another set of films are obtained in 10 to 15 minutes to evaluate evacuation of the opaque medium. Subtraction techniques may be used when fine ductal detail is desired. It is important to correlate the sialogram with the clinical findings. Ducts may be incompletely filled when obstructed by calculus (Fig. 36-24). Tumors in and adjacent to the parotid may displace the ducts; malignant tumor within the parotid gland characteristically causes irregular filling of the ducts. Normally the glands empty in 30 minutes. Follow-up films can be obtained if desired, to study emptying of the gland. If the contrast substance remains in the gland more than 24 hours, abnormality is indicated.

CT is also used to study salivary gland disease.[4, 21] It is most useful in differentiating masses in the parotid gland from those masses in the pharynx, and in detecting extension of a tumor beyond the limits of the gland. Although the parotid gland is not divided into lobes, it is useful to think of a superficial portion separated by the facial nerve from the deep portion. The facial nerve leaves the cranium through the stylomastoid foramen and enters the parotid from its posterior aspect on a line drawn from the styloid process to the posterolateral margin of the mandibular ramus. The course of the nerve has been studied on CT scans by Wiesenfeld and

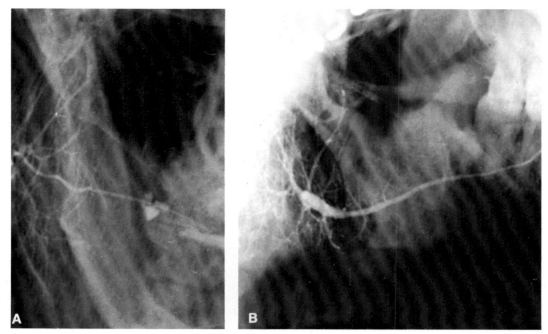

Figure 36–22.   Parotid sialogram—normal findings. (**A**) Frontal projection showing the treelike branching of the ducts, which are normal in caliber. (**B**) Oblique projection showing findings similar to those in *A*.

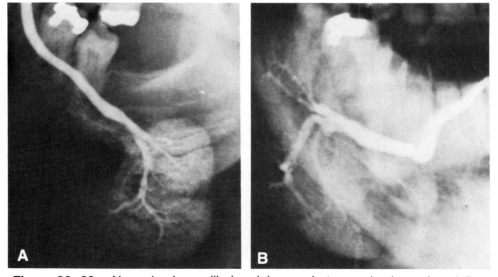

Figure 36–23.   Normal submandibular sialogram in two projections, *A* and *B*.

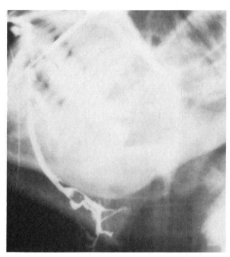

Figure 36–24. Sialogram showing small intraluminal defect in the submandibular duct; this proved to be a calculus. (Courtesy of June Unger, MD)

Ferguson.[58] It is represented by an arc with a radius of 8.5 mm extending from directly lateral to directly posterior to a point, the center of which is the most posterior part of the ramus of the mandible. It is at the level of the lateral mass of the atlas and the mastoid tip on the scan. The deep portion of the gland is medial to the facial nerve.

The superficial portion of the gland borders on the masseter muscle anteriorly, drapes around the sternocleidomastoid muscle posteriorly, and abuts the posterior belly of the digastric muscle posteromedially. The deep part extends posterior to the pterygoid muscles anterior to the stylopharyngeus aponeurosis.

If necessary, intravenous contrast can be used in conjunction with CT, particularly if the tumor is extraparotid. CT is used in conjunction with sialography when there is a problem in determining whether a tumor is present. Pantomography can also be used with sialography, but CT is a much more definitive examination.

MRI using surface coils is now being used extensively in the study of salivary gland disease. Advantages include multiplanar capabilities and lack of ionizing radiation; additionally, no contrast agents are needed and dental amalgam causes fewer problems than on CT. Furthermore, it is superior to CT in demonstrating tumor extension beyond the confines of the gland and in determining whether a tumor mass originated in the parotid or in the adjacent parapharyngeal space.[53] Gadolinium-enhanced MRI is useful in differentiating postoperative fibrosis from recurrent tumor.[55]

It may also permit histopathologic differentiation of certain parotid tumors.[45, 52]

PAROTID ULTRASONOGRAPHY

Parotid ultrasonography is also useful in the examination of the parotid gland.[9, 11] Calculi can be detected and their relationship to the duct often can be established. Inflammatory disease results in an increase in echogenicity and a coarsening of the parenchymal pattern of the gland.[59] Tumors are usually relatively hypoechoic, while abscesses are usually anechoic and may resemble cysts or sialoceles. Size, extent, and location in relation to the gland, adjacent vessels, and muscles can be determined. This is also a simple, noninvasive way to monitor tumor size following therapy. Ultrasound is also used to differentiate a parotid tumor from a superficial mass extrinsic to the gland. Deep tumors are best studied using MRI, but nearly 90% of parotid tumors arise in the superficial portion of the gland, so ultrasound may be very useful. As a rule, sialography is superior to ultrasound in the study of parotid infections, except for abscess when CT may also be useful (Fig. 36-25). Ultrasound may be useful in the study of Sjogren's syndrome but may be less effective in the study of inflammatory disease and sarcoidosis of the parotid.[3, 28]

SALIVARY GLAND TUMORS

Approximately 80% of salivary gland tumors occur in the parotids, 5% to 10% in the submandibular glands, and the remainder in the minor salivary glands. The incidence of malignancy in parotid tumors is about 15% to 20% as opposed to an incidence of 40% to 45% of malignancy in patients with submandibular tumors. MRI or CT may be helpful but is not definitive in differentiating benign from malignant tumors (Fig. 36-26). Generally, benign tumors are smooth and clearly defined while malignancies are poorly defined, irregular, and may invade adjacent fat and extend through fascial planes.[3] Malignant tumors tend to be less dense and, therefore, less opaque than benign tumors on CT. Fatty and vascular tumors may be identified specifically on MRI or CT.[36]

Sialographic signs of tumor include abrupt cut-off of ducts, lack of parenchymal filling, displacement and flattening of ducts, irregular pooling of contrast, and parotolymphatic backflow.[47] CT, in addition to sialography, often makes it possible to see the tumor better than on the sialogram alone, because small masses (< 2 cm) may not be detected on the sialogram.

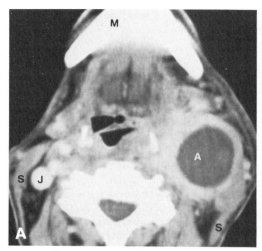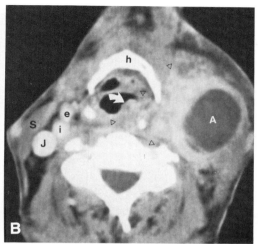

Figure 36–25.   Parotid abscess, CT with bolus contrast. (**A**) The abscess is defined clearly (A), with a moderately thick wall. The gland is virtually obliterated. Sternocleidomastoid muscle (S), jugular vein (J), mandible (M). (**B**) Lower section again shows the abscess (A). The parapharyngeal space is involved, and there is obliteration of soft tissue and fat planes (*arrowheads*) and encroachment on the airway (*curved arrow*). Jugular vein (J), internal carotid artery (i), external carotid artery (e), sternocleidomastoid muscle (S), and hyoid bone (h). (Courtesy of Richard Logan, MD)

OTHER SALIVARY GLAND DISEASES

Conditions such as duct stenosis, sialectasis (Fig. 36-27) and sialadenitis can be diagnosed most effectively using sialography. Calculi can be seen on ultrasound and on plain films, and can usually be related to the ducts on sonography. If necessary, sialography can be employed.[24]

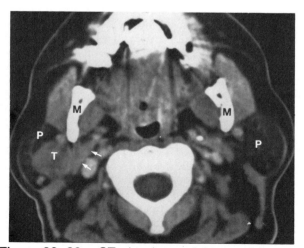

Figure 36–26.   CT showing a right parotid tumor (T), with extension into the deep lobe (*arrows*); parotid gland (P) showing a small amount of normal tissue anterolateral to the tumor. Mandible (M). (Courtesy of Richard Logan, MD)

Autoimmune diseases are a clinically heterogeneous group of salivary gland disorders (Sjögren's syndrome) that cause thinning of salivary duct walls. In this condition, the contrast material escapes through the wall of the diseased ducts to form small diffuse spherical collections termed *pseudosialectasis*.[49] The collections may be punctate, small (< 1 mm in diameter), or globular and larger (1 to 2 mm in diameter). In some instances, sonography shows sonolucent spaces compatible with the pseudosialectasis observed in Sjögren's syndrome, thus suggesting the diagnosis.[3] Larger collections are probably caused by secondary infections.

Sjögren's syndrome consists of keratoconjunctivitis, a connective tissue disease (usually rheumatoid arthritis), and xerostomia secondary to the salivary gland involvement. Mikulicz disease has similar histologic findings; some investigators believe that this term should be abandoned and the findings described below should be included under Sjögren's syndrome or autoimmune diseases.[35]

In the Mikulicz syndrome, sialadenitis, sialosis, and a multinodular gland may be found.[49] In sialadenitis, there is dilatation of the parotid (Stensen's) duct, often with pruning of distal ducts and acini. In sialosis, the gland is enlarged with sparse peripheral ducts. The multinodular gland is a very difficult problem. Parotid sarcoidosis results in granulomatous nodules that do not fill on sialography.[48] CT with sialography may be necessary to find the small nodules, which show lack of parenchymal filling. Metastases and multiple benign

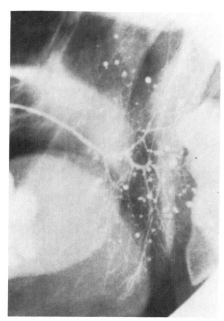

Figure 36–27. Parotid sialogram showing post-inflammatory sialectasis. Note numerous abnormal small globular dilatations manifested by collections of opaque medium involving the small ducts. (Courtesy of June Unger, MD)

tumors (usually Warthin tumors) can cause similar findings. Multiple small nodules can also be found in tuberculosis, actinomycosis, and cat scratch fever. Sarcoidosis often regresses on steroid therapy while the others do not. In some patients with sarcoidosis, there is diffuse enlargement of the gland and in others, a solitary mass. The parotid gland is involved in from 10% to 30% of patients with systemic sarcoidosis.

REFERENCES

1. BARRS DM, HELMS CA, KATZBERG RW, ET AL: Arthrotomography of the temporomandibular joint. Arch Otolaryngol 107:337, 1981
2. BECKER MH, KOPF AW, LANDE A: Basal cell nevus syndrome: Its roentgenologic significance. Am J Roentgenol 99:817, 1967
3. BRADUS RJ, HYBARGER P, GOODING GAW: Parotid gland: Ultrasound findings in Sjogren syndrome. Radiology 169:749, 1988
4. BRYAN RN, MILLER RH, FERREYRO RI, SESSIONS RB: Computed tomography of the major salivary glands. Am J Roentgenol 139:547, 1982
5. CLARK JL, UNNI KK, DAHLIN DC, ET AL: Osteosarcoma of the jaws. Cancer 51:2311, 1983
6. COHEN MA, MENDELSON DB: CT and MR imaging of myxofibroma of the jaws. J Comp Assist Tomogr 14:281, 1990
7. GIBILISCO JA ED: Stafne's Oral Radiographic Diagnosis. Philadelphia, W.B. Saunders, 1985
8. GIDDINGS NA, KENNED TL, KNIPE KL, ET AL: Aneurysmal bone cyst of the mandible. Arch Otolaryngol, Head & Neck Surg 115:865, 1989
9. GOODING GAW: Gray scale ultrasound of the parotid gland. Am J Roentgenol 134:469, 1980
10. GORLIN RJ, PINDBORG JJ, CLAUSEN FP, ET AL: The calcifying odontogenic cyst—a possible analog of the cutaneous calcifying epithelioma of Malherbe: An analysis of 15 cases. Oral Surg 15:1235, 1962
11. GRITZMANN N: Sonography of the salivary glands. Am J Roentgenol 153:161, 1989
12. HARINSTEIN D, BUCKINGHAM RB, BRAUM T, ET AL: Systemic joint laxity (the hypermobile joint syndrome) is associated with temporomandibular joint dysfunction. Arthritis Rheum 31:1259, 1988
13. HASSO AN, CHRISTIANSEN EL, ALDER ME: The temporomandibular joint. Radiol Clin North Am 27:301, 1989
14. HELMS CA, KAPLAN P: Diagnostic imaging of the temporomandibular joint: Recommendations for use of the various techniques. Am J Roentgenol 154:319, 1990
15. HELMS CA, MORRISH RB JR, KERCOS LT, ET AL: Computed tomography of the temporomandibular joint: Preliminary observations. Radiology 145:719, 1982
16. HERZOG S, MAFER M: Synovial chondromatosis of the TMJ: MR and CT findings. AJNR 11:742, 1990
17. HORNER K: Central giant cell granuloma of jaws. A clinico-radiological study. Clinic Radiol 40:622, 1989
18. HOUSTON IB, SHOTTS N: Rutherfurd's syndrome. A familial oculo-dental disorder. Acta Paediatr Scand 55:233, 1966
19. KAPLAN PA, HELMS CA: Current status of temporomandibular joint imaging for the diagnosis of internal derangements. Am J Roentgenol 152:697, 1989
20. KATZBERG RW, WESTESSON PL, TALLENTS RH, ET AL: Temporomandibular joint: MR assessment of rotational and sideways disk displacements. Radiology 169:741, 1988
21. KARENTAGER R, NOYEK AM, CHAPNIK JS, ET AL: Lipoma and liposarcoma of the parotid gland: High resolution preoperative imaging diagnosis. Laryngoscope 98:967, 1988
22. LAPAYOWKER MS, MILLER WT, LEVY WM, ET AL: Pigmental villonodular synovitis of the temporomandibular joint. Radiology 108:313, 1973
23. LARHEIM TA, KOLBENSVEDT A: Osseous temporomandibular joint abnormalities in rheumatic disease. Computed tomography versus hypocycloidal tomography. Acta Radiol 31:383, 1990
24. LARHEIM TA, SMITH HJ, ASPESTRAND F: Rheumatic disease of the temporomandibular joint: MR imaging and tomographic manifestations. Radiology 175:527, 1990
25. LUCAYA J, HERRERA M, VERA J: Unilateral hyperplasia of the coronoid process in a child. A cause of restricted opening of the mouth. Radiology 144:528, 1982

26. LYNCH TP, CHASE DC: Arthrography in the evaluation of the temporomandibular joint. Radiology 126:667, 1978

27. MANZIONE JV, KATZBERG RW, BRODSKY GT, ET AL: Internal derangements of the temporomandibular joint: Diagnosis by direct sagittal computed tomography. Radiology 150:111, 1984

28. MARCH DE, RAO VM, ZWILLENBERG D: Computed tomography of salivary glands in Sjogren's syndrome. Arch Otolaryngol, Head & Neck Surg 115:105, 1989

29. MUNK PL, HELMS CA: Coronoid process hyperplasia: CT studies. Radiology 171:783, 1989

30. MUNK PL, HELMS CA: Temporomandibular joint synovial osteochondromatosis: CT manifestations. J Canad Assoc Radiol 40:274, 1989

31. MURPHY WA: Arthrography of the temporomandibular joint. Radiol Clin North Am 19:365, 1981

32. NANCE EP, POWERS TA: Imaging of the temporomandibular joint. Radiol Clin North Am 28:1019, 1990

33. PAVSEK EJ: Mandibulofacial dysostosis (Treacher Collins syndrome). Am J Roentgenol 79:598, 1958

34. PINDBORG JJ: A calcifying epithelial odontogenic tumor. Cancer 11:838, 1958

35. RABINOV K, WEBER AL: Radiology of the Salivary Glands. Boston, G.K. Hall Medical Publishers, 1985

36. RAO VM, FAROLE A, KARASICK D: TM joint dysfunction: Correlation of MR imaging arthrography and arthroscopy. Radiology 174:663, 1990

37. ROBERTS D, SCHENCK J, JOSEPH P, ET AL: Temporomandibular joint: Magnetic resonance imaging. Radiology 155:829, 1985

38. ROLAND MN, PEARL N: Traumatic injuries to the teeth of children. Ann Radiol (Paris) 18:407, 1975

39. SCHELLHAS KP: Temporomandibular joint injuries. Radiology 173:211, 1989

40. SCHELLHAS KP, PIPER MA, OMLIE MR: Facial skeleton remodeling due to temporomandibular joint degeneration: Imaging study of 100 patients. Am J Roentgenol 155:373, 1990

41. SCHELLHAS KP, WILKES CH, FRITTS HM, ET AL: MR of osteochondritis dissecans and avascular necrosis of the mandibular condyle. AJNR 10:3, 1989

42. SCHWAIGHOFER BW, TANAKA TT, KLEIN MV, ET AL: MR imaging of the temporomandibular joint: A cadaver study of the value of coronal images. Am J Roentgenol 154:1245, 1990

43. SHAFER WG: Cysts, neoplasms, and allied conditions of odontogenic origin. Semin Roentgenol 6:403, 1971

44. SOM PM, BERGERSON RT: Head and Neck Imaging. 2nd edition, St. Louis, Mosby–Year Book, Inc., 1991

45. SOM PM, BILLER HF: High-grade malignancies of the parotid gland: Identification with MR imaging. Radiology 173:823, 1989

46. SOM PM, KHILNANI MT: Modification of the butterfly infusion set for sialography. Radiology 143:791, 1982

47. SOM PM, SHUGAR JMA: Paratolymphatic backflow: A new sign of malignancy. Ann Otol Rhinol Laryngol 90:64, 1981

48. SOM PM, SHUGAR JMA, BILLER HF: Parotid gland sarcoidosis and the CT sialogram. J Comput Assist Tomogr 5:674, 1981

49. SOM PM, SHUGAR JMA, TRAIN JS, BILLER JF: Manifestations of parotid gland enlargement: Radiologic, pathologic, and clinical correlations. Part I: The autoimmune pseudosialectasias. Radiology 141:415, 1981

50. SOM PM, SHUGAR JMA, TRAIN JS, BILLER JF: Manifestations of parotid gland enlargement: Radiologic, pathologic, and clinical correlations. Part II: The diseases of the Mikulicz syndrome. Radiology 141:421, 1981

51. STEINER RM, GOLDSTEIN BH, GOLD L: The medial mandibular bone concavity (Stafne's defect). Radiology 130:344, 1979

52. SWARTZ JN, ROTHMAN MI, MARLOWE FJ, ET AL: MR imaging of parotid mass lesions: attempts at histopathologic differentiation. J Comput Assist Tomogr 13:789, 1989

53. TABOR EK, CURTIN HD: MR of the salivary glands. Radiol Clin North Am 27:379, 1989

54. VIA WF JR: Radiology of the jaws: Diseases involving the teeth. Semin Roentgenol 6:370, 1971

55. VOGL TJ, DRESEL SHJ, SPATH M, ET AL: Parotid gland: Plain and gadolinium-enhanced MR imaging. Radiology 177:667, 1990

56. WASENKO JJ, ROSENBLOOM SA: Temporomandibular joint chondrosarcoma: CT demonstration. J Comp Assist Tomogr 14:1002, 1990

57. WESTESSON PL, ROHLIN M: Diagnostic accuracy of double-contrast arthrotomography: Correlation with postmortem morphology. Am J Roentgenol 143:655, 1984

58. WIESENFELD D, FERGUSON MB: The anatomy of the facial nerve in relation to CT/sialography of the parotid gland. Brit J Radiol 56:901, 1983

59. WITTICH GR, SCHEIBLE WF, HAJEK PC: Ultrasonography of the salivary glands. Radiol Clin North Am 23:29, 1985

Index

A

ISBN 0-397-51099-3

90000